ALREADY REGISTERED?

1. Log in at expertconsult.com
2. Scratch off your Activation Code below
3. Enter it into the "Add a Title" box
4. Click "Activate Now"
5. Click the title under "My Titles"

FIRST-TIME USER?

1. *REGISTER*
   - Click "Register Now" at expertconsult.com
   - Fill in your user information and click "Continue"
2. *ACTIVATE YOUR BOOK*
   - Scratch off your Activation Code below
   - Enter it into the "Enter Activation Code" box
   - Click "Activate Now"
   - Click the title under "My Titles"

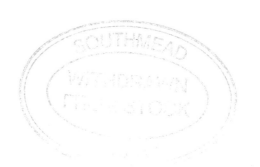
Plastic Surgery
THIRD EDITION
Volume Six
Hand and Upper Extremity

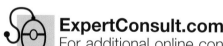

ExpertConsult.com
For additional online content visit expertconsult.com

Content Strategists: Sue Hodgson, Belinda Kuhn
Content Development Specialists: Louise Cook, Poppy Garraway, Alexandra Mortimer
Content Coordinators: Emma Cole, Trinity Hutton, Sam Crowe
Project Managers: Caroline Jones, Cheryl Brant
Design: Stewart Larking, Miles Hitchen
Illustration Manager: Jennifer Rose
Illustrator: Antbits
Marketing Manager: Helena Mutak
Technical Copyeditors: Darren Smith, Colin Woon
Video Reviewers: Leigh Jansen, James Saunders
Artwork Reviewer: Priya Chadha

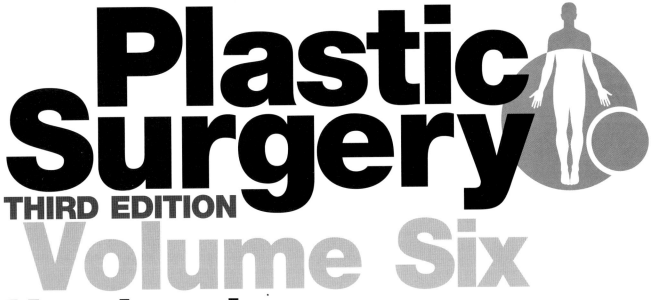

Plastic Surgery

THIRD EDITION

Volume Six

Hand and Upper Extremity

Editor in Chief

Peter C. Neligan

MB, FRCS(I), FRCSC, FACS
Professor of Surgery
Department of Surgery, Division of Plastic
Surgery
University of Washington
Seattle, WA, USA

Volume Editor

James Chang

MD
Professor and Chief
Division of Plastic and Reconstructive Surgery
Stanford University Medical Center
Stanford, CA, USA

Video Editor

Allen L. Van Beek

MD, FACS
Adjunct Professor
University Minnesota School of Medicine
Division Plastic Surgery
Minneapolis, MN, USA

ELSEVIER
SAUNDERS   London, New York, Oxford, St Louis, Sydney, Toronto

ELSEVIER
SAUNDERS

SAUNDERS an imprint of Elsevier Inc

Notices

Knowledge and best practice in this field are constantly changing. As new research and experience broaden our understanding, changes in research methods, professional practices, or medical treatment may become necessary.

Practitioners and researchers must always rely on their own experience and knowledge in evaluating and using any information, methods, compounds, or experiments described herein. In using such information or methods they should be mindful of their own safety and the safety of others, including parties for whom they have a professional responsibility.

With respect to any drug or pharmaceutical products identified, readers are advised to check the most current information provided (i) on procedures featured or (ii) by the manufacturer of each product to be administered, to verify the recommended dose or formula, the method and duration of administration, and contraindications. It is the responsibility of practitioners, relying on their own experience and knowledge of their patients, to make diagnoses, to determine dosages and the best treatment for each individual patient, and to take all appropriate safety precautions.

To the fullest extent of the law, neither the Publisher nor the authors, contributors, or editors, assume any liability for any injury and/or damage to persons or property as a matter of products liability, negligence or otherwise, or from any use or operation of any methods, products, instructions, or ideas contained in the material herein.

Volume 6 ISBN: 978-1-4557-1057-7
Volume 6 Ebook ISBN: 978-1-4557-4034-5
6 volume set ISBN: 978-1-4377-1733-4

 your source for books, journals and multimedia in the health sciences
www.elsevierhealth.com

Working together to grow
libraries in developing countries

www.elsevier.com | www.bookaid.org | www.sabre.org

ELSEVIER   BOOK AID
             International   Sabre Foundation

The
publisher's
policy is to use
paper manufactured
from sustainable forests

Printed in China
Last digit is the print number: 9 8 7 6 5 4 3 2 1

Contents

Volume One: Principles

Geoffrey C. Gurtner

Volume Six: Hand and Upper Extremity

James Chang

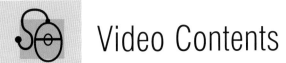

Video Contents

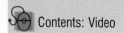

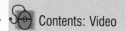

Foreword

In many ways, a textbook defines a particular discipline, and this is especially true in the evolution of modern plastic surgery. The publication of Zeis's *Handbuch der Plastischen Chirurgie* in 1838 popularized the name of the specialty but von Graefe in his monograph *Rhinoplastik*, published in 1818, had first used the title "plastic". At the turn of the last century, Nélaton and Ombredanne compiled what was available in the nineteenth century literature and published in Paris a two volume text in 1904 and 1907. A pivotal book, published across the Atlantic, was that of Vilray Blair, entitled *Surgery and Diseases of the Jaws* (1912). It was, however, limited to a specific anatomic region of the human body, but it became an important handbook for the military surgeons of World War I. Gillies' classic *Plastic Surgery of the Face* (1920) was also limited to a single anatomic region and recapitulated his remarkable and pioneering World War I experience with reconstructive plastic surgery of the face. Davis' textbook, *Plastic Surgery: Its Principles and Practice* (1919), was probably the first comprehensive definition of this young specialty with its emphasis on plastic surgery as ranging from the "top of the head to the soles of the feet." Fomon's *The Surgery of Injury and Plastic Repair* (1939) reviewed all of the plastic surgery techniques available at that time, and it also served as a handbook for the military surgeons of World War II. Kazanjian and Converse's *The Surgical Treatment of Facial Injuries* (1949) was a review of the former's lifetime experience as a plastic surgeon, and the junior author's World War II experience. The comprehensive plastic surgery text entitled *Plastic and Reconstructive Surgery*, published in 1948 by Padgett and Stephenson, was modeled more on the 1919 Davis text.

The lineage of the Neligan text began with the publication of Converse's five volume *Reconstructive Plastic Surgery* in 1964. Unlike his co-authored book with Kazanjian 15 years earlier, Converse undertook a comprehensive view of plastic surgery as the specialty existed in mid-20th century. Chapters were also devoted to pertinent anatomy, research and the role of relevant specialties like anesthesiology and radiology. It immediately became the bible of the specialty. He followed up with a second edition published in 1977, and I was the Assistant Editor. The second edition had grown from five to seven volumes (3970 pages) because the specialty had also grown. I edited the 1990 edition which had grown to eight volumes and 5556 pages; the hand section was edited by J. William Littler and James W. May. I changed the name of the text from *Reconstructive Plastic Surgery* to *Plastic Surgery* because in my mind I could not fathom the distinction between both titles. To the mother of a child with cleft lip, the surgery is "cosmetic," and many of the facelift procedures at that time were truly reconstructive because of the multiple layers at which the facial soft tissues were being readjusted. The late Steve Mathes edited the 2006 edition in eight volumes. He changed the format somewhat and V.R. Hentz was the hand editor. At that time, the text had grown to more than 7000 pages.

The education of the plastic surgeon and the reference material that is critically needed are no longer limited to the printed page or what is described in modern parlance as "hard copy". Certainly, Gutenberg's invention of movable type printing around 1439 allowed publication and distribution of the classic texts of Vesalius (*Fabrica*, 1543) and Tagliacozzi (*De Curtorum Chirurgia Per Insitionem* (1597) and for many years, this was the only medium in which surgeons could be educated. However, by the nineteenth century, travel had become easier with the development of reliable railroads and oceangoing ships, and surgeons conscientiously visited different surgical centers and attended organized meetings. The American College of Surgeons after World War II pioneered the use of operating room movies, and this was followed by videos. The development of the internet has, however, placed almost all information at the fingertips of surgeons around the world with computer access. In turn, we now have virtual surgery education in which the student or surgeon sitting at a computer is interactive with a software program containing animations, intraoperative videos with sound overlay, and access to the world literature on a particular subject. We are rapidly progressing from the bound book of the Gutenberg era to the currently ubiquitous hand held device or tablet for the mastery of surgical/knowledge.

The Neligan text continues this grand tradition of surgical education by bringing the reader into the modern communications world. In line with advances of the electronic era, there is extra online content such as relevant history, complete reference lists and videos. The book is also available as an e-book. It has been a monumental task, consuming hours of work by the editor and all of its participants. The "text" still defines the specialty of plastic surgery. Moreover, it ensures that a new generation of plastic surgeons will have access to all that is known. They, in turn, will not only carry this information into the future but will also build on it. Kudos to Peter Neligan and his colleagues for continuing the chronicle of the plastic surgery saga that has been evolving over two millennia.

Joseph G. McCarthy, MD
2012

Preface

I have always loved textbooks. When I first started my training I was introduced to Converse's *Reconstructive Plastic Surgery*, then in its second edition. I was over-awed by the breadth of the specialty and the expertise contained within its pages. As a young plastic surgeon in practice I bought the first edition of this book, *Plastic Surgery*, edited by Dr. Joseph McCarthy and found it an invaluable resource to which I constantly referred. I was proud to be asked to contribute a chapter to the second edition, edited by Dr. Stephen Mathes and never thought that I would one day be given the responsibility for editing the next edition of the book. I consider this to be the definitive text on our specialty so I took that responsibility very seriously. The result is a very changed book from the previous edition, reflecting changes in the specialty, changes in presentation styles and changes in how textbooks are used.

In preparation for the task, I read the previous edition from cover to cover and tried to identify where major changes could occur. Inevitably in a text this size, there is some repetition and overlap. So the first job was to identify where the repetition and overlap occurred and try to eliminate it. This allowed me to condense some of the material and, along with some other changes, enabled me to reduce the number of volumes from 8 to 6. Reading the text led me to another realization. That is that the breadth of the specialty, impressive when I was first introduced to it, is even more impressive now, 30 years later and it continues to evolve. For this reason I quickly realized that in order to do this project justice, I could not do it on my own. My solution was to recruit volume editors for each of the major areas of practice as well as a video editor for the procedural videos. Drs. Gurtner, Warren, Rodriguez, Losee, Song, Grotting, Chang and Van Beek have done an outstanding job and this book truly represents a team effort.

Publishing is at a crossroads. The digital age has made information much more immediate, much more easy to access and much more flexible in how it is presented. We have tried to reflect that in this edition. The first big change is that everything is in color. All the illustrations have been re-drawn

and the vast majority of patient photographs are in color. Chapters on anatomy have been highlighted with a red tone to make them easier to find as have pediatric chapters which have been highlighted in green. Reflecting on the way I personally use textbooks, I realized that while I like access to references, I rarely read the list of references at the end of a chapter. When I do though, I frequently pull some papers to read. So you will notice that we have kept the most important references in the printed text but we have moved the rest to the web. However, this has allowed us to greatly enhance the usefulness of the references. All the references are hyperlinked to PubMed and expertconsult facilitates a search across all volumes. Furthermore, while every chapter has a section devoted to the history of the topic, this is again something I like to be able to access but rarely have the leisure to read. That section in each of the chapters has also been moved to the web. This not only relieved the pressure on space in the printed text but also allowed us to give the authors more freedom in presenting the history of the topic. As well, there are extra illustrations in the web version that we simply could not accommodate in the printed version. The web edition of the book is therefore more complete than the printed version and owning the book, automatically gets one access to the web. A mouse icon 🖰 has been added to the text to mark where further content is available online. In this digital age, video has become a very important way to impart knowledge. More than 160 procedural videos contributed by leading experts around the world accompany these volumes. These videos cover the full scope of our specialty. This text is also available as an e-Book.

This book then is very different from its predecessors. It is a reflection of a changing age in communication. However I will be extremely pleased if it fulfils its task of defining the current state of knowledge of the specialty as its predecessors did.

Peter C. Neligan, MB, FRCS(I), FRCSC, FACS
2012

List of Contributors

Neta Adler, MD
Senior Surgeon
Department of Plastic and Reconstructive Surgery
Hadassah University Hospital
Jerusalem, Israel
Volume 3, Chapter 40 Congenital melanocytic nevi

Ahmed M. Afifi, MD
Assistant Professor of Plastic Surgery
University of Winsconsin
Madison, WI, USA
Associate Professor of Plastic Surgery
Cairo University
Cairo, Egypt
Volume 3, Chapter 1 Anatomy of the head and neck

Maryam Afshar, MD
Post Doctoral Fellow
Department of Surgery (Plastic and Reconstructive Surgery)
Stanford University School of Medicine
Stanford, CA, USA
Volume 3, Chapter 22 Embryology of the craniofacial complex

Jamil Ahmad, MD, FRCSC
Staff Plastic Surgeon
The Plastic Surgery Clinic
Mississauga, ON, Canada
Volume 2, Chapter 18 Open technique rhinoplasty
Volume 5, Chapter 8.3 Superior or medial pedicle

Hee Chang Ahn, MD, PhD
Professor
Department of Plastic and Reconstructive Surgery
Hanyang University Hospital, School of Medicine
Seoul, South Korea
Volume 6, Chapter 22 Ischemia of the hand
Volume 6, Video 22.01 Radial artery periarterial sympathectomy
Volume 6, Video 22.02 Ulnar artery periarterial sympathectomy
Volume 6, Video 22.03 Digital artery periarterial sympathectomy

Tae-Joo Ahn, MD
Jeong-Won Aesthetic Plastic Surgical Clinic
Seoul, South Korea
Volume 2, Video 10.01 Eyelidplasty non-incisional method
Volume 2, Video 10.02 Incisional method

Lisa E. Airan, MD
Assistant Clinical Professor
Department of Dermatology
Mount Sinai Hospital
Aesthetic Dermatologist
Private Practice
New York, NY, USA
Volume 2, Chapter 4 Soft-tissue fillers

Sammy Al-Benna, MD, PhD
Specialist in Plastic and Aesthetic Surgery
Department of Plastic Surgery
Burn Centre, Hand Centre, Operative Reference Centre for Soft Tissue Sarcoma
BG University Hospital Bergmannsheil, Ruhr University Bochum
Bochum, North Rhine-Westphalia, Germany
Volume 4, Chapter 18 Acute management of burn/electrical injuries

Amy K. Alderman, MD, MPH
Private Practice
Atlanta, GA, USA
Volume 1, Chapter 10 Evidence-based medicine and health services research in plastic surgery

Robert J. Allen, MD
Clinical Professor of Plastic Surgery
Department of Plastic Surgery
New York University Medical Centre
Charleston, SC, USA
Volume 5, Chapter 18 The deep inferior epigastric artery perforator (DIEAP) flap
Volume 5, Chapter 19 Alternative flaps for breast reconstruction
Volume 5, Video 18.02 DIEP flap breast reconstruction

Mohammed M. Al Kahtani, MD, FRCSC
Clinical Fellow
Division of Plastic Surgery
Department of Surgery
University of Alberta
Edmonton, AB, Canada
Volume 1, Chapter 33 Facial prosthetics in plastic surgery

Faisal Al-Mufarrej, MB, BCh
Chief Resident in Plastic Surgery
Division of Plastic Surgery
Department of Surgery
Mayo Clinic
Rochester, MN, USA
Volume 6, Chapter 20 Osteoarthritis in the hand and wrist

Gary J. Alter, MD
Assistant Clinical Professor
Division of Plastic Surgery
University of Califronia at Los Angeles School of Medicine
Los Angeles, CA, USA
Volume 2, Chapter 31 Aesthetic genital surgery

Al Aly, MD, FACS
Director of Aesthetic Surgery
Professor of Plastic Surgery
Aesthetic and Plastic Surgery Institute
University of California
Irvine, CA, USA
Volume 2, Chapter 27 Lower bodylifts

Khalid Al-Zahrani, MD, SSC-PLAST
Assistant Professor
Consultant Plastic Surgeon
King Khalid University Hospital
King Saud University
Riyadh, Saudi Arabia
Volume 2, Chapter 27 Lower bodylifts

Kenneth W. Anderson, MD
Marietta Facial Plastic Surgery & Aesthetics Center
Mareitta, GA, USA
Volume 2, Video 23.04 FUE FOX procedure

Alice Andrews, PhD
Instructor
The Dartmouth Institute for Health Policy and Clinical Practice
Lebanon, NH, USA
Volume 5, Chapter 12 Patient-centered health communication

Louis C. Argenta, MD
Professor of Plastic and Reconstructive Surgery
Department of Plastic Surgery
Wake Forest Medical Center
Winston Salem, NC, USA
Volume 1, Chapter 27 Principles and applications of tissue expansion

Charlotte E. Ariyan, MD, PhD
Surgical Oncologist
Gastric and Mixed Tumor Service
Memorial Sloan-Kettering Cancer Center
New York, NY, USA
Volume 3, Chapter 14 Salivary gland tumors

Stephan Ariyan, MD, MBA
Clinical Professor of Surgery
Plastic Surgery
Otolaryngology Yale University School of Medicine Associate Chief
Department of Surgery
Yale New Haven Hospital Director
Yale Cancer Center Melanoma Program
New Haven, CT, USA
Volume 1, Chapter 31 Melanoma
Volume 3, Chapter 14 Salivary gland tumors

Bryan S. Armijo, MD
Plastic Surgery Chief Resident
Department of Plastic and Reconstructive
Surgery
Case Western Reserve/University Hospitals
Cleveland, OH, USA
*Volume 2, Chapter 20 Airway issues and the
deviated nose*

Eric Arnaud, MD
Chirurgie Plastique et Esthétique
Chirurgie Plastique Crânio-faciale
Unité de chirurgie crânio-faciale du
departement de neurochirurgie
Hôpital Necker Enfants Malades
Paris, France
Volume 3, Chapter 32 Orbital hypertelorism

Christopher E. Attinger, MD
Chief, Division of Wound Healing
Department of Plastic Surgery
Georgetown University Hospital
Georgetown, WA, USA
Volume 4, Chapter 8 Foot reconstruction

Tomer Avraham, MD
Resident, Plastic Surgery
Institute of Reconstructive Plastic Surgery
NYU Medical Center
New York, NY, USA
*Volume 1, Chapter 12 Principles of cancer
management*

Kodi K. Azari, MD, FACS
Associate Professor of Orthopaedic Surgery
Plastic Surgery Chief
Section of Reconstructive Transplantation
Department of Orthopaedic Surgery and
Surgery
David Geffen School of Medicine at UCLA
Los Angeles, CA, USA
*Volume 6, Chapter 15 Benign and malignant
tumors of the hand*

Sérgio Fernando Dantas de Azevedo, MD
Member
Brazilian Society of Plastic Surgery
Volunteer Professor of Plastic Surgery
Department of Plastic Surgery
Federal University of Pernambuco
Permambuco, Brazil
*Volume 2, Chapter 26 Lipoabdominoplasty
Volume 2, Video 26.01 Lipobdominoplasty
(including secondary lipo)*

Daniel C. Baker, MD
Professor of Surgery
Insitiue of Reconstructive Plastic Surgery
New York University Medical Center
Department of Plastic Surgery
New York, NY, USA
*Volume 2, Chapter 11.5 Facelift: Lateral
SMASectomy*

Steven B. Baker, MD, DDS, FACS
Associate Professor and Program Director
Co-director Inova Hospital for Children
Craniofacial Clinic
Department of Plastic Surgery
Georgetown University Hospital
Georgetown, WA, USA
*Volume 3, Chapter 30 Cleft and craniofacial
orthognathic surgery*

Karim Bakri, MD, MRCS
Chief Resident
Division of Plastic Surgery
Mayo Clinic
Rochester, MN, USA
*Volume 6, Chapter 20 Osteoarthritis in the hand
and wrist*

Carla Baldrighi, MD
Staff Surgeon
Reconstructive Microsurgery Unit
Azienda Ospedaliera Universitaria Careggi
Florence, Italy
*Volume 6, Chapter 30 Growth considerations in
pediatric upper extremity trauma and
reconstruction
Volume 6, Video 30.01 Epiphyseal transplant
harvesting technique*

Jonathan Bank, MD
Resident, Section of Plastic and Reconstructive
Surgery
Department of Surgery
Pritzker School of Medicine
University of Chicago Medical Center
Chicago, IL, USA
*Volume 4, Chapter 12 Abdominal wall
reconstruction*

A. Sina Bari, MD
Chief Resident
Division of Plastic and Reconstructive Surgery
Stanford University Hospital and Clinics
Stanford, CA, USA
*Volume 1, Chapter 16 Scar prevention,
treatment, and revision*

Scott P. Bartlett, MD
Professor of Surgery
Peter Randall Endowed Chair in Pediatric
Plastic Surgery
Childrens Hospital of Philadelphia, University of
Philadelphia
Philadelphia, PA, USA
*Volume 3, Chapter 34 Nonsyndromic
craniosynostosis*

Fritz E. Barton, Jr., MD
Clinical Professor
Department of Plastic Surgery
University of Texas Southwestern Medical
Center
Dallas, TX, USA
*Volume 2, Chapter 11.7 Facelift: SMAS with skin
attached – the "high SMAS" technique
Volume 2, Video 11.07.01 The High SMAS
technique with septal reset*

Bruce S. Bauer, MD, FACS, FAAP
Director of Pediatric Plastic Surgery, Clinical
Professor of Surgery
Northshore University Healthsystem
University of Chicago, Pritzker School of
Medicine, Highland Park Hospital
Chicago, IL, USA
*Volume 3, Chapter 40 Congenital melanocytic
nevi*

Ruediger G.H. Baumeister, MD, PhD
Professor of Surgery Emeritus
Consultant in Lymphology
Ludwig Maximilians University
Munich, Germany
*Volume 4, Chapter 3 Lymphatic reconstruction of
the extremities*

Leslie Baumann, MD
CEO
Baumann Cosmetic and Research Institute
Miami, FL, USA
*Volume 2, Chapter 2 Non surgical skin care and
rejuvenation*

Adriane L. Baylis, PhD
Speech Scientist
Section of Plastic and Reconstructive Surgery
Nationwide Children's Hospital
Columbus, OH, USA
*Volume 3, Chapter 28 Velopharyngeal
dysfunction
Volume 3, Video 28 Velopharyngeal
incompetence (1-3)*

Elisabeth Beahm, MD, FACS
Professor
Department of Plastic Surgery
University of Texas MD Anderson Cancer
Center
Houston, TX, USA
*Volume 5, Chapter 10 Breast cancer: Diagnosis
therapy and oncoplastic techniques
Volume 5, Video 10.01 Breast cancer: diagnosis
and therapy*

Michael L. Bentz, MD, FAAP, FACS
Professor of Surgery Pediatrics and
Neurosurgery Chairman
Chairman of Clinical Affairs
Department of Surgery
Division of Plastic Surgery Vice
University of Winconsin School of Medicine and
Public Health
Madison, WI, USA
Volume 3, Chapter 42 Pediatric tumors

Aaron Berger, MD, PhD
Resident
Division of Plastic Surgery, Department of Surgery
Stanford University Medical Center
Palo Alto, CA, USA
Volume 1, Chapter 31 Melanoma

Pietro Berrino, MD
Teaching Professor
University of Milan
Director
Chirurgia Plastica Genova SRL
Genoa, Italy
Volume 5, Chapter 23 Poland's syndrome

Valeria Berrino, MS
In Training
Chirurgia Plastica Genova SRL
Genoa, Italy
Volume 5, Chapter 23 Poland's syndrome

Miles G. Berry, MS, FRCS(Plast)
Consultant Plastic and Aesthetic Surgeon
Institute of Cosmetic and Reconstructive Surgery
London, UK
Volume 2, Chapter 11.3 Facelift: Platysma-SMAS plication
Volume 2, Video 11.03.01 Facelift – Platysma SMAS plication

Robert M. Bernstein, MD, FAAD
Associate Clinical Professor
Department of Dermatology
College of Physicians and Surgeons
Columbia University
Director
Private Practice
Bernstein Medical Center for Hair Restoration
New York, NY, USA
Volume 2, Video 23.04 FUE FOX procedure
Volume 2, Video 23.02 Follicular unit hair transplantation

Michael Bezuhly, MD, MSc, SM, FRCSC
Assistant Professor
Department of Surgery, Division of Plastic and Reconstructive Surgery
IWK Health Centre, Dalhousie University
Halifax, NS, Canada
Volume 6, Chapter 23 Nerve entrapment syndromes
Volume 6, Video 23.01-04 Carpal tunnel and cubital tunnel releases in the same patient in one procedure with field sterility – local anaesthetic and surgery

Sean M. Bidic, MD, MFA, FAAP, FACS
Private Practice
American Surgical Arts
Vineland, NJ, USA
Volume 6, Chapter 16 Infections of the hand

Phillip N. Blondeel, MD, PhD, FCCP
Professor of Plastic Surgery
Department of Plastic and Reconstructive Surgery
University Hospital Gent
Gent, Belgium
Volume 5, Chapter 18 The deep inferior epigastric artery perforator (DIEAP) Flap
Volume 5, Chapter 19 Alternative flaps for breast reconstruction
Volume 5, Video 18.02 DIEP flap breast reconstruction

Sean G. Boutros, MD
Assistant Professor of Surgery
Weill Cornell Medical College (Houston)
Clinical Instructor
University of Texas School of Medicine (Houston)
Houston Plastic and Craniofacial Surgery
Houston, TX, USA
Volume 3, Video 7.02 Reconstruction of acquired ear deformities

Lorenzo Borghese, MD
Plastic Surgeon
General Surgeon
Department of Plastic and Maxillo Facial Surgery
Director of International Cooperation South East Asia
Pediatric Hospital "Bambino Gesu'"
Rome, Italy
Volume 4, Chapter 19 Extremity burn reconstruction
Volume 4, Video 19.01 Extremity burn reconstruction

Trevor M. Born, MD, FRCSC
Lecturer
Division of Plastic and Reconstructive Surgery
The University of Toronto
Toronto, Ontario, Canada
Attending Physician
Lenox Hill Hospital
New York, NY, USA
Volume 2, Chapter 4 Soft-tissue fillers

Gregory H. Borschel, MD, FAAP, FACS
Assistant Professor
University of Toronto Division of Plastic and Reconstructive Surgery
Assistant Professor
Institute of Biomaterials and Biomedical Engineering
Associate Scientist
The SickKids Research Institute
The Hospital for Sick Children
Toronto, ON, Canada
Volume 6, Chapter 35 Free functioning muscle transfer in the upper extremity

Kirsty U. Boyd, MD, FRCSC
Clinical Fellow – Hand Surgery
Department of Surgery – Division of Plastic Surgery
Washington University School of Medicine
St. Louis, MO, USA
Volume 1, Chapter 22 Repair and grafting of peripheral nerve
Volume 6, Chapter 33 Nerve transfers

James P. Bradley, MD
Professor of Plastic and Reconstructive Surgery
Department of Surgery
University of California, Los Angeles David Geffen School of Medicine
Los Angeles, CA, USA
Volume 3, Chapter 33 Craniofacial clefts

Burton D. Brent, MD
Private Practice
Woodside, CA, USA
Volume 3, Chapter 7 Reconstruction of the ear

Mitchell H. Brown, MD, Med, FRCSC
Associate Professor of Plastic Surgery
Department of Surgery
University of Toronto
Toronto, ON, Canada
Volume 5, Chapter 3 Secondary breast augmentation

Samantha A. Brugmann, PHD
Postdoctoral Fellow
Department of Surgery
Stanford University
Stanford, CA, USA
Volume 3, Chapter 22 Embryology of the craniofacial complex

Terrence W. Bruner, MD, MBA
Private Practice
Greenville, SC, USA
Volume 2, Chapter 28 Buttock augmentation
Volume 2, Video 28.01 Buttock augmentation

Todd E. Burdette, MD
Staff Plastic Surgeon
Concord Plastic Surgery
Concord Hospital Medical Group
Concord, NH, USA
Volume 1, Chapter 36 Robotics, simulation, and telemedicine in plastic surgery

Renee M. Burke, MD
Attending Plastic Surgeon
Department of Plastic Surgery
St. Alexius Medical Center
Hoffman Estates, IL, USA
Volume 3, Chapter 8 Acquired cranial and facial bone deformities
Volume 3, Video 8.01 Removal of venous malformation enveloping intraconal optic nerve

Charles E. Butler, MD, FACS
Professor, Department of Plastic Surgery
The University of Texas MD Anderson Cancer
Center
Houston, TX, USA
Volume 1, Chapter 32 Implants and biomaterials

Peter E. M. Butler, MD, FRCSI, FRCS, FRCS(Plast)
Consultant Plastic Surgeon
Honorary Senior Lecturer
Royal Free Hospital
London, UK
Volume 1, Chapter 34 Transplantation in plastic surgery

Yilin Cao, MD
Director, Department of Plastic and
Reconstructive Surgery
Shanghai 9th People's Hospital
Vice-Dean
Shanghai Jiao Tong University Medical School
Shanghai, The People's Republic of China
Volume 1, Chapter 18 Tissue graft, tissue repair, and regeneration
Volume 1, Chapter 20 Repair, grafting, and engineering of cartilage

Joseph F. Capella, MD, FACS
Chief, Post-Bariatric Body Contouring
Division of Plastic Surgery
Hackensack University Medical Center
Hackensack, NJ, USA
Volume 2, Chapter 29 Upper limb contouring
Volume 2, Video 29.01 Upper limb contouring

Brian T. Carlsen, MD
Assistant Professor of Plastic Surgery
Department of Surgery
Mayo Clinic
Rochester, MN, USA
Volume 6, Chapter 20 Osteoarthritis in the hand and wrist

Robert C. Cartotto, MD, FRCS(C)
Attending Surgeon
Ross Tilley Burn Centre
Health Sciences Centre
Toronto, ON, Canada
Volume 4, Chapter 23 Management of patients with exfoliative disorders, epidermolysis bullosa, and TEN

Giuseppe Catanuto, MD, PhD
Research Fellow
The School of Oncological Reconstructive
Surgery
Milan, Italy
Volume 5, Chapter 14 Expander/implant breast reconstructions
Volume 5, Video 14.01 Mastectomy and expander insertion: first stage
Volume 5, Video 14.02 Mastectomy and expander insertion: second stage

Peter Ceulemans, MD
Assistant Professor
Department of Plastic Surgery
Ghent University Hospital
Ghent, Belgium
Volume 4, Chapter 13 Reconstruction of male genital defects

Rodney K. Chan, MD
Staff Plastic and Reconstructive Surgeon
Burn Center
United States Army Institute of Surgical
Research
Fort Sam
Houston, TX, USA
Volume 3, Chapter 19 Secondary facial reconstruction

David W. Chang, MD, FACS
Professor
Department of Plastic Surgery
MD. Anderson Centre
Houston, TX, USA
Volume 4, Chapter 3 Lymphatic reconstruction of the extremities
Volume 4, Video 3.01 Lymphatico-venous anastomosis
Volume 6, Chapter 15 Benign and malignant tumors of the hand

Edward I. Chang, MD
Assistant Professor
Department of Plastic Surgery
The University of Texas M.D. Anderson Cancer
Center
Houston, TX, USA
Volume 3, Chapter 17 Carcinoma of the upper aerodigestive tract

James Chang, MD
Professor and Chief
Division of Plastic and Reconstructive Surgery
Stanford University Medical Center
Stanford, CA, USA
Volume 6, Introduction: Plastic surgery contributions to hand surgery
Volume 6, Chapter 1 Anatomy and biomechanics of the hand
Volume 6, Video 11.01 Hand replantation
Volume 6, Video 12.01 Debridement technique
Volume 6, Video 19.01 Extensor tendon rupture and end-side tendon transfer
Volume 6, Video 29.01 Addendum pediatric trigger thumb release

Robert A. Chase, MD
Holman Professor of Surgery – Emeritus
Stanford University Medical Center
Stanford, CA, USA
Volume 6, Chapter 1 Anatomy and biomechanics of the hand

Constance M. Chen, MD, MPH
Plastic and Reconstructive Surgeon
Division of Plastic and Reconstructive Surgery
Lenox Hill Hospital
New York, NY, USA
Volume 3, Chapter 9 Midface reconstruction

Philip Kuo-Ting Chen, MD
Director
Department of Plastic and Reconstructive
Surgery
Chang Gung Memorial Hospital and Chang
Gung University
Taipei, Taiwan, The People's Republic of China
Volume 3, Chapter 23 Repair of unilateral cleft lip

Yu-Ray Chen, MD
Professor of Surgery
Department of Plastic and Reconstructive
Surgery
Chang Gung Memorial Hospital
Chang Gung University
Tao-Yuan, Taiwan, The People's Republic of
China
Volume 3, Chapter 15 Tumors of the facial skeleton: Fibrous dysplasia

Ming-Huei Cheng, MD, MBA, FACS
Professor and Chief, Division of Reconstructive
Microsurgery
Department of Plastic and Reconstructive
Surgery
Chang Gung Memorial Hospital
Chang Gung Medical College
Chang Gung University
Taoyuan, Taiwan, The People's Republic of
China
Volume 3, Chapter 12 Oral cavity, tongue, and mandibular reconstructions
Volume 3, Video 12.02 Ulnar forearm flap for buccal reconstruction

You-Wei Cheong, MBBS, MS
Consultant Plastic Surgeon
Department of Surgery
Faculty of Medicine and Health Sciences,
University of Putra Malaysia
Selangor, Malaysia
Volume 3, Chapter 15 Tumors of the facial skeleton: Fibrous dysplasia

Armando Chiari Jr., MD, PhD
Adjunct Professor
Department of Surgery
School of Medicine of the Federal University of
Minas Gerais
Belo Horzonti, Minas Gerais, Brazil
Volume 5, Chapter 8.5 The L short scar mammaplasty

Ernest S. Chiu, MD, FACS
Associate Professor of Plastic Surgery
Department of Plastic Surgery
New York University
New York
USA
Volume 2, Chapter 9 Secondary blepharoplasty: Techniques

Hong-Lim Choi, MD, PhD
Jeong-Won Aesthetic Plastic Surgical Clinic
Seoul, South Korea
Volume 2, Video 10.01 Eyelidplasty non-incisional method
Volume 2, Video 10.02 Incisional method

Jong Woo Choi, MD, PhD
Associate Professor
Department of Plastic and Reconstructive
Surgery
Asan Medical Center
Ulsan University
College of Medicine
Seoul, South Korea
Volume 2, Chapter 10 Asian facial cosmetic surgery

**Alphonsus K. Chong, MBBS, MRCS,
MMed(Orth), FAMS(Hand Surgery)**
Consultant Hand Surgeon
Department of Hand and Reconstructive
Microsurgery
National University Hospital
Assistant Professor
Department of Orthopaedic Surgery
Yong Loo Lin School of Medicine
National University of Singapore
Singapore
Volume 6, Chapter 3 Diagnostic imaging of the hand and wrist
Volume 6, Video 3.01 Diagnostic imaging of the hand and wrist – Scaphoid lunate dislocation

David Chwei-Chin Chuang, MD
Senior Consultant, Ex-President, Professor
Department of Plastic Surgery
Chang Gung University Hospital
Tao-Yuan, Taiwan, The People's Republic of
China
Volume 6, Chapter 36 Brachial plexus injuries-adult and pediatric
Volume 6, Video 36.01-02 Brachial plexus injuries

Kevin C. Chung, MD, MS
Charles B. G. de Nancrede, MD Professor
Section of Plastic Surgery, Department of
Surgery
Assistant Dean for Faculty Affairs
University of Michigan Medical School
Ann Arbor, MI, USA
Volume 6, Chapter 8 Fractures and dislocations of the carpus and distal radius
Volume 6, Chapter 19 Rheumatologic conditions of the hand and wrist
Volume 6, Video 8.01 Scaphoid fixation
Volume 6, Video 19.01 Silicone MCP arthroplasty

Juan A. Clavero, MD, PhD
Radiologist Consultant
Radiology Department
Clínica Creu Blanca
Barcelona, Spain
Volume 5, Chapter 13 Imaging in reconstructive breast surgery

Mark W. Clemens, MD
Assistant Professor
Department of Plastic Surgery
Anderson Cancer Center University of Texas
Houston, TX, USA
Volume 4, Chapter 8 Foot reconstruction
Volume 5, Chapter 15 Latissimus dorsi flap breast reconstruction
Volume 5, Video 15.01 Latissimus dorsi flap technique

Steven R. Cohen, MD
Senior Clinical Research Fellow, Clinical
Professor
Plastic Surgery
University of California
San Diego, CA
Director
Craniofacial Surgery
Rady Children's Hospital, Private Practice,
FACES+ Plastic Surgery, Skin and Laser Center
La Jolla, CA, USA
Volume 2, Chapter 5 Facial skin resurfacing

Sydney R. Coleman, MD
Clinical Assistant Professor
Department of Plastic Surgery
New York University Medical Center
New York, NY, USA
Volume 2, Chapter 14 Structural fat grafting
Volume 2, Video 14.01 Structural fat grafting of the face

John Joseph Coleman III, MD
James E. Bennett Professor of Surgery,
Department of Dermatology and Cutaneuous
Surgery
University of Miami Miller School of Medicine
Miami, FA
Chief of Plastic Surgery
Department of Surgery
Indiana University School of Medicine
Indianapolis, IN, USA
Volume 3, Chapter 16 Tumors of the lips, oral cavity, oropharynx, and mandible

Lawrence B. Colen, MD
Associate Professor of Surgery
Eastern Virginia Medical School
Norfolk, VA, USA
Volume 4, Chapter 8 Foot reconstruction

E. Dale Collins Vidal, MD, MS
Chief
Section of Plastic Surgery
Dartmouth-Hitchcock Medical Center
Professor of Surgery
Dartmouth Medical School
Director of the Center for Informed Choice
The Dartmouth Institute (TDI) for Health Policy
and Clinical Practice
Hanover, NH, USA
Volume 1, Chapter 10 Evidence-based medicine and health services research in plastic surgery
Volume 5, Chapter 12 Patient-centered health communication

Shannon Colohan, MD, FRCSC
Clinical Instructor, Plastic Surgery
Department of Plastic Surgery
University of Texas Southwestern Medical
Center
Dallas, TX, USA
Volume 4, Chapter 2 Management of lower extremity trauma

Mark B. Constantian, MD, FACS
Active Staff
Saint Joseph Hospital
Nashua, NH (private practice)
Assistant Clinical Professor of Plastic Surgery
Division of Plastic Surgery
Department of Surgery
University of Wisconsin
Madison, WI, USA
Volume 2, Chapter 19 Closed technique rhinoplasty

Peter G. Cordeiro, MD, FACS
Chief
Plastic and Reconstructive Surgery
Memorial Sloan-Kettering Cancer Center
Professor of Surgery
Weill Cornell Medical College
New York, NY, USA
Volume 3, Chapter 9 Midface reconstruction
Volume 4, Chapter 14 Reconstruction of acquired vaginal defects

Christopher Cox, MD
Chief Resident
Department of Orthopaedic Surgery
Stanford University Medical School
Stanford, CA, USA
Volume 6, Chapter 5 Principles of internal fixation as applied to the hand and wrist
Volume 6, Video 5.01 Dynamic compression plating and lag screw technique

Albert Cram, MD
Professor Emeritus
University of Iowa
Iowa City Plastic Surgery
Coralville, IO, USA
Volume 2, Chapter 27 Lower bodylifts

Catherine Curtin, MD
Assistant Professor
Department of Surgery Division of Plastic
Stanford University
Stanford, CA, USA
*Volume 6, Chapter 37 Restoration of upper
extremity function*
*Volume 6, Video 37.01 1 Stage grasp IC 6 short
term*
*Volume 6, Video 37.02 2 Stage grasp release
outcome*

Lars B. Dahlin, MD, PhD
Professor and Consultant
Department of Clinical Sciences, Malmö-Hand
Surgery
University of Lund
Malmö, Sweden
*Volume 6, Chapter 32 Peripheral nerve injuries of
the upper extremity*
Volume 6, Video 32.01 Digital Nerve Suture
Volume 6, Video 32.02 Median Nerve Suture

Dai M. Davies, FRCS
Consultant and Institute Director
Institute of Cosmetic and Reconstructive
Surgery
London, UK
*Volume 2, Chapter 11.3 Facelift: Platysma-SMAS
plication*
*Volume 2, Video 11.03.01 Platysma SMAS
plication*

**Michael R. Davis, MD, FACS, LtCol,
USAF, MC**
Chief
Reconstructive Surgery and Regenerative
Medicine
Plastic and Reconstructive Surgeon
San Antonio Military Medical Center
Houston, TX, USA
*Volume 5, Chapter 1 Anatomy for plastic surgery
of the breast*

Jorge I. De La Torre, MD
Professor and Chief
Division of Plastic Surgery
University of Alabama at Birmingham
Birmingham, AL, USA
*Volume 5, Chapter 1 Anatomy for plastic surgery
of the breast*

A. Lee Dellon, MD, PhD
Professor of Plastic Surgery
Professor of Neurosurgery
Johns Hopkins University
Baltimore, MD, USA
*Volume 4, Chapter 6 Diagnosis and treatment of
painful neuroma and of nerve compression in the
lower extremity*
*Volume 4, Video 6.01 Diagnosis and treatment
of painful neuroma and of nerve compression in
the lower extremity*

Sara R. Dickie, MD
Resident, Section of Plastic and Reconstructive
Surgery
Department of Surgery
University of Chicago Medical Center
Chicago, IL, USA
*Volume 4, Chapter 9 Comprehensive trunk
anatomy*

Joseph J. Disa, MD, FACS
Attending Surgeon
Plastic and Reconstructive Surgery in the
Department of Surgery
Memorial Sloan Kettering Cancer Center
New York, NY, USA
Volume 3, Chapter 9 Midface reconstruction
*Volume 4, Chapter 14 Reconstruction of
acquired vaginal defects*

Risal Djohan, MD
Head of Regional Medical Practice
Department of Plastic Surgery
Cleveland Clinic
Cleveland, OH, USA
*Volume 3, Chapter 1 Anatomy of the head and
neck*

Erin Donaldson, MS
Instructor
Department of Otolaryngology
New York Medical College
Valhalla, NY, USA
*Volume 1, Chapter 36 Robotics, simulation, and
telemedicine in plastic surgery*

Amir H. Dorafshar, MBChB
Assistant Professor
Department of Plastic and Reconstructive
surgery
John Hopkins Medical Institute
John Hopkins Outpatient Center
Baltimore, MD, USA
Volume 3, Chapter 3 Facial fractures

Ivica Ducic, MD, PhD
Professor – Plastic Surgery
Director – Peripheral Nerve Surgery Institute
Department of Plastic Surgery
Georgetown University Hospital
Washington, DC, USA
*Volume 6, Chapter 23 Complex regional pain
syndrome in the upper extremity*

Gregory A. Dumanian, MD, FACS
Chief of Plastic Surgery
Division of Plastic Surgery, Department of
Surgery
Northwestern Feinberg School of Medicine
Chicago, IL, USA
*Volume 4, Chapter 11 Reconstruction of the soft
tissues of the back*
*Volume 6, Chapter 40 Treatment of the upper
extremity amputee*
*Volume 6, Video 40.01 Targeted muscle
reinnervation in the transhumeral amputee –
Surgical technique and guidelines for restoring
intuitive neural control*

William W. Dzwierzynski, MD
Professor and Program Director
Department of Plastic Surgery
Medical College of Wisconsin
Milwaukee, WI, USA
*Volume 6, Chapter 11 Replantation and
revascularization*

L. Franklyn Elliott, MD
Assistant Clinical Professor
Emory Section of Plastic Surgery
Emory University
Atlanta, GA, USA
*Volume 5, Chapter 16 The bilateral pedicled
TRAM flap*
*Volume 5, Video 16.01 Pedicle TRAM breast
reconstruction*

Marco Ellis, MD
Chief Resident
Division of Plastic Surgery
Northwestern Memorial Hospital
Northwestern University, Feinberg School of
Medicine
Chicago, IL, USA
Volume 2, Chapter 8 Blepharoplasty
Volume 2, Video 8.01 Periorbital rejuvenation

Dino Elyassnia, MD
Associate Plastic Surgeon
Marten Clinic of Plastic Surgery
San Francisco, CA, USA
*Volume 2, Chapter 12 Secondary deformities
and the secondary facelift*

Surak Eo, MD, PhD
Chief, Associate Professor
Plastic and Reconstructive Surgery
DongGuk University Medical Center
DongGuk University Graduate School of
Medicine
Gyeonggi-do, South Korea
*Volume 6, Video 34.01 EIP to EPL tendon
transfer*

Elof Eriksson, MD, PhD
Chief
Department of Plastic Surgery
Joseph E. Murray Professor of Plastic and
Reconstructive Surgery
Brigham and Women's Hospital
Boston, MA, USA
*Volume 1, Chapter 11 Genetics and prenatal
diagnosis*

Simon Farnebo, MD, PhD
Consultant Hand Surgeon
Department of Plastic Surgery, Hand Surgery
and Burns
Institution of Clinical and Experimental
Medicine, University of Linköping
Linköping, Sweden
*Volume 6, Chapter 32 Peripheral nerve injuries of
the upper extremity*
Volume 6, Video 32.01 Digital Nerve Suture
Volume 6, Video 32.02 Median Nerve Suture

Jeffrey A. Fearon, MD
Director
The Craniofacial Center
Medical City Children's Hospital
Dallas, TX, USA
Volume 3, Chapter 35 Syndromic craniosynostosis

John M. Felder III, MD
Resident Physician
Department of Plastic Surgery
Georgetown University Hospital
Washington, DC, USA
Volume 6, Chapter 23 Complex regional pain syndrome in the upper extremity

Evan M. Feldman, MD
Chief Resident
Division of Plastic Surgery
Baylor College of Medicine
Houston, TX, USA
Volume 3, Chapter 29 Secondary deformities of the cleft lip, nose, and palate
Volume 3, Video 29.01 Complete takedown
Volume 3, Video 29.02 Abbé flap
Volume 3, Video 29.03 Thick lip and buccal sulcus deformities
Volume 3, Video 29.04 Alveolar bone grafting
Volume 3, Video 29.05 Definitive rhinoplasty

Julius Few Jr., MD
Director
The Few Institute for Aesthetic Plastic Surgery
Clinical Associate
Division of Plastic Surgery
University of Chicago
Chicago, IL, USA
Volume 2, Chapter 8 Blepharoplasty
Volume 2, Video 8.01 Periorbital rejuvenation

Alvaro A. Figueroa, DDS, MS
Director
Rush Craniofacial Center
Rush University Medical Center
Chicago, IL, USA
Volume 3, Chapter 27 Orthodontics in cleft lip and palate management

Neil A. Fine, MD
Associate Professor of Clinical Surgery
Department of Surgery
Northwestern University
Chicago, IL, USA
Volume 5, Chapter 5 Endoscopic approaches to the breast
Volume 5, Video 5.01 Endoscopic transaxillary breast augmentation
Volume 5, Video 5.02 Endoscopic approaches to the breast
Volume 5, Video 11.02 Partial breast reconstruction with a latissimus D

Joel S. Fish, MD, MSc, FRCSC
Medical Director Burn Program
Department of Surgery, University of Toronto,
Division of Plastic and Reconstructive Surgery
Hospital for Sick Children
Toronto, ON, Canada
Volume 4, Chapter 23 Management of patients with exfoliative disorders, epidermolysis bullosa, and TEN

David M. Fisher, MB, BCh, FRCSC, FACS
Medical Director, Cleft Lip and Palate Program
Division of Plastic and Reconstructive Surgery
The Hospital for Sick Children
Toronto, ON, Canada
Volume 3, Video 23.02 Unilateral cleft lip repair – anatomic subunit approximation technique

Jack Fisher, MD
Department of Plastic Surgery
Vanderbilt University
Nashville, TN, USA
Volume 2, Chapter 23 Hair restoration
Volume 5, Chapter 8.1 Reduction mammaplasty
Volume 5, Chapter 8.2 Inferior pedicle breast reduction

James W. Fletcher, MD, FACS
Chief Hand Surgery
Department Plastic and Hand Surgery
Regions Hospital
Assistant Prof. U MN Dept of Surgery and Dept Orthopedics
St. Paul, MN, USA
Volume 6, Video 20.01 Ligament reconstruction tendon interposition arthroplasty of the thumb CMC joint

Joshua Fosnot, MD
Resident
Division of Plastic Surgery
The University of Pennsylvania Health System
Philadelphia, PA, USA
Volume 5, Chapter 17 Free TRAM breast reconstruction
Volume 5, Video 17.01 The muscle sparing free TRAM flap

Ida K. Fox, MD
Assistant Professor of Plastic Surgery
Department of Surgery
Washington University School of Medicine
Saint Louis, MO, USA
Volume 6, Chapter 33 Nerve transfers
Volume 6, Video 33.01 Nerve transfers

Ryan C. Frank, MD, FRCSC
Attending Surgeon
Plastic and Craniofacial Surgery
Alberta Children's Hospital
University of Calgary
Calgary, AB, Canada
Volume 2, Chapter 5 Facial skin resurfacing

Gary L. Freed, MD
Assistant Professor Plastic Surgery
Dartmouth-Hitchcock Medical Center
Lebanon, NH, USA
Volume 5, Chapter 12 Patient-centered health communication

Jeffrey B. Friedrich, MD
Assistant Professor of Surgery, Orthopedics and Urology (Adjunct)
Department of Surgery, Division of Plastic Surgery
University of Washington
Seattle, WA, USA
Volume 6, Chapter 13 Thumb reconstruction (non microsurgical)

Allen Gabriel, MD
Assitant Professor
Department of Plastic Surgery
Loma Linda University Medical Center
Chief of Plastic Surgery
Southwest Washington Medical Center
Vancouver, WA, USA
Volume 5, Chapter 2 Breast augmentation
Volume 5, Chapter 4 Current concepts in revisionary breast surgery
Volume 5, Video 4.01 Current concepts in revisionary breast surgery

Günter Germann, MD, PhD
Professor of Plastic Surgery
Clinic for Plastic and Reconstructive Surgery
Heidelberg University Hospital
Heidelberg, Germany
Volume 6, Chapter 10 Extensor tendon injuries and reconstruction

Goetz A. Giessler, MD, PhD
Plastic Surgeon, Hand Surgeon, Associate Professor of Plastic Surgery, Fellow of the European Board of Plastic Reconstructive and Aesthetic Surgery
BG Trauma Center Murnau
Murnau am Staffelsee, Germany
Volume 4, Chapter 4 Lower extremity sarcoma reconstruction
Volume 4, Video 4.01 Management of lower extremity sarcoma reconstruction

Jesse A. Goldstein, MD
Chief Resident
Department of Plastic Surgery
Georgetown University Hospital
Washington, DC, USA
Volume 3, Chapter 30 Cleft and craniofacial orthognathic surgery

Vijay S. Gorantla, MD, PhD
Associate Professor of Surgery
Department of Surgery, Division of Plastic and
Reconstructive Surgery
University of Pittsburgh Medical Center
Administrative Medical Director
Pittsburgh Reconstructive Transplantation
Program
Pittsburgh, PA, USA
*Volume 6, Chapter 38 Upper extremity
composite allotransplantation*
*Volume 6, Video 38.01 Upper extremity
composite allotransplantation*

Arun K. Gosain, MD
DeWayne Richey Professor and Vice Chair
Department of Plastic Surgery
University Hospitals Case Medical Center
Chief, Pediatric Plastic Surgery
Rainbow Babies and Children's Hospital
Cleveland, OH, USA
Volume 3, Chapter 38 Pierre Robin sequence

Lawrence J. Gottlieb, MD, FACS
Professor of Surgery
Director of Burn and Complex Wound Center
Director of Reconstructive Microsurgery
Fellowship
Section of Plastic and Reconstructive Surgery
Department of Surgery
University of Chicago
Chicago, IL, USA
*Volume 3, Chapter 41 Pediatric chest and trunk
defects*

Barry H. Grayson, DDS
Associate Professor of Surgery (Craniofacial
Orthodontics)
New York University Langone Medical Centre
Institute of Reconstructive Plastic Surgery
New York, NY, USA
Volume 3, Chapter 36 Craniofacial microsomia
Volume 3, Video 24.01 Repair of bilateral cleft lip

Arin K. Greene, MD, MMSc
Associate Professor of Surgery
Department of Plastic and Oral Surgery
Children's Hospital Boston
Harvard Medical School
Boston, MA, USA
Volume 1, Chapter 29 Vascular anomalies

James C. Grotting, MD, FACS
Clinical Professor of Plastic Surgery
University of Alabama at Birmingham;
The University of Wisconsin, Madison, WI;
Grotting and Cohn Plastic Surgery
Birmingham, AL, USA
Volume 5, Chapter 7 Mastopexy
Volume 5, Chapter 8.7 Sculpted pillar vertical
*Volume 5, Video 8.7.01 Marking the sculpted
pillar breast reduction*
Volume 5, Video 8.7.02 Breast reduction surgery

Ronald P. Gruber, MD
Associate Adjunct Clinical Professor
Division of Plastic and Reconstructive Surgery
Stanford University
Associate Clinical Professor
Division of Plastic and Reconstructive Surgery
University of California, San Francisco
San Francisco, CA, USA
Volume 2, Chapter 21 Secondary rhinoplasty

**Mohan S. Gundeti, MB, MCh, FEBU,
FRCS, FEAPU**
Associate Professor of Urology in Surgery and
Pediatrics, Director Pediatric Urology, Director
Centre for Pediatric Robotics and Minimal
Invasive Surgery
University of Chicago and Pritzker Medical
School Comer Children's Hospital
Chicago, IL, USA
*Volume 3, Chapter 44 Reconstruction of
urogenital defects: Congenital*
*Volume 3, Video 44.01 First stage hypospadias
repair with free inner preputial graft*
*Volume 3, Video 44.02 Second stage
hypospadias repair with tunica vaginalis flap*

Eyal Gur, MD
Head
Department of Plastic and Reconstructive
Surgery
The Tel Aviv Sourasky Medical Center
The Tel Aviv University School of Medicine
Tel Aviv, Israel
Volume 3, Chapter 11 Facial paralysis
Volume 3, Video 11.01 Facial paralysis

Geoffrey C. Gurtner, MD, FACS
Professor and Associate Chairman
Stanford University Department of Surgery
Stanford, CA, USA
*Volume 1, Chapter 13 Stem cells and
regenerative medecine*
*Volume 1, Chapter 35 Technology innovation in
plastic surgery*

Bahman Guyuron, MD
Kiehn-DesPrez Professor and Chairman
Department of Plastic Surgery
Case Western Reserve University School of
Medicine
Cleveland, OH, USA
*Volume 2, Chapter 20 Airway issues and the
deviated nose*
*Volume 3, Chapter 21 Surgical management of
migraine headaches*
Volume 2, Video 3.02 Botulinum toxin

Steven C. Haase, MD
Clinical Associate Professor
Department of Surgery, Section of Plastic
Surgery
University of Michigan Health
Ann Arbor, MI, USA
*Volume 6, Chapter 8 Fractures and dislocations
of the carpus and distal radius*

Robert S. Haber, MD, FAAD, FAAP
Assistant Professor, Dermatology and
Pediatrics
Case Western Reserve University School of
Medicine
Director
University Hair Transplant Center
Cleveland, OH, USA
*Volume 2, Video 23.08 Strip harvesting the
haber spreader*

Florian Hackl, MD
Research Fellow
Division of Plastic Surgery
Brigham and Women's Hospital
Harvard Medical School
Boston, MA, USA
*Volume 1, Chapter 11 Genetics and prenatal
diagnosis*

Phillip C. Haeck, MD
Private Practice
Seattle, WA, USA
*Volume 1, Chapter 4 The role of ethics in plastic
surgery*

Bruce Halperin, MD
Adjunct Associate Clinical Professor of
Anesthesia
Department of Anesthesia
Stanford University School of Medicine
Palo Alto, CA, USA
*Volume 1, Chapter 8 Patient safety in plastic
surgery*

Moustapha Hamdi, MD, PhD
Professor and Chairman of Plastic and
Reconstructive Surgery
Department of Plastic Surgery
Brussels University Hospital
Brussels, Belgium
*Volume 5, Chapter 21 Local flaps in partial
breast reconstruction*

Warren C. Hammert, MD
Associate Professor of Orthopaedic and
Plastic Surgery
Department of Orthopaedic Surgery
University of Rochester Medical Center
Rochester, NY, USA
*Volume 6, Chapter 7 Hand fractures and joint
injuries*

Dennis C. Hammond, MD
Clinical Assistant Professor
Department of Surgery
Michigan State University College of Human
Medicine
East Lansing
Associate Program Director
Plastic and Reconstructive Surgery
Grand Rapids Medical Education and Research
Center for Health Professions
Grand Rapids, MI, USA
*Volume 5, Chapter 8.4 Short scar periareolar
inferior pedicle reduction (SPAIR) mammaplasty*
Volume 5, Video 8.4.01 Spair technique

Scott L. Hansen, MD, FACS
Assistant Professor of Plastic and
Reconstructive Surgery
Chief, Hand and Microvascular Surgery
University of California, San Francisco
Chief, Plastic and Reconstructive Surgery
San Francisco General Hospital
San Francisco, CA, USA
*Volume 1, Chapter 24 Flap classification and
applications*

James A. Harris, MD
Cosmetic Surgeon
Private Practice
Hasson & Wong Aesthetic Surgery
Vancouver, BC, Canada
Volume 2, Video 23.05 FUE Harris safe system

Isaac Harvey, MD
Clinical Fellow
Department of Paediatric Plastic and
Reconstructive Surgery
Hospital for Sick Kids
Toronto, ON, Canada
*Volume 6, Chapter 35 Free functional muscle
transfers in the upper extremity*

Victor Hasson, MD
Cosmetic Surgeon
Private Practice
Hasson & Wong Aesthetic Surgery
Vancouver, BC, Canada
*Volume 2, Video 23.07 Perpendicular angle
grafting technique*

Theresa A Hegge, MD, MPH
Resident of Plastic Surgery
Division of Plastic Surgery
Southern Illinois University
Springfield, IL, USA
*Volume 6, Chapter 6 Nail and fingertip
reconstruction*

Jill A. Helms, DDS, PhD
Division of Plastic and Reconstructive Surgery
Department of Surgery
School of Medicine
Stanford University
Stanford, CA, USA
*Volume 3, Chapter 22 Embryology of the
craniofacial complex*

Ginard I. Henry, MD
Assistant Professor of Surgery
Section of Plastic Surgery
University of Chicago Medical Center
Chicago, IL, USA
*Volume 4, Chapter 1 Comprehensive lower
extremity anatomy, embryology, surgical exposure*

Vincent R. Hentz, MD
Emeritus Professor of Surgery and Orthopedic
Surgery (by courtesy)
Stanford University
Stanford, CA, USA
*Volume 6, Chapter 1 Anatomy and biomechanics
of the hand*
*Volume 6, Chapter 37 Restoration of upper
extremity function in tetraplegia*
*Volume 6, Video 37.01 1 Stage grasp IC 6 short
term*
*Volume 6, Video 37.02 2 Stage grasp release
outcome*

**Rebecca L. von der Heyde, PhD,
OTR/L, CHT**
Associate Professor
Program in Occupational Therapy
Maryville University
St. Louis, MO, USA
Volume 6, Chapter 39 Hand therapy
*Volume 6, Video 39.01 Hand therapy
Goniometric measurement*
Volume 6, Video 39.02 Threshold testing
*Volume 6, Video 39.03 Fabrication of a
synergistic splint*

Kent K. Higdon, MD
Former Aesthetic Fellow
Grotting and Cohn Plastic Surgery;
Current Assistant Professor
Vanderbilt University
Nashville, TN, USA
Volume 5, Chapter 7 Mastopexy
Volume 5, Chapter 8.1 Reduction mammaplasty
*Volume 5, Chapter 8.7 Sculpted pillar vertical
mammaplasty*

John Hijjawi, MD, FACS
Assistant Professor
Department of Plastic Surgery, Department of
General Surgery
Medical College of Wisconsin
Milwaukee, WI, USA
*Volume 4, Chapter 20 Cold and chemical injury
to the upper extremity*

Jonay Hill, MD
Clinical Assistant Professor
Anesthesiology Department
Anesthesia and Critical Care
Stanford University School of Medicine
Stanford, CA, USA
*Volume 6, Chapter 4 Anesthesia for upper
extremity surgery*

Piet Hoebeke, MD, PhD
Full Senior Professor of Paediatric Urology
Department of Urology
Ghent University Hospital
Ghent, Belgium
*Volume 4, Chapter 13 Reconstruction of male
genital defects*
*Volume 4, Video 13.01 Complete and partial
penile reconstruction*

William Y. Hoffman, MD
Professor and Chief
Division of Plastic and Reconstructive Surgery
University of California, San Francisco
San Francisco, CA, USA
Volume 3, Chapter 25 Cleft palate

Larry H. Hollier Jr., MD, FACS
Professor and Program Director
Division of Plastic Surgery
Baylor College of Medicine and Texas
Children's Hospital
Houston, TX, USA
*Volume 3, Chapter 29 Secondary deformities of
the cleft lip, nose, and palate*
Volume 3, Video 29.01 Complete takedown
Volume 3, Video 29.02 Abbé flap
*Volume 3, Video 29.03 Thick lip and buccal
sulcus deformities*
Volume 3, Video 29.04 Alveolar bone grafting
Volume 3, Video 29.05 Definitive rhinoplasty

Joon Pio Hong, MD, PhD, MMM
Chief and Associate Professor
Department of Plastic Surgery
Asian Medical Center University of Ulsan
School of Medicine
Seoul, Korea
*Volume 4, Chapter 5 Reconstructive surgery:
Lower extremity coverage*

Richard A. Hopper, MD, MS
Chief
Division of Pediatric Plastic Surgery
University of Washingtion
Surgical Director
Craniofacial Center
Seattle Childrens Hospital
Associate Professor
Division of Plastic Surgery
Seattle, WA, USA
Volume 3, Chapter 26 Alveolar clefts
Volume 3, Chapter 36 Craniofacial microsomia

Philippe Houtmeyers, MD
Resident
Plastic Surgery
Ghent University Hospital
Ghent, Belgium
*Volume 4, Chapter 13 Reconstruction of male
genital defects*
*Volume 4, Video 13.01 Complete and partial
penile reconstruction*

Steven E.R. Hovius, MD, PhD
Head
Department of Plastic, Reconstructive and
Hand Surgery
ErasmusmMC
University Medical Center
Rotterdam, The Netherlands
*Volume 6, Chapter 28 Congenital hand IV
disorders of differentiation and duplication*

Michael A. Howard, MD
Clinical Assistant Professor of Surgery
Division of Plastic Surgery
University of Chicago, Pritzker School of
Medicine
Northbrook, IL, USA
*Volume 4, Chapter 9 Comprehensive trunk
anatomy*

Jung-Ju Huang, MD
Assistant Professor
Division of Microsurgery
Plastic and Reconstructive Surgery
Chang Gung Memorial Hospital
Taoyuan, Taiwan, The People's Republic of
China
*Volume 3, Chapter 12 Oral cavity, tongue, and
mandibular reconstructions*
*Volume 3, Video 12.01 Fibula
osteoseptocutaneous flap for composite
mandibular reconstruction*
*Volume 3, Video 12.02 Ulnar forearm flap for
buccal reconstruction*

C. Scott Hultman, MD, MBA, FACS
Ethel and James Valone Distinguished
Professor of Surgery
Division of Plastic Surgery
University of North Carolina
Chapel Hill, NC, USA
*Volume 1, Chapter 5 Business principles for
plastic surgeons*

Leung-Kim Hung, MChOrtho (Liv)
Professor
Department of Orthopaedics and Traumatology
Faculty of Medicine
The Chinese University of Hong Kong
Hong Kong, The People's Republic of China
*Volume 6, Chapter 29 Congenital hand V
disorders of overgrowth, undergrowth, and
generalized skeletal deformities*

Gazi Hussain, MBBS, FRACS
Clinical Senior Lecturer
Macquarie Cosmetic and Plastic Surgery
Macquarie University
Sydney, Australia
Volume 3, Chapter 11 Facial paralysis

Marco Innocenti, MD
Director Reconstructive Microsurgery
Department of Oncology
Careggi University Hospital
Florence, Italy
*Volume 6, Chapter 30 Growth considerations in
pediatric upper extremity trauma and
reconstruction*
*Volume 6, Video 30.01 Epiphyseal transplant
harvesting technique*

Clyde H. Ishii, MD, FACS
Assistant Clinical Professor of Surgery
John A. Burns School of Medicine
Chief, Department of Plastic Surgery
Shriners Hospital
Honolulu Unit
Honolulu, HI, USA
*Volume 2, Chapter 10 Asian facial cosmetic
surgery*

Jonathan S. Jacobs, DMD, MD
Associate Professor of Clinical Plastic Surgery
Eastern Virginia Medical School
Norfolk, VA, USA
*Volume 2, Chapter 16 Anthropometry,
cephalometry, and orthognathic surgery*
*Volume 2, Video 16.01 Anthropometry,
cephalometry, and orthognathic surgery*

Jordan M.S. Jacobs, MD
Craniofacial Fellow
Department of Plastic Surgery
New York University Langone Medical Center
New York, NY, USA
*Volume 2, Chapter 16 Anthropometry,
cephalometry, and orthognathic surgery*
*Volume 2, Video 16.01 Anthropometry,
cephalometry, and orthognathic surgery*

**Ian T. Jackson, MD, DSc(Hon), FRCS,
FACS, FRACS (Hon)**
Emeritus Surgeon
Surgical Services Administration
William Beaumont Hospitals
Royal Oak, MI, USA
*Volume 3, Chapter 18 Local flaps for facial
coverage*

Oksana Jackson, MD
Assistant Professor of Surgery
Division of Plastic Surgery
University of Pennsylvania School of Medicine
Clinical Associate
The Children's Hospital of Philadelphia
Philadelphia, PA, USA
Volume 3, Chapter 43 Conjoined twins

Jeffrey E. Janis, MD, FACS
Associate Professor
Program Director
Department of Plastic Surgery
University of Texas Southwestern Medical
Center
Chief of Plastic Surgery
Chief of Wound Care
President-Elect
Medical Staff
Parkland Health and Hospital System
Dallas, TX, USA
Volume 4, Chapter 16 Pressure sores

Leila Jazayeri, MD
Resident
Stanford University Plastic and Reconstructive
Surgery
Stanford, CA, USA
*Volume 1, Chapter 35 Technology innovation in
plastic surgery*

Elizabeth B. Jelks, MD
Private Practice
Jelks Medical
New York, NY, USA
*Volume 2, Chapter 9 Secondary blepharoplasty:
Techniques*

Glenn W. Jelks, MD
Associate Professor
Department of Ophthalmology
Department of Plastic Surgery
New York University School of Medicine
New York, NY, USA
*Volume 2, Chapter 9 Secondary blepharoplasty:
Techniques*

Mark Laurence Jewell, MD
Assistant Clinical Professor of Plastic Surgery
Oregon Health Science University
Jewell Plastic Surgery Center
Eugene, OR, USA
*Volume 2, Chapter 11.4 Facelift: Facial
rejuvenation with loop sutures, the MACS lift and
its derivatives*

Andreas Jokuszies, MD
Consultant Plastic, Aesthetic and Hand
Surgeon
Department of Plastic, Hand and
Reconstructive Surgery
Hanover Medical School
Hanover, Germany
*Volume 1, Chapter 15 Skin wound healing:
Repair biology, wound, and scar treatment*

Neil F. Jones, MD, FRCS
Chief of Hand Surgery
University of California Medical Center
Professor of Orthopedic Surgery
Professor of Plastic and Reconstructive Surgery
University of California Irvine
Irvine, CA, USA
Volume 6, Chapter 22 Ischemia of the hand
*Volume 6, Chapter 34 Tendon transfers in the
upper extremity*
*Volume 6, Video 34.01 EIP to EPL tendon
transfer*

David M. Kahn, MD
Clinical Associate Professor of Plastic Surgery
Department of Surgery
Stanford University School of Medicine
Stanford, CA, USA
Volume 2, Chapter 21 Secondary rhinoplasty

Ryosuke Kakinoki, MD, PhD
Associate Professor
Chief of the Hand Surgery and Microsurgery
Unit
Department of Orthopedic Surgery and
Rehabilitation Medicine
Graduate School of Medicine
Kyoto University
Kyoto, Japan
*Volume 6, Chapter 2 Examination of the upper
extremity*
*Volume 2, Video 2.01-2.17 Examination of the
upper extremity*

Alex Kane, MD
Associate Professor of Surgery
Washington University School of Medicine
St. Louis, WO, USA
Volume 3, Chapter 23 Repair of unilateral cleft lip

Gabrielle M. Kane, MBBCh, EdD, FRCPC
Medical Director, Associate Professor
Department of Radiation Oncology
Associate Professor
Department of Medical Education and
Biomedical Informatics
University of Washington School of Medicine
Seattle, WA, USA
*Volume 1, Chapter 28 Therapeutic radiation:
Principles, effects, and complications*

Michael A. C. Kane, MD
Attending Surgeon Manhattan Eye, Ear and
Throat Institute
Department of Plastic Surgery
New York, NY, USA
Volume 2, Chapter 3 Botulinum toxin (BoNT-A)

Dennis S. Kao, MD
Hand Fellow
Department of Plastic Surgery
Medical College of Wisconsin
Milwaukee, WI, USA
*Volume 4, Chapter 20 Cold and chemical injury
to the upper extremity*

Sahil Kapur, MD
Resident, Plastic and Reconstructive Surgery
Department of Surgery, Division of Plastic and
Reconstructive Surgery
University of Wisconsin
Madison, WI, USA
Volume 3, Chapter 42 Pediatric tumors

Leila Kasrai, MD, MPH, FRCSC
Head, Division of Plastic Surgery
St Joseph's Hospital
Toronto, ON, Canada
Volume 2, Video 22.01 Setback otoplasty

Abdullah E. Kattan, MBBS, FRCS(C)
Clinical Fellow
Division of Plastic Surgery
Department of Surgery
University of Toronto
Toronto, ON, Canada
*Volume 4, Chapter 23 Management of patients
with exfoliative disorders, epidermolysis bullosa,
and TEN*

David L. Kaufman, MD, FACS
Private Practice Plastic Surgery
Aesthetic Artistry Surgical and Medical Center
Folsom, CA, USA
Volume 2, Chapter 21 Secondary rhinoplasty

Lindsay B. Katona, BA
Research Associate
Thayer School of Engineering
Dartmouth College
Hanover, NH, USA
*Volume 1, Chapter 36 Robotics, simulation, and
telemedicine in plastic surgery*

Henry K. Kawamoto, Jr., MD, DDS
Clinical Professor
Division of Plastic Surgery
University of California at Los Angeles
Los Angeles, CA, USA
Volume 3, Chapter 33 Craniofacial clefts

Jeffrey M. Kenkel, MD, FACS
Professor and Vice-Chairman
Rod J Rohrich MD Distinguished Professorship
in Wound Healing and Plastic Surgery
Department of Plastic Surgery
Southwestern Medical School
Director
Clinical Center for Cosmetic Laser Treatment
Dallas, TX, USA
*Volume 2, Chapter 24 Liposuction: A
comprehensive review of techniques and safety*

Carolyn L. Kerrigan, MD, MSc
Professor of Surgery
Section of Plastic Surgery
Dartmouth Hitchcock Medical Center
Lebanon, NH, USA
*Volume 1, Chapter 10 Evidence-based medicine
and health services research in plastic surgery*

Marwan R. Khalifeh, MD
Instructor of Plastic Surgery
Department of Plastic Surgery
Johns Hopkins University School of Medicine
Washington, DC, USA
*Volume 4, Chapter 12 Abdominal wall
reconstruction*

Jae-Hoon Kim, MD
April 31 Aesthetic Plastic Surgical Clinic
Seoul, South Korea
*Volume 2, Video 10.03 Secondary rhinoplasty:
septal extension graft and costal cartilage strut
fixed with K-wire*

**Timothy W. King, MD, PhD, MSBE,
FACS, FAAP**
Assistant Professor of Surgery and Pediatrics
Director of Research
Division of Plastic Surgery, Department of
Surgery
University of Wisconsin School of Medicine and
Public Health
Madison, WI, USA
Volume 1, Chapter 32 Implants and biomaterials

Brian M. Kinney, MD, FACS, MSME
Clinical Assistant Professor of Plastic Surgery
University of Southern California School of
Medicine
Los Angeles, CA, USA
*Volume 1, Chapter 7 Photography in plastic
surgery*

Richard E. Kirschner, MD
Chief, Section of Plastic and Reconstructive
Surgery
Director, Ambulatory Surgical Services
Director, Cleft Lip and Palate Center
Co-Director Nationwide Children's Hospital
Professor of Surgery and Pediatrics
Senior Vice Chair, Department of Plastic Surgery
The Ohio State University College of Medicine
Columbus, OH, USA
Volume 3, Chapter 28 Velopharyngeal dysfunction
*Volume 3, Video 28.01-28.03 Velopharyngeal
incompetence*

Elizabeth Kiwanuka, MD
Division of Plastic Surgery
Brigham and Women's Hospital
Harvard Medical School
Boston, MA, USA
*Volume 1, Chapter 11 Genetics and prenatal
diagnosis*

Grant M. Kleiber, MD
Plastic Surgery Resident
Section of Plastic and Reconstructive Surgery
University of Chicago Medical Center
Chicago, IL, USA
*Volume 4, Chapter 1 Comprehensive lower
extremity anatomy, embryology, surgical exposure*

Mathew B. Klein, MD, MS
David and Nancy Auth-Washington Research
Foundation Endowed Chair for Restorative
Burn Surgery
Division of Plastic Surgery
University of Washington
Program Director and Associate Professor
Division of Plastic Surgery
Harborview Medical Center
Seattle, WA, USA
Volume 4, Chapter 22 Reconstructive burn surgery

Kyung S Koh, MD, PhD
Professor of Plastic Surgery
Asan Medical Center, University of Ulsan
School of Medicine
Seoul, Korea
*Volume 2, Chapter 10 Asian facial cosmetic
surgery*

John C. Koshy, MD
Postdoctoral Research Fellow
Division of Plastic Surgery
Baylor College of Medicine
Houston, TX, USA
*Volume 3, Chapter 29 Secondary deformities of
the cleft lip, nose, and palate*
Volume 3, Video 29.01 Complete takedown
Volume 3, Video 29.02 Abbé flap
*Volume 3, Video 29.03 Thick lip and buccal
sulcus deformities*
Volume 3, Video 29.04 Alveolar bone grafting
Volume 3, Video 29.05 Definitive rhinoplasty

Evan Kowalski, BS
Section of Plastic Surgery
University of Michigan Health System
Ann Arbor, MI, USA
Volume 6, Video 19.02 Silicone MCP arthroplasty

Stephen J. Kovach, MD
Assistant Professor of Surgery
Division of Plastic and Reconstructive Surgery
University of Pennsylvannia Health System
Assistant Professor of Surgery
Department of Orthopaedic Surgery
University of Pennsylvannia Health System
Philadelphia, PA, USA
Volume 4, Chapter 7 Skeletal reconstruction

Steven J. Kronowitz, MD, FACS
Professor, Department of Plastic Surgery
MD Anderson Cancer Center
The University of Texas
Houston, TX, USA
*Volume 1, Chapter 28 Therapeutic radiation
principles, effects, and complications*

Todd A. Kuiken, MD, PhD
Director
Center for Bionic Medicine
Rehabilitation Institute of Chicago
Professor
Department of PMandR
Fienberg School of Medicine
Northwestern University
Chicago, IL, USA
*Volume 6, Chapter 40 Treatment of the upper
extremity amputee*
*Volume 6, Video 40.01 Targeted muscle
reinnervation in the transhumeral amputee*

Michael E. Kupferman, MD
Assistant Professor
Department of Head and Neck Surgery
Division of Surgery
The University of Texas MD Anderson Cancer
Center
Houston, TX, USA
*Volume 3, Chapter 17 Carcinoma of the upper
aerodigestive tract*

Robert Kwon, MD
Plastic Surgeon
Regional Plastic Surgery Center
Richardson, TX, USA
Volume 4, Chapter 16 Pressure sores

**Eugenia J. Kyriopoulos, MD, MSc, PhD,
FEBOPRAS**
Attending Plastic Surgeon
Department of Plastic Surgery and Burn Center
Athens General Hospital "G. Gennimatas"
Athens, Greece
*Volume 5, Chapter 21 Local flaps in partial
breast reconstruction*

Donald Lalonde, BSC, MD, MSc, FRCSC
Professor Surgery
Division of Plastic Surgery
Saint John Campus of Dalhousie University
Saint John, NB, Canada
*Volume 6, Chapter 24 Nerve entrapment
syndromes*
*Volume 6, Video 24.01 Carpal tunnel and cubital
tunnel releases*

Wee Leon Lam, MB, ChB, M Phil, FRCS
Microsurgery Fellow
Department of Plastic and Reconstructive
Surgery
Chang Gung Memorial Hospital
Taipei, Taiwan, The People's Republic of China
*Volume 6, Chapter 14 Thumb and finger
reconstruction – microsurgical techniques*
Volume 6, Video 14.01 Trimmed great toe
Volume 6, Video 14.02 Second toe for index
*Volume 6, Video 14.03 Combined second and
third toe for metacarpal hand*

Julie E. Lang, MD, FACS
Assistant Professor of Surgery
Department of surgery
Director of Breast Surgical Oncology
University of Arizona
Tucson, AZ, USA
*Volume 5, Chapter 10 Breast cancer: Diagnosis
therapy and oncoplastic techniques*
*Volume 5, Video 10.01 Breast cancer: diagnosis
and therapy*

Patrick Lang, MD
Plastic Surgery Resident
University of California
San Francisco, CA, USA
*Volume 1, Chapter 24 Flap classification and
applications*

Claude-Jean Langevin, MD, DMD
Assistant Professor University of Central Florida
Department of Surgery MD Anderson Cancer
Center
Plastic and Reconstructive Surgeon
University of Central Florida
Orlando, FL, USA
Volume 2, Chapter 13 Neck rejuvenation

Laurent Lantieri, MD
Department of Plastic Surgery
Hôpital Européen Georges Pompidou
Assistance Publique Hôpitaux de Paris
Paris Descartes University
Paris, France
Volume 3, Chapter 20 Facial transplant
Volume 3, Video 20.1 and 20.2 Facial transplant

Michael C. Large, MD
Urology Resident
Department of Surgery, Division of Urology
University of Chicago Hospitals
Chicago, IL, USA
*Volume 3, Chapter 44 Reconstruction of
urogenital defects: Congenital*
*Volume 3, Video 44.01 First stage hypospadias
repair with free inner preputial graft*
*Volume 3, Video 44.02 Second stage
hypospadias repair with tunica vaginalis flap*

Don LaRossa, MD
Emeritus Professor of Surgery
Division of Plastic and Reconstructive Surgery
Perelman School of Medicine
University of Pennsylvania
Philadelphia, PA, USA
Volume 3, Chapter 43 Conjoined twins

Caroline Leclercq, MD
Consultant Hand Surgeon
Institut de la Main
Paris, France
*Volume 6, Chapter 17 Management of
Dupuytren's disease*

Justine C. Lee, MD, PhD
Chief Resident
Section of Plastic and Reconstructive Surgery
Department
University of Chicago Medical Center
Chicago, IL, USA
*Volume 3, Chapter 41 Pediatric chest and trunk
defects*

W. P. Andrew Lee, MD
The Milton T. Edgerton, MD, Professor and
Chairman
Department of Plastic and Reconstructive
Surgery
Johns Hopkins University School of Medicine
Baltimore, MD, USA
*Volume 1, Chapter 34 Transplantation in plastic
surgery*
*Volume 6, Chapter 38 Upper extremity
composite allotransplantation*
*Volume 6, Video 38.01 Upper extremity
composite tissue allotransplantation*

Valerie Lemaine, MD, MPH, FRCSC
Assistant Professor of Plastic Surgery
Department of Surgery
Division of Plastic Surgery
Mayo Clinic
Rochester, MN, USA
*Volume 1, Chapter 10 Evidence-based medicine
and health services research in plastic surgery*

**Ping-Chung Leung, SBS, OBE, JP, MBBS,
MS, DSc, Hon DSocSc, FRACS, FRCS,
FHKCOS, FHKAM (ORTH)**
Professor Emeritus
Orthopaedics and Traumatology
The Chinese University of Hong Kong
Hong Kong, The People's Republic of China
*Volume 6, Chapter 29 Congenital hand V
disorders of overgrowth, undergrowth, and
generalized skeletal deformities*

Benjamin Levi, MD
Post Doctoral Research Fellow
Division of Plastic and Reconstructive Surgery
Stanford University
Stanford, CA
House Officer
Division of Plastic and Reconstructive Surgery
University of Michigan
Ann Arbor, MI, USA
*Volume 1, Chapter 13 Stem cells and
regenerative medicine*

L. Scott Levin, MD, FACS
Chairman of Orthopedic Surgery
Department of Orthopaedic Surgery
University of Pennsylvania School of Medicine
Philadelphia, PA, USA
Volume 4, Chapter 7 Skeletal reconstruction

Bradley Limmer, MD
Assistant Clinical Professor
Department of Internal Medicine
Division of Dermatology
Associate Clinical Professor
Department of Plastic and Reconstructive
Surgery
Surgeon, Private Practice
Limmer Clinic
San Antonio, TX, USA
*Volume 2, Video 23.02 Follicular unit hair
transplantation*

Bobby L. Limmer, MD
Professor of Dermatology
University of Texas
Surgeon, Private Practice
Limmer Clinic
San Antonio, TX, USA
*Volume 2, Video 23.02 Follicular unit hair
transplantation*

Frank Lista, MD, FRCSC
Medical Director
Burn Program
The Plastic Surgery Clinic
Mississauga, ON, Canada
*Volume 5, Chapter 8.3 Superior or medial
pedicle*

Wei Liu, MD, PhD
Professor of Plastic Surgery
Associate Director of National Tissue
Engineering Research Center
Department of Plastic and Reconstructive
Surgery
Shanghai 9th People's Hospital
Shanghai Jiao Tong University School of
Medcine
Shanghai, The People's Republic of China
*Volume 1, Chapter 18 Tissue graft, tissue repair,
and regeneration*
*Volume 1, Chapter 20 Repair, grafting, and
engineering of cartilage*

Michelle B. Locke, MBChB, MD
Honourary Lecturer
University of Auckland Department of Surgery
Auckland City Hospital Support Building
Grafton, Auckland, New Zealand
*Volume 2, Chapter 1 Managing the cosmetic
patient*

Sarah A. Long, BA
Research Associate
Thayer School of Engineering
Dartmouth College
San Mateo, CA, USA
*Volume 1, Chapter 36 Robotics, simulation, and
telemedicine in plastic surgery*

Michael T. Longaker, MD, MBA, FACS
Deane P. and Louise Mitchell Professor and
Vice Chair
Department of Surgery
Stanford University
Stanford, CA, USA
*Volume 1, Chapter 13 Stem cells and
regenerative medicine*

Peter Lorenz, MD
Chief of Pediatric Plastic Surgery, Director
Craniofacial Surgery Fellowship
Department of Surgery, Division of Plastic
Surgery
Stanford University School of Medicine
Stanford, CA, USA
*Volume 1, Chapter 16 Scar prevention,
treatment, and revision*

Joseph E. Losee, MD, FACS, FAAP
Professor of Surgery and Pediatrics
Chief, Division Pediatric Plastic Surgery
Children's Hospital of Pittsburgh
University of Pittsburgh Medical Center
Pittsburgh, PA, USA
Volume 3, Chapter 31 Pediatric facial fractures

Albert Losken, MD, FACS
Associate Professor Program Director
Emory Division of Plastic and Reconstructive
Surgery
Emory University School of Medicine
Atlanta, GA, USA
*Volume 5, Chapter 11 The oncoplastic approach
to partial breast reconstruction*

Maria M. LoTempio, MD
Assistant Professor in Plastic Surgery
Medical University of South Carolina
Charleston, SC
Adjunct Assistant Professor in Plastic Surgery
New York Eye and Ear Infirmary
New York, NY, USA
*Volume 5, Chapter 19 Alternative flaps for breast
reconstruction*

Otway Louie, MD
Assistant Professor
Division of Plastic and Reconstructive Surgery
Department of Surgery
University of Washington Medical Center
Seattle, WA, USA
Volume 4, Chapter 17 Perineal reconstruction

David W. Low, MD
Professor of Surgery
Division of Plastic Surgery
University of Pennsylvania School of Medicine
Clinical Associate
The Children's Hospital of Philadelphia
Philadelphia, PA, USA
Volume 3, Chapter 43 Conjoined twins

Nicholas Lumen, MD, PhD
Assistant Professor of Urology
Urology
Ghent University Hospital
Ghent, Belgium
*Volume 4, Chapter 13 Reconstruction of male
genital defects*
*Volume 4, Video 13.01 Complete and partial
penile reconstruction*

Antonio Luiz de Vasconcellos Macedo, MD
General Surgery
Director of Robotic Surgery
President of Oncology
Board of Albert Einstein Hospital
Sao Paulo, Brazil
*Volume 5, Chapter 20 Omentum reconstruction
of the breast*

Gustavo R. Machado, MD
University of California Irvine Medical Center
Department of Orthopaedic Surgery, Orange,
CA, USA
*Volume 6, Video 34.01 EIP to EPL tendon
transfer*

Susan E. Mackinnon, MD
Sydney M. Shoenberg, Jr. and Robert H.
Shoenberg Professor
Department of Surgery, Division of Plastic and
Reconstructive Surgery
Washington University School of Medicine
St. Louis, MO, USA
*Volume 1, Chapter 22 Repair and grafting of
peripheral nerve*
Volume 6, Chapter 33 Nerve transfers
Volume 6, Video 33.01 Nerve transfers

Ralph T. Manktelow, BA, MD, FRCS(C)
Professor
Department of Surgery
University of Toronto
Toronto, ON, Canada
Volume 3, Chapter 11 Facial paralysis

Paul N. Manson, MD
Professor of Plastic Surgery
University of Maryland Shock Trauma Unit
University of Maryland and Johns Hopkins
Schools of Medicine
Baltimore, MD, USA
Volume 3, Chapter 3 Facial fractures

Daniel Marchac, MD
Professor
Plastic, Reconstructive and Aesthetic
College of Medicine of Paris Hospitals
Paris, France
Volume 3, Chapter 32 Orbital hypertelorism

Malcom W. Marks, MD
Professor and Chairman
Department of Plastic Surgery
Wake Forest University School of Medicine
Winston-Salem, NC, USA
*Volume 1, Chapter 27 Principles and applications
of tissue expansion*

Timothy J. Marten, MD, FACS
Founder and Director
Marten Clinic of Plastic Surgery
Medical Director
San Francisco Center for the Surgical Arts
San Francisco, CA, USA
*Volume 2, Chapter 12 Secondary deformities
and the secondary facelift*

Mario Marzola, MBBS
Private Practice
Norwood, SA, Australia
Volume 2, Video 23.01 Donor closure tricophytic technique

Alessandro Masellis, MD
Plastic Surgeon
Department of Plastic Surgery and Burn Therapy
Ospedale Civico ARNAS Palermo
Palermo, Italy
Volume 4, Chapter 19 Extremity burn reconstruction

Michele Masellis, MD, PhD
Plastic Surgeon
Former Chief
Professor Emeritus
Department of Plastic Surgery and Burn Unit
ARNAS Civico Hospital
Palermo, Italy
Volume 4, Chapter 19 Extremity burn reconstruction

Jaume Masia, MD, PhD
Professor and Chief
Plastic Surgery Department
Hospital de la Santa Creu i Sant Pau
Universidad Autónoma de Barcelona
Barcelona, Spain
Volume 5, Chapter 13 Imaging in reconstructive breast surgery

David W. Mathes, MD
Associate Professor of Surgery
Department of Surgery, Division of Plastic and Reconstructive Surgery
University of Washington School of Medicine
Chief of Plastic Surgery
Puget Sound Veterans Affairs Hospital
Seattle, WA, USA
Volume 1, Chapter 34 Transplantation in plastic surgery

Evan Matros, MD
Assistant Attending Surgeon
Department of Surgery
Memorial Sloan-Kettering Cancer Center
Assistant Professor of Surgery (Plastic)
Weill Cornell University Medical Center
New York, NY, USA
Volume 1, Chapter 12 Principles of cancer management

G. Patrick Maxwell, MD, FACS
Clinical Professor of Surgery
Department of Plastic Surgery
Loma Linda University Medical Center
Loma Linda, CA, USA
Volume 5, Chapter 2 Breast augmentation
Volume 5, Chapter 4 Current concepts in revisionary breast surgery

Isabella C. Mazzola
Milan, Italy
Volume 1, Chapter 2 History of reconstructive and aesthetic surgery

Riccardo F. Mazzola, MD
Professor of Plastic Surgery
Postgraduate School Plastic Surgery
Maxillo-Facial and Otolaryngolog
Department of Specialistic Surgical Science
School of Medicine
University of Milan
Milan, Italy
Volume 1, Chapter 2 History of reconstructive and aesthetic surgery

Steven J. McCabe, MD, MSc
Assistant Professor
Department of Bioinformatics and Biostatistics
University of Louisville School of Public Health and Information Sciences
Louisville, KY, USA
Volume 6, Chapter 18 Occupational hand disorders

Joseph G. McCarthy, MD
Lawrence D. Bell Professor of Plastic Surgery,
Director Institute of Reconstructive Plastic Surgery and Chair
Department of Plastic Surgery
New York University Langone Medical Center
New York, NY, USA
Volume 3, Chapter 36 Craniofacial microsomia

Mary H. McGrath, MD, MPH
Plastic Surgeon
Division of Plastic Surgery
University of California San Francisco
San Francisco, CA, USA
Volume 1, Chapter 3 Psychological aspects of plastic surgery

Kai Megerle, MD
Research Fellow
Division of Plastic and Reconstructive Surgery
Stanford Medical Center
Stanford, CA, USA
Volume 6, Chapter 10 Extensor tendon injuries

Babak J. Mehrara, MD, FACS
Associate Member, Associate Professor of Surgery (Plastic)
Memorial Sloan-Kettering Cancer Center
Weil Cornell University Medical Center
New York, NY, USA
Volume 1, Chapter 12 Principles of cancer management

Bryan Mendelson, FRCSE, FRACS, FACS
Private Plastic Surgeon
The Centre for Facial Plastic Surgery
Melbourne, Australia
Volume 2, Chapter 6 Anatomy of the aging face

Constantino G. Mendieta, MD, FACS
Private Practice
Miami, FL, USA
Volume 2, Chapter 28 Buttock augmentation
Volume 2, Video 28.01 Buttock augmentation

Frederick J. Menick, MD
Private Practitioner
Tucson, AZ, USA
Volume 3, Chapter 6 Aesthetic nasal reconstruction
Volume 3, Video 6.01 Aesthetic reconstruction of the nose – The 3-stage folded forehead flap for cover and lining,
Volume 3, Video 6.02 Aesthetic reconstruction of the nose-First stage transfer and intermediate operation

Ursula Mirastschijski, MD, PhD
Assistant Professor
Department of Plastic, Hand and Reconstructive Surgery, Burn Center Lower Saxony, Replantation Center
Hannover Medical School
Hannover, Germany
Volume 1, Chapter 15 Skin wound healing: Repair biology, wound, and scar treatment

Takayuki Miura, MD
Emeritus Professor of Orthopedic Surgery
Department of Orthopedic Surgery
Nagoya University School of Medicine
Nagoya, Japan
Volume 6, Chapter 29 Congenital hand V: Disorders of overgrowth, undergrowth, and generalized skeletal deformities

Fernando Molina, MD
Professor of Plastic, Aesthetic and Reconstructive Surgery
Reconstructive and Plastic Surgery
Hospital General "Dr. Manuel Gea Gonzalez"
Universidad Nacional Autonoma de Mexico
Mexico City, Mexico
Volume 3, Chapter 39 Treacher-Collins syndrome

Stan Monstrey, MD, PhD
Professor in Plastic Surgery
Department of Plastic Surgery
Ghent University Hospital
Ghent, Belgium
Volume 4, Chapter 13 Reconstruction of male genital defects
Volume 4, Video 13.01 Complete and partial penile reconstruction

Steven L. Moran, MD
Professor and Chair of Plastic Surgery
Division of Plastic Surgery, Division of Hand and Microsurgery
Professor of Orthopedics
Rochester, MN, USA
Volume 6, Chapter 20 Management of osteoarthritis of the hand and wrist

Luis Humberto Uribe Morelli, MD
Resident of Plastic Surgery
Unisanta Plastic Surgery Department
Sao Paulo, Brazil
Volume 2, Chapter 26 Lipoabdominoplasty
Volume 2, Video 26.01 Lipobdominoplasty
(including secondary lipo)

Robert J. Morin, MD
Plastic Surgeon and Craniofacial Surgeon
Department of Plastic Surgery
Hackensack University Medical Center
Hackensack, NJ
New York Eye and Ear Infirmary
New York, NY, USA
Volume 3, Chapter 8 Acquired cranial and facial
bone deformities

Steven F. Morris, MD, MSc, FRCS(C)
Professor of Surgery
Professor of Anatomy and Neurobiology
Dalhousie University
Halifax, NS, Canada
Volume 1, Chapter 23 Vascular territories

Colin Myles Morrison, MSc (Hons),
FRCSI (Plast)
Consultant Plastic Surgeon
Department of Plastic and Reconstructive
Surgery
St. Vincent's University Hospital
Dublin, Ireland
Volume 2, Chapter 13 Neck rejuvenation
Volume 5, Chapter 18 The deep inferior
epigastric artery perforator (DIEAP) flap

Wayne A. Morrison, MBBS, MD, FRACS
Director
O'Brien Institute
Professorial Fellow
Department of Surgery
St Vincent's Hospital
University of Melbourne
Plastic Surgeon
St Vincent's Hospital
Melbourne, Australia
Volume 1, Chapter 19 Tissue engineering

Robyn Mosher, MS
Medical Editor/Project Manager
Thayer School of Engineering (contract)
Dartmouth College
Norwich, VT, USA
Volume 1, Chapter 36 Robotics, simulation, and
telemedicine in plastic surgery

Dimitrios Motakis, MD, PhD, FRCSC
Plastic and Reconstructive Surgeon
Private Practice
University Lecturer
Department of Surgery
University of Toronto
Toronto, ON, Canada
Volume 2, Chapter 4 Soft-tissue fillers

A. Aldo Mottura, MD, PhD
Associate Professor of Surgery
School of Medicine
National University of Córdoba
Cordoba, Argentina
Volume 1, Chapter 9 Local anesthetics in plastic
surgery

Hunter R. Moyer, MD
Fellow
Department of Plastic and Reconstructive
Surgery
Emory University, Atlanta, GA, USA
Volume 5, Chapter 16 The bilateral Pedicled
TRAM flap

Gustavo Muchado, MD
Plastic surgeon
Division of Plastic and Reconstructive Surgery
and Department of Orthopaedic Surgery
University of California Irvine Medical Center
Orange, CA, USA
Volume 6, Video 34.01 EIP to EPL tendon
transfer

Reid V. Mueller, MD
Associate Professor
Division of Plastic and Reconstructive Surgery
Oregon Health and Science University
Portland, OR, USA
Volume 3, Chapter 2 Facial trauma: soft tissue
injuries

John B. Mulliken, MD
Director, Craniofacial Centre
Department of Plastic and Oral Surgery
Children's Hospital
Boston, MA, USA
Volume 1, Chapter 29 Vascular anomalies
Volume 3, Chapter 24 Repair of bilateral cleft lip

Egle Muti, MD
Associate Professor of Plastic Reconstructive
and Aesthetic Surgery
Department of Plastic Surgery
University of Turin School of Medicine
Turin, Italy
Volume 5, Chapter 23.1 Congenital anomalies of
the breast
Volume 5, Video 23.01.01 Congenital anomalies
of the breast: An example of tuberous breast
type 1 corrected with glandular flap type 1

Maurice Y. Nahabedian, MD
Associate Professor Plastic Surgery
Department of Plastic Surgery
Georgetown University and Johns Hopkins
University
Northwest, WA, USA
Volume 5, Chapter 22 Reconstruction of the
nipple-areola complex
Volume 5, Video 11.01 Partial breast
reconstruction using reduction mammaplasty
Volume 5, Video 11.03 Partial breast
reconstruction with a pedicle TRAM

Foad Nahai, MD, FACS
Clinical Professor of Plastic Surgery
Department of Surgery
Emory University School of Medicine
Atlanta, GA, USA
Volume 2, Chapter 1 Managing the cosmetic
patient

Fabio X. Nahas, MD, PhD
Associate Professor
Division of Plastic Surgery
Federal University of São Paulo
São Paulo, Brazil
Volume 2, Video 24.01 Liposculpture

Deepak Narayan, MS, FRCS (Eng),
FRCS (Edin)
Associate Professor of Surgery
Yale University School of Medicine
Chief
Plastic Surgery
VA Medical Center
West Haven, CT, USA
Volume 3, Chapter 14 Salivary gland tumors

Maurizio B. Nava, MD
Chief of Plastic Surgery Unit
Istituto Nazionale dei Tumori
Milano, Italy
Volume 5, Chapter 14 Expander/implant
reconstruction of the breast
Volume 5, Video 14.01 Mastectomy and
expander insertion: first stage
Volume 5, Video 14.02 Mastectomy and
expander insertion: second stage

Carmen Navarro, MD
Plastic Surgery Consultant
Plastic Surgery Department
Hospital de la Santa Creu i Sant Pau
Universidad Autónoma de Barcelona
Barcelona, Spain
Volume 5, Chapter 13 Imaging in reconstructive
breast surgery

Peter C. Neligan, MB, FRCS(I), FRCSC,
FACS
Professor of Surgery
Department of Surgery, Division of Plastic
Surgery
University of Washington
Seattle, WA, USA
Volume 1, Chapter 1 Plastic surgery and
innovation in medicine
Volume 1, Chapter 25 Flap pathophysiology and
pharmacology
Volume 3, Chapter 10 Cheek and lip
reconstruction
Volume 4, Chapter 3 Lymphatic reconstruction of
the extremities
Volume 3, Video 11.01-03 (1) Facial paralysis (2)
cross fact graft, (3) gracilis harvest
Volume 3, Video 18.01 Facial artery perforator
flap
Volume 4, Video 3.02 Charles Procedure
Volume 5, Video 18.01 SIEA
Volume 5, Video 19.01-19.03 Alternative free
flaps

Jonas A Nelson, MD
Integrated General/Plastic Surgery Resident
Department of Surgery
Division of Plastic Surgery
Perelman School of Medicine
University of Pennsylvania
Philadelphia, PA, USA
Volume 5, Video 17.01 The muscle sparing free TRAM flap

David T. Netscher, MD
Clinical Professor
Division of Plastic Surgery
Baylor College of Medicine
Houston, TX, USA
Volume 6, Chapter 21 The stiff hand and the spastic hand

Michael W. Neumeister, MD
Professor and Chairman
Division of Plastic Surgery
SIU School of Medicine
Springfield, IL, USA
Volume 6, Chapter 6 Nail and fingertip reconstruction

M. Samuel Noordhoff, MD, FACS
Emeritus Superintendent
Chang Gung Memorial Hospitals
Taipei, Taiwan, The People's Republic of China
Volume 3, Chapter 23 Repair of unilateral cleft lip

Christine B. Novak, PT, PhD
Research Associate
Hand Program, Division of Plastic and Reconstructive Surgery
University Health Network, University of Toronto
Toronto, ON, Canada
Volume 6, Chapter 39 Hand therapy

Daniel Nowinski, MD, PhD
Director
Department of Plastic and Maxillofacial Surgery
Uppsala Craniofacial Center
Uppsala University Hospital
Uppsala, Sweden
Volume 1, Chapter 11 Genetics and prenatal diagnosis

Scott Oates, MD
Professor
Department of Plastic Surgery
The University of Texas MD Anderson Cancer Center
Houston, TX, USA
Volume 6, Chapter 15 Benign and malignant tumors of the hand

Kerby Oberg, MD, PhD
Associate Professor
Department of Pathology and Human Anatomy
Loma Linda University School of Medicine
Loma Linda, CA, USA
Volume 6, Chapter 25 Congenital hand 1: embryology, classification, and principles

James P. O'Brien, MD, FRCSC
Associate Professor of Surgery
Dalhousie University
Halifax Nova Scotia
Clinical Associate Professor of Surgery
Memorial University
St. John's Newfoundland
Vice President Research
Innovation and Development
Horizon Health Network
New Brunswick, NB, Canada
Volume 6, Chapter 24 Nerve entrapment syndromes

Andrea J. O'Connor, BE(Hons), PhD
Associate Professor of Chemical and Biomolecular Engineering
Department of Chemical and Biomolecular Engineering
University of Melbourne
Melbourne, VIC, Australia
Volume 1, Chapter 19 Tissue engineering

Rei Ogawa, MD, PhD
Associate Professor
Department of Plastic
Reconstructive and Aesthetic Surgery Nippon Medical School
Tokyo, Japan
Volume 1, Chapter 30 Benign and malignant nonmelanocytic tumors of the skin and soft tissue

Dennis P. Orgill, MD, PhD
Professor of Surgery
Division of Plastic Surgery, Brigham and Women's Hospital
Harvard Medical School
Boston, MA, USA
Volume 1, Chapter 17 Skin graft

Cho Y. Pang, PhD
Senior Scientist
Research Institute
The Hospital for Sick Children
Professor
Departments of Surgery/Physiology
University of Toronto
Toronto, ON, Canada
Volume 1, Chapter 25 Flap pathophysiology and pharmacology

Ketan M. Patel, MD
Resident Physician
Department of Plastic Surgery
Georgetown University Hospital
Washington DC, USA
Volume 5, Chapter 22 Reconstruction of the nipple-areola complex

William C. Pederson, MD, FACS
President and Fellowship Director
The Hand Center of San Antonio
Adjunct Professor of Surgery
The University of Texas Health Science Center at San Antonio
San Antonio, TX, USA
Volume 6, Chapter 12 Reconstructive surgery of the mutilated hand

José Abel de la Peña Salcedo, MD
Secretario Nacional
Federación Iberolatinoamericana de Cirugía Plástica, Estética y Reconstructiva
Director del Instituto de Cirugia Plastica, S.C.
Hospital Angeles de las Lomas
Col.Valle de las Palmas
Huixquilucan, Edo de Mexico, Mexico
Volume 2, Chapter 28 Buttock augmentation
Volume 2, Video 28.01 Buttock augmentation

Angela Pennati, MD
Assistant Plastic Surgeon
Unit of Plastic Surgery
Istituto Nazionale dei Tumori
Milano, Italy
Volume 5, Chapter 14 Expander/implant breast reconstructions
Volume 5, Video 14.01 Mastectomy and expander insertion: first stage
Volume 5, Video 14.02 Mastectomy and expander insertion: second stage

Joel E. Pessa, MD
Clinical Associate Professor of Plastic Surgery
UTSW Medical School
Dallas, TX
Hand and Microsurgery Fellow
Christine M. Kleinert Hand and Microsurgery
Louisville, KY, USA
Volume 2, Chapter 17 Nasal analysis and anatomy

Walter Peters, MD, PhD, FRCSC
Professor of Surgery
Department of Plastic Surgery
University of Toronto
Toronto, ON, Canada
Volume 5, Chapter 6 Iatrogenic disorders following breast surgery

Giorgio Pietramaggiori, MD, PhD
Plastic Surgery Resident
Department of Plastic and Reconstructive Surgery
University Hospital of Lausanne
Lausanne, Switzerland
Volume 1, Chapter 17 Skin graft

John W. Polley, MD
Professor and Chairman
Rush University Medical Center
Department of Plastic and Reconstructive Surgery
John W. Curtin – Chair
Co-Director, Rush Craniofacial Center
Chicago, IL, USA
Volume 3, Chapter 27 Orthodontics in cleft lip and palate management

Bohdan Pomahac, MD
Assistant Professor
Harvard Medical School
Director
Plastic Surgery Transplantation
Medical Director
Burn Center
Division of Plastic Surgery
Brigham and Women's Hospital
Boston, MA, USA
Volume 1, Chapter 11 Genetics and prenatal diagnosis

Julian J. Pribaz, MD
Professor of Surgery Harvard Medical School
Division of Plastic Surgery
Brigham and Women's Hospital
Boston, MA, USA
Volume 3, Chapter 19 Secondary facial reconstruction

Andrea L. Pusic, MD, MHS, FRCSC
Associate Attending Surgeon
Department of Plastic and Reconstructive
Memorial Sloan-Kettering Cancer Center
New York, NY, USA
Volume 1, Chapter 10 Evidence-based medicine and health services research in plastic surgery
Volume 4, Chapter 14 Reconstruction of acquired vaginal defects

Oscar M. Ramirez, MD, FACS
Adjunct Clinical Faculty
Plastic Surgery Division
Cleveland Clinic Florida
Boca Raton, FL, USA
Volume 2, Chapter 11.8 Facelift: Subperiosteal facelift
Volume 2, Video 11.08.01 Facelift: Subperiosteal mid facelift endoscopic temporo-midface

William R. Rassman, MD
Director
Private Practice
New Hair Institution
Los Angeles, CA, USA
Volume 2, Video 23.04 FUE FOX procedure

Russell R. Reid, MD, PhD
Assistant Professor of Surgery, Bernard Sarnat Scholar
Section of Plastic and Reconstructive Surgery
University of Chicago
Chicago, IL, USA
Volume 1, Chapter 21 Repair and grafting of bone
Volume 3, Chapter 41 Pediatric chest and trunk defects

Neal R. Reisman, MD, JD
Chief of Plastic Surgery, Clinical Professor
Plastic Surgery
St. Luke's Episcopal Hospital
Baylor College of Medicine
Houston, TX, USA
Volume 1, Chapter 6 Medico-legal issues in plastic surgery

Dominique Renier, MD, PhD
Pediatric Neurosurgeon
Service de Neurochirurgie Pédiatrique
Hôpital Necker-Enfants Malades
Paris, France
Volume 3, Chapter 32 Orbital hypertelorism

Dirk F. Richter, MD, PhD
Clinical Director
Department of Plastic Surgery
Dreifaltigkeits-Hospital Wesseling
Wesseling, Germany
Volume 2, Chapter 25 Abdominoplasty procedures
Volume 2, Video 25.01 Abdominoplasty

Thomas L. Roberts III, FACS
Plastic Surgery Center of the Carolinas
Spartanburg, SC, USA
Volume 2, Chapter 28 Buttock augmentation
Volume 2, Video 28.01 Buttock augmentation

Federico Di Rocco, MD, PhD
Pediatric Neurosurgery
Hôpital Necker Enfants Malades
Paris, France
Volume 3, Chapter 32 Orbital hypertelorism

Natalie Roche, MD
Associate Professor
Department of Plastic Surgery
Ghent University Hospital
Ghent, Belgium
Volume 4, Chapter 13 Reconstruction of male genital defects
Volume 4, Video 13.01 Complete and partial penile reconstruction

Eduardo D. Rodriguez, MD, DDS
Chief, Plastic Reconstructive and Maxillofacial Surgery, R Adams Cowley Shock Trauma Center
Professor of Surgery
University of Maryland School of Medicine
Baltimore, MD, USA
Volume 3, Chapter 3 Facial fractures

Thomas E. Rohrer, MD
Director, Mohs Surgery
SkinCare Physicians of Chestnut Hill
Clinical Associate Professor
Department of Dermatology
Boston University
Boston, MA, USA
Volume 2, Video 5.02 Facial resurfacing

Rod J. Rohrich, MD, FACS
Professor and Chairman Crystal Charity Ball
Distinguished Chair in Plastic Surgery
Department of Plastic Surgery
Professor and Chairman Betty and Warren
Woodward Chair in Plastic and Reconstructive Surgery
University of Texas Southwestern Medical Center at Dallas
Dallas, TX, USA
Volume 2, Chapter 17 Nasal analysis and anatomy
Volume 2, Chapter 18 Open technique rhinoplasty

Joseph M. Rosen, MD
Professor of Surgery
Division of Plastic Surgery, Department of Surgery
Dartmouth-Hitchcock Medical Center
Lyme, NH, USA
Volume 1, Chapter 36 Robotics, simulation, and telemedicine in plastic surgery

E. Victor Ross, MD
Director of Laser and Cosmetic Dermatology
Scripps Clinic
San Diego, CA, USA
Volume 2, Chapter 5 Facial skin resurfacing

Michelle C. Roughton, MD
Chief Resident
Section of Plastic and Reconstructive Surgery
University of Chicago Medical Center
Chicago, IL, USA
Volume 4, Chapter 10 Reconstruction of the chest

Sashwati Roy, PhD
Associate Professor of Surgery
Department of Surgery
The Ohio State University Medical Center
Columbus, OH, USA
Volume 1, Chapter 14 Wound healing

J. Peter Rubin, MD, FACS
Chief of Plastic Surgery
Director, Life After Weight Loss Body Contouring Program
University of Pittsburgh
Pittsburgh, PA, USA
Volume 2, Chapter 30 Post-bariatric reconstruction
Volume 2, Video 30.01 Post bariatric reconstruction – bodylift procedure
Volume 5, Chapter 25 Contouring of the arms, breast, upper trunk, and male chest in the massive weight loss patient
Volume 5, Video 25.01 Brachioplasty part 1: contouring of the arms
Volume 5, Video 25.02 Bracioplasty part 2: contouring of the arms

Alesia P. Saboeiro, MD
Attending Physician
Private Practice
New York, NY, USA
Volume 2, Chapter 14 Structural fat grafting
Volume 2, Video 14.01 Structural fat grafting of
the face

Justin M. Sacks, MD
Assistant Professor
Department of Plastic and Reconstructive
Surgery
The Johns Hopkins University School of
Medicine
Baltimore, MD, USA
Volume 3, Chapter 17 Carcinoma of the upper
aerodigestive tract
Volume 6, Chapter 15 Benign and malignant
tumors of the hand

Hakim K. Said, MD
Assistant Professor of Surgery
Division of Plastic Surgery
University of Washington
Seattle, WA, USA
Volume 4, Chapter 17 Perineal reconstruction

Michel Saint-Cyr, MD, FRCSC
Associate Professor Plastic Surgery
Department of Plastic Surgery
University of Texas Southwestern Medical
Center
Dallas, TX, USA
Volume 4, Chapter 2 Management of lower
extremity trauma
Volume 4, Video 2.01 Alternative flap harvest

Cristianna Bonneto Saldanha, MD
Resident
General Surgery Department
Santa Casa of Santos Hospital
São Paulo, Brazil
Volume 2, Chapter 26 Lipoabdominoplasty
Volume 2, Video 26.01 Lipobdominoplasty
(including secondary lipo)

Osvaldo Ribeiro Saldanha, MD
Chairman of Plastic Surgery
Unisanta
Santos
Past President of the Brazilian Society of
Plastic Surgery (SBCP)
International Associate Editor of Plastic and
Reconstructive Surgery
São Paulo, Brazil
Volume 2, Chapter 26 Lipoabdominoplasty
Volume 2, Video 26.01 Lipobdominoplasty
(including secondary lipo)

Osvaldo Ribeiro Saldanha Filho, MD
São Paulo, Brazil
Volume 2, Chapter 26 Lipoabdominoplasty
Volume 2, Video 26.01 Lipobdominoplasty
(including secondary lipo)

Douglas M. Sammer, MD
Assistant Professor of Plastic Surgery
Department of Plastic Surgery
University of Texas Southwestern Medical
Center
Dallas, TX, USA
Volume 6, Chapter 19 Rheumatologic conditions
of the hand and wrist

Joao Carlos Sampaio Goes, MD, PhD
Director Instituto Brasileiro Controle Cancer
Chairman
Department Plastic Surgery and Mastology of
IBCC
Sao Paulo, Brazil
Volume 5, Chapter 8.6 Periareolar technique with
mesh support
Volume 5, Chapter 20 Omentum reconstruction
of the breast

Michael Sauerbier, MD, PhD
Chairman and Professor
Department for Plastic, Hand and
Reconstructive Surgery
Cooperation Hospital for Plastic Surgery of the
University Hospital Frankfurt
Academic Hospital University of Frankfurt a.
Main
Frankfurt, Germany
Volume 4, Chapter 4 Lower extremity sarcoma
reconstruction
Volume 4, Video 4.01 Management of lower
extremity sarcoma reconstruction

Hani Sbitany, MD
Plastic and Reconstructive Surgery
Assistant Professor of Surgery
University of California
San Francisco, CA, USA
Volume 1, Chapter 24 Flap classification and
applications

Tim Schaub, MD
Private Practice
Arizona Center for Hand Surgery, PC
Phoenix, AZ, USA
Volume 6, Chapter 16 Infections of the hand

Loren S. Schechter, MD, FACS
Assistant Professor of Surgery
Chief, Division of Plastic Surgery
Chicago Medical School
Chicago, IL, USA
Volume 4, Chapter 15 Surgery for gender identity
disorder

Stephen A. Schendel, MD
Professor Emeritus of Surgery and Clinical
Adjunct Professor of Neurosurgery
Department of Surgery and Neurosurgery
Stanford University Medical Center
Stanford, CA, USA
Volume 3, Chapter 4 TMJ dysfunction and
obstructive sleep apnea

Saja S. Scherer-Pietramaggiori, MD
Plastic Surgery Resident
Department of Plastic and Reconstructive
Surgery
University Hospital of Lausanne
Lausanne, Switzerland
Volume 1, Chapter 17 Skin graft

Clark F. Schierle, MD, PhD
Vice President
Aesthetic and Reconstructive Plastic Surgery
Northwestern Plastic Surgery Associates
Chicaho, IL, USA
Volume 5, Chapter 5 Endoscopic approaches to
the breast

Stefan S. Schneeberger, MD
Visiting Associate Professor of Surgery
Department of Plastic Surgery
Johns Hopkins Medical University
Baltimore, MD, USA
Associate Professor of Surgery
Center for Operative Medicine
Department for Viszeral
Transplant and Thoracic Surgery
Innsbruck Medical University
Innsbruck, Austria
Volume 6, Chapter 38 Upper extremity
composite allotransplantation

Iris A. Seitz, MD, PhD
Director of Research and International
Collaboration
University Plastic Surgery
Rosalind Franklin University
Clinical Instructor of Surgery
Chicago Medical School
University Plastic Surgery, affiliated with
Chicago Medical School, Rosalind Franklin
University
Morton Grove, IL, USA
Volume 1, Chapter 21 Repair and grafting of
bone

Chandan K. Sen, PhD, FACSM, FACN
Professor and Vice Chairman (Research) of
Surgery
Department of Surgery
The Ohio State University Medical Center
Associate Dean
Translational and Applied Research
College of Medicine
Executive Director
OSU Comprehensive Wound Center
Columbus, OH, USA
Volume 1, Chapter 14 Wound healing

Subhro K. Sen, MD
Clinical Assistant Professor
Division of Plastic and Reconstructive Surgery
Robert A. Chase Hand and Upper Limb
Center, Stanford University Medical Center
Palo Alto, CA, USA
Volume 1, Chapter 14 Wound healing
Volume 6, Chapter 4 Anesthesia for upper
extremity surgery
Volume 6, Video 4.01 Anesthesia for upper
extremity surgery

Joseph M. Serletti, MD, FACS
Henry Royster – William Maul Measey
Professor of Surgery and Chief
Division of Plastic Surgery
Vice Chair (Finance)
Department of Surgery
University of Pennsylvania
Philadelphia, PA, USA
Volume 5, Chapter 17 Free TRAM breast
reconstruction
Volume 5, Video 17.01 The muscle sparing free
TRAM flap

Randolph Sherman, MD
Vice Chair
Department of Surgery
Cedars-Sinai Medical Center
Los Angeles, CA, USA
Volume 6, Chapter 12 Reconstructive surgery of
the mutilated hand

Kenneth C. Shestak, MD
Professor of Plastic Surgery
Division of Plastic Surgery
University of Pittsburgh
Pittsburgh, PA, USA
Volume 5, Chapter 9 Revision surgery following
breast reduction and mastopexy
Volume 5, Video 7.01 Circum areola mastopexy

Lester Silver, MD, MS
Professor of Surgery
Department of Surgery/Division of Plastic
Surgery
Mount Sinai School of Medicine
New York, NY, USA
Volume 3, Chapter 37 Hemifacial atrophy

Navin K. Singh, MD, MSc
Assistant Professor of Plastic Surgery
Department of Plastic Surgery
Johns Hopkins University School of Medicine
Washington, DC, USA
Volume 4, Chapter 12 Abdominal wall
reconstruction

Vanila M. Singh, MD
Clinical Associate Professor
Stanford University Medical Center
Department of Anesthesiology and Pain
Management
Stanford, CA, USA
Volume 6, Chapter 4 Anesthesia for upper
extremity surgery

Carla Skytta, DO
Resident
Department of Surgery
Doctors Hospital
Columbus, OH, USA
Volume 3, Chapter 5 Scalp and forehead
reconstruction

Darren M. Smith, MD
Resident
Division of Plastic Surgery
University of Pittsburgh Medical Center
Pittsburgh, PA, USA
Volume 3, Chapter 31 Pediatric facial fractures

**Gill Smith, MB, BCh, FRCS(Ed),
FRCS(Plast)**
Consultant Hand, Plastic and Reconstructive
Surgeon
Great Ormond Street Hospital
London, UK
Volume 6, Chapter 26 Congenital hand II Failure
of formation (transverse and longitudinal arrest)

Paul Smith, MBBS, FRCS
Honorary Consultant Plastic Surgeon
Great Ormond Street Hospital London, UK
Volume 6, Chapter 26 Congenital hand II Failure
of formation (transverse and longitudinal arrest)

Laura Snell, MSc, MD, FRCSC
Assistant Professor
Division of Plastic Surgery
University of Toronto
Toronto, ON, Canada
Volume 4, Chapter 14 Reconstruction of
acquired vaginal defects

Nicole Z. Sommer, MD
Assistant Professor of Plastic Surgery
Southern Illinois University School of Medicine
Springfield, IL, USA
Volume 6, Chapter 6 Nail and fingertip
reconstruction

David H. Song, MD, MBA, FACS
Cynthia Chow Professor of Surgery
Chief, Section of Plastic and Reconstructive
Surgery
Vice-Chairman, Department of Surgery
The University of Chicago Medicine & Biological
Sciences
Chicago, IL, USA
Volume 4, Chapter 10 Reconstruction of the
chest

Andrea Spano, MD
Senior Assistant Plastic Surgeon
Unit of Plastic Surgery
Istituto Nazionale dei Tumori
Milano, Italy
Volume 5, Chapter 14 Expander/implant breast
reconstructions
Volume 5, Video 14.01 Mastectomy and
expander insertion: first stage
Volume 5, Video 14.02 Mastectomy and
expander insertion: second stage

Scott L. Spear, MD, FACS
Professor and Chairman
Department of Plastic Surgery
Georgetown University Hospital
Georgetown, WA, USA
Volume 5, Chapter 15 Latissimus dorsi flap
breast reconstruction
Volume 5, Chapter 26 Fat grafting to the breast
Volume 5, Video 15.01 Latissimus dorsi flap
technique

Robert J. Spence, MD
Director
National Burn Reconstruction Center
Good Samaritan Hospital
Baltimore, MD, USA
Volume 4, Chapter 21 Management of facial
burns
Volume 4, Video 21.01 Management of the
burned face intra-dermal skin closure
Volume 4, Video 21.02 Management of the
burned face full-thickness skin graft defatting
technique

Samuel Stal, MD, FACS
Professor and Chief
Division of Plastic Surgery, Baylor College of
Medicine and Texas Children's Hospital
Houston, TX, USA
Volume 3, Chapter 29 Secondary deformities of
the cleft lip, nose, and palate
Volume 3, Video 29.01 Complete takedown
Volume 3, Video 29.02 Abbé flap
Volume 3, Video 29.03 Thick lip and buccal
sulcus deformities
Volume 3, Video 29.04 Alveolar bone grafting
Volume 3, Video 29.05 Definitive rhinoplasty

Derek M. Steinbacher, MD, DMD
Assistant Professor
Plastic and Carniomaxillofacial Surgery
Yale University, School of Medicine
New Haven, CT, USA
Volume 3, Chapter 34 Nonsyndromic
craniosynostosis

Douglas S. Steinbrech, MD, FACS
Gotham Plastic Surgery
New York, NY, USA
Volume 2, Chapter 9 Secondary blepharoplasty:
Techniques

Lars Steinstraesser, MD
Heisenberg-Professor for Molecular Oncology
and Wound Healing
Department of Plastic and Reconstructive
Surgery, Burn Center
BG University Hospital Bergmannsheil, Ruhr
University
Bochum, North Rhine-Westphalia, Germany
Volume 4, Chapter 18 Acute management of
burn/electrical injuries

Phillip J. Stephan, MD
Clinical Instructor
Department of Plastic Surgery
University of Texas Southwestern
Wichita Falls, TX, USA
Volume 2, Chapter 24 Liposuction: A comprehensive review of techniques and safety

Laurie A. Stevens, MD
Associate Clinical Professor of Psychiatry
Columbia University College of Physicians and Surgeons
New York, NY, USA
Volume 1, Chapter 3 Psychological aspects of plastic surgery

Alexander Stoff, MD, PhD
Senior Fellow
Department of Plastic Surgery
Dreifaltigkeits-Hospital Wesseling
Wesseling, Germany
Volume 2, Chapter 25 Abdominoplasty procedures
Volume 2, Video 25.01 Abdominoplasty

Dowling B. Stough, MD
Medical Director
The Dermatology Clinic
Clinical Assistant Professor
Department of Dermatology
University of Arkansas for Medical Sciences
Little Rock, AR, USA
Volume 2, Video 23.09 Tension donor dissection

James M. Stuzin, MD
Associate Professor of Surgery (Plastic)
Voluntary
University of Miami Leonard M. Miller School of Medicine
Miami, FL, USA
Volume 2, Chapter 11.6 Facelift: The extended SMAS technique in facial rejuvenation
Volume 2, Video 11.06.01 Facelift – Extended SMAS technique in facial shaping

John D. Symbas, MD
Plastic and Reconstructive Surgeon
Private Practice
Marietta Plastic Surgery
Marietta, GA, USA
Volume 5, Chapter 16 The bilateral pedicled TRAM flap
Volume 5, Video 16.01 Pedicle TRAM breast reconstruction

Amir Taghinia, MD
Instructor in Surgery
Harvard Medical School
Staff Surgeon
Department of Plastic and Oral Surgery
Children's Hospital
Boston, MA, USA
Volume 6, Chapter 27 Congenital hand III disorders of formation – thumb hypoplasia
Volume 6, Video 27.01 Congenital hand III disorders of formation – thumb hypoplasia
Volume 6, Video 31.01 Vascular anomalies of the upper extremity

David M.K. Tan, MBBS
Consultant
Department of Hand and Reconstructive Microsurgery
National University Hospital
Yong Loo Lin School of Medicine
National University Singapore
Kent Ridge, Singapore
Volume 6, Chapter 3 Diagnostic imaging of the hand and wrist
Volume 6, Video 3.01 Diagnostic imaging of the hand and wrist – Scaphoid lunate dislocation

Jin Bo Tang, MD
Professor and Chair
Department of Hand Surgery
Chair
The Hand Surgery Research Center
Affiliated Hospital of Nantong University
Nantong, The People's Republic of China
Volume 6, Chapter 9 Flexor tendon injuries and reconstruction
Volume 6, Video 9.01 Flexor tendon injuries and reconstruction – Partial venting of the A2 pulley
Volume 6, Video 9.02 Flexor tendon injuries and reconstruction – Making a 6-strand repair
Volume 6, Video 9.03 Complete flexor-extension without bowstringing

Daniel I. Taub, DDS, MD
Assistant Professor
Oral and Maxillofacial Surgery
Thomas Jefferson University Hospital
Philadelphia, PA, USA
Volume 2, Chapter 16 Anthropometry, cephalometry, and orthognathic surgery
Volume 2, Video 16.01 Anthropometry, cephalometry, and orthognathic surgery

Peter J. Taub, MD, FACS, FAAP
Associate Professor, Surgery and Pediatrics
Division of Plastic and Reconstructive Surgery
Mount Sinai School of Medicine
New York, NY, USA
Volume 3, Chapter 37 Hemifacial atrophy

Sherilyn Keng Lin Tay, MBChB, MRCS, MSc
Microsurgical Fellow
Department of Plastic Surgery
Chang Gung Memorial Hospital
Taoyuan, Taiwan, The People's Republic of China
Specialist Registrar
Department of Reconstructive and Plastic Surgery
St George's Hospital
London, UK
Volume 1, Chapter 26 Principles and techniques of microvascular surgery

G. Ian Taylor, AO, MBBS, MD, MD (HonBrodeaux), FRACS, FRCS (Eng), FRCS (Hon Edinburgh), FRCSI (Hon), FRSC (Hon Canada), FACS (Hon)
Professor
Deparment of Plastic Surgery
Royal Melbourne Hospital
Professor
Department of Anatomy
University of Melbourne
Melbourne, Australia
Volume 1, Chapter 23 Vascular territories

Oren M. Tepper, MD
Assistant Professor
Plastic and Reconstructive Surgery
Montefiore Medical Center
Albert Einstein College of Medicine
New York, NY, USA
Volume 3, Chapter 36 Craniofacial microsomia

Chad M. Teven, BS
Research Associate
Section of Plastic and Reconstructive Surgery
University of Chicago
Chicago, IL, USA
Volume 1, Chapter 21 Repair and grafting of bone

Brinda Thimmappa, MD
Adjunct Assistant Professor
Department of Plastic and Reconstructive Surgery
Loma Linda Medical Center
Loma Linda, CA
Plastic Surgeon
Division of Plastic and Maxillofacial Surgery
Southwest Washington Medical Center
Vancouver, WA, USA
Volume 3, Chapter 4 TMJ dysfunction and obstructive sleep apnea

Johan Thorfinn, MD, PhD
Senior Consultant of Plastic Surgery, Burn Unit Co-Director
Department of Plastic Surgery, Hand Surgery, and Burns
Linköping University Hospital
Linköping, Sweden
Volume 6, Chapter 32 Peripheral nerve injuries of the upper extremity
Volume 6, Video 32.01-02 Peripheral nerve injuries (1) Digital Nerve Suture (2) Median Nerve Suture

Charles H. Thorne, MD
Associate Professor of Plastic Surgery
Department of Plastic Surgery
NYU School of Medicine
New York, NY, USA
Volume 2, Chapter 22 Otoplasty

Michael Tonkin, MBBS, MD, FRACS (Orth), FRCS Ed Orth
Professor of Hand Surgery
Department of Hand Surgery and Peripheral
Nerve Surgery
Royal North Shore Hospital
The Childrens Hospital at Westmead
University of Sydney Medical School
Sydney, Australia
*Volume 6, Chapter 25 Congenital hand 1
Principles, embryology, and classification*
*Volume 6, Chapter 29 Congenital hand V
Disorders of Overgrowth, Undergrowth, and
Generalized Skeletal Deformities (addendum)*

Patrick L Tonnard, MD
Coupure Centrum Voor Plastische Chirurgie
Ghent, Belgium
*Volume 2, Video 11.04.01 Loop sutures MACS
facelift*

Kathryn S. Torok, MD
Assistant Professor
Division of Pediatric Rheumatology
Department of Pediatrics
Univeristy of Pittsburgh School of Medicine
Childrens Hospital of Pittsburgh
Pittsburgh, PA, USA
Volume 3, Chapter 37 Hemifacial atrophy

Ali Totonchi, MD
Assistant Professor of Surgery
Division of Plastic Surgery
MetroHealth Medical Center
Case Western Reserve University
Cleveland, OH, USA
*Volume 3, Chapter 21 Surgical management of
migraine headaches*

Jonathan W. Toy, MD
Body Contouring Fellow
Division of Plastic and Reconstructive Surgery
University of Pittsburgh
University of Pittsburgh Medical Center Suite
Pittsburg, PA, USA
*Volume 2, Chapter 30 Post-bariatric
reconstruction*
*Volume 5, Chapter 25 Contouring of the arms,
breast, upper trunk, and male chest in the
massive weight loss patient*

Matthew J. Trovato, MD
Dallas Plastic Surgery Institute
Dallas, TX, USA
Volume 2, Chapter 29 Upper limb contouring
Volume 2, Video 29.01 Upper limb contouring

Anthony P. Tufaro, DDS, MD, FACS
Associate Professor of Surgery and Oncology
Departments of Plastic Surgery and Oncology
Johns Hopkins University
Baltimore, MD, USA
*Volume 3, Chapter 16 Tumors of the lips, oral
cavity, oropharynx, and mandible*

Joseph Upton III, MD
Clinical Professor of Surgery
Department of Plastic Surgery
Children's Hospital Boston
Shriner's Burn Hospital Boston
Beth Israel Deaconess Hospital
Harvard Medical School
Boston, MA, USA
*Volume 6, Chapter 27 Congenital hand III
disorders of formation – thumb hypoplasia*
*Volume 6, Chapter 31 Vascular anomalies of the
upper extremity*
*Volume 6, Video 27.01 Congenital hand III
disorders of formation – thumb hypoplasia*
*Volume 6, Video 31.01 Vascular anomalies of
the upper extremity*

Walter Unger, MD
Clinical Professor
Department of Dermatology
Mount Sinai School of Medicine
New York, NY
Associate Professor (Dermatology)
University of Toronto
Private Practice
New York, NY, USA
Toronto, ON, Canada
Volume 2, Video 23.06 Hair transplantation

Francisco Valero-Cuevas, PhD
Director
Brain-Body Dynamics Laboratory
Professor of Biomedical Engineering
Professor of Biokinesiology and Physical
Therapy
By courtesy Professor of Computer Science
and Aerospace and Mechanical Engineering
The University of Southern California
Los Angeles, CA, USA
*Volume 6, Chapter 1 Anatomy and biomechanics
of the hand*

Allen L. Van Beek, MD, FACS
Adjunct Professor
University Minnesota School of Medicine
Division Plastic Surgery
Minneapolis, MN, USA
Volume 2, Video 3.01 Botulinum toxin
Volume 2, Video 4.01 Soft tissue fillers
Volume 2, Video 5.01 Chemical peel
*Volume 2, Video 18.01 Open technique
rhinoplasty*

Nicholas B. Vedder
Professor of Surgery and Orthopaedics
Chief of Plastic Surgery Vice Chair, Department
of Surgery
University of Washington
Seattle, WA, USA
*Volume 6, Chapter 13 Thumb reconstruction:
non microsurgical techniques*

Valentina Visintini Cividin, MD
Assistant Plastic Surgeon
Unit of Plastic Surgery
Istituto Nazionale dei Tumori
Milano, Italy
*Volume 5, Chapter 14 Expander/implant
reconstruction of the breast*
*Volume 5, Video 14.01 Mastectomy and
expander insertion: first stage*
*Volume 5, Video 14.02 Mastectomy and
expander insertion: second stage*

Peter M. Vogt, MD, PhD
Professor and Chairman
Department of Plastic Hand and Reconstructive
Surgery
Hannover Medical School
Hannover, Germany
*Volume 1, Chapter 15 Skin wound healing:
Repair biology, wound, and scar treatment*

Richard J. Warren, MD, FRCSC
Clinical Professor
Division of Plastic Surgery
University of British Columbia
Vancouver, BC, Canada
Volume 2, Chapter 7 Forehead rejuvenation
Volume 2, Chapter 11.1 Facelift: Principles
*Volume 2, Chapter 11.2 Facelift: Introduction to
deep tissue techniques*
Volume 2, Video 7.01 Modified Lateral Brow Lift
*Volume 2, Video 11.1.01 Parotid masseteric
fascia*
Volume 2, Video 11.1.02 Anterior incision
Volume 2, Video 11.1.03 Posterior Incision
Volume 2, Video 11.1.04 Facelift skin flap
Volume 2, Video 11.1.05 Facial fat injection

Andrew J. Watt, MD
Plastic Surgeon
Department of Surgery
Division of Plastic and Reconstructive Surgery
Stanford University Medical Center
Stanford University Hospital and Clinics
Palo Alto, CA, USA
*Volume 6, Chapter 17 Management of
Dupuytren's disease*
*Volume 6, Video 17.01 Management of
Dupuytren's disease*

Simeon H. Wall, Jr., MD, FACS
Private Practice
The Wall Center for Plastic Surgery
Gratis Faculty
Division of Plastic Surgery
Department of Surgery
LSU Health Sciences Center at Shreveport
Shreveport, LA, USA
Volume 2, Chapter 21 Secondary rhinoplasty

Derrick C. Wan, MD
Assistant Professor
Department of Surgery
Stanford University School of Medicine
Stanford, CA, USA
*Volume 1, Chapter 13 Stem cells and
regenerative medicine*

Renata V. Weber, MD
Assistant Professor Surgery (Plastics)
Division of Plastic and Reconstructive Surgery
Albert Einstein College of Medicine
Bronx, NY, USA
Volume 1, Chapter 22 Repair and grafting of peripheral nerve

Fu Chan Wei, MD
Professor
Department of Plastic Surgery
Chang Gung Memorial Hospital
Taoyuan, Taiwan, The People's Republic of China
Volume 1, Chapter 26 Principles and techniques of microvascular surgery
Volume 6, Chapter 14 Thumb and finger reconstruction – microsurgical techniques
Volume 6, Video 14.01 Trimmed great toe
Volume 6, Video 14.02 Second toe for index
Volume 6, Video 14.03 Combined second and third toe for metacarpal hand

Mark D. Wells, MD, FRCS, FACS
Clinical Assistant Professor of Surgery
The Ohio State University
Columbus, OH, USA
Volume 3, Chapter 5 Scalp and forehead reconstruction

Gordon H. Wilkes, MD
Clinical Professor and Divisional Director
Division of Plastic Surgery
University of Alberta Faculty of Medicine
Alberta, AB, Canada
Volume 1, Chapter 33 Facial prosthetics in plastic surgery

Henry Wilson, MD, FACS
Attending Plastic Surgeon
Private Practice
Plastic Surgery Associates
Lynchburg, VA, USA
Volume 5, Chapter 26 Fat grafting to the breast

Scott Woehrle, MS, BS
Physician Assistant
Department of Plastic Surgery
Jospeh Capella Plastic Surgery
Ramsey, NJ, USA
Volume 2, Chapter 29 Upper limb contouring
Volume 2, Video 29.01 Upper limb contouring

Johan F. Wolfaardt, BDS, MDent (Prosthodontics), PhD
Professor
Division of Otolaryngology-Head and Neck Surgery
Department of Surgery
Faculty of Medicine and Dentistry
Director of Clinics and International Relations
Institute for Reconstructive Sciences in Medicine
University of Alberta
Covenant Health Group
Alberta Health Services
Alberta, AB, Canada
Volume 1, Chapter 33 Facial prosthetics in plastic surgery

S. Anthony Wolfe, MD
Chief
Division of Plastic Surgery
Miami Children's Hospital
Miami, FL, USA
Volume 3, Chapter 8 Acquired cranial and facial bone deformities
Volume 3, Video 8.01 Removal of venous malformation enveloping intraconal optic nerve

Chin-Ho Wong, MBBS, MRCS, MMed (Surg), FAMS (Plast. Surg)
Consultant
Department of Plastic Reconstructive and Aesthetic Surgery
Singapore General Hospital
Singapore
Volume 2, Chapter 6 Anatomy of the aging face

Victor W. Wong, MD
Postdoctoral Research Fellow
Department of Surgery
Stanford University
Stanford, CA, USA
Volume 1, Chapter 13 Stem cells and regenerative medecine

Jeffrey Yao, MD
Assistant Professor
Department of Orthopaedic Surgery
Stanford University Medical Center
Palo Alto, CA, USA
Volume 6, Chapter 5 Principles of internal fixation as applied to the hand and wrist

Akira Yamada, MD
Assistant Professor
Department of Plastic and Reconstructive Surgery
Osaka Medical College
Osaka, Japan
Volume 3, Video 7.01 Microtia: auricular reconstruction

Michael J. Yaremchuk, MD, FACS
Chief of Craniofacial Surgery-Massachusetts General Hospital
Program Director-Plastic Surgery Training Program
Massachusetts General Hospital
Professor of Surgery
Harvard Medical School
Boston, MA, USA
Volume 2, Chapter 15 Skeletal augmentation
Volume 2, Video 15.01 Midface skeletal augmentation and rejuvenation

David M. Young, MD
Professor of Plastic Surgery
Department of Surgery
University of California
San Francisco, CA, USA
Volume 1, Chapter 24 Flap classification and applications

Peirong Yu, MD
Professor
Department of Plastic Surgery
The University of Texas M.D. Anderson Cancer Center
Houston, TX, USA
Volume 3, Chapter 13 Hypopharyngeal, esophageal, and neck reconstruction
Volume 3, Video 13.01 Reconstruction of pharyngoesophageal defects with the anterolateral thigh flap

James E. Zins, MD
Chairman
Department of Plastic Surgery
Dermatology and Plastic Surgery Institute
Cleveland Clinic
Cleveland, OH, USA
Volume 2, Chapter 13 Neck rejuvenation

Christopher G. Zochowski, MD
Chief Resident
Department of Plastic and Reconstructive Surgery
Case Western Reserve University
Cleveland, OH, USA
Volume 3, Chapter 38 Pierre Robin sequence

Elvin G. Zook, MD
Professor Emeritus
Division of Plastic Surgery
Southern Illinois University School of Medicine
Springfield, IL, USA
Volume 6, Chapter 6 Nail and fingertip reconstruction

Ronald M. Zuker, MD, FRCSC, FACS, FRCSEd(Hon)
Staff Plastic Surgeon
The Hospital for Sick Children
Professor of Surgery
Department of Surgery
The University of Toronto
Toronto, ON, Canada
Volume 3, Chapter 11 Facial paralysis

Acknowledgments

Editing a textbook such as this is an exciting, if daunting job. Only at the end of the project, over 4 years later, does one realize how much work it entailed and how many people helped make it happen. Sue Hodgson was the Commissioning Editor who trusted me to undertake this. Together, over several weekends in Seattle and countless e-mails and phone calls, we planned the format of this edition and laid the groundwork for a planning meeting in Chicago that included the volume editors and the Elsevier team with whom we have worked. I thank Drs. Gurtner, Warren, Rodriguez, Losee, Song, Grotting, Chang and Van Beek for tirelessly ensuring that each volume was as good as it could possibly be.

I had a weekly call with the Elsevier team as well as several visits to the offices in London. I will miss working with them. Louise Cook, Alexandra Mortimer and Poppy Garraway have been professional, thorough, and most of all, fun to work with. Emma Cole and Sam Crowe helped enormously with video content. Sadly, Sue Hodgson has left Elsevier, however Belinda Kuhn ably filled her shoes and ensured that we kept to our timeline, didn't lose momentum, and that the final product was something we would all be proud of.

Several residents helped, in focus groups to define format and style as well as specifically engaging in the editing process. I thank Darren Smith and Colin Woon for their help as technical copyeditors. Thanks to James Saunders and Leigh Jansen for reviewing video content and thanks also to Donnie Buck for all of his help with the electronic content. Of course we edited the book, we didn't write it. The writers were our contributing authors, all of whom engaged with enthusiasm.

I thank them for defining Plastic Surgery, the book and the specialty.

Finally, I would like to thank my residents and fellows, who challenge me and make work fun. My partners in the Division of Plastic Surgery at the University of Washington, under the leadership of Nick Vedder, are a constant source of support and encouragement and I thank them. Finally, my family, Kate and David and most of all, my wife Gabrielle are unwavering in their love and support and I will never be able to thank them enough.

Peter C. Neligan, MB, FRCS(I), FRCSC, FACS
2012

This volume represents the current generation's brightest minds in hand and microvascular surgery. I am indebted to my colleagues and friends from around the globe for their hard work and eloquent writing, and to our talented staff at Elsevier who have made this project into a reality. It is our hope that this text will serve as a guide for the optimal treatment of all of our patients. I am fortunate to have two families to thank: the students, residents, fellows, and faculty at Stanford University who stimulate and enrich me intellectually; and my own loved ones, my wife Dr. Harriet Walker Roeder, and girls Julia, Kathleen, and Cecilia who sustain me in every way.

James Chang, MD
2012

Dedicated to the memory of Stephen J. Mathes

Plastic surgery contributions to hand surgery

James Chang

Although references to surgery of the hand date back to Hippocrates in ancient Greece, the dedicated specialty of hand surgery is relatively young. The Second World War is thought to be the major driving event for the development of hand surgery as a separate surgical discipline. This modern specialty was founded by a combination of general surgeons, plastic surgeons, orthopedic surgeons, vascular surgeons, and neurosurgeons. Hand surgery has remained unique in that it is a regional specialty instead of a tissue specialty – its practitioners are ideally trained in managing problems affecting all component tissues of the hand. This introduction chronicles the role plastic surgery has played in the development of hand surgery as a surgical specialty. Furthermore, it predicts how plastic surgery will influence the future direction of hand surgery.

Origins of hand surgery

Henry C Marble, in Flynn's classic textbook, *Hand Surgery*, found the earliest references to surgery of the hand by Hippocrates (460–377 BC) in ancient Greece.[1] In his writings, Hippocrates described methods to reduce wrist fractures and also highlighted the importance of well-fitting, clean dressings to the hand. A later Greek physician, Heliodorus, described his technique for amputation of a finger with specific reference to dissecting adequate skin flaps with which to cover the remaining bone. While Galen (131–201 AD) confused tendons with nerves and cautioned against suturing tendons for fear of "nervous spasms,"[2] Avicenna (981–1038 AD),[3] an Arabian physician, wrote detailed descriptions of tendon repair in medieval times. Other references to hand surgery have been found in history, but comprehensive care of the hand was not truly developed until the 20th century.

An understanding of human anatomy has been critical to both plastic surgery and hand surgery, and therefore, the history of anatomy has paralleled the development of these two surgical disciplines. J William Littler reviewed the influence of famed anatomists on hand surgery.[4] Perhaps these anatomists were drawn to the hand as the most intricate of body parts – the ultimate challenge to their craft. In the Renaissance period, Leonardo da Vinci (1452–1519) used his artistic genius to create extraordinarily accurate representations of the hand. His knowledge of anatomy was acquired from over 100 human dissections and ultimately resulted in a collection of 779 anatomical drawings.[5]

Andreas Vesalius (1514–64) *(Figs 1 and 2)* published his monumental work *De Corporis Humani Fabrica* in 1543 with many engravings dedicated to the hand.[6] Like da Vinci, Vesalius relied on his own dissections of cadavers rather than accepting the dogma found in previous medical texts. His observations refuted the inaccuracies found in the earlier writings of Galen and his disciples. Modern-day hand surgeons J William Littler and Robert A Chase have both credited Sir Charles Bell (1774–1842) as the foremost anatomist of the hand.[7] His *Fourth Bridgewater Treatise – The Hand: Its Mechanism and Vital Endowments as Evincing Design* (1834) remains a classic essay on the anatomic and functional aspects of the hand.[8]

In addition to anatomy, two more recent achievements allowed hand surgery to develop into a unique specialty in the modern era. On October 16, 1846 at the Massachusetts General Hospital, Dr. William Morton delivered sulfuric ether fumes to a patient undergoing excision of a neck mass by Dr. John Collins Warren.[9] For the first time, adequate anesthesia was performed, thus allowing the possibility of more complex reconstructive procedures in both plastic surgery and hand surgery.

The second major achievement was an understanding of microbiology with resulting advances in sterile technique and antibiotics.[10] In the 1860s, Louis Pasteur's work with fermentation introduced the field of bacteriology. Semmelweis, in Vienna, and Lister, in England, developed antiseptic surgery

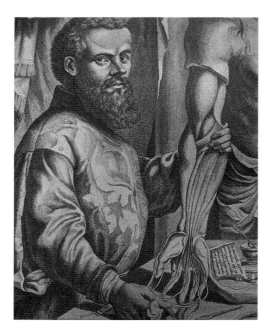

Fig. 1 Andreas Vesalius, master anatomist, at the age of 28. (Reproduced from Haeger K. The Illustrated History of Surgery. Gothenburg, Sweden: AB Nordbok, 1988.)

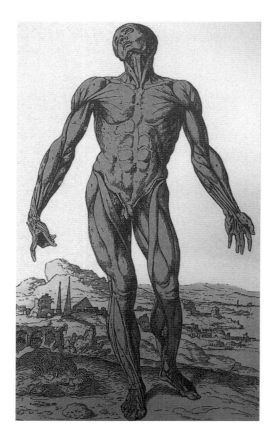

Fig. 2 An example of the anatomic illustrations of Stephan van Calcar in the monumental text of Vesalius, *De Humani Corporis Fabrica* (1543). (Reproduced from Haeger K. The Illustrated History of Surgery. Gothenburg, Sweden: AB Nordbok, 1988.)

with the early use of carbolic acid as a disinfectant. In the 20th century, several Nobel Prizes marked the importance of the development of antibiotics. Paul Erlich, a German bacteriologist, developed the principle of "antimicrobial chemotherapy" and received the Nobel Prize in 1908. Another German, Gerhard Domagk, received the Nobel Prize in 1939 for discovering the antibacterial effects of sulfa drugs. Finally, Alexander Fleming shared the Nobel Prize in 1945 for discovering the ability of a mold, *Penicillium notatum* to halt the growth of staphylococcus bacteria. With penicillin and later antibiotics, plastic surgeons and hand surgeons had an armamentarium of agents to control infections.

Over the course of this history, how has plastic surgery contributed to the development and progress of hand surgery? Like hand surgery, plastic surgery became a separate surgical specialty in the US only in the 20th century with the founding of the American Association of Oral and Plastic Surgeons (later shortened to the American Association of Plastic Surgeons) in 1921. The American Board of Plastic Surgery was not established until 1938. However, plastic surgery has profoundly influenced hand surgery, and this influence has predated formal associations and boards. In other words, surgeons throughout history have used plastic surgery principles before they were known as "plastic surgeons." Therefore, early plastic surgery contributions to hand surgery are best chronicled by reviewing the development of plastic surgery principles and how they have been applied to hand surgery.

Principles of plastic surgery and their application to hand surgery

Sushruta, a Hindu surgeon in India around the first century AD, performed reconstruction of the nose using pedicled flaps from the face – either forehead or cheek. He described the operation as follows:

The physician should take the leaf of a tree the same size as the nose and apply it to the cheek in such a way that a stem is still adherent. Then he stitches the cheek with needle and thread, scarifies the stump of the nose and quickly but carefully places the flap in the nose. After the transplanted piece has grown, the stem is cut off. In like manner the flap might be turned up from the upper or lower arm and attached to the nose – with the arm over the head.[11]

This description included the basic plastic surgery principles of precise patterning of the defect, preparation of the recipient bed, and the use of local and distant flaps, all which have had obvious applicability to soft-tissue reconstruction of the hand.

Another famed surgeon, Ambrose Paré (1510–90), offered principles that allowed for optimal care of battlefield wounds, including the upper extremity: "to enlarge the wound for drainage; to remove bone splinters and foreign bodies from wounds; to control hemorrhage with ligatures; not to encourage suppuration; and to amputate through sound tissues."[12] Paré's use of ligatures during amputation controlled hemorrhage and saved countless lives on the battlefield *(Figs 3 and 4)*. His principles of wound care would later be applied directly to the enormous number of battlefield casualties of World War II. In addition, Paré popularized the anatomic

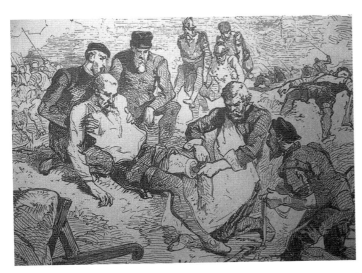

Fig. 3 Ambrose Paré applying a ligature during battlefield amputation. (Reproduced from Haeger K. The Illustrated History of Surgery. Gothenburg, Sweden: AB Nordbok, 1988.)

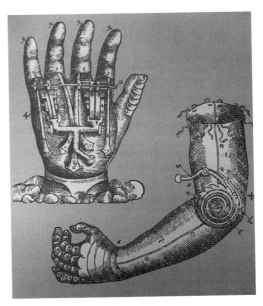

Fig. 4 Examples of Paré's designs for prostheses. (Reproduced from Haeger K. The Illustrated History of Surgery. Gothenburg, Sweden: AB Nordbok, 1988.)

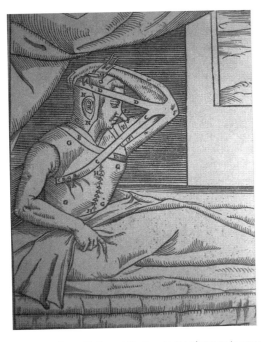

Fig. 5 Tagliacozzi's immobilization device after arm-to-nose pedicled transfer. (Reproduced from Haeger K. The Illustrated History of Surgery. Gothenburg, Sweden: AB Nordbok, 1988.)

drawings of Vesalius amongst surgeons, and even designed elaborate prostheses for upper extremity amputees, victims of the French wars of the 1500s. Paré was perhaps the quintessential upper extremity trauma surgeon.

Gaspare Tagliacozzi (1545–99) did not invent the Italian method of nasal reconstruction, which has been generally attributed to Branca. However, Tagliacozzi, a professor of medicine and anatomy in Bologna, did popularize this technique of attaching a medial upper arm skin flap to the nasal defect. In addition, specialized leather band contraptions were devised to immobilize the patient during the period of

flap revascularization *(Fig. 5)*. His detailed textbook, *De Chirugia Curtorum per Insitionem*, was published in 1597 and allowed later generations of surgeons to learn techniques for the transfer of distant pedicled flaps.[13]

As plastic surgeons became more adept at tissue transfer, these innovations were applied to reconstruction of the hand. Carl Nicoladoni (1849–1903) pioneered work on reconstruction of the thumb. Nicoladoni reported on a case of total skin avulsion of the thumb that he treated by a skin flap from the patient's left pectoral region – similar to the thoracoepigastric or random pattern chest flaps still used today.[14] In 1903, his paper, "Further experience with thumb reconstruction," described the pedicled toe transfer to the thumb that continues to bear his name. Microsurgeons today have obviated the need for the uncomfortable positioning of this transfer; nevertheless, Nicoladoni deserves credit for the ingenuity behind the toe-to-hand transfer. Plastic surgeon George H Monks (1853–1933) transferred a composite skin island flap from the forehead on the superficial temporal arteriovenous pedicle to a lower-eyelid defect.[15] The use of island flaps would later be applied to the hand with the neurovascular island flaps of Littler, and, more recently, with the dorsal metacarpal artery flaps. Even Sir Harold Gillies (1882–1960) who, with Millard, codified the principles of plastic surgery and was one of history's most influential plastic surgeons, turned from the head and neck to the hand and devised a method to lengthen the stump of a thumb, the Gillies "cocked-hat" flap.[16]

Vilray P Blair (1871–1955) was one of the founding fathers of American plastic surgery.[17] In addition to a large body of work in cleft lip repair and maxillofacial surgery, Blair made two significant contributions to plastic surgery that translated directly to hand surgery. Blair helped redefine the delay phenomenon of Tagliacozzi in a 1921 article, "The delayed transfer of long pedicled flaps in plastic surgery." Blair and his disciple, James Barrett Brown (1899–1971), described a new technique of harvesting skin for skin grafting in a paper published in *Surgery, Gynecology, and Obstetrics* entitled "The use and uses of large split skin grafts of intermediate thickness."[18] This simple and reproducible method of harvesting split-thickness skin improved on the previous techniques of Thiersch and would have a tremendous impact on the reconstruction of hand burns and other wounds in World War II.

Origins of modern hand surgery

With this historical background in wound management, flap transfer, and skin grafting, plastic surgeons were poised to contribute to the founding of modern hand surgery. World War II was the crucible in which hand surgery became a separate specialty. Prior to the outbreak of this war, two surgeons were instrumental in hand surgery's early development. In 1939, Allen B. Kanavel published his *Infections of the Hand,*[19] and for the first time, a comprehensive approach to the myriad of hand infections and treatments was described. Even at that early time, Kanavel stressed the importance of hospitalization for hand infections, intravenous hydration, and placing the hand at rest.

Sterling Bunnell (1882–1957) has been widely regarded as the father of hand surgery. The first edition of Bunnell's comprehensive textbook, *Surgery of the Hand,*[20] was published in 1944, and remained the classic reference for many years. He was a general surgeon but believed in the importance of plastic surgery principles, and as the consummate hand surgeon, was able to apply plastic, orthopedic, and vascular principles equally to hand surgery. Marble recounted Bunnell's mastery:

> He insisted on all of the teachings of the past masters, stressing particularly the gentle handling of the tissues. He called this atraumatic surgery. He exercised his skill also in plastic, bone, tendon, nerve, blood vessel, and muscle surgery to reconstruct crippled hands. He showed that tendons could be grafted to substitute for lost ones, and could be transferred to give function to useless digits or joints. He taught that nerves could be grafted and that whole fingers could be moved about for better function. Thus he opened the door for the complete reconstruction of the injured hand.[21]

The specialty of hand surgery in the US really developed in the field hospitals and regional medical referral centers established during the Second World War. During those years, massive numbers of surviving casualties with upper extremity injuries, an organized resuscitation and transportation service, and increasing sophistication within the fields of general surgery, plastic surgery, orthopedic surgery, vascular surgery, and neurosurgery together formed the critical mass necessary for accelerated technical and educational development.

The high volume of hand injuries requiring care in World War II was unprecedented. Unlike the trench warfare of World War I when head and neck wounds were common, World War II involved open warfare with rapid movements and grenades, leading to a greater likelihood of upper extremity injuries. In the early years of the war, soldiers with injured hands and upper extremities were placed into individual hospitals and distributed somewhat arbitrarily on to orthopedic, general surgery, plastic surgery, and neurosurgery wards

depending on the nature of the injury and the availability of beds. It became evident that specialized interdisciplinary care of the hand patient was necessary. In a masterpiece of organizational effort, regional hand referral centers were established in US military hospitals. Colonel JJ Reddy and Colonel FV Kilgore together established the first ward designated for hand surgery at Cushing General Hospital in Framingham, Massachusetts.[22] Plastic surgeon Captain (later Major) J William Littler was assigned to this ward and supervised the first service specifically dedicated to care of the injured hand. Joint conferences involving plastic surgery, orthopedic surgery, and neurosurgery were established and, within a short time, four complete wards dedicated to hand surgery were in operation.

Dr. Littler's unit was used as a model by Surgeon General Norman T Kirk to establish nine military referral centers throughout the US.[23] Sterling Bunnell served as civilian surgical consultant to the Secretary of War and visited each referral center to teach hand surgery.

Simultaneously, advances in plastic surgery had provided effective and reliable methods of wound coverage ranging from split- and full-thickness skin grafts to local and distant pedicled flaps. This ability to cover wounds was critical to the development of hand surgery. Because wound coverage was a priority, the regional hand centers established across the US were situated in hospitals that had been already designated as plastic surgery centers.

Plastic surgeons were instrumental in this early phase of development in American hand surgery because of their expertise in wound care and trauma reconstruction. In March 1945, Lieutenant Colonel Eugene M Bricker outlined in an Army memorandum the principles of plastic surgery relevant to hand surgery:

1. Conservative, careful and thorough debridement of the primary wound is essential. Primary closure is not advised in an evacuation hospital, but skin flaps can be dressed back into place.

2. Splint purposefully, maintaining the palmar arch and flexion of the metacarpophalangeal joints.

3. Bring about delayed closure as early as possible, preferably on the third or fourth day, by simple closure, split graft or pedicle graft, according to the necessities of the case.

4. Use traction only when it is urgently indicated, and then for a minimum length of time.

5. Concentrate on maintenance of such function as remains following certain severe types of injury. Restoration of the injured part should not be attempted, and healing should be accomplished as rapidly as possible. Amputation of an irreparably damaged finger is justified.

6. Institute active motion as early as possible, and supplement by occupational therapy when healing has occurred.

7. Try to prevent edema and infection in open wounds. Proper debridement, proper dressings, proper splinting, and effective elevation of the hand will prevent this development.

8. Manage an open wound aseptically as long as it remains open. Aseptic management implies the use of masks and

of instruments or gloves, whether or not the wound is infected.[24]These principles served as the foundation for acute treatment of traumatic hand injuries.

Developments after World War II

Immediately after World War II, plastic surgeons continued to have a profound influence on hand surgery. In 1946, plastic surgeon Darrel T Shaw and general surgeon Robert Lee Payne published a landmark paper entitled, "One stage tubed abdominal flaps."[25] This paper described an axial flap based on the superficial inferior epigastric vessels for composite tissue transfer to the hand. The development of reliable composite tissue transfer allowed early coverage of extensive hand and upper extremity defects. Sir Archibald McIndoe, a disciple of Gillies, established several burn facilities in England and refined techniques in burn excision and reconstruction of the hand.[26]

The patients wounded during the battles of World War II returned to the US for further reconstructive surgery by an increasingly better-trained cadre of hand surgeons. In order to coordinate this explosive growth in hand surgery, representatives from general surgery, plastic surgery, and orthopedic surgery combined to form the American Society for Surgery of the Hand in 1946.[27] The first annual meeting was held on January 20, 1946 at the Blackstone Hotel in Chicago, Illinois, with Sterling Bunnell as the first president. Plastic surgeons figured prominently – of the 35 founding members, 13 (37%) came from plastic surgery backgrounds.[28]

Hand surgery underwent another period of accelerated productivity during the Korean War. By that time, the US military had experience in organizing regional referral centers for reconstruction of the hand. Dr. J William Littler took on Bunnell's former role and was appointed as Hand Surgery Civilian Consultant to the Military.[29] Littler's unrivaled experience from World War II and then the Korean conflict allowed him to become perhaps the most famous of plastic hand surgeons. His achievements have included the Littler digital neurovascular transfer and countless other surgical innovations bearing his name, in addition to his legendary anatomic sketches of the hand and long list of trainees who have become distinguished hand surgeons themselves. Other plastic surgeons who were involved in the Korean War effort included Robert A Chase and Earle Peacock. Robert A Chase returned from his military duty to embark on a lifelong effort of developing educational aids related to functional anatomy of the hand. Earle Peacock contributed original laboratory work on wound healing, particularly related to flexor tendon wound healing.

The era of microsurgery

Hand surgery underwent an intense period of laboratory and clinical activity in the 1960s and 1970s devoted to microsurgery and free tissue transfer. In 1963, Goldwyn et al. presented their work on abdominal free flaps in dogs, based on the inferior epigastric vessels.[30] This investigative work was further developed by Krizek et al. in 1965.[31] Together, these plastic surgeons, along with O'Brien,[32] Taylor et al.[33] and many others throughout the world, established the possibility of free tissue transfer that liberated the hand surgeon from the anatomic limitations of local tissue transfer.

Replantation of fingers and other body parts came into reality via an international effort of plastic surgeons, orthopedic surgeons, and general surgeons. The first successful replantation of an upper arm amputation by Malt and McKhann was carried out in 1962, and the first successful replantation of an amputated thumb was performed in 1968 by Komatsu and Tamai. Since then, replantation teams have been organized in major hospitals, and microsurgical techniques have become an integral part of the training of hand surgeons. The techniques of replantation in the upper extremity have been extrapolated to successful replantation of other parts of the body, including the lower limb, the scalp, the ear, portions of the lip and nose, and the penis, and have led directly to the further evolution of elective microsurgical free tissue transfer. In addition, plastic surgeons have devised innovations to improve the success rates of replantation, including the use of Y-shaped interposition vein grafts in multiple-digit replantations[34] and replantation of fingers distal to the proximal interphalangeal joint.[35]

Plastic surgeon Harry J Buncke helped pioneer the toe-to-thumb transplant in animal models, and eventually in humans. His efforts in the past 40 years have made him one of the fathers of American microsurgery.[36] Beyond the earlier work of Littler on thumb reconstruction, plastic surgeons have continued to contribute greatly to the refinement of various operations, including the toe-to-hand transfer[37,38] and the great-toe wraparound free flap of Morrison et al.[39]

Critical to reconstruction of the hand with both pedicled flaps and free flaps has been a detailed knowledge of anatomy as it relates to vascular distributions to muscle and skin. McCraw et al. popularized the use of musculocutaneous flaps[40] and Mathes and Nahai developed an atlas of these muscle and musculocutaeous flaps which has been an invaluable reference for the reconstructive surgeon.[41] Ian Taylor and his plastic surgery colleagues have described the vascular territories of skin flaps. Taylor's angiosome theory, where the body is divided into different vascular territories to the skin, originating from deeper source arteries, has allowed surgeons to design flaps with reliable perfusion. In addition, second-generation flaps, based on smaller vessels, may be possible with an understanding of this intricate anatomy.

Plastic surgeons have also continued to be involved in the political and educational development of hand surgery. In 1970, a second hand organization – the American Association for Hand Surgery (AAHS) – was founded.[42] By the fall of 1971, there were 65 full members. As in the American Society for Surgery of the Hand, plastic surgeons played an instrumental role. The first meeting in 1971 immediately preceded the annual American Society of Plastic and Reconstructive Surgeons meeting. This arrangement symbolized the influence and participation of plastic surgeons in the AAHS that continues today.

Recent developments

In recent years, significant contributions to hand surgery have been made by plastic surgeons. One area of intense study in the past several decades has been peripheral nerve repair and reconstruction. Millesi et al.[43] published a landmark paper in 1972 on interfascicular nerve grafting of median and ulnar nerves. Since then, nerve grafting, as well as autogenous vein grafting of nerve defects, has helped improve results of nerve reconstruction.[44,45] Mackinnon and Hudson[46] have examined the possibility of immunosuppression for allograft nerve transplantation to bridge extensive defects where autogenous donor nerve may not be sufficient, and more recently pioneered the field of nerve transfers.[47] Several plastic surgeons, including Terzis et al.[48] and Hentz and Narakas,[49] have published reports of their considerable experience on reconstruction of brachial palsy injury. Their dedication to the comprehensive reconstruction and rehabilitation of these devastating injuries has resulted in improved surgical outcomes.

Beyond replantation, more intricate microvascular operations have been undertaken by plastic hand surgeons to restore form and function to the hand. Although the indications are limited, microvascular transfer of a toe metatarsophalangeal joint to recreate a metacarpophalangeal joint has been shown to be possible.[50] Further advances in microsurgical reconstruction of the hand include functional free muscle transfer. Manktelow and McKee's landmark paper in 1978 introduced the concept of a free gracilis or free pectoralis major muscle transfer with motor nerve coaptation to restore active finger flexion.[51]

Plastic surgeons have also been at the forefront of congenital hand surgery.[52] Graham Lister published one of the first significant series of toe-to-hand microvascular transfers in children, ushering in a new era of complex reconstruction for congenital hand problems.[53] Other authors, including Gilbert[54] and Buck-Gramcko,[55] have also published their series. More recently, Neil Jones has added his work on pediatric toe-to-hand transfers to previous contributors, thus refining these technically challenging procedures.[56] In addition, Joseph Upton et al.[57] reported on their unrivalled experience with excision and reconstruction of vascular anomalies in the upper extremity.

The plastic surgery techniques of flap dissection have been used to develop newer flaps intrinsic to the hand and upper extremity such as vascularized bone flaps from the distal radius. There is much excitement in using these pedicled bone flaps for revascularization of the scaphoid in scaphoid nonunion and avascular necrosis, or revascularization of the lunate in Kienbock's disease.[58] These second-generation flaps may lead to other intrinsic flaps that will also be useful for bone and ligament reconstruction.

Plastic surgeons know of their legacy of involvement in the field of organ transplantation. Much of the pioneering work on allograft rejection and homograft tolerance by Sir Peter Medawar and others was derived from experimentation with skin grafts in various animal models.[59] Joe Murray, the only plastic surgeon ever to receive the Nobel Prize, received it for his work on transplantation, including the first human kidney transplantation in 1954.[60] With newer immunosuppressive agents and greater acceptance of the risks of transplantation, human hand allograft transplantation has now become a reality.[61] While the ultimate success of these early operations remains to be seen, reaching these new frontiers in hand reconstruction as well as in other forms of composite tissue allotransplantation is now possible.

Future directions

An accomplished hand and plastic surgeon once wrote:

I learned about hand surgery's battle against scar adherence and contraction and that the Z-plasty can be a major and intriguing weapon in that battle in other parts of the body as well as in the hand. I thought a lot about the Z-plasties that year and used them often, in multiple parts of the body, always trying to pick the optimum size and the best orientation, trying to decide which of the two parallel sides of the Z-plasty's diamond would be most advantageous for mimicking the wrinkle lines, and trying to avoid running into features not to be moved or, occasionally, to something on or in one of the flaps … Ever since, I have looked upon the Z-plasty as a little bit of magic.[62]

That surgeon was Leonard T Furlow Jr, who took the z-plasty from the scarred hand to the cleft palate. It is an excellent example of the intellectual interplay between plastic surgery and hand surgery.

Current plastic surgery research has focused on growth factor technology to inhibit scarring or to augment bone growth, wound healing,[63] and angiogenesis. Tissue engineering may allow formation of ample supplies of bone, cartilage,[64] even muscle, skin, and nerve. Virtual reality surgery will help plastic surgeons model and practice complex reconstructive procedures prior to undertaking them. In the next decade, hand surgeons will acquire an armamentarium that includes bone substitutes, tissue-engineered bone, cartilage and nerve, and three-dimensional computer models for complex intracarpal abnormalities. Throughout the chapters of this hand volume, you will find new, pioneering translational work that shapes the future of hand and upper extremity surgery. As in microsurgery, plastic surgeons will lead the way for this new technical revolution in hand surgery.

Access the complete references list online at **http://www.expertconsult.com**

2. Kleinert HE, Spokevicius S, Papas NH. History of flexor tendon repair. *J Hand Surg.* 1995;20A:S46.
   This paper by Kleinert et al. describes the evolution of flexor tendon repair over time from secondary repair of tendon laceration in zone II to the current techniques of primary repair.

20. Bunnell S. *Surgery of the Hand*, Philadelphia: Lippincott; 1944.
   This is the first edition of the first modern textbook in hand surgery, written by Sterling Bunnell, widely regarded as the father of American hand surgery.

39. Morrison WA, O'Brien BM, Macleod AM. Thumb reconstruction with a free neurovascular wrap-around flap from the big toe. *J Hand Surg* 1980;5A:575.

    This original description of the great toe wrap-around flap represents a significant refinement of the great toe transfer, resulting in a narrower thumb and preservation of a portion of the length of the great toe donor site.

47. Tung TH, Mackinnon SE. Nerve transfers: indications, techniques, and outcomes. *J Hand Surg* 2010;35:332.

    This review article describes current state of the art for new techniques in nerve transfers. Nerve transfers represent a developing field in hand surgery whereby fascicular dissection of nerves allows precise transfer of specific nerve branches to reinnervate other nerve–muscle units.

56. Chang J, Jones NF. Radiographic Analysis of Growth in Pediatric Toe-to-Hand Transfer. *Plast Reconstr Surg.* 2002;109:576.

    This article reviews a large clinical experience with pediatric toe-to-hand transfers. Radiographic analysis of the transferred toes was performed, with comparison to the opposite toe as a growth control. The authors showed that, with careful preservation of the growth plates, growth of these transferred toes is maintained over time.

1

Anatomy and biomechanics of the hand

James Chang, Francisco Valero-Cuevas, Vincent R. Hentz, and Robert A. Chase

SYNOPSIS

- Introduction – history to anatomy and biomechanics of the hand
- Skin, subcutaneous tissue, and fascia
- Bones and joints
  - Hand elements
  - The wrist
  - Joint motion
  - The thumb
- Muscles and tendons
  - Extrinsic extensors
  - Pronators and supinators
  - Extrinsic flexors
  - The retinacular system
  - Intrinsic muscles
- Blood supply
- Peripheral nerves

Introduction

During the Renaissance, Vesalius corrected early misconceptions and brought gross anatomy into proper focus. Since that time, many investigators have embellished the basic structural studies with functional, physiologic, and philosophical observations. The forearm and hand have been prominently included in those observations. Sir Charles Bell (1834),[2] in his thought-provoking volume, *The Hand – Its Mechanism and Vital Endowments as Evincing Design*, presented a concept of hand anatomy that places it in proper context with the position of humans in the animal kingdom. Frederick Wood-Jones (1920) probed more extensively into comparative anatomy

and anthropology in his excellent work, *The Principles of Anatomy as Seen in the Hand*.[3] Duchenne (1867) carried out detailed analysis of muscular function by isolated electrical stimulation, described in his classic volume, *Physiologie des Mouvements*.[4]

Allen B Kanavel (1925) published his monograph, *Infections of the Hand*, which reported detailed analysis of the spaces and synovial sheaths.[5] *Surgery of the Hand* by Sterling Bunnell (1944) became an indispensable reference during World War II.[6] Emanuel B Kaplan (1953) produced the nicely illustrated, detailed volume, *Functional and Surgical Anatomy of the Hand*.[7] Detailed studies of the integration of the intrinsic and extrinsic muscles operating the polyarticular digits may be found in the work of Landsmeer,[8–11] Kaplan,[12] Eyler and Markee,[13] Stack,[14] Tubiana and Valentin,[15] and others. More recently, newer flaps intrinsic to the hand and upper extremity have been developed from more detailed investigation into vascular anatomy.[16,17] Lastly, Berger,[18] Viegas *et al.*,[19] and others have expanded our knowledge of the ligamentous anatomy of the wrist.

As a functional puppet, the hand responds to human desires; its motor performance is initiated by the contralateral cerebral cortex. The conscious demands relayed to the hand and forearm from the central nervous controlling mechanism are sent as movement commands. At subconscious levels, such a movement command is broken down, regrouped, coordinated, and sent on as a signal for fixation, graded contraction, or relaxation of a specific muscular unit. The degree of contraction or relaxation is then modified by relayed evidence that the motion created is that desired by the person. The modifying factors arrive centrally from a multiplicity of sensory sources such as the eye, peripheral sensory end organs, and muscle or joint sensory endings.

The surgeon planning reconstructive surgery on the upper extremity must be aware not only of the complex anatomy of the hand and arm, but also of the physiologic interplay of balanced muscular functions under the influence of complex central nervous coordination. The maintenance of physiologic viability by the central and peripheral circulatory and

This chapter has attempted to preserve the character and style of the original edition by master anatomist, Robert A Chase MD.[1] In addition, we have updated the text with more recent anatomic findings, clinical pearls, basic concepts in biomechanics, and full-color illustrations.

lymphatic systems must also concern the reconstructive surgeon.

This chapter will address the fundamentals of hand and upper extremity anatomy. It will highlight clinical pearls, new anatomic descriptions that may aid surgery of the hand, and the fundamentals of biomechanics relevant to the hand surgeon.

Skin, subcutaneous tissue, and fascia

There is great disparity in the character of the skin and soft-tissue envelope covering the dorsum of the hand and that covering the palm. Dorsal skin is thin and pliable, anchored to the deep investing fascia by loose, areolar tissue. These characteristics, coupled with the fact that the major venous and lymphatic drainage in the hand courses dorsally, serve to explain why hand edema is first evident dorsally. The prominent, visible veins in the subcutaneous tissue make it the standard site in which to evaluate venous filling and limb venous pressure on physical examination. The same characteristics make the dorsum of the hand vulnerable to skin avulsion injuries.

Palmar skin, in contrast, is characterized by a thick dermal layer and a heavily cornified epithelial surface. The skin is not as pliable as dorsal skin, and it is held tightly to the thick fibrous palmar fascia by diffusely distributed vertical fibers between the fascia and dermis. Stability of palmar skin is critical to hand function. At the same time, if scar fixation or loss of elasticity occurs in palmar skin, contractures and functional loss result. The skin of the palm is laden with a high concentration of specialized sensory end organs and sweat glands. The surgeon must understand the relationship of the palmar skin creases and the underlying joints in order to plan precise placement of skin incisions for exposure of joints and their related structures (Box 1.1 and Fig. 1.1).

Examination of hand skin during normal ranges of motion in various planes is important in planning incisions or geometrically rearranging lacerations that might result in disabling scar contractures. Most loss of elasticity and some longitudinal shortening are compensated for adequately by mobility and elasticity of the uninjured dorsal skin. On the palmar aspect, however, scar shortening and inelasticity of the skin may result in contracture. The nature of palmar skin, its stabilizing fixation to the palmar fascia, and its position on the concave side of the hand are the bases for such contractures. Littler outlined the specific sites in the palm where a longitudinal scar would impede extension.[21] For example, in each digit the geometry has been worked out by noting each joint axis and the kissing surfaces of the palmar skin in full flexion. These diamond-shaped skin surfaces should not be shortened and rendered inelastic by longitudinal scars if limitation of extension is to be avoided (Fig. 1.2).

The palmar fascia consists of resistant fibrous tissue arranged in longitudinal, transverse, oblique, and vertical fibers (Fig. 1.3). The longitudinal fibers concentrate at the proximal origin of the palmar fascia at the wrist, taking origin from the palmaris longus when it is present (in about 80–85% of individuals). The fascia at this level is separable from the underlying flexor retinaculum/carpal ligament, being identified by the longitudinal orientation of its fibers in contrast to the transverse fibers of the retinaculum. The palmar fascia fibers fan out from this origin, concentrating in flat bundles to each of the digits. Generally, the fibers spread at the base of each digit and send minor fibers to the skin and the bulk of fibers distal into the fingers, where they attach to tissues making up the fibrous flexor sheath of the digits. There are attachments of the fascia to the volar plate and intermetacarpal ligaments at each side of the flexor tendon sheath at the level of the metacarpal heads.

Transverse fibers are concentrated in the midpalm and the web spaces. The midpalmar transverse fibers, although intimately associated with the longitudinal bundles, lie deep to them and are inseparable from the vertical fibers that concentrate into septa between the longitudinally oriented structures

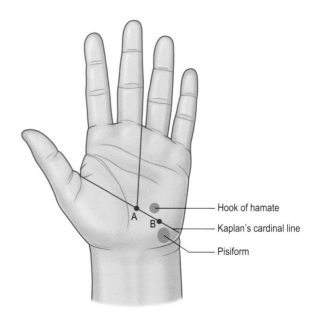

Fig. 1.1 Kaplan's cardinal line, along with lines from the ulnar aspect of the middle finger and the ulnar aspect of the ring finger. Point A corresponds with the motor branch of the median nerve and point B with the motor branch of the ulnar nerve.

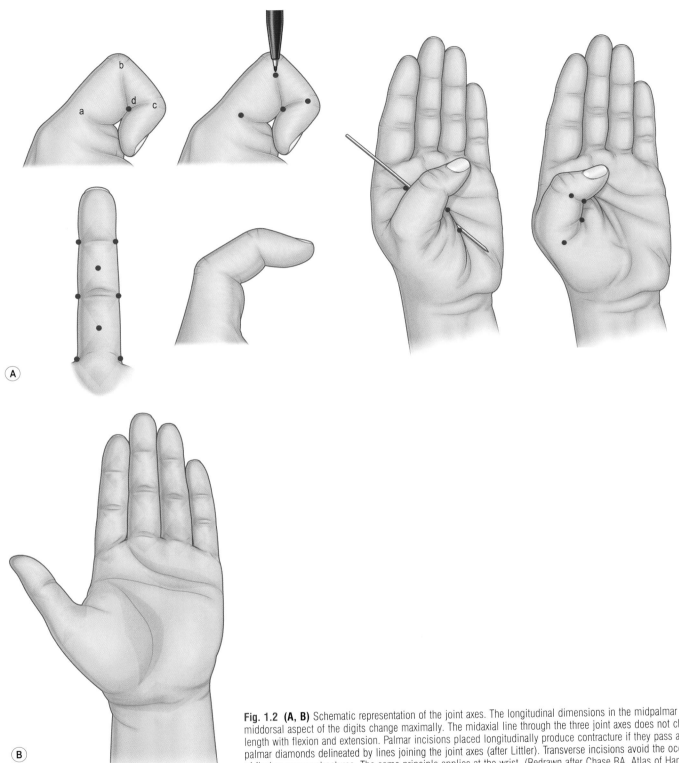

Fig. 1.2 (A, B) Schematic representation of the joint axes. The longitudinal dimensions in the midpalmar and middorsal aspect of the digits change maximally. The midaxial line through the three joint axes does not change in length with flexion and extension. Palmar incisions placed longitudinally produce contracture if they pass across the palmar diamonds delineated by lines joining the joint axes (after Littler). Transverse incisions avoid the occurrence of flexion scar contractures. The same principle applies at the wrist. (Redrawn after Chase RA. Atlas of Hand Surgery, vol 1. Philadelphia: WB Saunders, 1973.)

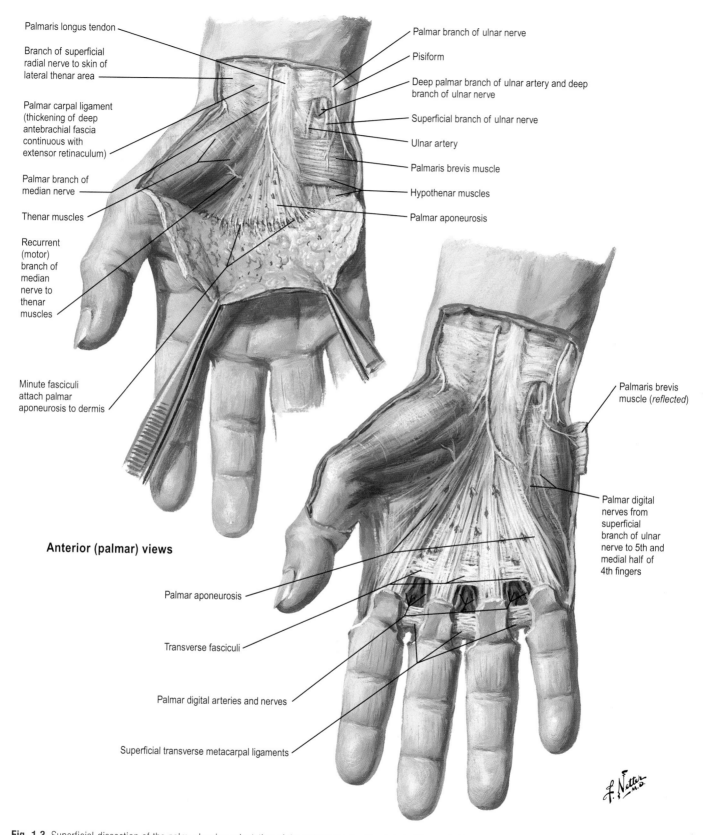

Palmaris longus tendon

Branch of superficial radial nerve to skin of lateral thenar area

Palmar carpal ligament (thickening of deep antebrachial fascia continuous with extensor retinaculum)

Palmar branch of median nerve

Thenar muscles

Recurrent (motor) branch of median nerve to thenar muscles

Minute fasciculi attach palmar aponeurosis to dermis

Palmar branch of ulnar nerve

Pisiform

Deep palmar branch of ulnar artery and deep branch of ulnar nerve

Superficial branch of ulnar nerve

Ulnar artery

Palmaris brevis muscle

Hypothenar muscles

Palmar aponeurosis

Palmaris brevis muscle (reflected)

Palmar digital nerves from superficial branch of ulnar nerve to 5th and medial half of 4th fingers

Anterior (palmar) views

Palmar aponeurosis

Transverse fasciculi

Palmar digital arteries and nerves

Superficial transverse metacarpal ligaments

Fig. 1.3 Superficial dissection of the palm, showing orientation of the palmar fascia. (Reprinted with permission from www.netterimages.com © Elsevier Inc. All Rights Reserved.)

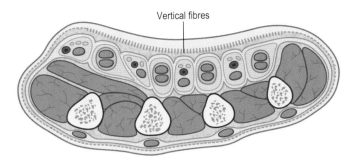

Vertical fibres

Fig. 1.4 The palmar fascia with its longitudinal, transverse, and vertical fibers. The longitudinal fibers take origin in the palmaris longus (when present). Transverse fibers are concentrated in the distal palm supporting the web skin and in the midpalm as the transverse palmar ligament. Vertical fibers extend superficially as multiple, tiny tethering strands to stabilize the thick palmar skin. The deep vertical components concentrate in septa between the longitudinally oriented structures in the fingers. (Redrawn after McCarthy JG. Plastic Surgery. Philadelphia: WB Saunders, 1990.)

passing to the fingers. This system of palmar transverse fibers makes up what Skoog (1967) called the transverse palmar ligament.[22] In fact, the transverse fibers form the roof of tunnels at this point that act as pulleys for the flexor tendons proximal to the level of the digital pulleys. Longitudinal fibers pass toward the palmar surface of the thumb, but these fibers are generally less numerous and sometimes difficult to identify. The thumb fibers blend into the deep fascia overlying the thenar muscles. The ulnar extreme palmar fascia blends with the hypothenar fascia. The proximal one-third of this border is the attachment site of the palmaris brevis muscle. Laterally, the muscle attaches to the hypothenar skin and hypothenar fascia.

The vertical fibers of the palmar fascia, which lie superficially to the tough triangular membrane made up by the longitudinal and transverse fibers, consist of abundant vertical fibers to the palm skin dermis *(Fig. 1.4)*. Deep to the palmar fascia, the vertical fibers coalesce into septa, or the "perforating fibers of Legueu and Juvara,"[23] forming compartments for flexor tendons to each digit and separate compartments for the neurovascular bundles together with the lumbrical muscles. There are eight such compartments, which extend proximally to about the midpalm. Proximal to this, there is a common central compartment.[24] The marginal septa extend more proximally than the seven intermediate septa closing the central compartment laterally and medially. The major septum between the index flexor tendons and the neurovascular and lumbrical space to the third interspace attaches to the third metacarpal, dividing the thenar or adductor space from the midpalmar space. Knowledge of these vertical compartments aids dissection and identification of structures in operations such as trigger-finger release and Dupuytren's fasciectomy *(Fig. 1.5)*.

In the fingers, two important bands of fascia are named Grayson's ligaments and Cleland's ligaments. Grayson's ligaments are volar to the neurovascular bundles and are quite flimsy. The much stouter Cleland's ligaments are dorsal to the neurovascular bundles. These two fascial sheets help contain and protect the ulnar and radial digital arteries and nerves *(Fig. 1.6)*.

Bones and joints

Hand elements

The ability of the hand to resist and create powerful gross action, combined with its capacity to perform intricate fine movements in multiple planes, reflects the masterful construction of its supporting architecture. Reducing the hand to its supporting skeleton and its restraining ligaments reveals the architectural basis for its varied function. A study of the range of joint motions in the hand and forearm with all motor elements removed discloses the full range and limitations that the skeleton imposes on hand function.

The hand skeleton is divisible into four elements:

1. The fixed unit of the hand, consisting of the second and third metacarpals and the distal carpal row.

2. The thumb and its metacarpal with a wide range of motion at the carpometacarpal joint. Five intrinsic muscles and four extrinsic muscles are specifically influential on thumb positioning and activity.

3. The index digit with independence of action within the range of motion allowed by its joints and ligaments. Three intrinsic and four extrinsic muscles allow such digital independence.

4. The third, fourth, and fifth digits with the fourth and fifth metacarpals. This unit functions as a stabilizing vise to grasp objects for manipulation by the thumb and index finger, or in concert with the other hand units in powerful grasp *(Fig. 1.7)*.

The distal row of carpal bones forms a solid architectural arch with the capitate bone as a keystone. The articulations of the distal carpals with one another, the intercarpal ligaments, and the important transverse carpal ligament (flexor retinaculum) maintain a strong, fixed transverse carpal arch. Projecting distally from the central third of this arch are the fixed central metacarpals, the second and third. Littler called this "the fixed unit of the hand." It forms a fixed transverse arch of carpal bones and a fixed longitudinal arch created by the anatomic convexity of the metacarpals. As a stable foundation, this unit creates a supporting base for the three other mobile units. This central beam moves as a unit at the wrist under the influence of the prime wrist extensors (the extensor carpi radialis longus and brevis) and the prime wrist flexor, the flexor carpi radialis. These major wrist movers insert on the second and third metacarpals. Thus, the fixed central unit is positioned for activity of the adaptive elements of the hand around it.

The distal row of carpal bones constitutes a fixed transverse arch. At the level of the metacarpal heads, the transverse arch of the hand becomes mobile, which is possible because the first metacarpal moves through a wide range of motion at the saddle-like carpometacarpal joint. The loose capsular ligaments and the shallow saddle articulation between the first metacarpal and the trapezium allow circumduction of the mobile first metacarpal. Its range of motion is checked by these capsular ligaments, including the volar beak ligament, and by its attachment to the fixed hand axis through the adductor pollicis, the first dorsal interosseous, and the fascia and skin of the first web space. The mobile fourth and fifth metacarpal heads move dorsally and palmarly in relation to

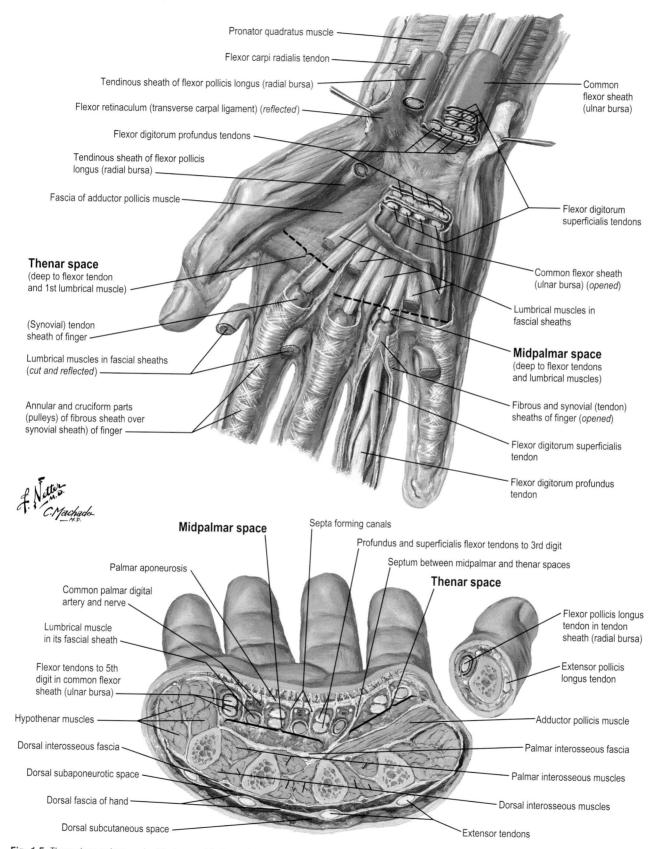

Pronator quadratus muscle

Flexor carpi radialis tendon

Tendinous sheath of flexor pollicis longus (radial bursa)

Flexor retinaculum (transverse carpal ligament) (reflected)

Flexor digitorum profundus tendons

Tendinous sheath of flexor pollicis longus (radial bursa)

Fascia of adductor pollicis muscle

Thenar space
(deep to flexor tendon and 1st lumbrical muscle)

(Synovial) tendon sheath of finger

Lumbrical muscles in fascial sheaths (cut and reflected)

Annular and cruciform parts (pulleys) of fibrous sheath over synovial sheath) of finger

Common flexor sheath (ulnar bursa)

Flexor digitorum superficialis tendons

Common flexor sheath (ulnar bursa) (opened)

Lumbrical muscles in fascial sheaths

Midpalmar space
(deep to flexor tendons and lumbrical muscles)

Fibrous and synovial (tendon) sheaths of finger (opened)

Flexor digitorum superficialis tendon

Flexor digitorum profundus tendon

Midpalmar space

Septa forming canals

Profundus and superficialis flexor tendons to 3rd digit

Septum between midpalmar and thenar spaces

Thenar space

Palmar aponeurosis

Common palmar digital artery and nerve

Lumbrical muscle in its fascial sheath

Flexor tendons to 5th digit in common flexor sheath (ulnar bursa)

Hypothenar muscles

Dorsal interosseous fascia

Dorsal subaponeurotic space

Dorsal fascia of hand

Dorsal subcutaneous space

Flexor pollicis longus tendon in tendon sheath (radial bursa)

Extensor pollicis longus tendon

Adductor pollicis muscle

Palmar interosseous fascia

Palmar interosseous muscles

Dorsal interosseous muscles

Extensor tendons

Fig. 1.5 These deep palmar and midpalmar axial views of the hand reinforce the concept of distinct anatomic compartments separated by fascia. (Reprinted with permission from www.netterimages.com © Elsevier Inc. All Rights Reserved.)

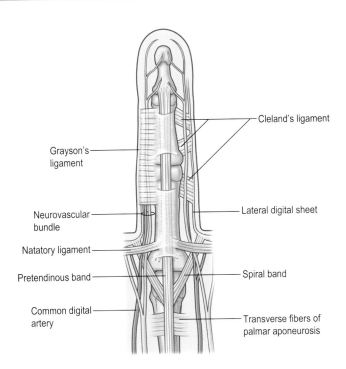

Cleland's ligament

Grayson's ligament

Neurovascular bundle

Lateral digital sheet

Natatory ligament

Pretendinous band

Spiral band

Common digital artery

Transverse fibers of palmar aponeurosis

Fig. 1.6 The components of the digital fascia that help to anchor the axial plane skin are Grayson's ligaments palmar to the neurovascular bundles and Cleland's ligaments dorsal to the bundles. (Redrawn after McCarthy JG. Plastic Surgery. Philadelphia: WB Saunders, 1990.)

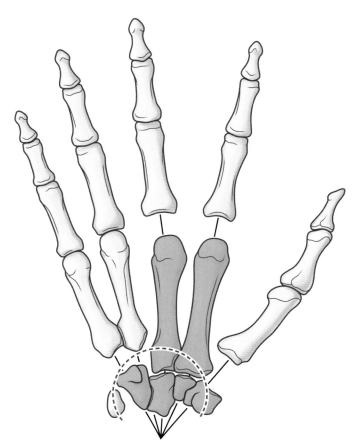

Fig. 1.7 Exploded view of the functional elements of the hand: (1) the thumb and its metacarpal with a wide range of motion at the carpometacarpal joint; (2) the index digit with independence of action in several planes; (3) the third, fourth, and fifth digits with the fourth and fifth metacarpals; and (4) the fixed unit consisting of the carpals with the fixed transverse carpal arch and the second and third metacarpals forming a fixed longitudinal arch. (Redrawn after McCarthy JG. Plastic Surgery. Philadelphia: WB Saunders, 1990.)

the central hand axis by limited mobility at the carpometacarpal joints. These metacarpal heads are tethered to the central metacarpals by the intermetacarpal ligaments. The latter unite adjacent metacarpophalangeal volar plates, which are an intimate part of the joint capsules.

When the head of the first metacarpal is palmar-abducted by thenar muscles innervated by the median nerve, and the fourth and fifth metacarpals are palmar-abducted by the hypothenar muscles innervated by the ulnar nerve, a volar, concave, transverse metacarpal arch is created, approximating a semicircle. The mobile metacarpal heads are pulled dorsally by extrinsic extensor tendons when the thenar and hypothenar muscles relax. It is obvious that a flaccid paralysis of the intrinsic muscles of the hand in median and ulnar nerve palsy will produce a flattened or even reversed transverse metacarpal arch. The active production of a semicircular transverse arch by the thenar and hypothenar muscles creates the proper circumferential arrangement of the metacarpophalangeal joints for convergence of the fingers in flexion. In this position the fingers, flexing at the metacarpophalangeal joints only, converge, forming with the thumb a cone, the apex of which lies over the anatomic center of the hand *(Fig. 1.8)*. A vertical line dropped from the apex of the cone to the center of its base will strike the third metacarpophalangeal joint. This point at the apex of the transverse metacarpal arch is the anatomic center of the hand. With the fingers fully abducted, the tips form radii of equal length from the anatomic center of the hand. The same radius projected proximally falls at the wrist joint.

The most important single motor operating the central hand beam at the wrist level is the extensor carpi radialis brevis, which works against gravity, positioning the pronated

hand into extension. In the absence of any other motors it pulls the central third metacarpal into extension, making it the apex of the passively created transverse metacarpal arch.

The wrist

The wrist joint is the site for major postural change between the arm beam and the working hand end piece *(Fig. 1.9)*. It has a multiarticulated architecture that creates a potentially wide range of motion in flexion, extension, radial deviation, ulnar deviation, and circumduction. The distal radioulnar joint allows pronation and supination of the hand as the radius rotates around the head of the ulna. The proximal row of carpal bones (scaphoid, lunate, triquetrum, pisiform) articulates with the distal radius and ulna, providing the ability to flex and extend the hand and perform radial and ulnar deviation. The distal carpal row (trapezium, trapezoid, capitate, and hamate), along with the second and third metacarpals, forms the "fixed unit" of the hand.

The radiocarpal joint includes the carpal bones and the distal radius *(Fig. 1.10)*. The principal articulation of the carpus is with the distal surface of the radius. The articular

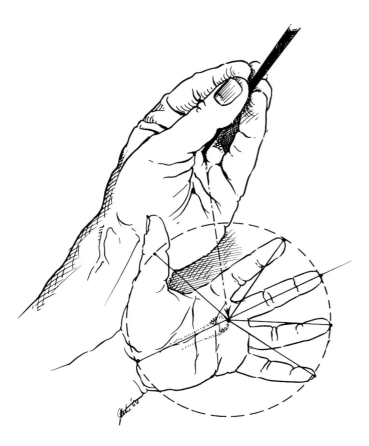

Fig. 1.8 When the adaptive arch is semicircular, the fingers converge in a cone over the anatomic center of the hand – the long-finger metacarpophalangeal joint. (From McCarthy JG. Plastic Surgery. Philadelphia: WB Saunders, 1990.)

surface of the radius slopes in several planes. In the radial-to-ulnar plane, the radius exhibits an average slope of 22°. In the dorsal-to-palmar plane, the articular surface of the radius slopes 12° with the dorsal surface more distal than the palmar surface. Fractures of the distal radius frequently result in a loss of the normal radiocarpal configuration in one or both planes. A loss of the normal dorsal-to-palmar tilt of the articular surface will result in a change in the biomechanical properties of the wrist joint, which may lead to degenerative arthritis.

The relationship of the length of the radius to the length of the ulna is fairly constant in individuals, and is termed ulnar variance. The distal ulna will complete the curve of the articular surface of the radius. If the end of the ulna falls short of this curvature, the condition is termed ulnar negative variance. If the ulna extends distal to this imaginary extension, the condition is termed ulnar positive variance. Either condition may lead to wrist problems. Ulnar negative variance is associated with a higher incidence of Kienbock's disease, avascular necrosis of the lunate. Ulnar positive variance greater than 2–3 mm is associated with ulnar impaction *(Fig. 1.11)*.

Gilula and others have described several anatomic features that denote normal extracarpal and intracarpal architecture.[25] A line that follows the proximal articular contours of the proximal row of carpal bones circumscribes a smooth arc, termed the greater arc *(Fig. 1.12)*. A disruption in the smooth appearance of this arc is one of the signs of carpal abnormality, such as abnormal rotation of one of the bones of the proximal carpal row, as would be seen with disruption of the scapholunate ligament. Similarly, the joint line between the proximal

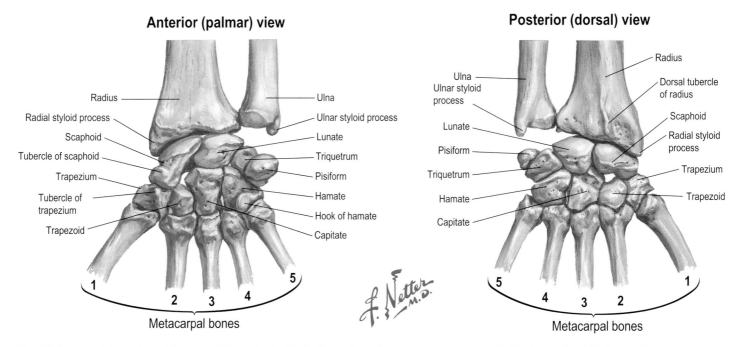

Anterior (palmar) view

Radius — Ulna
Radial styloid process — Ulnar styloid process
Scaphoid — Lunate
Tubercle of scaphoid — Triquetrum
Trapezium — Pisiform
Tubercle of trapezium — Hamate
Trapezoid — Hook of hamate
— Capitate

1   5
2   3   4

Metacarpal bones

Posterior (dorsal) view

Ulna — Radius
Ulnar styloid process — Dorsal tubercle of radius
Lunate — Scaphoid
Pisiform — Radial styloid process
Triquetrum — Trapezium
Hamate — Trapezoid
Capitate —

5   1
4   3   2

Metacarpal bones

Fig. 1.9 Palmar and dorsal views of the bones of the wrist. (Reprinted with permission from www.netterimages.com © Elsevier Inc. All Rights Reserved.)

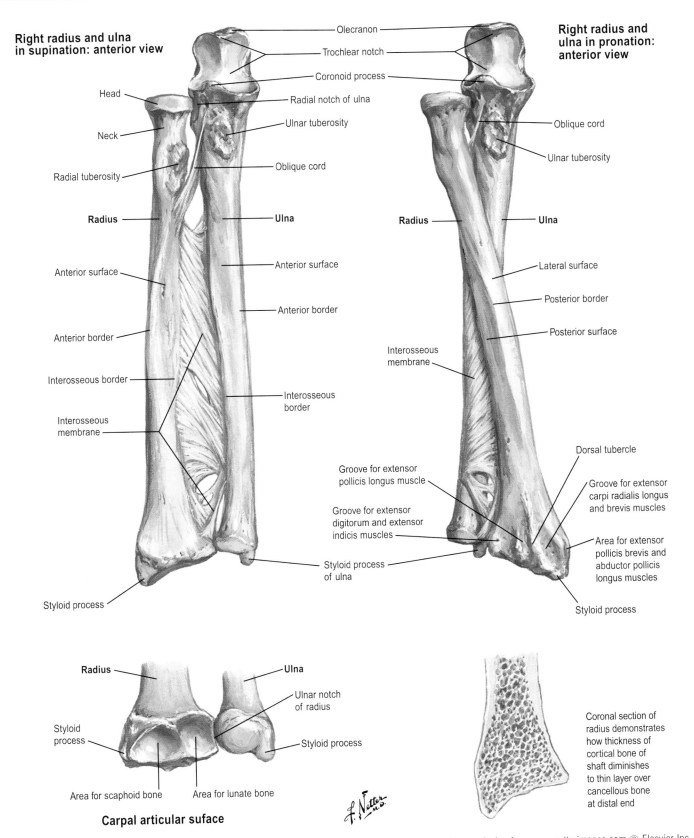

Right radius and ulna in supination: anterior view

Olecranon

Trochlear notch

Coronoid process

Head

Radial notch of ulna

Neck

Ulnar tuberosity

Radial tuberosity

Oblique cord

Radius

Ulna

Anterior surface

Anterior surface

Anterior border

Anterior border

Interosseous border

Interosseous border

Interosseous membrane

Right radius and ulna in pronation: anterior view

Oblique cord

Ulnar tuberosity

Radius

Ulna

Lateral surface

Posterior border

Posterior surface

Interosseous membrane

Dorsal tubercle

Groove for extensor pollicis longus muscle

Groove for extensor carpi radialis longus and brevis muscles

Groove for extensor digitorum and extensor indicis muscles

Area for extensor pollicis brevis and abductor pollicis longus muscles

Styloid process of ulna

Styloid process

Styloid process

Radius

Ulna

Styloid process

Ulnar notch of radius

Styloid process

Area for scaphoid bone

Area for lunate bone

Coronal section of radius demonstrates how thickness of cortical bone of shaft diminishes to thin layer over cancellous bone at distal end

Carpal articular suface

J. Netter m.d.

Fig. 1.10 Relationship of the radius and ulna at the proximal and distal radioulnar joints. (Reprinted with permission from www.netterimages.com © Elsevier Inc. All Rights Reserved.)

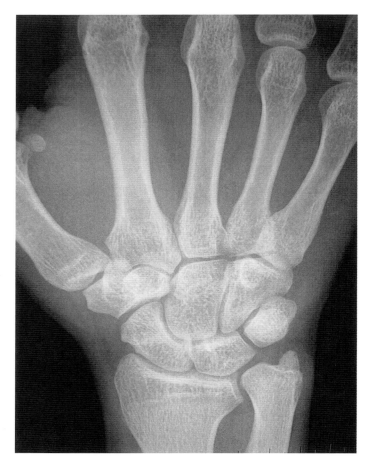

Fig. 1.11 X-ray of ulnar positive variance: this patient has ulnar-sided wrist pain due to ulnar impaction syndrome.

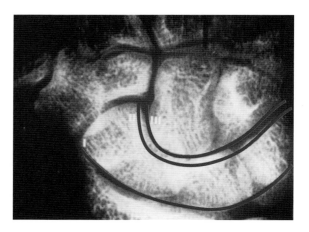

Fig. 1.12 Gilula's lines showing the greater arc and lesser arc of the carpal bones. (Reproduced from Hentz VR, Chase RA. Hand Surgery: A Clinical Atlas. Philadelphia: WB Saunders, 2001.)

and distal row of carpal bones circumscribes another smooth arc, termed the lesser arc. The presence of abnormalities in either of these arcs may be an indication of carpal pathology, either acute or chronic.

The scaphoid and lunate bones of the proximal carpal row form the convex articular counterparts of the concave distal radius for the major wrist articulation. In fact, the articular

surface of the radius is divided into scaphoid and lunate fossae **(Box 1.2)**. The triquetrum articulates with the lunate in the proximal row, and with the hamate across the midcarpal joint. The pisiform is essentially a floating bone, unimportant for carpal stability.

All four of the bones in the distal carpal row present articular surfaces for junction with the metacarpals. The distal carpal row forms a solid architectural arch with the central capitate as the keystone. The nature of the articulations of the distal carpals with one another, and of the carpal ligament (flexor retinaculum), is such that they make up a strong and fixed transverse carpal arch **(Box 1.3)**.

The complex motions of the wrist are a product of the sums of the movements of the carpal bones in various planes and degrees of rotation relative to one another. The motion of any one carpal bone is a consequence of several factors. First is the contour of the bone and the arrangements of its articular surfaces. The second is the degree of freedom afforded by intrinsic ligaments, which are ligaments originating from one carpal bone and inserting on another carpal bone, and by extrinsic ligaments, which are ligaments arising from the radius or ulna and attaching to a carpal bone or bones. This complex set of ligaments and the shape of the intercarpal and radiocarpal articulations control movement because no muscles arise or insert on any of the carpal bones except for the pisiform.

This unique adaptation of nature avoids the need for a thickly muscled wrist and hand unit. It permits great flexibility in positioning the hand in space without the need for sets of muscle agonists and antagonists to control the several degrees of freedom of movement.

The proximal row of carpal bones is anchored to the radius by a series of stout palmar ligaments arising primarily from the radius and by an additional set of stout ligaments arising from the ulna and the palmar portion of the triangular fibrocartilage complex. The triangular fibrocartilage complex separates the distal end of the ulna from the ulnar-sided carpal bones and serves to suspend the distal ulna to the radius at the distal radioulnar joint. These primary extrinsic palmar lunotriquetral ligament is also composed of dorsal, proximal, and palmar portions. There is less motion between these two carpal bones. Disruption of either the scapholunate or lunotriquetral ligaments may lead to wrist instability as the normal restraints on synchronous motion are removed.

Joint motion

The bony anatomy of the hand is presented in *Figure 1.14*. Normal metacarpophalangeal joint motion in the fingers ranges from 0 to 90°. Lateral activity in the metacarpophalangeal joints is limited by the rein-like collateral ligaments. These ligaments are loose and redundant when the metacarpophalangeal joints are in extension, allowing maximal medial and lateral deviation. As the metacarpophalangeal joint is flexed, the cam effect of the eccentrically placed ligaments and the epicondylar bowing of the collateral ligaments result in tightening and strict limitation of lateral mobility *(Fig. 1.15)*. The fingers that have been fixed in extension during a period of healing have had the stage set for collateral ligament shrinkage and locking of the metacarpophalangeal joints in hyperextension.

The proximal interphalangeal joint can be pushed to 110° of flexion, but extension usually cannot be carried beyond 5° of hyperextension because of the ligamentous volar plate, which is an inseparable part of the joint capsule. The medial and lateral collateral ligaments are a part of the capsule. They are radially fixed in a manner that allows no medial or lateral deviation of the joint in any position. The shape of the articular joint surface also strongly contributes to this stability in lateral motion.

The distal interphalangeal joints of the fingers can be pushed into about 90° of flexion before they are limited by the dorsal joint capsule and extensor mechanism. The distal interphalangeal joints extend to 30° of hyperextension. There is no lateral mobility in these joints with the collateral ligaments intact. The collateral ligaments of the distal interphalangeal joints are simply thickened medial and lateral portions of the joint capsule.

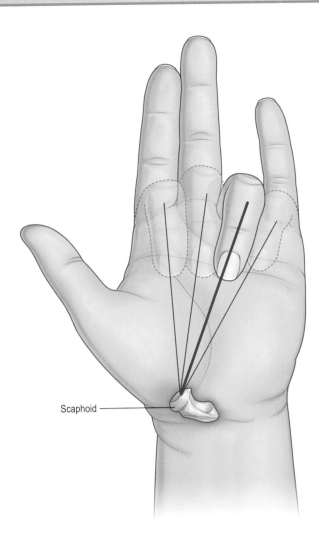

Scaphoid

Fig. 1.13 Each finger in correct alignment points to the tubercle of the scaphoid when flexed individually. (Redrawn after Chase RA. Atlas of Hand Surgery, vol. 1. Philadelphia: WB Saunders, 1973.)

ligaments take the form of an inverted "V" with its apex pointed distally. Dorsally, the extrinsic radiocarpal ligament complex is thinner and is primarily a condensation of capsular tissues, except for two stout structures, the dorsal intercarpal ligament joining the distal pole of the scaphoid and the triquetrum, and the dorsal radiocarpal ligament. According to work by Viegas, these two dorsal ligaments form a unique lateral "V" configuration that allows variation in length by changing the angle of the "V" while maintaining a stabilizing force on the scaphoid during wrist range of motion.[27]

The intrinsic ligaments are broad, stout structures that link one carpal bone to another, either within the proximal or distal row, or linking one carpal row to the other. The two most significant intrinsic ligaments are the scapholunate ligament and the lunotriquetral ligament. The scapholunate ligament anchors the scaphoid to the lunate to allow these two carpal bones to move in synchrony. Berger has subdivided this U-shaped structure into three regions: dorsal, proximal, and palmar.[28] The dorsal region is thick and controls scapholunate stability. The proximal portion, composed mainly of fibrocartilage, and the palmar region, with thin and obliquely oriented fibers, are less important for stability.[29] The

Biomechanical concept: joint motion

Brand and Hollister, in their textbook, *Clinical Mechanics of the Hand*, discuss how joints move.[30] An axis of rotation of a joint refers to a line fixed to the proximal bone about which the motion of the distal bone appears to be a pure rotation. For the simple (hinge type) interphalangeal joints of the fingers, the motion occurs only in flexion and extension; the axis of rotation is perpendicular to the sagittal plane and is located in the distal head of the phalanx proximal to the joint. A related concept is that of the degrees of freedom of a joint. The degrees of freedom of a joint are the minimum number of axes of rotation that can be used to describe completely the motion of the bone distal to the joint. The wrist as a whole, for example, has two degrees of freedom (flexion–extension and radial–ulnar deviation), represented by two nearly perpendicular axes of rotation.[31] The kinematics of more complex joints such as the thumb carpometacarpal joint[32] or the intercarpal joints[33] is still the subject of research and thought to have at least two degrees of freedom with nonintersecting, nonperpendicular axes of rotation.

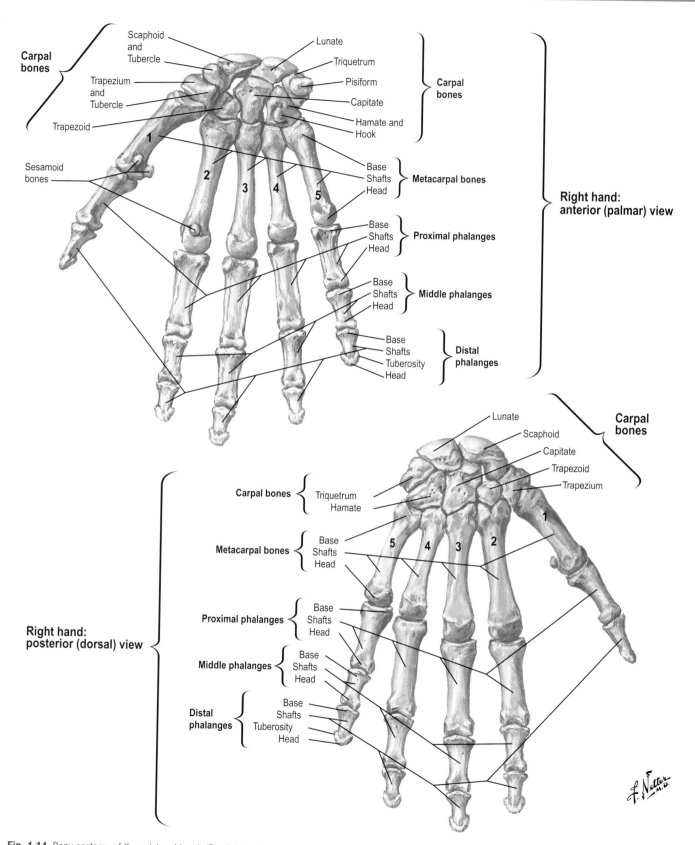

Fig. 1.14 Bony anatomy of the wrist and hand. (Reprinted with permission from www.netterimages.com © Elsevier Inc. All Rights Reserved.)

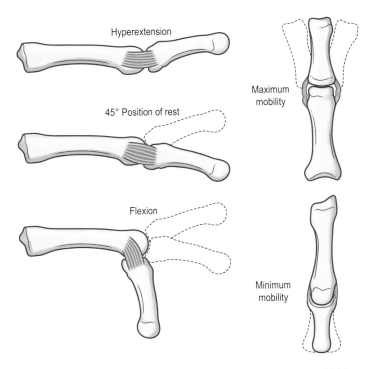

Fig. 1.15 **(A–D)** The true collateral ligaments of the metacarpophalangeal joint are loose in extension but tight in flexion of the joint as a result of the cam effect of the metacarpal head in relationship to the proximal phalanx. This accounts for the lack of lateral mobility of the joint when it is flexed. (Redrawn after Chase RA. Atlas of Hand Surgery, vol. 1. Philadelphia: WB Saunders, 1973.)

The proximal and distal interphalangeal joints are hinge joints: any lateral motion is limited in all phases of flexion and extension by radially oriented collateral ligaments, which are tight at any angle. The metacarpophalangeal joints, in contrast, allow motion through several axes. The capsule, including the collateral ligaments and volar plate, is quite lax, allowing medial and lateral deviation, flexion, extension, and thereby circumduction and a small degree of distraction. In the absence of other sources of stabilization, upon cutting of the collateral ligaments the metacarpophalangeal joint becomes a flail, unstable mechanism. Nature, fortunately, has created another source of lateral stability – the interosseous muscles. By virtue of the selective variable pull, the interossei normally influence lateral motion in the metacarpophalangeal joint to the extent allowed by the unyielding collateral ligaments. If the collateral ligaments are sacrificed, the interossei remain the sole source of lateral stability. When there is intrinsic (ulnar) paralysis, if the collateral ligaments are sacrificed, all lateral stability is lost and disastrous ulnar deviation occurs. At the interphalangeal joints lateral stability is again dependent on the collateral ligaments, but at this level there is no second line of defense. The collateral ligaments of the interphalangeal joints, therefore, cannot be sacrificed without creating a lateral instability that is curable only by fusion of the interphalangeal joints.

The volar plates of the metacarpophalangeal joints are the sites of insertion of the intermetacarpal ligaments, which limit separation or fanning of the metacarpal heads. The volar plate is fixed to that portion of the capsule that originates from the proximal phalanx, and therefore the plate moves with the proximal phalanx in flexion and extension. The volar plates

to the proximal and distal interphalangeal joints are also stout structures that may become scarred in cases of fracture/dislocation and may ultimately lead to joint flexion contractures *(Box 1.4)*.

The thumb

The thumb occupies the extreme radial position in the transverse arch of the hand.

The column of bones making up the thumb architectural base comprises the two phalanges, the metacarpal, and the trapezium. Its formula differs from that of the remaining digits by virtue of its two named phalanges rather than three. From a functional point of view, however, the thumb metacarpal can be compared to a proximal phalanx and the trapezium to a grossly foreshortened metacarpal. This suggests that the thumb is a digit recessed by a short metacarpal (the trapezium) with the proximal phalanx loosely syndactylized to the second metacarpal. There is no clear evidence to support this point of view phylogenetically, but it seems sensible in understanding the gross anatomy of the thumb's architecture. Like the finger metacarpophalangeal joints, the thumb's metacarpotrapezial joint has the greatest degree of freedom of any in the digital rays. The metacarpotrapezial joint is a synovial joint separated and distinct from the general intercarpal joints of the wrist. The trapezium itself articulates with the trapezoid and scaphoid with ligamentous restraints that sharply limit trapezial motion in relationship to the carpus *(Fig. 1.16)*.

The uniquely wide range of thumb motion as compared with that of the remaining digits is attributable largely to the joint between the base of the first metacarpal and the trapezium. In simplest terms, it is described as a biconcave double saddle joint with a permissively loose capsule. That combination allows movements best described as flexion, extension, adduction, and abduction through infinite combinations that result in circumduction. The thumb rotates as a cone with its apex at a point where the axes of flexion–extension and abduction-adduction cross within the carpometacarpal joint.[35–37]

The first carpometacarpal joint is best described as a double saddle where one saddle sits atop another, allowing three degrees of motion: (1) flexion-extension; (2) abduction-adduction; and (3) medial rotation-lateral rotation.[38] As the thumb rocks along the central ridge of the trapezial saddle in abduction and adduction, the metacarpal saddle's extensions over the trapezial saddle engage the trapezial saddle's medial or lateral condylar parts along the central axis. The axis line is curved in such a way that when the metacarpal is adducted, it locks into medial rotation, and when it is abducted, it locks into lateral rotation. This accounts for the sweep of the thumb

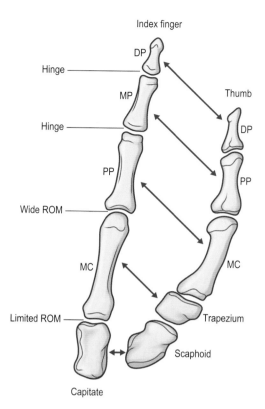

Fig. 1.16 The osteoarticular column of the thumb as compared with that of a finger. The trapezium in this comparison is the equivalent of a foreshortened metacarpal, and the metacarpotrapezial joint of the fingers. FDP, flexor digitorum profundus; FDS, flexor digitorum superficialis. (Redrawn after Chase RA. Anatomy of the thumb. In: Strickland J (ed.) The Thumb. Edinburgh: Churchill Livingstone, 1989.)

In the figure labels: Index finger; DP; Hinge; MP; Thumb; Hinge; DP; PP; PP; Wide ROM; MC; MC; Limited ROM; Trapezium; Scaphoid; Capitate

in adduction to abduction along the transverse arch of the metacarpal heads. This mandatory rotation into medial rotation on adduction helps to position the thumb for pulp-to-pulp opposition of the thumb to the fingers. In neutral position the axis of the trapezium, represented by its central ridge, sits at about 60° from a line through the heads of the central stable second and third metacarpals. The base of the first metacarpal has a quadrilateral articular surface that is a complementary match to the articular surface of the trapezium. Its concavity is slightly exaggerated on the ulnar volar side by a protrusion or "beak" for insertion of the important anterior oblique carpometacarpal ligament, commonly referred to as the "volar beak" ligament. As in some other joints in the body (e.g., the shoulder), stability and close coaptation of the joint surfaces between the trapezium and the first metacarpal are dependent on the presence of operational muscles and tendons. As noted above, there is a lot of slack in the joint capsule, allowing a wide range of motion, including joint distraction of up to 3 mm.[39]

An important stabilizing capsular ligament for the first carpometacarpal joint is the anterior oblique carpometacarpal ligament or volar beak ligament referred to above. It extends like the leg of a person seated in the trapezial saddle extending from the "beak" of the first metacarpal to the anterior crest of the trapezium and adjacent intercarpal ligaments. It retains the fragment of bone fractured free from the base of the metacarpal as the metacarpal displaces radially in Bennett's fracture. In advanced metacarpotrapezial joint arthritis it weakens

and attenuates, as also does the intermetacarpal ligament, allowing radial subluxation of the metacarpotrapezial joint.[40]

The ligament at the radial border of the joint is like a radial collateral ligament and is referred to as the dorsoradial or anteroexternal ligament. Thus, the radial side of the joint support is the right anteroexternal ligament, which inserts close to but beneath the insertion of the abductor pollicis longus on the radial base of the first metacarpal. It forms part of the joint capsule and then attaches to the anterior crest of the trapezium. Dorsally, one sees the posterior oblique ligament crossing the dorsal joint capsule from the radially positioned posteroexternal tubercle of the trapezium to attach to the ulnar base of the first metacarpal.

There is a stout intermetacarpal ligament between the base of the first metacarpal and the adjacent base of the second metacarpal, and good evidence that this ligament together with the anterior oblique ligament is a key to prevention of radial subluxation of the metacarpotrapezial joint, as seen in arthroses of the joint.[41] Function and range of motion within the limits imposed by these ligaments are influenced by the extrinsic and intrinsic muscles of the thumb and the external forces applied to the thumb. Bettinger and Berger have updated this ligamentous anatomy to include 16 different ligaments that are thought to stabilize the trapezium and trapeziometacarpal joint.[42]

The first metacarpophalangeal joint differs from other metacarpophalangeal joints in several respects in both anatomic make-up and function. Generally, the first metacarpophalangeal joint range of motion in flexion and extension, as well as abduction and adduction, is less than that in the finger metacarpophalangeal joints. The metacarpal and proximal phalanx are more stout in order to accommodate to greater forces normally borne by the thumb in pinching and grasping. The head of the first metacarpal is different because the radial articular prominence is larger than the ulnar. The articular surface of the proximal phalanx is fashioned reciprocally to match. The collateral ligaments are similar to those of finger metacarpophalangeal joints. The metacarpophalangeal portion is taut in flexion and looser in extension. In extension, the portion of the fanlike collateral ligaments to the palmar plate is taut; thus, adduction and abduction are limited in both extension and flexion.[43] Some pronation but no supination is allowed at the metacarpophalangeal joint when it is in extension. In supination, the joint locks into a stable position for secure grasping.

The sturdy fibrocartilaginous volar plate of the metacarpophalangeal joint extends from the palmar base of the proximal phalanx to the neck of the metacarpal. It regularly incorporates two sesamoid bones, one medial and one lateral to the flexor pollicis longus.

The nature of the condyle of the proximal phalanx of the interphalangeal joint to the thumb is such that, upon flexion of the joint, pronation of the distal phalanx occurs.

Muscles and tendons

Extrinsic extensors

Extensor muscles lie on the dorsum of the forearm and hand and are innervated by the radial nerve **(Figs 1.17–1.19)**. The

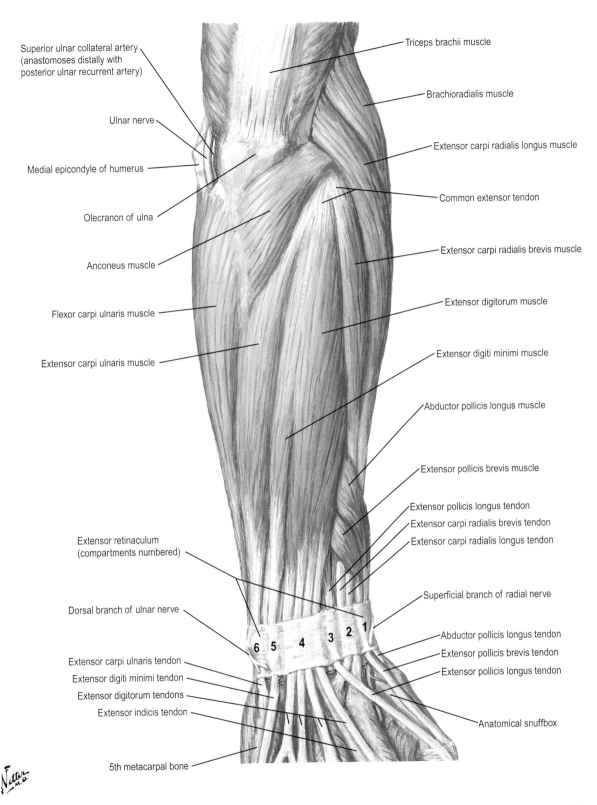

Superior ulnar collateral artery
(anastomoses distally with
posterior ulnar recurrent artery)

Ulnar nerve

Medial epicondyle of humerus

Olecranon of ulna

Anconeus muscle

Flexor carpi ulnaris muscle

Extensor carpi ulnaris muscle

Extensor retinaculum
(compartments numbered)

Dorsal branch of ulnar nerve

Extensor carpi ulnaris tendon
Extensor digiti minimi tendon
Extensor digitorum tendons
Extensor indicis tendon

5th metacarpal bone

Triceps brachii muscle

Brachioradialis muscle

Extensor carpi radialis longus muscle

Common extensor tendon

Extensor carpi radialis brevis muscle

Extensor digitorum muscle

Extensor digiti minimi muscle

Abductor pollicis longus muscle

Extensor pollicis brevis muscle

Extensor pollicis longus tendon
Extensor carpi radialis brevis tendon
Extensor carpi radialis longus tendon

Superficial branch of radial nerve

Abductor pollicis longus tendon
Extensor pollicis brevis tendon
Extensor pollicis longus tendon

Anatomical snuffbox

6 5   4   3   2 1

Fig 1.17 The anatomy of the extensor muscles: superficial to deep. (Reprinted with permission from www.netterimages.com © Elsevier Inc. All Rights Reserved.)

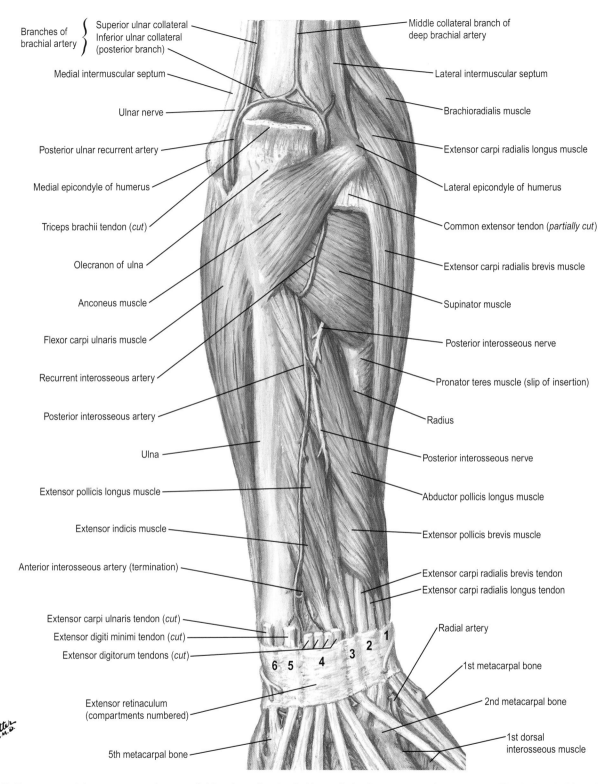

Branches of brachial artery
{ Superior ulnar collateral
Inferior ulnar collateral (posterior branch)

Medial intermuscular septum

Ulnar nerve

Posterior ulnar recurrent artery

Medial epicondyle of humerus

Triceps brachii tendon (*cut*)

Olecranon of ulna

Anconeus muscle

Flexor carpi ulnaris muscle

Recurrent interosseous artery

Posterior interosseous artery

Ulna

Extensor pollicis longus muscle

Extensor indicis muscle

Anterior interosseous artery (termination)

Extensor carpi ulnaris tendon (*cut*)

Extensor digiti minimi tendon (*cut*)

Extensor digitorum tendons (*cut*)

Extensor retinaculum (compartments numbered)

5th metacarpal bone

Middle collateral branch of deep brachial artery

Lateral intermuscular septum

Brachioradialis muscle

Extensor carpi radialis longus muscle

Lateral epicondyle of humerus

Common extensor tendon (*partially cut*)

Extensor carpi radialis brevis muscle

Supinator muscle

Posterior interosseous nerve

Pronator teres muscle (slip of insertion)

Radius

Posterior interosseous nerve

Abductor pollicis longus muscle

Extensor pollicis brevis muscle

Extensor carpi radialis brevis tendon

Extensor carpi radialis longus tendon

Radial artery

1st metacarpal bone

2nd metacarpal bone

1st dorsal interosseous muscle

Fig 1.18 The anatomy of the extensor muscles: superficial to deep. (Reprinted with permission from www.netterimages.com © Elsevier Inc. All Rights Reserved.)

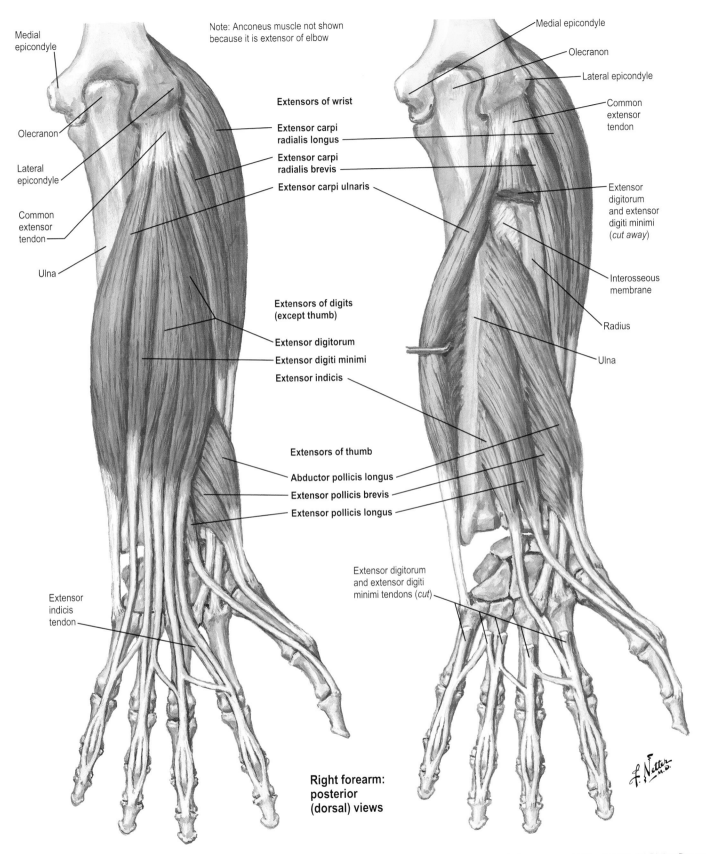

Note: Anconeus muscle not shown
because it is extensor of elbow

Medial epicondyle

Olecranon

Lateral epicondyle

Common extensor tendon

Ulna

Extensors of wrist

Extensor carpi radialis longus

Extensor carpi radialis brevis

Extensor carpi ulnaris

Extensors of digits (except thumb)

Extensor digitorum

Extensor digiti minimi

Extensor indicis

Extensors of thumb

Abductor pollicis longus

Extensor pollicis brevis

Extensor pollicis longus

Extensor indicis tendon

Medial epicondyle

Olecranon

Lateral epicondyle

Common extensor tendon

Extensor digitorum and extensor digiti minimi (*cut away*)

Interosseous membrane

Radius

Ulna

Extensor digitorum and extensor digiti minimi tendons (*cut*)

Right forearm: posterior (dorsal) views

Fig 1.19 (A, B) The anatomy of the extensor muscles: superficial to deep. (Reprinted with permission from www.netterimages.com © Elsevier Inc. All Rights Reserved.)

brachioradialis is a flexor of the elbow joint but is included with the extensor muscles because it is supplied by the radial nerve. The brachioradialis and the extensor carpi radialis longus originate from the lateral supracondylar ridge of the humerus. The four superficial extensors (extensor carpi radialis brevis, extensor digitorum communis, extensor digiti minimi, and extensor carpi ulnaris) originate from the common extensor tendon which is attached to the supracondylar ridge and the lateral epicondyle.

The extensors can be divided by function. The extensor carpi radialis longus and brevis and the extensor carpi ulnaris serve to extend the wrist. The extensor digitorum communis, extensor indicis proprius, and the extensor digiti minimi are finger extensors. Three extrinsic extensors assist in thumb motion: abductor pollicis longus, extensor pollicis brevis, and extensor pollicis longus.

Biomechanical concept: muscle structure

Muscles are composed of tissue that can actively contract under the influence of the brain and spinal cord to produce hand and finger motion and forces by pulling on bones via tendons.[44,45] Muscle tissue is composed of parallel arrangements of muscle fibers that can actively shorten and passively resist stretching, but cannot actively lengthen. The muscles of the hand anchor to bone at either end, typically by a short tendon at their origin (proximal end) and a long tendon at their insertion (distal end). Muscle fibers run along the length of the muscle attaching to tendon at either end. The aponeurosis is the transitional region where the contractile fibers of the muscle interdigitate with the collagen fibers that form the tendon. Tendons are stout parallel bundles of collagen fibers that often cross multiple joints of the hand before inserting into bone. Some tendons of the hand are atypical as they bifurcate or combine before inserting into bone to form the extensor mechanism (or extensor hood) of the fingers. The lumbrical muscle is atypical as it both originates from and inserts on to tendon (the flexor profundus tendon and the extensor mechanism, respectively) and has no direct bony attachment.

Striated muscle fibers are themselves parallel assemblies of similarly long cells with multiple nuclei containing sarcomeres, the fundamental contractile unit of muscle tissue. At the biochemical level, sarcomeres are interdigitated filaments of f-actin and myosin proteins. Muscle activation and contraction occur when a neural command causes the release of calcium ions inside the muscle cell to cause the free end of the myosin filaments to "ratchet" past the f-actin filaments to increase the overlap between them by metabolizing adenosine triphosphate, an important source of energy fueling cellular processes. The maximal force a muscle can produce is proportional to the number of parallel muscle fibers that compose it (physiological cross-sectional area), and the angle the fibers make with the line of action of the tendons (pennation angle). Mammalian muscle tissue is considered to produce a maximal stress of around 35 N/cm², which is a remarkable ratio of force per unit weight that is difficult to match artificially. In addition, the connective tissue that holds together the muscle fibers grants muscle tissue passive viscoelastic properties.

The extensor retinaculum prevents bowstringing of tendons across the wrist *(Fig. 1.20)*. Six extensor compartments exist: (1) abductor pollicis longus and extensor pollicis brevis; (2) extensor carpi radialis longus and extensor carpi radialis brevis; (3) extensor pollicis longus; (4) extensor digitorum communis and extensor indicis proprius; (5) extensor digiti minimi; and (6) extensor carpi ulnaris.

Extension of the phalanges of the fingers and thumb is dependent both on long extensors at the metacarpophalangeal joints and on an interplay between the long extensors and intrinsic muscles at the interphalangeal joints. The extensor digitorum is a series of tendons with a common muscle belly that enters into the central extensor of each of the fingers. There are intertendinous bridges between these separate tendons over the dorsum of the hand. Independent long extensor power is supplied to the index finger through the extensor indicis and to the little finger through the extensor digiti minimi. In each case the independent extensor lies on the ulnar side of the long extensor tendon to these two fingers from the extensor digitorum.

Biomechanical concept: the extensor mechanism of the fingers *(Fig. 1.21)*

The extensor hood of the fingers is an example of tendons bifurcating and recombining in an intricate network that results in complex muscle actions. For example, extensor muscles can flex the proximal interphalangeal joints, and intrinsic muscles can simultaneously flex the metacarpophalageal joint and extend the interphalangeal joints.[46] The effect of each muscle at each joint, however, may depend on finger posture and the distribution of tendon tension. Detailed cadaver studies have shown that, although the change in length of the different components of the extensor hood is relatively small,[47,48] their spatial orientation varies considerably from one finger configuration to another, and it has been suggested that the extensor mechanism may act as a floating net to amplify tendon forces[49,50] or to coordinate joint motion.[51,52] However, the anatomy of the insertion of the extrinsic and intrinsic muscles is quite complex and shows variations in the geometry of muscle bellies and insertion tendons.[53,54] Further work is necessary to understand fully the anatomy and function of the extensor hood.

Each of the three extrinsic muscles to the thumb on its extensor surface inserts on one of the thumb bones. The abductor pollicis longus inserts on the metacarpal where it primarily radially abducts the metacarpal, but since it bridges the wrist it secondarily radially deviates the wrist. The extensor pollicis brevis inserts on the proximal phalanx, so that it primarily acts as an extensor of the metacarpophalangeal joint but acts at the other joints with the abductor pollicis longus. The extensor pollicis longus inserts on the distal phalanx and is the primary extensor of the interphalangeal joint. It secondarily acts to extend and dorsally abduct the other two thumb joints.

Pronators and supinators

The pronator teres originates from the common flexor origin and inserts at the midportion of the radius *(Fig. 1.22)*. It is

Posterior (dorsal) view

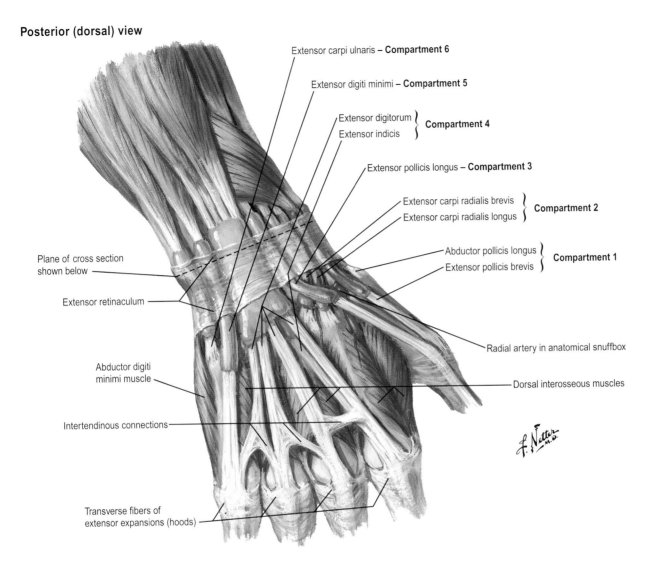

Extensor carpi ulnaris – **Compartment 6**

Extensor digiti minimi – **Compartment 5**

Extensor digitorum
Extensor indicis } **Compartment 4**

Extensor pollicis longus – **Compartment 3**

Extensor carpi radialis brevis
Extensor carpi radialis longus } **Compartment 2**

Abductor pollicis longus
Extensor pollicis brevis } **Compartment 1**

Plane of cross section shown below

Extensor retinaculum

Radial artery in anatomical snuffbox

Abductor digiti minimi muscle

Dorsal interosseous muscles

Intertendinous connections

Transverse fibers of extensor expansions (hoods)

Cross section of most distal portion of forearm

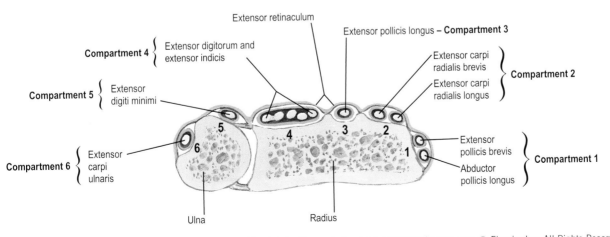

Extensor retinaculum

Extensor pollicis longus – **Compartment 3**

Compartment 4 { Extensor digitorum and extensor indicis

Extensor carpi radialis brevis
Extensor carpi radialis longus } **Compartment 2**

Compartment 5 { Extensor digiti minimi

Compartment 6 { Extensor carpi ulnaris

Extensor pollicis brevis
Abductor pollicis longus } **Compartment 1**

Ulna

Radius

Fig. 1.20 The extensor retinaculum and extensor compartments. (Reprinted with permission from www.netterimages.com © Elsevier Inc. All Rights Reserved.)

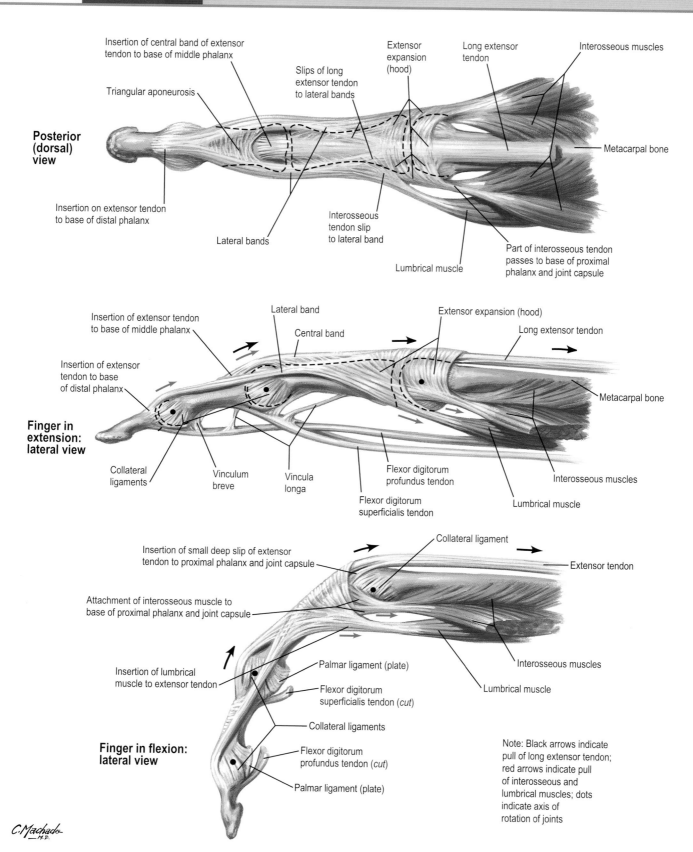

Posterior (dorsal) view

Insertion of central band of extensor tendon to base of middle phalanx

Triangular aponeurosis

Slips of long extensor tendon to lateral bands

Extensor expansion (hood)

Long extensor tendon

Interosseous muscles

Metacarpal bone

Insertion on extensor tendon to base of distal phalanx

Lateral bands

Interosseous tendon slip to lateral band

Lumbrical muscle

Part of interosseous tendon passes to base of proximal phalanx and joint capsule

Finger in extension: lateral view

Insertion of extensor tendon to base of middle phalanx

Insertion of extensor tendon to base of distal phalanx

Lateral band

Central band

Extensor expansion (hood)

Long extensor tendon

Metacarpal bone

Collateral ligaments

Vinculum breve

Vincula longa

Flexor digitorum profundus tendon

Flexor digitorum superficialis tendon

Interosseous muscles

Lumbrical muscle

Finger in flexion: lateral view

Insertion of small deep slip of extensor tendon to proximal phalanx and joint capsule

Attachment of interosseous muscle to base of proximal phalanx and joint capsule

Insertion of lumbrical muscle to extensor tendon

Palmar ligament (plate)

Flexor digitorum superficialis tendon (cut)

Collateral ligaments

Flexor digitorum profundus tendon (cut)

Palmar ligament (plate)

Collateral ligament

Extensor tendon

Interosseous muscles

Lumbrical muscle

Note: Black arrows indicate pull of long extensor tendon; red arrows indicate pull of interosseous and lumbrical muscles; dots indicate axis of rotation of joints

C. Machado M.D.

Fig. 1.21 The extensor mechanism of the fingers. (Reprinted with permission from www.netterimages.com © Elsevier Inc. All Rights Reserved.)

Right forearm: anterior view

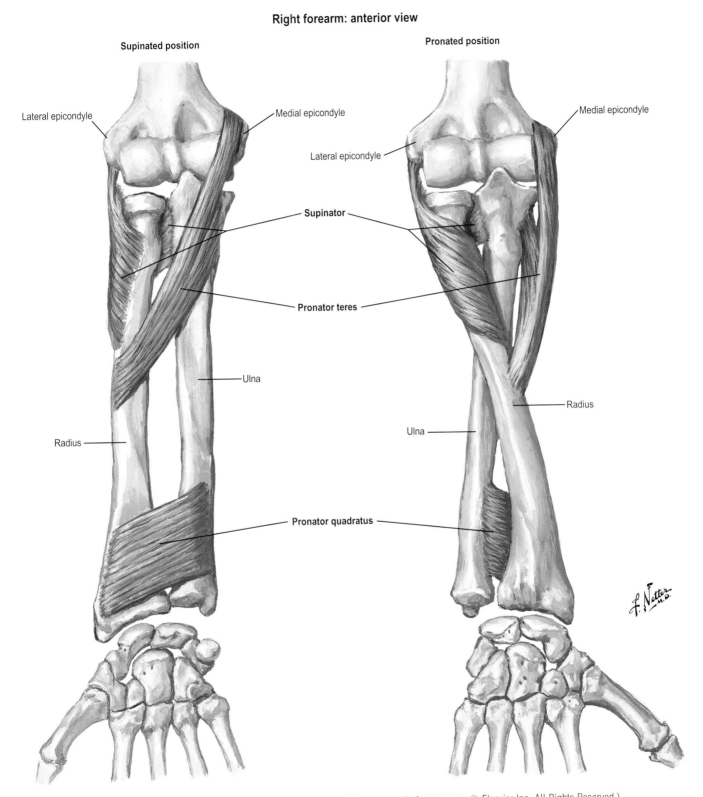

Supinated position

Pronated position

Lateral epicondyle

Medial epicondyle

Medial epicondyle

Lateral epicondyle

Supinator

Pronator teres

Ulna

Radius

Radius

Ulna

Radius

Pronator quadratus

Fig. 1.22 The forearm pronators and supinators. (Reprinted with permission from www.netterimages.com © Elsevier Inc. All Rights Reserved.)

innervated by the median nerve and is a primary forearm pronator and a weak forearm flexor. The pronator quadratus is a short wide muscle that spans transversely across the distal radius and ulna. It is also innervated by the median nerve and is a forearm pronator. The supinator originates from the lateral epicondyle of the humerus and inserts on the proximal third of the radius. It is innervated by the deep branch of the radial nerve and is a primary supinator, assisted by the biceps brachii.

Extrinsic flexors

Flexion of the phalanges into the palm is a complicated motion representing the sum of actions of the long flexors (profundus and superficialis) and long extensors (extensor digitorum, extensor digiti minimi, and extensor indicis), modified and enhanced by the intrinsic muscles (interossei and lumbricals) *(Figs 1.23–1.27)*. The long flexors to the fingers are responsible for flexion of the interphalangeal joints and are supplements to active flexion of the metacarpophalangeal joints and the wrist joint.[55]

Biomechanical concept: muscle force production

Muscles can produce force in different ways.[56] Concentric contractions occur when muscle fibers can shorten to induce tendon stretch, tendon excursion, and/or joint motion. Eccentric contractions occur when tendon forces overpower the passive and active force the muscle can produce and the muscle fibers lengthen during muscle activation. Isometric contractions occur when the muscle is not allowed to shorten (calling this state of the muscle a "contraction," when in reality it remains the same length, is a historical artifact). The structural and biochemical properties of the sarcomere make the exact magnitude of muscle force for a given level of neural excitation a function of length of the fibers, velocity at which fibers shorten or lengthen, and its previous activation history. The force–length relationship of muscle (sometimes called the Blix curve) indicates that there is an optimal length of the fiber at which maximal force can be produced, and drops at longer or shorter fiber lengths *(Fig. 1.28)*. Thus, the length at which the muscle is placed in reconstructive surgeries or tendon transfers can greatly influence the force the muscle can produce postoperatively. The force–velocity relationship of muscle indicates that muscle force drops greatly from its isometric level when muscle fibers shorten rapidly during concentric contractions, and rises to a plateau almost double its isometric level when muscle fibers lengthen rapidly during eccentric contractions *(Fig. 1.29)*.

The flexors are located on the volar side of the forearm and wrist and are innervated by the median nerve, except the flexor carpi ulnaris, and the flexor digitorum profundus to the ring and small fingers, which are innervated by the ulnar nerve *(Figs 1.23–1.27)*. The flexor carpi radialis, flexor carpi ulnaris, and palmaris longus provide wrist flexion. The digital flexors (flexor digitorum superficialis, flexor digitorum profundus, and flexor pollicis longus) pass through the carpal tunnel to provide dual flexion to the fingers and single flexion to the thumb.

Box 1.5 **Clinical pearl: independent and common flexor muscles**

The flexor profundi to the third, fourth, and fifth fingers work from a common muscle belly. Acting in unison, they fit the architectural concept of this unit as a stable vise for grasping objects. The independent function of the index profundus frees the index finger for use with the thumb to manipulate an object grasped by the viselike ulnar unit. Independence of action is well developed in the superficialis muscles and the intrinsic muscles.

The flexor digitorum superficialis tendon lies palmar (superficial) to the profundus tendon in the palm.[57] It flattens, then splits at the level of the proximal phalanx, and its two tails surround the profundus, decussating behind the profundus to insert on the middle phalanx. The flexor digitorum profundus perforates the flexor digitorum superficialis to run superficially along the length of the proximal and middle phalanges to insert at the base of the distal phalanx. These flexors contribute most of the force for digital flexion. The flexor digitorum profundus of the index finger is unique in that it has an independent muscle belly. The flexor pollicis longus inserts at the distal phalanx of the thumb *(Box 1.5)*.

In the finger and distal palm, the flexor tendons pass through a fitted fibrous flexor sheath that has thickened areas. The tendons at this level are surrounded by synovial sheaths. The flexor pollicis longus is the interphalangeal flexor of the thumb equivalent to the finger profundi. The flexor digitorum profundus is the only muscle that flexes the distal interphalangeal joint. Testing for profundus function requires observation of active flexion of the distal interphalangeal joint. Selected flexion of one or more of the metacarpophalangeal joints, or either the proximal or distal interphalangeal joint, depends on

Biomechanical concept: the shape of hand muscles

Many muscles of the hand depart from the simple fusiform (fish-like) shape seen in most textbooks. Many are flat, while others have multiple bellies. The interosseous muscles, for example, are bipennate. That is, a central common tendon is pulled on by fibers originating in different bones. The opposite arrangement is also found in muscles like the flexor superficialis of the fingers, which originate in a short belly that leads to a tendon that inserts in a second larger belly that then subdivides into four branches, each with a superficialis tendon to each finger. While it is possible to find muscle fibers that fire only when one finger is being flexed,[58,59] the degree to which force production in each belly is independent of the others is still unknown. Moreover, most extrinsic flexor and extensor muscles have tendons that are connected by thin strands of collagen at the level of the metacarpals that prevent independent motions of the fingers (try to extend the ring finger with all other fingers flexed). Other muscles such as the adductor pollicis have a fan-shaped origin where the resultant force at the insertion tendon depends on the distribution of force among muscle fibers. Whether or not muscle fibers fire in synchrony to produce a consistent resultant force, or if the fibers can be subdivided in functional regions to produce different resultant forces, is still unknown.

Text continued on page 28

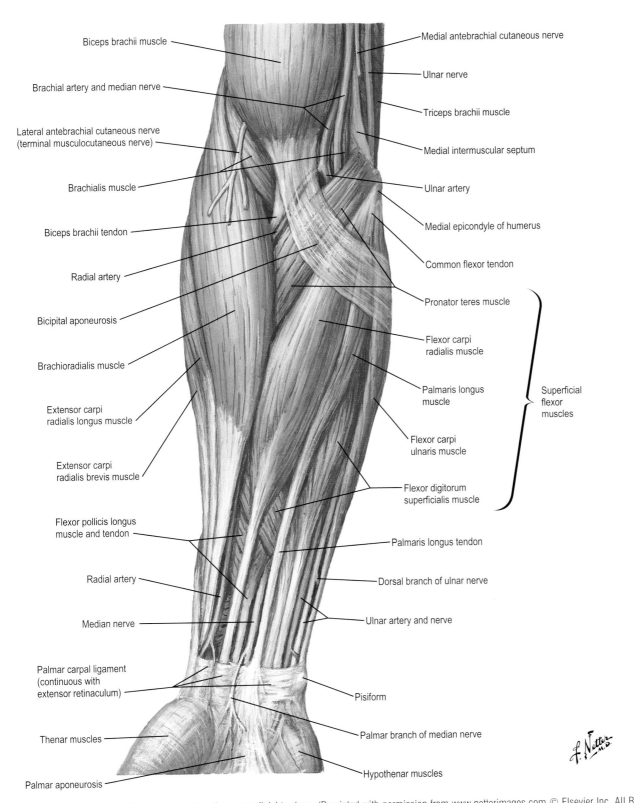

Biceps brachii muscle

Brachial artery and median nerve

Lateral antebrachial cutaneous nerve
(terminal musculocutaneous nerve)

Brachialis muscle

Biceps brachii tendon

Radial artery

Bicipital aponeurosis

Brachioradialis muscle

Extensor carpi
radialis longus muscle

Extensor carpi
radialis brevis muscle

Flexor pollicis longus
muscle and tendon

Radial artery

Median nerve

Palmar carpal ligament
(continuous with
extensor retinaculum)

Thenar muscles

Palmar aponeurosis

Medial antebrachial cutaneous nerve

Ulnar nerve

Triceps brachii muscle

Medial intermuscular septum

Ulnar artery

Medial epicondyle of humerus

Common flexor tendon

Pronator teres muscle

Flexor carpi
radialis muscle

Palmaris longus
muscle

Flexor carpi
ulnaris muscle

Flexor digitorum
superficialis muscle

Superficial
flexor
muscles

Palmaris longus tendon

Dorsal branch of ulnar nerve

Ulnar artery and nerve

Pisiform

Palmar branch of median nerve

Hypothenar muscles

Fig 1.23 The anatomy of the flexor muscles, from superficial to deep. (Reprinted with permission from www.netterimages.com © Elsevier Inc. All Rights Reserved.)

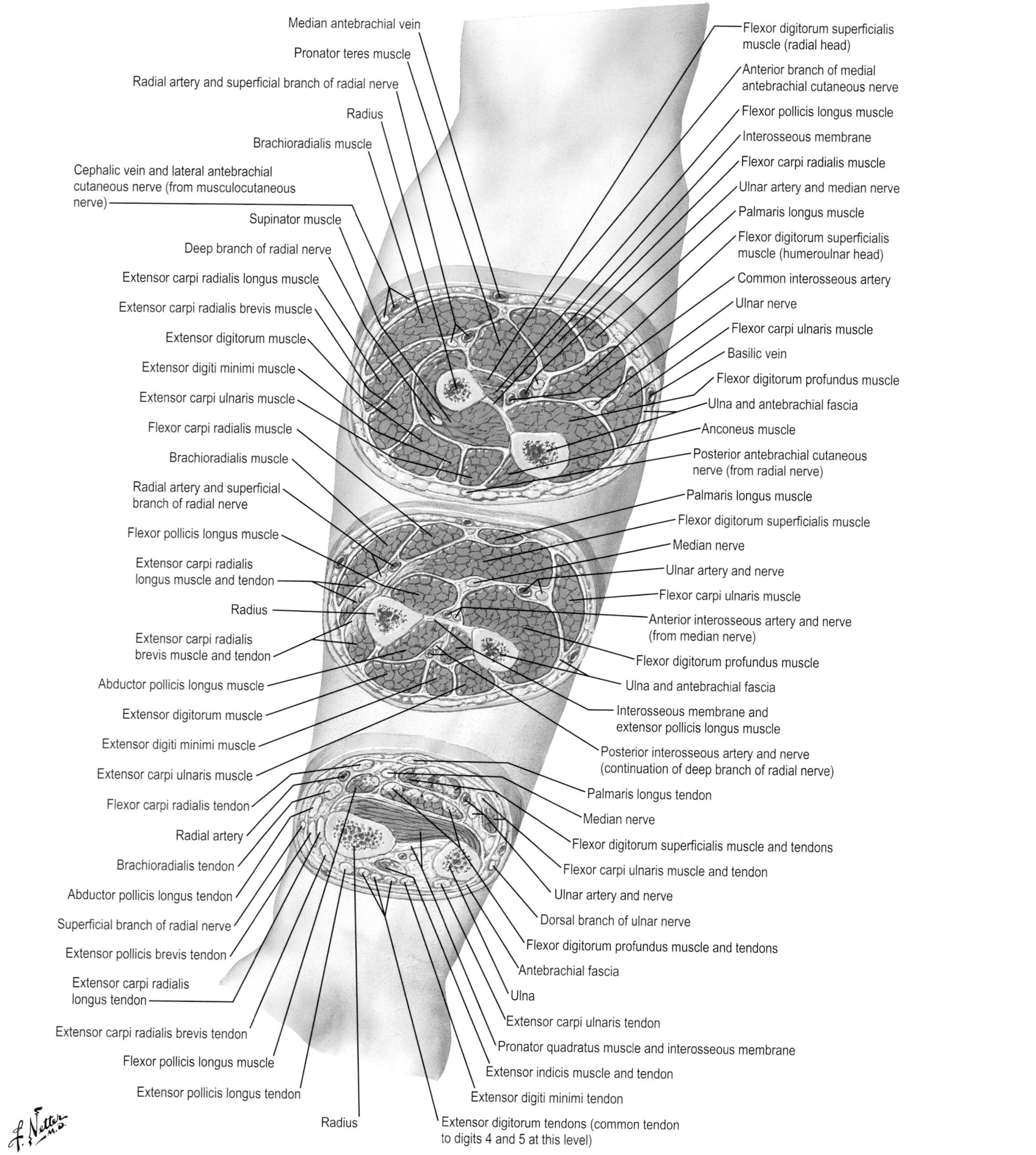

Median antebrachial vein

Pronator teres muscle

Radial artery and superficial branch of radial nerve

Radius

Brachioradialis muscle

Cephalic vein and lateral antebrachial cutaneous nerve (from musculocutaneous nerve)

Supinator muscle

Deep branch of radial nerve

Extensor carpi radialis longus muscle

Extensor carpi radialis brevis muscle

Extensor digitorum muscle

Extensor digiti minimi muscle

Extensor carpi ulnaris muscle

Flexor carpi radialis muscle

Brachioradialis muscle

Radial artery and superficial branch of radial nerve

Flexor pollicis longus muscle

Extensor carpi radialis longus muscle and tendon

Radius

Extensor carpi radialis brevis muscle and tendon

Abductor pollicis longus muscle

Extensor digitorum muscle

Extensor digiti minimi muscle

Extensor carpi ulnaris muscle

Flexor carpi radialis tendon

Radial artery

Brachioradialis tendon

Abductor pollicis longus tendon

Superficial branch of radial nerve

Extensor pollicis brevis tendon

Extensor carpi radialis longus tendon

Extensor carpi radialis brevis tendon

Flexor pollicis longus muscle

Extensor pollicis longus tendon

Radius

Flexor digitorum superficialis muscle (radial head)

Anterior branch of medial antebrachial cutaneous nerve

Flexor pollicis longus muscle

Interosseous membrane

Flexor carpi radialis muscle

Ulnar artery and median nerve

Palmaris longus muscle

Flexor digitorum superficialis muscle (humeroulnar head)

Common interosseous artery

Ulnar nerve

Flexor carpi ulnaris muscle

Basilic vein

Flexor digitorum profundus muscle

Ulna and antebrachial fascia

Anconeus muscle

Posterior antebrachial cutaneous nerve (from radial nerve)

Palmaris longus muscle

Flexor digitorum superficialis muscle

Median nerve

Ulnar artery and nerve

Flexor carpi ulnaris muscle

Anterior interosseous artery and nerve (from median nerve)

Flexor digitorum profundus muscle

Ulna and antebrachial fascia

Interosseous membrane and extensor pollicis longus muscle

Posterior interosseous artery and nerve (continuation of deep branch of radial nerve)

Palmaris longus tendon

Median nerve

Flexor digitorum superficialis muscle and tendons

Flexor carpi ulnaris muscle and tendon

Ulnar artery and nerve

Dorsal branch of ulnar nerve

Flexor digitorum profundus muscle and tendons

Antebrachial fascia

Ulna

Extensor carpi ulnaris tendon

Pronator quadratus muscle and interosseous membrane

Extensor indicis muscle and tendon

Extensor digiti minimi tendon

Extensor digitorum tendons (common tendon to digits 4 and 5 at this level)

Fig 1.24 The anatomy of the flexor muscles, from superficial to deep. (Reprinted with permission from www.netterimages.com © Elsevier Inc. All Rights Reserved.)

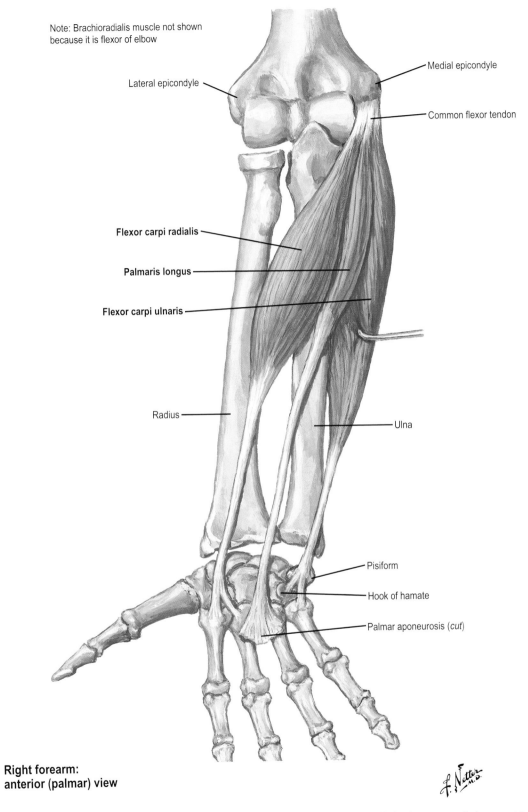

Note: Brachioradialis muscle not shown
because it is flexor of elbow

Medial epicondyle

Lateral epicondyle

Common flexor tendon

Flexor carpi radialis

Palmaris longus

Flexor carpi ulnaris

Radius

Ulna

Pisiform

Hook of hamate

Palmar aponeurosis (*cut*)

**Right forearm:
anterior (palmar) view**

Fig 1.25 The anatomy of the flexor muscles, from superficial to deep. (Reprinted with permission from www.netterimages.com © Elsevier Inc. All Rights Reserved.)

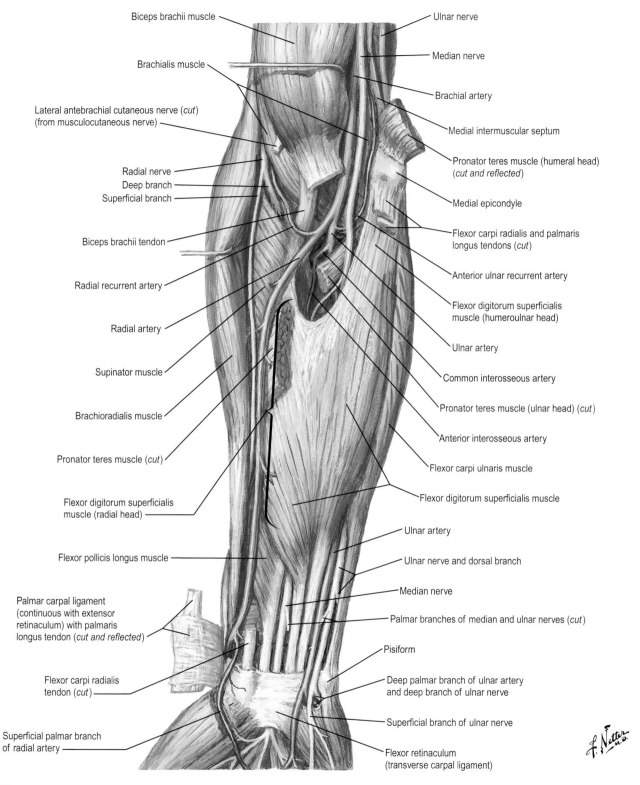

Biceps brachii muscle

Brachialis muscle

Lateral antebrachial cutaneous nerve (cut)
(from musculocutaneous nerve)

Radial nerve
Deep branch
Superficial branch

Biceps brachii tendon

Radial recurrent artery

Radial artery

Supinator muscle

Brachioradialis muscle

Pronator teres muscle (cut)

Flexor digitorum superficialis
muscle (radial head)

Flexor pollicis longus muscle

Palmar carpal ligament
(continuous with extensor
retinaculum) with palmaris
longus tendon (cut and reflected)

Flexor carpi radialis
tendon (cut)

Superficial palmar branch
of radial artery

Ulnar nerve

Median nerve

Brachial artery

Medial intermuscular septum

Pronator teres muscle (humeral head)
(cut and reflected)

Medial epicondyle

Flexor carpi radialis and palmaris
longus tendons (cut)

Anterior ulnar recurrent artery

Flexor digitorum superficialis
muscle (humeroulnar head)

Ulnar artery

Common interosseous artery

Pronator teres muscle (ulnar head) (cut)

Anterior interosseous artery

Flexor carpi ulnaris muscle

Flexor digitorum superficialis muscle

Ulnar artery

Ulnar nerve and dorsal branch

Median nerve

Palmar branches of median and ulnar nerves (cut)

Pisiform

Deep palmar branch of ulnar artery
and deep branch of ulnar nerve

Superficial branch of ulnar nerve

Flexor retinaculum
(transverse carpal ligament)

Fig 1.26 The anatomy of the flexor muscles, from superficial to deep. (Reprinted with permission from www.netterimages.com © Elsevier Inc. All Rights Reserved.)

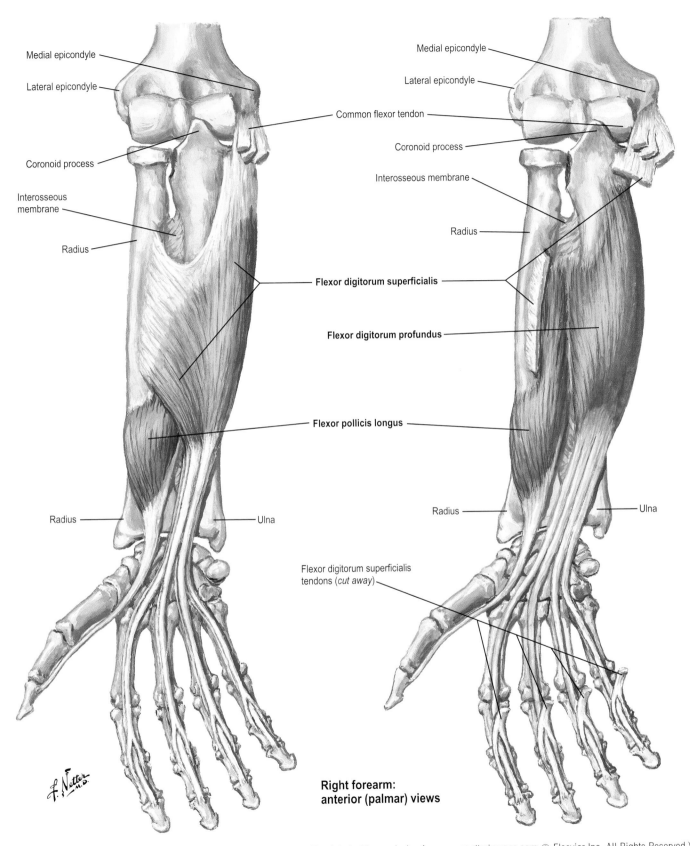

Fig 1.27 The anatomy of the flexor muscles, from superficial to deep. (Reprinted with permission from www.netterimages.com © Elsevier Inc. All Rights Reserved.)

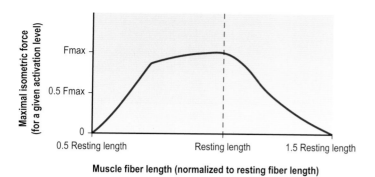

Fig. 1.28 The Blix curve. The maximal force is plotted on the vertical axis, and the muscle fiber length is plotted on the horizontal axis. There is an optimal length of the fiber at which maximal force can be produced, and this drops at longer or shorter fiber lengths.

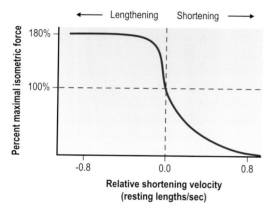

Fig. 1.29 The force–velocity curve. The percentage of maximal isometric force is plotted on the vertical axis, and the relative shortening velocity is plotted on the horizontal axis. Therefore, muscle force drops from its isometric level when muscle fibers shorten rapidly during concentric contractions and rises to a plateau almost double its isometric level when muscle fibers lengthen rapidly during eccentric contractions.

combined with either a contraction or fixation of the lateral bands, results in extension of the proximal interphalangeal joint. This effect is easily aborted by the intact flexor superficialis, whose prime flexion function is exerted on the proximal interphalangeal joint. Absence of the superficialis, whether occasioned by injury or by tendon graft replacement of the profundus only, results not infrequently in flexion of the distal interphalangeal joint with recurvatum deformity at the proximal interphalangeal joint. This can be corrected by fusion of the distal interphalangeal joint, making the profundus a functional superficialis, or by tenodesis or capsulodesis of the proximal interphalangeal joint in mild flexion. It is wise to keep in mind the innumerable functional circumstances that can be created by selective interplay of multiple motor forces exerted through a series of interdependent joints.[60]

Biomechanical concept: moment arms

The moment arm of a tendon about an axis of rotation of a joint is defined as the shortest distance between the axis of rotation and the tendon as it crosses the joint **(Fig. 1.30)**. This distance can vary with joint angle because of the suspension system of pulleys guiding flexor tendons, and/or the curved but not circular contour of the joint surfaces guiding extensor tendons.[60] The greater the moment arm, the greater the excursion of a tendon (and change in length of a muscle) that accompanies a given angle of rotation of the joint. Similarly, the moment of force (rotational action) of a tendon force about an axis of rotation increases with the magnitude of the moment arm of the tendon. These relationships between moment arm and tendon excursion/force assume hinge-type joints without sliding actions, which holds well for most finger joints. Note that a tendon that crosses a joint with multiple degrees of freedom (such as the thumb carpometacarpal joint) will have simultaneous and different actions about each axis of rotation.

stabilizing fixation of the remainder by flexor–extensor interplay. Elimination of any single motor element reduces the selective adaptability of a finger.

As noted above, a muscle may positively influence any joint between its site of origin and its insertion. The flexor digitorum profundus muscle originates in the forearm, and its tendon therefore bridges the wrist joint, the metacarpophalangeal joint, the proximal interphalangeal joint, and the distal interphalangeal joint before it inserts on the distal phalanx. It may flex any of these joints, depending on the dynamic fixation of the others. Fixation of the distal interphalangeal joint converts the profundus tendon into a functional superficialis tendon by recessing its prime site of action to the proximal interphalangeal joint. By combined fixation of any of the joints, the profundus tendon may primarily flex any selected one.

It is intriguing to realize that under certain conditions the flexor profundus may accentuate extension of the proximal interphalangeal joint. The profundus pulling primarily at the distal interphalangeal joint may flex it acutely. In flexing the distal interphalangeal joint, the insertion of the extensor mechanism is advanced distally. This advancement,

The gross anatomic configuration and function of the extrinsic digital flexor tendons have been known since antiquity. The great growth in our knowledge and understanding of functional biomechanics, muscle physiology, tendon nutrition, and blood supply has influenced the management of problems involving these important flexor tendons. The long flexor tendons cross multiple joints. The tendon-muscle unit has an effect on each joint it crosses, which is altered by the positioning of the other joints in the linkage system. Thus, the influence of the long flexor tendon on one joint in the system is augmented by the function of its antagonists at each of the other joints it crosses. For example, a digital flexor tendon aids in flexing the wrist, but its flexion capability within the digit at the metacarpophalangeal joints and interphalangeal joints is increased by wrist extension using wrist extensors, which in fact are antagonists to the digital flexors at the wrist. This is the simplified definition of synergistic function – finger flexion augmented by wrist extension, and vice versa.

Synergistic and antagonistic groups of muscles in hand function must be considered when functional substitution by tendon transfers is contemplated. Obviously, certain groups of muscles have developed functional synergism, which makes readjustment natural when one group is transferred to

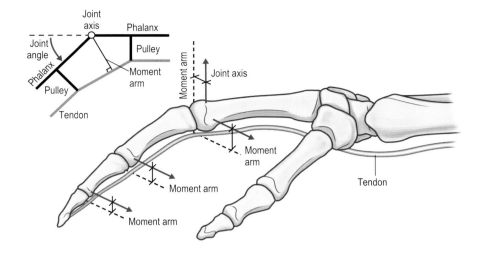

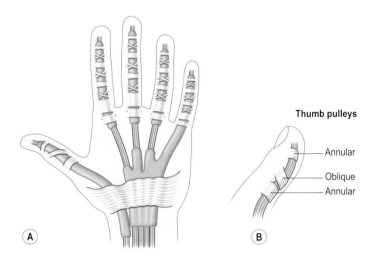

Fig. 1.30 The moment arm is defined as the shortest distance between the axis of rotation and the tendon as it crosses the joint.

take on the function of the other. Examples of such natural synergism are the united functions of the wrist flexors and digital flexors or the wrist extensors and digital flexors.

In its course from forearm to fingers, the digital profundus flexor crosses the palmar aspect of the wrist joint, the metacarpophalangeal joint, and the interphalangeal joints. The relationship of the tendon to the joint axes is maintained by retinacular structures, or pulleys. This prevents the bowstring effect, which would allow the tendon to move away from the joint axis, changing the moment arm and therefore the force exerted at that joint by the flexor tendon. The finely balanced relationship between the flexor muscle-tendon unit at each joint in the series may be disrupted by such a change. Such alterations can be compensated for, to some extent, by graded, proportional changes in the controlled power of antagonists, but the physiologic balance may be interfered with.

The retinacular system

The large, restraining pulley at the wrist, which serves all the long digital flexors, is the transverse carpal ligament *(Fig. 1.31)*. It bridges the volar surface of the carpals from the pisiform and hook of the hamate medially to the scaphoid tubercle and trapezium laterally. It confines the nine extrinsic flexor tendons and the median nerve within the carpal tunnel, and prevents bowstringing of the flexor tendons at the wrist.

Three pulleys housing the flexor pollicis longus within the thumb are regularly present. The proximal annular pulley is at the level of the metacarpophalangeal joint arising from the volar plate and base of the proximal phalanx. The distal annular pulley is located over the volar plate of the interphalangeal joint. Between the two is a single oblique pulley that originates proximally on the ulnar side of the middle phalanx, where it also gains fibers from the adductor pollicis before it extends to the middle one-third of the radial palmar surface of the middle phalanx. The oblique pulley must be preserved in order to prevent bowstringing of the flexor pollicis longus tendon.

Four or five discrete annular pulleys and three cruciate bands are ordinarily present in the fingers *(Fig. 1.32)*. The most proximal pulley (A1) begins 0.5 cm proximal to the

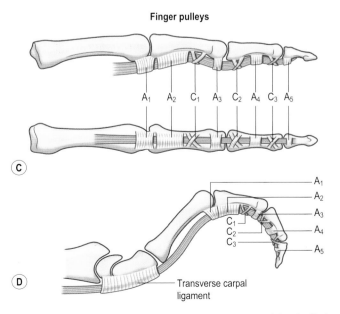

Fig. 1.31 (A–D) The flexor tendon pulley system for fingers and thumb. (Redrawn after Chase RA. Atlas of Hand Surgery, vol. II. Philadelphia: WB Saunders, 1984.)

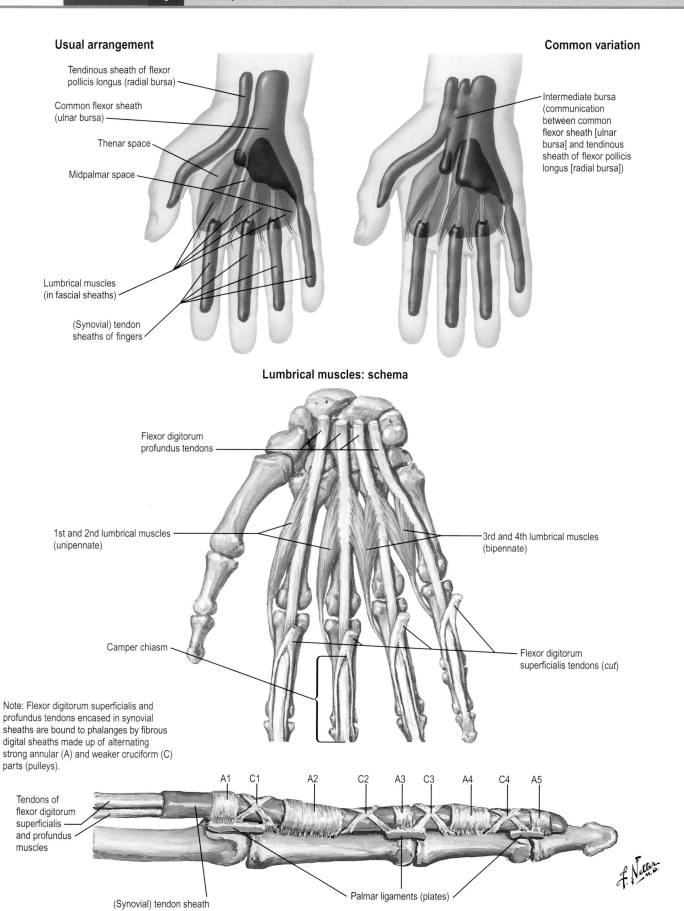

Usual arrangement

Tendinous sheath of flexor pollicis longus (radial bursa)

Common flexor sheath (ulnar bursa)

Thenar space

Midpalmar space

Lumbrical muscles (in fascial sheaths)

(Synovial) tendon sheaths of fingers

Common variation

Intermediate bursa (communication between common flexor sheath [ulnar bursa] and tendinous sheath of flexor pollicis longus [radial bursa])

Lumbrical muscles: schema

Flexor digitorum profundus tendons

1st and 2nd lumbrical muscles (unipennate)

3rd and 4th lumbrical muscles (bipennate)

Camper chiasm

Flexor digitorum superficialis tendons (*cut*)

Note: Flexor digitorum superficialis and profundus tendons encased in synovial sheaths are bound to phalanges by fibrous digital sheaths made up of alternating strong annular (A) and weaker cruciform (C) parts (pulleys).

A1   C1   A2   C2   A3   C3   A4   C4   A5

Tendons of flexor digitorum superficialis and profundus muscles

(Synovial) tendon sheath

Palmar ligaments (plates)

Fig. 1.32 Orientation of the flexor tendon sheaths, flexor tendons, and pulleys. (Reprinted with permission from www.netterimages.com © Elsevier Inc. All Rights Reserved.)

metacarpophalangeal joint. It is anchored to the volar plate and the proximal phalanx. Just distal to it is the second annular band (A2), which is the largest pulley, extending to nearly the proximal one-half of the proximal phalanx. The first cruciform band (C1) lies distal to A2 and well proximal to the proximal interphalangeal joint. The third annular pulley (A3) lies over the proximal interphalangeal joint arising from its volar plate. The second cruciate ligament (C2) is at the base of the middle phalanx. The fourth annular pulley (A4) lies over the middle one-third of the middle phalanx, and just distal to it is the third cruciate (C3). Often it is possible to identify thickening of the sheath over the distal interphalangeal joint, which, when present, is designated the fifth annular pulley (A5).

The pulleys are strategically placed to maintain the relationship of the flexor tendons to the axis of each finger joint, thus preventing the bowstring effect. The A2 and A4 pulleys are crucial to prevent bowstringing. The gaps between pulleys allow unrestrained flexion and extension of the joints by folding and pleating of the thin sheath between pulleys.

The synovial sheaths are closed sacs around the tendons composed of a visceral layer on the tendon surface and a parietal layer on the fibrous sheath surface. The thumb synovial sheath is continuous from the wrist to the distal extreme of the flexor pollicis longus. The digital synovial sheaths for the index, long, and ring fingers usually start at the level of the distal palmar crease and extend to the distal interphalangeal joints. Often the little-finger sheath extends more proximally to communicate with a common sheath around the finger flexors and then across the wrist to the distal forearm, where tendons pass through the carpal tunnel.

During embryonic development, synovial sacs form where the flexor tendons are subject to restraint by retinacula. The tendon invaginates into the sac, creating a two-layered, closed synovial membrane around the tendon. The tendon carries its segmental nutrient vessels, and thus with invagination a mesentery-like mesotenon is formed. As time passes, and where the tendon has great excursion in relationship to adjacent bone, the mesentery refines itself to tiny, flexible bands, or vincula. At the sites of insertion, where differential motion between the bone and tendon is least, the mesenteric configuration persists, as it does for flexor tendons in the hand outside the confining tunnels. The vincula brevia form the residual mesotenon at the sites of insertion of the profundus and superficialis tendons on the phalanges. The vincula longa are the flexible, vessel-carrying bands to each tendon in the area where the complete mesotenon has disappeared *(Fig. 1.33)*.

Because the cell population of tendons is sparse, metabolic demand is low and cells can survive with minimal nutritional support. The longitudinal blood supply to a tendon comes from its musculotendinous junction and its insertion site into bone. The segmental blood supply derives from the mesotenon where a mesotenon exists and from the vincula within the digital sheaths. It is now clear that synovial fluid within the sheath supplies nutrition to the tendon much as synovial fluid in a joint supports cartilage. This fact has altered thinking about the necessity for adhesion formation to ensure cell survival within a lacerated tendon stripped of blood supply or within tendon grafts.

On the basis of the anatomy of the flexor tendons and the associated synovial and fibrous sheaths, the area traversed by the tendons is divided into clinically important zones *(Fig. 1.34)*.

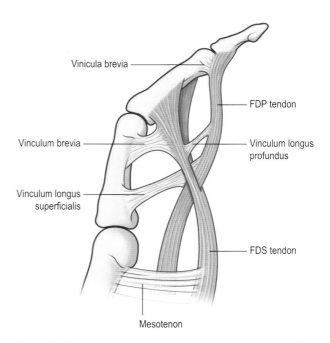

Fig. 1.33 The common configuration of the vincula. (Redrawn after Chase RA. Atlas of Hand Surgery, vol. II. Philadelphia: WB Saunders, 1984.)

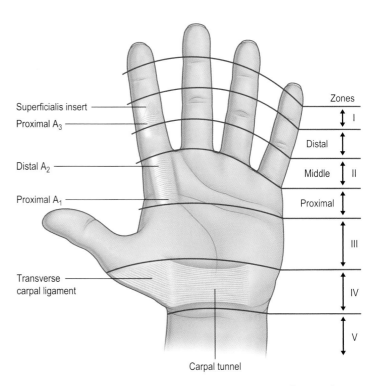

Fig. 1.34 Flexor tendon zones are classified for their relevance to flexor tendon injuries. (Redrawn after Chase RA. Atlas of Hand Surgery, vol. II. Philadelphia: WB Saunders, 1984.)

- Zone 1 is the area traversed by the flexor digitorum profundus distal to the insertion of the flexor digitorum superficialis on the middle phalanx.
- Zone 2 extends from the proximal end of zone 1 to the proximal end of the digital fibrous sheath.

- Zone 3 is the area traversed by the flexor tendons in the palm and is free of fibrous pulleys. It extends, therefore, from the proximal end of the finger pulley system (Al) to the distal end of the wrist retinaculum, the transverse carpal ligament.
- Zone 4 is the carpal tunnel. It extends from the distal to the proximal borders of the transverse carpal ligament.
- Zone 5 extends from the proximal border of the transverse carpal ligament to the musculotendinous junctions of the flexor tendon (*Box 1.6*).

A knowledge of the classical anatomy of the synovial sheaths and potential anatomic spaces in the hand is essential for proper diagnosis and treatment of serious hand infections. The flexor tendons are shrouded in synovial sheaths, particularly where there is flexion mobility in the longitudinal arch of each ray and at the wrist. The synovial sheath of the flexor pollicis longus generally extends from the flexor insertion to a point proximal to the wrist flexor retinaculum. The same is true of the synovial sheath around the little-finger flexors, but as the little-finger sheath approaches the proximal palm just distal to the carpal tunnel, it expands to encompass the flexors of the ring, long, and index fingers. At this point it is referred to as the ulnar bursa. Each index, long, and ring finger has a flexor synovial sheath from the point of insertion of the profundus tendon to the level of the distal palmar crease in the palm. The deep space beneath the flexor tendons is divided into two compartments by the heavy vertical septum from the palmar fascia to the third metacarpal. Ulnar to the septum is the midpalmar space, and radial to it lies the thenar space. The thenar space straddles the adductor pollicis muscle like two legs extending between the adductor and deep flexors on the palmar side, and between the adductor and the first dorsal interosseous on the dorsal side. Infection starting in the digital synovial sheaths may extend proximally to the deep palmar spaces.

Intrinsic muscles

Intrinsic muscles arise and insert within the hand (*Figs 1.35 and 1.36*). They can be divided into four groups. The thenar muscles are a group of four muscles consisting of the abductor pollicis brevis, flexor pollicis brevis, opponens pollicis brevis, and the adductor pollicis brevis. The abductor pollicis brevis, opponens pollicis brevis, and superficial head of flexor pollicis brevis are median-innervated whereas the adductor pollicis brevis and the deep head of the flexor pollicis brevis are ulnar-innervated.

The hypothenar muscles are all innervated by the ulnar nerve. These four muscles include the palmaris brevis, abductor digiti minimi, flexor digiti minimi brevis, and opponens digiti minimi.

Lumbricals originate from flexor digitorum profundus tendons and insert on the radial aspect of the extensor mechanisms, distal to the metacarpophalangeal joint. They contribute to the flexion of metacarpophalangeal joints and the extension of the interphalangeal joints. The index and middle-finger lumbricals are innervated by the median nerve, whereas the ring and small-finger lumbricals are innervated by the ulnar nerve. The tiny lumbrical muscles harmonize function between the lateral band interphalangeal extensor mechanism and the flexor digitorum profundus. They have a moving site of origin from the profundus tendon. As the flexor profundus contracts, the lumbrical origin moves proximally. At the same time, the lumbrical insertion moves distally as the extensor is advanced by interphalangeal flexion. The separation of its insertion and origin makes the lumbrical more effective in flexing the metacarpophalangeal joint. Conversely, with a change in balance of power, the lumbrical tends to pull the profundus distally as it shortens the lateral bands. This combination of profundus relaxation and lateral band pull results in extension at the interphalangeal joints.

All interossei are ulnar-innervated. There are three volar muscles and four dorsal muscles. The interossei originate from the metacarpals and form the lateral bands with the lumbricals. The interosseous muscles function as ulnar and radial deviators of the fingers as well as flexors of the metacarpophalangeal joints and extensors of the interphalangeal joints. The dorsal interossei act as abductors from the axis of the hand, which falls in the middle of the long finger. The long finger moves both radially and ulnarly under the influence of the second and third dorsal interossei. The abductor digiti minimi is the dorsal interosseous equivalent of the little finger. The palmar interossei adduct the fingers to the hand axis.

The pull of all the interossei palmar to the axis of the metacarpophalangeal joints and dorsal to the interphalangeal joint axis acts to flex the metacarpophalangeal joints and extend the interphalangeal joints. The position assumed is called the "intrinsic plus" posture (*Fig. 1.37 and Box 1.7*).

With the hand axis or fixed unit in position, the metacarpal arch is adjusted primarily by the thenar and the hypothenar muscle groups. The median nerve generally innervates all the thenar muscles on the radial side of the flexor pollicis longus. These two and one-half muscles (the abductor pollicis brevis, opponens pollicis, and superficial head of the flexor pollicis brevis) are positioning muscles that act to bring the first metacarpal into palmar abduction, thus increasing the concavity of the transverse metacarpal arch. This in turn prepares the thumb for proper pulp-to-pulp opposition with the fingers.

The thumb is steadied in position by contraction of the antagonist muscles to the abductors and the thumb adductor. Both the adductors and the abductors support flexion of the metacarpophalangeal joint to prevent recurvatum at this joint

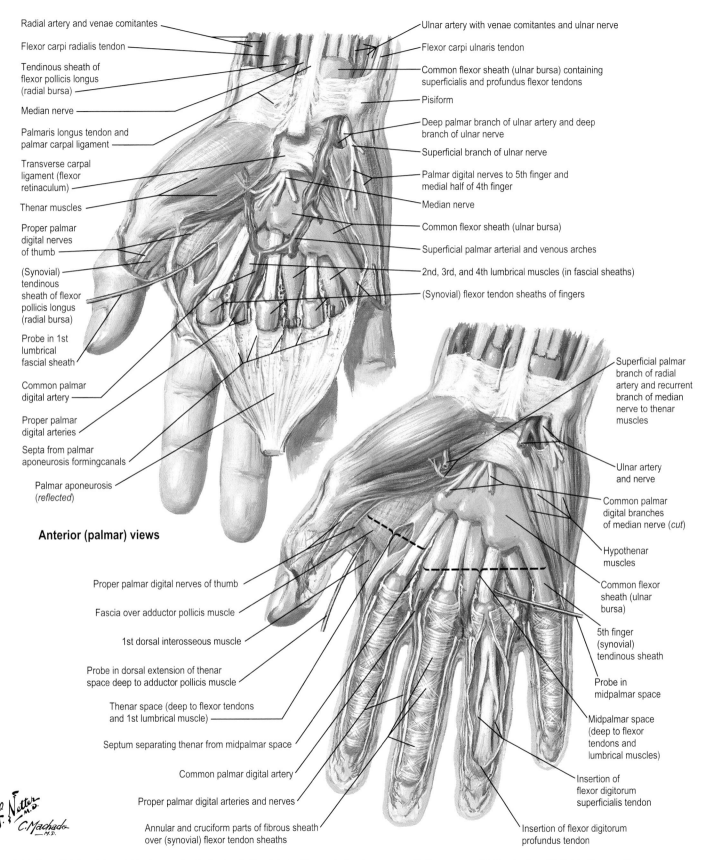

Radial artery and venae comitantes

Flexor carpi radialis tendon

Tendinous sheath of flexor pollicis longus (radial bursa)

Median nerve

Palmaris longus tendon and palmar carpal ligament

Transverse carpal ligament (flexor retinaculum)

Thenar muscles

Proper palmar digital nerves of thumb

(Synovial) tendinous sheath of flexor pollicis longus (radial bursa)

Probe in 1st lumbrical fascial sheath

Common palmar digital artery

Proper palmar digital arteries

Septa from palmar aponeurosis formingcanals

Palmar aponeurosis (*reflected*)

Ulnar artery with venae comitantes and ulnar nerve

Flexor carpi ulnaris tendon

Common flexor sheath (ulnar bursa) containing superficialis and profundus flexor tendons

Pisiform

Deep palmar branch of ulnar artery and deep branch of ulnar nerve

Superficial branch of ulnar nerve

Palmar digital nerves to 5th finger and medial half of 4th finger

Median nerve

Common flexor sheath (ulnar bursa)

Superficial palmar arterial and venous arches

2nd, 3rd, and 4th lumbrical muscles (in fascial sheaths)

(Synovial) flexor tendon sheaths of fingers

Anterior (palmar) views

Proper palmar digital nerves of thumb

Fascia over adductor pollicis muscle

1st dorsal interosseous muscle

Probe in dorsal extension of thenar space deep to adductor pollicis muscle

Thenar space (deep to flexor tendons and 1st lumbrical muscle)

Septum separating thenar from midpalmar space

Common palmar digital artery

Proper palmar digital arteries and nerves

Annular and cruciform parts of fibrous sheath over (synovial) flexor tendon sheaths

Superficial palmar branch of radial artery and recurrent branch of median nerve to thenar muscles

Ulnar artery and nerve

Common palmar digital branches of median nerve (*cut*)

Hypothenar muscles

Common flexor sheath (ulnar bursa)

5th finger (synovial) tendinous sheath

Probe in midpalmar space

Midpalmar space (deep to flexor tendons and lumbrical muscles)

Insertion of flexor digitorum superficialis tendon

Insertion of flexor digitorum profundus tendon

Fig. 1.35 Superficial and deep intrinsic muscles in the hand. (Reprinted with permission from www.netterimages.com © Elsevier Inc. All Rights Reserved.)

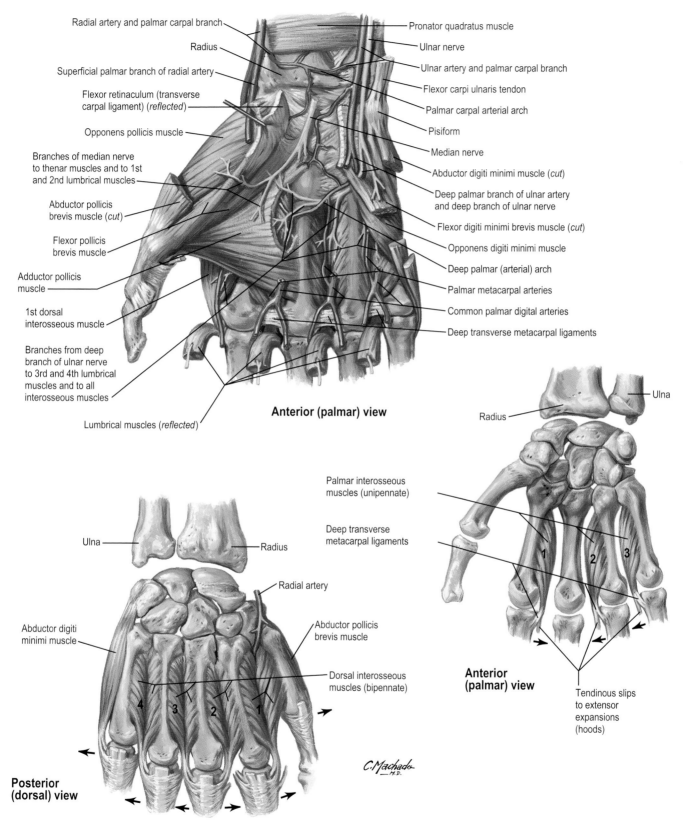

Radial artery and palmar carpal branch

Radius

Superficial palmar branch of radial artery

Flexor retinaculum (transverse carpal ligament) (*reflected*)

Opponens pollicis muscle

Branches of median nerve to thenar muscles and to 1st and 2nd lumbrical muscles

Abductor pollicis brevis muscle (*cut*)

Flexor pollicis brevis muscle

Adductor pollicis muscle

1st dorsal interosseous muscle

Branches from deep branch of ulnar nerve to 3rd and 4th lumbrical muscles and to all interosseous muscles

Lumbrical muscles (*reflected*)

Pronator quadratus muscle

Ulnar nerve

Ulnar artery and palmar carpal branch

Flexor carpi ulnaris tendon

Palmar carpal arterial arch

Pisiform

Median nerve

Abductor digiti minimi muscle (*cut*)

Deep palmar branch of ulnar artery and deep branch of ulnar nerve

Flexor digiti minimi brevis muscle (*cut*)

Opponens digiti minimi muscle

Deep palmar (arterial) arch

Palmar metacarpal arteries

Common palmar digital arteries

Deep transverse metacarpal ligaments

Anterior (palmar) view

Ulna

Radius

Abductor digiti minimi muscle

Radial artery

Abductor pollicis brevis muscle

Dorsal interosseous muscles (bipennate)

4   3   2   1

Posterior (dorsal) view

Palmar interosseous muscles (unipennate)

Deep transverse metacarpal ligaments

1   2   3

Ulna

Radius

Anterior (palmar) view

Tendinous slips to extensor expansions (hoods)

C. Machado M.D.

Note: Arrows indicate action of muscles.

Fig. 1.36 Superficial and deep intrinsic muscles in the hand. (Reprinted with permission from www.netterimages.com © Elsevier Inc. All Rights Reserved.)

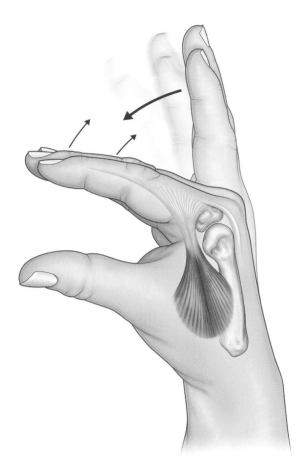

Fig. 1.37 All interossei act as prime flexors of the metacarpophalangeal joints since they pass palmar to the joint axis. Extensions into the lateral bands result in extension of the interphalangeal joints. (Redrawn after Chase RA. Atlas of Hand Surgery, vol. 1. Philadelphia: WB Saunders, 1973.)

Box 1.7 **Clincal pearl: examination of intrinsic muscles**

Examination of the hand for finger intrinsic function requires little more than an understanding of the anatomy described above and its related function. Function of the interossei may be assessed by asking the patient to adduct and abduct the fingers from the hand axis in the middle of the long finger. The ability to flex the metacarpophalangeal joints with the interphalangeal joints extended ("intrinsic plus" posture) confirms interosseous function. Paralysis is reflected by clawing of the fingers with hyperextension of the metacarpophalangeal joints and flexion of the interphalangeal joints on attempts actively to extend the fingers ("intrinsic minus").

Lumbrical function is best refle cted by having the patient fully flex the finger (extrinsic flexor function), then move the finger smoothly into extension at the interphalangeal joints while holding active flexion at the metacarpophalangeal joint.

Tightness or contracture of the interossei results in inability actively or passively to flex the interphalangeal joints while the metacarpophalangeal joint is extended. Inability to flex the interphalangeal joints may be a result of fixation of the extrinsic extensor tendons proximal to the metacarpophalangeal joint. Testing to differentiate these two possible etiologies is done by passively extending, then passively flexing, the metacarpophalangeal joint while assessing the degree of passive extension of the interphalangeal joints. If the interphalangeal joints passively extend when the metacarpophalangeal joint is extended, the interosseous muscle and tendon are short. If, by contrast, the interphalangeal joints extend when the metacarpophalangeal joint is passively flexed, the extrinsic extensor is adherent proximal to the metacarpophalangeal joint *(Fig. 1.38)*.

extension and dorsal abduction function, with resultant adduction contracture that becomes fixed after an extended period of unopposed adduction. The ulnar nerve innervates the hypothenar muscle group, which serves further to develop the concavity of the transverse metacarpal arch *(Box 1.8)*.

Blood supply

The vascular inflow to the upper arm and hand is a continuation of the axillary artery to the brachial artery. The brachial artery is palpable just medial to the biceps tendon at the level of the elbow. The brachial artery branches into the radial and ulnar arteries at the bicipital aponeurosis of the elbow *(Fig. 1.39)*. Supplementary arteries in the forearm include the anterior interosseous artery, the posterior interosseous artery, and the median artery.

The radial artery continues distally in the forearm between the brachioradialis and flexor carpi radialis muscles. At the wrist, the radial artery is located near the styloid process of the radius, and then travels dorsally, crossing the "anatomic snuffbox" deep to the tendons of the abductor pollicis longus, extensor pollicis brevis, and extensor pollicis longus. In the hand, it penetrates between the first and second metacarpal bones, through an arcade in the first dorsal interosseous muscle, to enter the palm and form the deep palmar arch. A superficial branch of the radial artery arises at the level of the distal radius before the artery enters the "snuffbox" and courses over or through the abductor pollicis brevis to contribute to the superficial palmar arch. This branch contributes blood supply to the skin over the thenar area and the underlying intrinsic muscles of the thumb.

on pinching, which may occur with paralysis of either or both (Froment's sign). With graded relaxation of the abductors, the adductor will dominate and pull the thumb against the side of the hand.

The carpometacarpal joint is a saddle joint with a lax capsule. This allows a wide range of circumduction motion and even a small degree of distraction of the joint on traction. Stability of the thumb root is heavily dependent on the muscles affecting it. The radial-innervated extensor pollicis longus and brevis and abductor pollicis longus secure the metacarpal dorsally. Opposing this to achieve stability are two groups of intrinsic muscles that, together with the extensor and dorsal abductor, triangulate the metacarpal. These two intrinsic groups are the median-innervated palmar abductors (the abductor pollicis brevis, opponens pollicis, and superficial head of the flexor pollicis brevis) and the ulnar-innervated adductors (the adductor pollicis, first dorsal interosseus, and deep head of the flexor pollicis brevis).

When there is paralysis of any of the three major motor nerves, thumb stability is compromised. In median nerve palsy, the positioning muscles of the thenar eminence are lost, resulting in inability to oppose the thumb for pulp-to-pulp opposition with other digits. Ulnar nerve palsy results in adduction weakness and imbalance of the structures influencing the metacarpophalangeal joint. Radial nerve palsy destroys

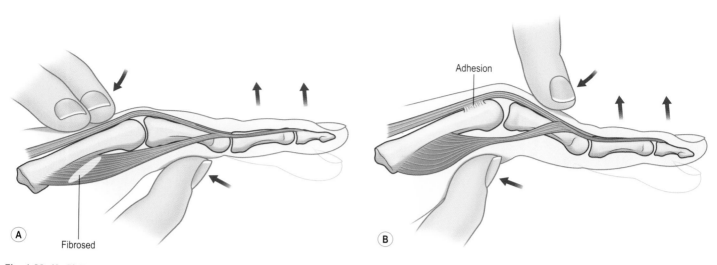

Fig. 1.38 (A, B) Testing for tightness or shortening of the interosseous muscles as a cause of passive extension contracture of the interphalangeal joint. The metacarpophalangeal joint is passively extended and the interphalangeal joints passively extend. If the cause of extensor tightness at the interphalangeal joint is a result of long extensor adhesions to the metacarpal, the interphalangeal joints will passively extend on passive flexion of the metacarpophalangeal joint. (Redrawn after Chase RA. Atlas of Hand Surgery, vol. II. Philadelphia: WB Saunders, 1984.)

Box 1.8 Clinical pearl: dynamics of hand function:

The central backbone of the hand is positioned in extension by the very important extensor carpi radialis brevis and longus. Flexion is effected by the flexor carpi radialis. All three muscles insert on the central two metacarpals (the second and third). These key motors are responsible for positioning the hand axis in preparation for operation of the adaptive hand elements around it. There are numerous other modifying motors to adjust the hand axis in the exact position desired, such as the flexor carpi ulnaris and extensor carpi ulnaris, which produce ulnar deviation. The fixed unit of the hand is extended from the radius at the radiocarpal joint. The entire complex is a beam attached to the ulna by the distal radioulnar joint, the interosseous membrane, and the proximal radioulnar articulation. Rotation around the fixed ulna in supination and pronation is largely under the influence of the median-innervated pronator teres and pronator quadratus and the radial-innervated supinator. The biceps and brachioradialis augment supination.

The ulnar artery is the other major branch of the brachial artery. Soon after the takeoff of the ulnar artery, the common interosseous artery originates and itself branches into the anterior and posterior interosseous arteries. The ulnar artery continues in the forearm under the flexor carpi ulnaris muscle. At the wrist, it lies radial to the pisiform and ulnar to the hook of the hamate and travels into the hand through Guyon's canal, deep to the palmaris brevis and the hypothenar fascia. Here it divides into a deep palmar branch and a superficial palmar branch. The superficial branch becomes the dominant contributor to the superficial palmar arch. The superficial arch crosses the palm at the level of the fully abducted thumb. The deep branch contributes to the deep palmar arch.

In general, the blood supply of the hand is conveniently divided into palmar vessels, which are subdivided into a superficial and a deep layer, and a single dorsal layer *(Fig. 1.40).*[61] For example, the superficial vascular arch and its branches constitute the superficial group, the deep arch and the palmar metacarpal branches make up the deep layer, and the dorsal arch with its dorsal metacarpal branches forms the dorsal distribution *(Box 1.9).*

The superficial palmar arch gives rise to three common digital arteries and multiple branches to intrinsic muscles and skin. The deep vascular arch lies at the proximal ends of the metacarpals deep to all the flexor tendons. It arises chiefly from the radial artery and becomes an arch by anastomosis with the deep branch of the ulnar artery. The deep arch is the major source of blood supply to the thumb and to the radial side of the index finger. This blood supply comes from the first of the four palmar metacarpal arteries. The first metacarpal artery is the prime source of blood supply to the radial and ulnar proper digital arteries of the thumb and the radial proper digital artery of the index finger. These digital arteries generally receive collateral branches from the superficial palmar arch as well. After giving its branch to the index finger, the first metacarpal artery becomes the primary source of blood supply to the thumb and is frequently called the princeps pollicis *(Box 1.10).*

The dorsal arteries originate proximally from the posterior interosseous artery and a dorsal perforating branch of the anterior interosseous artery. These arteries are joined by branches from the radial and ulnar arteries to form a dorsal carpal arch. Dorsal metacarpal arteries arise from this arch and extend distally to the margins of the fingers.[62–65] These dorsal arteries are joined by a varying number of vessels perforating from the deep palmar metacarpal arteries. In fact, the dominant supply to the dorsal metacarpal arteries may come from these perforators. Dorsal arteries to the thumb come from branches of the radial artery before it plunges through the first dorsal interosseous arcade. Thus, the dorsal arterial blood supply of the thumb is similar to that of the fingers *(Box 1.11).*

Veins generally follow the arterial pattern in the deep system as venae comitantes. An abundant superficial system of venous drainage also exists *(Fig. 1.41).* Ultimately, these superficial veins contribute to the cephalic and basilic veins

Anterior view

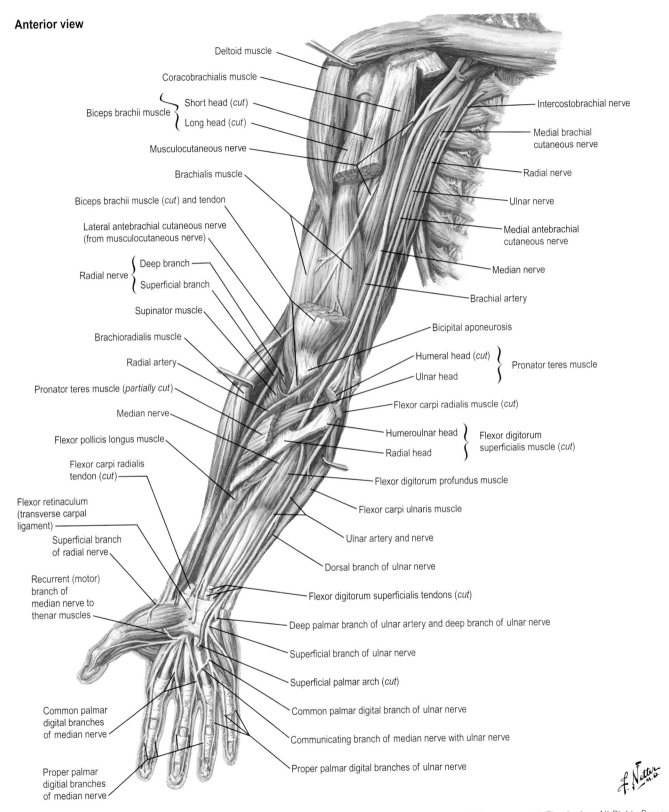

Deltoid muscle

Coracobrachialis muscle

Biceps brachii muscle { Short head (*cut*)
Long head (*cut*)

Musculocutaneous nerve

Brachialis muscle

Biceps brachii muscle (*cut*) and tendon

Lateral antebrachial cutaneous nerve
(from musculocutaneous nerve)

Radial nerve { Deep branch
Superficial branch

Supinator muscle

Brachioradialis muscle

Radial artery

Pronator teres muscle (*partially cut*)

Median nerve

Flexor pollicis longus muscle

Flexor carpi radialis
tendon (*cut*)

Flexor retinaculum
(transverse carpal
ligament)

Superficial branch
of radial nerve

Recurrent (motor)
branch of
median nerve to
thenar muscles

Common palmar
digital branches
of median nerve

Proper palmar
digitial branches
of median nerve

Intercostobrachial nerve

Medial brachial
cutaneous nerve

Radial nerve

Ulnar nerve

Medial antebrachial
cutaneous nerve

Median nerve

Brachial artery

Bicipital aponeurosis

Humeral head (*cut*) } Pronator teres muscle
Ulnar head

Flexor carpi radialis muscle (*cut*)

Humeroulnar head } Flexor digitorum
Radial head } superficialis muscle (*cut*)

Flexor digitorum profundus muscle

Flexor carpi ulnaris muscle

Ulnar artery and nerve

Dorsal branch of ulnar nerve

Flexor digitorum superficialis tendons (*cut*)

Deep palmar branch of ulnar artery and deep branch of ulnar nerve

Superficial branch of ulnar nerve

Superficial palmar arch (*cut*)

Common palmar digital branch of ulnar nerve

Communicating branch of median nerve with ulnar nerve

Proper palmar digital branches of ulnar nerve

Fig. 1.39 Upper arm vascular anatomy and surrounding structures. (Reprinted with permission from www.netterimages.com © Elsevier Inc. All Rights Reserved.)

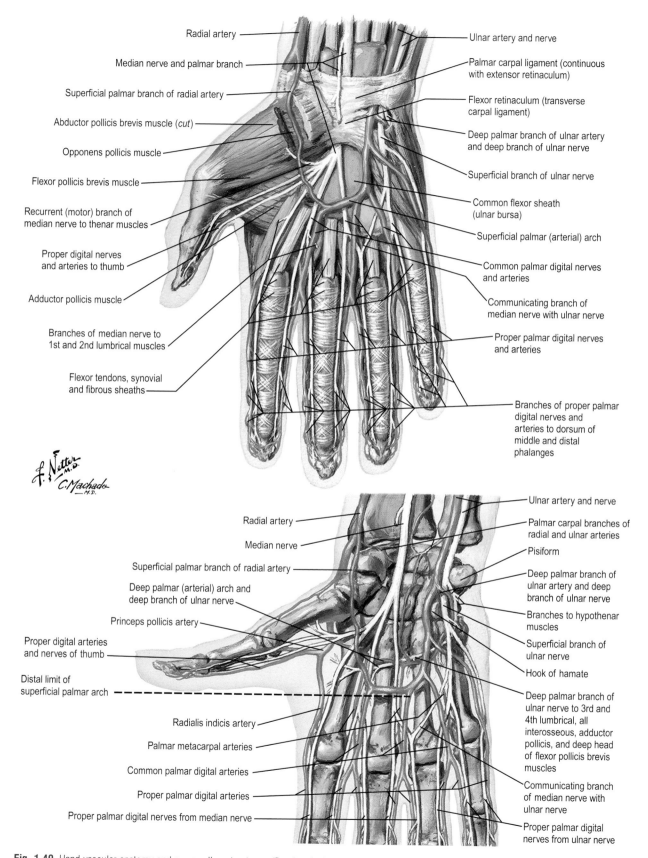

Fig. 1.40 Hand vascular anatomy and surrounding structures. (Reprinted with permission from www.netterimages.com © Elsevier Inc. All Rights Reserved.)

Anterior (palmar) view

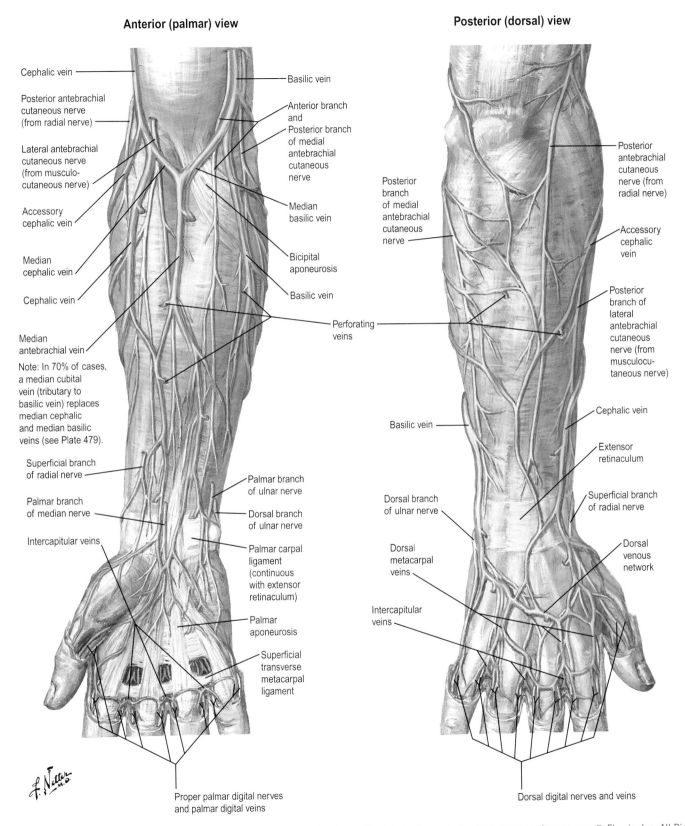

Cephalic vein

Posterior antebrachial cutaneous nerve (from radial nerve)

Lateral antebrachial cutaneous nerve (from musculo-cutaneous nerve)

Accessory cephalic vein

Median cephalic vein

Cephalic vein

Median antebrachial vein

Note: In 70% of cases, a median cubital vein (tributary to basilic vein) replaces median cephalic and median basilic veins (see Plate 479).

Superficial branch of radial nerve

Palmar branch of median nerve

Intercapitular veins

Basilic vein

Anterior branch and Posterior branch of medial antebrachial cutaneous nerve

Median basilic vein

Bicipital aponeurosis

Basilic vein

Perforating veins

Palmar branch of ulnar nerve

Dorsal branch of ulnar nerve

Palmar carpal ligament (continuous with extensor retinaculum)

Palmar aponeurosis

Superficial transverse metacarpal ligament

Proper palmar digital nerves and palmar digital veins

Posterior (dorsal) view

Posterior branch of medial antebrachial cutaneous nerve

Basilic vein

Dorsal branch of ulnar nerve

Dorsal metacarpal veins

Intercapitular veins

Posterior antebrachial cutaneous nerve (from radial nerve)

Accessory cephalic vein

Posterior branch of lateral antebrachial cutaneous nerve (from musculocutaneous nerve)

Cephalic vein

Extensor retinaculum

Superficial branch of radial nerve

Dorsal venous network

Dorsal digital nerves and veins

Fig. 1.41 The superficial and deep venous drainage system of the hand and arm. (Reprinted with permission from www.netterimages.com © Elsevier Inc. All Rights Reserved.)

Box 1.9 Clinical pearl: the Allen's test

This test may be used to assess the competence of the major arterial contributors to blood supply in the hand and the functional efficiency of the vascular arches in the hand. Palpate the radial and ulnar pulses at the wrist and prepare to compress these arteries. Have the patient make a very tight fist. Compress the arteries and ask the patient to extend the digits. The hand will be blanched white. Release pressure on one of the arteries and observe the return of a red flush on the hand. Normally, the flush is immediate and progresses across the whole hand without delay. This confirms the patency of the artery and the competence of circulatory collaterals through the vascular arches. The test may be performed to confirm the competence of each of the two major arteries before surgery or to check their competence after repair, thrombectomy, manipulation, or injury.

The Allen's test principle may be used in clinically assessing the competence of the two proper digital arteries in the fingers. It may be done by observing return of color after compression of both arteries and release of one to the digit. Compress one artery, then the other, and then both to note the individual proper artery contribution to cutaneous blood supply. The technique may be useful when one is planning an island pedicle flap from a donor finger whose digital artery may have been damaged by an injury proximal to the finger.

Box 1.10 Clinical pearl: the relative size of digital vessels

Although two digital arteries (radial and ulnar) usually perfuse each finger, there are differences in the diameter of the radial versus ulnar digital arteries.[62] In the thumb, the ulnar digital artery is usually much larger. The index finger is similarly ulnar-dominant whereas the small finger is radial-dominant. The arteries to the middle and ring fingers do not have appreciable size differences between radial and ulnar sides. This anatomic variation may be important in finding adequate vessels for microanastomosis during replantation or revascularization.

Box 1.11 Clinical pearl: dorsal metacarpal artery flaps

The dorsal arterial circulation of the hand is the source of multiple intrinsic hand flaps. The radial artery and the dorsal carpal arch give off the first and second metacarpal arteries which run in the intermetacarpal spaces between the thumb and index finger, and the index finger and middle finger respectively. The third metacarpal artery is much smaller and is less reliable for flap transfer. Although multiple uses and variations have been described, the simplest method to catalogue these flaps is by artery and by direction of flow. Therefore, both the first and second dorsal metacarpal arteries may be used in an anterograde or retrograde fashion.

The first dorsal metacarpal artery (FDMA) has been found to originate from the dorsal radial artery, just distal to the extensor pollicis longus tendon. In a series of 30 hand dissections, 90% of hands had superficial or fascial FDMAs, 40% of hands had a deep intramuscular branch, and 30% had both vessels present.[63] The external diameter averaged 1.0–1.5 mm at the largest part. This vessel can be used to harvest a pedicled island flap of skin from the dorsum of the index proximal phalanx innervated by a branch of the radial sensory nerve.[64] In the anterograde fashion, this flap may reach about the dorsum of the radial two-thirds of the hand, and even to a portion of the volar hand. The reach of the FDMA flap can be extended distally if designed in a retrograde fashion.[65]

The second dorsal metacarpal artery (SDMA) was found in 29 of 30 (97%) hands dissected. The origin of this vessel varied, including from the dorsal carpal arch, radial artery, FDMA, and the posterior interosseus artery. Once the SDMA reached the index finger extensor tendons, the vessel passed deep to the tendons and within the fascia of the second dorsal interosseous muscle. The SDMA branched and became superficial at the level of the metacarpophalangeal joints. The pedicle, being more central than the FDMA, can nearly reach the entire dorsum of the hand and can also be extended in a retrograde fashion, to reach the level of the proximal interphalangeal joints of the index and middle fingers.[66]

---

of the upper extremities. Lymphatic drainage terminates in the axillary, supraclavicular, and subclavicular nodes.

Peripheral nerves

The peripheral nerves to the upper extremity have anatomic relationships of great importance to the surgeon. For example, one needs to know the anatomic availability for nerve block and sites where nerves are subject to compression or injury. Sites of particular susceptibility to injury coincide quite accurately with the sites chosen for anesthesia.

With the ability to perform fascicular and group fascicular repair of nerves in addition to epineurial repair, it is important for surgeons to understand the generic internal structure of peripheral nerves. The epineurium is the tubular fibrous support structure surrounding the entire nerve; it also courses between the fascicles. Subdivisions consisting of multiple fascicles within the nerve are covered by epineurium. Each fascicle is covered by perineurium. Within each fascicle are separate axons, some myelinated and some unmyelinated. Motor, sensory, and sympathetic fibers are present within each peripheral nerve. Blood vessels are found on the epineurial surface and in the internal supporting structure of the nerve. The internal topography is plexus-like, as described in detail in the classic monograph by Sunderland.[66]

The radial nerve arises from the posterior cord of the brachial plexus (C6–8). As the nerve passes the distal humerus, muscular branches innervate the brachioradialis and extensor carpi radialis longus muscles (Fig. 1.42). The radial nerve divides into terminal deep and superficial branches at the proximal forearm (Fig. 1.43). The deep posterior interosseous nerve supplies the supinator as well as muscles in all the extensor compartments: extensor carpi radialis brevis, extensor digitorum communis, extensor digiti minimi, extensor carpi ulnaris, extensor indicis proprius, extensor pollicis longus, extensor pollicis brevis, and abductor pollicus longus muscles. Finally, the deep posterior interosseous nerve terminates to supply carpal joint sensation.

The dorsal or superficial branch of the radial nerve courses through the forearm in relationship to the brachioradialis muscle on the radial side of the arm. The nerve crosses the "anatomic snuffbox" between the extensor pollicis brevis and the extensor pollicis longus in the loose subcutaneous tissue. It divides into multiple branches, which give sensibility to the dorsum of the hand over the radial two-thirds, the dorsum of the thumb, and the index, long, and half of the ring finger proximal to the distal interphalangeal joint.

The median nerve arises from the lateral and medial cords of brachial plexus (C5–T1) (Fig. 1.44). In the forearm,

Text continued on page 44

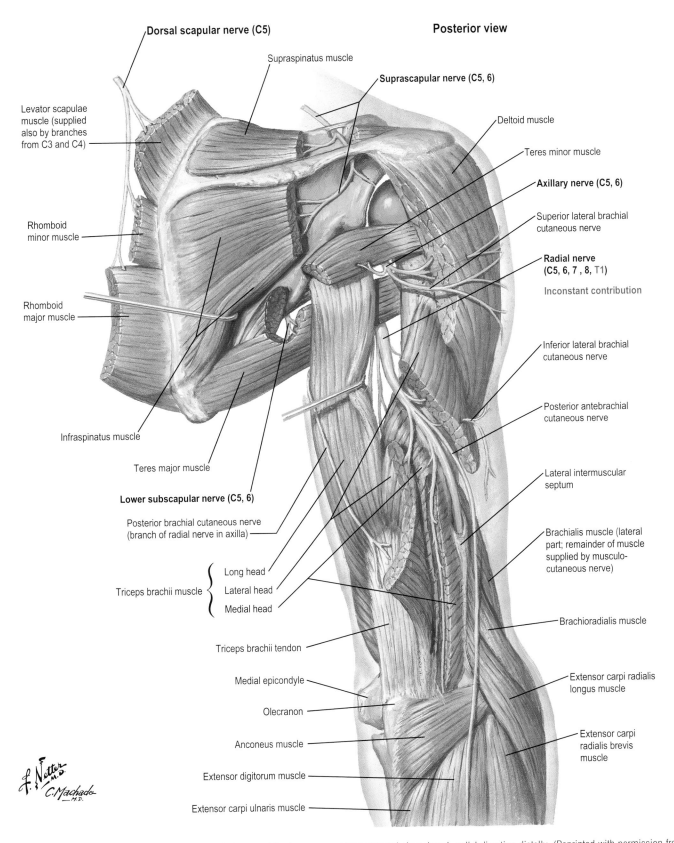

Dorsal scapular nerve (C5)

Posterior view

Supraspinatus muscle

Suprascapular nerve (C5, 6)

Levator scapulae muscle (supplied also by branches from C3 and C4)

Deltoid muscle

Teres minor muscle

Axillary nerve (C5, 6)

Superior lateral brachial cutaneous nerve

Rhomboid minor muscle

Radial nerve (C5, 6, 7 , 8, T1)
Inconstant contribution

Rhomboid major muscle

Inferior lateral brachial cutaneous nerve

Posterior antebrachial cutaneous nerve

Infraspinatus muscle

Lateral intermuscular septum

Teres major muscle

Lower subscapular nerve (C5, 6)

Brachialis muscle (lateral part; remainder of muscle supplied by musculo-cutaneous nerve)

Posterior brachial cutaneous nerve (branch of radial nerve in axilla)

Long head
Lateral head
Medial head

Triceps brachii muscle

Brachioradialis muscle

Triceps brachii tendon

Medial epicondyle

Extensor carpi radialis longus muscle

Olecranon

Anconeus muscle

Extensor carpi radialis brevis muscle

Extensor digitorum muscle

Extensor carpi ulnaris muscle

Fig. 1.42 The proximal radial nerve wraps posteriorly around the humerus and then proceeds in a dorsal–radial direction distally. (Reprinted with permission from www.netterimages.com © Elsevier Inc. All Rights Reserved.)

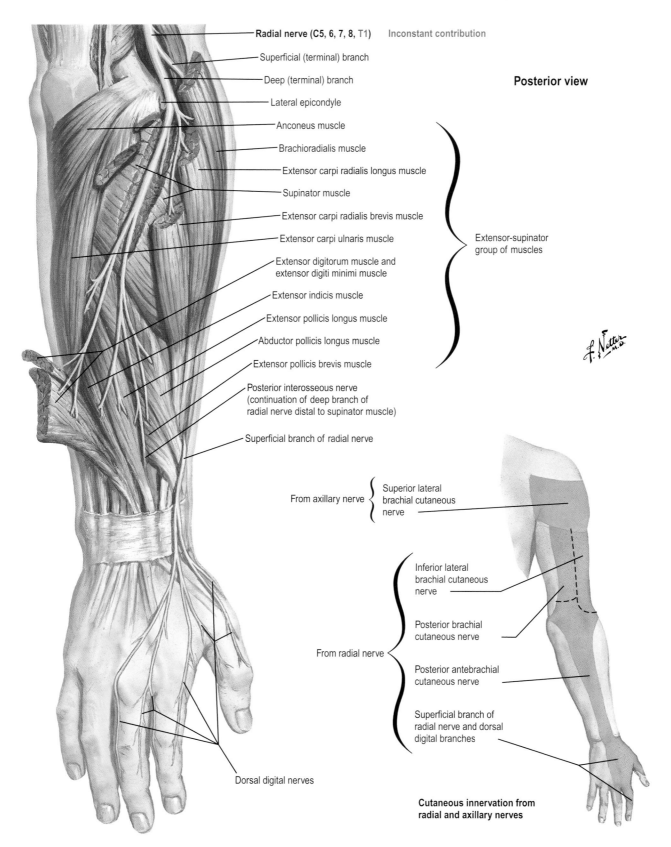

Radial nerve (C5, 6, 7, 8, T1)   Inconstant contribution

Superficial (terminal) branch

Deep (terminal) branch

Lateral epicondyle

Anconeus muscle

Brachioradialis muscle

Extensor carpi radialis longus muscle

Supinator muscle

Extensor carpi radialis brevis muscle

Extensor carpi ulnaris muscle

Extensor digitorum muscle and
extensor digiti minimi muscle

Extensor indicis muscle

Extensor pollicis longus muscle

Abductor pollicis longus muscle

Extensor pollicis brevis muscle

Posterior interosseous nerve
(continuation of deep branch of
radial nerve distal to supinator muscle)

Superficial branch of radial nerve

Extensor-supinator
group of muscles

Posterior view

Dorsal digital nerves

From axillary nerve { Superior lateral
brachial cutaneous
nerve

Inferior lateral
brachial cutaneous
nerve

Posterior brachial
cutaneous nerve

From radial nerve {

Posterior antebrachial
cutaneous nerve

Superficial branch of
radial nerve and dorsal
digital branches

Cutaneous innervation from
radial and axillary nerves

Fig. 1.43 The radial nerve in the forearm innervates the extensor muscles and then lends sensibility to the radial dorsal aspect of the hand. (Reprinted with permission from www.netterimages.com © Elsevier Inc. All Rights Reserved.)

Anterior view

Note: Only muscles innervated by median nerve shown

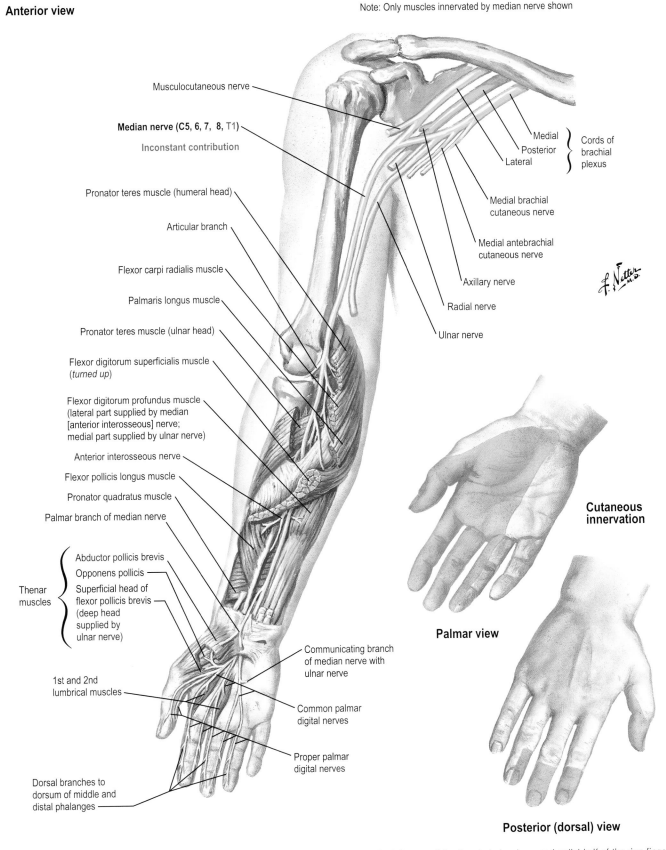

Musculocutaneous nerve

Median nerve (C5, 6, 7, 8, T1)

Inconstant contribution

Pronator teres muscle (humeral head)

Articular branch

Flexor carpi radialis muscle

Palmaris longus muscle

Pronator teres muscle (ulnar head)

Flexor digitorum superficialis muscle
(*turned up*)

Flexor digitorum profundus muscle
(lateral part supplied by median
[anterior interosseous] nerve;
medial part supplied by ulnar nerve)

Anterior interosseous nerve

Flexor pollicis longus muscle

Pronator quadratus muscle

Palmar branch of median nerve

Thenar muscles
- Abductor pollicis brevis
- Opponens pollicis
- Superficial head of
  flexor pollicis brevis
  (deep head
  supplied by
  ulnar nerve)

1st and 2nd
lumbrical muscles

Dorsal branches to
dorsum of middle and
distal phalanges

Medial
Posterior
Lateral } Cords of
brachial
plexus

Medial brachial
cutaneous nerve

Medial antebrachial
cutaneous nerve

Axillary nerve

Radial nerve

Ulnar nerve

Communicating branch
of median nerve with
ulnar nerve

Common palmar
digital nerves

Proper palmar
digital nerves

**Cutaneous
innervation**

Palmar view

Posterior (dorsal) view

Fig. 1.44 The median nerve classically lends sensibility to the palmar aspect and the distal dorsum of the thumb, index, long, and radial half of the ring fingers. Intrinsic muscles radial to the flexor pollicis longus and the two radial lumbricals receive motor innervation from the median nerve. (Reprinted with permission from www.netterimages.com © Elsevier Inc. All Rights Reserved.)

muscular branches supply the pronator teres, flexor carpi radialis, palmaris longus, and flexor digitorum superficialis muscles. The anterior interosseous branch of the median nerve innervates the flexor pollicis longus, flexor digitorum profundus (index and middle finger), and pronator quadratus muscles, and provides wrist sensation. Proximal to the wrist and running between the flexor carpi radialis and palmaris longus tendons, the palmar cutaneous branch provides lateral palmar sensation. As the median nerve passes through the carpal tunnel, the recurrent motor branch innervates the thenar muscles (abductor pollicis brevis, opponens pollicis, and flexor pollicis brevis (superficial head). Sensory branches supply digital nerves to the thumb, index, and middle fingers, as well as the radial aspect of the ring finger.

Lastly, the ulnar nerve enters the upper extremity as a branch of the medial cord of the brachial plexus (C8–T1) **(Fig. 1.45)**. Muscular branches innervate the flexor carpi ulnaris and flexor digitorum profundus muscles to the ring and small fingers. The palmar cutaneous branch of the ulnar nerve provides sensation to hypothenar eminence and medial portion of the palm. The dorsal branch of the ulnar nerve courses around the ulnar aspect of the forearm in its distal one-fourth after branching from the main trunk at a variable site in the distal one-third of the forearm. It passes from its position deep to the flexor carpi ulnaris out through the dorsal fascia to become subcutaneous. This sensory nerve branches to innervate the dorsum of the ulnar portion of the dorsum of the hand, the dorsum of the little finger, and at least part of the dorsum of the ring finger. In contrast, the main sensory branch forms the ulnar digital nerve to the small finger and the common digital nerve which divides into the small-finger radial digital nerve and the ring-finger ulnar digital nerve. The deep motor branch of the ulnar nerve passes through the pisohamate and opponens tunnel in company with the deep branch of the ulnar artery. It courses with the deep vascular arch across the depths of the palm, giving off motor branches to the four hypothenar muscles (abductor digiti minimi, opponens digiti minimi, flexor digiti minimi brevis, and palmaris brevis), all the interossei, the two ulnar lumbricals, and the thumb intrinsics ulnar to the flexor pollicis longus – the adductor pollicis brevis and the flexor pollicis brevis (deep head).

Essentially the flexor pollicis longus divides the hand into a median and ulnar-innervated portion from the motor standpoint. The ulnar nerve is far less important from the standpoint of hand sensation but is very important for its motor innervation of all the hypothenar muscles and interossei. In addition, it innervates the thumb adductor, the deep head of the flexor pollicis brevis, and the two ulnar lumbricals. Classically, all the intrinsic muscles on the radial side of the flexor pollicis longus are median nerve-innervated (the abductor pollicis brevis, opponens, and superficial head of the flexor pollicis brevis). All other intrinsic muscles in the hand receive their innervation from the ulnar nerve. The two tiny radial lumbricals (median nerve innervated) are the only exceptions to this axiom **(Boxes 1.12 and 1.13)**.

Box 1.13 **Clinical pearl: crowded areas with unyielding boundaries**

Flexion and extension motions in the hand occur at two levels, the wrist and the finger joints. Flexion at these joints would surely create volar bowstringing at the long flexor tendons unless it were prevented by fixed retinacular conduits at these points. At the wrist the flexor retinaculum is the fixed roof of the carpal tunnel. The fibrous flexor sheath in the digits forms a fitted pulley system with condensed thickening in the areas of greatest fulcrum responsibility. At the wrist and in the digital fibrosynovial sheaths, anatomic structures create full occupancy. Any addition, whether it be more structures, postinjury or inflammatory swelling of the contents, or inflammatory tightening of the sheath, sets the stage for an inflammatory reaction and adhesion formation.

At the wrist, the median nerve passes beneath the flexor retinaculum and the transverse carpal ligament as the most superficial structure in this crowded space. It is subject to compression injury when swelling occurs within the carpal tunnel.

Just proximal to the wrist, the ulnar nerve passes from beneath the flexor carpi ulnaris along the radial side of the easily palpable pisiform. At this point the nerve enters a fibromusculofascial space that is tubular in configuration, crossing the entire length of the carpus. This is Guyon's tunnel, which is quite separate from the carpal tunnel, through which the median nerve and longitudinal structures to the digits pass. Guyon's tunnel starts at a hiatus formed by the distal edge of the volar carpal ligament superficially and the proximal edge of the transverse carpal ligament deeply. The pisiform forms the ulnar side of the tunnel, and fibers from the volar carpal ligament that plunge down to join the underlying transverse carpal ligament form the radial wall. There is no fibrous roof on the proximal part of the tunnel until the pisohamate arcade fibers are encountered distally. The roof of the tunnel, therefore, consists of a thick layer of fascia continuous with the hypothenar fascia and generally a part of the palmaris brevis muscle. Through this rather soft hiatus, the superficial branch of the ulnar artery and the arterial branches to the palmaris brevis and overlying skin pass, together with the superficial branches of the ulnar nerve. Within Guyon's tunnel the ulnar nerve lies ulnar to the artery, and the division of the ulnar nerve into its deep motor branch and two superficial branches is evident. After the superficial branches of the artery and nerve emerge through the roof of the tunnel, the deep artery and deep branch of the ulnar nerve enter the pisohamate tunnel beneath the pisohamate arcade. Although the tunnel of Guyon is devoid of a thick, fibrous roof, it is nonetheless covered by palmaris brevis fascia, creating an unyielding space, and its contents are therefore subject to compression from a variety of causes. Repeated trauma, as when one uses the heel of the hand to pound objects, may result in swelling of the tissues and resultant hypertrophy and fibrosis or hemorrhage in the tunnel, which may squeeze the nerve or artery, or both. Ganglia, tumors, or displaced bone may cause compression in the ulnar tunnel, just as occurs with the median nerve in the carpal tunnel.

Box 1.12 **Clinical pearl: median and ulnar nerve lacerations**

The ulnar and median nerves are frequently injured just proximal to the wrist. The nerves are quite superficial and it is a region where injuries to all structures are frequent. Median palsy alone results in anesthesia over the important exploring and manipulating digits (the thumb, index, and long fingers, and part of the ring finger) on the palmar surface. The median positioning muscles of the thumb become paralyzed, resulting in an inability to position the thumb for pulp-to-pulp opposition with other digits. In addition, the two radial lumbricals are paralyzed, but this may be barely perceptible functionally. There is a constant midvolar blood vessel on the median nerve that helps in its identity and in achieving very accurate axial rotation to perfect end-to-end opposition.

The ulnar nerve divides into a deep motor branch and a superficial sensory branch just beyond the pisiform. Occasionally, stab wounds of the hand result in transection of the motor branch with no sensory loss. A guide to proper fascicular orientation in the ulnar nerve is the fact that one can identify that portion destined to be the deep or superficial branches well above the wrist.

Ulnar Nerve

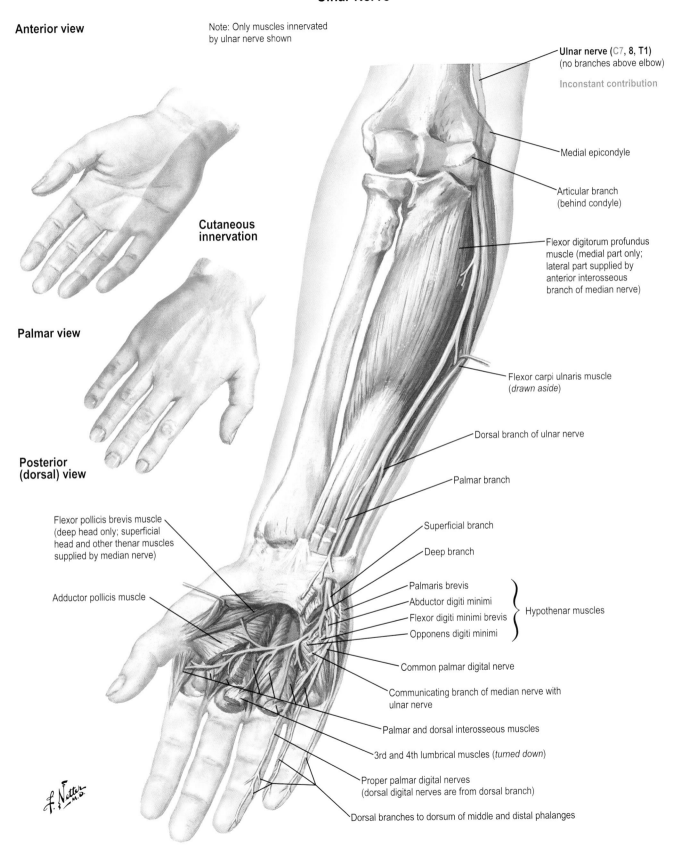

Anterior view

Note: Only muscles innervated by ulnar nerve shown

Cutaneous innervation

Palmar view

Posterior (dorsal) view

Ulnar nerve (C7, 8, T1) (no branches above elbow)

Inconstant contribution

Medial epicondyle

Articular branch (behind condyle)

Flexor digitorum profundus muscle (medial part only; lateral part supplied by anterior interosseous branch of median nerve)

Flexor carpi ulnaris muscle (*drawn aside*)

Dorsal branch of ulnar nerve

Palmar branch

Superficial branch

Deep branch

Flexor pollicis brevis muscle (deep head only; superficial head and other thenar muscles supplied by median nerve)

Adductor pollicis muscle

Palmaris brevis
Abductor digiti minimi
Flexor digiti minimi brevis
Opponens digiti minimi
} Hypothenar muscles

Common palmar digital nerve

Communicating branch of median nerve with ulnar nerve

Palmar and dorsal interosseous muscles

3rd and 4th lumbrical muscles (*turned down*)

Proper palmar digital nerves (dorsal digital nerves are from dorsal branch)

Dorsal branches to dorsum of middle and distal phalanges

Fig. 1.45 The ulnar nerve classically gives sensory innervation to the little finger and the ulnar half of the ring finger. All hypothenar muscles, all interossei, the two ulnar lumbricals, the adductor pollicis, and the ulnar half of the flexor pollicis brevis are usually innervated by the ulnar nerve. (Reprinted with permission from www.netterimages.com © Elsevier Inc. All Rights Reserved.)

Conclusion

In the human hand, the complicated motor balance at each joint resulting from contraction, fixation, or relaxation of opposing muscle groups is worthless in the absence of the precisely fitted elements in the skeletal architecture. The skeletal framework with its restraining ligaments is beautifully designed but is useless without proper dynamic motor tension. The anatomic presence of both architecture and functioning muscles is only serviceable when there is integrity of the central nervous control mechanisms. As a unified inter-related melding of these elements emerges, hand function becomes the marvelous adaptable fact that it is in humans. Its function is modified and further refined by sensory integrity. Sensation is protective and influential on central motor function. Moreover, special sensation as it resides in the hand makes the hand a special sense organ with which human beings explore their environment. From a practical standpoint, surgeons need repeatedly to remind themselves of the anatomic basis for diagnosis and management of surgical problems in the hand.

Access the complete references list online at **http://www.expertconsult.com**

2. Bell C. *The Hand - Its Mechanism and Vital Endowments as Evincing Design*. London: William Pickering; 1834.

   This treatise by Sir Charles Bell is a literary classic that should be read by any student of hand surgery and anatomy.

6. Bunnell S. *Surgery of the Hand*. Philadelphia: J. B. Lippincott; 1944.

   This is the first edition of the first modern textbook in hand surgery, written by Sterling Bunnell, widely regarded as the father of American hand surgery.

18. Berger RA. The gross and histologic anatomy of the scapholunate interosseous ligament. *J Hand Surg*. 1996;21:170.

    In this journal article, Dr. Berger clearly describes the unique anatomy of the scapholunate interosseous ligament. He discusses clinical implications of the anatomy for injury patterns and repair/reconstruction.

23. Legueu F, Juvara E. Des aponèvroses de la paume de la main. *Bull Mem Soc Anat Paris*. 1892;67:383.

    In this original manuscript, Legueu and Juvara perform anatomic dissections to outline the palmar aponeurosis of the hand. The vertical fibers that bear the authors' names are described. These vertical fibers separate the neurovascular and flexor tendon compartments within the palm.

26. Gelberman RH, Menon J. The vascularity of the scaphoid bone. *J Hand Surg* 1980;5:508.

    The authors perform dye injection studies to determine the vascular anatomy to the scaphoid. The relative decreased blood flow to the proximal pole has implications for poor healing of scaphoid fractures in this region.

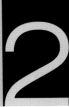

Examination of the upper extremity

Ryosuke Kakinoki

SYNOPSIS

- Physical examination of the upper extremity starts with a detailed and accurate patient history.
- Physical examination of the upper extremity consists of inspection, palpation, measurement of length, girth and ranges of motion, assessment of stability, and detailed assessment of the associated nerve and vascular systems.
- Thorough understanding of the anatomy, physiology and biomechanics of the upper extremity is essential to perform a physical examination correctly and to make a correct diagnosis of pathologic conditions of the upper extremity.
- Examiners must master correct physical examination techniques based on the anatomic, physiologic and biomechanical rationale.
- Even if a patient's complaint focuses on only the hand, the entire upper extremity should be examined.
- It is essential to master correct techniques of physical examination to identify the pathologic conditions of patients.
- Each technique of physical examination is based on the anatomic, physiologic and biomechanical rationale of the musculoskeletal, nerve or vascular systems.
- Examiners should have their own routine protocol of examination of the upper extremity so not to leave a part unexamined.
- Comparison of the affected upper extremity with the contralateral unaffected one helps examiners identify pathologic conditions of the affected one.
- Imaging tools such as X-rays, CT or MRI should be used to confirm the diagnosis drawn from the physical examinations or to choose the most possible diagnosis among the several differential diagnoses.

Obtaining a patient history

The patient history can be the most important tool in developing an accurate diagnosis. The history should not only detail the patient's current complaint, but should also document other elements of the patient's history which may be of great significance for interpreting the patient's current problem and choosing between treatment options. A patient history should include information on the patient's demographics, current complaint, medical history, allergies, medications, and socio-economic status. The time course of the patient history interview should be documented.

Patient demographics

The patient's name, age, occupation, hand dominance and hobbies should be documented. Information about previous injuries or diseases should be obtained, regardless of whether they seem to be related to the patient's current complaint.

Current complaint

All information on the patient's current problem, including symptoms of pain, numbness, tingling (paresthesia), weakness, dislocation, coldness, clumsiness or poor coordination and clicking or snapping, should be documented. Each symptom should be characterized according to its location, intensity, duration, frequency, radiation and associated symptoms. The patient history should include information on activities or treatments that aggravate or ameliorate the symptoms. It is also important to record the time and place at which the initial injury occurred and the mechanism by which it was incurred.

In trauma cases, the following data are especially significant:

1. The time of the injury and the interval between the injury and the patient's presentation should be determined. The interval between an injury and revascularization of amputated fingers has a great effect on the outcome of replantation surgery.

2. The environment in which the injury occurred is important. Whether an injury occurred in a dirty or a clean environment may determine whether infection is likely to be present.

3. The mechanism of injury is also important. For example, information on the posture of the fingers and hand at the time of a tendon laceration is helpful for locating a transected tendon stump.

4. Any previous treatment associated with the injury is documented.

In nontrauma cases, the following data are especially significant:

1. The time at which symptoms such as pain, abnormal sensation, swelling or stiffness began and the subsequent progression of the symptoms is critical.

2. The effects of the symptoms on the patient's daily life, hobby or job are unique to that patient.

3. One must also ascertain whether or not the symptoms are limited to one part of the body.

4. Activities or postures that aggravate or ameliorate the symptoms are also discussed.

5. The association between time and the intensity of symptoms must be carefully documented (e.g., whether pain increases just after waking up in the morning or during the night).

Medical history

The patient's health status may influence diagnosis and treatment. Before starting treatment, it is essential to determine whether the patient has diabetes, or cardiac, pulmonary and/or renal disease and whether the patient has a history of rheumatologic disease. Documentation on the family's medical history may be helpful for making an accurate diagnosis and for choosing an appropriate treatment modality if the disease is hereditary. Patients and their families should be questioned about previous problems associated with bleeding and anesthesia. It is also important to determine the course of any prior surgery.

Allergies and medications

The patient history should include data on any medications that the patient is taking. Previous allergic reactions to foods or medications should be noted. People who are allergic to shellfish are often allergic to contrast media that contain iodine.

Social history

Social history includes the patient's use of tobacco and alcohol. The amount of tobacco and alcohol used should be documented. Substance abuse and infection with hepatitis virus or HIV should also be noted. The patient's hobbies or sports should be documented because these activities often determine the most appropriate treatment.

Physical examination of the hand

Accurate diagnosis of hand problems depends on a systematic, careful physical examination. Physical examination should be performed routinely following a specific protocol. Even if the patient complains of a problem limited to the hand, the physical examination should start at the neck and shoulder region because the hand is suspended by the bones of the forearm, which connect proximally to the elbow joint, which in turn is stabilized by the humerus and the shoulder joint. In addition, numbness of the hand may be associated with cervical problems. The following eight elements (inspection, palpation, measurement of range of motion, stability assessment, musculotendinous assessment, nerve assessment, vascular assessment, and specific tests) should be included in the examination procedure for patients with problems of the upper extremities. An understanding of the interrelationships among these elements is helpful for drawing accurate diagnostic conclusions. Repeated physical examinations reveal how symptoms change over time, which is important for assessing the effectiveness of the treatment.

Inspection

When inspecting the upper extremities, it is essential to compare the affected extremity with the contralateral extremity because the latter can be used as a normal reference if the injury is unilateral.

Discoloration

An abnormal skin color or a change in the color of the skin of the upper extremity is indicative of a wide variety of problems. Infections often cause swelling and patches of redness with proximal streaking. Vascular problems caused by arterial inflow insufficiency often present as pale colored and the distal part of the upper limb appears to have shrunk, whereas those caused by venous outflow insufficiency present as a purple or dark red discoloration and a swollen limb. The color of a hematoma can be used to estimate the interval since the trauma occurred. A fresh hematoma has purple or blue patches, which then become green and finally yellow.

Deformity

Fractures, tumors, arthritis and some infectious conditions can cause deformities of the upper extremity. Fractures of the phalanges of the fingers frequently result in angular rotation or malrotation of the fingers. When the fingers are held up, the point at which the long axes of the fingers converge corresponds with the position of the scaphoid tubercle. However, the long axis of a malrotated finger deviates from the position of the scaphoid.

Muscular atrophy

It is important to determine whether atrophied muscles are innervated by specific peripheral nerves. If the atrophic muscles are innervated by a specific nerve, the atrophy may have been caused by a peripheral nerve disorder. Muscular atrophy may occur under systemic neural or muscular patho-logical conditions; in most of these cases, the atrophy is symmetrical in the bilateral extremities. Generally, neurogenic diseases involve muscles in the distal part of the extremity and muscular diseases involve the proximal part of the extremity. The girths of the arm (a portion measured should be noted, like the arm girth 20 cm distal to the acromion) and forearm (a portion with the maximum diameter of the forearm) of both upper extremities should be measured routinely because this often reveals a loss of muscle mass, which may not be obvious to the eye.

Trophic changes

Trophic changes are associated with an abnormality of the sympathetic nervous system. Increased hair growth or abnormal perspiration of the hands is often observed in chronic regional pain syndrome.

Swelling

Swelling can be identified by comparison with the uninvolved extremity. Localized swelling indicates recent trauma or inflammation. Diffuse swelling is often caused by infection. General swelling may originate from a lymphatic or venous obstruction. Swelling of the dorsum of the hand is also common.

Skin creases

Disappearance of skin creases is indicative of loss of motion of the joint under the creases and can be helpful in determining the validity of a complaint of an inability to move the fingers or upper extremities. Clear finger creases over joints that a patient claims he or she is unable to flex or extend indicate that the patient moves the joint. In such cases, the patient may be malingering or may have a psychosis in which he or she cannot recognize motion of the joint.

Palpation

Palpation is a powerful maneuver for identifying masses, abnormal skin temperature, areas of tenderness, crepitance, clicking or snapping and effusion. Masses in the deep layer can be detected by palpation before they emerge as masses under the skin. When performing palpation, special attention should be paid to differences in hardness or mobility relative to that of the surrounding tissue. For example, subtle palpation can identify a palmar bowstring of a flexor tendon in a patient who complains of lack of finger flexion after an injury of the flexor pulleys.

Range of motion assessment

Both passive and active ranges of motion should be documented. The range of motion of both the contralateral healthy limb and the affected limb should be measured and compared. The range of motion may be affected by the posture of the adjacent joints. For example, active and passive distal interphalangeal (DIP) joint flexion is limited when the proximal interphalangeal (PIP) joint of the same finger is extended. When the wrist joint is flexed, the active range of finger flexion

decreases. The range of motion of a joint should be measured in a posture that permits maximum motion.

The passive range of motion is measured by holding the patient's structures proximal and distal to the joint in question and then moving the joint from one limit of motion to the other in the absence of any muscular contraction by the patient. A limited range of passive motion is associated with joint stiffness and soft tissue contracture.

The active range of motion of a joint is that which occurs when the patient contracts his or her muscles. The active range of motion is affected by tendon excursion, the posture of the hand and fingers, nerve function and muscular strength.

Stability assessment

The tightness of the ligaments around a joint, morphology of the surface of a joint and musculotendinous balance around a joint are useful indices of joint stability. When assessing joint stability, the biomechanical and physiological properties of the ligaments should be taken into consideration and the stress forces applied should be appropriate for the ligament in question. For example, the straight portions of the bilateral collateral ligaments of the finger metacarpal (MP) joints tighten when the joint is in the flexed position *(Fig. 2.1)*, whereas those of the PIP joints tighten when the joints are in an extended position. The stability of ligaments is tested by holding the portions distal and proximal to the joint and gently moving the joint passively to stress the ligaments that stabilize the joint. It is useful to measure the opening angle of the affected joint under stress using X-rays and to compare the opening angle of the affected joint with that of the corresponding healthy joint of the opposite hand *(Fig. 2.2)*. The tear of the ulnar collateral ligament of the thumb MP joint is known to be *Stener lesion*. The radial collateral ligament instability of the thumb MP joint demonstrates palmar dislocation and ulnar deviation of the thumb MP joint. The radial

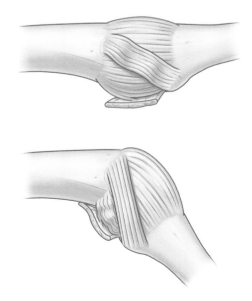

Fig. 2.1 The collateral ligament of the MP joint. The proper portion of the collateral ligament is relaxed when the joint is extended (top) and is tight when the MP joint is flexed (bottom). The smaller accessory portion has the opposite effect.

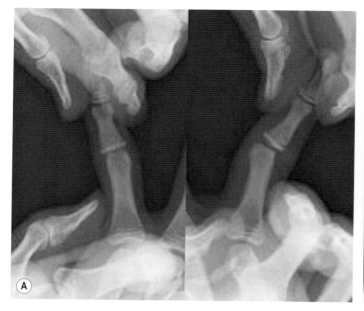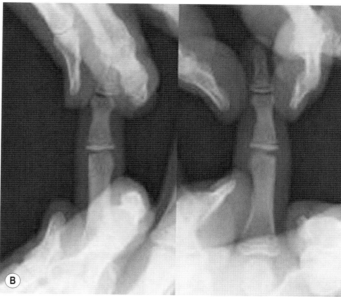

Fig. 2.2 Rupture of the radial collateral ligament of the index finger PIP joint. Measure the opening angle of the affected joint under the radial and ulnar stress forces on X-ray films and compare the angle with that of the corresponding normal joint of the opposite hand. **(A)** Affected finger. **(B)** Normal opposite finger.

collateral ligament courses from the distal-palmar to proximal-dorsal direction, the line of which is almost perpendicular to the sagittal axial line of the thumb, the MP joint has tendency to be dislocated palmarly, when the ligament is not functioning. Because the force vector of the adductor pollicis muscle is more transverse to the axial line than that of the thumb abductor muscles, which is more parallel to the axis of the thumb, the thumb MP joint with the radial collateral ligament insufficiency demonstrates ulnar deviation. On the other hand, the long-lasting ulnar collateral ligament insufficiency of the thumb MP joint may also show palmar dislocation.

Assessment of the stability of wrist joints is complex and difficult. The stability of the wrist joint is determined by the stability of the radiocarpal, ulnocarpal, distal radioulnar and midcarpal joints. Special tests for assessing the stability of specific ligaments or imaging tools such as X-rays, CT or MRI may be helpful in making a diagnosis.

Musculotendinous assessment

The integrity of the tendon and the strength of the muscle should be considered when conducting a musculotendinous assessment.

Posture

When musculotendinous units are examined, it should be kept in mind that the muscle strength and ranges of motion of the hand and digits change depending on the posture of the wrist, forearm or digits. For example, the range of motion of the DIP joint of a finger is less when the PIP joint is passively extended than when the PIP joint is flexed.

Motion

There are many muscles and tendons in the hand. When the origin and insertion of a muscle are both distal to the wrist joint, the muscle is called an intrinsic muscle. When a muscle extends across the wrist joint, it is called an extrinsic muscle. Other muscles often compensate for a nonfunctioning muscle, in which case the nonfunctioning muscle appears to function. To evaluate muscle function, each muscle should be evaluated in a posture or situation in which the cooperative muscles do not function. For example, the extensor pollicis longus (EPL) can compensate for impaired thumb adduction. Even when the thumb adductors do not function because of ulnar nerve palsy, patients may be able to adduct the thumb using a functional EPL.

The presence of abnormal muscles or an abnormal linkage of tendons should sometimes be considered. The flexion function of the PIP joint of a finger is generally accepted to be independent of that of the other fingers because the flexor digitorum superficialis (FDS) tendon of each finger has its own muscle belly. The motion of the FDS tendon of the small finger is often linked to that of the ring and/or the long finger and the PIP joint flexion of the small finger often coordinates with that of the ring and/or long fingers.[1] The extensor digitorum manus brevis is sometimes present in the middle finger and causes dorsal wrist pain.[2]

Power

Muscle power is classed according to the Medical Research Council scale, which ranges from zero to five (0–5) *(Table 2.1)*.[3] Grip strength is a good indicator of the global muscle strength of the upper extremity. Grip strength is measured using a dynamometer with the shoulder and elbow joints stabilized. The patient grips the dynamometer with the elbow

Table 2.1 Medical research council scale

Grade	Physical examination findings
0	No contraction
1	Flicker or trace contraction
2	Active movement with gravity eliminated
3	Active movement against gravity
4	Active movement against gravity and resistance
5	Normal power

Reproduced with permission from: Seddon HJ. Peripheral Nerve Injuries. Medical Research Council Special Report Series, 282. London: HMSO; 1954.[3]

straightened beside the trunk in the standing position or flexed 90° in the sitting position.

In clinical settings, it is very important to distinguish nerve palsy from tendon laceration or rupture. The milking test and dynamic tenodesis effects (described later) can be used to distinguish between the two.

Tests for specific muscles

Extrinsic muscles

The flexor digitorum profundus (FDP) muscle

Video 1

Flexor profundus test
This test is used to assess the continuity and muscle power of each of the FDP tendons. The patient's hand is placed palm upward on a table. The examiner holds the proximal and middle phalanges of the target finger down to keep the MP and PIP joints in extension and asks the patient to flex the DIP joint. The test should be performed on each finger.

The flexor digitorum superficialis (FDS) muscle

Video 2

Flexor sublimis test
This test is used to assess the continuity and muscle power of each of the FDS tendons. The FDS tendons insert on the proximal half of the palmar surface of the middle phalanx of the fingers. Because each FDS tendon has its own muscle belly, its function is independent of the FDS of the adjacent fingers. The patient's hand is placed palm upward on a table. The examiner holds the distal phalanges of all fingers down except that of the finger to be tested to keep the MP, PIP and DIP joints of the other fingers in full extension. The patient is asked to flex the finger to be tested. Each finger is tested individually. Because the FDP muscles share a common origin, holding the DIP joint of a finger in full extension may prevent motion of all FDPs. However, because each FDS has an individual origin, the FDS moves but the FDP does not when the other fingers are kept fully extended.

The flexor pollicis longus (FPL) muscle

The FPL inserts on the palmar surface of the distal phalanx of the thumb and can be tested by asking the patient to flex the IP joint of the thumb.

The extensor pollicis brevis (EPB) and the abductor pollicis longus (APL) muscles

The EPB inserts at the dorsal base of the proximal phalanx of the thumb. It is sometimes connected to the EPL. The APL has several tendons and inserts at the dorsolateral base of the thumb metacarpus and trapezium. Both tendons pass through the first dorsal component at the wrist (the APL tendon lies radial to the EPB in the compartment). When the patient abducts the thumb maximally, the EPB and APL tendons as well as the EPL tendon merge under the skin over the radio-dorsal side of the wrist and create the snuffbox. The EPB and APL tendons are palpable as taut tendons in the radiopalmar border of the snuffbox.

The extensor carpi radialis longus (ECRL) and brevis (ECRB) muscles

The ECRL and ECRB tendons insert at the dorsal bases of the second and third metacarpal bones, respectively. The function of these muscles is to extend the wrist joint. Because the functional axis of the ECRL deviates radially, the ECRL extends the wrist dorsoradially. When the ECRB does not function, extension of the wrist deviates radially because of the intact ECRL tendon. The extensor digitorum communis (EDC) tendon also may function as a wrist extensor. To remove the EDC contribution to wrist extension, the patient is asked to make a fist and then extend the wrist. Making a fist eliminates EDC function.

The extensor pollicis longus (EPL) muscle

Video 3

The EPL passes through the third dorsal compartment, turns radially at the Lister's tubercle and inserts at the dorsal base of the distal phalanx of the thumb. The EPL extends the IP joint of the thumb. The hand is placed palm down on a table with the thumb adducted. The patient is asked to lift only the thumb off the surface of the table, keeping the thumb adducted. The taut EPL tendon is palpable in the radiodorsal aspect of the wrist.

The extensor digitorum communis (EDC) muscles

Video 4

The EDC tendons pass through the fourth extensor compartment and insert at the dorsal base of the middle phalanges of the fingers. They mainly extend the MP joint, while the intrinsic extensors extend the PIP and DIP joints. EDC function is examined by asking the patient to lift the MP joints of four fingers (the index to the small finger) keeping the PIP and DIP joints flexed.

The extensor indicis proprius (EIP) muscle

The EIP tendon passes through the fourth extensor compartment at the wrist deep to the EDC tendon and merges with the ulnar side of the index finger EDC tendon over the MP joint. The function of the EIP is to extend the MP joint of the index finger, which is isolated from the extension of the MP joints of the other fingers. The EIP is functional if the patient can straighten the index finger completely when the other fingers are flexed in a fist.

The extensor digiti minimi (EDM) muscle

The EDM tendon passes the fifth extensor compartment and merges with the ulnar side of the small finger EDC tendon at the MP joint level. Because the EDM tendon is usually divided into two tails distally, both tails of the tendon must be transected when the tendon is transferred. This tendon is evaluated by asking the patient to straighten the small finger when the other fingers are flexed into a fist.

The extensor carpi ulnaris (ECU) muscle

The ECU tendon passes through the sixth extensor compartment and inserts on the dorsal base of the fifth metacarpal bone. The function of this tendon is ulnar deviation of a wrist that is held extended. The wrist cannot be extended dorsally only by the ECU. This tendon is evaluated by asking the patient to make a fist and to lift and deviate the wrist ulnarly. The tendon is palpable radial to the ulnar styloid process.

Intrinsic muscles

The thenar muscles

The thenar muscles cover the metacarpal of the thumb and consist of three muscles: the abductor pollicis brevis, the flexor pollicis brevis and the opponens pollicis. The muscles move the thumb into opposition, enabling the thumb to touch the fingertips when the nails are parallel. These muscles are evaluated by asking the patient to place the dorsum of the hand flat on a table and to raise the thumb until it is perpendicular to the palm. The patient is then asked to resist a downward force by the examiner on the thumb.

The adductor pollicis muscle (ADP)

The ADP muscle arises from the third metacarpal and inserts to the ulnar base of the proximal phalanx of the thumb. Some fibers of the ADP extend dorsally to form an extensor apparatus for the thumb. Together with the first dorsal interosseous muscle, the ADP approximates the thumb to the second metacarpal.

The interosseous and lumbrical muscles

The interosseous and lumbrical muscles flex the MP joints and extend the PIP and DIP joints of the fingers. In addition, four dorsal interosseous muscles abduct the thumb and the radial three fingers and three palmar interosseous muscles adduct the fingers. The second and third dorsal interosseous muscles are evaluated by asking the patient to place the hand flat on a table and then to stretch the long finger upward (i.e., to hyperextend it) and to deviate it radially and ulnarly. Patients with ulnar nerve palsy cannot do this because of loss of power in the interosseous muscles (the *Pitres–Testut sign*). The first palmar interosseous and the second dorsal interosseous muscles are tested by the *"crossing fingers" sign*. The patient is asked to cross a flexed long finger over the index finger or to cross a flexed index finger over the long finger when the palm and the ring and little fingers are placed flat on a table. (Finger abduction refers to movement away from the long finger; finger adduction refers to movement toward the long finger.)

The hypothenar muscles

The hypothenar muscles: the abductor digiti minimi, the flexor digiti minimi, the opponens digiti minimi and the palmaris brevis muscle, abduct the small finger, moving it away from the other fingers.

Nerve assessment

Evaluation of peripheral nerves should include both motor and sensory function. To evaluate the motor function of the hand, it is necessary to understand not only the anatomy and

biomechanics of the muscles of the upper extremity but also the peripheral innervation of the muscles. An understanding of the order in which branches of the nerve trunk innervate muscles is important for assessing nerve recovery after a nerve injury or a compression neuropathy.

Sensibility testing also relies on knowledge of peripheral nerve anatomy. It is essential to understand which parts of the hand are innervated by which peripheral nerves. Peripheral nerve palsy should be diagnosed using motor and sensory evaluation. When the outcome of a motor assessment does not coincide with that of a sensory assessment, abnormal innervation of muscles or an unusual anastomosis between peripheral nerves should be considered. The Martin–Gruber connection is an abnormal innervation of the median nerve to the motor branch of the ulnar nerve. Patients with cubital tunnel syndrome and this nerve connection may have a sensory palsy of the ulnar nerve without motor palsy.

Comprehensive sensibility evaluation includes static and dynamic two-point discrimination (2 PD) testing, Semmes–Weinstein monofilament testing, vibrotactile threshold testing, and cold-heat testing. The 2 PD test evaluates the tactile sensation of the skin and assesses density of the perception receptors in the skin. Stimuli generated by the static 2 PD test are mainly sensed by Merkel cells (slow-adapting mechanoreceptors), while the main receptors of stimuli generated by the moving 2 PD test are Meissner corpuscles (quick-adapting receptors). In the static 2PD test, a caliper is applied longitudinally to the digit and the smallest distance between the tips of the caliper that the patient can distinguish is measured.[4] The moving 2PD test is the smallest perceived distance between the tips of a caliper that is moved longitudinally along the ulnar or radial aspect of the finger.[5] The normal distance is 3 mm for the moving 2PD test and 6 mm for the static 2PD test of the fingertips (see specific tests). The Semmes–Weinstein test evaluates the pressure perception of the skin of the fingers and assesses the threshold of the perception receptors in the skin. This test is conducted by touching the fingers with filaments of various diameters (see specific tests).[6] The vibrotactile test also assesses the threshold of the perception receptors and is performed using two types of tuning forks with 30 cycles per second (cps) and 250 cps. The vibrating forks are touched on area examined and whether patients can recognize the vibration is examined. Main receptors of stimuli generated by the tuning forks with 250 cps are Pacinian corpuscles, while those by the forks with 30 cps are Meissner corpuscles. In the cold-heat test, the perception of heat is evaluated by touching the skin with a test tube containing water at 40–45°C and the perception of cold is tested using a test tube containing water at 10°C. Stimuli of the cold-heat test are mainly sensed by free nerve endings of the skin *(Table 2.2)*.

Vascular assessment

There are two types of vascular problems: arterial and venous insufficiency. Vascular problems are assessed according to the color, capillary refill, pressure (turgor) and temperature of the affected part.

Arterial interruption causes a pale white or grayish discoloration of the affected area. Venous blockage results in blood congestion, which causes a purple-blue discoloration.

Table 2.2 Specific sensory testing and main receptors

Test	Perception	Main receptor	Type of adaptation	Evaluation of innervation
Static 2PD	Tactile	Merkel cell	Slowly	Density
Moving 2PD	Tactile	Meissner corpuscle	Quickly	Density
Tune fork (250 cps)	Vibration	Pacinian corpuscle	Quickly	Threshold
Tune fork (30 cps)	Vibration	Meissner corpuscle	Quickly	Threshold
S-W test	Pressure	Merkel cell	Slowly	Threshold

cps, cycles per second.
(Reproduced with permission from Bell-Krotosoki J, Tomancik E. The repeatability of testing with Semmes-Weinstein monofilaments. J Hand Surg 1987;12A:155–161.)

Capillary refill is indicative of the circulation status of the digits. When the fingertip or nail bed is depressed, the area under pressure turns white. When the pressure is released, the area should turn pink within 2 seconds. A delay in refill is indicative of an arterial inflow problem. Prompt refilling may indicate venous congestion. A decrease in skin pressure or temperature may also indicate vascular problems.

The Allen's test is helpful for determining if there is an intact circulatory connection between the radial and ulnar arteries in the hand. If there is an intact circulatory path between the two arteries, the hand may be nourished by either of the arteries. In this test, the examiner presses down on the radial and ulnar arteries at the wrist to occlude them, while the patient repeatedly makes and releases a tight fist to exsanguinate the hand. The patient then opens the hand and the examiner releases the pressure on one of the arteries at the wrist. If the released artery has an intact circulatory path in the hand, the palm and fingers should turn pink within 2–5 seconds. The test should then be repeated releasing the pressure on the other artery (see specific tests). This test is essential for assessing the vascularity of the hand before harvesting radial or ulnar forearm flaps. If both arteries are not patent, pedicled forearm flap elevation may compromise the vascularity of the hand.

To assess the circulatory connection between the radial and ulnar palmar digital arteries, the same maneuver is performed at the base of the fingers and thumb (digital Allen's test). If there is no circulatory connection between the palmar digital arteries, pedicled island flap harvest should be avoided.[7]

Special provocative tests for the hand

Range of motion assessment

Flexor profundus test

Purpose: This test is used to assess the continuity, excursion and muscle power of each of the FDP tendons.
Maneuver: The patient's hand is placed palm up on a table. The examiner presses down on the proximal and middle phalanges of the target finger to keep the MP and PIP joints in extension and asks the patient to flex the DIP joint. The test should be performed on each finger.

Flexor sublimis test

Purpose: This test is used to assess the continuity, excursion and muscle power of each of the flexor digitorum superficialis tendons.

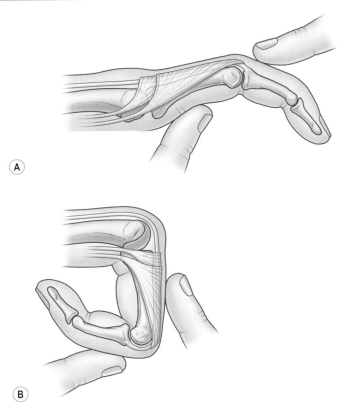

Fig. 2.3 Intrinsic tightness test. If there is a tightness of the interosseous muscles, the PIP joint can be more easily flexed when the MP joint is held flexed than when the MP joint is extended. **(A)** The MP joint is extended. **(B)** The MP joint is flexed.

Maneuver: The patient's hand is placed palm up on a table. The examiner presses down on the distal phalanges of all fingers except that of the finger to be tested to keep the MP, PIP and DIP joints of the other fingers in full extension. The patient is then asked to flex the finger to be tested. Each finger is tested individually.

Intrinsic tightness test (Bunnell)

Purpose: This test assesses the contracture of the interosseous muscles.
Maneuver: The PIP joint is more easily flexed when the MP joint is flexed than when it is extended (0 degree extended position) if tightness of the interosseous muscles is present *(Fig. 2.3)*.[8] The test should be performed using radial and

ulnar deviation of the finger to distinguish between tightness of the radial and ulnar lateral bands.

Extrinsic tightness test

In contrast, the PIP joint is more easily flexed when the MP joint is kept extended than when it is flexed signifying that tightness of the extrinsic muscles is present.[9]

Lumbrical muscle tightness test

The lumbrical muscle connects the flexor digitorum profundus tendon and the radial lateral band of each extensor tendon. The PIP and DIP joints are apt to be extended when a patient with lumbrical muscle tightness intends to flex a finger. The finger flexion is thus blocked (paradoxical movement of the finger) *(Fig. 2.4)*.

Stability assessment

Scaphoid shift test (Watson)

Video 12

Purpose: This test was originally developed to detect loosening or disruption of the scapholunate interosseous ligament. This test can also be used to detect a scaphoid fracture or scapholunate advanced collapse (SLAC) arthritis.
Maneuver: When the wrist deviates radially, the scaphoid rotates palmarly and the palmar prominence of the tubercle of the scaphoid thus becomes evident. However, when the wrist deviates ulnarly, the scaphoid rotates dorsally and the bony prominence is less evident. The examiner holds the dorsum of the patient's hand with his or her fingers and places his or her thumb onto the radial palmar wrist to palpate the bony prominence of the scaphoid tubercle. When the examiner holds the patient's hand and deviates the wrist radially and ulnarly, he or she will feel the motion of the bony prominence under his or her thumb. When the examiner feels the palmar movement of the bony prominence of the scaphoid tubercle when moving the patient's wrist from the ulnar to

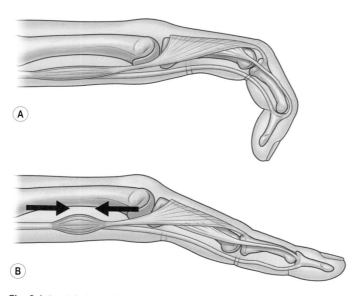

Ⓐ

Ⓑ

Fig. 2.4 Lumbrical muscle tightness test. Because the lumbrical muscle connects the flexor digitorum profundus tendon and the radial lateral band of the extensor tendon, the PIP and DIP joint are apt to be extended when the patient intends to flex the finger (paradoxical movement).

the radial deviation, he or she pushes dorsally up on the tubercle against the force of the palmar movement. If scapholunate ligament insufficiency is present, the examiner will feel a clunk on the thumb over the distal tubercle. If the scaphoid tubercle does not move despite deviation of the wrist, the scaphoid may be fractured. If pain is produced by this maneuver, a scaphoid fracture or scapholunate arthritis is indicated.[10]

Finger extension test

Purpose: To detect the pre-dynamic rotary subluxation of the scaphoid (dorsal wrist syndrome).
Maneuver: When being asked to extend the DIP and PIP joints of all fingers fully, keeping the wrist and the MP joints of all fingers in a full-flexed position, patients with overloaded scapholunate ligaments (pre-dynamic rotary subluxation of the scaphoid) experience pain around the scapholunate joint in the dorsal wrist.[11]

Triquetrolunate ballottement test and the lunotriquetral shuck test

Purpose: To evaluate the stability of the lunotriquetral ligament.
Maneuver: The examiner places his or her thumb dorsally over the triquetrum and the index finger palmarly over the pisiform bone to keep the triquetrum–pisiform unit between the thumb and index finger. The examiner then places his or her opposite thumb on the dorsum of the lunate and pushes it palmarly down. If there is triquetrolunate ligament incompetence, the examiner will feel palmar movement of the lunate and the patient will complain of pain in the wrist *(Fig. 2.5)*.[12] The lunotriquetral shuck test is similar to the triquetrolunate ballottement test. The patient is asked to place the elbow on a table with the forearm in neutral rotation. The examiner's thumb is placed over the dorsal side of the lunate just beyond the radiolunate joint. The examiner's opposite thumb pushes the palmar side of the pisiformis dorsally to load the pisotriquetral joint.[13] In lunotriquetral ligament incompetence, the triquetrum-pisiform unit is moved dorsally and the patient will complain of pain in the lunotriquetral joint *(Fig. 2.6)*.

Distal radioulnar joint instability test

Purpose: To evaluate the integrity of the deep layer of the dorsal or palmar distal radioulnar ligaments.
Maneuver: The deep layers of the dorsal and palmar ligaments of the distal radioulnar joint (DRUJ) comprise the triangular ligament of the triangular fibrocartilage complex (TFCC) and play a primary role to stabilize the DRUJ. The deep dorsal ligament becomes taut when the forearm is supinated and the deep palmar ligament is taut when the forearm is pronated. The deep layers of the palmar and dorsal ligaments thus restrict dorsal and palmar shift of the ulna head, respectively. The examiner sits opposite the patient at a table. The patient's elbow is flexed 90° and placed on the table. The patient's forearm is fully pronated and the examiner places his or her thumb on the palmar aspect of the ulnar head and pushes dorsally upward. This maneuver should be repeated on the healthy wrist. If abnormal dorsal movement of the distal ulna is felt with the thumb, insufficiency of the deep layer of the palmar distal radioulnar ligament (palmar portion of the triangular ligament of the TFCC) is present. Next, the

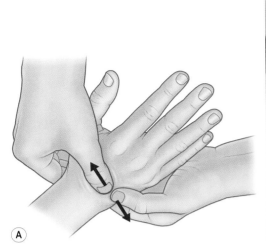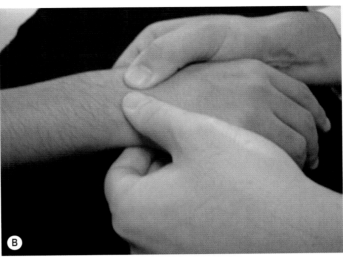

Fig. 2.5 (A,B) Triquetrolunate ballottement test.

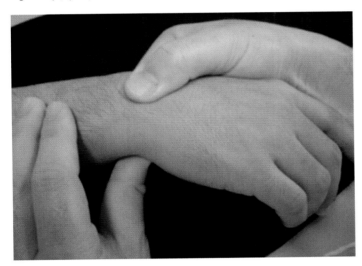

Fig. 2.6 Lunotriquetral shuck test.

patient's forearm is fully supinated and the examiner places his or her thumb on the dorsum of the distal ulna and pushes palmarly down. If abnormal palmar movement of the distal ulna compared with that of the opposite wrist is felt with the thumb, insufficiency of the deep layer of the dorsal distal radioulnar ligament (dorsal portion of the triangular ligament of the TFCC) is present *(Fig. 2.7)*.[14]

Ulnocarpal abutment test

Purpose: To evaluate TFCC injuries.
Maneuver: The examiner places a thumb on the patient's distal ulna and holds the patient's hand with the remaining four fingers. The patient's forearm is stabilized by the examiner's opposite hand. The patient's wrist is fully deviated ulnarly and the forearm is pronated and supinated. A patient with a TFCC injury may complain of ulnar wrist pain and a click or pop may be felt when the examiner's thumb is placed on the ulnocarpal joint *(Fig. 2.8)*.

Pisiformis gliding test

Purpose: To evaluate arthritis in the pisotriquetral joint.

Maneuver: The examiner palpates the pisiform and pushes it down against the triquetrum and applies shear force between the two bones. If there is arthritis in the pisotriquetral joint, the patient will feel pain in the joint during this procedure *(Fig. 2.9)*.

Extensor carpi ulnaris (ECU) synergy test

Purpose: To detect ECU tendinitis.
Maneuver: The patient's forearm is held fully supinated. The examiner asks the patient to abduct all fingers and applies a counterforce to the index and small fingers sufficient to prevent abduction of the index and small fingers. A patient with ECU tendinitis will experience pain in the sixth extensor compartment *(Fig. 2.10)*.[15]

Midcarpal instability test

Purpose: To evaluate midcarpal stability.
Maneuver: The examiner places a thumb on the dorsal midcarpal joint and holds the patient's affected hand with the remaining four fingers. The patient's forearm is stabilized by the examiner's opposite hand. A patient with midcarpal instability will complain of pain in the midcarpal joint when the wrist is deviated ulnarly or radially. Patients with dorsal intercalary segmental instability (DISI) often complain of pain in the ulnodorsal portion of the midcarpal joint, and a click or pop may be felt when the wrist is deviated ulnarly.

Musculotendinous assessment

Dynamic tenodesis effect

Purpose: To evaluate the continuity and mobility of the extrinsic tendons of the hand.
Maneuver: The examiner asks the patient to place an elbow flexed at 90° on a table. If the hand is relaxed, it should flex palmarly and the fingers and thumb should be extended if there are no contractures of the joints and nothing prevents the tendons from sliding in the hand and forearm. When the patient's wrist is held fully extended, the thumb and fingers flex. This phenomenon is called a positive dynamic tenodesis effect. This test is useful for distinguishing nerve palsy from tendon laceration. Because the FPL tendon is intact in patients

Video
13

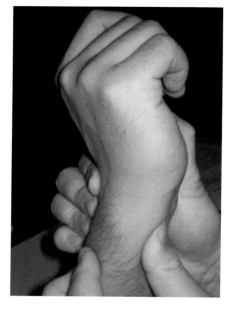

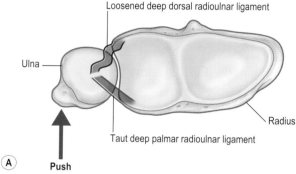

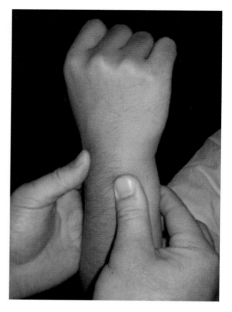

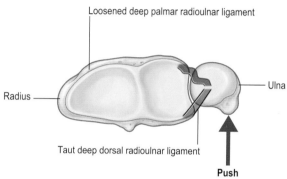

Fig. 2.7 Distal radioulnar joint (DRUJ) instability test. **(A)** Examination for the palmar instability of the DRUJ. The examiner pushes the ulna head from the palmar side when the forearm is pronated to examine the deep palmar distal RU ligament. The deep palmar ligament is taut in the forearm pronated. **(B)** Examination for the dorsal instability of the DRUJ. The examiner pushes the ulna head from the dorsal side when the forearm is supinated to examine the deep dorsal distal RU ligament. The deep dorsal ligament is taut in the forearm supinated.

with anterior interosseous syndrome, it would show the positive dynamic tenodesis effect. However, in patients with FPL rupture, the thumb does not flex when the wrist is held in the extended position. This maneuver is also used to determine the appropriate tension of transferred or transplanted tendons.

Milking test of the finger and thumb flexor tendons

Purpose: To evaluate the continuity and excursion of the extrinsic flexors of the thumb and fingers. This test and the dynamic tenodesis test are useful for distinguishing nerve palsy from tendon rupture.
Maneuver: The patient is asked to place the dorsum of the forearm and the hand on a table and to relax. The examiner pushes down on the musculotendinous junctions of the flexor tendons around the palmar aspect of the middle forearm. If the tendons have normal excursion and no adhesions, the fingers and thumb flex as the forearm is pushed down.

Finkelstein test

Purpose: To detect de Quervain's tendinitis (tendinitis in the first extensor compartment).

Maneuver: The patient places the hand on a table with the thumb up. The examiner pushes down on the proximal phalanx of the thumb. A patient with de Quervain's tendinitis will experience pain or discomfort in the first extensor compartment of the wrist.

Eichoff test

Purpose: To detect de Quervain's tendinitis (tendonitis in the first extensor compartment).
Maneuver: The patient is asked to hold the thumb with the four flexed fingers of the affected hand. The hand is deviated ulnarly by the examiner. A patient with de Quervain's tendinitis will experience pain or discomfort in the first extensor compartment of the wrist.

Nerve assessment

Tinel's sign

Purpose: To detect nerve regeneration.
Maneuver: When the examiner taps on a peripheral nerve distal to a nerve injury such as a compression neuropathy or

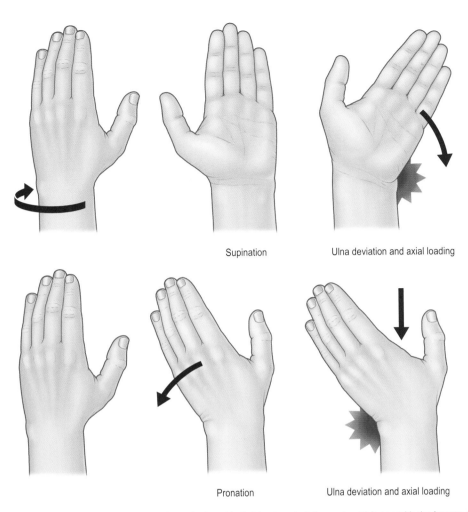

Supination   Ulna deviation and axial loading

Pronation   Ulna deviation and axial loading

Fig. 2.8 Ulnocarpal abutment test. The wrist is subjected to ulnar deviation and axial forces with the forearm fully supinated or pronated.

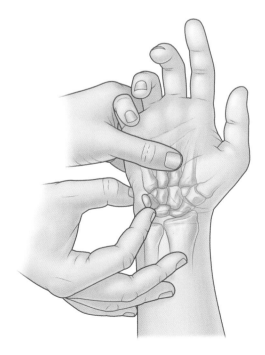

Fig. 2.9 Pisiform gliding test.

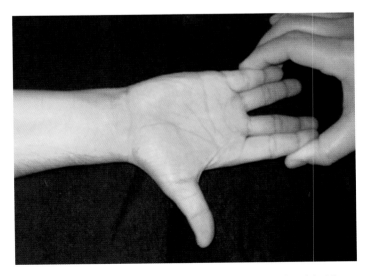

Fig. 2.10 Extensor carpi ulnaris synergy test. The patient is asked to abduct the fingers with the forearm fully supinated. The examiner applies counterforce to the index and little fingers.

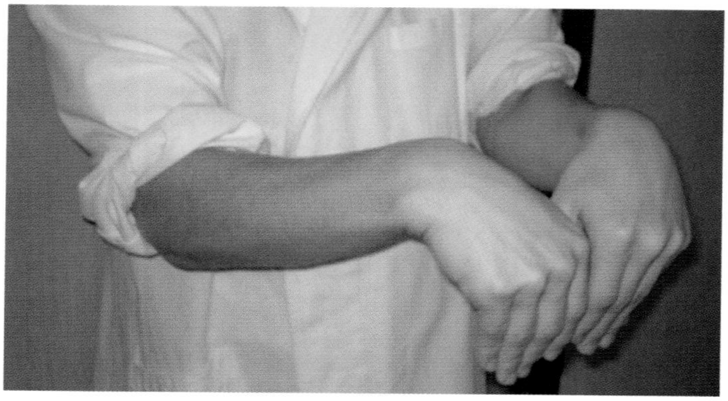

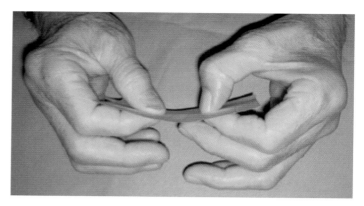

Fig. 2.11 Phalen test.

Fig. 2.12 *Froment's sign.* A patient with left ulnar nerve palsy attempts to hold the paper by flexing the thumb IP joint using the flexor pollicis longus and hyperextending the thumb MP joint to stabilize it. He also demonstrates flexion of the PIP joint and hyperextension of the DIP joint of the index finger to compensate for weakness of MP joint flexion of the finger (*Jeanne's sign*).

a laceration, the patient will experience tingling that radiates distally along the course of the nerve. This phenomenon is called a *Tinel's sign*. The most distal point of the pain indicates the site at which axon sprouting has occurred. Peripheral nerve recovery after a nerve injury can be assessed by observing the advancement of *Tinel's sign* along the nerve (approximately 1 mm/day of advancement).

Phalen's test

Purpose: This test is used as a provocative test specific to carpal tunnel syndrome.

Maneuver: With the elbow in neutral position, the patient's wrist is held in maximum palmar flexion for up to 2 min. This increases pressure on the carpal tunnel and provokes paresthesia in the area innervated by the median nerve in patients with carpal tunnel syndrome *(Fig. 2.11)*. Maximum extension of the wrist also increases pressure on the carpal tunnel. This is called the reverse Phalen's test.

Froment's test

Purpose: To assess the motor function of the ulnar nerve.

Maneuver: The patient is asked to hold a piece of paper between the ulnar tip of the thumb and the radial tip of the index fingers. The examiner slowly pulls the paper away from the patient while encouraging the patient to hold on it. Patients with normal strength of the first dorsal interosseous and adductor pollicis muscles keep the IP joint of the thumb extended. If the patient has weakness of thumb adduction caused by ulnar nerve palsy, the patient attempts to hold the paper by flexing the thumb IP joint using the flexor pollicis longus and (hyper)extends the thumb MP joint to stabilize it (*Jeanne's sign*). Such patients also flex the PIP joint and hyperextend the DIP joint of the index finger to compensate for weakness of MP joint flexion of the index finger *(Fig. 2.12)*.

Jeanne's sign

Purpose: To assess the motor function of the ulnar nerve.

Maneuver: When patients with ulnar nerve dysfunction attempt a lateral or key pinch of the thumb, they hyperextend the thumb MP joint, which locks it to compensate for the lateral instability of the joint secondary to weakness of the thumb adductors *(Fig. 2.12)*.

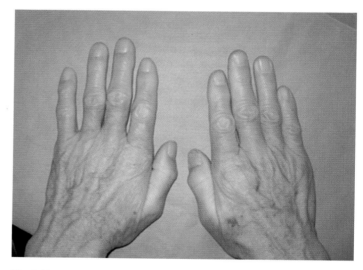

Fig. 2.13 *Wartenberg's sign.* A patient with left ulnar nerve palsy demonstrates inability to perform adduction of the left little finger when he attempts to adduct all fingers.

Wartenberg's sign

Purpose: To assess the motor function of the ulnar nerve.

Maneuver: The patient is asked to keep the fingers adducted with the MP, PIP and DIP joints fully extended. If the patient has motor dysfunction of the ulnar nerve, the small finger deviates away from the ring finger because the third palmar interosseous muscle does not function and the extensor digiti minimi muscle abducts the small finger *(Fig. 2.13)*.

Other signs associated with ulnar nerve palsy

Duchenne's sign: If the FDP muscles are functioning and the intrinsic muscles are paralyzed (low-level ulnar nerve palsy), the ring and little fingers show hyperextension of the MP joint and flexion of the PIP and DIP joints (claw finger deformity).

André–Thomas sign: A conscious effort to extend the fingers by tenodesing the extensor tendons with palmar flexion of the wrist only increases the claw deformity.

Bouvier maneuver: When hyperextension of the MP joint of the ring and little fingers is corrected, the flexion of the PIP and DIP joints of the fingers is reduced.

The Pitres–Testut sign: this sign reveals the function of the second and third interosseous muscles. The patient is asked to place the hand flat on a table and then to stretch the long finger upward (i.e., to hyperextend it) and to deviate it radially and ulnarly. See the section on interosseous and lumbrical muscles.

The "crossed fingers" sign: The function of the first palmar interosseous and the second dorsal interosseous muscles is evaluated by this sign. The patient is asked to cross a flexed long finger over the index finger or to cross a flexed index finger over the long finger when the palm and the ring and little fingers are placed flat on a table. See the section of interosseous and lumbrical muscles.

Video 6

Semmes–Weinstein monofilament test

Purpose: To evaluate the pressure perception threshold of the skin (A-β nerve fiber function). Stimuli generated by this test are mainly sensed by Merkel cells (slow-adapting mechanoreceptors).

Maneuver: Filaments of various diameters are used. The patient places a finger on a table with the palm up and closes his or her eyes. The tip of a filament is held vertically against the skin of the finger and sufficient force is applied to bend the filament before allowing it to return to the vertical position. The filament should remain in contact with the skin surface after the force is released. If the patient senses the pressure applied by the filament, other filaments of decreasing diameter are used until the patient no longer senses the pressure. The size of the smallest-diameter filament that can be sensed by the patient is recorded (*Table 2.3*).[6]

Video 9

Two-point discrimination (2PD) test

Purpose: To evaluate the tactile sensation of the skin (A-β nerve fiber function) and assess density of the perception receptors of the skin.

Maneuver: In the static 2PD test, a caliper is applied longitudinally to the digit and the smallest distance between the tips of the caliper that the patient is able to distinguish is measured. In the dynamic 2PD test, the distance between the tips

of a caliper that is moved longitudinally along the ulnar or radial aspect of the finger is measured.[5] The normal distance is 3 mm for the moving 2PD test and 6 mm for the static 2PD test. Although it is known that the main receptors for the static 2 PD test are Merkel cells (slow-adapting mechanoreceptors) and those for the moving 2 PD test are Meissner corpuscles (quick-adapting mechanoreceptors), the results of the 2PD test reflect the functions of multiple sensory receptors in the skin. It is thus difficult to detect the initial stage of a neuropathological status by using this test. This test is best for evaluation nerve lacerations.

Moberg pick-up test

Purpose: To generally evaluate the motor and sensory function of the hand. This test is applied to patients with median nerve injuries or injuries of both the ulnar and median nerves.

Maneuver: Small items such as a button, a key and a paperclip are placed on a cloth mat. The patient is asked to pick up each item and put it into a small box as quickly as possible with their eyes open and again with their eyes closed. The times required to finish these tasks are measured (*Fig. 2.14*).[4]

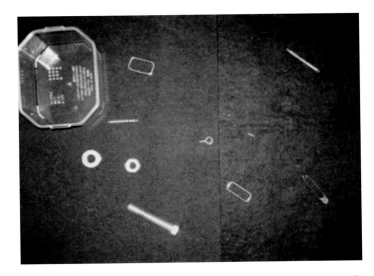

Fig. 2.14 Moberg pick-up test. A patient with eyes open or closed picks up small items on a cloth mat and puts them into the box. The time required to finish the task is recorded.

Table 2.3 Semmes–Weinstein test

Evaluator size	Pressure force (*g*)	Color	Interpretation
1.65–2.83	0.008–0.07	Green	Normal
3.32–3.61	0.16–0.4	Blue	Normal
3.84–4.31	0.6–2	Purple	Diminished light touch sensation
4.56–4.93	4–8	Red	Diminished protective sensation
5.07–6.45	10–180	Red	Loss of protective sensation
6.65	300	Red	Deep pressure sensation only

Reproduced with permission from: Bell-Krotosoki J, Tomancik E. The repeatability of testing with Semmes–Weinstein monofilaments. J Hand Surg 1987; 12A:155–161.[6]

Vascular assessment

Allen's test

Video
10

Purpose: To assess the blood supply of the radial and ulnar arteries to the hand.

Maneuver: The patient places the dorsum of the hand on a table. The examiner pushes down on the patient's radial and ulnar arteries at the wrist to occlude both arteries. The patient is then asked to make and release a tight fist repeatedly to exsanguinate the hand, after which the fingers are held in a relaxed position. The examiner releases the pressure on the radial artery while keeping pressure on the ulnar artery. The time taken for blood to return to the hand and fingers is noted. A normal interval for this process is 2–5 seconds. The procedure is repeated for the ulnar artery.[7]

Digital Allen's test

Purpose: To assess the blood supply of the radial and ulnar palmar digital arteries to the finger.

Maneuver: The patient is asked to place the dorsum of the finger to be tested flat on a table. The examiner presses down on the ulnar and radial side of the patient's fingertip with his or her two fingers and moves them proximally to exanguinate the finger to be tested. The examiner then releases the pressure on the radial palmar digital artery while maintaining pressure on the ulnar digital artery.

Video
11

The time taken for blood to return to the finger is noted. A normal interval for this process is ≤3 seconds. The procedure is repeated for the palmar ulnar digital artery of the finger. A delay in the return of blood to the finger indicates that the blood flow of the radial or ulnar palmar digital arteries is impaired.

Physical examination specific to the forearm

The main functions of the forearm are to transmit force between the elbow and hand and to enable pronation and supination. According to a cadaveric study, 80% of an axial load applied to the wrist is transmitted to the radius and 20% is transmitted to the ulna. The axial force is distributed to the radiocapitellar and ulnohumeral joints in a 60:40 ratio, respectively. Some 20% of an axial force applied to the radius is therefore transferred to the ulna through the interosseous membrane (IOM).[16] After resection of the radial head, 90% of an axial load applied to the forearm is transferred through the IOM.[17]

The interosseous membrane of the forearm (IOM)

The IOM is divided into three portions. Each portion contains several fibers that connect the radius and the ulna *(Fig. 2.15)*.[18]

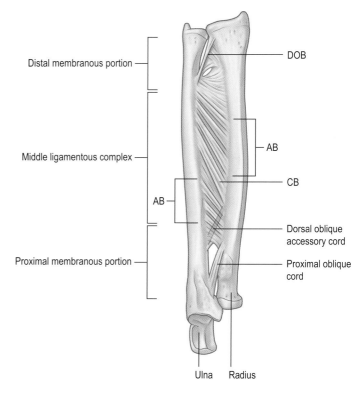

Fig. 2.15 Interosseous membrane of the forearm. DOB, dorsal oblique band; CB, central band; (DL)AB, distal ligament of accessory band; (PL)AB, proximal ligament of accessory band.

Distal membranous portion

Dorsal oblique band (DOB): This band functions as a stabilizer of the DRUJ, in particular by restricting a palmar shift of the ulna in the supination position.[19]

Middle ligamentous portion

a. Central band (CB): This is the strongest fiber of the IOM and extends from the proximal radius to the distal ulna. When the radial head removed, the CB carries 71% of the overall mechanical stiffness of the forearm.[17]

b. Distal ligament of accessory band (DLAB)

c. Proximal ligament of accessory band (PLAB)

Proximal membranous portion

a. Distal oblique accessory cord (DOAC)

b. Proximal oblique cord (POC): a stabilizer of the proximal radioulnar joint

Among these fibers, the DOB and CB are isometric components and their lengths do not change during forearm rotation. By contrast, the POC is shorter when the forearm is in a neutral or supination position than when it is in a pronation position. The length of the DOAC shortens as the forearm is rotated from pronation to supination.[20]

Measurement of forearm rotation

The patient should be seated on a chair with the elbow joints tucked in lateral to the abdomen. The patient is asked to grasp a pen in each hand and to rotate the forearm. The angle between the pen and a line perpendicular to the floor should be measured.

Measurement of the muscle strength of the forearm

Supination

The main supinators of the forearm are the supinator muscle and the biceps brachii muscle. The extensor carpi radialis longus (ECRL) and brachioradialis (BR) muscles act as the forearm supinators when the forearm is pronated.

Pronation

The main pronators are the pronator teres and pronator quadratus (PQ) muscles. The flexor carpi radialis and palmaris longus muscles also act as forearm pronators. The BR muscle is a forearm pronator when the forearm is in the supinated position. A recent study revealed that the PQ is responsible for 20% of forearm pronation, except when in the fully pronated position.[21] The muscle power of the PQ should be measured when the elbow joint is fully flexed to eliminate the effects of the other pronators.

Pronation or supination strength is evaluated with the elbow joint at 90° of flexion. Pronation strength is measured by grasping the wrist with the forearm in a neutral or supination position. To test supination strength, the forearm should be in a neutral or pronation position.

Physical examinations specific to the elbow

Bony landmarks of the elbow

The medial epicondyle, lateral epicondyle and the tip of the olecranon are located along a straight line (Hüter's line) when the elbow is extended and form an equilateral triangle (Hüter's triangle) when the elbow is flexed (*Fig. 2.16*). This feature is helpful for identifying a deformity of the distal humerus and elbow joint caused by fracture, malunion, dislocation or growth disturbances.

On the lateral aspect, the capitellum of the humerus and the radial head are easily palpable. The extensor muscles originate from the lateral epicondyle. The radial nerve is palpable in the interface between the BR muscle and the brachialis muscle.

On the anterior aspect, the cubital fossa is bordered by the BR muscle laterally and the pronator teres muscle medially. The musculocutaneous nerve is located deep to the brachioradialis muscle and medial to the biceps brachii tendon. The pulsation of the brachial artery is palpable, as it lies medial to the biceps brachii tendon and deep to the lacertus fibrosus. The median nerve is located just medial to the brachial artery

under the lacertus fibrosus, which can cause median nerve palsy (pronator teres syndrome).

In the medial aspect, the ulnar nerve groove is palpable between the medial epicondyle and the ulna. The ulna nerve is sometimes palpated as a strand in the posterior aspect of the groove. In some patients with ulnar nerve palsy, a dislocated ulnar nerve is palpable over the epicondyle when the elbow is flexed.

On the posterior aspect, the olecranon and olecranon fossa of the humerus are easily palpated. The triceps brachii tendon is attached to the olecranon.

Lateral ligament complex

The lateral ligament complex consists of the following four ligaments (*Fig. 2.17*).

Lateral ulnar collateral ligament

The lateral ulnar collateral ligament originates from the lateral epicondyle, blends with the fibers of the annular ligament and terminates at the tubercle of the crest of the supinator. It functions as a primary stabilizer of the joint when a varus stress is applied.

Radial collateral ligament

This structure originates from the lateral epicondyle and terminates in the annular ligament. The ligament is located near the axis of the elbow joint and is uniformly taut during elbow motion.

Annular ligament

This ligament originates from the anterior margin of the sigmoid notch and inserts on the posterior notch of the sigmoid of the ulna to connect the radial head to the ulna.

Accessory collateral ligament

The ligament blends with the inferior margin of the annular ligament to support the annular ligament during varus stress.

Medial collateral ligament complex

The medial collateral ligament complex consists of three portions: the anterior bundle, the posterior bundle and the transverse ligament. The transverse ligament is not considered functional. The posterior bundle is clinically insignificant with regard to the stability of the elbow joint. Contracture of the posterior bundle generates extension contracture of the elbow joint. The anterior bundle functions as the prime stabilizer of the elbow joint against valgus stress (*Fig. 2.18*).

Instability of the elbow joint

The elbow joint is stabilized by the medial collateral ligament (MCL) complex, the lateral collateral ligament (LCL) complex, the joint capsule and the osteochondral articulation.

The MCL, joint capsule and osteochondral articulation contribute equally to restrain valgus displacement of the elbow joint when the joint is extended. The MCL contributes more

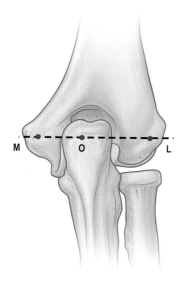

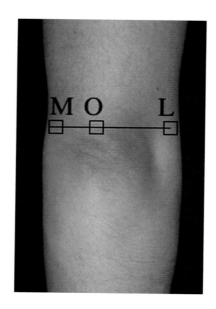

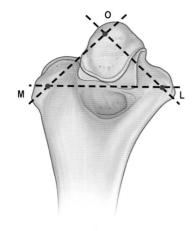

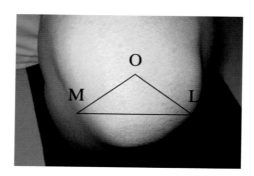

Fig. 2.16 Bony landmarks of the elbow. The medial (M) epicondyle, (L) lateral epicondyle and the tip of the (O) olecranon locate on a straight line when the elbow is extended and form an equilateral triangle when the elbow is flexed.

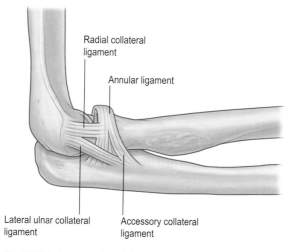

Radial collateral ligament

Annular ligament

Lateral ulnar collateral ligament

Accessory collateral ligament

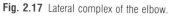

Fig. 2.17 Lateral complex of the elbow.

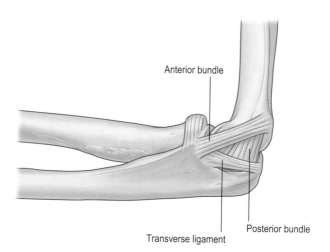

Anterior bundle

Posterior bundle

Transverse ligament

Fig. 2.18 Medial complex of the elbow.

than the osteochondral articulation to restrain valgus stress when the joint is flexed. The osteochondral articulation contributes more than the LCL to restrain varus displacement, especially in the flexed position.[22]

When examining instability of the elbow joint, the elbow should be placed in a position in which other factors that affect its stability (articulation and tension of the joint capsule) are minimized. To assess collateral ligament integrity, the elbow should be flexed by about 15°. This position relaxes the anterior capsule and unlocks the olecranon from the fossa.

Varus instability of the elbow is therefore assessed with the humerus in full internal rotation and varus stress is applied to the slightly flexed joint. By contrast, valgus instability of the elbow is evaluated with the humerus in full external rotation while valgus stress is applied to the joint in slight flexion (*Fig. 2.19*).

Posterolateral rotatory instability (PLRI)

Insufficiency (loosening, rupture or laceration) of the lateral ulnar collateral ligament causes posterolateral instability of the elbow joint. PLRI is evaluated using the pivot shift test maneuver.[23]

The pivot shift test maneuver

The patient is placed in a supine position with the shoulder and elbow flexed at 90°. The examiner stands cephalad to the patient. The examiner grasps the patient's forearm in a fully supinated position and extends the elbow slowly, applying valgus and axial compressions to the joint. If the patient has lateral collateral ligament insufficiency, these maneuvers cause rotatory subluxation in the ulnohumeral joint. The examiner continues to extend the elbow slowly. As the elbow joint approaches extension, the radial head is suddenly dislocated anteriorly. The prominence of the radial head disappears and a skin dimple appears. The dislocated radial head is repositioned by flexion of the elbow (*Fig. 2.20*).

Measurement of malrotation of the distal humerus

Patients in whom fractures of the distal humerus have not been treated correctly often demonstrate malrotation of the distal humerus, which restricts the functional arc of the shoulder joint. Malrotation of the distal humerus is easily assessed. The patient is asked to stand and flex the trunk more than 90° forward. The patient is then asked to extend both shoulder joints maximally with the elbow joints in 90° of flexion. The angles formed between the floor and the forearms are measured. The malrotation angle of the affected distal humerus can be measured by comparing it with that of the contralateral normal side (*Fig. 2.21*).

Physical examination of thoracic outlet syndrome

Thoracic outlet syndrome (TOS) is a broad term that refers to compression of the neurovascular structures in the area just above the first rib and behind the clavicle resulting in

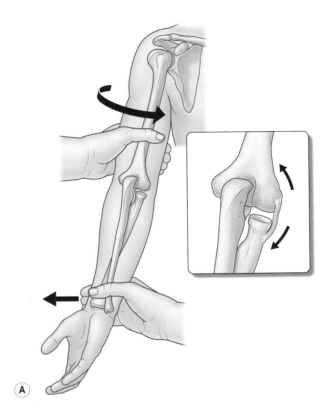
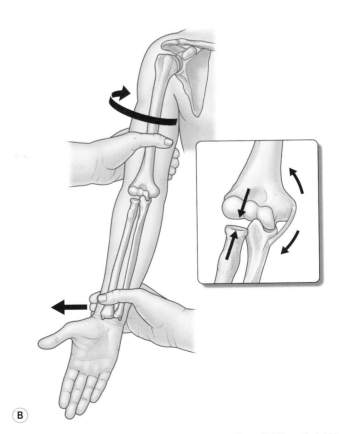

Fig. 2.19 Assessment of the lateral instability of the elbow. **(A)** Varus instability of the elbow is examined with the humerus in full internal rotation. **(B)** Valgus instability is assessed with the humerus in full external rotation.

Subluxation

Axial compression   Valgus

Supination

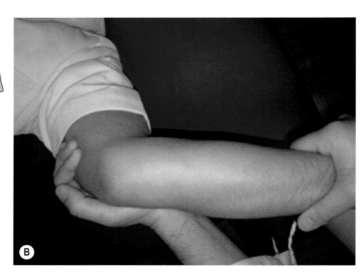

(A)

(B)

Fig. 2.20 Pivotal shift test of the elbow. **(A,B)** Subluxation.

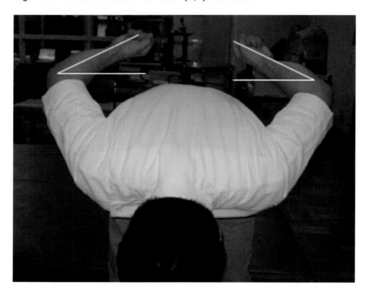

Fig. 2.21 Assessment of malrotation of the humerus. The patient is asked to stand and flex the trunk more than 90° forward with the bilateral shoulder joints extended maximally and the elbow joints in 90° of flexion. The angles formed between the floor and the forearms are measured.

upper extremity symptoms. It represents a constellation of symptoms.

Classification

TOS is usually classified into two groups: neurogenic group and vascular group. The neurogenic group is caused by compression or irritation of the brachial plexus trunks and comprises 90% of the TOS. The neurogenic type can be divided into three types, depending on involvement of cervical nerve roots; the upper type (C5, C6, C7 spinal nerve involvement), lower type (C8, T1 spinal nerve involvement) and the combined type. The lower and combined types comprise 85–90% of all patients with TOS. 40–50% of TOS is associated with

distal compression neuropathies, such as carpal tunnel, pronator teres, cubital tunnel and radial tunnel syndromes.[24]

The vascular group is subtyped into the venous type and arterial type. The venous type comprises 70–80% of the vascular group of TOS. The symptom include pain, swelling, distended vein and discoloration of the affected upper limb. Compression of the subclavian vein does not occur in the interscalene space because it passes anterior to the anterior scalene muscle, but usually occurs at the area between the anterior scalene insertion to the first rib and at the costocoracoid ligament and subclavius tendon insertion of the first rib. This type sometimes develops into thrombosis formation in the subclavian vein (Paget–Schroetter syndrome). The arterial type comprises only 20–30% of the vascular group and occurs direct pressure of the cervical rib, or an abnormal middle scalene muscle to the first rib, or anomalous band-like structure under the subclavian artery.[24]

Anatomy

The brachial plexus trunks and subclavian vessels are subject to compression or irritation in three spaces at the thoracic outlet region. The most important of these spaces is the interscalene space (triangle), which is also the most proximal. This space is bordered by the anterior scalene muscle anteriorly, the middle scalene muscle posteriorly, and the medial surface of the first rib inferiorly. This area may be small at rest and may become even smaller in the posture with elevation or hyperabduction of the upper limb, which moves the scapula posteroinferiorly, resulting in the access of the clavicle to the first rib. The anomalous structures, such as fibrous bands, cervical ribs, and anomalous muscles, may constrict this space further. The second space is the costoclavicular space, which is bordered anteriorly by the middle third of the clavicle, posteromedially by the first rib, and posterolaterally by the upper border of the scapula. The last space is the subpectoralis minor space beneath the coracoid process just deep to the pectoralis minor tendon *(Fig. 2.22)*. Trauma to the neck, shoulder girdle, and upper extremity, particularly the lower trunk

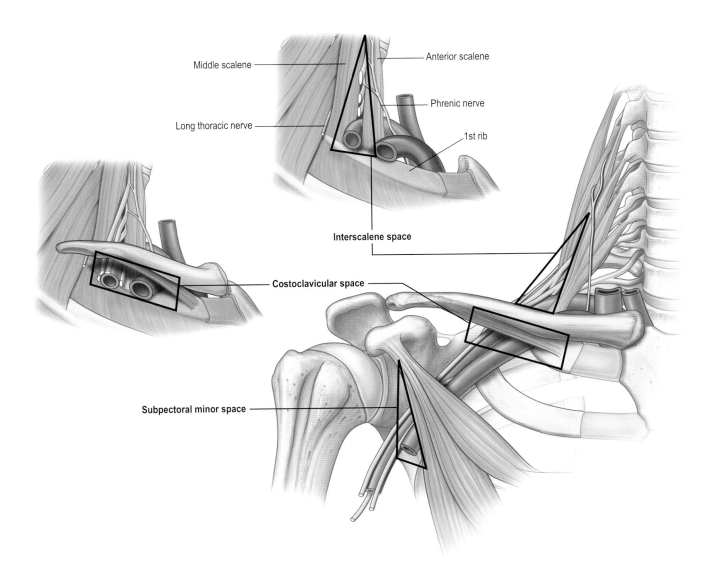

Middle scalene

Anterior scalene

Phrenic nerve

Long thoracic nerve

1st rib

Interscalene space

Costoclavicular space

Subpectoral minor space

Fig. 2.22 The three spaces that potentially entrap the neurovascular bundle in patients with the thoracic outlet syndrome.

and C8–T1 spinal nerves, is thought to play an important role in developing the symptoms of thoracic outlet syndrome. The trauma can be a single blow or a repetitive, strenuous type. The initiation of the symptoms has 70–80% history of trauma.[24]

Provocative maneuver

Adson test

The patient is asked to inhale deeply with the chin up and tilt the neck toward the involved arm holding the breath. If the radial artery pulsation disappears or is diminished, the test is positive.[25] This test is considered sensitive to compression in the interscalenus space *(Fig. 2.23)*.

The neck tilting

The patient is asked to inhale deeply and tilt the neck to the opposite direction of the involved arm holding the breath. In patients with TOS, this action produces arm heaviness, numbness and tingling in the fingers or/and arm, with some pain.

The costoclavicular compression test

The patient is asked to inhale deeply and hold the breath. The examiner depresses the patient's shoulder of the involved limb. Patients with TOS complain of symptoms such as heaviness, pain, numbness or tingling in the limb and the pulsation of the radial artery is often diminished. This maneuver calls attention to compression in the costoclavicular space *(Fig. 2.24)*.

Wright test

The examiner holds the patient's arm in 90° abduction with the elbow 90° flexed, and rotates the arm externally. If the pulsation is diminished and the symptoms are provoked by this maneuver, the test is positive.[26] Entrapment of the neurovascular bundle at the subpectoralis minor space or the costoclavicular space can make the test positive *(Fig. 2.25)*.

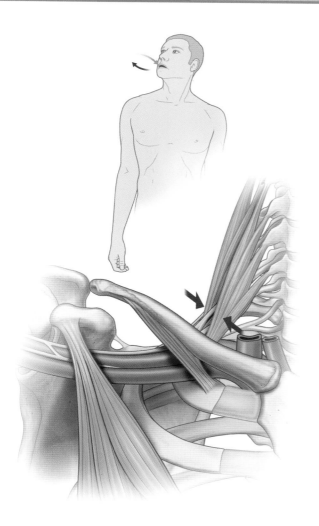

Fig. 2.23 Adson test is sensitive to entrapment of the neurovascular bundle in the interscalene space (arrows) by Adson test.

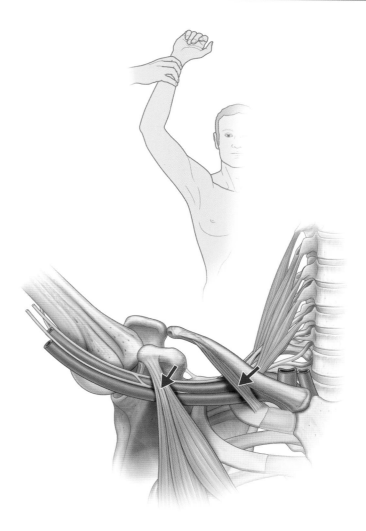

Fig. 2.25 The neurovascular bundle can be potentially entrapped in the costoclavicular space (red arrow) and the subpectoralis minor space (black arrow) by Wright test.

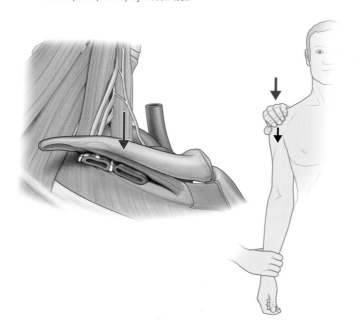

Fig. 2.24 The costoclavicular compression test is considered to detect the entrapment in the costoclavicular space (arrow).

Roos extended arm stress test

Video 17

The patient is asked to hold both arms with the shoulders in 90°-abduction and 90°-external rotation position and open and close the hands repetitively. If the patient develops any fatigue, pain, numbness or tingling in the hand or arm within three minutes, the test is positive.[27]

Morley's test

The patient complains of pain, numbness, tingling or uncomfortable feelings when the examiner pushes the patient's brachial plexus in the supraclavicular fossa.

These provocative tests should be performed on the bilateral upper limbs and the outcomes of the involved limb should be compared with those of the opposite one, because the tests can be positive in a normal person.

Physical examination of the upper extremity in children

Communication with very young children is often difficult or impossible and young children are not able to articulate their symptoms. A fatty subcutaneous tissue layer often prevents doctors from identifying a deformity or swelling. It is often difficult to locate the source of pain because children tend to complain that the pain is everywhere. Questioning of the parents and family of the patient is sometimes helpful for making a diagnosis. Physical examination should include observing the child's activities when he or she is held by a parent or is playing. Valuable information in terms of the usage and dexterity of the upper extremity can be obtained by observing children playing with age-appropriate toys or props. The affected limb should be examined from the tip of fingers to the hemithorax, which should be compared with the contralateral limb to confirm the anomaly. The physical examination should include not only a musculoskeletal examination but also a nervous system examination. Primitive reflexes, including the Moro reflex, the systemic tonic neck response, the mouth lip reflex and palmar grasp stimulation are used to assess neuromuscular function in newborns. As these patients age, gross movement patterns and integration of the affected hand into functional activities can be assessed.

Access the complete reference list online at **http://www.expertconsult.com**

2. Ranade AV, Rai R, Prabhu LV, et al. Incidence of extensor digitorum brevis manus muscle. *Hand (NY)*. 2008;3:320–323.

   Small vestigial extensor tendons are sometimes found in the long and ring fingers besides the extensor digitorum communis tendons, which are called the extensor digitorum brevis manus. This muscle is often found as a soft tissue mass and sometimes causes pain in the dorsum of the hand.

10. Watson HK, Ryu J, Akelman E. Limited triscaphoid intercarpal arthrodesis for rotatory subluxation of the scaphoid. *J Bone Joint Surg*. 1968;68:245–349.

    Watson described his original maneuver of the so-called "scaphoid test" in this article. This maneuver has been modified by several authors and is now recognized as the "scaphoid shift test", which is a useful physiological examination to identify the instability of the scapholunate ligament complex.

14. Kleinman WB. Stability of the distal radioulnar joint: Biomechanics, pathophysiology, physical diagnosis and restoration of function what we have learned in 25 years. *J Hand Surg*. 2007;32A:1086–1106.

    The author describes detailed anatomy and biomechanics of the ulnar side of the wrist, including the TFCC. The deep layer of the distal radioulnar ligament plays an important role to stabilize the distal radioulnar joint. The dorsal deep layer of the ligament becomes tight in the supinated forearm and the palmar deep layer increases the strain in the pronated forearm.

17. Hotchkiss RN, An KN, Sowa DT, et al. An anatomic and mechanical study of the interosseous membrane of the forearm: pathomechanics of proximal migration of the radius. *J Hand Surg*. 1989;14A:256–261.

    When the radial head was resected, 90% of the axial load applied to the wrist joint was transmitted to the ulna through the interosseous membrane. The central band of the interosseous membrane provided 71% of the overall mechanical stiffness of the forearm.

23. O'Driscoll SW, Bell DF, Morrey BF. Posterolateral rotatory instability of the elbow. *J Bone Joint Surg*. 1991;73A:440–446.

    The authors addressed grades of dislocation of the joint caused by lateral ligament insufficiency (from instability of the joint to complete dislocation) and described a maneuver of the pivot shift test that was provocative of the elbow dislocation due to the lateral ligament instability.

3

Diagnostic imaging of the hand and wrist

Alphonsus K. Chong and David M.K. Tan

SYNOPSIS

- Radiographs form the cornerstone of diagnostic imaging of the hand and wrist, and are usually the first imaging modalities performed following clinical evaluation.
- The keys to obtaining the most information from radiographs are ordering the correct radiographs for the situation, and ensuring the radiograph is appropriately taken.
- A systematic and careful examination of the radiograph is necessary to glean the often subtle findings in the hand and wrist.
- Clinical evaluation with plain radiographs often provides sufficient information for clinical decision-making.
- Computed tomography (CT) scans, ultrasound, magnetic resonance imaging (MRI) and other advanced imaging modalities can supplement information from plain radiographs in selected situations. On occasion, they may be the primary imaging performed.
- These advanced imaging modalities allow today's clinician to visualize disorders that would previously have required open surgery or biopsy.

 Access the Historical Perspective section online at
http://www.expertconsult.com

- Technological advances in many advanced imaging modalities like ultrasound, CT, and MRI, has led to them being applied for use in the hand and wrist. This increases clinician choices for diagnostic imaging of a suspected clinical condition.
- The radiograph, despite its simplicity and age, still forms the foundation of imaging of hand and wrist conditions. In many clinical situations, an appropriately chosen and well-taken set of radiographs may be all the diagnostic imaging required.
- The key to obtaining the most information from a radiograph is to understand which radiographs are appropriate for each clinical situation, and how to obtain good-quality radiographs for evaluation.
- Advanced imaging modalities may then be ordered to provide additional information for decision-making.
- This chapter will equip the reader with practical information about the different imaging modalities available for the hand and wrist.
- It will start from the foundation of radiographs, covering the appropriate views, how they are taken, and how best to evaluate them. From this foundation, the advanced imaging techniques will be described in turn, emphasizing their applications in the hand and wrist.

Introduction

- A proper and directed history-taking followed by a careful examination of both hands and wrists forms the foundation of a clinical differential diagnosis in hand conditions.
- Appropriate investigations are then ordered to help confirm the clinical diagnosis.
- Diagnostic imaging modalities are often the first-line investigations ordered, as many clinical conditions in the hand and wrist can be seen visually.

Radiography

Radiography is the cornerstone in diagnostic imaging of the hand and wrist. It should be the first imaging modality for the diagnosis of most hand and wrist disorders.[2] The plain radiograph is cheap in relation to other imaging modalities, technically easy to perform, and widely available. The correct radiograph taken in an appropriate manner provides much imaging information to the attending clinician. In many hand and wrist conditions, radiography may also be the only imaging modality required for definitive diagnosis and assessment.

Evaluation of the hand

The three basic radiographs to evaluate the hand are: posteroanterior, oblique, and true lateral views. The radiographs should be performed in a standardized fashion to allow proper evaluation *(Figs 3.1 and 3.2)*. Specialized views are required to assess specific areas not well seen in the above views. The posteroanterior hand view provides a useful overview of the skeletal structure of the hand. Fractures, osseous tumors, and even soft-tissue masses *(Fig. 3.3)* can be seen on this view. The oblique view of the hand is useful to assess the metacarpals, as a true lateral view of the hand will lead to an overlapping of the second to fifth metacarpals. In the common boxer's or fifth metacarpal neck fracture, this view allows an assessment of the amount of angulation of the fracture.

In hand radiographs, begin by assessing the overall alignment of the metacarpals and phalanges. The individual bones should then be evaluated in terms of cortical shape and integrity, as well as bony quality. Fractures are usually easy to detect, although a careful review is necessary in the case of undisplaced or minimally displaced fractures. Osseous tumors are identified by an area of different lucency in the bone. There may be changes in the outline of the bone. Enchondromas are common benign bony tumors in the hand. They can result in pathological fractures, so an assessment of the bone for such pathology should be done, particularly if the trauma resulting in the injury is trivial *(Fig. 3.4)*. Osteomyelitis typically occurs in the hand following open injuries *(Fig. 3.5)*.

The joints should then be assessed, starting from the carpometacarpal joints (CMCJs) and working distally. The CMCJs may be dislocated following injury. These injuries are uncommon but are difficult to diagnose. In a normal hand X-ray the second to fifth CMCJs should be clearly visible on the posteroanterior view *(Fig. 3.6)*.[3] The loss of these features in the second to fifth CMCJs is usually due to a fracture dislocation of one or more of the CMCJs. However, an improperly performed hand radiograph can also give this impression.

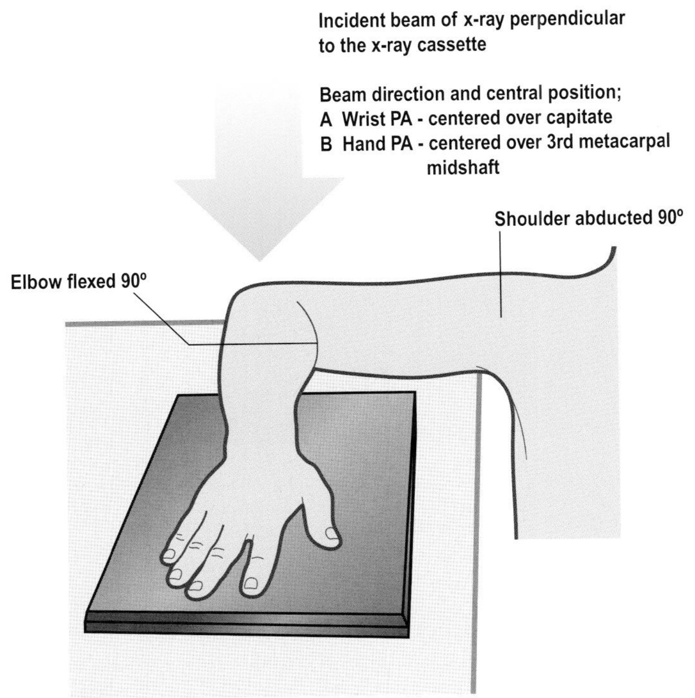

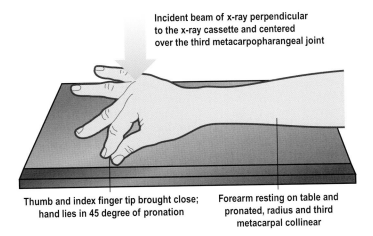

Fig. 3.1 The posteroanterior (PA) radiograph of the hand and wrist is taken in the position shown. For the hand radiograph, the beam is centered over the midshaft of the third metacarpal. For the wrist radiograph, it is centered over the capitate.

Incident beam of x-ray perpendicular to the x-ray cassette

Beam direction and central position;
A Wrist PA - centered over capitate
B Hand PA - centered over 3rd metacarpal midshaft

Shoulder abducted 90°

Elbow flexed 90°

Incident beam of x-ray perpendicular to the x-ray cassette and centered over the third metacarpopharangeal joint

Thumb and index finger tip brought close; hand lies in 45 degree of pronation

Forearm resting on table and pronated, radius and third metacarpal collinear

Fig. 3.2 The oblique hand radiograph is taken with the hand positioned as shown. This position provides a good nonoverlapping view of the metacarpals. The view is not adequate for assessment of the digits; separate lateral views of the digits should be performed if necessary.

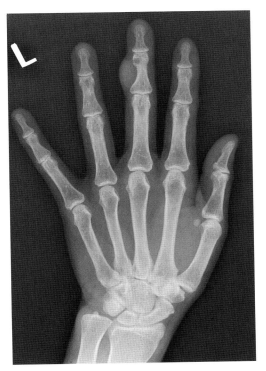

Fig. 3.3 This female patient presented with a soft-tissue mass over the ulnar side of the middle finger. The radiograph shows the outline of the soft-tissue mass with scalloping of the ulnar border of the middle phalanx. Histology of the mass showed this to be a pigmented villonodular synovitis.

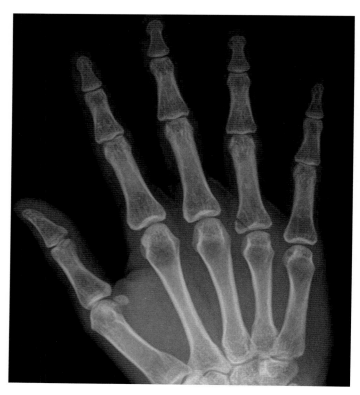

Fig. 3.4 This nurse presented with pain at the base of her right ring finger after transferring a patient from his bed to a chair. The radiograph shows a partial articular fracture of the base of the proximal phalanx of the right ring finger. The area of lucency just at the fracture site and minor trauma were suspicious for a pathological fracture.

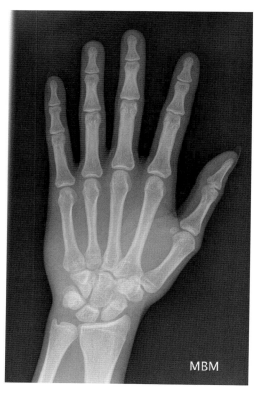

Fig. 3.6 In a normal hand radiograph, the second to fifth carpometacarpal joints should be well visualized, as shown. The articular surfaces should be profiled without overlap, parallel to each other, and have distinct cortical rims.

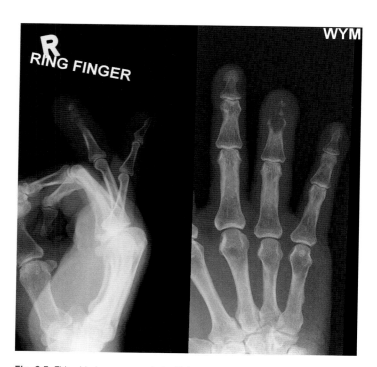

Fig. 3.5 This elderly man presented with increasing pain and redness in the finger. The radiograph shows a destructive lesion of the distal phalanx and head of the middle phalanx. This is consistent with osteomyelitis. A differential diagnosis would be that of a malignant bone tumor. These are much rarer, and usually due to metastatic disease in terminally ill patients.

Fisher *et al.* described a systematic approach to evaluating the posteroanterior view of the hand for dislocations of the fourth and fifth CMCJs.[3] In subluxation of the fifth CMCJ, the base of the fifth metacarpal is usually offset ulnarly compared to the hamate *(Fig. 3.7)*. Several views have been suggested to confirm this diagnosis. The true lateral of the hand provides a useful way to assess the CMCJ for any signs of dislocation and oblique views may also be helpful[4,5]; if the diagnosis is still uncertain, a CT scan of the hand including the CMCJs will confirm the diagnosis.[6] The more distal joints are then evaluated, from the metacarpophalangeal joints to the proximal interphalangeal joints and distal interphalangeal joints. A normal joint should be completely congruent with a visible joint space.

Osteoarthritis commonly affects the interphalangeal joints and thumb CMCJs. It is often demonstrable on radiographs by narrowing of the joint space, subchondral sclerosis, osteophytes, and deformity *(Fig. 3.8)*.

Special views in the hand

A true lateral radiograph of the finger is needed to complete an assessment of the digit. Hand radiographs alone are insufficient for assessment. This is because the oblique view of the hand does not provide an adequate lateral profile of the digit and interphalangeal joint spaces to supplement the posteroanterior view. With only a posteroanterior view, subtle fractures, fracture displacement, or joint subluxation of the fingers may not be apparent.

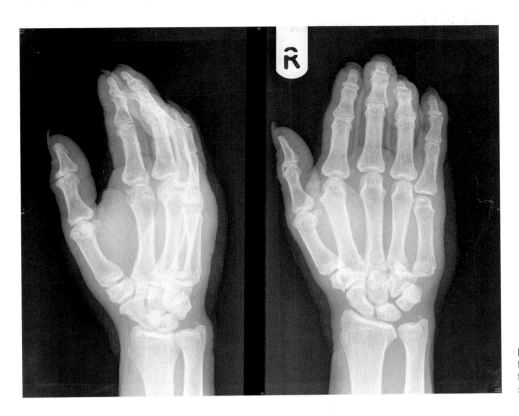

Fig. 3.7 This radiograph shows a dislocation of the fifth carpometacarpal joint. Note the ulnar offset of the fifth metacarpal with loss of the normal articular space.

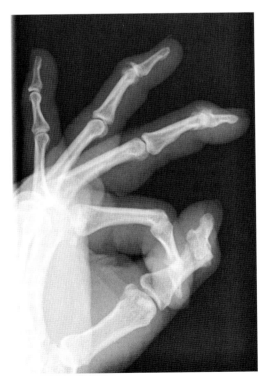

Fig. 3.8 Osteoarthritis of the distal interphalangeal joints of middle and ring fingers. There is loss of joint space, and osteophytes are clearly seen on this lateral view.

To assess the thumb, specialized views are also necessary as the thumb lies in an oblique plane relative to the other digits in the usual hand radiograph. A true posteroanterior and lateral view of the thumb is obtained to allow proper radiographic assessment of the thumb. One common condition in the thumb for which radiographs are performed is that of basal joint or trapeziometacarpal joint (TMCJ) arthritis *(Fig. 3.9)*. This condition is graded radiologically using the Eaton classifcation.[7] However, the irregular saddle shape of the trapezium makes visualization of the bone difficult. Multiple and specialized views of the TMCJ will help *(Box 3.1)*.[8] The thumb base is also the site of a fracture subluxation of the first CMCJ, also known as a "Bennett's fracture."

The ulnar collateral ligament of the thumb metacarpophalangeal joint is commonly injured in forceful thumb abduction.[9] Less commonly the radial collateral ligament may also be injured. Lateral stress application during the posteroanterior thumb radiograph can be helpful to assess if the ligament injuries are complete or partial. Ultrasonography and MRI are alternatives to assess this injury.[10,11]

Pediatric hand radiographs

Evaluation of the pediatric hand, especially after injury, is often more difficult than in adults. There are several reasons for this. Firstly, clinical evaluation in children is more difficult, the more so the younger the child. It may not be possible to localise the site of the problem clearly, e.g., the site of injury following trauma. Secondly, the staggered ossification of the various carpal bones *(Fig. 3.10)* and the presence of the growth

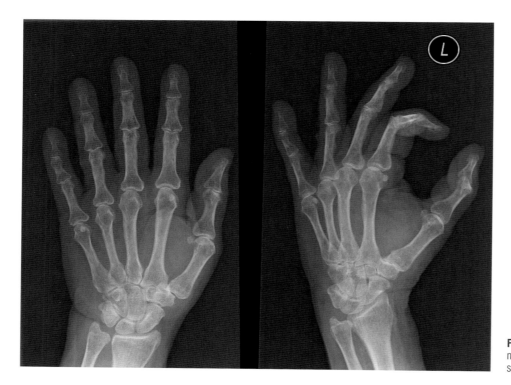

Fig. 3.9 The trapeziometacarpal joint shows narrowing of the joint space with osteophytes and joint subluxation.

Box 3.1 **Special views for the trapeziometacarpal joint (TMCJ)**

The true anteroposterior view of the TMCJ (Roberts view) is taken with the thumb dorsum on the cassette with the forearm in maximum pronation and the beam angled 15° from the vertical. The Betts/Gedda view of the thumb (true lateral of TMCJ) may help to improve the assessment of the classification of TMCJ arthritis.[8] This is performed with the palm on the cassette, and the forearm slightly pronated. The beam is angled about 5–10° in a distal to proximal projection.

plate may confuse the examiner as to whether a fracture is present or not. Finally, in the young child, proper standardized views may be difficult to obtain. Where the clinical suspicion remains high and the films obtained are inadequate, the radiograph should be repeated, either the same day or at another time when the patient is more cooperative. Similar views taken of the opposite uninjured limb are also helpful for evaluation.

Growth plate-related injuries are common in children. These injuries can be classified according to the system described by Salter and Harris **(Fig. 3.11)**.[12] The Salter–Harris type II fracture injury is the most common type of growth plate injury seen in the hand.

Wrist evaluation

A properly performed set of orthogonal wrist radiographs forms the basis of an effective evaluation of the wrist.[13,14] This is especially important when indices are being measured. The wrist has numerous asymmetrically arranged bones, so a methodical assessment of the bones, joints, and overall alignment of the wrist is necessary.

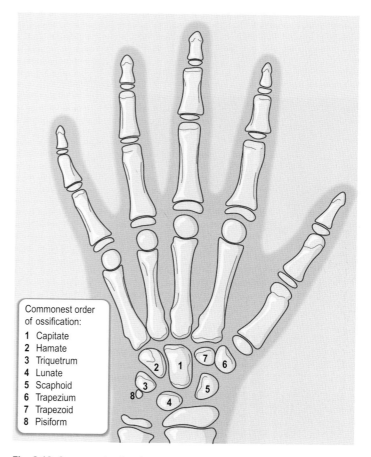

Commonest order of ossification:
1 Capitate
2 Hamate
3 Triquetrum
4 Lunate
5 Scaphoid
6 Trapezium
7 Trapezoid
8 Pisiform

Fig. 3.10 Commonest order of ossification: capitate, hamate, triquetrum, lunate, scaphoid, trapezium, trapezoid, and pisiform. Note the position of the growth plates on the proximal ends of the phalanges and first metacarpal. In the remaining ulnar four metacarpals, the growth plate is on the distal end of the bone.

Obtaining proper views for wrist radiographs *(Figs 3.1, 3.12, and see Fig. 3.17, below)* requires careful positioning which may be difficult to achieve in patients with pain or limitations in motion of the affected upper limb *(Box 3.2)*.

The wrist radiograph is first evaluated by checking the overall alignment of the bones of the wrist, starting with the distal radius and ulna, progressing to the carpal bones and metacarpal bases. Gilula described three smooth arcs made by the articular surfaces of the proximal and distal carpal row bones in a normal wrist posteroanterior radiograph *(Fig. 3.13)*.[15] A loss of the normal contour usually indicates a disruption in the normal arrangement of these carpal bones. A

common cause of this is a perilunate dislocation *(Fig. 3.14)*. Lunotriquetral (LT) instability is another cause of the loss of the normal Gilula's lines. Care must be taken when interpreting these findings in an asymptomatic patient as radial or ulnar deviation of the wrist can introduce a break in the arcs.[16]

Box 3.2 **Assessing quality of wrist radiographs**

There are criteria for acceptable wrist views. The posteroanterior view is assessed using the position of the ulnar styloid and extensor carpi ulnaris tendon groove.[13] The lateral view is assessed using the radioulnar overlap and scaphopisocapitate relationships.[14]

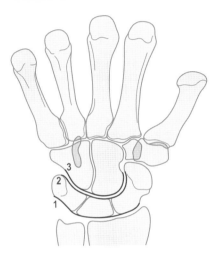

Fig. 3.13 In a normal posteroanterior wrist radiograph, three smooth curved nonoverlapping lines can be drawn on the proximal and distal cortical surfaces of the proximal carpal bones (lines 1 and 2) and proximal surface of the distal carpal row (line 3). A disruption or stepoff indicates a loss of the normal carpal bone relationships.

Fig. 3.11 (A–E) The Salter–Harris classification of epiphyseal plate injuries. (Redrawn after Salter RB, Harris R. Injuries involving the epiphyseal plate. J Bone Joint Surg Am 1963;45:587–621.)

Most common

Crush injury of growth plate

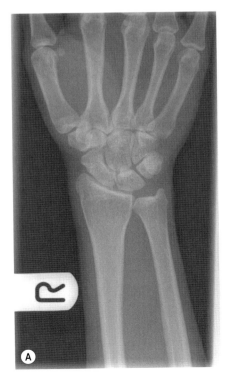

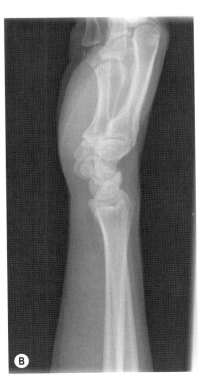

Fig. 3.12 Normal wrist radiograph. **(A)** In the posteroanterior view, note the lateral position of the ulnar styloid and position of the extensor carpi ulnaris groove. It lies radial to the straight line that passes tangential to the radial edge of the ulnar styloid at the fovea. This indicates a good posteroanterior view. **(B)** On the lateral view, there is good radioulnar overlap.

The overall relationship between the different bones can also be assessed using two common parameters: the carpal height ratio and ulnar variance. These provide a quantitative assessment of the structural integrity of the carpal rows, and the relationship of the distal radius and ulna articular surfaces respectively.

The carpal height ratio *(Fig. 3.15)*[17,18] gives a measure of the distance between the distal articular surface of the radius to the proximal articular surface of the third metacarpal base. A loss of this distance is seen in collapse of a carpal bone, for example Kienbock's disease (avascular necrosis (AVN) of the lunate) or in malrotation of the carpal bones, for example in rheumatoid arthritis or scapholunate (SL) dissociation. A ratio is used instead of actual dimensions to correct for variability in carpal bone sizes.

The ulnar variance provides a measure of the height difference between distal radius and ulnar articular surfaces. There are several ways to measure the ulnar variance.[19,20] We prefer the technique of the perpendiculars *(Fig. 3.16)*. It is easy to perform and has been shown to have higher intra- and inter-observer reliability.[21]

A proper lateral radiograph of the wrist *(Fig. 3.12 and 3.17)* is the first necessary imaging for the evaluation of a suspected distal radioulnar joint (DRUJ) instability. Radiographic findings associated with this injury include widening of the DRUJ, a fracture of the ulnar styloid base, or a displaced fracture from the ulna fovea. On the lateral view, there is loss of the normal radioulnar overlap. A comparison radiograph of the contralateral normal wrist is helpful if the findings are unclear. The application of volar or dorsal-directed stress is also helpful in cases of suspected DRUJ instability *(Fig. 3.18)*.

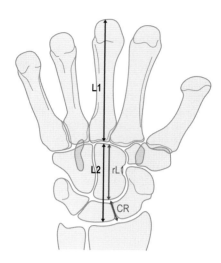

Fig. 3.15 (1) Carpal height ratio = carpal height (L2)/third metacarpal length (L1). Nnormal is 0.54 ± 0.03. (2) Revised carpal height ratio = carpal height (L2)/ heights of capitate (rL1). (3) Capitate–radius index (CR). This is the shortest line between two eccentric arches of the carpal rows. The line is moved until the shortest distance is measured. Mean CR index 0.999 ± 0.034. Values less than 0.92 are abnormal.

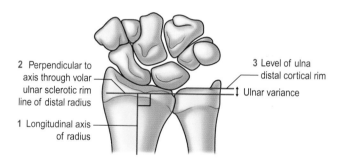

Fig. 3.16 Ulnar variance is measured on a true neutral posteroanterior view of the wrist. First a line along the longitudinal axis of the radius is drawn. Next a line perpendicular to this line through the volar ulnar sclerotic rim of the distal radius is drawn. Finally a line parallel to this second line at the level of the distal cortical rim of the ulna is drawn. The distance between these two parallel lines is the ulnar variance.

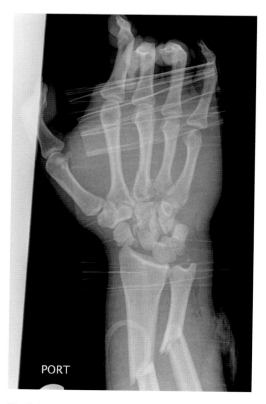

Fig. 3.14 This radiograph shows a perilunate fracture dislocation with disruption of the normal smooth carpal arcs. There are associated radioulnar shaft fractures.

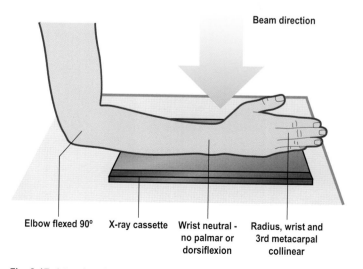

Fig. 3.17 A true lateral view of wrist is taken in the position shown.

Fractures involving the forearm bones are the commonest fractures encountered in the emergency room.[22] Of these, distal radius fractures form one of the largest groups of fractures. Loss of the normal distal radius indices (*Figs 3.19 and 3.20*) due to fracture displacement can affect final outcome. Intra-articular distal radius fractures are commonly treated with plates and screws close to the articular surface. Conventional wrist views do not allow accurate assessment of screw position, particularly to check if the screws are in the radiocarpal joint. This is because standard views do not

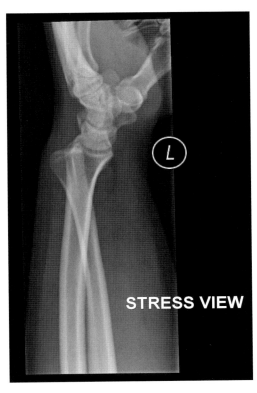

Fig. 3.18 Stress view true lateral of the wrist. Notice the loss of radioulnar overlap due to the dorsal subluxation of the distal radioulnar joint. The pisiform lies between the volar aspect of the scaphoid and capitate, so the view is accurate.

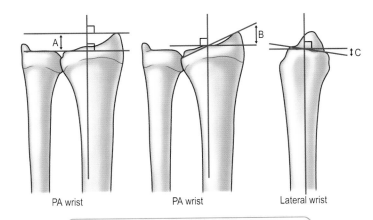

A: Radial height. Normal = 11-12mm, Range = 8-18mm
B: Radial inclination. Normal = 22-23°, Range = 13-30°
C: Volar tilt. Normal = 11-12°, Range = 0-28°

Fig. 3.19 Normal distal radius indices. (A) Radial height: normal = 11–12 mm, range = 8–18 mm. (B) Radial inclination: normal = 22–23°, range = 13–30°. (C) Volar tilt: normal = 11–12°, range = 0–28°. PA, posteroanterior.

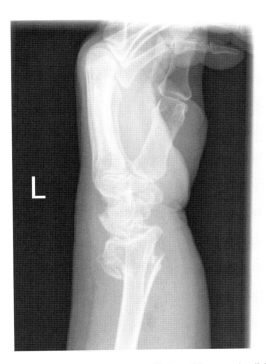
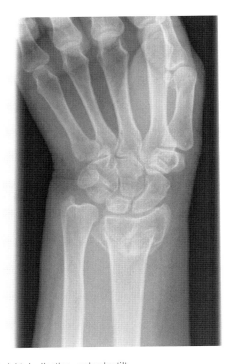

Fig. 3.20 Distal radius fracture with loss of the normal radial height, inclination, and volar tilt.

compensate for the normal anatomic tilt of the radius. Lateral radiographs angled 11° posteroanterior and 22° *(Fig. 3.21)* enable tangential X-ray exposure to the articular surface and facilitate this assessment after fixation.

Scaphoid fractures are the commonest carpal bone injuries. The shape of the scaphoid bone does not lend itself well to interrogation by just two orthogonal views, so a "scaphoid series" of X-rays is usually done *(Fig. 3.22 and Box 3.3)*.

Fractures of the hook of the hamate are uncommon but disabling. A carpal tunnel view is helpful to diagnose this injury *(Fig. 3.23)*, although a CT scan can also provide the definitive diagnosis.

Injuries to the wrist ligaments, for example the SL ligament, can lead to carpal instability. In severe cases, this can be seen on the usual wrist views as loss of the normal relationships between the carpal bones. In SL instability, this is typically seen as a dorsal intercalated segmental instability deformity *(Fig. 3.24)* with an increase in the SL angle, and dorsal tilt in the radiolunate angles *(Fig. 3.25)*. However, in milder forms of instability, application of loads and/or positioning of the wrist are necessary to bring out these dynamic changes in carpal relationships. The clenched-fist posteroanterior views of the wrist are one technique used to diagnose dynamic carpal instability *(Fig. 3.26)*.

Ulnar abutment syndrome is a common cause of ulnar-sided wrist pain. The use of a clenched-fist pronated view of the wrist enhances the ulnar variance and may demonstrate the abutment *(Fig. 3.27)*.[23]

Video 1

The availability of fluoroscopy in many clinics and operating rooms allows the dynamic assessment of many hand and wrist conditions. Smaller, lower cost and radiation[24] mini c-arms have also lowered the barrier to acquiring such facilities. The clinician can operate the c-arm to obtain the best

Box 3.3　Scaphoid series

The scaphoid view of the wrist addresses the normal foreshortening of the scaphoid seen on the conventional posteroanterior wrist radiograph. The view is taken with the wrist ulnarly deviated and the X-ray tube angled 20–30°. Several other views are helpful for assessment of the scaphoid: a pronated oblique view (to view the distal third and tubercle of the scaphoid better), a supinated view (to assess the dorsoradial ridge of scaphoid and pisiotriquetral articulation), and a lateral view to help assess a humpback deformity.

Box 3.4　Special view for ulnar abutment syndrome

Ulnar abutment syndrome is a common cause of ulnar-sided wrist pain. The use of a clenched-fist pronated view of the wrist enhances the ulnar variance and may demonstrate the abutment *(Fig. 3.27)*.[23]

view and view changes in the relationships of the bones "live" with motion, loading, or application of stress. Fluoroscopy is helpful for assessing carpal instability, including SL injuries[25] (see video), guiding percutaneous insertion of implants, and assessing the position of implants *(Box 3.4)*.[26]

Ultrasonography

Diagnostic ultrasound has advanced much recently. New ultrahigh-frequency probes and smaller probe sizes allow higher-quality images of the hand and wrist.[27] Ultrasound's safety, portability, and relatively low cost have led to wider use, especially by clinicians operating the machines themselves.[28] One additional advantage over other forms of imaging, like CT scanning or MRI, is that it allows dynamic and real-time assessment. The addition of Doppler imaging enhances the information provided by the ultrasound study.[27]

Ultrasound uses the acoustic properties of generated sound waves to form images.[28] The ultrasound transducer generates the sound waves in pulses. When the transducer is applied over the surface of the part to be examined, the sound waves pass through tissues. At the junction of two tissues, an acoustic interface occurs. When the sound waves meet an acoustic interface, some of the sound wave energy is reflected, while the rest continue to be transmitted deeper. The greater the differences in material properties of the adjacent tissues, the more energy is reflected. The reflected sound wave is received in the transducer. This is then converted to an electrical signal for processing. The greater the sound reflected, the larger the amplitude of the reflected wave, and consequently, the brighter the image.

Ultrasound has its disadvantages *(Table 3.1)*. It only allows a small field of view, so is best used for a focused examination of a small area. Differentiation of different soft-tissue tumors of the hand and wrist, apart from ganglia, is also inadequate.[29] The problem of anisotropy can lead to reduced echogenicity when tendons are being imaged. Anisotropy is a phenomenon where the echogenicity of the tendon changes when the incidence of the sound beam changes. This can lead to the operator mistaking anisotropy for pathology like tendon

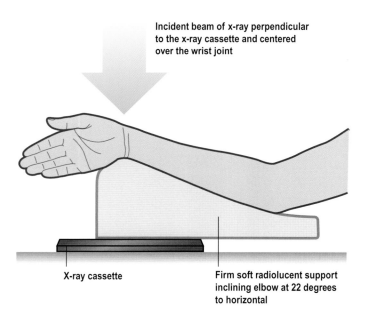

Incident beam of x-ray perpendicular to the x-ray cassette and centered over the wrist joint

X-ray cassette

Firm soft radiolucent support inclining elbow at 22 degrees to horizontal

Fig. 3.21 Position of the limb and direction of X-ray beam for an anatomical tilt lateral view of the distal radius. This view is very helpful for assessing screw position when applying plates and screws close to the articular surface in distal radius fractures.

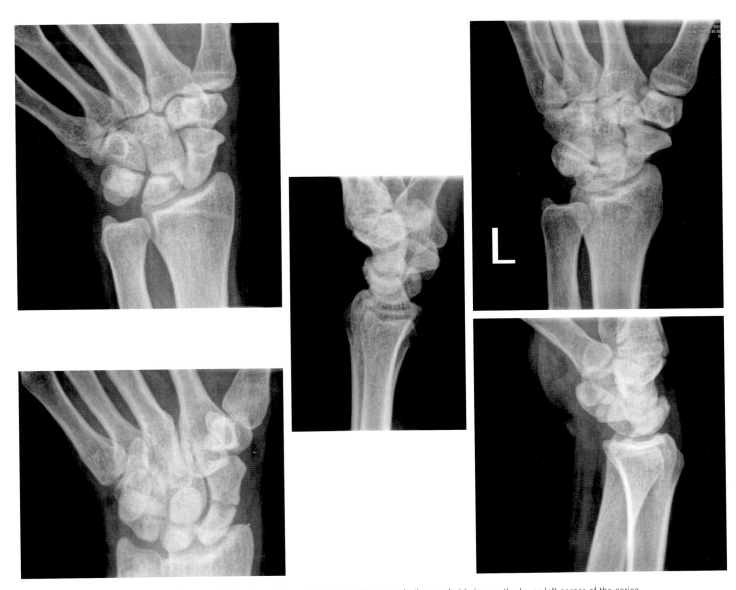

Fig. 3.22 Scaphoid series to assess for a scaphoid fracture. Notice the fracture is best seen in the scaphoid view on the lower left corner of the series.

degeneration. A careful complete assessment of suspected tendon lesions will detect this phenomenon.[30]

One major advantage of musculoskeletal ultrasound is the ability to do real-time and dynamic assessments. An area in the hand and wrist where this is particularly useful is in the assessment of tendons. For example, flexor tendon bowstringing due to pulley rupture can be dynamically demonstrated on ultrasound by the patient. Tendinopathy, partial and complete tendon tears, or lacerations can be demonstrated *(Fig. 3.28)*. Ultrasound has also been shown to be able to detect changes in trigger finger[31] and DeQuervain's tenosynovitis.[32] In trigger finger, ultrasound has also been used to guide steroid injection and percutaneous release.[33,34]

Diagnostic ultrasonography has also been applied to other wrist and hand disorders. Carpal ligament injuries and triangular fibrocartilage (TFCC) tears can be assessed using ultrasonography.[35] For TFCC tears, ultrasonography has been

Table 3.1 Advantages and disadvantages of ultrasound

Advantages	Disadvantages
No ionizing radiation	Very limited field of view
Allows real-time and dynamic assessment by operator	Highly operator-dependent
Relatively cheap to acquire and operate	Limited usefulness for assessment of soft-tissue masses

shown to have good correlation with MRI.[36] Ultrasonography of the carpal tunnel may be helpful to assess carpal tunnel syndrome. The median nerve is enlarged in carpal tunnel syndrome, with changes in the echogenity of the nerve. The most consistent finding across the studies is the increase of the cross-sectional area of the median nerve at the level

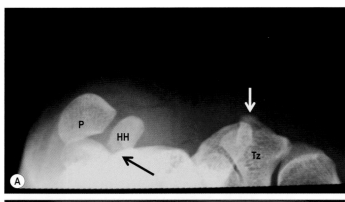

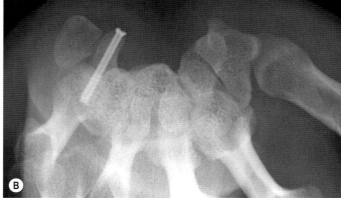

Fig. 3.23 (A) Carpal tunnel view of the wrist demonstrating several structures: trapezium (Tz), pisiform (P) and hook of hamate (HH). A fracture across the hook of the hamate is indicated by the black arrow. The trapezial ridge (indicated by white arrow) is an unusual site for fractures that is best seen on this projection. **(B)** Same patient with carpal tunnel view of the same wrist following open reduction and screw fixation. Notice that the fracture line is no longer visible.

of the pisiform bone.[37] Ultrasound is also useful for clinical assessment if other causes of carpal tunnel syndrome are suspected (e.g., mass lesions in the carpal tunnel or tenosynovitis).

Computed tomography

CT is a key advanced imaging modality for the assessment of hand and wrist disorders, particularly those affecting the bones and joints. Advances in CT scanning technology have resulted in shorter scanning times, and allow manipulation and reformatting of the CT data for image reconstruction in multiple planes and the development of three-dimensional images. The advantages and disadvantages of CT are shown in *Table 3.2*.

Fractures and dislocations

CT is useful in evaluation of the hand and wrist for bony and joint injuries that are not well visualized or assessed using radiographs. Examples of these include scaphoid fractures, CMCJ injuries (see discussion in radiography section, above), and other articular fractures *(Fig. 3.29)*.

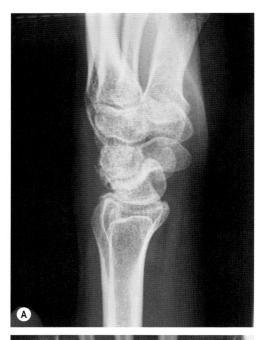

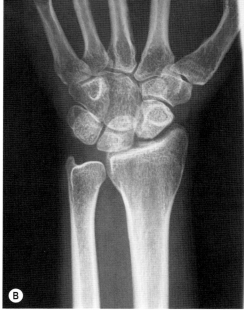

Fig. 3.24 (A) DISI is the acronym for dorsal intercalated segmental instability. The term "intercalated segment" refers to the proximal carpal row bones. This row has no direct musculotendinous insertions, hence it is "intercalated." "Dorsal" refers to the dorsiflexion of the lunate seen in the radiograph. A scapholunate dissociation is the commonest cause of a DISI deformity, and will show an increased scapholunate angle as above. **(B)** On the posteroanterior view, the scaphoid will appear flexed and foreshortened with a positive cortical ring sign as seen.

Scaphoid fractures are often difficult to detect on plain radiology after an acute injury. A repeat radiograph several weeks later, or other radiological investigations like CT scan, MRI, and bone scans, is often employed to detect an occult scaphoid fracture.[38] In one study, multidetector CT was shown to be as effective as MRI in the detection of such occult fractures.[39] In the management of scaphoid fractures, CT scan is useful in

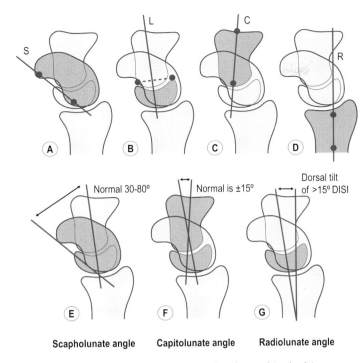

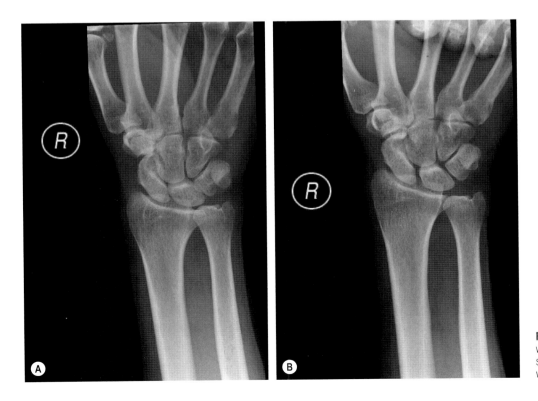

Scapholunate angle   Capitolunate angle   Radiolunate angle

Fig. 3.25 Carpal indices. Axes are drawn based on the true lateral wrist radiograph. **(A)** The scaphoid (S) is represented by a tangential line that connects the two palmar convexities of the bone; **(B)** the lunate (L) axis is perpendicular to a line that joins the two distal horns of the bone; **(C)** the capitate (C) axis is determined by the center of the two proximal and distal articular surfaces; and **(D)** the axis of the radius (R) is obtained by tracing perpendicular lines to its distal third and connecting the center of these lines. **(E)** Normal scapholunate angles. **(F)** Normal capitolunate angles. **(G)** Normal radiolunate angles. DISI, dorsal intercalated segmental instability.

evaluating fracture union,[40] as plain radiography has been shown to have poor interobserver agreement for assessing scaphoid union.[41] CT scans along the long axis of the scaphoid[42] improve the ability to evaluate the scaphoid for fractures, and assess for any displacement or humpback deformity.[43] CT scan is also useful for the evaluation of other carpal fractures.[44]

Wrist radiographs provide a first evaluation of the distal radius fractures. In an acute fracture, patient positioning is hindered by pain, and suboptimal radiographs are common. Radiography can over- and underestimate the articular stepoff in 30% of intra-articular fractures.[45] CT scans of the wrist can improve assessment, which has an impact on clinical decision-making *(Fig. 3.30)*. CT scanning and three-dimensional reconstruction are also helpful in complex fractures of the distal radius and ulna to help in surgical planning. In distal radius malunion, CT is recommended to assess the deformity[46] and as a basis for computer-assisted surgical techniques.[47,48]

CT is also helpful in suspected DRUJ instability. A proper lateral view of the wrist is the key initial imaging. There are several pitfalls associated with this. Proper positioning of the wrist for a proper lateral wrist radiograph or stress views may not be possible because of pain or other factors. The instability may be subtle, manifesting only in certain wrist positions or under load. Bilateral axial cut CT scans of the wrists in the neutral, pronated, and supinated position provide critical information to allow better evaluation of these injuries *(Fig. 3.31)*. For CT evaluation of DRUJ instability, different radiographic parameters have been described.[49–52] Our institution uses the subluxation ratio method described by Park and Kim.[53]

Fig. 3.26 These radiographs show a patient with dynamic scapholunate instability. The scapholunate interval is normal on an unloaded wrist **(A)**, but widens on clenching the fist **(B)**.

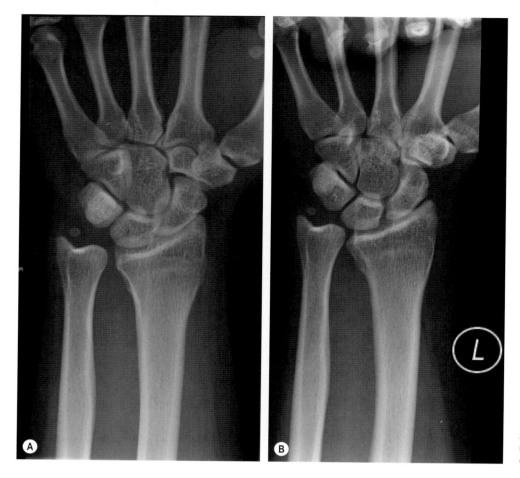

Fig. 3.27 This patient presented with signs and symptoms of ulnar carpal abutment. The positive ulnar variance **(A)** is increased with the pronated clenched-fist view **(B)**.

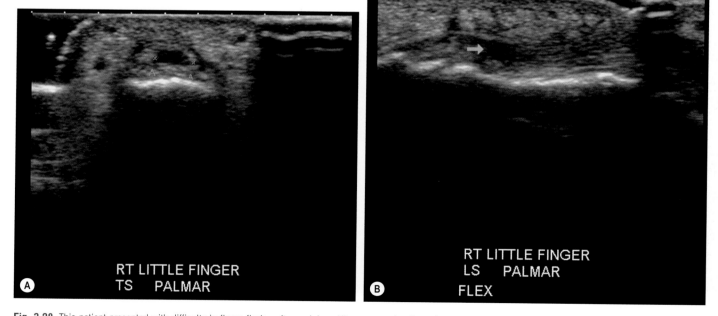

Fig. 3.28 This patient presented with difficulty in finger flexion after an injury. Ultrasonography showed a partial tear of flexor tendon at the level of the head of middle phalanx, more obvious on flexion against resistance (dark area, arrowed on longitudinal section image and between calipers on transverse section image). (Courtesy of Dr. Ian Tsou, Singapore.)

Table 3.2 Advantages and disadvantages of computed tomography (CT)

Advantages	Disadvantages
Quick scanning with modern machines	Inferior to magnetic resonance imaging for imaging of soft tissue
Capacity to image in any anatomic plane (multiplanar imaging) and three-dimensional reconstruction	Requires expose to ionizing radiation
Excellent for assessing complex or poorly visualized fractures in the hand and wrist	Prone to artifacts from patient movement and implants
CT angiography can be performed at the same sitting to assess the vascular tree	

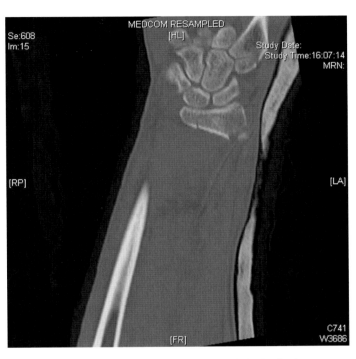

Fig. 3.30 Coronal computed tomography (CT) image of distal radius fracture. Extension into the radiocarpal joint is seen here but not on the plain radiograph. CT is helpful for the assessment of intra-articular distal radius fractures with respect to articular involvement and incongruity, fragment number, and fragment orientation.

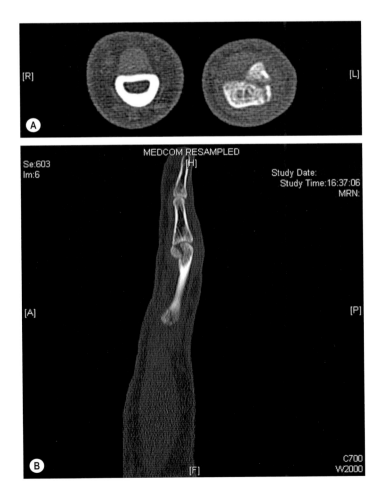

Fig. 3.29 This displaced fracture of the radial condyle of the proximal phalanx (small finger) is well visualized on the computed tomography **(A)** and **(B),** but obscured on plain radiograph. There is a concomitant fracture of phalanx base, seen in **(B).**

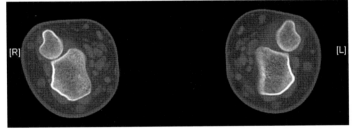

Fig. 3.31 Axial computed tomography cut of distal radioulnar joint in neutral position shows dorsal subluxation of the left joint (right image). This can be quantified by the use of indices.

Other applications of CT

CT is also helpful for the evaluation for bony tumors in the hand. CT can help characterize the bony tumor and assess for bony destruction. In these situations, MRI is often complementary. Fine-cut CTs are the modality of choice for osteoid osteoma.[54]

There are limitations to the use of CT. Soft-tissue resolution is limited, so it is less useful than MRI for imaging soft-tissue disorders . Artifacts from various sources, including patient movement and metal implants, hinder evaluation. Software techniques can be used to limit these artifacts, but often at the cost of resolution at the site of interest.[55]

The usefulness of CT is often enhanced when coupled with volume-rendering techniques. These allow clearer imaging of subtle fractures and complex injuries. They are also helpful in the evaluation of suspected infections or neoplastic disease. After operative fixation of fractures, volume rendering can improve the quality of imaging by eliminating streak artifacts.[56] Using intravenous contrast, CT angiography can be performed (see section on vascular imaging techniques for the upper extremity, below).

Magnetic resonance imaging

MRI of the hand and wrist has come to the forefront in the last decade. It is the preferred modality for imaging soft tissue, particularly those associated with trauma and neoplastic conditions. Larger more powerful magnets, improved gradient strength and speed, dedicated coils providing favorable signal-to-noise ratios, and the capability of supporting small fields of view enable visualization of pathology in exquisite anatomic detail. The advantages and disadvantages of MRI are shown in *Table 3.3*.

Basics

MRI employs magnetic fields and radiowaves rather than ionizing radiation. The magnetic field is generated by an electromagnetic coil with field strengths ranging from 1.5 to 3.0 Tesla (T) (15 000–30 000 gauss). Gradient (secondary) magnets finetune and focus the MRI on specific areas of interest. MRI coils send and receive radiofrequency pulses that are used to create images. In general, the smaller the coil and the more centrally located an anatomic structure is within the coil, the sharper the image and the higher the signal-to-noise ratio.

MR differentiates tissues such as fat, muscle, bone, blood, and water on the basis of their innate magnetic characteristics and the varying tissue concentration of hydrogen ions (protons). Each proton spins like a top, around an axis. In the absence of a magnetic field, their axes are randomly oriented and produce no net magnetic effect. In the MRI scanner, the magnetic field generated causes the axes of rotation of the protons to align themselves with the longitudinal axes of the magnet. Gradient magnets change the alignment of the rotating protons whilst radiofrequency pulses from the coils excite the protons to a higher energy level. Cessation of radiofrequency stimulation induces a tiny current within the surrounding coil which can be detected and amplified to give a signal. The time taken for a proton to become magnetized is known as the T_1 relaxation time and the time taken for the proton to be demagnetized is known as the T_2 relaxation time. The amount of energy released by a tissue is directly proportional to its concentration of protons. It is also the varying concentration of protons between different tissues that allows them to be magnetized and demagnetized differentially. This is the basis of differentiating the soft tissues. The relevant signals of different tissues on T_1- and T_2-weighted images are shown in *Table 3.4*. Different MRI sequences are used to enhance visualization in the area of interest. Common sequences useful in MRI of the hand and wrist are shown in *Table 3.5*.

Water can be categorized into free water and bound water. Free water is found mostly in extracellular fluid whilst bound water is mostly in intracellular fluid. Free water has long T_1 and T_2 relaxation times. Hence it typically shows low signal intensity on T_1-weighted images and high signal intensity on T_2-weighted images. Water that is not free is usually bound to proteins which inhibit motion. This preferentially shortens the T_1 relaxation time more than the T_2 relaxation time, hence the T_1 signal is usually of intermediate to high intensity. Examples of proteinaceous fluid include abscesses, synovial fluid, and purulent collections.

Clinical applications of MRI

MRI for soft-tissue masses

MRI is the preferred modality for imaging soft-tissue masses in the hand and wrist. The majority of soft-tissue masses in the hand and wrist are benign.[57] MRI characteristics of the common tumors are well described in literature and references.[58–60] MRI, with its multiplanar imaging capability,

Table 3.3 Advantages and disadvantages of magnetic resonance imaging (MRI)

Advantages	Disadvantages
Capacity to image in any anatomic plane (multiplanar imaging)	The high cost of equipment
High soft-tissue contrast with indication of tissue composition	Image artifacts from motion and ferromagnetic objects
No ionizing radiation	Inferior to computed tomography for imaging of cortical bone
Acquisition of three-dimensional volume data using gradient echo sequences	Contraindicated in patients with cardiac pacemakers, aneurysm clips, metallic foreign body, claustrophobia
Noninvasive imaging of blood vessels and other structures without the use of contrast (e.g., MR arthrography)	

Table 3.4 Signal intensities of tissues on T_1- and T_2-weighted magnetic resonance images

Tissue	Signal T_1-weighted image	Signal T_2-weighted image
Fluid (free water)	Low	High
Fluid (proteinaceous)	Intermediate	High
Fat	High	High
Muscle	Intermediate	Intermediate
Cartilage	Intermediate	High
Cortical bone	Low	Low
Bone marrow (yellow)	High	Intermediate
Bone marrow (red)	Low	Intermediate

Table 3.5 Terminology of pulse sequences and enhancements

Fat suppression (FS)	Fat signal is visible on most MRI images. Controlling the fat signal is critical in determining the contrast and clarity of pathology. FS is employed in pulse sequences of the musculoskletal system, allowing the cancellation or reduction of fat signals
Fast spin echo (FSE)	Fast or turbo spin echo sequences permit acquisition of images with contrast properties similar to those from routine spin-echo sequences, but with a shorter acquisition time.[57] With FSE, the signal from fat is much brighter than that seen with ordinary spin-echo images, necessitating fat suppression
Short tau inversion recovery (STIR)	Typically a T_1-weighted sequence employed in musculoskeletal MRI.[58] Pathology is seen as a high signal against a muted background. Examples include bone marrow edema, inflammation from trauma, infective or neoplastic processes, and ligament tears. It is the most sensitive sequence for the detection of bone marrow or soft-tissue abnormalities. STIR is usually combined with FSE to quicken acquisition and has a relatively poor signal-to-noise ratio. The FS T_2-weighted sequence is less sensitive but without these disadvantages
Gradient echo (GRE)	Conventional spin-echo techniques utilize radiofrequency pulses directed at 90° to the direction of the magnetic field and subsequently followed by a refocusing pulse at 180°. The angle of the focusing pulse is known as the flip angle. In a GRE sequence, the flip angle ranges from 0 to 90°, there is no refocusing pulse, and the gradient magnets create a dephasing pulse followed by a rephasing pulse from the opposite direction, which generates the "echo." Using very low flip angles allows suppression of T_1-weighted images and rapid acquisition of T_2-weighted images; conversely larger flip angles (70°) tend to result in T_1-weighted focused images. GRE sequences enable much thinner slices than possible with routine spin-echo techniques, with no slice gaps and with greater rapidity of acquisition times. These sequences are preferred for joint imaging and cartilage lesions[59]
Contrast enhancement	Two forms of intravenous contrast media are chelated gadolinium (Gd-DTPA) and iron oxide particles. Gd-DTPA causes an increased signal in T_1-weighted images due to a paramagnetic effect. Gd-DTPA is water-soluble and considered a "positive" agent used to produce contrast between areas of high uptake and the surrounding tissue. Iron oxide particles are "negative" agents because they exert a ferromagnetic effect and give reduced signals in areas of increased uptake. Contrast may also be injected into a joint to perform an MR arthrogram, most commonly that of the wrist

MRI, magnetic resonance imaging.

tissue characterization of lesions, and ability to define relationship of lesions to surrounding tissue and vessels (including tumor invasion), allows one in many circumstances to arrive at a specific diagnosis.

Ganglion cysts

Ganglia show low to intermediate signals on T_1-weighted images and high signals on T_2-weighted images. They may be uniloculated or multiloculated and contain proteinaceous synovial fluid. This accounts for its isointense or slightly hypointense signal on T_1-weighted images compared to muscle *(Fig. 3.32)*. Demonstration of a stalk can usually reveal its site of origin. Hemorrhage into a ganglion cyst can result in high signal intensity on T_1-weighted images. A ganglion shows no enhancement on administration of intravenous gadolinium; however its capsule and septa will usually show enhancement. Ganglion cysts occurring in "classical" locations such as the dorsum of the wrist can usually be diagnosed clinically and do not require MRI.

Giant cell tumors of the tendon sheath (GCTTS)

Synonymous with focal pigmented villonodular synovitis, these benign tumors of synovial origin typically occur in the digits over the volar aspect, and arise from the tendon sheath,

joint capsule, fascia, or ligaments. They contain multinucleated giant cells and have intra- and extracellular hemosiderin deposition. On MRI, GCTTS appear as solid masses, hypointense on both T_1- and T_2-weighted images. The low signal is due to the paramagnetic effect of hemosiderin deposition. On T_1-and T_2-weighted images, these masses appear isointense with skeletal muscle. Uniform enhancement is seen following administration of intravenous gadolinium contrast *(Fig. 3.33)*.

Lipomas

Lipomas are less common in the hand and wrist than in other parts of the body. In the hand, they usually occur over the palmar aspect, either in the thenar or hypothenar eminence or in the mid palmar space. They show the same homogeneous high signal intensity as fat on T_1-weighted images and superficial lipomata can appear inconspicuous. They show low signals on short tau inversion recovery (STIR) and T_2-weighted sequences. The presence of distinct nodules or solid components may suggest a liposarcoma.

Hemangiomas

Hemangiomas are benign tumors classified into capillary, cavernous, and venous types. T_1-weighted signal intensity varies from low, to high, depending on the amount of fat contained.

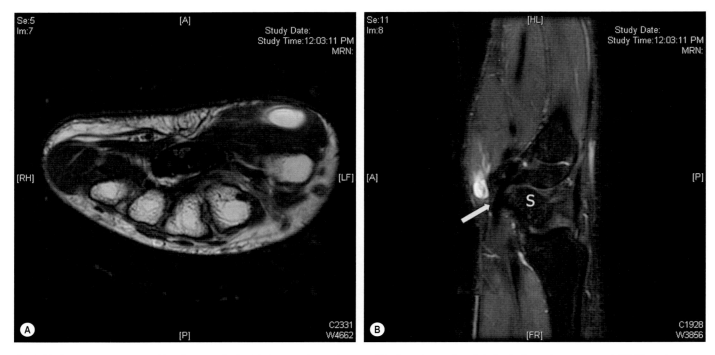

Fig. 3.32 This patient presented with a firm mass in the left thenar eminence that was difficult to characterize clinically. Radiographs were normal. **(A)** Magnetic resonance imaging shows a mass with typical high signal intensity during the T2-weighted sequence. **(B)** A sagittal fat suppression short tau inversion recovery sequence shows the stalk of the ganglion connecting to the sheath of the flexor carpi radialis (indicative arrow) with the scaphoid (S) in close relation.

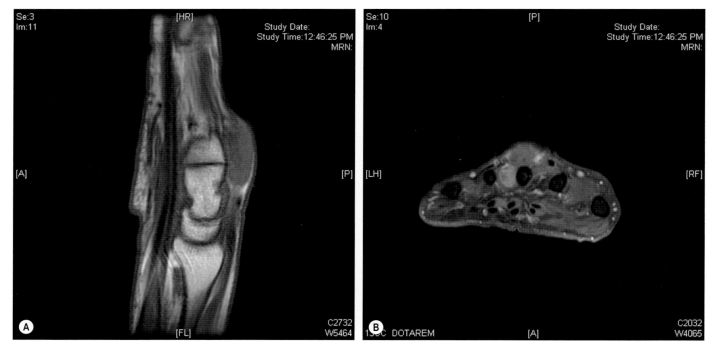

Fig. 3.33 This man presented with a firm painless enlarging mass over the dorsum of the left hand. Magnetic resonance imaging shows a low signal intensity mass over the third carpometacarpal junction, seen on **(A)** sagittal T1-weighted sequence and **(B)** axial T2-weighted sequence.

On T_2-weighted sequences, they tend to be lobulated with well-defined borders and very high signal intensity from pooled blood. A lace-like pattern of enhancement may be seen on T_1-weighted images due to fibrofatty elements. Signal voids may be present on all MR sequences as a consequence of phleboliths within the hemangiomas. The heterogeneous nature of hemangiomas thus makes preoperative diagnosis by MRI less certain.[57]

Enchondromas

Enchondromas are the most common benign tumors of bone that are found in the hand. Problems associated with enchondromas are pathological fractures and the rare occurrence of malignant transformation. Radiography demonstrates a lytic expansile lesion with a clear zone of transition and speckled calcifications. Cortical thinning is present and may be associated with a pathological fracture. On MRI, they appear as high-signal-intensity lobulated tumors on fat suppression (FS) STIR and T_2-weighted sequences. They show low to intermediate signal intensity on T_1-weighted sequences.

MRI for wrist and hand trauma

This application of MRI has become more widespread in the last two decades, in particular for ligamentous injuries. A further advantage of MRI is its superior imaging of bone marrow and vascularity of bone with a wide range of applications, including diagnosing AVN, marrow edema, and inflammation, as well as infection.

Occult scaphoid and carpal fractures

MRI is the most sensitive and specific imaging modality for occult scaphoid fractures, although its cost may be greater or equitable compared to the classic diagnostic algorithm.[61,62] An area of a linear band of low signal intensity on T_1-weighted sequences, coupled with an area of high signal intensity on FS T_2-weighted sequences or STIR sequences, has the highest combined sensitivity and specificity. Cortical fracture lines are best seen on a STIR or gradient echo (GRE) sequence. Use of MRI for diagnosis of radiographically occult fractures is not limited to the scaphoid, but includes other carpal bone fractures which are difficult to image on radiography.[63] The added value of using MRI for detection of occult carpal bone fractures is that it also demonstrates ligament injuries which can clinically mimic carpal fractures (*Fig. 3.34*).

Bone bruising, a term synonymous with bone contusion, exhibits exactly the same MRI findings as occult fractures do with the exception of a cortical break. This diagnosis is made in the setting of a positive history of preceding trauma and positive MRI findings, as described above.

Ligamentous injuries of the hand and wrist

Suspected ligamentous injures of the hand and wrist are probably the commonest indication for ordering an MRI. SL and LT ligament tears as well as tears of interphalangeal or metacarpophalangeal joint ligaments are frequent clinical problems. Another large group of wrist pathologies; ulnar-sided wrist pain, including but not limited to tears of the TFCC,

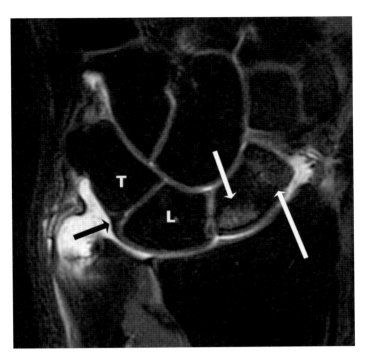

Fig. 3.34 This patient presented with persistent dorsoradial-sided wrist pain after a fall. He had initially been seen by a general physician and diagnosed as having a sprain. Magnetic resonance imaging coronal fast spin echo proton density sequences with fat suppression showed two areas (white arrows) of high signal intensity in the scaphoid proximal pole and waist (associated with fracture). The signal enhancement in the proximal pole is due to an injury of the scapholunate ligament, noting a normal ligamentous structure of the lunotriquetral ligament (black arrow).

ulnocarpal abutment, DRUJ and tendinitis, is considered separately in the next section.

An intact ligament is shown as a homogeneous black signal or band on a proton density-weighted GRE sequence or a T_1-weighted spin echo sequence on coronal slices. An abnormal ligament shows increased signal intensity on T_2-weighted sequences or STIR sequences, segmental defect, increased length, thickening, thinning, and nonvisualization.[64] MR arthrography can be performed with saline or dilute gadolinium injected into the joint, enhancing the detection of ligaments and TFCC perforations.

Thumb ulnar collateral ligament injuries

A poorly treated complete tear of the ulnar collateral ligament of the thumb metacarpophalangeal joint can lead to painful and chronic instability. MRI is valuable in assessing for complete ligamentous disruption, a diagnosis that may be difficult to make in early or acute presentations (*Fig. 3.35*). Such imaging helps exclude a Stener lesion,[65] where the adductor aponeurosis becomes interposed between the two ends of the ruptured ligament, preventing ligament healing.

Scapholunate interosseous ligament injury

This is the commonest intrinsic wrist ligament injury. Presentations vary from occult SL joint ganglions, dynamic SL instability, to static SL dissociation. SL dissociation is the

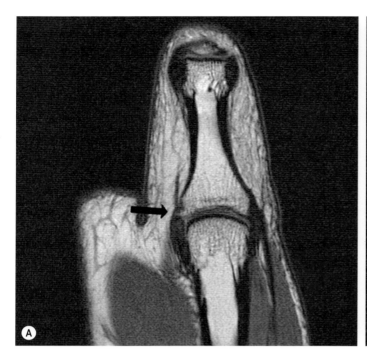
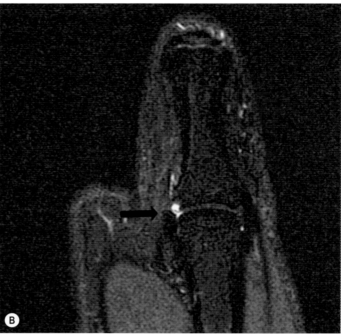

Fig. 3.35 This 15-year-old girl presented with pain at the ulnar aspect of the metacarpophalangeal joint of her right thumb after an abduction injury from a fall. Plain posteroanterior and lateral radiographs showed no abnormalities. Clinical assessment for joint instability was difficult because of her anxiety and pain and a magnetic resonance imaging scan was performed. The coronal fast spin echo proton density sequence, a variant form of gradient echo sequences, reveals a distal avulsion/rupture **(A)** of the ulnar collateral ligament (black arrow). The radial collateral ligament on the other hand is intact and smoothly inserts or joins the base of the proximal phalanx of the thumb. **(B)** The short tau inversion recovery sequence shows bright signal intensity at the site of rupture seen on the proton density sequence, correlating with an acute tear or rupture of the ligament.

commonest cause of carpal instability. Early recognition of SL instability allows treatment and prevention of late arthritis. Features which support a tear of the SL ligament include widening of the SL interval, fluid signal traversing the SL or LT ligaments on the fat-suppressed fast spin echo (FSE) T_1-weighted sequence, or STIR sequence *(Fig. 3.36)*. Proton density sequences as well as T_2-weighted sequences with FS can also reveal morphological abnormalities and absence of the SL ligament. The same criteria also apply for evaluating the less common LT ligament injuries.

MRI for evaluating ulnar-sided wrist pain

Ulnar-sided wrist pain is common and a challenging problem. Common causes of ulnar-sided wrist pain are injuries to the TFCC, LT ligament injuries, and ulnocarpal abutment syndrome. Other differentials include fractures and nonunion of fractures, especially of the ulnar styloid, DRUJ problems, and tendinopathies.

TFCC tears

TFCC injuries are classified into two groups: those occurring acutely and degenerative lesions. In the latter group, lesions occur in the central portion of the TFCC and the incidence increases with advancing age. Acute traumatic tears of the TFCC usually occur following a forced axial load of the wrist in an extended and ulnar-deviated position. Acute tears of the TFCC resulting in detachment from the fovea or detachment from its radial border can result in DRUJ instability. The gold standard for evaluation of TFCC injuries is arthroscopy. MRI

has been increasingly used for imaging the TFCC. The sequence which best demonstrates the TFCC is the FS FSE T_1-weighted and GRE T_2 sequence.[66] GRE sequences which mimic FS FSE T_1-weighted sequences such as the proton density-weighted GRE sequence depicts TFCC disruptions even more distinctly *(Fig. 3.37)*. With the advent of 3.0-T MRI machines, the sensitivity and specificity of MRI for detection of TFCC lesions exceed that of 1.5-T machines.[67,68]

Ulnocarpal abutment

This is a degenerative condition related to excessive load-bearing across the ulnar side of the wrist. An ulna positive variance may be present. Radiography may be normal or may show subchondral cyst formation in the lunate and/or triquetrum. Stress films can demonstrate dynamic increase in ulnar length relative to the radius (pronated grip film of the wrist). MRI shows foci of low signal intensities in the lunate and triquetrum and occasionally in the ulnar head, reflecting chondromalacia. On FS STIR or FS T_2-weighted sequences, these same areas show bright signal intensities from bone marrow edema or secondary to the presence of cyst formation *(Fig. 3.38)*.

DRUJ instability and tendinopathies

CT is the preferred imaging modality for DRUJ instability and subluxation. MRI however allows visualization of the ligaments and the insertion of the TFCC into the fovea, which contributes to stability of the DRUJ. Furthermore, high signal intensities on FS STIR sequence will suggest reactive marrow edema from persistent DRUJ instability and synovitis. The relationship of the ulnar head to the distal end of the radius

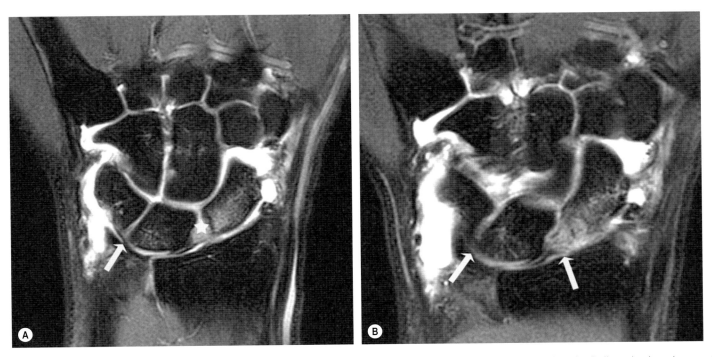

Fig. 3.36 This patient presented with right-sided wrist pain. He had tenderness over the scapholunate junction over the dorsum of the wrist. Radiography showed a normal scapholunate angle on lateral wrist projections and no widening of the scapholunate interval on posteroanterior projections of the wrist. Magnetic resonance imaging coronal fast spin echo proton density sequences with fat suppression **(A)** showed widening of the scapholunate (SL) interval (star) with absence of the membranous portion of the ligament. The membranous portion of the lunotriquetral (LT) ligament is intact (white arrow). The next sequence shows a more dorsal section of the proximal carpal row with an intact LT ligament (white arrow) and disrupted SL ligament with abnormal fluid signal traversing it and a thickened and fibrillar morphology (white arrow) **(B).**

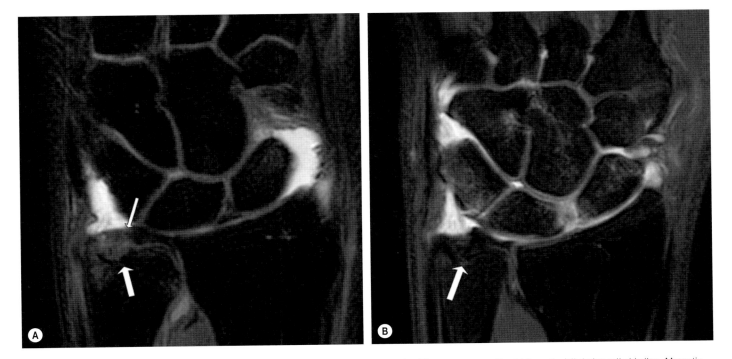

Fig. 3.37 This 27-year-old male presented with right ulnar-sided wrist pain of 1 year's duration. There was a preceding history of a fall during rollerblading. Magnetic resonance imaging proton density-weighted sequences show that the portion of the triangular fibrocartilage (small arrow) that inserts into the fovea (big arrow) has been avulsed off its insertion **(A).** In a different patient, the triangular fibrocartilage with its insertion into the fovea preserved (white arrow) is shown **(B).** This patient had instead a scapholunate ligament injury.

and DRUJ subluxation is best assessed on an axial FSE T_1-weighted sequence. A halo of high signal enhancement can be seen in tendinopathies on axial slices during an FS STIR sequence or an FS T_2-weighted sequences. In addition, there may be thickening of the tendon and abnormal signal within the tendon itself on coronal slices.

MRI for evaluation of fracture nonunion

Scaphoid fractures are prone to nonunion. Radiography to assess for fracture healing lacks a high degree of sensitivity and specificity. The MRI criterion to assess union is the presence on T_1-weighted sequences of normal signal intensity crossing the previous fracture line.[69] Nonunion is shown by the presence of high signal intensity at the fracture line on FS STIR or FS T_2-weighted sequences or the GRE equivalents.

MRI for AVN in scaphoid fracture nonunion

The proximal pole of the scaphoid is prone to AVN following a fracture due to its retrograde vascular axis pattern.[70] Radiographs can show changes associated with AVN, including sclerosis of the proximal fragment, osseous absorption, and cysts. MRI can detect AVN at an earlier stage. Knowing the vascularity of the proximal fragment guides clinical decision-making, including whether to use vascularized or nonvascularized grafts. Low signal intensity of the proximal fragment on T_1-weighted sequences indicates replacement of the normal marrow with fibrous tissue. High signal intensity of the proximal pole on gadolinium contrast-enhanced study suggests that vascularity is preserved. This finding has not been consistently proven in all studies, and the relative enhancement should be significantly greater than the surrounding carpal bones.[69]

Kienbock's disease

Idiopathic AVN of the lunate is relatively uncommon when compared with postraumatic AVN of the scaphoid. A negative ulnar variance has been shown to be associated with an increased risk of Kienbock's disease. MRI is of value in detecting early disease, prognosticating, and for monitoring revascularization of the lunate following treatment.[71] AVN of the lunate is suggested by low signal intensity on T_1-weighted sequence as marrow is replaced by fibrous tissue. Areas of high signal intensity may be seen on FS T_2-weighted sequence or FSE FS STIR sequences, suggesting marrow edema or neovascularization *(Fig. 3.39)*. Low signal intensity on such sequences likely indicates established ischemic necrosis without any further bone reactive changes.

Osteomyelitis

Osteomyelitis of the hand and wrist bones is relatively uncommon. It is usually a consequence of previous surgical intervention for fractures or other procedures. Traditionally, either scintigraphy or MRI has been used when plain film radiography has been negative in suspected osteomyelitis. MRI has

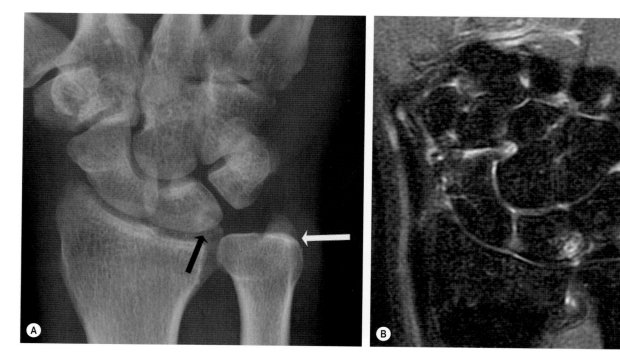

Fig. 3.38 This patient presented with persistent right ulnar-sided wrist pain of 6 months' duration and he complained of inability, in particular in hammering objects. He had tenderness over the ulnar fovea and a positive ulnocarpal grind. Plain film radiography **(A)** showed no fractures of the ulnar styloid. There was however a subchondral cyst seen in the proximal ulnar corner of the lunate (black arrow) and there was positive ulnar variance (white arrow). On magnetic resonance imaging, the fat suppression short tau inversion recovery sequence showed high signal intensity in the same corresponding area of the lunate **(B)**. Note that the triangular fibrocartilage and the ulnar head (white arrows) show no signal enhancement which would typify more advanced involvement.

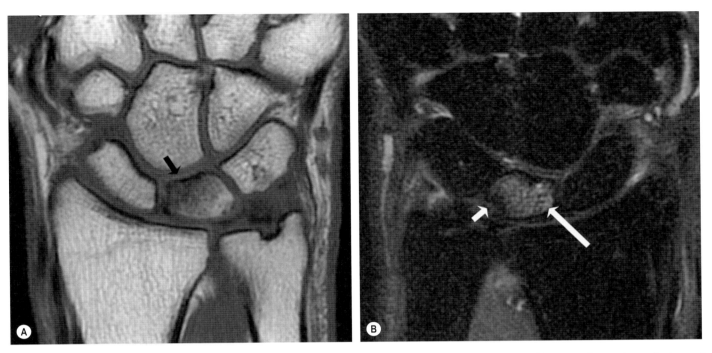

Fig. 3.39 A karate enthusiast presented with right wrist central dorsal pain of gradual onset that was associated with morning stiffness as well as weakness of grip over the passage of time. Radiography was normal aside from the suggestion of an area of faint linear sclerosis in the lunate. Magnetic resonance imaging fast spin echo T_1-weighted sequence showed loss of normal marrow signal affecting the radial corner of the lunate **(A).** Fast spin echo fat suppression short tau inversion recovery sequences showed diffuse marrow enhancement, sparing only the proximal ulnar tip of the lunate **(B).**

the advantage of discriminating marrow abnormalities from joint and soft-tissue changes. Areas of marrow involvement will show low signal on T_1-weighted sequence and high signal intensity on T_2-weighted sequence.

Vascular imaging techniques for the upper extremity

Digital subtraction angiography (DSA) is the gold standard for vascular imaging of the extremities.[72,73] Improvements in CT angiography and magnetic resonance angiography (MRA) make them increasingly viable alternatives in vascular imaging of the upper extremity. Arterial imaging of the upper limb is usually performed in two different clinical settings: the detection of extremity vasculary injury following trauma to the limb, and assessment of vascular disorders involving the upper limb.

The indications for angiography following trauma are: decreased or absent pulse or blood pressure, cold limb, bruit or murmur, uncontrolled bleeding or increasing hematoma, neurologic deficit, and proximity of the injury to vascular structures.[74] When the clinical condition warrants immediate surgery, conventional angiography is contraindicated. Knife injuries (80%) and blunt trauma (67%) are more likely to be associated with vascular abnormalities, followed by gunshot wounds (44%).[74]

DSA has a role in the assessment of the vascular tree in peripheral arteriosclerotic disease, connective tissue diseases, thoracic outlet syndrome, and Raynaud's phenomenon. It is also useful for assessing arteriovenous fistulae and vascular tumors and malformation of the upper limb.

CT angiography (CTA) is less invasive than DSA and can additionally assess vessel wall and extraluminal pathology. The data obtained allow reconstruction in three-dimensional and multiple planes. The advancements in CT technology, new protocols, and availability of CTs in proximity of many emergency departments have made CTA an increasingly attractive option for the assessment of the extremity vascular tree following trauma.[75,76] In extremity trauma, CTA can identify arterial injuries, including pseudoaneurysm, active arterial hemorrhage, arteriovenous fistulae, occlusion, intimal injury, or vasospasm.[77] Venous injury may also be assessed. CTA has also been shown to be useful in the evaluation of suspected extremity vascular trauma in pediatric patients.[78] In pediatric patients, CTA allows imaging of the vascular tree where DSA is often not possible.

The indications for CTA are similar to that of DSA. There are limitations with use of CTA for evaluation following trauma. For example, differentiation of a tapered contour deformity of CTA, which may variously represent dissection, intimal injury, vasospasm, or adjacent hematoma, is difficult.[75] Imaging of the distal vascular tree is also difficult. DSA also offers an advantage where there is a possibility of endovascular treatment, for example in an arteriovenous fistula. The sensitivity and specificity of CT arteriography have been

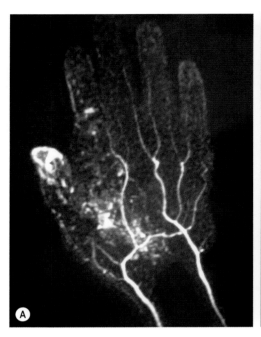
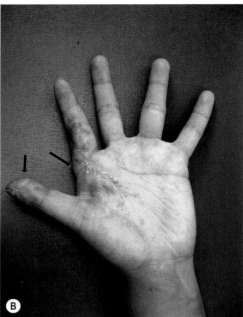

Fig. 3.40 This 23-year-old female had a previous excision of arteriovenous malformation more than 5 years ago and now presents with skin changes suggestive of recurrence. Magnetic resonance angiography delineates the palmar arch well and in addition shows blushes of bright signal intensity over the thumb pulp, the first web area, and over the index finger **(A)**. This correlated well with the pigmented changes seen on the clinical photo **(B)**.

shown to be 95.1% and 98.7% in cases of suspected vascular injury following blunt or penetrating injury.[79]

MRA offers advantages over conventional DSA for extremity vascular imaging. MRA is less invasive, does not require iodinated contrast, and can simultaneously demonstrate extraluminal disease.[80] The angiographic effect in MRA is created by various techniques with or without contrast enhancement with gadolinium chelate agent. The use of contrast-enhanced MRA with a dedicated surface coil enables quick and high-quality examination of the hand vascular tree.[81]

MRA of the wrist and hand has a potential number of indications for its use and has been employed successfully in imaging of vascular malformations, vascular trauma, and vascular occlusion.[82] MRA is performed making use of a coronal volume three-dimensional spoiled GRE time-of-flight sequence and dynamic administration of intravenous gadolinium contrast with image acquisition using a wrist coil. The inherent contrast from protons in flowing blood relative to the saturated protons in the stationary soft tissue produces the image which is formulated based on an MR algorithm which deletes the signal from the soft tissue. MRA has the potential to depict pathologic change in vessels of up to 1 mm in diameter and can reliably show the superficial and deep palmar arches of the hand *(Fig. 3.40)*. Some of the disadvantages of MRA include the inferior resolution of vasculature at 1 mm diameter or less, susceptibility to motion artifacts, as well as flow artifacts at sites of severe stenosis or thrombosis where a high signal intensity may be mistaken for flowing blood. MRA is useful in patients with renal impairment where

intravascular ionic contrast could cause further nephrotoxic damage, as well as in pediatric patients.

Radionuclide imaging

Radionuclide imaging is a highly sensitive imaging modality[83] with applications in hand and wrist conditions. It can be positive even when conventional imaging techniques are unable to visualize the condition. The main limitation of radionuclide imaging is its lack of specificity. This is because the tracers used reflect function.[84] The imaging detail required to differentiate physiological and pathological processes is often lacking in these scans. Therefore it is most useful as a screening tool. The most common radionuclide musculoskeletal imaging is bone scintigraphy with technetium-99m-labelled diphosphonates. The three-phase bone scan is highly sensitive for osteomyelitis. However, similar findings can be mimicked by conditions such as tumors, fractures, and joint neuropathy. The use of indium-111-labeled autologous leukocytes can improve its specificity.[85] Bone scintigraphy is also useful for diagnosis of complex regional pain syndrome (reflex sympathetic dystrophy),[86] occult fractures of the scaphoid,[87] and metastatic disease.[88] Newer modalities, such as the combination of scintigraphy with morphologic information, e.g., single-photon emission CT/CT can improve diagnostic yields in the extremity.[89]

Video 3.1 Intraoperative fluoroscopic assessment showing scapholunate instability. Notice the scapholunate intervals widen on ulnar deviation.

Access the complete references list online at **http://www.expertconsult.com**

3. Fisher MR, Rogers LF, Hendrix RW. Systematic approach to identifying fourth and fifth carpometacarpal joint dislocations. *AJR Am J Roentgenol.* 1983;140:319–324.

12. Salter RB, Harris R. Injuries Involving the Epiphyseal Plate. *J Bone Joint Surg Am.* 1963 1963;45:587–621.

    This classic instructional lecture course provides an excellent overview of the growth plate, its injury patterns, mechanisms and prognosis,as well as radiographic features.

15. Gilula LA. Carpal injuries: analytic approach and case exercises. *AJR Am J Roentgenol.* 1979;133:503–517.

28. Smith J, Finnoff JT. Diagnostic and interventional musculoskeletal ultrasound: part 1. *Fundamentals. PM R.* 2009;1:64–75.

    The principles of medical ultrasonography as applied to the musculoskeletal system are covered in this first part of a two-part comprehensive review. Part 2 covers clinical applications of ultrasonography.

44. Kaewlai R, Avery LL, Asrani AV, et al. Multidetector CT of Carpal Injuries: Anatomy, Fractures, and Fracture-Dislocations1. *Radiographics.* 2008;28:1771–1784.

53. Park MJ, Kim JP. Reliability and Normal Values of Various Computed Tomography Methods for Quantifying Distal Radioulnar Joint Translation. *J Bone Joint Surg Am.* 2008;90:145–153.

60. Ergun T, Lakadamyali H, Derincek A, et al. Magnetic Resonance Imaging in the Visualization of Benign Tumors and Tumor-like Lesions of Hand and Wrist. *Curr Probl Diagnost Radiol.* 2010;39:1–16.

    This review provides a practical approach to MR evaluation of benign tumors of the hand and wrist. A comprehensive list of conditions is covered, with descriptions and images of the MRI findings.

66. Nakamura T, Yabe Y, Horiuchi Y. Fat suppression magnetic resonance imaging of the triangular fibrocartilage complex. Comparison with spin echo, gradient echo pulse sequences and histology. *J Hand Surg Br.* 1999;24:22–26.

80. Stepansky F, Hecht EM, Rivera R, et al. Dynamic MR Angiography of Upper Extremity Vascular Disease: Pictorial Review. *Radiographics.* 2008;28:e28–e.

    MRA is rapidly becoming a viable alternative to digital subtraction angiography. This article reviews MRA techniques and protocols, and shows examples of upper extremity pathology diagnosed with MRA.

83. Love C, Din AS, Tomas MB, et al. Radionuclide bone imaging: an illustrative review. *Radiographics.* 2003;23:341–358.

    Bone scintigraphy is one of the most frequently performed radionuclide procedures. This article reviews the basic principles, protocols, normal findings, and applications of bone scintigraphy.

4

Anesthesia for upper extremity surgery

Jonay Hill, Vanila M. Singh, and Subhro K. Sen

SYNOPSIS

- Optimal perioperative anesthetic outcomes are achieved by a thorough understanding of anatomy, pharmacology, techniques, and potential complications.
- Local anesthetics (LA) make regional anesthesia possible by preventing the propagation of nerve conduction and by inhibiting or relieving pain.
- Ultrasound guidance in the use of regional anesthesia has decreased the need for high volumes of anesthetic.

Introduction

The goal of anesthesia for hand and upper extremity procedures is to provide a comfortable and safe experience for the patient during surgery. Many options are available for anesthesia, with respective benefits and risks. The decision regarding which anesthetic technique is chosen depends on various factors, including the extent, site, and expected duration of surgery; need for sedation; general medical health of the patient, and personal preference.

General anesthesia techniques can be applied for hand and upper extremity procedures the same as for procedures elsewhere. In addition, regional anesthesia techniques can be applied for procedures involving the upper extremity when used in the proper setting and patient population. Adjunctive measures are used to augment local anesthetics to provide longer duration of action, lower risk of adverse systemic effects, and less bleeding at the surgical site.

Optimal perioperative anesthetic outcomes are achieved by a thorough understanding of anatomy, pharmacology, techniques, potential complications, and general pain management.

Anatomy

The brachial plexus arises from the ventral rami of nerves C5–8 and T1, with variable contributions from C4 and T2 *(Fig. 4.1)*. These rami unite and diverge forming the roots, trunks, divisions, cords, and terminal nerves of the brachial plexus. C5 and C6 roots form the superior trunk, C7 becomes the middle trunk, and C8 and T1 form the inferior trunk between the anterior and middle scalene muscles. The three trunks then divide into anterior and posterior divisions, coursing over the first rib and lateral to the subclavian artery. The divisions then reunite to form cords. The anterior divisions of the superior and middle trunk form the lateral cord, while the anterior division of the inferior trunk forms the medial cord. The posterior divisions of all three trunks form the posterior cord. The cords are named according to their anatomic relationship with the axillary artery. The cords then divide once again to become the terminal branches of the brachial plexus. The lateral cord gives rise to the musculocutaneous nerve and contributes to the median nerve. The medial cord also contributes to the median nerve and gives rise to the ulnar nerve and the medial brachial and antebrachial cutaneous nerves. The posterior cord becomes the axillary and radial nerves.[1]

Additional nerves outside the brachial plexus can be important for complete anesthesia of the upper extremity. The supraclavicular nerve (C3–4) provides sensory innervation to the "cape" of the shoulder, and the intercostobrachial nerve (T2) innervates the skin of the medial upper arm and axilla.

Knowledge of brachial plexus anatomy and the dermatomes supplied *(Figs 4.2, 4.3)*, enables selective regional anesthesia.

Perineurial environment

The axillary sheath is the connective tissue surrounding the neurovascular structures of the brachial plexus. It originates

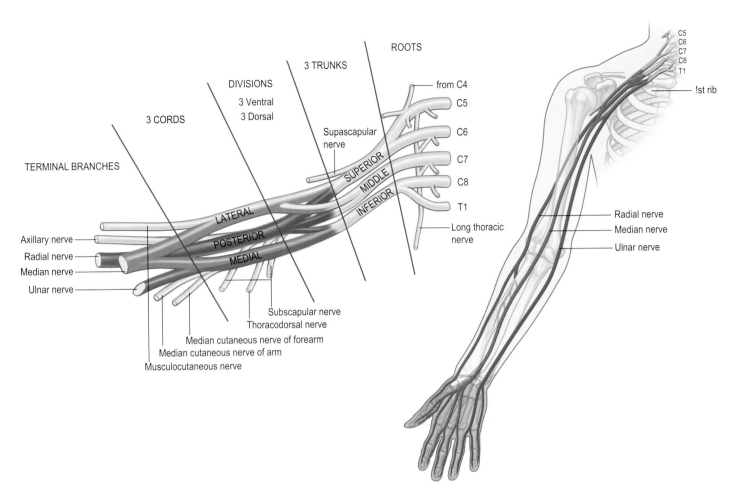

ROOTS

from C4

C5

C6

C7

C8

T1

3 TRUNKS

Supascapular nerve

SUPERIOR

MIDDLE

INFERIOR

Long thoracic nerve

DIVISIONS

3 Ventral

3 Dorsal

3 CORDS

LATERAL

POSTERIOR

MEDIAL

TERMINAL BRANCHES

Axillary nerve

Radial nerve

Median nerve

Ulnar nerve

Subscapular nerve

Thoracodorsal nerve

Median cutaneous nerve of forearm

Median cutaneous nerve of arm

Musculocutaneous nerve

C5

C6

C7

C8

T1

!st rib

Radial nerve

Median nerve

Ulnar nerve

Fig. 4.1 Brachial plexus anatomy.

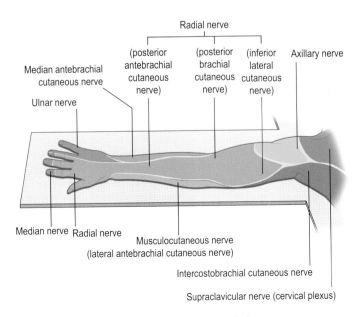

Radial nerve

(posterior antebrachial cutaneous nerve)

(posterior brachial cutaneous nerve)

(inferior lateral cutaneous nerve)

Axillary nerve

Median antebrachial cutaneous nerve

Ulnar nerve

Median nerve   Radial nerve

Musculocutaneous nerve (lateral antebrachial cutaneous nerve)

Intercostobrachial cutaneous nerve

Supraclavicular nerve (cervical plexus)

Fig. 4.2 Upper extremity nerve innervation (arm pronated).

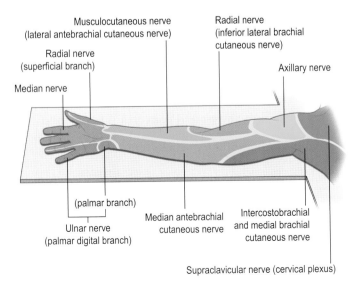

Musculocutaneous nerve (lateral antebrachial cutaneous nerve)

Radial nerve (superficial branch)

Median nerve

Radial nerve (inferior lateral brachial cutaneous nerve)

Axillary nerve

(palmar branch)

Ulnar nerve (palmar digital branch)

Median antebrachial cutaneous nerve

Intercostobrachial and medial brachial cutaneous nerve

Supraclavicular nerve (cervical plexus)

Fig. 4.3 Upper extremity nerve innervation (arm supinated).

as a continuation of the prevertebral fascia and joins the fascia of the biceps and brachialis muscles distally. This connective tissue extends inward, forming septa between components of the plexus and creating fascial compartments for each nerve.[2] Controversy exists regarding the ability of the septae to limit the spread of local anesthetics within the sheath. Some investigators report that these fascial compartments limit the circumferential spread of local anesthetics and that injected solutions spread longitudinally up and down the nerve and remain compartmentalized. This concept provides a rational explanation for the occurrence of a rapid and profound block of one nerve, yet partial or absent block in other nerves during brachial plexus blockade.[3] Other investigators propose that these septa are incomplete and form small bubble-like pockets when solution is injected. They found that single injections of dye solutions into the axillary sheath resulted in immediate staining of median, radial, and ulnar nerves, despite the presence of septa. These data demonstrate that there are connections between compartments within the sheath, and may explain why single injection techniques have success rates comparable with multiple injection techniques during blockade of the brachial plexus.[4]

Microneuroanatomy

Peripheral nerves are composed of fascicles of individual nerve fibers surrounded by endoneurium. Groups of fascicles are contained within the epineurium. As the nerve travels away from the spinal cord, fascicle numbers increase, while fascicle size decreases.[5] The nerve roots contain large fascicles, demonstrating a monofascicular or oligofascicular pattern, while a multifascicular pattern is found more distally.[6,7] While the amount of neural tissue remains constant, the amount of non-neural connective tissue increases from proximal to distal. The ratio of neural to non-neural tissue changes from 1:1 in the proximal plexus to 1:2 in the more distal plexus.[2,7] The presence of non-neural tissue may explain why injections within the epineurium rarely result in neural injury.[6]

Sonoanatomy

The shape and echogenicity of a nerve determine its ultrasound appearance. Structures that strongly reflect ultrasound waves generate large signal intensities and appear white or hyperechoic. In contrast, hypoechoic structures weakly reflect ultrasound waves and appear darker.[8] Peripheral nerves show a mixture of hypoechoic and hyperechoic structures constituting a typical "honeycomb" structure.[9] Hypoechoic structures seen with ultrasound correspond to neural tissue, while hyperechoic areas correlate with connective tissue.[10] Ultrasound imaging of the proximal brachial plexus usually shows hypoechoic structures reflecting an oligofascicular pattern. Distal brachial plexus structures display a more hyperechoic, honeycomb appearance, reflecting a multifascicular pattern.[7]

Pharmacology of local anesthetics

Local anesthetics (LA) make regional anesthesia possible by preventing the propagation of nerve conduction and inhibiting or relieving pain.[11] LA are primarily weak bases that attach to sites of the sodium channel in nerves and prevent the movement of the sodium ion through the nerve pores, which temporarily halts nerve conduction.[12]

Local anesthetics are classified as amides or esters, based on the chemical structure. Most local anesthetics used in regional anesthesia are amides (e.g., "-caines"). The structure of a typical local anesthetic consists of a lipophilic head, a hydrophilic tail, and a chain linking the head and tail which is either an amide or ester and determines the classification of the type of LA. Alteration of the structure of the LA affects the various actions of the LA itself and is important when making the choice of which LA to use. For example, increasing the alkyl substitution on the aromatic ring increases its lipid solubility, thereby increasing its potency. Allergic reactions to local anesthetics are more common with esters and rare with amides.

Pharmacokinetics

Local anesthetics differ from other drugs because they are directly delivered at their site of action. Efficacy depends on the amount of LA that reaches the nerve and proximity to the nerve. Diffusion of local anesthetic is dependent on the amount of connective tissue and adipose tissue that is present in the area of the block.

Toxicity

Local anesthetic toxicity has been a concern since its first use in nerve blockade. Regardless of which local anesthetic is injected, traditional methods have required large volumes for successful regional anesthesia such as with brachial plexus blockade or Bier blocks. Frequent aspiration and incremental dosing are imperative, as is communication with the patient to detect early signs of potential intravenous injection before progression to signs and symptoms of toxicity. Factors such as drug dose, rate of absorption, biotransformation, and elimination of the drug from the circulation are determinants of the plasma concentration of local anesthetics. Fortunately, one of the benefits of ultrasound guidance in the use of regional anesthesia has been the decreased need for large volumes.[13]

High plasma levels may be a consequence of direct intravascular injection, plasma absorption, and/or certain underlying medical conditions of the patient (i.e., hypoproteinemia in renal or hepatic disease). Elevated intravascular levels of LA may result in minor CNS symptoms such as dizziness, ringing in the ears, and may proceed to more intense symptoms of loss of consciousness, and seizures. At even higher levels, cardiac arrhythmias ensue, including complete cardiovascular collapse. Use of LA in regional anesthesia demands an appreciation of these toxicities. Understanding agent specific toxic levels is vital – as much as the preparation for these unintended events.

Adjuncts such as epinephrine affect absorption and elimination. The use of epinephrine as a marker of intravascular injection is warranted in almost all situations. Exceptions include those cases where the vasoconstriction resulting from epinephrine may in fact compromise the blood flow to the area.

Physicians must be prepared with monitors, emergency drugs, and airway supplies to facilitate treatment of LA related toxicity. Toxicity related to LA can include but is not limited to oxygen desaturation, hypotension, bradycardia, and seizures. The extent of toxicity is determined by the specific drug's intrinsic properties as well as the plasma level of the LA. The safety of LA is an essential aspect of regional anesthesia and is dependent on the skill of the physician, placement of the needle, the drug utilized, and patient health. All of these factors must be considered when determining the appropriate procedure and LA dose.[14]

Bupivacaine has been in use for many years and has the highest cardiotoxicity potential due to its intrinsic properties. Although the cardiac system is generally resistant to the effects of LA, bupivacaine is the notable exception. An overdose is more likely to result in cardiovascular collapse compared with other LA. This cardiac collapse is difficult to treat traditionally with ACLS/CPR alone. Recent case studies have demonstrated that IV infusion of Intralipid, an emulsified fat, may be successful in ameliorating cardiotoxicity associated with local anesthetics by acting as a "sink."

Vasoconstrictors

With the addition of vasoconstrictors such as epinephrine or phenylephrine to the LA anesthetic solution, the systemic absorption rate of an LA can be decreased.[14] The dose of bupivacaine increases from 3.5 to 4.0 mg/kg. This action of epinephrine is more significant with lidocaine as the upper limit increases from 3.0 to 7.0 mg/kg. Vasoconstrictors allow the physician to identify an intravascular injection sooner rather than later, due to the development of tachycardia with an intravascular injection.[15] The block can be halted immediately, possibly preventing a more serious intravascular complication. Vasoconstrictors result in decreased plasma uptake and increased duration of local anesthetic effect.[16]

LA selection

The choice of a LA depends on toxicity (as discussed previously), duration of effect, and time to onset *(Table 4.1)*.

Duration is important when considering surgical times when the block is the primary anesthetic. In such instances, the longer acting agents such as ropivacaine or bupivacaine have the distinct advantage as they often can outlast the surgery and offer the greater benefits of postoperative pain management.

Time to onset is also an important factor. Most of the time, regional anesthesia is done prior to the surgery and a fast time to onset is highly desirable. Each LA has its own time to onset or latency. Various factors can shorten this latency, including the addition of bicarbonate, higher dose, and needle location. The recent use of ultrasound allows for a more precise needle placement, which in turn allows for quicker onset.

Table 4.1 Commonly used agents in upper extremity regional anesthesia

Lidocaine	Most widely used LA
	Prototype amide
	Can be used in almost any peripheral block
	1.5% or 2% with or without epinephrine is most commonly used for surgical anesthesia
Mepivacaine	Intermediate duration
	Similar to lidocaine
	Less vasodilation
	Ineffective as topical agent
	1.5% mepivacaine is the most commonly used agent in regional anesthesia
Bupivacaine	One of the most commonly used LA in regional and infiltration anesthesia
	Long-acting
	High quality sensory anesthesia relative to motor blockade
	Most commonly used for epidural and spinal
	Refractory cardiac arrest with 0.75% concentration. Interaction with cardiac Na+ channels "fast in, slow out"
	Disruption of atrioventricular nodal conduction
	Depression of myocardial contractility
	Indirect effects mediated by CNS
	Limitations on total dose of bupivacaine given
Ropivacaine	Developed due to cardiotoxicity related to bupivacaine
	Long-acting
	Slightly less potent than bupivacaine
	Higher concentrations fastens its onset and density of block
	Reduced CNS/CV toxicity compared to bupivacaine

The choice of local anesthetic affects the quality of the block, time to onset, and duration of action *(Table 4.2)*.[15] Quicker onset generally leads to quicker clearance. Lidocaine and mepivacaine, agents with intermediate duration, have a short latency period which is further shortened by the addition of bicarbonate as mentioned above. In comparison, bupivacaine and ropivacaine, two long acting agents used commonly in regional anesthesia, have a longer latency period, and are not able to mix with bicarbonate due to precipitation concerns. In order to obtain both the quicker onset characteristic and the longer duration, some may consider mixing two agents together to achieve the quicker onset effect and the longer duration of anesthesia/analgesia. These mixtures can be about 50:50, however, it can vary depending on the experience and training of the anesthesiologist. The toxicity of mixtures are additive and the mixture does not lower the overall toxicity.[17]

Another consideration is the differential blockade, as nerves are blocked unequally and at different rates. Nerve blockade proceeds in the following order: sympathetic nerves, pin-prick sensation, touch, temperature, and finally motor.[18] This is an important attribute of bupivacaine, as one

Table 4.2 Comparative pharmacology and current use of local anesthetics

Classification and compounds	pKa	Non-ionized (%) at pH 7.4	Potency[a]	Max. dose (mg) for infiltration[b]	Duration after infiltration (min)	Topical	Infiltration	Intravenous regional	Peripheral block	Epidural	Spinal[c]
Esters											
Procaine	8.9	3	1	500	45–60	No	Yes	No	Yes	No	Yes
Chloroprocaine	8.7	5	2	600	30–60	No	Yes	No	Yes	Yes	Yes (?)
Tetracaine	8.5	7	8	–	–	Yes	No	No	No	No	Yes
Amides											
Lidocaine	7.9	24	2	300	60–120	Yes	Yes	Yes	Yes	Yes	Yes (?)
Mepivacaine	7.6	39	2	300	90–180	No	Yes	No	Yes	Yes	Yes (?)
Prilocaine	7.9	24	2	400	60–120	No	Yes	Yes	Yes	Yes	Yes (?)
Bupivacaine, levobupivacaine	8.1	17	8	150	240–480	No	Yes	No	Yes	Yes	Yes
Ropivacaine	8.1	17	6	200	240–480	No	Yes	No	Yes	Yes	Yes

[a]Relative potencies vary based on experimental model or route of administration. [b]Dosage should take into account the site of injection, use of a vasoconstrictor, and patient-related factors. [c]Use of lidocaine, mepivacaine, prilocaine, and chloroprocaine for spinal anesthesia is controversial and evolving (see text).

can provide improved analgesia without much motor blockade in the postoperative period if an infusion is run at analgesic doses. Optimally, an LA with sensory selectivity is desired.

Regional anesthesia techniques

Regional anesthesia has been shown to be an excellent anesthetic modality for upper extremity surgery. This relates to long lasting pain relief, reduced opioid-related side-effects during the first 24 hours after surgery, and expedited hospital discharge.[2,19] Despite this, many patients still receive other types of anesthesia for a variety of reasons. Alternatives to regional anesthesia include general anesthesia, monitored anesthetic care (MAC), Bier block or simple local anesthetic infiltration without blockade of the brachial plexus. The factors involved in determining suitability of an anesthetic include patient preference, surgeon preference, relative and absolute contraindications to regional anesthesia, as well as type of surgery. General anesthesia has been utilized for many years with a safety record that has improved significantly over the past decades.[20] Due to respiratory depression, general anesthesia requires airway management not routine in regional anesthesia, local anesthesia or in monitored anesthetic care. Additionally, patients who undergo general anesthesia may experience hemodynamic variations that may be significant in those with cardiac disease. All patients who will undergo any type of anesthesia need to have standard ASA monitors, which include pulse oximetry, blood pressure monitoring, and electrocardiogram monitoring as well as intravascular access established in the nonoperative limb.

The use of ultrasound guided blocks has gained significant momentum in the last decade. The benefits of ultrasound include shortened time to onset, enhanced visualization of the nerve target and surrounding structures such as arteries,

veins, muscle, and other soft tissues, needle visualization, visualization of the local anesthetic and its spread, and anomalies of anatomy.[21] Combining the traditional technique of peripheral nerve stimulation with ultrasound has not demonstrated notable benefits, although that has been a common practice, particularly for difficult cases. Surprisingly, there have been no studies that demonstrate improved safety with ultrasound over the technique of peripheral nerve stimulation.[22,23]

Digital block

Digital nerve blockade is easy to perform and provides useful anesthesia for a variety of surgical procedures or injuries isolated to a digit. Many techniques for performing digital nerve blocks have been described. These techniques rely on anesthesia of the volar common digital nerves derived from the median and ulnar nerves as well as the dorsal digital branches of the radial nerve.

The authors' preferred technique for digital blockade involves volar and dorsal injections. The hand is placed palm up and the skin is cleansed. With a 25-gauge or 27-gauge needle, 5 mL of local anesthetic, usually 1% lidocaine or 0.25% bupivacaine, is injected into the subdermal space directly overlying the A1 pulley of the involved finger. A wheal is slowly raised. The hand is then turned palm down and an additional 2–3 mL of local anesthetic is injected into the subcutaneous tissue over the dorsum of the finger, just distal to the metacarpophalangeal joint.

The use of epinephrine in digital blocks has been a controversial subject. Despite the admonition against epinephrine use in numerous medical textbooks, no case of digital gangrene has been reported in the literature resulting solely from the use of epinephrine with a local anesthetic. A number of studies have demonstrated epinephrine can be safely used as an adjunct for digital block anesthesia. Lalonde *et al.*

performed a randomized, prospective, blinded study with over 3000 consecutive cases and showed no cases of infarction, necrosis or tissue loss.[24] Epinephrine can be added to local anesthetics to lengthen the duration of action, lessen bleeding, reduce the need for a tourniquet, and reduce the risk of adverse systemic effects.[25]

Wrist block

When the entire hand requires anesthesia, a wrist block is appropriate. A wrist block is the technique of blocking the median, ulnar and radial nerves at the level of the wrist. Similar to the digital block, it is easy to perform, has minimal complications, and is highly effective.

The patient should be supine with the arm abducted and wrist in slight dorsiflexion. The median nerve is located between the tendons of the palmaris longus (PL) and the flexor carpi radialis (FCR). The palmaris longus tendon is usually the more prominent of the two; the median nerve passes just radial to it. The ulnar nerve passes between the ulnar artery and tendon of the flexor carpi ulnaris (FCU). The tendon of the flexor carpi ulnaris is superficial to the ulnar nerve. The superficial branch of the radial nerve runs along the medial aspect of the brachioradialis muscle. It then passes between the tendon of the brachioradialis and radius to pierce the fascia on the dorsal aspect. Just above the radial styloid process, it gives digital branches for the dorsal skin of the thumb, index finger, and lateral half of the middle finger.

The median nerve is blocked by inserting a 25-gauge needle between the tendons of the palmaris longus and flexor carpi radialis at a 30° angle. The needle is inserted until it pierces the deep fascia. Piercing of the deep fascia may be appreciated with a fascial "click." Local anesthetic, 3–5 mL, is injected. There should be no resistance to the injection as the local anesthetic travels up and down the carpal tunnel.

The ulnar nerve is anesthetized by transversely inserting the needle under the tendon of the FCU muscle close to its distal attachment proximal to the ulnar styloid. The needle is advanced 5–10 mm past the FCU tendon. The syringe is aspirated to confirm that it is not intravascular in the ulnar artery. Local anesthetic solution, 3–5 mL is then injected. A subcutaneous injection of 2–3 mL of local anesthesia just above the tendon of the FCU is also advisable in blocking the cutaneous branches of the ulnar nerve.

The radial nerve is essentially anesthetized with a field block. This blockade requires a more extensive infiltration because of the less predictable anatomic location and division into multiple, smaller, cutaneous branches. Local anesthetic, 5 mL is injected subcutaneously just above the radial styloid, aiming medially. The infiltration is then extended laterally, using an additional 5 mL of local anesthetic.

Intravenous regional anesthesia (Bier block)

A Bier block is indicated for brief surgery of the hand or forearm (up to 1 h). This technique relies on diffusion of local anesthetic from the venous system to nearby nerves. The operative extremity is exsanguinated using an Esmarch bandage. A double tourniquet is inflated sequentially from distal to proximal. The distal tourniquet is then deflated to allow local anesthetic to penetrate that area. Local anesthetic

solution is then injected through a small IV catheter placed in the hand of the arm to be anesthetized. A total of 50 mL of 0.5% lidocaine is commonly used. Of note, the patient should have a separate IV on the nonoperative limb to be available for sedation and/or emergency access. Anesthesia onset is within minutes. Patients may complain of tourniquet pain after 30 min, at which time the distal cuff is inflated and the proximal cuff is released. At the conclusion of surgery, the tourniquet is deflated, and there is a rapid resolution of anesthesia. To prevent local anesthetic toxicity, the tourniquet should not be deflated before 30 min have elapsed after drug infusion. Advantages of a Bier block include its safety profile, simplicity and reliability. However, its use is limited to short procedures due to tourniquet discomfort, and it offers no postoperative analgesia.

Interscalene block

Indications for an interscalene block include surgery of the shoulder, distal clavicle, acromioclavicular joint, and proximal humerus. The block is performed at the level of C5–C7 nerve roots, providing anesthesia to the shoulder and upper arm. Proximal spread of local anesthetic to C3–4 will also anesthetize the cape of the shoulder. Ulnar nerve distribution is usually spared with this technique. The nerve roots lie in a groove between the anterior and middle scalene muscles, posterolateral to the sternocleidomastoid muscle and phrenic nerve.

To perform the block, the patient is placed in a semi-recumbent position. When using the nerve stimulation technique, the interscalene groove is palpated at the level of C6 and the needle is advanced in a slight postero-caudad direction. A twitch of the bicep, tricep, or distal muscle is sought. When using ultrasound, the C5–7 roots form a characteristic "stoplight" appearance as they lie sequentially between the scalene muscles. The nerves are identified, and local anesthetic is deposited circumferentially around the nerves (Fig. 4.4).

Complications and side-effects specific to this block are ipsilateral phrenic nerve palsy, Horner's syndrome, hoarseness from blockade of the recurrent laryngeal nerve, and vascular puncture or injection; the carotid artery, internal and external jugular veins, and vertebral artery are in close proximity to the nerves of interest.

Supraclavicular block

The supraclavicular approach to the brachial plexus provides more reliable and effective regional anesthesia to the upper extremity than other approaches.[26] Indications for the supraclavicular approach include surgery of the upper extremity including the arm, elbow, and hand. Though the supraclavicular block can also be used for shoulder surgery, it may require some supplementation of the supraclavicular nerve (C3–C4).[2]

With ultrasound assistance, it is easy to appreciate the continuum that exists within the brachial plexus. Moving the ultrasound probe up or down, the brachial plexus will change a block from an interscalene block to a supraclavicular block. With the gain in popularity with ultrasound, there

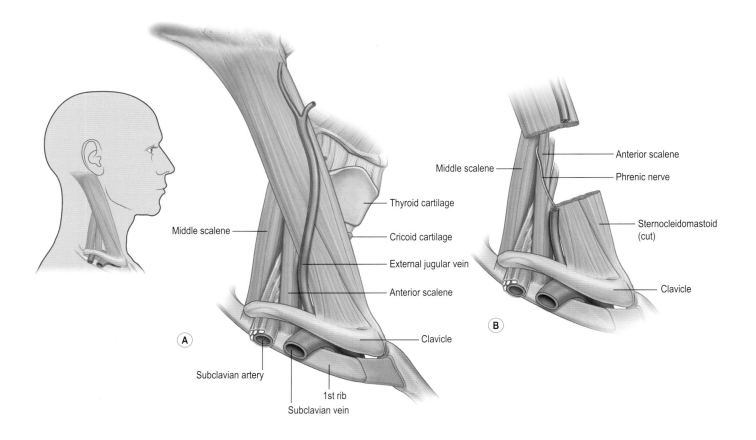

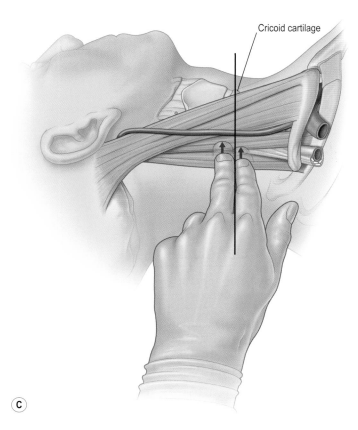

Fig. 4.4 (A,B) Interscalene block, functional anatomy and **(C)** technique.

has been a resurgence in the supraclavicular block as the concerns of pneumothorax have diminished. In a recent study of 510 patients who underwent ultrasound guided supraclavicular blocks, none were found to have a pneumothorax.[27]

The supraclavicular block is performed with the probe placed in the supraclavicular fossa. The sonoanatomy includes the subclavian artery, which is the primary landmark in this block. The brachial plexus (trunks and/or divisions of the plexus) lies superior (posterior) and lateral to the artery in a majority of patients and appears as a "bunch of grapes" or several round structures with a dark interior (hypoechoic) and a bright outline (hyperechoic outer circle). Once an adequate view is identified, the area is prepped and draped in a sterile fashion. The needle is then aligned with the probe in what is referred to as an "in-plane" technique. The needle appears on screen to move in a lateral to medial fashion. Once the needle is seen, placement should be carefully done with frequent aspiration. It may take 2–3 needle placements to ensure adequate coverage of the brachial plexus *(Fig. 4.5)*.

The most common side-effects include hemi-diaphragmatic paresis secondary to phrenic nerve block, ipsilateral Horner's syndrome, ipsilateral nasal congestion. Other risks include infection, bleeding, nerve injury, and pneumothorax.

Nerve stimulation technique of the supraclavicular block is less frequently performed due to the concerns and risk of pneumothorax. There are other suitable alternatives if the ultrasound view is difficult to obtain.

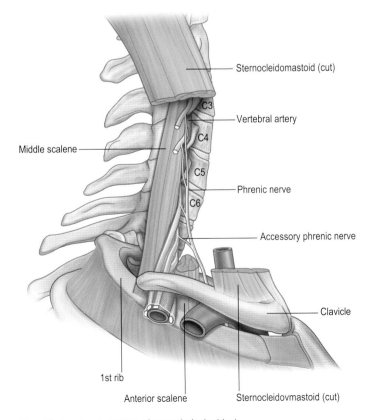

Fig. 4.5 Functional anatomy of supraclavicular block.

Labels: Sternocleidomastoid (cut); C3; Vertebral artery; C4; Middle scalene; C5; Phrenic nerve; C6; Accessory phrenic nerve; Clavicle; 1st rib; Anterior scalene; Sternocleidovmastoid (cut)

Infraclavicular block

Indications for an infraclavicular block are the same as for the supraclavicular approach. The main difference is that the infraclavicular approach generally preserves pulmonary function by avoiding a block of the diaphragm, which is possible with the supraclavicular approach. The infraclavicular approach is a block of the brachial plexus at the level the lateral, medial and posterior cords. These cords are named for their relationship to the axillary artery, although this relationship can have many variations.[28] In the United States, the most common approach for the infraclavicular block is using the coracoid process as a landmark, both with ultrasound guidance, as well as with peripheral nerve stimulation. Ultrasound guided infraclavicular blocks are performed with the probe placed just medial to the coracoid process and below the clavicle. Important sonoanatomy includes the axillary artery with the three cords surrounding the artery in a U-shaped fashion. The approach includes an in-plane technique with the needle aligned with the probe in a 45° angle aiming in a cephalad to caudad direction. The needle is placed just posterior to the axillary artery, which, when the LA is injected, provides coverage to all three cords in a U-shaped spread *(Fig. 4.6)*.

Use of the nerve stimulator with the infraclavicular approach is quite common and may be considered to be less difficult by some than ultrasound guided infraclavicular block. In order to perform the infraclavicular block, the coracoid process is identified and marked. Once this is achieved, the physician will measure 2 cm medial and 2 cm inferior – this marks the nerve stimulator needle entry point. The nerve stimulator is turned to 1.0 mA. The needle is advanced in a direction that is perpendicular to the floor. It is important to note as with other blocks, there should be frequent aspiration throughout the block in order to minimize the risk of intravascular injection. As the needle is advanced, stimulation of the posterior cord is sought (extension of the elbow, wrist or fingers) and maintained at 0.5 mA. If the correct stimulation of muscle groups is not achieved, the needle's direction should be redirected by 5° at a time. Some anesthesiologists may seek both the medial and lateral cord if the posterior cord is difficult to find in order to improve success rates. The risks of the infraclavicular block include infection, bleeding, nerve injury, and pneumothorax.

Axillary block

An axillary block is indicated for surgery of the hand and forearm. It is performed at the level of the terminal branches of the brachial plexus. The radial, median, and ulnar nerves are positioned around the axillary artery, and the musculocutaneous nerve resides in the coracobrachialis muscle, lateral to the neurovascular bundle. The distribution of anesthesia includes the entire arm, except for the medial strip of skin in the upper arm, which is supplied by the intercostobrachial nerve from T2 *(Fig. 4.7)*.

For this block, the arm is abducted and the elbow flexed. When using the nerve stimulation technique, the axillary artery is palpated high in the axilla and the needle is directed lateral, medial, and posterior to the artery to stimulate the median, ulnar, and radial nerves, respectively. Obtaining two

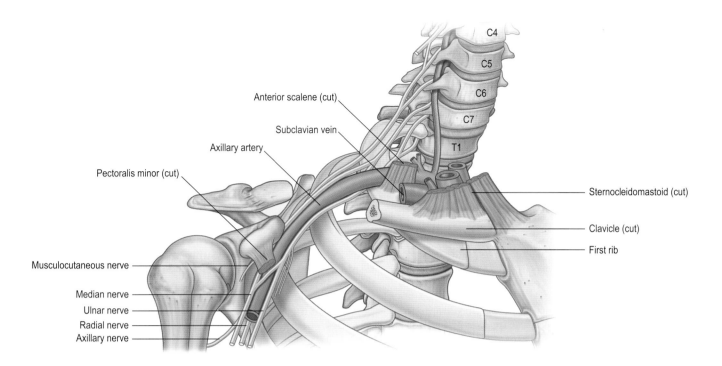

Fig. 4.6 Functional anatomy of infraclavicular block.

or more separate twitches, and therefore injecting local anesthetic near two or more nerves, improves block success.[29] The musculocutaneous nerve is then blocked by directing the needle laterally into the coracobrachialis muscle, obtaining a twitch of the bicep muscle, and depositing additional local anesthetic. When using ultrasound, the probe is placed transversely on the upper arm near the axilla, perpendicular to the axillary artery. The artery and nerves of interest are visualized. The needle is advanced in a lateral to medial direction, and local anesthetic is deposited around each nerve.

The axillary approach to the brachial plexus has potential benefits for certain patient populations such as patients with pulmonary disease, because the phrenic nerve will not be affected. This block may also be superior in patients with coagulopathies, since the area is superficial and easily compressible if vascular puncture occurs. One disadvantage of this block is that the needle must be repositioned multiple times to adequately block all of the nerves, potentially increasing the risk of vascular puncture or causing more patient discomfort. Additionally, the arm must be abducted in order to have adequate access to the upper arm and axilla, which may be difficult in some patients such as those with injuries.

Complications

Complications associated with regional anesthesia present a rare but significant risk to patients undergoing surgery of the upper extremity. Serious complications include neurologic injury, seizures, and cardiac arrest. Other risks associated with regional anesthesia are hematoma, infection, and block-specific complications such as pneumothorax. A large French prospective study reported an incidence of severe complications related to peripheral nerve blocks to be <5/10 000 and an incidence of serious neurologic injury to be 2.4/10 000.[30]

Peripheral nerve injury

Peripheral nerve injury can present as pain, sensory disturbances, or motor deficits. Most of these are transient, with 95% resolving within 4–6 weeks and over 99% resolving within 1 year.[2,29] Nerve damage can be classified as mechanical, chemical, or ischemic. Recovery and prognosis are related to the location of injury. If the axon is damaged, recovery is slow and often incomplete, relying on collateral reinnervation or axonal regrowth. Damage to the myelin sheath disrupts the nerve action potential and tends to have faster recovery and a better prognosis. Mechanical injury from needles or catheters can disrupt the axon, although nerves tend to move away from approaching needles.[31] Local anesthetics can cause chemical injury to nerves through cellular cytotoxic effects, dependent on the concentration and duration of exposure.[30] Finally, ischemic injury may be caused by vascular injury, prolonged tourniquet use, or the use of vasoconstrictors. Ischemia causes metabolic stress and is associated with axonal damage and a poorer prognosis.

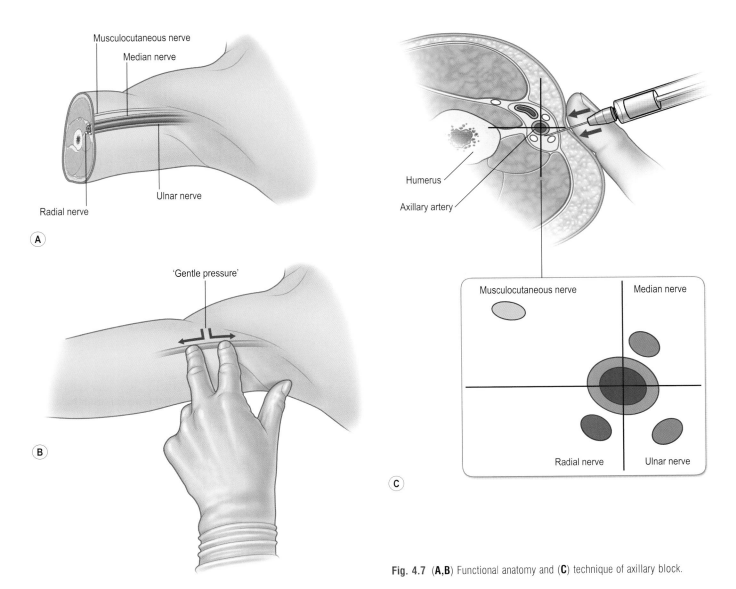

Fig. 4.7 (**A,B**) Functional anatomy and (**C**) technique of axillary block.

Evaluation and management

A suspected peripheral nerve injury warrants an immediate evaluation, including a complete history and physical examination to screen for any pre-existing problems and to determine the location of the lesion. The 2008 American Society of Regional Anesthesia and Pain Medicine (ASRA) Practice Advisory on Neurologic Complications recommends that a complete or progressive deficit should be evaluated immediately by a neurologist or peripheral nerve surgeon. Mild or resolving symptoms without evidence of a neural deficit can be monitored and may only require patient reassurance. However, if symptoms fail to improve, a neurological consultation is recommended. Incomplete lesions with evidence of a neural deficit should initially be evaluated by a neurologist and may require referral to a peripheral nerve surgeon if symptoms persist or worsen.[31] Neurologic tests such as nerve conduction studies, electromyography, and MRI may be helpful in establishing the degree of nerve damage, location, and prognosis.

Local anesthetic toxicity

Local anesthetics used for peripheral nerve blocks have the potential to cause serious harm. Systemic absorption of local anesthetic from an appropriately placed and dosed nerve block may result in mild symptoms, while an unintentional intravascular injection can lead to severe neurologic or cardiac toxicity causing major disability or even death. Risk factors that increase the potential for local anesthetic systemic toxicity (LAST) include local anesthetic potency and dose, peripheral nerve block location and technique, and patient risk factors such as age, pre-existing disease, and medications. Methods to prevent LAST revolve around avoiding intravascular injection and limiting the total dose of local anesthetic. Intravascular injection can be limited or avoided by incrementally injecting local anesthetic to monitor for symptoms of systemic absorption, aspirating prior to injection, and using an intravascular marker such as epinephrine. If systemic toxicity does occur, the classic symptoms present as auditory changes, circumoral numbness, metallic taste, and agitation. Symptoms may then progress to seizures, CNS depression, and finally, cardiac excitation followed by depression. However, cardiac toxicity may occur simultaneously or even before neurological symptoms. The treatment of LAST is circulatory and airway support to minimize hypoxia and acidosis. Seizures can be controlled with benzodiazepines, although succinylcholine may be necessary for persistent seizures. Cardiac arrest requires rapid restoration of cardiac output and oxygen delivery. If standard ACLS measures such as epinephrine or amiodarone fail to provide an adequate response, lipid emulsion therapy should be administered. Cardiac arrest refractory to vasopressor and lipid emulsion therapy should prompt institution of cardiopulmonary bypass.[32]

Vascular injury

Vascular complications include hematomas, vasospasm from arterial puncture or local anesthetic induced vasoconstriction, and arterial dissection from intramural injection. Hematomas have the potential to cause ischemic injury to nearby neural structures from compression, although they are usually small and inconsequential.[33] The severity of symptoms and progression are related to the rate and duration of hematoma formation. Risk factors include the extent of arterial injury (number of needle punctures,) intrinsic vascular elasticity, and presence of diabetes, hypertension, or anticoagulation.[34] The presence of a hematoma should prompt evaluation of neurological function. Surgical decompression and evacuation may be necessary for severe cases, although conservative management is often appropriate.

When considering peripheral nerve blocks in the anticoagulated patient, significant blood loss, rather than neural deficits, may be the most serious complication. The expansile nature of the neurovascular sheath may decrease the chance of irreversible neural ischemia. Although neuraxial regional anesthesia presents significant risk to the anticoagulated patient, the risk after peripheral techniques remains undefined. Published case reports of clinically significant bleeding after peripheral regional anesthesia techniques demonstrate that all patients presenting with neurodeficits had complete recovery within 6 months to 1 year.[35] The 2010 ASRA Guidelines on Regional Anesthesia in the Anticoagulated Patient suggest that brachial plexus blockade in this patient population is not contraindicated, but should be evaluated on a case-by-case basis with increased caution.[2]

Infection

Infectious complications associated with regional anesthesia of the upper extremity are rare. Localized infection and bacteremia have been reported after both single-shot and continuous catheter techniques. One study reported catheter tip colonization in 29% of peripheral catheters, with 3% resulting in local inflammation.[36,37] Patient risk factors for infectious complications include underlying sepsis, diabetes, immunocompromised status, steroid therapy, localized bacterial infection, chronic catheter maintenance (>48 h), and ICU admission.[38,39] A careful evaluation of the risk-to-benefit ratio should be made prior to placing nerve blocks in infected or immunocompromised patients.[2,37]

Outcomes

Upper extremity surgery can be performed successfully under both general anesthesia (GA) and regional anesthesia (RA). The potential benefits of RA techniques in outpatient surgery include improved clinical outcomes, patient satisfaction, efficiency, and reduced cost.[40] However, GA is still widely used for outpatient surgery, and many of the newer anesthetic agents are short-acting with fewer side-effects and better recovery profiles as compared with older agents. Additionally, many anesthesiologists are more familiar and comfortable with providing GA compared with RA.[41,42]

Clinical outcomes and patient satisfaction

Several studies comparing regional anesthesia to general anesthesia for upper extremity surgery have demonstrated more favorable clinical outcomes with regional anesthesia, in terms of improved pain control, less nausea and vomiting, and fewer opioid-related side-effects. Other benefits include patients feeling more alert, tolerating oral intake sooner, and ambulating sooner.[40,41]

While improved clinical outcomes have been shown for RA in the immediate postoperative period, long-term benefits are still undefined. In a study comparing RA to GA in patients undergoing outpatient hand and wrist surgery, patients having RA had better initial analgesia and faster recovery but both groups had a similar degree of pain and need for oral analgesics 48 hours postoperatively.[40] In another study comparing RA to GA in ambulatory hand surgery, patients in the RA group had significantly less postoperative pain before hospital discharge, but on postoperative days 1, 7, and 14, there were no differences in pain, opioid consumption, adverse effects, pain-disability index, or satisfaction.[41] Improved functional capacity has been demonstrated in patients having lower extremity surgery with continuous RA techniques. A study of patients undergoing outpatient shoulder and foot surgery under RA with continuous outpatient perineural infusions of local anesthetics demonstrated optimized functional recovery, analgesia, and patient satisfaction for 3 days postoperatively.[43] Further studies are necessary to determine if RA for upper extremity surgery has a benefit after the immediate postoperative period in terms of pain control, adverse effects, and functional capacity.

Patient satisfaction, although difficult to define, is usually high, with both regional and general anesthesia. Improved patient satisfaction with RA techniques may be a result of improved analgesia and fewer side-effects.[44] Studies showing lower patient satisfaction with RA techniques often cite tourniquet pain and discomfort during the nerve block placement, as causes of dissatisfaction.[45]

Operating room cost and efficiency

Several investigators have sought to determine if regional anesthesia is superior to general anesthesia in terms of operating room (OR) efficiency and costs. Some potential areas to improve efficiency and reduce costs are OR utilization time and recovery room time.

Some studies suggest that in order to save OR time through the use of regional anesthesia techniques, nerve blocks must be performed outside the operating room. In this case, the cost of valuable OR time is spared and efficiency is maximized because patients are ready for surgery as soon as they enter the operating room.[41] Others have reported similar OR times for RA versus GA techniques even when the blocks were performed in the operating room. This was attributed to the combination of fast-acting local anesthetics, the ability for surgeons to prepare the patients while the nerve blocks took full effect, and faster emergence time compared to GA.[40]

Patients having RA for upper extremity surgery who experience superior pain control and fewer side-effects may potentially have a shorter PACU stay. A meta-analysis of RA versus GA for ambulatory anesthesia showed that patients receiving RA had an increased ability to bypass the PACU and/or a decreased PACU time.[44]

To date, studies demonstrating an overall cost reduction for intraoperative and postoperative care during upper extremity surgery have compared GA to intravenous regional anesthesia (Bier block). The IVRA group had significant cost-savings attributed to lower anesthetic drug and equipment costs, shorter OR times, shorter PACU times, and shorter nursing times.[46,47] In contrast, a retrospective comparison of costs for RA and GA techniques demonstrated a cost disadvantage for brachial plexus regional anesthesia, although recovery room costs were not included in this analysis.[48] More research is needed to determine if RA techniques for upper extremity surgery show a significant cost reduction when compared with other anesthetic techniques.

Special considerations

Cardiac patients

Patients with cardiac disease, including those with cardiac dysfunction and low ejection fractions, conduction abnormalities or ongoing ischemia, should be given consideration for regional anesthesia for upper extremity cases when indicated. Regional anesthesia allows patients the usual advantages of perioperative analgesia and possibly avoidance of general anesthesia.[20] General anesthesia, while very safe, can cause hemodynamic variations during the induction of anesthesia, intubation, emergence from anesthesia and possibly during surgical stimulation or bleeding. In this patient population, variations in blood pressure and heart rate can have significant consequences. The prospect of regional anesthesia and analgesia allows the patient to avoid hemodynamic fluctuations, thus minimizing risk.

Patients with cardiac disease may be anticoagulated for a variety of reasons. In these patients, the risks and benefits of the block must take into consideration the possibility of an increased likelihood of bleeding during a nerve block with a resultant hematoma and nerve compression.

Pediatric patients

The pediatric population warrants special considerations when considering the type of anesthetic for surgery. These include anatomic and physiologic differences when compared with adult counterparts. Regional anesthesia offers the advantage of intraoperative and postoperative analgesia for the pediatric population. While still receiving a general anesthesia in most cases, the pediatric patient may benefit from a regional anesthetic as a result of decreased requirements for inhalational agents, leading to improved respiratory status.[49] Improved respiratory status decreases the chance of laryngospasm on emergence. There are additional benefits of comfort for the patient's family, observing a more comfortable and pain-free child in the recovery room. Overall, there is less stress for all involved.[50]

The types of blocks performed on pediatric patients are generally performed with the patient under GA. It is not until the child is older and demonstrating a level of maturity that the block can be performed on the awake patient. When a block is performed on an asleep patient, there is an elevated risk of nerve injury as the patient cannot relay the sensation of paresthesias and pain from the rare event of neural trauma. Overall, regional anesthetic techniques are considered safe with an extremely low incidence of complications.[51]

Ultrasound guidance is strongly recommended when considering regional anesthesia as part of the anesthetic in infants and children. The increased assistance provided in locating sonographic landmarks and nerve targets are of great benefit.[52–54]

Perioperative pain management

For upper extremity surgery, the use of regional anesthesia with local anesthetics is primarily motivated by the desire to avoid general anesthesia. It has resulted in lower postoperative opiate usage and therefore alleviation of opiate-related side-effects.[55] This approach has become, in many ways, the standard of care in upper extremity cases.

Peripheral catheters

Peripheral nerve blockade is safe and provides postoperative analgesia through the use of long-acting local anesthetics and/or continuous infusions through peripheral nerve catheters.[56] Peripheral nerve catheters are usually placed preoperatively by the anesthesiologist when the initial nerve block is performed. Alternatively, a catheter may be placed in the postoperative period if the patient experiences severe pain. Continuous catheters do not delay discharge in outpatient surgery as they can be managed at home by the patient.

Preemptive analgesia

Preemptive analgesia is a pain management technique initiated prior to incision, which continues during the surgical procedure to reduce ongoing changes that occur in the body as a result of surgical incision and stimulation.[57] The rationale is that by preemptively blocking the nociceptive transmission onslaught that occurs with surgical incision, there will be less pain in the postoperative period and thus less need for consumption of opiates with fewer side-effects. The duration of treatment includes the entire time that the noxious stimulation of surgery and its inflammatory injuries occur (intraoperative and early postoperative period).[57]

Opiate-related side-effects of sedation, nausea, respiratory depression, ileus and urinary retention can impact patient safety and satisfaction, discharge or patient admission, particularly in the outpatient setting, thereby affecting cost issues. Multimodal analgesic regimens have been developed featuring the peripheral nerve block in order to improve perioperative outcomes for minimally invasive procedures.

There has been much controversy surrounding the relevance and effectiveness of preemptive analgesia. Although the benefits have been established to some degree in animal studies, it has had questionable effect in human studies to date.[58] Many physicians practice with the belief that there is some preemptive analgesic effect. Some suggest that there is greater complexity in pain pathways than our understanding, and that studies are too simplistic. However, there is little doubt that excellent pain management in the pre- and post-surgical area contributes to an overall improved pain experience. A meta-analysis demonstrated that analgesia in the preoperative period lowered opiate consumption when the preemptive treatment was epidural analgesia, local infiltration, and systemic NSAIDs.[59] The findings were equivocal with opioids and NMDA receptors alone. Certain studies go further to demonstrate that the preemptive analgesia associated with ketamine or a cox-2 analgesic gives additional benefit pre-incision.

One such study looked at patients about to undergo upper limb surgery under axillary brachial plexus blockade.[60] The study examined the addition of a long-acting NSAID, ampiroxicam, versus placebo given 3 h prior to surgery. A significant improvement occurred in patients who received the NSAID when compared to those in the placebo group. The treated patients consumed significantly less opiates and therefore were less likely to develop narcotic side-effects such as sedation, nausea, constipation, or urinary retention. Nociceptive afferent transmission is known to be sensitive to inflammation and NSAIDs are postulated to have this effect via their anti-inflammatory action. Another study retrospectively reviewed a multimodal, preemptive pathway for patients undergoing major knee or hip surgery featuring peripheral nerve blocks, found that patients were better able to participate in postoperative rehabilitation, were eligible for hospital discharge sooner, initiated earlier ambulation, experienced lower perioperative pain scores, and experienced

Table 4.3 Risk factors for severe postoperative pain

Preoperative pain
Prior use of opiates
Female gender
Nonlaparoscopic surgery
Knee and shoulder surgery
Psychosocial vulnerability
Repeat surgery
Intensity of early postoperative pain
Surgical approach with risk of nerve damage

reduced postoperative nausea and vomiting when compared with more traditional PCA measures.[61] These findings advocate for the preemptive multimodal analgesic regimen.

Chronic postoperative pain

The development of postoperative pain after surgery is due to complex pathways – endocrine, metabolic, and inflammatory – that trigger a prolonged state of excitation of the spinal cord.[62] Various chemicals released during and soon after surgical incision may induce conversion of high threshold nociceptors into low threshold receptors, via a process called peripheral sensitization. This complex process eventually leads to release of cellular mediators in the recuperative period resulting in central sensitization and chronic pain.[63] Chronic pain is, among other factors, linked to patients with severe postoperative pain.[15,64] While the development of chronic pain following surgery has lacked a spotlight in the medical literature, it is a reality that needs to be considered particularly in patients who may be at higher risk of developing chronic pain.[65] Inadequately treated postoperative pain is a major source of patients' dissatisfaction with their overall surgical experience.[66] Severe pain in the postoperative period correlates to a greater likelihood of developing chronic pain.[67] There are a number of risk factors[68] for developing severe postoperative pain *(Table 4.3)*.

It is imperative that postoperative pain be treated effectively, possibly with a multimodal approach which considers preemptive analgesia and its potential benefits. It is crucial to identify those patients that have a greater likelihood of developing severe postoperative pain, not only to minimize the likelihood of developing chronic pain, but also to improve the patient's experience in the perioperative period.

Access the complete references list online at **http://www.expertconsult.com**

2. Neal JM, Gerancher JC, Hebl JR, et al. Upper extremity regional anesthesia: essentials of our current understanding, 2008. *Reg Anesth Pain Med.* 2009;34(2): 134–170.

   This article provides a comprehensive review of upper extremity regional anesthesia, including relevant anatomy, pharmacology, techniques, and complications. This review also summarizes the essential scholarly works available on upper extremity regional anesthesia and identifies informational gaps where further study is warranted.

6. Moayeri N, Bigeleisen PE, Groen GJ. Quantitative architecture of the brachial plexus and surrounding compartments, and their possible significance for plexus blocks. *Anesthesiology.* 2008;108(2):299–304.

8. Sites BD, Brull R, Chan VW, et al. Artifacts and pitfall errors associated with ultrasound-guided regional anesthesia. Part I: understanding the basic principles of ultrasound physics and machine operations. *Reg Anesth Pain Med.* 2007;32(5):412–418.

This article presents the basics of ultrasound used for regional anesthesia. By understanding basic ultrasound physics most relevant to regional anesthesia and recognizing brachial plexus ultrasound anatomy, physicians can improve their ability to visualize target nerves, position of needles, and real-time spread of local anesthetic, thus improving nerve block efficiency, success, and safety.

15. Bridenbaugh PO, Cousins MJ. *Neural blockade in clinical anesthesia and management of pain.* 3rd edn. Philadelphia: Lippincott-Raven; 1998:xxii, 1177.

This book chapter presents a review of the clinical pharmacology of local anesthetics, including factors that influence their usefulness and toxicity. Additionally, the various local anesthetics are reviewed for their specific activity, physiochemical structure, and applicability in clinical practice. These drugs, integral to the practice of regional anesthesia, are presented in a totality essential to the understanding of their role in practice.

18. Raj PP. *Textbook of regional anesthesia.* New York: Churchill Livingstone; 2002:xix, 1083.

19. Klein SM, Evans H, Nielsen KC, et al. Peripheral nerve block techniques for ambulatory surgery. *Anesth Analg.* 2005;101(6):1663–1676.

21. Neal JG, Cox MJ, Drake DB, et al. The ASRA evidence-based medicine assessment of ultrasound-guided regional anesthesia and pain medicine: Executive summary. *Reg Anesth Pain Med.* 2010; 35(2 Suppl):S1–S9.

29. Sorenson EJ. Neurological injuries associated with regional anesthesia. *Reg Anesth Pain Med.* 2008;33(5): 442–448.

This article provides a concise review of neurological injuries associated with regional anesthesia, including mechanisms, diagnosis, and management. Although neurologic injury is rare, every anesthesiologist and surgeon employing regional anesthesia techniques for their patients must be able to recognize a potential injury and institute treatment if necessary.

44. Liu SS, Strodtbeck WM, Richman JM, et al. Comparison of regional versus general anesthesia for ambulatory anesthesia: a meta-analysis of randomized controlled trials A. *Anesth Analg.* 2005;101(6):1634–1642.

60. Hebl JR, Dilger JA, Byer DE, et al. A pre-emptive multimodal pathway featuring peripheral nerve block improves perioperative outcomes after major orthopedic surgery. *Reg Anesth Pain Med.* 2008;33(6):510–517.

5

Principles of internal fixation as applied to the hand and wrist

Jeffrey Yao and Christopher Cox

SYNOPSIS

- Most minimally or nondisplaced fractures can be managed nonoperatively.
- Careful preoperative planning facilitates safe and expeditious surgery.
- Ligamentotaxis relies on the application of linear traction to indirectly reduce fragments via the intact periosteum and soft tissues.
- A myriad of fracture fixation options are available; selecting the most appropriate depends on a careful assessment of the fracture and patient related factors.
- Postoperative care should allow for early mobilization if fixation permits.

Introduction

Fracture care was significantly advanced in the 20th century with the introduction of new techniques and instrumentation for internal and external fixation.[1] Today's capable hand surgeon must be well versed in the spectrum of available techniques of fracture fixation to provide optimum care for the myriad of bony injuries that occur within the purview of a hand surgery practice. Fixation of fractures in the hand is notoriously difficult given the relatively small size of the osseous structures and complexity of the surrounding anatomy.[2] The aim of this chapter is not to review every possible technique of fracture fixation in the hand, but rather, to present basic concepts and general techniques useful in routine fracture care.

Much of the credit for these advances in fracture management should go to the Arbeitsgemeinschaft fur Osteosynthesefragen (AO) who devised a set of principles *(Table 5.1)* that, in its modified form, provides the basic tenets that underlie appropriate fracture care.[3]

Patient selection

Fracture assessment

Any consideration of fracture fixation must begin with a careful, complete history and physical examination. Was this the sequelae of high or low energy trauma? Is this an isolated injury or is the patient polytraumatized? Are there open wounds? Does the patient require early return to functional activities or are their daily demands limited? How much time has elapsed since the fracture and the current presentation? Is there angular or rotational displacement? The vast majority of fractures that are non- or minimally displaced are amenable to treatment with nonoperative methods.

Host factors

The decision to treat a fracture with internal fixation requires a commitment from the patient to comply and participate in appropriate postoperative care. Failure to comply with splinting regimens, follow-up care, therapy recommendations, or weight-bearing restrictions may result in compromised outcomes.

Certain host factors imply an increased susceptibility to wound healing problems or infection. Systemic factors include: diabetes mellitus,[4] an immunocompromised state, advanced age, and smoking, amongst many others. Local factors include: skin quality, volume/quality of soft tissues available for closure, type of hardware elected, and tension across the wound. Failure to recognize and address these factors may result in compromised outcomes. Patients with elevated risk for wound problems should be counseled accordingly and managed with alternative strategies where appropriate.

Table 5.1 Arbeitsgemeinschaft fur Osteosynthesefragen (AO) principles

Anatomical fracture reduction
Appropriate stability of the fixation construct
Preservation of blood supply and soft tissue attachments to fracture fragments
Early and safe mobilization

Preoperative imaging

Radiographic assessment requires a minimum of two orthogonal views with the X-ray beam centered near the fracture to minimize distortion. Factors to carefully evaluate include:

1. Location of fracture (articular, metaphyseal, diaphyseal)
2. Pattern (transverse, oblique, spiral)
3. Presence of comminution
4. Displacement
5. Angulation (sagittal, coronal, and axial (rotational) planes)
6. Potential deforming forces acting across the fracture site.

Occasionally, as with a complex or suspected occult fracture, three-dimensional imaging with computed tomography (CT) scans or magnetic resonance imaging (MRI) may be indicated. After careful consideration of the fracture pattern in the context of the injured patient, a decision must be made regarding nonoperative versus operative treatment.

Treatment/surgical technique

Preoperative planning

Once a decision has been made to treat a fracture operatively, the surgeon begins the planning phase. Similar to the "reconstructive ladder" concept for management of soft tissue defects, the surgeon should, in general, use the simplest method that will reliably produce excellent clinical results. Planning should include every detail of the planned operation. This includes patient positioning, operating room setup, implants needed, operative approach, type of imaging (fluoroscopy) desired, and consideration of backup plans. Time spent planning pays off by saving operative time, decreasing staff frustration, and ensuring that the appropriate tools are present for the safest, most successful and most efficient surgery possible.

Fracture reduction

Fracture reduction may be obtained by numerous means. If done in a closed fashion, this reduction is usually in the form of pulling linear traction across the fracture site. This utilizes the phenomenon of ligamentotaxis,[5,6] whereby any intact periosteum and/or ligaments help realign attached bony fragments as they are stretched. When open reduction is elected,

reduction is obtained usually through a combination of external manipulation and instruments placed within the fracture site. The reduction may be held with reduction forceps or provisional Kirschner wires. The concept of reducing the number of fragments by temporary or final fixation of fragments to other fragments is critical in achieving a satisfactory reduction in the face of comminution. Forceps or wires used for temporary fixation should be carefully thought out so as to not interfere with the planned definitive fixation.

Hints and tips

Reduction forceps

Reduction forceps may be useful to attain and maintain fracture reduction in fixation of larger fragments. One tine of the forceps is introduced firmly onto a fragment and the other tine is used to tease another fragment into the appropriately reduced position. Careful pronation and supination movements while applying the forceps may allow for the restoration of length to difficult fractures. One has to take care not to crush or shatter the fragments with excessive compression of the clamps.

Hints and tips

Kirschner wires (K-wires)

These are discussed in detail, in a separate section below. In fracture reduction, K-wires can be used to temporarily secure fractures that are already reduced. Alternatively, they may be applied in a unicortical fashion and utilized as "joysticks" or "handles" to manipulate pieces into the appropriate position. After attaining this position, they are often advanced across the fracture to transition them from a reduction aid into a tool of temporary or definitive fixation.

Hints and tips

Kapandji (intrafocal) pinning[7-11]

This is a special type of utilization of K-wire commonly utilized in distal radial fractures. The wire is introduced through the fracture site (intrafocally). The pin is then tilted in the desired direction of the reduction, then advanced through the far cortex. This has particular applicability to the restoration of volar tilt and radial inclination in distal radial fracture. This may be employed as either definitive or temporary fixation.

Hints and tips

Temporary/supplemental external fixation

For select, extremely difficult fractures, an external fixator may be utilized to apply ligamentotaxis to assist with fracture reduction while other methods are utilized.

Intraoperative imaging

Fluoroscopy provides a valuable adjunct to many fracture fixation surgeries. A complete review of fluoroscopic physics and principles is beyond the scope of this chapter, but a few points are worth mentioning. For upper extremity surgery, either an image intensifier or a "mini" fluoroscopic unit may be employed. For the vast majority of hand surgery cases a "mini" fluoro provides adequate visualization with greater mobility and less radiation.[12–15]

Many different operating room setups may be employed, but patient positioning should be confirmed preoperatively to allow for adequate fluoroscopic visualization during surgery. We typically position the mini-fluoroscopic unit parallel to the bed, oriented from the foot toward the axilla, so that the patient's arm can be adducted off of the hand table to provide unobstructed views.

The region being examined should always be centered on the detector of the fluoroscopic unit to minimize the distortion from the "parallax" effect. Multiple views are helpful to determine fracture reduction or hardware position in all planes. It may also be helpful to orient the beam directly down a placed K-wire or screw to precisely visualize its placement. Specific knowledge of certain anatomic regions may also be helpful. For instance, in the distal radius, inclining the wrist approximately 20–30° from a true lateral can provide better visualization of the cortex of the lunate facet to evaluate for screw penetration into the radiocarpal joint.[16] Live, dynamic fluoroscopy may be useful to examine for stability across a fracture site with controlled motion or in other, select instances.

Fixation options

Absolute versus relative stability

> ### Key concept
>
> #### Absolute versus relative stability
>
> Bone healing following fracture fixation depends on the stability of the fixation technique chosen. With absolute stability, very rigid, internal fixation is utilized. This typically is in the form of lag screws or compression plates. This requires anatomical reduction of fracture fragments and is often the goal with articular fractures and simple diaphyseal fractures. Interfragmentary compression, as discussed below, facilitates healing with this type of fixation. Typically, absolute stability is possible only with simple fracture patterns or with minimally comminuted fractures with relatively large comminuted fragments (i.e., a "butterfly" segment). *Primary bone healing* with absolute stability is achieved histologically with "cutting cones" *(Fig. 5.1)* that facilitate direct healing of one fragment to another. No fracture callus is observed.

The concept of relative stability is important either when treating comminuted diaphyseal fractures where anatomical reduction is deemed impossible or in cases where closed reduction is elected. With relative stability, the primary focus is on achieving anatomical alignment of the neighboring articular surfaces in the coronal, sagittal, and axial planes. Some

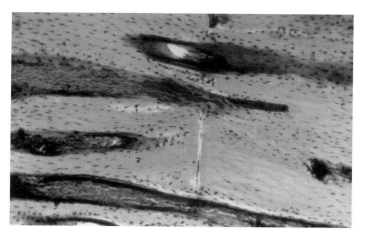

Fig. 5.1 Compressed osteotomy site. Note the migration of osteocytes across the fracture line, an example of contact healing (H&E: magnification ×100).

micro-motion occurs at the fracture site, and, in fact, is conducive to this type of healing (*secondary bone healing*). Stability, however, must be adequate to maintain the alignment. In contrast to primary bone healing via absolute stability, secondary bone healing occurs via progression through cartilaginous intermediaries and fracture callus is observed. Relative stability is typically achieved with external fixation, bridge plating, or intramedullary fixation. This concept, in general, is not commonly applied to articular fractures.

Interfragmentary compression

Interfragmentary compression is a critical component of fixation when the surgeon attempts to achieve absolute stability.[17,18] This compression, when combined with anatomical reduction, leads to microscopic interdigitation of fracture ends, thus minimizing the distance required for cells to travel from one side of the fracture to the other. This may be achieved via a variety of methods discussed below, including lag screws, compression plates, and tension bands. Interfragmentary compression may be detrimental in certain situations. For instance, in highly comminuted fractures, overzealous compression may lead to excessive shortening.

Kirschner wires

Kirschner wires (K-wires) are simple, yet versatile tools to assist with fracture fixation. They may be inserted in either a closed or open fashion and appropriate insertion causes minimal tissue trauma. They may be implemented either as temporary or definitive fixation *(Fig. 5.2).*[19] When used for definitive fixation, relative stability is generally attained and healing occurs with callus formation. Insertion of K-wires may be either directly across a fracture site or in an intramedullary fashion. The main limitation of K-wires is that they do not allow for interfragmentary compression and may loosen over time, leading to implant migration.

Sizes of Kirschner wires are usually reported either in terms of inches or millimeters. For instance a 0.062-inch K-wire is the same thing as a 1.6 mm K-wire. Sizes typically utilized in hand surgery range from 0.035 inches (0.9 mm) to 0.079 inches (2.0 mm), although larger wires may be used for

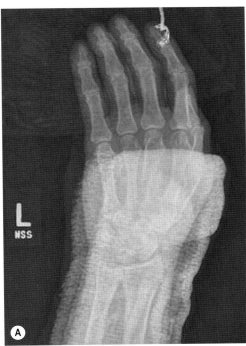

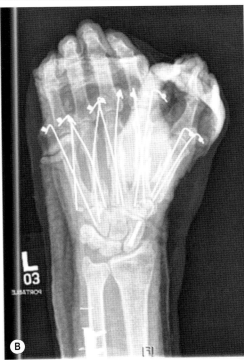

Fig. 5.2 (A,B) This 75-year-old was polytraumatized after being run over by a truck. He sustained fractures of all metacarpals. Relative stability through usage of multiple K-wires was elected to minimize further soft tissue disruption.

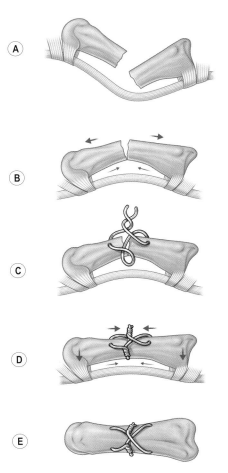

Fig. 5.3 Tension band technique. **(A)** Transverse midshaft proximal phalangeal fracture with volar angulation and displacement. **(B)** Reduction without fixation allows compression of the volar cortex during digital flexion but unacceptable dorsal cortical instability, causing an unacceptable gap. **(C)** A figure-of-eight tension band wire is applied dorsal to the central axis of the proximal phalanx. **(D)** The loops on either side of the tension band are tightened simultaneously to achieve symmetric tension on both sides of the fracture. After the tension band wire is applied, the compressive forces created during digital flexion are evenly distributed across the entire fracture site. The tension band wire absorbs an amount of tension equal to the compression at the fracture site. **(E)** Dorsal view of the tightened tension band wire. Holes may be drilled in the bone, and the ends of the wire loops may be inserted into these holes to minimize soft tissue irritation. (Redrawn after Freeland AE: Hand Fractures: Repair, Reconstruction and Rehabilitation. Philadelphia: Churchill Livingstone; 2000:42).

Tension band constructs

Each bone is subject to axial forces, which differ from one side of the bone to the other. This produces one side of the bone subject to compression forces and the opposite side to tension forces. A tension band,[20–23] either in the form or a wire construct or a plate, aims to convert these tension forces into compression forces to assist with fracture healing *(Fig. 5.3)*. This concept is most applicable to simple, transverse fractures in the diaphyseal region and requires an intact cortex on the compression side.

To accomplish this conversion of forces into compression, the tension band must be placed on the tension surface. Fortunately, in the hand, this is on the dorsal side of the metacarpals and the phalanges, allowing easy surgical access. As

select indications. Most wires are available in either smooth or threaded varieties. Smooth wires allow for easy removal in a clinic setting, but are also more prone to unintended migration. Threaded wires have a tendency to follow prior tracts within bone; advancing them with the drill on reverse somewhat negates this tendency.

Table 5.2 Techniques for internal fixation

	Interosseous wire (gauge)	Kirschner wire (diameter, inches)	Interosseous (lag) screw (mm)	Plate (mm)
Distal phalanx	28	0.028/0.035	1.3/1.5	NA
Middle phalanx	28	0.035	1.3/1.5	1.3/1.5
Proximal phalanx	26/28	0.045	1.5/2.0	1.5/2.0
Metacarpal	26	0.045/0.062	1.5/2.0	2.0
Carpal	24/26	0.045/0.062	1.5/2.0/2.4	2.0/2.4

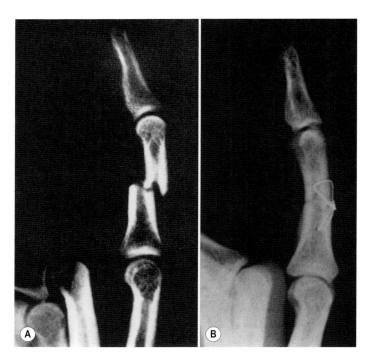

Fig. 5.4 (A) A displaced transverse fracture of the mid-diaphysis of the middle phalanx resulting from a glancing blow to the dorsum of the long finger. **(B)** Application of a tension band wire resulting in good interdigitation of the fracture so that it was held securely against rotational forces. (From Freeland AE, Jabaley ME, Hughes JL. Stable Fixation of the Hand and Wrist. New York: Springer-Verlag; 1985:89).

a twist on either side of the bone, combine K-wires with the intraosseous wires, or many other techniques.

In the hand, 28-gauge wire is adequate for a tension band in small phalanges; 26-gauge wire serves in larger phalanges and metacarpals. Rotation may be controlled and stability augmented by accurately interdigitating the jagged edges of fracture fragments together *(Table 5.2)*.

A specific form of intraosseous wiring,[24] the 90–90 technique *(Fig. 5.5)*, is useful, especially for arthrodesis, replantation, and transverse fractures. Although not a tension band, strictly speaking, it is a rigid enough construct that it will permit immediate motion.

External fixation

External fixation provides a useful, versatile option for fracture stabilization. This typically consists of pins placed on either side of the fracture with the fragments connected to each other through an external apparatus. This may be employed as either temporary or definitive fixation. Reduction is achieved through *ligamentotaxis*.[5,25,26] While this may be used with any fracture, it serves a particular purpose when there is severe fracture comminution *(Fig. 5.6)* and/or an element of soft tissue loss requiring reconstruction, thus increasing the risk of infection with internal implants. External fixators can typically be inserted through small incisions away from the fracture site, thus avoiding violation of the fracture hematoma. Knowledge of local anatomy together with proper techniques of pin insertion should be used to avoid damage to neurovascular structures. For instance, when placing an external fixator for distal radius fracture, great care should be taken to avoid damage to the radial sensory nerve. Most authors advocate using an open approach and identifying the radial sensory nerve in this instance although other have advocated a more dorsal position of the pins.[27]

Two main categories of external fixators exist: nonbridging and bridging. Nonbridging fixators[28] only span the fracture site, while bridging fixators also span a joint. Bridging fixators are more often used with metaphyseal fractures. Bridging fixators may also be combined with limited internal fixation for comminuted articular fractures.[11,29] When bridging joints, great care must be taken to avoid unwanted over-distraction.[30] Some specialized bridging fixators are hinged to allow mobilization of the spanned joint.[31] Relative stability is achieved with any method of external fixation and healing occurs with abundant callus via secondary bone healing.

the patient actively flexes the fingers, the force of flexion on the annular pulleys is transmitted directly to the attached bone, and the vectors of force are through the volar cortex toward one another. Because the tension band fixes the dorsal cortex stably, the effect is to force the volar cortices against each other and, by this process, produce further compression of the fragments, thus attaining absolute stability.

The exact configuration of the wires may vary with the individual fracture, but most commonly consists of a "figure of 8" construct with dorsally crossed wires *(Fig. 5.4)*. Typically, this is employed by passing the wire either through a drill hole or under a tendinous origin/insertion on each side of the fracture. The wire can then be twisted to reduce and compress the fracture. Depending on the specific situation, one may use

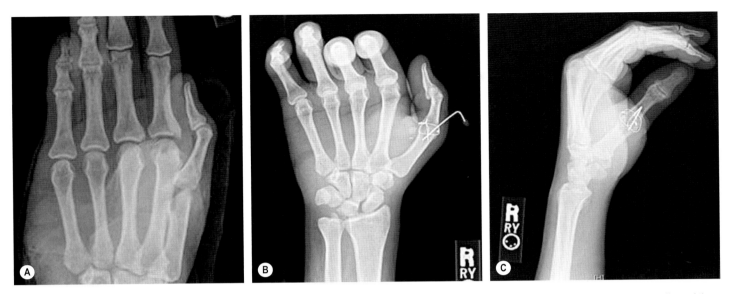

Fig. 5.5 (A–C) This 37-year-old male had a saw injury to the palm of the hand. In addition to multiple tendon injuries, he sustained a severe injury to the cartilage of the thumb metacarpophalangeal joint. A primary fusion was elected with usage of 90–90 interosseous wires and a supplemental K-wire.

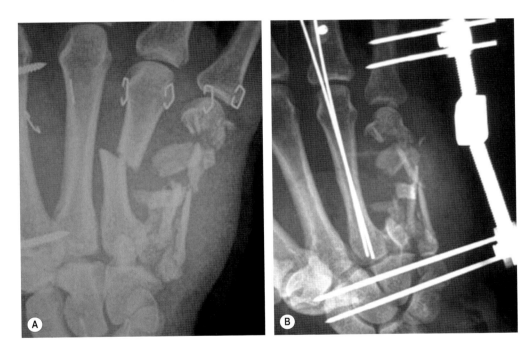

Fig. 5.6 (A,B) A spanning external fixator has been applied to this highly comminuted 5th metacarpal shaft fracture.

Interfragmentary lag screws

Lag screws *(Figs 5.7, 5.8)* provide compression between two fragments to achieve absolute stability. These may be used alone, in combination with another method of fixation, or through a plate. Lag screws are most useful in simple oblique or spiral fractures,[32] but also may be used to piece together comminuted fractures. The utility of lag screws is very limited in the fixation of transverse fractures as proper orientation perpendicular to the fracture is difficult.

Technique is of paramount importance in the proper insertion of lag screws, particularly in the small bones of the hand that are unforgiving to improper technique.

First, a proper site of insertion is selected. Ideally, lag screws should be positioned perpendicular to the fracture site. Long spiral fractures may be fixed with lag screws in different planes, but perpendicular to the fracture at each position. Screws placed too close to fracture edges may lead to fracture propagation.

Second, the near cortex is overdrilled with a drill size equivalent or slightly larger than the outer thread diameter of the planned screw. This allows the screw to "glide" through the near cortex as the screw is tightened.

Next, the far cortex is drilled with a smaller drill size equivalent to the core diameter of the planned screw. Tapping may be done at this stage. However, most modern screws are self-tapping.

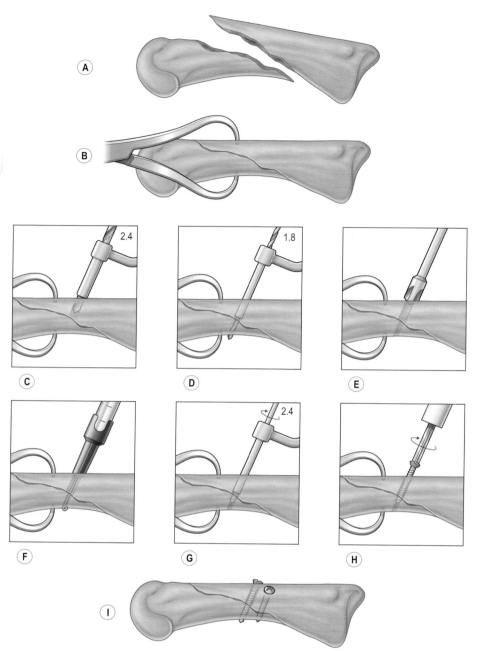

Fig. 5.7 Lag screw technique. **(A,B)** A long oblique metacarpal fracture is reduced and secured with a pointed reduction forceps. **(C)** A glide hole is drilled perpendicular to the fracture in the near cortex with a 2.4 mm drill bit. A drill guide is used to protect adjacent soft tissue and to prevent skating of the drill bit on the bone. The opposite end of this double-ended drill guide inserts into the 2.4 mm gliding hole. It has an internal diameter of 1.8 mm. **(D)** A concentric 1.8 mm core hole is drilled in the opposite cortex. **(E)** A countersink fashions an area in the proximal half of the dorsal cortex to correspond to and seat the screw head. **(F)** A depth gauge determines the appropriate screw length. **(G)** A 2.4 mm tap threads the core hole of the opposite cortex. A tap sleeve is used to protect the adjacent soft tissues (This step may be omitted for self-tapping screws). **(H)** A 2.4 mm screw is applied. As the screw glides through the proximal hole, its head engages the proximal cortex. **(I)** A second screw is applied in a manner similar to the first but in a plane perpendicular to the long metacarpal axis, thus satisfying the need for a neutralization screw. (Redrawn after Freeland AE. Hand Fractures: Repair, Reconstruction and Rehabilitation. Philadelphia: Churchill Livingstone; 2000:42).

The near cortex is then countersunk. This increases the contact area of the screw head on the near cortex, thus distributing the forces more evenly and avoiding the high contact pressure that may lead to fracture propagation from the drill site into the fracture site. Countersinking also decreases the prominence of the screw head, decreasing irritation of the overlying soft tissues.

Finally, the screw length is measured and the appropriate length screw is inserted. Compression across the fracture site is frequently observed. Care should be taken to avoid over-compression.

Another type of compression screw is the headless, variable pitch screw *(Fig. 5.9)*. This screw has threads of varying pitches. The coarser threads within one fragment lead to more

travel per turn within that fragment compared with the finer pitch threads in the other fragment. Thus, as the screw is tightened, compression is achieved.

Compression plating

Compression plating is a method of obtaining absolute stability and interfragmentary compression through a specific method of plate application. This particular plating method is typically employed for oblique or transverse fractures, but also may be used for segmental fractures or minimally comminuted fractures.

For transverse fractures *(Fig. 5.10)*, the fracture is provisionally reduced and the plate is affixed to one side of the

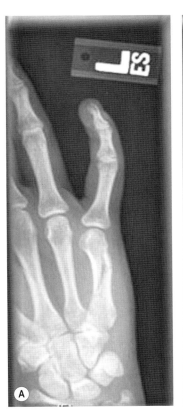
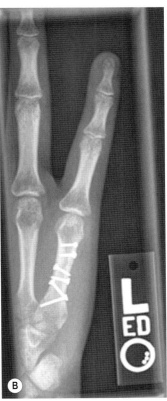

Fig. 5.8 (A,B) This 25-year-old hairdresser sustained a comminuted fracture of the small finger metacarpal shaft during an altercation with angular and rotational deformity. Absolute stability was achieved through usage of multiple lag screws. Note that the screws are placed in different planes, but perpendicular to the fracture at each site.

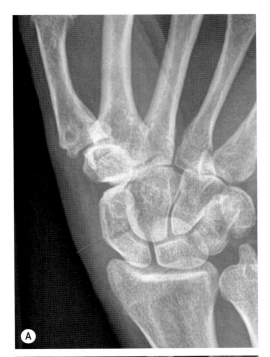
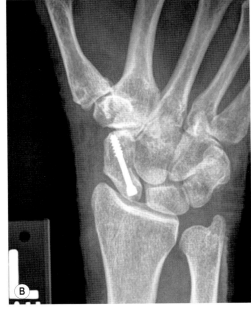

Fig. 5.9 (A,B) A scaphoid waist fracture has been secured with a variable pitch screw achieving interfragmentary compression and absolute stability.

fracture in a neutralization fashion (holes drilled centrally within the screw holes of the plate). Next, a hole is drilled eccentrically (portion of screw hole farther away from the fracture) on the opposite side of the fracture. As the screw head engages the plate it slides down the incline of the screw hole in the plate, thus causing the screw/bone complex to translate toward the fracture site, leading to interfragmentary compression.

In oblique fractures *(Fig. 5.11)*, the plate should be affixed first to the side of the fracture that allows for an acute angle (or axilla) to be created between the undersurface of the plate and the fragment. This allows for the second fragment to be compressed into the axilla, thus entrapping the fragment and assisting with reduction and compression. If the opposite sequence was done and an obtuse angle was created, further compression would lead to shortening and displacement of the fracture. An angled lag screw through the plate may be added to provide further interfragmentary compression following the compression plating.

Bridge plating

Bridge plating *(Fig. 5.12)* is a useful method of relative stability for stabilization of comminuted diaphyseal fractures where anatomic restoration is either not possible or would require

extensive dissection to do so.[33] Ideally, the fracture site should not be opened with this technique to avoid unnecessary surgical trauma to the surrounding soft tissues and allow for the preservation of vascularity to the comminuted fragments. Its usage is very similar to that of an external fixator. The principal goal is overall restoration of alignment of the proximal and distal articular surfaces. Healing is indirect via callus formation. Alternatively, if inadequate bone is thought to be present to allow healing, this technique may be combined with a bone grafting procedure to stimulate healing.

Video 1

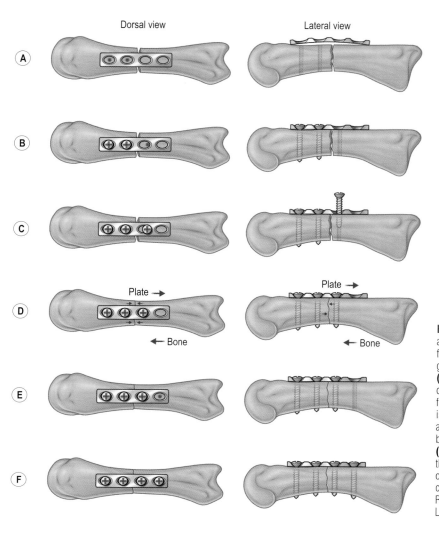

Fig. 5.10 Compression plate. This illustration demonstrates the application of a mini compression plate to a reduced transverse fracture of the mid-metacarpal shaft. **(A)** The straight miniplate has a graduated bend of about 5° centered at the middle of the plate. **(B)** Two neutral (centered) screws secure the plate to the left (distal) of the fracture. **(C)** A drill hole is placed eccentrically away from the fracture site in the first plate hole to the right of the fracture. A screw is inserted in the eccentric drill hole. **(D)** As the screw is tightened and the screw head engages the plate, translation of the plate and bone in opposite directions causes compression at the fracture site. **(E)** After compression is obtained, a neutral drill hole is centered in the remaining plate holes. If further compression is desired a second offset hole may be used instead. **(F)** A neutral screw is inserted, completing the fixation. (Redrawn after Freeland AE, Hand Fractures, Repair, Reconstruction and Rehabilitation. Philadelphia: Churchill Livingstone; 2000:53).

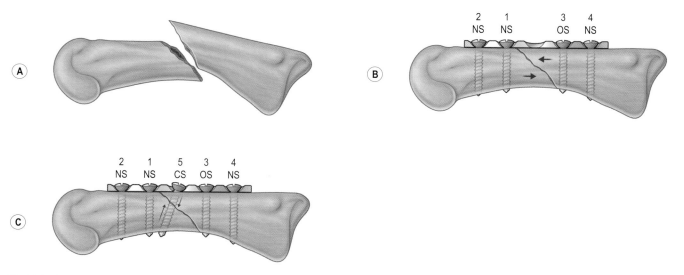

Fig. 5.11 Compression plate: compression screw (CS) within the plate. **(A)** Lateral view of a short oblique mid-diaphyseal metacarpal fracture in the coronal plane. **(B)** The fracture is reduced and a tension band plate is applied, compressing the fracture. It is essential to place the offset mini compression screw (OS) eccentrically away from the triangle of bone that is compressed into the "axilla" of the miniplate. **(C)** A large screw is placed across the fracture site, adding compression and stability. (Redrawn after Freeland AE. Hand Fractures, Repair, Reconstruction and Rehabilitation. Philadelphia: Churchill Livingstone; 2000:55).

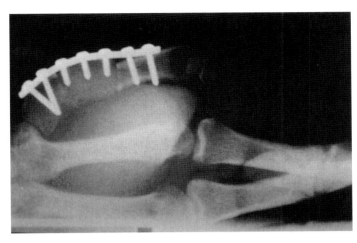

Fig. 5.12 Bridge plate. A complicated fracture in the first metacarpal with comminution and bone loss has been excised and filled with an autogenous graft. This plate provides a modicum of compression and screws through it further stabilize the graft. (From Freeland AE, Jabaley ME, Hughes JL. Stable Fixation of the Hand and Wrist. New York: Springer-Verlag; 1986:248).

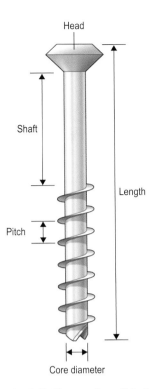

Fig. 5.13 Diagram of a partially threaded cancellous screw.

Locked plating

Locking plates allow for the creation of angular stable constructs to be created. This may occur by various mechanisms. Special threads on the sides of the screw head allow for interdigitation with threads located within the screw hole of the plate *(Fig. 5.13)*. The resultant angular stable construct is no longer reliant on screw thread purchase within bone and may present an advantage in osteoporotic bone or in low-density metaphyseal bone. Failure of this construct is not at the screw-plate interface, but rather would represent catastrophic failure of the entire construct from the bone. Furthermore, because purchase within the far cortex is not mandatory, screws may be used in a unicortical fashion, thus avoiding soft tissue irritation in the tissues overlying the far side of the fracture.

Locked plates may be applied in a variety of methods, depending on the particular fracture pattern. Compression, if desired, may be achieved through lag screws (either outside or through the plate) or usage of nonlocked eccentrically placed compression screws (depending on plate selected).

Postoperative care

Immobilization following fracture fixation may be done for several reasons including: need to protect the soft tissues during initial healing, desire to mitigate the possibility of secondary loss of reduction, and as treatment for associated injuries in the polytraumatized patient. Immobilization, however, is not without risks. Certain joints, such as the proximal interphalangeal joints of the fingers and the elbow are notoriously more prone to problematic stiffness than other joints.

Joint immobilization following fracture fixation may result in increased stiffness due to either tendon adhesions or capsular contraction. In the setting of articular fractures, unwanted alterations in cartilage physiology occur with immobilization.

Several studies have shown a protective effect of early motion on cartilage following articular injury.[34,35] Furthermore, some degree of micromotion across the fracture site may be beneficial for fracture healing, as illustrated in the examples of bridge plating and external fixation. This micromotion facilitates callous formation through the secondary bone healing pathway.

Where possible, fixation should be stable enough to allow for early postoperative motion without allowing unintended motion across the fracture site. The decision whether to add supplemental splint or cast immobilization following fracture fixation should consider the need for soft tissue protection, level of stability attained, and presence of associated injuries.

Summary

The hand surgeon must be familiar with various aspects of proper fracture care. Decisions regarding optimal treatment rely heavily on careful consideration of patient related factors and on a detailed analysis of fracture morphology. Once operative management is chosen, a myriad of options are available. Comprehensive preoperative planning should be done to shorten operative times and ensure that adequate instrumentation is present. The level of stability desired, planned operative sequence, and desired implants should all be included in the preoperative plan. A thorough understanding of the key concepts underlying proper operative fracture care aids the hand surgeon in optimizing surgical outcomes.

Access the complete reference list online at **http://www.expertconsult.com**

2. Henry MH. Fractures of the proximal phalanx and metacarpals in the hand: preferred methods of stabilization. *J Am Acad Orthop Surg*. 2008;16(10): 586–595.

   This is a concise review article, which summarizes many options for fracture fixation in the proximal phalanx and metacarpals with case examples.

5. Agee JM. Distal radius fractures. Multiplanar ligamentotaxis. *Hand Clin*. 1993;9(4):577–585.

   This classic article describes the use of ligamentotaxis in multiple planes to achieve optimal reduction of distal radius fractures. The author has developed innovative external fixators that use the concepts described in this article.

9. Kapandji A. [Intra-focal pinning of fractures of the distal end of the radius 10 years later]. *Ann Chir Main*. 1987;6(1):57–63.

   This is a report of some refinements to the author's originally published technique of intrafocal pinning for distal radius fractures. This is a useful technique to understand, even in this era of volar plate fixation of the distal radius.

16. Soong M, Got C, Katarincic J, Akelman E. Fluoroscopic evaluation of intra-articular screw placement during locked volar plating of the distal radius: a cadaveric study. *J Hand Surg Am*. 2008;33(10):1720–1723.

17. Bagby GW, Janes JM. The effect of compression on the rate of fracture healing using a special plate. *Am J Surg*. 1958;95(5):761–771.

23. Pehlivan O, Kiral A, Solakoglu C, et al. Tension band wiring of unstable transverse fractures of the proximal and middle phalanges of the hand. *J Hand Surg Br*. 2004;29(2):130–134.

24. Lister G. Intraosseous wiring of the digital skeleton. *J Hand Surg Am*. 1978;3(5):427–435.

29. Weil WM, Trumble TE. Treatment of distal radius fractures with intrafocal (Kapandji) pinning and supplemental skeletal stabilization. *Hand Clin*. 2005;21(3):317–328.

32. Horton TC, Hatton M, Davis TR. A prospective randomized controlled study of fixation of long oblique and spiral shaft fractures of the proximal phalanx: closed reduction and percutaneous Kirschner wiring versus open reduction and lag screw fixation. *J Hand Surg Br*. 2003;28(1):5–9.

   In this prospective, randomized clinical trial, K-wiring and lag screw fixation of proximal phalangeal fractures were compared. The series is limited by the uniqueness of each fracture, nevertheless, worthwhile conclusions may be drawn from this study.

33. Hanel DP, Lu TS, Weil WM. Bridge plating of distal radius fractures: the Harborview method. *Clin Orthop Relat Res*. 2006;445:91–99.

   In this retrospective study, the authors describe their method of bridge plating of the distal radius, including a summary of indications for this technique. Their experience is derived from patients in an extremely busy trauma center.

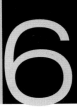

Nail and fingertip reconstruction

Michael W. Neumeister, Elvin G. Zook, Nicole Z. Sommer, and Theresa A. Hegge

SYNOPSIS

- Fingertip and nail bed injuries are the most common injuries of the hand.
- Common primary injuries include subungual hematomas, nail bed lacerations and fractures of the distal phalanx.
- Common secondary nail deformities seen after nail bed injury include nail ridging, splitting, nonadherence, absence, cornified nail bed, hook and spikes, or cysts.
- It is important to have a thorough understanding of the anatomy of the fingertip in order to adequately manage common injuries and deformities of the fingertip and nail.
- The purpose of the current chapter is to provide the reader with a comprehensive review of the pathophysiology, diagnosis, and treatment of nail and fingertip injuries and their management.

Introduction

The perionychium develops near the end of the 1st trimester.[1] A thickened area of epidermis on the dorsal distal phalanx of each finger and toe proximally invades the underlying dermis to form the nail groove. The deep layer of epidermal cells proliferates to form the nail matrix. Cells within the superficial layer of the nail matrix differentiate into hard keratin, forming the nail. At approximately 14 weeks, proliferation of the deeper layers of the nail matrix pushes the nail distally across the nail bed while firm attachment is maintained between the nail and nail bed.[2] Folds of epidermis lateral and proximal to the developing nail form the nail folds. Nails reach the tips of the fingers and toes at about 32 and 36 weeks of intrauterine life, respectively.[3]

Basic science/disease process

Anatomy

Topography of the nail was first described by Zaias.[4] A standardized nomenclature for the anatomy of the nail was proposed by Zook et al.[5] to improve communication between physicians regarding nail pathology, injury, and treatment (Fig. 6.1A,B). The entire nail structure, including the nail fold, paronychium, hyponychium, nail bed (germinal and sterile matrices), and nail, is referred to as the perionychium. The paronychium refers to the lateral skin surrounding the nail bed and nail. The skin over the dorsum of the nail fold is referred to as the nail wall. Extension of the nail wall distally onto the dorsum of the nail forms the eponychium. The eponychium is attached to the nail by a cornified material known as the nail vest, or cuticle. The white, convex opacity extending distally from beneath the eponychium is the lunula, which is the distal visible extent of the germinal matrix. The white color remains after removal of the nail and is thought to be secondary to retention of nuclei of the germinal cells to this level in the nail. The mass of keratin beneath the distal aspect of the nail and at the distal edge of the nail bed is the hyponychium (Fig. 6.1C).

The nail bed consists of the germinal and sterile matrices. The germinal matrix makes up the ventral floor of the proximal nail fold. The sterile matrix consists of the soft tissue immediately beneath the nail distal to the germinal matrix.

Vascularity

The nail unit is supplied by branches of the common volar digital arteries. According to Flint,[6] the digital arteries form three arterial anastomoses over the dorsal surface of the distal phalanx. A superficial arcade supplies the nail fold, and

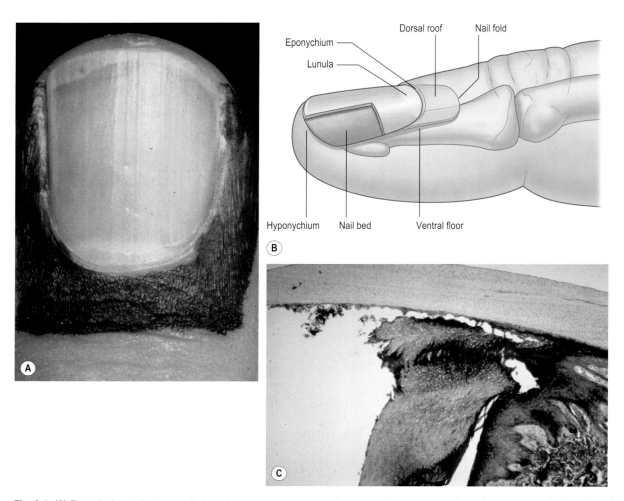

Fig. 6.1 (A) The nail, the sterile and germinal matrices, and the surrounding tissue marked here compose the perionychium. **(B)** A lateral view of the nail bed showing the ventral floor (germinal matrix), the nail bed (sterile matrix), and the dorsal roof of the nail fold. **(C)** The keratinous plug is shown at the hyponychium. (© Southern Illinois University School of Medicine.)

proximal and distal arcades wrap around the waist of the distal phalanx to supply the sterile matrix as well as the pulp space. On dissection of 10 amputated digits, Zook et al.[5] found two consistent dorsal arterial branches of the digital arteries. The first branch was seen at the base of the nail fold and the second branch at the level of the lunula. Venous drainage of the perionychium coalesces laterally and dorsally, proximal to the nail fold, drains in a random fashion over the dorsum of the digit, and becomes large enough for vessel anastomosis at the level of the distal interphalangeal joint.[7]

Lymphatics roughly parallel the veins and are most numerous at the free edge of the nail (hyponychium). The density of hyponychial lymphatics is greater than in any other dermal area of the body.[8] This explains the low subungual infection rate, considering the heavy exposure of the hyponychial region to pathogenic organisms with use of the nails and fingertips to scratch frequently contaminated areas.

Nerve supply

The common volar digital nerves branch dorsally, just distal to the distal interphalangeal joint, to supply the periony-chium. Zook et al.[5] reported the most common distribution of branching (70%) to be a proximal fascicle into the deep nail bed at the level of the lunula and a distal branch to the hypo-nychial area. Wilgis and Maxwell[9] reported innervation by three nerve branches including two dorsal branches, as well as a branch to the pulp.

Physiology

Nail growth averages about 0.1 mm a day,[4,10] and fingernails grow faster than toenails at a rate of 4:1.[11] The rate of growth changes by season (growth is increased in the summer) as well as by age (growth is twice as rapid before the age of 30 years than after 80 years).[11] Nail growth is also affected by comorbid conditions of the individual, including endocrine, vascular, infectious, and nutritional disorders.[12] The rate of complete nail progression from the nail fold to the free margin has been reported to be between 70 and 140 days.[4] Baden[10] described a 21-day delay in growth after injury, during which time the nail thickens proximally but does not grow distally. Distal growth of a thicker than normal nail proceeds for the next 50 days; followed by growth of a thinner than normal nail for 30 days. Therefore, it is normal for an injury-induced lump to be present on the growing nail. Nail growth is not normal for approximately 100 days after injury. The nail is not fixed to underlying tissues by some mysterious glue but is fixed by virtue of its being a continuous chain of cells from the germinal layer into the nail, each cell attached to the one in front, behind, and beside it.

The nail is produced by cells from three areas of the perionychium: the germinal matrix, the sterile matrix, and the dorsal roof of the nail fold (*Fig. 6.2*). The germinal matrix produces the majority of the nail volume (90%) by gradient parakeratosis.[4] The sterile matrix and the dorsal roof of the proximal nail fold produce the remaining nail cells. The sterile matrix adds cells to the volar surface of the nail, accounting for the attachment of the nail to the matrix. The addition of ventral nail during distal growth usually results in a thicker nail distally and compensates for the dorsal wear.[13,14] There are longitudinal ridges in the sterile matrix that increase the surface for attachment. The dorsal roof of the nail fold adds flattened cells to the dorsal surface of the nail, producing the shine of the nail.[15] Loss of the dorsal roof causes a dull-appearing nail. ⊛ FIG **6.2** APPEARS ONLINE ONLY

Function

The function of nails was described in 1724 as "weapons to defend us from trouble … from small creatures, that often make their habitation upon our bodies and to allay the uneasy titillation by scratching."[13] Accordingly, fingernails are used for scratching as well as in defense. The nail protects the fingertip and contributes to tactile sensation.[16] Counterpressure between the nail and the volar skin and pulp aids in delicate and precise touch. Picking up small objects is difficult if the nail is absent. Two-point discrimination will frequently double when the nail is lost. Incompletely attached or split nails are often painful, especially in individuals who work with their hands.

Acute injury

Epidemiology

Injury to the fingertip and nail bed is the most common injury of the hand because of their prominent position.[17] The long finger is the most commonly injured, followed by the ring, index, and small fingers and the thumb with equal frequency bilaterally. The majority of injuries occur between the ages of 4 and 30 years; 75% occur in males.[17] Fractures of the distal phalanx are present in 50% of nail bed injuries, and most injuries occur to the middle or distal third of the nail bed.

Injury is caused by a deforming force, which compresses the nail bed between the nail and the distal phalanx. A subungual hematoma results from injury to the nail bed, causing bleeding beneath the nail. The most common injury to the nail bed is the simple laceration (*Fig. 6.3A*).[17] A simple laceration is common when the object causing the injury is small or sharp. The stellate laceration (*Fig. 6.3B*) is seen after compression with larger objects causing a bursting injury. Severe crush of the nail bed (*Fig. 6.3C*) is commonly caused by a wider, greater force of compression. Avulsion injuries (*Fig. 6.3D*) are the least common.[17] ⊛ FIG **6.3** APPEARS ONLINE ONLY

Subungual hematoma

Subungual hematoma formation causes separation of the nail from the nail bed. The pressure of the bleeding in this closed space frequently results in throbbing pain. Hematoma drainage is thus indicated for pain relief.

Treatment/surgical technique

Drainage is performed with a heated (red-hot), sterile paper clip or battery-operated cautery. The heated object burns a hole through the nail and is cooled by the underlying hematoma. The hole is made large enough to ensure prolonged drainage of the hematoma. A small hematoma will be incorporated into the nail and travel distally with nail growth.

The extent of underlying nail bed injury is difficult to assess with a subungual hematoma. If there is minimal disruption of the nail bed, normal nail growth is expected. However, if a significant disruption of the nail bed is present, there is higher risk of nail deformity if the nail bed is not repaired.

Therefore, whether a subungual hematoma should be drained with the nail left intact or the nail removed and the nail bed repaired is debatable. In the past, removal of the nail for inspection of the nail bed with repair as needed was advocated for hematomas undermining more than 25% of the nail. Simon and Wolgin[18] examined the nail beds of 47 patients presenting to the emergency department with a subungual hematoma and found that a hematoma >50% had a 60% incidence of laceration requiring repair. Repair of the nail bed was advocated with a hematoma >50% and an associated distal phalanx fracture. At the University of Pittsburgh, a 2-year prospective, observational study was designed to examine the outcome of 48 patients with subungual hematomas treated with drainage alone. No complications of nail deformity were found with this treatment, regardless of the size of hematoma or presence of fracture.[19] Roser and Gellman[20] compared three treatment groups in a prospective study of 52 children with subungual hematomas. A total of 26 fingers were treated with nail removal and repair of the nail bed. Drainage only was performed in 11 fingers, and 16 of 27 fingers were observed. No notable difference in outcome was found between the groups, regardless of hematoma size. It was concluded that nail removal and nail bed exploration are not justified in children with subungual hematoma with an intact nail and nail margin. Leaving the nail in place is recommended for most subungual hematomas with an intact nail. Exceptions may include children or patients with concern for an optimally aesthetic nail. If the nail is broken or the edge disrupted, removal of the nail and exploration of the nail bed are advised.

> **Hints and tips: Nail bed repair**
>
> Be conservative with the placement of sutures. The goal is simple – re-approximation. Tension on the nail bed suture line will lead to excessive scarring.

Lacerations

Avulsion of the nail, or nonadherence of the nail to the nail bed, is an indication for nail removal. Any loose nail as well as enough nail to allow adequate exposure and repair of the nail bed laceration should be removed. Complete removal of the nail is not always necessary. With middle to distal nail bed injuries, it may be possible to leave the nail in place within the nail fold.

Treatment/surgical technique

Exploration of the nail bed is performed with digital block, anesthesia, and tourniquet (e.g., a half-inch Penrose drain). The nail plate is gently removed from the nail bed with a small periosteal elevator or iris scissors. Careful removal of the nail is important to avoid further injury to the nail bed. Once removed, the nail is scraped to remove residual soft tissue, then soaked in povidone-iodine (Betadine) solution. The nail bed is examined with loupe magnification. It is better to leave ragged edges and allow the replaced nail to mold the edges than to débride and cause tension on closure. Careful undermining of the edges may assist in reducing tension on closure. A double-armed 7–0 chromic suture on an ophthalmic needle is recommended. The suture is cut in half to provide a second stitch because the needle is commonly bent during the repair.

Meticulous repair of the more complex stellate laceration and crush injury is more difficult. The severe crush injury may appear to be missing fragments. However, these fragments are often present, attached to the undersurface of the nail. Small fragments should be gently removed with a periosteal elevator and used as a nail bed graft. A split- or full-thickness nail bed graft up to 1 cm in diameter will usually survive, even when it is placed directly on the distal phalanx cortex.[6] Blood supply to the graft is established by inosculation and vascular ingrowth from the periphery.

Avulsion injuries commonly present with nail bed fragments attached to the nail. To avoid further injury to the nail bed, leaving the large nail bed fragment on the nail is recommended. The edges of the nail are trimmed a few millimeters to expose the nail bed for suturing into the defect.

Avulsion of the bed often occurs at the level of the germinal matrix and proximal nail fold, leaving a distally based nail bed flap of germinal or sterile matrix (*Fig. 6.4A*). The nail bed remains attached to the nail, avulsing the germinal matrix off the bone and out of the nail fold (*Fig. 6.4B*). The nail and germinal matrix must be separated and the germinal matrix replaced and sutured back into the nail fold (*Fig. 6.4C*). The nail fold is exposed with unilateral or bilateral incisions perpendicular to the lateral corners of the eponychium. The incisions should be made at a 90° angle to the eponychium to prevent a notch deformity (*Fig. 6.4D*). If the laceration occurs at the junction of the ventral and dorsal roof of the nail fold, suture approximation may not be possible. In this case, a horizontal mattress stitch is placed through the proximal end of the avulsed nail bed and brought out through the nail wall. This will secure the nail bed within the nail fold. The eponychial incisions are then reapproximated with 5–0 or 6–0 nylon after nail bed repair.

Loss of small areas of nail bed may be replaced with split-thickness nail bed grafts from adjacent uninjured nail bed, harvested carefully with a No. 15 scalpel blade (*Fig. 6.5A,B*). A split-thickness nail bed graft may be harvested from an adjacent noninjured finger (risky) or an amputated finger. A split toenail bed graft may also be used acutely and avoids the possible deformity of an adjacent nail (*Fig. 6.5C–H*).[21]

On completion of the nail bed repair, the nail is removed from the povidone-iodine solution and a hole made in the nail away from the site of injury. The hole allows drainage of the subungual space after reinsertion of the nail into the nail fold. The nail is placed within the nail fold to mold the edges of the repair, to act as a splint for tuft or phalangeal fractures, to prevent formation of synechiae between the nail fold and the injured nail bed, and to protect the tender fingertip. The nail is held in place with a 5–0 nylon suture placed distally through the nail and hyponychial region. On rare occasions with severe injury to the fingertip, a mattress suture may be placed proximally through the nail fold. If the nail is not available or is in small fragments, a piece of silicone sheeting (reinforced 0.020-inch-thickness Silastic) may be shaped to fit beneath the nail fold and secured proximally through the nail fold (*Fig. 6.6*). Unlike the nail, the Silastic sheet is soft and easily slips from beneath the nail fold if it is secured only distally. Nonadherent gauze may also be placed within the nail fold if no nail or silicone sheet is available. ⊛ FIG **6.6** APPEARS ONLINE ONLY

Hints and tips: Nail plate replacement

Trim the nail plate of sharp contours. Place the nail plate under the eponychial fold for a distance of 2–3 mm. An absorbable suture can be used to hold the nail plate in place as an alternative to nylon. This will avoid painful suture removal.

Postoperative care

The fingertip is dressed with nonadherent gauze, 2-inch roll gauze, and a four-prong splint to protect the repair. At 3–7 days after repair, the holding suture is removed, especially if it is in the proximal nail fold position. The authors have observed stitch track formation in the nail fold if the stitch is left in place longer than 7–10 days. If not disturbed, the nail will frequently adhere to the nail bed for 1–3 months as the new nail forms beneath. Fingertip tenderness is usually less with the nail replaced.

Distal phalanx fractures

Diagnosis/patient presentation

Distal phalanx fractures are found in approximately 50% of nail bed injuries and result in a higher incidence of secondary nail deformities.[17] Therefore, radiographs of the distal phalanx are recommended.

Treatment/surgical technique

Treatment of nondisplaced distal fractures consists of nail bed repair and replacement of the nail. The nail acts as an excellent splint for the fracture. Small, displaced tuft fractures and most stable distal fractures can be reduced with reapproximation of the nail bed and replacement of the nail. Larger displaced fractures or unstable fractures require longitudinal or cross K-wire fixation. Care must be taken to put the pin in the medullary cavity of the bone (see *Fig. 6.9*).

Secondary procedures

Reconstruction

The manual laborer may be bothered by a painful nonadherent, split, or hooked nail, which hinders productivity at work. Another patient may be concerned with the aesthetics

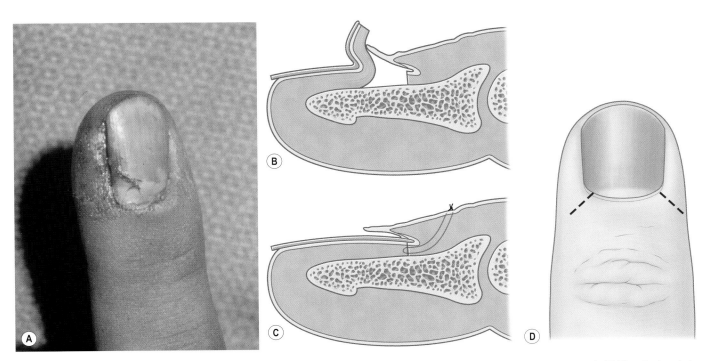

Fig. 6.4 (A) When the proximal nail is flipped out of the nail fold and is lying on top of it, one must remove the nail and explore the nail bed. **(B)** There is almost always a nail bed laceration with stripping of the germinal matrix up with the nail or a Salter fracture of the distal phalanx. **(C)** The laceration must be replaced and repaired. **(D)** Radial incisions are made in the eponychium to access the nail fold. It is almost impossible to replace the nail in the nail fold without its total removal and then sliding it back. (© Southern Illinois University School of Medicine.)

of a nail deformity, such as nail ridges, grooves, or absence of the nail. Goals for reconstruction should be based on the concerns and wishes of each patient. Reconstruction can often improve function and appearance of the nail but often does not produce a normal nail. The best chance for restoring a normal nail is at the initial repair.

The majority of nail deformities are secondary to scarring of the nail bed and subsequent disruption of nail growth. As with other scars, it is recommended to wait at least 8–12 months after injury before consideration of reconstruction. With scar remodeling, small nail deformities may resolve significantly or completely. Common secondary nail deformities seen after nail bed injury include nail ridging, splitting, nonadherence, absence, cornified nail bed, hook and spikes, or cysts.

Nail ridge

Introduction

Nail ridges are secondary to an irregularly healed distal phalanx fracture or scar within the nail bed. Nail ridges may also be secondary to a K-wire placed between the sterile matrix and the periosteum on reduction of a phalanx fracture *(Fig. 6.7)*. Longitudinal irregularities result in longitudinal ridges or grooves. Transverse irregularities beneath the nail bed result in corresponding transverse grooves or ridges or distal nonadherence. Correction of this deformity requires excision of the scar or irregular bone edge to form a flat, smooth nail bed surface.[6,16] A defect that cannot be reapproximated primarily requires use of a nail bed graft. FIG **6.7** APPEARS ONLINE ONLY

Transverse nail ridges may also develop secondary to hypoxia from ischemic injury or tourniquet hemostasis. The ridges resolve with correction of the inciting factor and subsequent new nail growth.

Split nail

Introduction

A split nail is often secondary to longitudinal scarring of the germinal or sterile matrix. Unlike the germinal and sterile matrices, the scar does not produce nail cells, resulting in splitting of the nail. Scar within the germinal matrix can split the nail from its most proximal aspect. Scar within the sterile matrix disrupts the progressive addition of nail cells to the volar nail, leading to detachment of the nail plate *(Fig. 6.8)*. Other causes of split nails include bone spurs beneath the nail bed, eponychial pterygium resulting from failure of the dorsal roof matrix to detach from the nail, and scar formation between the dorsal roof and ventral floor of the nail fold. Although longitudinal splits are most common, a horizontal split has been reported; it caused a diagonal scar in the matrix and formation of a portion of the nail on each side *(Fig. 6.9)*. The nail was produced within both folds, forming a horizontally split nail. FIGS **6.8**, **6.9** APPEAR ONLINE ONLY

Treatment/surgical technique

Scar must be minimized to allow normal nail production. Scar within the sterile matrix can occasionally be treated with excision and primary closure. The excised defect is frequently too wide to be approximated without tension and requires repair

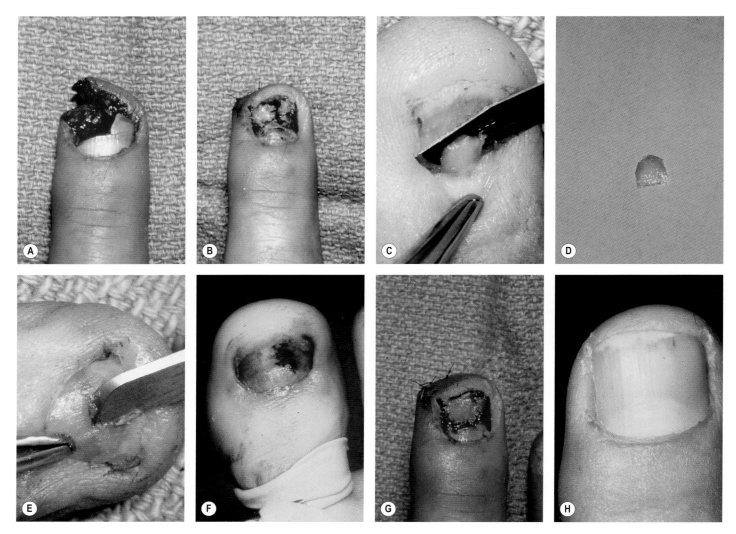

Fig. 6.5 (A) A crushing injury to the tip of the finger with laceration of the surrounding skin. **(B)** After the skin is sutured, an area of cortex is seen. **(C)** A split-thickness sterile matrix graft is removed from an adjoining area on the finger or toe. Back-and-forth sawing with a scalpel blade will remove a small fragment of nail bed, which is slightly curved after the nail has been removed. The white line of the sharp edge of the blade should always be able to be seen so that the graft is not taken too thick with a resultant deformity. **(D)** The fragment of nail bed taken. **(E)** If a larger piece of nail bed graft is needed, it may be taken from proximal to distal; the tip of the knife blade is used to dissect up the split-thickness layer of nail bed. **(F)** The large toe after removal of the split-thickness nail bed graft. **(G)** A split-thickness nail bed graft is sutured into place over the periosteum without any manipulation of the cortex. **(H)** One year later, good regrowth of the nail and adherence are shown. (© Southern Illinois University School of Medicine.)

with a split-thickness sterile nail bed graft from the same digit or a toe. In germinal matrix injuries, Johnson[22] recommended releasing incisions in the lateral paronychial folds with bilateral central advancement of the germinal matrix, but the authors' experience with this technique has been disappointing in traumatic deformities. Replacement of germinal matrix with sterile matrix will not be successful because sterile matrix grafts do not produce a nail. Split-thickness germinal matrix grafts also do not produce hard nail growth. The germinal matrix defect requires repair with a full-thickness germinal matrix nail bed graft.[21,23] The second-toe germinal matrix is a good option with its similar shape and size; the large toe is a second choice *(Fig. 6.10)*. The patient is warned that use of the toenail germinal matrix will eliminate hard nail growth on the toe. This second-toe nail defect is frequently more acceptable to patients than a defect of the great toenail. In the case of an existing bone spur, the nail bed

is lifted free and the spur is removed with rongeurs to produce a flat surface, and the nail bed is replaced.

Pterygium

Splitting of the nail may also be caused by a pterygium. A pterygium of the eponychium results from adherence of the eponychium or dorsal roof of the nail fold to the nail plate or nail bed during healing. A web between the eponychium and nail bed will result in splitting of the nail as it grows distally from the nail fold *(Fig. 6.11)*. FIG **6.11** APPEARS ONLINE ONLY

Treatment/surgical technique

Simple pterygia are amenable to warm water soaks until the eponychium can be bluntly separated from the nail. Sharp dissection of the eponychium from the dorsal nail is performed if blunt dissection is unsuccessful. Separation between

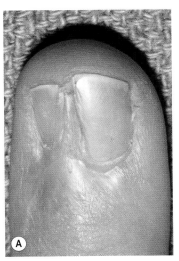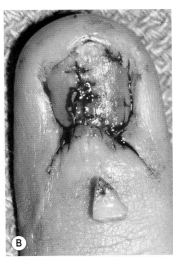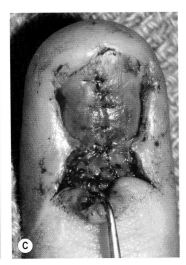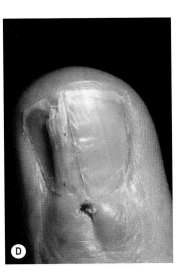

Fig. 6.10 (A) Avulsion of a portion of the germinal matrix with a split nail. **(B)** The sterile matrix has been reapproximated after resection of the scar, and a toe germinal matrix graft is shown before insertion in the germinal matrix. **(C)** Insertion of the germinal matrix graft as a free graft into the sterile matrix. **(D)** At 6 months, the graft of germinal matrix is shown to be growing nail. (© Southern Illinois University School of Medicine.)

the dorsal roof and nail is then maintained with nonadherent gauze or a Silastic sheet. This allows epithelialization of the undersurface of the nail fold. If adherence persists between the dorsal roof and the ventral floor (matrix) of the nail fold, it must be divided surgically. Once the nail fold has been redesigned, maintenance of the separation must be achieved with nail, silicone sheet, or gauze until healing occurs. If a large raw surface is present after freeing, a split-thickness sterile matrix graft is placed on the raw surface of the dorsal roof. If the scar has replaced normal germinal matrix, a full-thickness germinal matrix graft is necessary.

Nonadherence (onycholysis)

Introduction

Nonadherence of the nail is the most common nail deformity after trauma and is often found distal to transverse or diagonally oriented nail bed scars or bone irregularities. The most common cause of nonadherence is nail bed scarring. The scar interrupts the progressive addition of nail cells from the sterile matrix to the volar nail plate, causing detachment of the nail. The nail is unable to reattach to the nail bed distally.[24]

Distal nonadherence may lead to problems with subungual hygiene, an unstable nail when picking up small objects, pain from repeated avulsions when catching the nail on objects, or may be of no consequence except for aesthetic concerns.

Treatment/surgical technique

Nonadherence secondary to a nail bed scar is corrected with scar excision and primary closure or closure with a split-thickness sterile matrix graft from the adjacent nail bed or toenail bed.[24–26]

Malalignment of distal phalanx fractures may cause nonadherence. Prevention begins with accurate alignment of the fracture at initial repair. Secondary deformities caused by bone exostosis, bone angulation, or nonunion will require

revision. The exostosis should be removed to form a flat surface for the sterile matrix and subsequent nail adherence. Bone angulation may require osteotomy of the distal phalanx to re-form a flat surface.

Absence

Introduction

Causes of nail absence include trauma, infection, and burn, which destroy nail matrix. Absence is also rarely seen as a congenital deformity known as anonychia.

Treatment/surgical technique

Free partial and composite nonvascularized nail grafts have been described by McCash[27] and Lille et al.[28] for reconstruction of absent nails. Both germinal and sterile matrices are needed for total reconstruction of a nail bed. Zook recommended a full-thickness second-toe germinal and sterile matrix graft to approximate the width of the fingernail. To match the length of the fingernail, a split-thickness sterile matrix graft from another toe is placed distal to the free composite graft. The large toenail is used for thumbnail reconstruction. Results can be unpredictable and at times unsuccessful secondary to nontake or shrinkage of the graft. Patients should be informed of the risk of toenail deformity and a possible suboptimal outcome.

The most reliable and normal-appearing nail is constructed with a free vascularized dorsal tip of the toe.[29–32] This procedure can be technically difficult, requiring microsurgical skills, and produces scarring of the foot from harvest of the vascular pedicle.

Skin grafts, as opposed to nail bed grafts, have been used with some success to mimic the nail. This method has been advocated for treatment of traumatic nail absence and congenital nail absence in which multiple digits are involved *(Fig. 6.12)*. The scar is excised from the fingertip in the shape of a larger than normal nail (10% larger), and replaced with

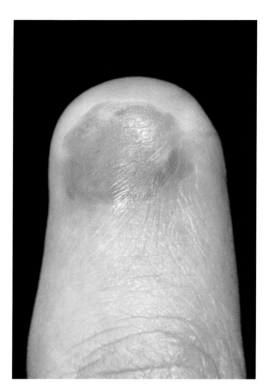

Fig. 6.12 A nail-shaped split-thickness skin graft is placed on the dorsum of the finger to mimic a nail. (© Southern Illinois University School of Medicine.)

a similarly shaped split- or full-thickness skin graft. Full-thickness grafts can be placed proximally and distally to simulate a white lunula and hyponychia, respectively. An artificial nail can then be fixed to the healed skin with glue, but patients may have difficulties maintaining the nail in place with glue alone. To aid in nail adherence, Bunke and Gonzales[33] reconstructed the proximal fold using a prosthesis wrapped in split-thickness skin graft and buried it under the dorsal finger skin. Artificial nails were then secured beneath the new fold. Unfortunately, the fold was only temporary and slowly disappeared with time. Baruchin et al.[34] described an osseointegrated anchorage device to secure the artificial nail.

Cornified nail bed

Introduction

With ablation of the germinal matrix, nail production ceases. However, an intact sterile matrix will continue to produce varying amounts of keratinous material, resulting in a cornified nail bed.

Treatment/surgical technique

The treatment is excision of the sterile matrix and replacement with a split-thickness skin graft.

Overproduction of keratinous material from the sterile matrix can also occur beneath a nail from chronic repetitive partial avulsion, allowing build-up beneath the distal nail, leading to nonadherence. Treatment includes removal of the nail to a point just proximal to this area of overproduction. The keratinous material is scraped from the nail bed with a scalpel blade. The nail is then able to adhere to the nail bed during distal growth. The process may need to be repeated if

overproduction on the exposed nail bed occurs more quickly than nail growth *(Fig. 6.13)*. Sterile matrix grafts may be necessary if scraping is unsuccessful *(Fig. 6.14)*. ⊚ FIGS **6.13**, **6.14** APPEAR ONLINE ONLY

Nail spikes and cysts

Introduction

On elimination of the nail bed or amputation of the distal phalanx, care must be taken to excise the germinal matrix completely. Any residual matrix allows continued production of nail cells. Cells produced within a closed space form nail cysts. Cells that grow distally form nail spikes.

Treatment/surgical technique

Treatment is complete surgical removal of the cyst or spike and of the residual matrix.

Hooked nail

Introduction

The hooked nail is a nail that hooks volarly during distal growth. This deformity is commonly seen after tight closure of tip amputations. On closure, the nail bed is pulled around the tip of the finger. Healing of a distal amputation site by secondary intention may also pull the nail bed volarly over the tip. Because the growing nail follows the direction of the nail bed, the nail grows in a hooked fashion, curving around the fingertip.

Treatment/surgical technique

This deformity can be avoided during repair of the acute injury by following two rules. The nail bed should never be pulled over the tip of the distal phalanx. If bone support is missing, support beneath the nail bed must be replaced or the nail bed shortened to match the length of the remaining distal phalanx.

Correction of the hooked nail secondary to the distal nail being pulled over the tip comprises release of contracted soft tissue, return of the nail bed to its normal position, and replacement of fingertip soft tissue. A full-thickness skin graft, V-Y advancement flap, cross-finger flap, or proximal thenar crease flap can be used to augment the tip and reposition the nail bed on the dorsum of the distal phalanx.[35] When bony support is missing, the options are either to shorten the nail bed or add bony support to maintain length. Nonvascularized bone grafts have been placed distally with successful initial support of the nail bed. However, they often resorb with time, and the correction is lost.[6] Osteotomy and distraction of the distal phalanx with placement of a bone graft between the distracted segments has been proposed to decrease the incidence of graft resorption but may be technically difficult.

Bubak et al.[36] described a repair of a hooked nail deformity using a composite second-toe graft for tip support. A fish-mouth incision is made in the hyponychium and carried proximally on the lateral aspects of the digit until the nail bed is released. An elliptical, transverse wedge of skin and pulp is excised from the second toe and placed beneath the released nail bed. Good results were reported with a 2-year follow-up.

Free vascularized second-toe tip (bone, soft tissue, and nail bed) transfer has been presented as a more permanent yet more complex option.[30]

Eponychial deformities

Introduction

Eponychial deformities may be secondary to trauma, burns, tumor, or infection, all of which cause direct destruction of the tissue as well as lead to scar contracture on healing. Loss of eponychium is more of an aesthetic defect than a functional defect. Notching or loss of the eponychium exposes more of the proximal nail and can result in loss of the nail shine. Although the shine of the nail is lost, there is no effect on nail growth.

Treatment/surgical technique

Reconstruction of the nail fold is difficult because of its three-dimensional structure. Multiple local rotation flaps have been described. Reconstruction of a nail fold with both inner and outer surfaces has been described with use of rotation flaps lined with split-thickness skin grafts.[16] Hayes[37] used distally based ulnar finger flaps for creation of the nail fold without reconstruction of the inner surface. Kasai and Ogawa[38] modified Hayes' technique of distally based ulnar finger flaps by using the local tissue to reconstruct the inner surface. The scarred eponychial tissue is incised proximally and turned over distally to form the nail roof. An ulnar, dorsal flap is then raised on a distal base and placed on top of the new roof to form the new eponychium, with split-thickness skin grafting of the donor site. Achauer and Welk[39] described a one-stage reconstruction of the burn-scarred eponychium with dorsal transposition of bilateral proximally based lateral digit flaps.

A composite eponychial graft of skin and dorsal roof from the first or second toe to the eponychial defect is recommended. This eponychial graft has been found to improve appearance as well as to restore the shine to the nail (*Fig. 6.15*).

Hyponychial defects

Introduction

The keratinous plug of the hyponychium may hypertrophy secondary to acute or chronic trauma to the distal nail and hyponychium. When this occurs, it sometimes protrudes beyond the nail and causes pain when it is bent or pressed with use of the finger. It may also produce an unsightly protrusion from under the nail (*Fig. 6.16*). ⊛ FIG **6.16** APPEARS ONLINE ONLY

Treatment/surgical technique

Adequate treatment of the hypertrophic hyponychium requires accurate determination of the cause, which is often acute or chronic irritation. If irritation cannot be avoided and symptoms persist, excision of the hypertrophic hyponychium and coverage with a split-thickness sterile matrix graft have resulted in a high incidence of symptom relief. The split-thickness sterile matrix graft is carried out in the same manner as with replacement for avulsion of a portion of the sterile matrix or scar excision.

Pigmented lesions

Introduction

The differential diagnosis for pigmentation of the nail bed is complex; it includes subungual hematoma, foreign body, onychomycosis nigricans, junctional nevi, pyogenic granuloma, paronychia, vascular lesion, melanonychia striata, melanoma *in situ*, and malignant melanoma.[40] Although most pigmented lesions of the nail are benign, they should be evaluated carefully to rule out malignancy.

Patient presentation

The history of the pigmentation is important. Trauma may cause bands of pigment, especially in darkly pigmented individuals. Development of pigment in adults, even without a known history of trauma, is often secondary to a subungual

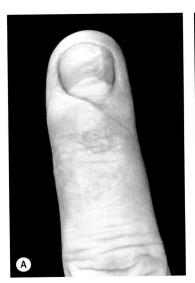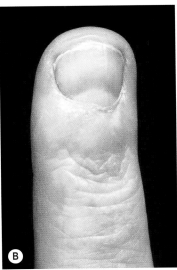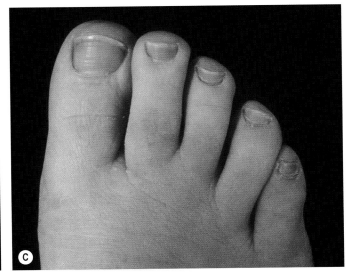

Fig. 6.15 **(A)** Loss of eponychium secondary to trauma with resultant irregularity and roughness of the nail. **(B)** One year after a full-thickness composite graft of second-toe dorsal roof transfer to the finger. Note the improvement in the contour and shine of the dorsum of the nail. **(C)** The eponychial graft was taken from the second toe and here shows essentially no deformity. (© Southern Illinois University School of Medicine.)

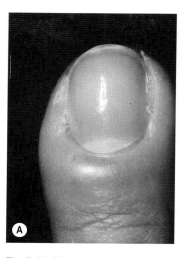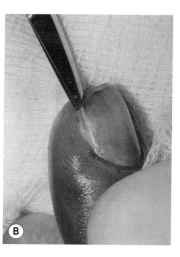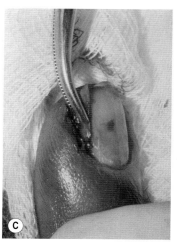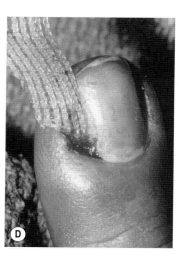

Fig. 6.17 (A) A swollen, inflamed paronychium known as a paronychia. **(B)** The side of the nail, which is undermined by the infection, is separated from the nail bed and the lateral aspect of the dorsal roof of the nail fold. **(C)** This fragment of nail is removed, giving adequate drainage to the infection. **(D)** A piece of water-soluble gauze is placed as a drain. (© Southern Illinois University School of Medicine.)

hematoma, but the differential diagnosis of malignant melanoma must be considered. These suspicious areas can be monitored by scratching the nail at the proximal and distal edges of the pigment with a scalpel blade or 18-gauge needle *(Fig. 6.17)*. Distal migration of pigmentation over 3–4 weeks, together with the scratch marks suggests a hematoma. However, if the scratch marks move distally, away from the pigment, this suggests foreign body, nevus, or melanoma.

Melanonychia striata is defined as any linear tan-brown-black pigment of the nail bed that is carried into the nail as growth occurs. This pigmentation is caused by focal increase in the number or function of melanocytes. Melanonychia striata is common in individuals with darkly pigmented skin but uncommon in those with fair skin *(Fig. 6.18)*.

Subungual nevi produce pigmentation within the nail bed and the ventral nail *(Fig. 6.19)*. These pigmented nevus cells are derived from neural crest cells and are frequently present at birth or shortly thereafter. The nail is frequently pigmented with elevation and ridging *(Fig. 6.20)*.

Fleegler and Zeinowicz[41] recommended nail bed biopsy of dark streaks present at or shortly after birth because of the danger of malignant degeneration at puberty. Melanocytic hyperplasia without atypia can be observed. However, complete excision with reconstruction of the nail bed is advised if atypical cells are found.

Pincer nail

Introduction

Pincer nail deformity is described as lateral hooking or excessive transverse curvature of the nail plate, unilaterally or bilaterally *(Fig. 6.21)*. The progressive tubing of the nail eventually pinches off the nail bed and hyponychium, resulting in an unaesthetic, painful nail *(Fig. 6.22)*. Pincer nail is most commonly seen in middle-aged to elderly women. The cause of the pincer nail is not known. ⊛ FIG **6.22** APPEARS ONLINE ONLY

Treatment/surgical technique

Previous treatments have included resection of a wedge of the phalanx to flatten the nail edges and release of the nail bed

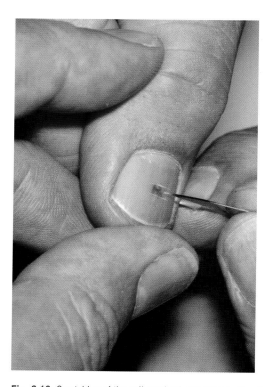

Fig. 6.18 Scratching of the nail proximal and distal to the pigment to determine whether the pigment is in the nail or in the nail bed. (© Southern Illinois University School of Medicine.)

with a medial longitudinal nail bed incision and split-thickness skin graft coverage of the resultant triangular defect.[42] They have been largely unsuccessful. Brown *et al.*[43] have advocated the use of dermal graft strips between the lateral nail bed and the distal phalanx periosteum for elevation of the lateral borders of the nail bed. The nail is removed, and incisions are made at the tip of the digit to allow freeing and elevation of the paronychial folds from the periosteum. The dermal grafts are placed within this space to maintain the elevation and to flatten the nail bed. Human dermis (AlloDerm) is currently

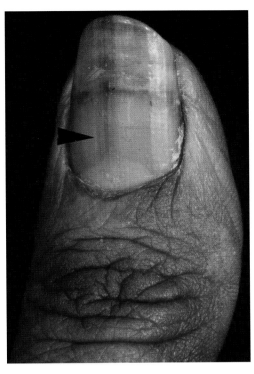

Fig. 6.19 The melanocytic streaks in an African American patient after trauma to the perionychium (arrowhead). (© Southern Illinois University School of Medicine.)

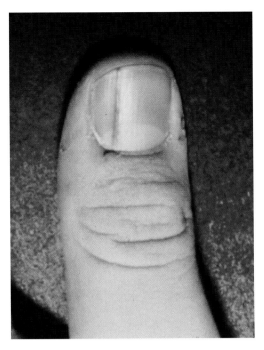

Fig. 6.20 A newly occurring pigmented streak that originates in the germinal matrix or proximal to the observable pigment. (© Southern Illinois University School of Medicine.)

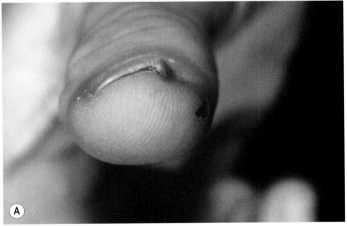

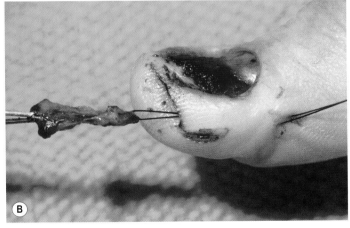

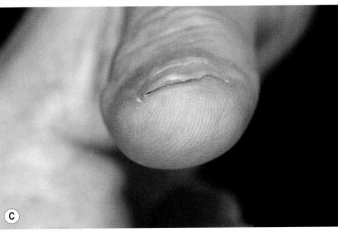

Fig. 6.21 **(A)** A unilateral pincer nail. **(B)** The perionychium is freed from the bone, and a graft of dermis or dermal substitute is placed into the tunnel to flatten the nail bed. **(C)** One year after correction. (© Southern Illinois University School of Medicine.)

being used at the authors' institution in place of the dermal strips with equally good correction of pincer nail.

The pain from a pincer nail deformity may be severe enough to warrant surgical ablation of the nail bed if other forms of reconstruction are unsuccessful.

Local flap reconstruction of finger tip injuries

Introduction

The challenging reconstructive treatment of the defects in the fingers requires a sound working knowledge of the variety of flaps. As the hand surgeons weigh the pros and cons of each possible flap to obtain definitive closure, they must also integrate the priorities of function, contour, and stability, as well as the anticipation for further reconstructive surgery in choosing the flap of choice. Flaps selection is based on the characteristics of the defect, including size, shape, and location and the availability of donor sites as well as the goals of reconstruction.

Reconstructive principles

The principles of wound management in the traumatized digit or hand include irrigation, debridement, and restoration of vascularity, stabilization of fractures and then repair of specialized tissues such as nerve or tendon followed by the definitive soft tissue coverage. The skin of the hand and the fingers varies from palmar to dorsal sides. The palmar aspect is covered with a glabrous skin notable for its limited sheer, high friction coefficient and characteristic "finger print" papillary ridges. Numerous fibrous septae compartmentalize subcutaneous tissue of the palm with fibers from the underlying dermis to the musculoskeletal structures below. The mid-axial line of each digit is formed by connecting the lateral volar finger crease at the distal interphalangeal joint (DIP), proximal interphalangeal joint (PIP) and metacarpal phalangeal (MCP) joint. It is at this line that the transition from the glabrous to nonglabrous skin of the hand occurs. The dorsal skin is relatively soft, pliable, and thin. It is devoid of the fibrous septae observed in the volar skin.[13] The importance of understanding the difference of glabrous and nonglabrous skin comes to light when one observes one of the dictums of reconstructive surgeons to replace "like with like." Local flaps that include glabrous skin should be used for glabrous defects. On the other hand, defects of the dorsal aspect of the skin can be readily closed with dorsal quality skin.

Flap selection

Today, a multitude of flaps permits optimal outcomes of both recipient and donor site. Each flap has its inherent advantages and disadvantages. Ultimately, flap selection is dependent upon variables such as size, shape, location of the defect, and the characteristics of the tissue that was lost. The hand surgeon must select the most ideal flap to restore as many of the native skin characteristics that were present prior

to the tissue lost, and to provide the quickest means of wound closure.

Fingertip injuries should be thoroughly irrigated and debrided of foreign material and nonviable tissue before closure is attempted. If the entire defect cannot be closed primarily, one can close most of the wound and allow the rest to heal by secondary intention. The wound should be closed with a chromic or other resorbable suture. Nylon sutures in the fingertip are not usually necessary as they are uncomfortable to remove in the early follow-up periods. The wound is dressed with Xeroform® or other minimal adherence dressing. Daily dressing changes permits rapid wound healing. Early motion is encouraged to prevent stiffness at the DIP or PIP joints. Larger wounds can heal by secondary intention if bone, tendon or neurovascular structures are not exposed. Wounds up to 2–3 cm may be allowed to heal by re-epithelization, but both surgeon and patient must be aware that closure may take 4–6 weeks *(Fig. 6.23)*. Previously, authors advocated that defects >1 cm should be closed with local flaps.[44] However, secondary intention offers many advantages over flap closure, including improved contour, sensation, and lack of donor site morbidity.[45]

Skin grafting

Patient selection

When the extent of the defect is limited to skin, a split- or full-thickness skin graft may be used for coverage of a well vascularized bed. Graft contraction is expected. Although re-innervation is poor with split-thickness grafts, protective sensation may be possible if full thickness grafts are used.[44,46] Distal fingertip amputations often comprise skin, subcutaneous fat and a portion of the nail bed. The amputated part may be replaced as a composite graft after defatting.[47] The overall success rate of composite grafts is poor in the adult population and better in children <10 years of age. A composite graft that is placed on a fingertip but does not revascularize should be left as a biologic dressing to allow healing from below the eschar. This often leads to an adequately contoured fingertip.

Treatment/surgical technique

Local flaps

Numerous flaps have been described for fingertip coverage. The utilization of local flaps leaves donor site morbidity, and this must be taken into account before the flap is elevated.

Volar V-Y advancement (Atasoy, Kleinert)

Fingertip defects with exposed bone may be closed primarily with a volar V-Y advancement flap if the defect measures ≤1 cm and is oriented in a more dorsal oblique transverse fashion.[46] The flap is oriented in a triangular fashion with the base of the triangle at the wound edge and the apex at the DIP crease *(Fig. 6.24)*.[48,49] This skin is incised down through the dermis and then scissor dissection is used to release fibrous septae that anchor glabrous skin to the deeper musculoskeletal structures.[46] The most distal corners of the flap must be freed by 2–3 mm in order to allow adequate release of the flap distally. Similarly, the apex of the flap at the DIP joint must be released significantly to permit distal migration of the flap.[50]

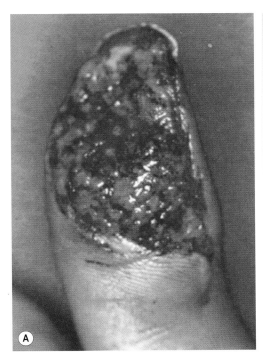

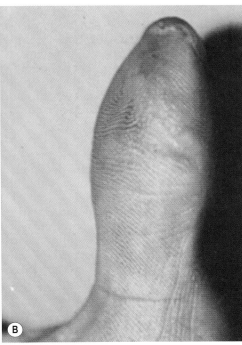

Fig. 6.23 (A) Large soft tissue defect of the volar aspect of the thumb allowed to heal by secondary intent. **(B)** 4-year follow-up of healed thumb showing good contour.

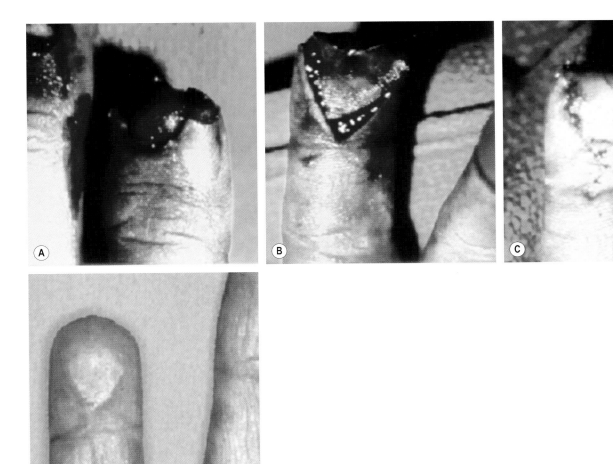

Fig. 6.24 (A–D) Distal defects of the fingertip that require flap coverage can sometimes be closed with volar V-Y flaps. The flap is designed with the apex down to the DIP joint. Flaps can be transposed distally from point 0.5 cm to 1 cm in length.

The flap is elevated with its neurovascular pedicles on either side of the flap in the plane of flexor tendon sheath; 0.75–1 cm of length can be obtained with a volar V-Y advancement flap. Functional and cosmetic results are extremely good as this flap remains one of the most important tools in treatment of fingertip injury closure.[44,46,48,49]

Lateral V-Y advancement flaps (Kutler)

Transverse and oblique defects can be covered with sensate vascularized skin using V-Y advancement flaps on the lateral aspect of the digits *(Fig. 6.25)*.[46] Often bilateral flaps are required in order to get sufficient closure of the soft tissue defect of the distal aspect of the fingertip. The lateral V-Y flaps are elevated in a similar fashion as to the volar V-Y flap; however, they are based laterally and medially instead of volarly. Unlike the volar V-Y flap, however, lateral V-Y advancement has limited mobility of around 0.5 cm but up to 1 cm can be achieved on occasion. The flap is elevated on the plane of the deeper musculoskeletal structures.[50]

The visor flap

The visor flap is indicated for closure of transverse distal fingertip amputations that have exposed bone.[50,51] In an attempt to preserve length the visor flap utilizes the skin on the dorsal aspect of the finger to close up the most distal aspect of the amputation site. The visor flap involves raising a rectangular shaped flap from the dorsal aspect of the skin at the level of the paratenon just proximal to the defect *(Fig. 6.26)*. The width of the flap is approximately that of the defect on the fingertip. The flap is again elevated at the paratenon level and transferred distally in a visor type fashion as a bipedicled axial flap. The flap is sensate and vascularized by branches of the volar lateral

and medial digital arteries and nerves, respectively.[51] Back cuts in the dorsal aspect of the skin may be required to allow appropriate transposition of the bipedicled flap. The donor site is closed with a skin graft. The "dog ears" are left in place and should resolve over a period of months. The visor flap provides acceptable sensation, good cosmetic appearance and preservation of length of the digit without violating normal adjacent digits or creating volar scars.

Homodigital flaps

Homodigital flaps take advantage of the fact that the finger can remain viable on one digital artery alone. The other artery can provide the blood supply for an axial flap that can be either proximally or distally based *(Fig. 6.27)*. The digital nerve should remain *in situ* to preserve sensation to the distal aspect of the finger. Arterial perforator flaps involve small perforators arising from the digital artery. Small islands of tissue can be isolated on the perforator while the remaining aspect of the artery provides length to the pedicle, ultimately creating an arc of rotation of up to 180° *(Fig. 6.28A) (Fig. 6.28B–D)*.[52,53] The donor site may be closed with a skin graft if primary closure is not possible. Distally based homodigital flaps take advantage of the communication with the contralateral digital artery.[54] These flaps may be somewhat precarious as they require retrograde venous flow and may have limited communication with the contralateral vessels. ⊛ FIG 6.28B, C, D, E APPEARS ONLINE ONLY

Heterodigital flaps

The cross finger flap

The cross finger flap utilizes the skin from the dorsal aspect of the adjacent finger as part of a two-stage technique. The

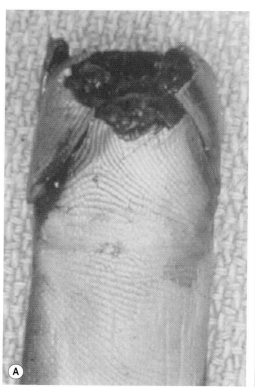

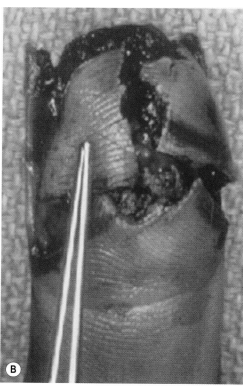

Fig. 6.25 Some distal fingertips are amenable to laterally V-Y flaps limited length is gained with these flaps up to 0.5–0.75 cm.

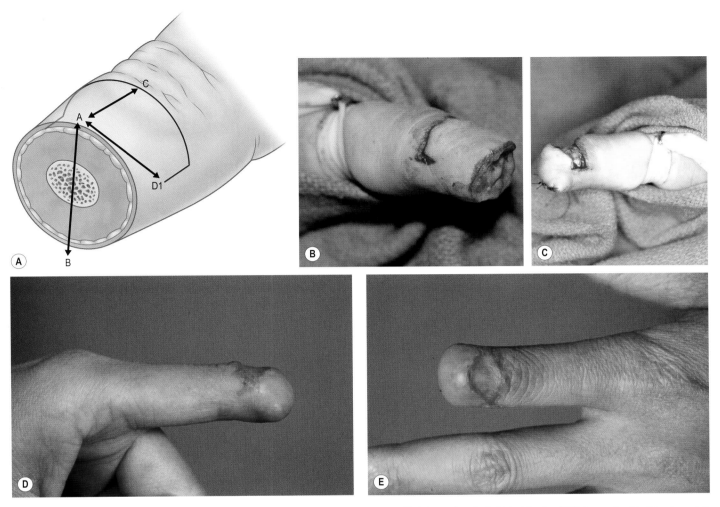

Fig. 6.26 (A) The visor flap is designed over the dorsum of the digit. The height of the defect **(AB)** is equal to the height of the flap **(AC)** the proximal incision is carried down to the mid axial line on either side of the dorsum of the finger. A back cut to D1 can be made but only through the dermis in order to protect the neurovascular structures supplying the flap. **(B)** Clinical picture of the design of the visor flap. **(C)** The flap was transposed over the distal aspect of the amputated stump. The donor defect is closed with a split thickness skin graft or a full thickness graft. **(D,E)** Lateral and AP view of the visor flap after it is transposed and healed.

inner cross finger flap is most applicable for volar defects of the distal aspect of an adjacent finger. The flap is normally taken from the dorsal radial surface over the middle phalanx of the adjacent digits.[44,46,50] The flap is designed slightly larger than the defect to ensure complete coverage. Vascularity of the flap arises from the digital artery and vena comitantes that send branches dorsally beyond the PIP joint. The flap is elevated superficial to the extensor paratenon and flipped over like a page in a book to cover the volar defect of the adjacent finger *(Fig. 6.29)*. The base of the flap remains intact with the donor finger while the donor defect on the dorsal aspect of the middle phalanx is covered with a full thickness or split thickness skin graft. The flap is sutured in the chromic sutures and the fingers are immobilized for 2–3 weeks. The flap is then divided and inset. The dorsal cutaneous branches of the digital nerve can be incorporated into the flap and coapted to the recipient digital nerve to improve reinnervation potential.[50]

The reverse cross finger flap is utilized to cover dorsal defects of the adjacent digit. In the reverse cross finger flap, the dorsal skin is elevated but left with an intact base at the lateral border away from the defect. The subcutaneous tissue is then elevated at the level of the paratenon and turned over 180° like a page of a book to cover the dorsal defect of the involved finger *(Fig. 6.30)*. The elevated full-thickness skin flap on the opposite side of the donor finger is then replaced in its original position.[44] A skin graft is still required at the recipient site to cover the adipofascial flap that overlies the dorsal defect. Both cross finger and reverse cross finger flaps provide tissue with reliable blood supply to defects measuring up to 3 cm in size. Following division and insetting of the flaps, mobilization and aggressive therapy may be warranted to prevent stiffness or contractures.

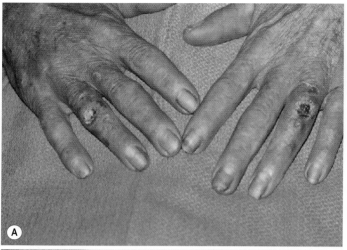

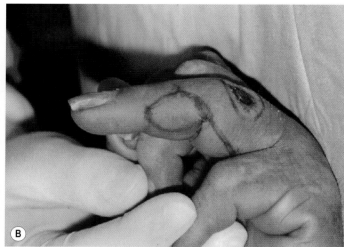

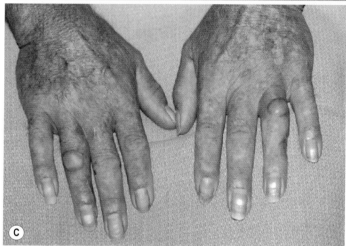

Fig. 6.27 (A) Dorsal defects of the fingers with exposed bone or flap closure **(B)** A homodigital island flap is designed involving the nondominant side of the right finger. **(C)** The healed flap over the dorsal aspect of the fingers. The flap was based on the ulnar digital artery.

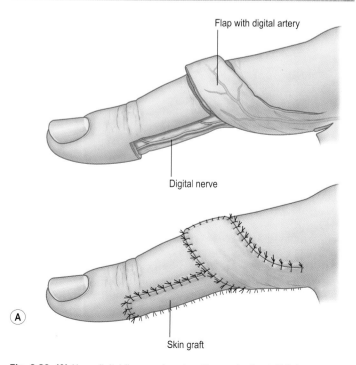

Fig. 6.28 (A) Homodigital flaps are based on the nondominant digital artery to the fingers and used to transpose either on a retrograde or an antegrade fashion.

Thenar crease flap

Smaller fingertip defects with exposed bone may be closed with a thenar crease flap. The flap itself is designed based on the radial aspect of the palmar thenar crease. It is most often utilized for the index and long fingers because of their proximity to the thumb.[44,46] The thenar crease flap is designed in a two-stage fashion. At the initial phase the flap can be elevated measuring up to $1\frac{1}{2} \times 1$ cm *(Fig. 6.31)*. Care must be taken not to injure the neurovascular bundles that lie immediately beneath the fasciocutaneous thenar crease flap. The injured finger must be flexed at the PIP and often the DIP joint in order to allow flap inset with chromic sutures and the donor site closed primarily *(Fig. 6.32)*. After 2 weeks, the flap is divided.[55] Sensation is reported to be better than skin grafting to the affected digit or with cross finger flaps.[56] Care must be taken when utilizing this flap in the elderly, as permanent stiffness or PIP joint contractures may arise. Aggressive therapy is required following the flap division and inset. ⊛ FIG **6.32** APPEARS ONLINE ONLY

Littler neurovascular island flap

This neurovascular island flap utilizes the donor skin from the ulnar aspect of the long or ring finger to provide sensate vascularized tissue to a given recipient site *(Fig 6.33)*.[46] However,

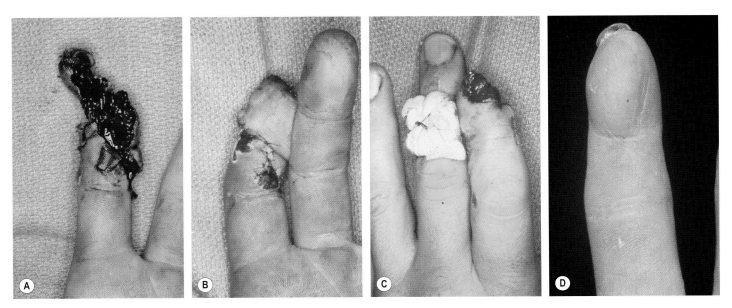

Fig. 6.29 (A) Mutilated fingertip with exposed bone requiring soft tissue coverage **(B)** Cross finger flap from the adjacent digit is used to cover the volar defect of the index finger. The flap is elevated at the level of the paratenon and the donor site is then closed with a full thickness skin graft. **(C)** 2–3 weeks later the flap is divided and inset.

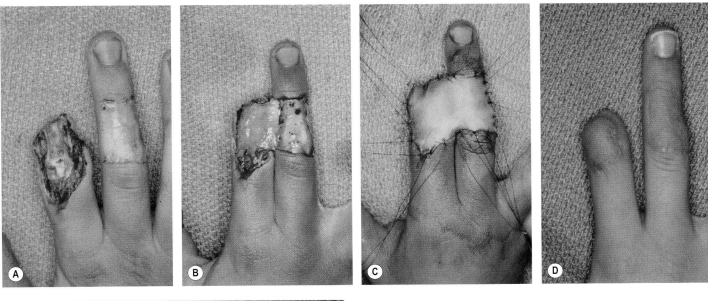

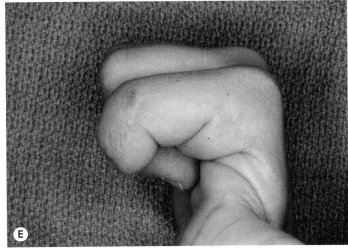

Fig. 6.30 (A) The dorsal aspect of the index finger has exposed tendon a reverse cross finger flap is designed the dorsal skin of the long finger is de-epithelialized. **(B)** The flap is elevated at the level of the paratenon and transposed like a page in a book over the dorsal aspect of the index finger. **(C)** Both digits are covered with a full thickness skin graft and then the flaps are then divided and then inset 2–3 weeks later. **(D,E)** Final outcome of the reverse cross finger flap and donor site is shown.

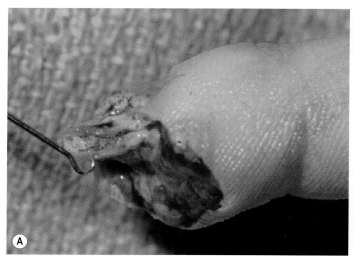
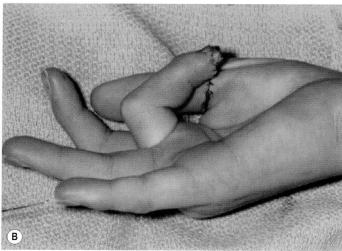

Fig. 6.31 (A) The long finger has a distal amputation with exposed bone to preserve length. The defect will be closed with a thenar crease flap. **(B)** The thenar crease flap can be designed with approximately 1 cm width and based radially. The recipient finger needs to be flexed at the PIP joint to have the flap inset.

donor site compromise may be significant resulting in stiff fingers with contractures making this flap less desirable than others for fingertip or thumb pulp reconstruction. Arteriograms have been advocated prior to performing this flap to make sure to two arteries supply the donor finger because the dissection of the flap requires extension beyond the bifurcation of the common digital artery. The contralateral branch will need to be ligated and divided. Dividing this contralateral branch in a finger that does not have another means of circulation can result in significant digital ischemia. Therefore, before ligating and dividing the contralateral branch, a temporary clip should be applied, the tourniquet released, and the viability of the finger verified.[57] ⊛ FIG **6.33** APPEARS ONLINE ONLY

The flap may be tunneled through a subcutaneous plane to the defect on the volar aspect of the thumb or alternatively, through a zig-zag Brunner type incision to allow easy transposition of the flap without fear of compression or compromise to the pedicle. The donor site is closed with a split thickness skin graft. Creating chevron incisions lateral to the DIP and PIP creases are important to prevent contractures at these joints following healing of the skin graft. Protective sensation has been observed with two-point discrimination averaging 6–7 mm.[48] Although there is a potential for cortical relearning or plasticity, most patients perceive the sensation as that of the donor site and not the recipient site. Cortical relearning may only be present in 25–40% of individuals.[46,58,59]

Dorsal metacarpal artery flaps

Foucher described the first dorsal metacarpal artery flap for reconstruction of thumb defects involving the volar thumb pulp *(Fig. 6.34)*. This is also known as a kite flap because of its distinct appearance of a distal skin paddle pedicled on a tail of neurovascular structures. This flap utilizes the skin and subcutaneous tissue of the proximal phalanx of the index finger and is based on the neurovascular bundle that rests within or under the fascia of the first dorsal interosseous muscle *(Fig. 6.35)*.[60] The first dorsal metacarpal artery supplies vascularity in the vena comitantes and some superficial veins supply the venous outflow of the flow. Branches of the superficial radial nerve provide sensibility to this flap. The flap is elevated at the plane above the paratenon so that the donor site can accept the split thickness graft for closure. The rest of the pedicle is dissected and the flap can either be transposed through a tunnel or through a zig-zag incision into the volar thumb defect.[50] Although this flap provides protective sensation, cortical relearning and the need for harvesting tissue from an undamaged digit may still result in morbidity. ⊛ FIG **6.34** APPEARS ONLINE ONLY

A reverse dorsal metacarpal artery flap is also been described based on perforators from the palmar system to the dorsal system *(Fig. 6.36)*.[50] These perforators arise between the metacarpophalangeal joints. This flap is a reverse-flow island flap where the skin paddle is taken from the dorsum of the hand closer to the wrist. It is elevated off the fascia of the interosseous muscles and transposed to resurface distal finger defects. In order to get adequate pedicle length to cover the distal finger, the pedicle should be dissected down in to the web space. This flap is not typically used for distal fingertips but for dorsal defects of the finger as the dissection is somewhat tedious between the digits. ⊛ FIG **6.36** APPEARS ONLINE ONLY

> ### Hints and tips: Reverse dorsal metacarpal artery flap
>
> To gain pedicle length, continue the dissection between the proximal phalanges on either side. The pedicle is easily mobilized to reach the volar or dorsal finger tip area.

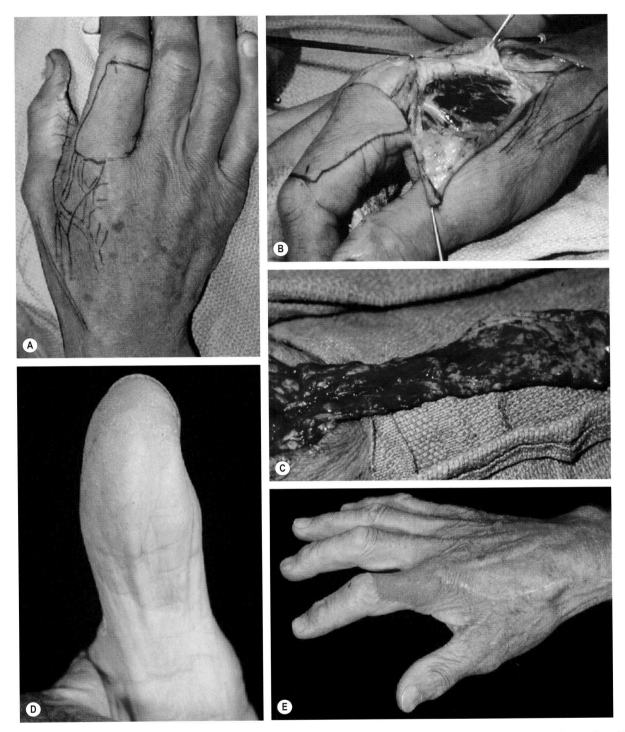

Fig. 6.35 **(A)** First dorsal metacarpal artery flap is designed over the dorsal aspect of the index finger. **(B,C)** First dorsal metacarpal artery lies within the fascia of the first dorsal interosseous muscle. The pedicle is elevated with the fascia and care is taken to keep the superficial veins to allow appropriate drainage of the flap. **(D,E)** Final appearance of the defect on the thumb as well as the donor site.

Bonus images for this chapter can be found online at **http://www.expertconsult.com**

Fig. 6.2 Components of the nail are produced in three areas. (© Southern Illinois University School of Medicine.)

Fig. 6.3 (A) Of nail bed injuries; 36% are classified as simple lacerations; **(B)** 27% as stellate lacerations; **(C)** 22% as crushing injuries of the nail bed; **(D)** 15% as avulsions of the germinal or sterile matrix. (© Southern Illinois University School of Medicine.)

Fig. 6.6 An example of a stitch in the silicone sheeting to hold it in place. (© Southern Illinois University School of Medicine.)

Fig. 6.7 A longitudinal pin was placed to maintain fracture reduction but was between the periosteum and sterile matrix, causing scarring in the ridge. (© Southern Illinois University School of Medicine.)

Fig. 6.8 (A) A split nail may occur within the sterile matrix with minimal problems. **(B)** An injury to the germinal matrix can cause a split in the entire nail, causing significant pain secondary to trauma and disfigurement. (© Southern Illinois University School of Medicine.)

Fig. 6.9 (A) A horizontal laceration in the sterile matrix with a resultant transverse scar can cause a separation so that two nails grow out. If the volar nail is adequate, surgical removal of the dorsal nail-producing matrix will correct the problem. **(B)** The patient's index finger postoperatively. (© Southern Illinois University School of Medicine.)

Fig. 6.11 (A) A split of the nail due to scarring between the dorsal roof and the ventral floor of the nail fold. **(B)** End-on view of the nail deformity. **(C)** With the two portions of nail removed, the cicatrix between the dorsal roof and the ventral floor of the nail fold can be seen. **(D)** The cicatrix is divided with the resultant defect on the dorsal roof. **(E)** A split-thickness sterile matrix graft is removed from the sterile matrix and sutured in place on the dorsal roof of the nail fold. **(F)** The patient is seen 1 year later not with a perfect nail but with a reduced functional problem and

improved appearance. **(G)** An end-on view of the nail showing flattening. (© Southern Illinois University School of Medicine.)

Fig. 6.13 (A) Nonadherence of nail to the sterile matrix thought to be due to an episode of pulling the nail free from the nail bed traumatically and then repeated attempts to clean under the nail. **(B)** The area of nonadherence is marked on the nail. **(C)** That area of nail is removed, showing the hyperkeratinous sterile matrix. **(D)** The hypertrophic keratinous material is scraped off with a scalpel blade to bare the vascular sterile matrix. **(E)** The patient 1 year later with improved adherence of the nail. (© Southern Illinois University School of Medicine.)

Fig. 6.14 (A) Nonadherence of the nails to the nail bed after a crushing injury and then application of artificial nails. The cause of the detachment could be either of these. **(B)** Great toe donor site. **(C)** A split-thickness sterile matrix graft from the large toe is placed over the defect. **(D)** The patient 1 year later with much improved attachment. (© Southern Illinois University School of Medicine.)

Fig. 6.16 (A) A hypertrophic hyponychium (arrowhead) causing pain and discomfort with upper traction on the nail. **(B)** Dorsal view of the same patient. **(C)** Same patient with relief of pain after resection of the hypertrophic hyponychium and a split-thickness sterile matrix graft in its place. **(D)** Same patient, dorsal view with hyponychial attachment. (© Southern Illinois University School of Medicine.)

Fig. 6.22 (A) A bilateral pincer nail or trumpet nail before freeing of the perionychium and insertion of dermal grafts. **(B)** One year after grafting. (© Southern Illinois University School of Medicine.)

Fig. 6.28 (B,C) Exposed PIP joint necessitates closure, the homodigital flap is elevated, care is taken to incorporate the digital artery proper into the flap. **(C,D)** The flap is transposed and the donor site closed with a full thickness skin

graft. **(E)** Healed flap, dorsal aspect of the finger.

Fig. 6.32 (A) The distal fingertips with exposed bone to the index and long fingers in a 23-year-old woman. **(B)** A thenar crease flap is elevated based on the radial aspect of the MP joint of the thumb. The index finger is flexed at the PIP joint and the flap is inset onto the defect of the fingertip. Heterodigital flap is elevated on the index finger and transposed to the tip of the long finger. **(C)** Flaps are divided and definitively inset after 2–3 weeks time to provide appropriate coverage for the distal fingertips of the index and long fingers.

Fig. 6.33 (A) The Littler neurovascular island flap utilizes the skin subcutaneous tissue and neurovascular bundle from the nondominant side of the long or ring fingers. The dissection is carried down into the palm and the flap is transposed to the defect on the thumb. **(B)** The flap is elevated on the neurovascular bundle involving the nondominant side of the long finger. **(C)** The donor defect is closed with a full thickness graft. The flap is transposed onto the dorsum of the thumb. **(D)** The healed defect on the thumb with the neurovascular island flap well inset compromised to the donor finger that may result in contractures if the flap is harvested in a more volar aspect of the finger.

Fig. 6.34 Significant defect of the volar pulp of the thumb with exposed bone and tendon.

Fig. 6.36 (A) Dorsal defects of the finger with a designed reversed dorsal metacarpal artery flap. **(B)** The flap is based between the metacarpal heads as perforators from the palmar side communicate with the dorsal metacarpal arteries. The venous drainage is retrograde. **(C)** The flap is tunneled and inset into place to the dorsal aspect of the finger. This flap can be carried out to the distal aspect of the finger if further dissection is carried down within the webspace.

Access the complete references list online at **http://www.expertconsult.com**

5. Zook EG, Van Beek AL, Russell RC, et al. Anatomy and physiology of the perionychium: a review of the literature and anatomic study. *J Hand Surg Am.* 1980;5:528–536.

    This article offers complete analysis of the normal architecture of the nail bed unit called the perionychium. They compile the literature review with their own cadaveric dissection as a precursor to the concept of applied anatomy in nail bed repair and reconstruction.

8. Zook EG, Brown RE. Injuries of the fingernail. In: Green DP, Hotchkiss RN, Pederson WC, eds. *Operative hand surgery.* 4th ed. New York: Churchill Livingstone; 1999:1353–1380.

16. Ashbell TS, Kleinert HE, Putcha SM, et al. The deformed fingernail, a frequent result of failure to repair nail bed injuries. *J Trauma.* 1967;7:177–190.

17. Zook EG, Guy RJ, Russell RC. A study of nail bed injuries: causes, treatment and prognosis. *J Hand Surg Am.* 1984;9:247–252.

24. Zook EG, Russell RC. Reconstruction of a functional and esthetic nail. *Hand Clin.* 1990;6:59–68.

    This article is an extensive review of the options to correct a variety of nail deformities. All pictures are clinical photographs, with excellent long-term follow-up.

25. Yong FC, Teoh LC. Nail bed reconstruction with split thickness nail bed grafts. *J Hand Surg Br.* 1992;17:193–197.

26. Pessa JE, Tsai TM, Li Y, et al. The repair of nail deformities with the nonvascularized nail bed graft: indications and results. *J Hand Surg Am.* 1990;15:466–470.

33. Bunke HJ, Gonzales RI. Fingernail reconstruction. *Plast Reconstr Surg.* 1962;30:452–461.

39. Achauer BM, Welk RA. One-stage reconstruction of the post-burn nailfold contracture. *Plast Reconstr Surg.* 1990;85:938–941.

   This article describes reconstruction of the eponychium for burn reconstruction. Various local flaps are described with indications and outcomes.

45. Russell R. Fingertip injuries. In: May Jr JW, Littler JW, eds. *The hand.* Philadelphia: WB Saunders; 1990: 4477.

46. Ganchi PA, Lee WPA. Fingertip reconstruction. In: Mathes SJ, ed. Plastic surgery. Vol 7. Philadelphia: Elsevier; 2006:153.

50. Neumeister MW. Intrinsic flaps of the hand. In: Guyron B, ed. *Plastic surgery, indications and practice.* Philadelphia: WB Saunders; 2009:1001.

   A review of the vast variety of flaps used for closure of the finger. Technical details and indications are provided.

59. Ghavami A. Soft tissue coverage of the hand and upper extremity. In: Janis J, ed. *Essentials of plastic surgery.* St. Louis: Quality Medical; 2007:620.

60. Omokawa S, Takaala Y, Ryu J, et al. The anatomical basis for reverse first to fifth dorsal metacarpal arterial flaps. *J Hand Surg* 2005;30B:40–44.

   Many local or regional flaps require flexion of the PIP joint to permit tension free coverage. The article describes the practical anatomy and defining features of the reverse dorsal artery metacarpal arterial flaps.

7

Hand fractures and joint injuries

Warren C. Hammert

SYNOPSIS

- Diagnosis of hand fractures and joint injuries requires history, examination, and adequate imaging studies.
- Treatment decisions are based on fracture geometry, stability, and individual patient needs.
- Nonoperative principles include reduction, maintenance of reduction through casting or splinting, followed by protected motion.
- Operative treatment includes closed reduction with or without percutaneous pinning, external fixation, and open reduction and internal fixation.
- Rehabilitation is an important aspect of caring for patients with hand fractures and joint injuries and involves splinting and restoring motion.
- Secondary procedures may be considered when the desired outcome is not achieved. These include correction of malunion, tenolysis, and capsulotomy.

Introduction

Fractures of the phalanges and metacarpals are the most common fractures in the upper extremity and have been reported to account for 10% of all fractures.[1] Appropriate diagnosis and treatment can minimize deformity and maximize function. Although many of these fractures can be managed nonoperatively, appropriate follow-up is crucial for a good outcome. These injuries can result in time away from work and activities and can be complicated by stiffness and weakness. The goal of the treating physician should be to minimize deformity and maximize function. Operative indications depend on multiple factors, including stability, location, geometry, configuration, and associated injuries, but ultimately, is chosen when the anticipated outcome is better than nonoperative management.[2]

The goal of treatment of fractures in the hand is to reduce and stabilize the fracture, maintain the reduction and begin rehabilitation to restore function. The treating physician must take into account the vocation and avocation of the injured patient, as this may affect the treatment.

Anatomy

The metacarpals and proximal and middle phalanges are anatomically divided into the head, neck, shaft, and base. The distal phalanx is divided into the tuft, shaft, and base. The carpometacarpal (CMC) joints of the index and middle fingers have little mobility, while the ring and small fingers have some motion to allow for grasp and power grip. The metacarpophalangeal (MCP) joints are stabilized by the volar plate and the collateral ligaments: the proper collateral ligaments are thicker and run between the head of the metacarpal and the base of the middle phalanx, while the accessory collateral ligaments are thinner and have a more vertical direction, running from the metacarpal head to the volar plate. The cam shape of the metacarpal head contributes to the tightening of the collateral ligaments when the joint is flexed, stabilizing the joint and decreasing abduction and adduction. The thick intermetacarpal ligaments stabilize the second through fifth metacarpals distally, often providing stability with fractures of the metacarpal shaft.

The proximal phalanx acts as an intercalated segment, with tendons running on all sides, but nothing inserting on this bone. The collateral ligaments of the proximal interphalangeal (PIP) joint contain a proper and accessory component, with insertions into the base of the middle phalanx and the volar plate, respectively. They function to provide lateral stability. The head is bicondylar in shape (as opposed to the cam shape of the metacarpal head) and the collateral ligaments of the PIP joint are tightest with the joint in extension. The middle phalanx has insertions of the extensor mechanism (central slip) and flexor (flexor digitorum superficialis – FDS). The distal interphalangeal (DIP) joint is similar anatomically similar to the PIP joint and the distal phalanx contains the insertion of the terminal portion of the extensor mechanism and the flexor digitorum profundus (FDP).

The volar plates of the MCP joints differ from the IP joints in that the MCP joints have more of an accordion like structure, allowing for the volar plate to be compressed with flexion and expanded with extension. The volar plates of the IP joints have stout proximal extensions known as checkrein ligaments. When contracted, these can contribute to PIP flexion contractures.

The thumb has a greater degree of motion at the CMC joint, allowing for opposition to the fingers. The shape of the metacarpal head (greater diameter on ulnar aspect), allows for pronation of the thumb to assist with opposition.

Classification of fractures and dislocations

Fractures of the phalanges and metacarpals may occur through the joints (articular) or along the shaft (extra-articular). Articular fractures are more common in the PIP and DIP joints than the MCP joints. They may occur through the head or the base. Fractures through the head of the phalanges are classified as unicondylar or bicondylar and can occur in the sagittal or coronal plane. Fractures through the shaft can occur as transverse, oblique, or spiral planes. In addition, fractures can be classified as comminuted when there are multiple fragments.

The angular deformity of the fracture is dependent upon the forces acting on the distal bones. Metacarpal fractures most commonly have an apex dorsal configuration secondary to the pull of the interosseous muscles, while fractures of the proximal phalanx tend to have apex volar configuration due to the interosseous muscles. Fractures of the middle phalanx have a variable deformity, depending of the location of the fracture. Those proximal to the insertion of the FDS have dorsal angulation due to flexion of the distal portion of the bone from the FDS, while fractures distal to the FDS insertion have apex volar angulation due to flexion of the proximal fragment (*Fig. 7.1*).

For a dislocation to occur, the stabilizing structures (collateral ligaments, volar plate, dorsal capsule) must be disrupted. Dislocations are described by the location of the distal bone and are classified as dorsal, volar, radial, or ulnar.

Fracture dislocations commonly occur at the PIP joints of the fingers, and the base of the thumb and ring/small metacarpals. PIP joint and ulnar sided CMC joint fracture dislocations are most commonly dorsal. Thumb CMC joint fracture dislocations are referred as Bennett or Rolando, depending on the configuration and size of the fractured segments.

Fracture stabilization/fixation and return to function

The goal of fracture treatment in the hand is to reduce the fracture and maintain the reduction while restoring motion. Prolonged immobilization will lead to stiffness and should be avoided. Open reduction requires exposure of the fracture sites and stripping of the periosteum. This will provide scaring and

potentially impede motion, so when open reduction is performed, fixation should be stable enough to allow early motion.

For nondisplaced fractures, often protection with buddy straps and active motion without resistance is adequate. For displaced or unstable fractures, reduction and fixation is necessary. Rigid internal fixation with plates and/or screws can provide an anatomic reduction, and the fractures can heal by primary bone healing, but this is not always necessary. This can be particularly problematic for proximal and middle phalanx fractures as there are tendons on all sides that must glide for full motion. The presence of plates and screws in this area will produce scarring and often require removal to maximize motion and ultimately function.

Functionally stable fixation implies the fracture is stable enough to begin motion. This can often be accomplished by closed reduction with percutaneous Kirschner wire (K-wire) insertion. The K-wires can be removed, leaving no internal hardware and minimizing additional scarring.

Pediatric fractures

Pediatric fractures, or fractures in patients with open growth plates require special attention. The physes are located in the metacarpal neck regions in the index, long, ring, and small fingers and at the metacarpal base in the thumb. The physes of the phalanges are located at the base. Growth plate fractures are described by the Salter–Harris classification (*Fig. 7.2*) and (*Table 7.1*), with type II being the most common.

General principles include early reduction and stabilization. An initial reduction attempt should be completed for displaced fractures, but remanipulating a fracture involving the growth plate should be minimized as this can lead to physeal arrest and premature closure of the growth plate. Generally, the use of plates and screws is avoided and hardware is removed when the fracture is healed. Stabilization of fractures occurs with smooth K-wires and if necessary to cross the physis, effort should be made to minimize the number of passes and thus further injury to the growth plate.

Open fractures

Open fractures of the distal phalanx are treated with irrigation and debridement. If the circulation is intact and the patient is immunocompetent, antibiotics are not necessary. Fractures of

Table 7.1 Classification of Salter–Harris fractures

Type 1	Fracture is confined to the physis, often with normal radiographs
Type 2	Fracture starts in the physis and extends through the shaft (away from the joint)
Type 3	Fracture starts in the physis and extends into the joint
Type 4	Fracture starts in the shaft and extends through the physis and into the joint
Type 5	The physis is crushed, and there may be sheering through the physis

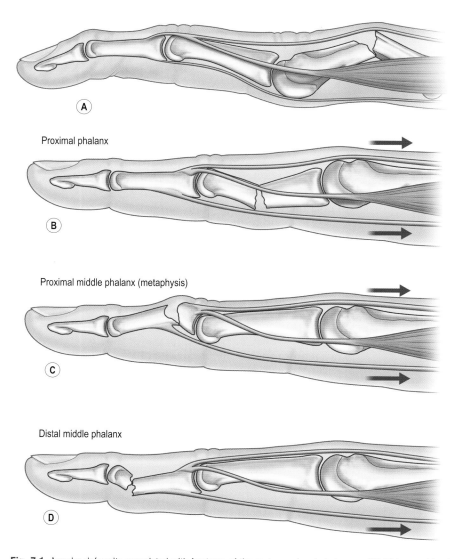

Fig. 7.1 Angular deformity associated with fractures of the metacarpal and phalanges. **(A)** Metacarpal fractures typically have apex dorsal angulation secondary to the location of the interosseous muscles while the proximal phalanx fractures **(B)** have an apex volar angulation. The angulation of middle phalanx fractures is dependent o the location of the fracture, relative to the insertion of the FDS tendon: fractures proximal to the insertion **(C)** will have apex dorsal angulation while those distal **(D)** will have apex volar angulation.

other bones in the hand are treated with antibiotics in addition to irrigation and debridement. Cephalosporins are generally used and with crush injuries or heavy contamination, an aminoglycoside is added. Bite wounds (human or animal) should have penicillin added to cover anaerobes (*Eikenella* in human bites) and *Pasteurella* in animal bites (see Ch. 16).

Diagnosis

The diagnosis of hand injuries begins with a history, including hand dominance and occupation as well as the mechanism of injury. The appearance of the hand should be evaluated with the fingers extended as well as flexed. The alignment of the digits may appear normal with the fingers in extension, only to notice a rotational deformity when the digits are flexed *(Fig. 7.3)*.

Specific areas of edema, ecchymosis or tenderness are noted as well as any wounds that may be present. While general screening radiographs of the hand may be beneficial for initial evaluation, specific X-rays provide better detail and should be used once the diagnosis is made (radiographs of the injured finger are preferred over radiographs of the hand for phalangeal fractures). Three views of the injured part are required to adequately evaluate a fracture in the hand.

Occasionally, additional studies will be necessary for diagnosis or to further define the injury. For example, a collateral ligament injury at the metacarpophalangeal (MCP) of the thumb may not be apparent with plain radiographs, but will become apparent with stress views when the joint space is increased. Magnetic resonance imaging (MRI) can also be used to evaluate collateral ligament injuries and determine if a Stener lesion is present, guiding treatment. Computerized tomography (CT) scans can be used to determine bony

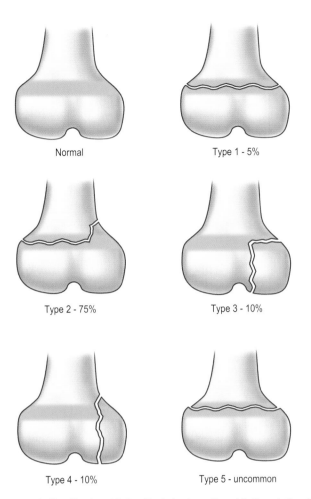

Fig. 7.2 Classification of Salter–Harris fractures. Type 1 is through the physis. Type 2 extends from the physis toward the shaft. Type 3 extends from the physis toward the joint. Type 4 starts in the shaft and extends through the physis and into the joint. Type 5 is a crush injury of the physis.

Normal

Type 1 - 5%

Type 2 - 75%

Type 3 - 10%

Type 4 - 10%

Type 5 - uncommon

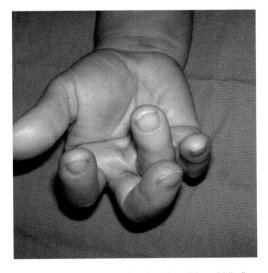

Fig. 7.3 Clinical example of malrotation of the middle finger secondary to a metacarpal fracture.

alignment/fracture configuration and may be helpful in some joint injuries.

Treatment: fingers

Once the diagnosis of a fracture has been made, a decision must be made regarding the best treatment. Options include protection with early motion, immobilization alone or following reduction by closed or open techniques. The goal should be to reduce the fracture, maintain the reduction and return the patient to function with early motion, while minimizing stiffness.

Phalangeal fractures and dislocations

Fractures of the *distal phalanx* are one of the most common fractures encountered.[3] They can involve the tuft, shaft, or base, often extending into the articular surface of the DIP joint. Tuft fractures are often associated with nail bed injuries and repair of the nail bed often reduces and stabilizes the fracture. Shaft fractures are often stable and patients may function well after healing with a fibrous union. For those cases where the fibrous union is symptomatic, correction of the nonunion/ fibrous union can be performed.

DIP joint

Bony mallet fractures involve the dorsal aspect of the base of the distal phalanx. The dorsal aspect contains the terminal extensor tendon and the goal of treatment should be to allow healing of a congruent joint without an extension lag. Most of these can be treated with a splint, maintaining the alignment of the joint.[4,5] These fractures tend to have palpable and sometimes visible prominence along the dorsal aspect of the finger following healing, even when the radiographic alignment is anatomical, but this typically does not adversely affect their function. Fractures with volar subluxation of the distal phalanx should be reduced and often require pinning of the joint to maintain the reduction.[6] Several techniques have been described, but all involve reduction of the joint surface.[7–9] Attempted screw placement into the fragment is difficult, even when the fragment appears large on radiograph, and often results in fragmentation of the dorsal bone. Surgical treatment of stable fractures without subluxation is generally reserved for patients who cannot wear the splint continuously during the healing process, as complications such as pin breakage, pin tract infections and subsequent osteomyelitis can occur and the risks must be carefully considered.

DIP joint dislocations are typically in a dorsal direction (distal phalanx is dorsal to the middle phalanx) *(Fig. 7.4)*. Acute dislocations can often be managed by closed reduction. Flexing the wrist and MCP joints to take the tension off the flexor tendons, and applying distal pressure to the base of the distal phalanx will often reduce the joint. If this is unsuccessful, it is often due to tissue interposed in the joint – most commonly the volar plate – and an open reduction is necessary.[10] This can be completed through a volar zig-zag incision or midlateral incisions. The joint is exposed and any intervening tissue is removed, taking care to avoid damaging the

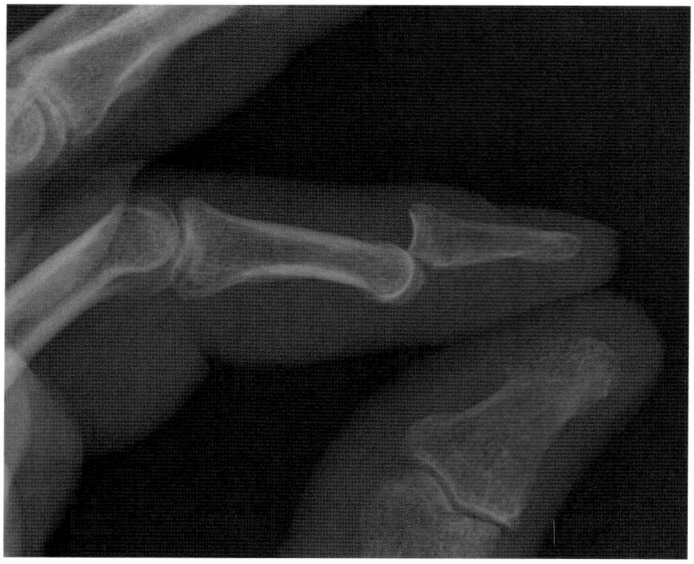

Fig. 7.4 Radiograph of DIP dorsal dislocation of index finger.

articular cartilage, and the joint is reduced. Late presentation of DIP joint dislocations will usually require open reduction, using the same technique. Following reduction, these injuries are typically stable and early motion can be started using a dorsal blocking splint.

Fractures involving the proximal aspect of the DIP joint can occur as isolated middle phalanx articular fractures, involving one or both condyles and may extend proximally into the shaft (diaphysis). Stable fractures can be managed with protective splinting and followed closely with radiographs. If alignment is maintained, buddy taping and range of motion (ROM) exercises can begin around 3 weeks and continued for an additional 3 weeks or until radiographic healing is present. Unstable or displaced fractures should be reduced and stabilized either with K-wires or screws.

Middle phalanx shaft fractures

Treatment of middle phalanx shaft fractures depends on stability and fracture pattern (transverse versus oblique/spiral). Stable, nondisplaced fractures can be managed with a short period of immobilization (typically 2–3 weeks) followed by protected motion with buddy taping. They should be followed closely, checking for displacement and clinical signs of malrotation. This should be checked with the fingers in flexion. Any evidence of malrotation is an indication for reduction and stabilization.

Oblique fractures tend to be unstable, even following reduction, and often result in shortening, which is poorly tolerated by the extensor mechanism. Spiral fractures shorten and rotate. Therefore, these fractures are usually best treated with stabilization. Stiffness is common following these injuries, making postoperative rehabilitation important to optimize the outcome. Plate and screw fixation can provide good stability and allow early motion, but hardware tends to irritate extensor tendons, often resulting on adhesions, and necessitation removal. Lag screws are better tolerated than plates, but still require soft tissue dissection, which can result

in adhesions and limit postoperative motion. K-wire fixation can often be accomplished with minimal soft tissue stripping and can easily be removed following healing, but the fixation is not rigid, so the rehabilitation program cannot be as aggressive. These fractures take a longer to heal due to the higher ratio of cortical to cancellous bone (in comparison to the proximal phalanx and metacarpal), but are usually stable enough to remove the K-wires between 4 and 6 weeks. Radiographic healing may take up to 4 months. A removable splint for protection and protected motion with buddy strapping is instituted to maximize motion.

PIP joint injuries

Injuries around the PIP joint are challenging to treat and good outcomes can be difficult to obtain. Stiffness is common and causes difficulty with gripping and grasping activities, as well as fine dexterity. The small size of the articular fracture fragments can make it difficult to maintain reduction. The goal in treating injuries of the PIP joint is to create a congruent joint and begin a rehabilitation program aimed at restoring motion.

The PIP joint functions as a hinge joint with approximately 100° of motion in the sagittal plane (flexion–extension) and minimal motion in the coronal or axial planes. The base of the middle phalanx is a biconcave surface with a central ridge. The volar lateral aspects of the bone are the sites of insertion of the proper collateral ligaments. The volar plate is a fibrocartilaginous structure, which provides additional stability to the joint. It has thicker fibers that insert laterally and thinner fibers, which insert centrally, to the base of the middle phalanx and proximal extensions, which attach to the periosteum on the proximal phalanx. The volar base of the middle phalanx and its curvature play an important role in stability, preventing dorsal subluxation of the middle phalanx.

The head of the proximal phalanx contains two condyles, separated by a groove or sulcus. There is a slight difference on the size of each condyle, allowing the fingers to converge in flexion. The index and middle have a slightly larger radial condyle while the small finger has a slightly larger ulnar condyle.

Injuries involving the PIP joint can involve the volar base of the middle phalanx, the head of the proximal phalanx, a pure dislocation, or any combination of these. Fractures involving the base of the middle phalanx include dorsal base fractures (involving the insertion of the central slip of the extensor mechanism), the volar base, resulting dorsal subluxation of the middle phalanx, avulsion of the collateral ligaments, or pilon type of fracture involving the dorsal and volar margins, with a depressed central articular fragment (*Fig. 7.5*). Fractures involving the proximal phalanx head can involve one or both condyles and can occur with or without proximal extension.

Pure dislocations result from hyperextension and an axial load. They are often dorsal dislocations and are managed similar to the DIP joint, with an initial trial of closed reduction (with the wrist and fingers flexed and distal pressure on the base of the middle phalanx). When successful, a dorsal blocking splint and early active flexion can produce good results. When reduction cannot be completed by closed means, open reduction is indicated, either through a volar or mid-lateral approach.[11]

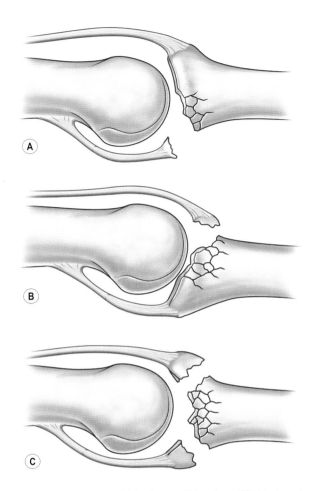

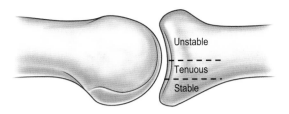

Fig. 7.6 Stability of PIP fracture dislocations. Fractures involving <30% of the articular surface are typically stable. Those involving 30–50% are tenuous and those involving >50% are unstable and have resultant dorsal subluxation.

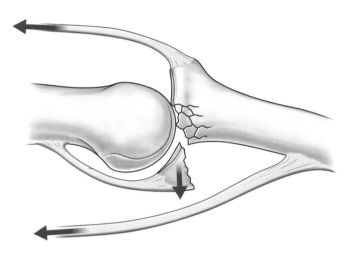

Fig. 7.7 The lateral "V" sign indicating dorsal subluxation of the middle phalanx and associated hinging with flexion.

Fig. 7.5 Classification of PIP joint fracture dislocations. **(A)** Volar base fracture resulting in dorsal subluxation of the middle phalanx. **(B)** Dorsal base fracture resulting in volar subluxation of the middle phalanx. **(C)** Pilon type fracture with dorsal and volar base fractures and comminuted, depressed central articular surface.

Volar dislocations are less common, but can lead to late deformities if not recognized and treated.[12] The central slip is often injured and can result in late boutonniere deformities. Following reduction, splinting the PIP joint in extension and active flexion of the DIP joint will allow gliding of the lateral bands. Active flexion can be started following three weeks, as further immobilization of the PIP joint may result in permanent stiffness. Irreducible dislocations are due to an interposed central slip or collateral ligament and require open reduction through a dorsal approach, allowing direct inspection of the central slip.

Middle phalanx base articular fractures

Fracture dislocations of the PIP joint result from an axial load in a dorsal direction or longitudinal direction when the finger is slightly flexed. These injuries are classified according to the amount of the articular surface involved. Fractures involving <30% of the articular surface of the base of the middle phalanx are typically stable and can be managed nonoperatively. Fractures involving 30–50% of the articular surface are tenuous and often are unstable. Fractures involving >50% are

unstable and result in dorsal subluxation of the middle phalanx *(Fig. 7.6)*.[13]

Lateral radiographs should be carefully evaluated for the "V sign", indicative of dorsal subluxation *(Fig. 7.7)*. The two condyles of the proximal phalanx should be superimposed and the base of the middle phalanx should be collinear with the head of the proximal phalanx. There should be a smooth curvature of the joint surface, with a consistent space between the proximal and middle phalanx. If there is convergence of the joint space creating a dorsal "V", the patient may be able to flex the digit at the PIP joint, but this occurs through a hinge process rather than rotation, and the joint surface will degenerate.

Treatment is directed at recreating a congruent joint surface and restoring motion. Stable fractures and those which are classified as tenuous but maintain reduction and a congruent joint with <30° of flexion, can be managed nonoperatively with a dorsal extension block splint. Active flexion is initiated and extension is allowed short of the point of subluxation. These patients should be followed closely to ensure that subluxation of the joint does not develop. Unstable fractures, or those which a congruent joint cannot be established with <30° of flexion, require operative treatment.

A variety of techniques have been described, including extension block pinning,[14,15] open reduction and internal fixation,[16] volar plate arthroplasty,[17,18] replacement arthroplasty,[19,20] and external fixation.[21–23] All of these techniques have case reports or small series illustrating good outcomes, but there are no prospective studies indicating one technique is better than others for a particular injury.

External fixation

A variety of devices have been described for management of PIP joint fracture dislocations.[21–24] The common principle is to produce distraction across the joint, allowing alignment to be maintained through ligamentotaxis. In addition, some devices provide a volar directed force on the middle phalanx to assist in maintaining alignment. They all allow immediate PIP joint motion. Careful attention should be paid to the fragments along the volar base of the middle phalanx as dorsal subluxation can recur if these do not heal in proper position (the volar lip of the base of the middle phalanx is a restraint to dorsal subluxation, so healing of the fracture fragments must recreate the normal curvature).

External fixation systems can be fabricated from K-wires with or without the use of rubber bands or commercially available devices can be used. Figure 7.10 illustrates and example of a PIP joint fracture dislocation in the small finger managed with an external fixator fabricated from K-wires.

Technique of external fixation

A 0.045-inch K-wire is inserted through the head of the proximal phalanx, perpendicular to the joint surface *(Fig. 7.8)*. A second 0.045-inch K-wire is inserted through the distal shaft of the middle phalanx, parallel to the DIP joint surface. The proximal wire is bent distally along the radial and ulnar aspects, paralleling the digit. Distal to the second wire, a dorsal proximal bend is created, followed by a dorsal distal bend. The bends should be at the same level on both the radial and ulnar sides. This creates a groove in the proximal wire for the distal wire to be positioned, allowing slight distraction across the joint, which will aid the reduction via ligamentotaxis. Increasing or decreasing the first bend on the proximal wire can adjust the distraction across the joint. This can be performed under local anesthesia and immediate motion is initiated. The fixator is left in place for approximately six weeks and rehabilitation focuses on motion of the PIP and DIP joints. The joint surface will remodel over time.

Internal fixation

Internal fixation of middle phalanx base fractures can be demanding, but good results can be obtained. Postoperative rehabilitation is critical to a good outcome, so the patient must be compliant or the result can be a good radiograph with a stiff nonfunctional finger. Larger fragments can often be stabilized with small screws, reconstructing the volar base of the middle phalanx *(Fig. 7.9)*. Dorsal fragments can be stabilized with screws or K-wires to reinsert the central slip. Comminution at the base of the middle phalanx creates a greater challenge and the surgeon should be prepared for this as often what appears as a large piece on X-ray is found to be multiple smaller pieces. If the articular surface can be reduced, a cerclage wire may be used to hold the bone fragments in place *(Fig. 7.10)*.[25] This may provide adequate stability to allow early motion. ⊕ FIGS **7.9**, **7.10** APPEAR ONLINE ONLY

If the remaining fragments are too small to stabilize, they can be excised and the joint surface is reconstructed. The two most common methods to accomplish this are by advancing the volar plate (volar plate arthroplasty) or replacement of the volar base of the middle phalanx. This can be accomplished by using a portion of the hamate (hemi-hamate replacement arthroplasty, HHRA).

The volar plate arthroplasty was described by Eaton and Malerich in 1980[18] and involves removing the comminuted portion of bone along the volar aspect of the base of the middle phalanx, creating a trough parallel to the dorsal surface of the middle phalanx, and advancing the volar plate to resurface the joint. The volar plate is attached to the bone, either through drill holes or with a permanent suture at the lateral aspect. The joint is temporarily pinned in slight flexion. At 3 weeks, the pin is removed and motion is begun.[17] The volar plate serves to prevent dorsal subluxation of the middle phalanx. The results with this technique can be unpredictable as stiffness and recurrent dorsal subluxation can occur. Long-term follow-up of Dr Eaton's patients have been published with good results,[26] but there are few recent reports of this procedure.

More recently, the hemi-hamate replacement arthroplasty has been described (Hastings *et al.* ASSH annual meeting, 1999) and subsequently published. The dorsal distal portion of the hamate has similar anatomy to the volar base of the middle phalanx. Osseous cuts must be precise and the curvature of the volar base of the middle phalanx must be reproduced or persistent dorsal subluxation will occur. This can be rigidly fixed and early motion can be instituted. Published series have shown promising results.[20,27]

Technique of HHRA

The procedure can be performed under regional or general anesthesia. The finger is approached from the volar aspect with a Bruner incision from the palmodigital crease to the DIP flexion crease *(Fig. 7.11)*. Skin flaps are elevated and retracted. The digital neurovascular bundles are freed so they are not under tension when the joint is exposed. A radial or ulnar based flap of the flexor sheath is created between the A-2 and A-4 pulleys. The collateral ligaments are released from the middle phalanx, leaving a small stump for later repair, and the volar plate is released from fragments at the base of the middle phalanx. The neurovascular bundles are inspected to make sure they will not tether as the joint is exposed. The flexor tendons are retracted and the joint is shot gunned open exposing the joint. If resistance is encountered, it is usually due to the collateral ligaments; these are inspected, ensuring complete release from the middle phalanx.

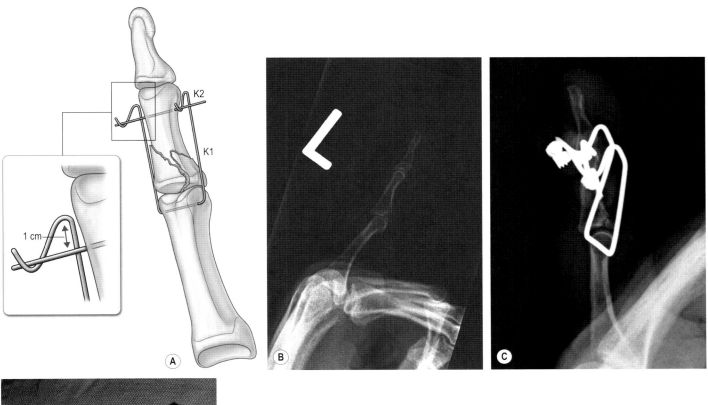

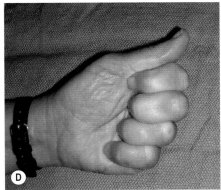

Fig. 7.8 (A) Fabrication of external fixator from K-wires. Preoperative radiograph **(B)** of PIP fracture dislocation involving the small finger, **(C)** Radiograph with external fixator in place, allowing motion. **(D)** Postoperative results in flexion.

Once the joint is exposed, the loose fragments are removed and a smooth surface is created along the joint surface and along the volar margin of the middle phalanx. This will be the site of insertion of the hemi-hamate graft. Care must be taken to preserve as much of the dorsal cortex as possible as this becomes prone to fracture if insufficient bone remains. The defect for the graft should be large enough to allow fixation of the graft with at least two, and preferably three screws. The dimensions of the defect are measured so an appropriate size graft can be obtained.

Next, a dorsal transverse incision is outlined proximal to the base of the ring and small metacarpals to expose the distal aspect of the hamate. Fluoroscopy can be used to confirm the correct location of the incision. Care is taken to preserve the dorsal sensory branch of the ulnar nerve and a transverse capsulotomy is performed exposing the joint. The dimensions of the graft are outlined and the graft is harvested slightly larger than necessary, so it can be trimmed to the appropriate dimensions. The axial and sagittal cuts are made using a small saw. A portion of the dorsal hamate can be removed proximal to the axial cut to facilitate the coronal cut. This can be completed with a curved osteotome. The graft is removed and the donor site is closed. The graft is placed along the base of the middle phalanx and provisionally fixed with small K-wires. This step is crucial as proper positioning is necessary for a good outcome. The graft must be placed so the normal curvature of the middle phalanx base is recreated. If the graft is positioned too vertically, dorsal subluxation of the middle phalanx will occur. The joint is reduced and visualized with fluoroscopy. The joint should now appear congruent, with appropriate curvature of the middle phalanx base and without evidence of the dorsal "V." The cartilage on the graft is typically thicker than the middle phalanx, so images may appear as if the graft is not in proper position. This can be ignored since direct visualization will ensure alignment of the joint surface. The joint is opened and the K-wires are replaced with small screws (1.0–1.5 mm), rigidly securing the graft to the middle phalanx. The joint is reduced and fluoroscopy is used to confirm appropriate length of the screws and position of the graft.

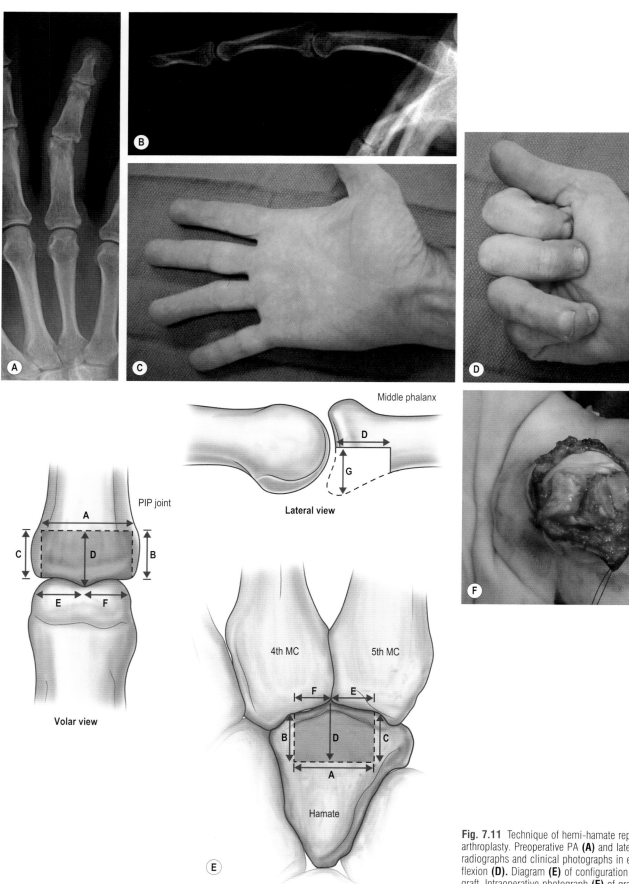

Fig. 7.11 Technique of hemi-hamate replacement arthroplasty. Preoperative PA **(A)** and lateral **(B)** radiographs and clinical photographs in extension **(C)** and flexion **(D)**. Diagram **(E)** of configuration of hemi-hamate graft. Intraoperative photograph **(F)** of graft secured (note articular wear on the head of the proximal phalanx due to delay in presentation.

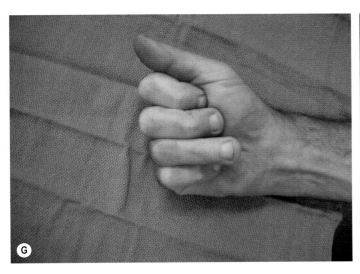

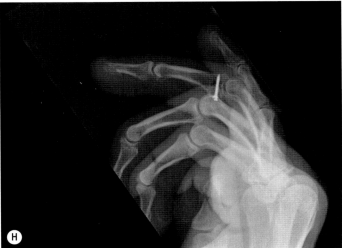

Fig. 7.11, cont'd Postoperative clinical photograph **(G)** and lateral radiograph **(H)**.

The volar plate is repositioned, but does not need to be secured to the graft. The collateral ligaments can be repaired to the residual stumps on the base of the middle phalanx. The stability of the reconstructed PIP joint (and prevention of dorsal subluxation) is created by the shape and position of the hemi-hamate graft. The flexor sheath can be placed dorsal to the flexor tendons and secured to the opposite side. The skin is closed, the tourniquet is deflated and perfusion of the digit is evaluated. Occasionally, the vessels are in spasm, but the perfusion should be restored within a few minutes. A volar splint is placed from the forearm to the fingertips.[19,28] Rehabilitation is begun around day five with attention to edema control and motion. A figure of eight splint is used to prevent the final 10–15° of extension. A removable wrist is used for comfort to support the donor site.

The average arc of motion at the PIP joint has been reported between 65° and 100° (average 85) with return to light activities at one month and return to manual labor at 2 months.[20,27]

If the entire base of the middle phalanx is involved, replacement arthroplasty can be considered, but there are only a few case reports of this technique. Hemiarthroplasty has been reported, but currently, the use of the PyroCarbon and surface replacement arthroplasty requires special approval and is not available for routine use in the PIP joint.

Hints and tips

- Postoperative therapy and a motivated patient are critical to obtain a good result following PIP joint fracture dislocations
- The patient should be informed that the goal is to create a stable joint with motion, but the return of motion to the pre-injury level is rare
- Some degree of post-traumatic PIP joint arthritis is inevitable, but this does not always correlate with functional outcomes

Proximal phalanx head fractures

Fractures involving the head of the proximal phalanx are intra-articular and anatomic reduction and early motion of these injuries is the goal. Fractures can involve one or both condyles and classification systems have been described.[29] These fractures are often unstable and require treatment. Stable, nondisplaced fractures can be treated with a short period of immobilization with frequent radiographic evaluation. Motion is typically started at three weeks and the finger is protected with buddy taping to an adjacent digit. Displaced or unstable fractures require reduction and stabilization.[29] Fixation is dependent on the size of the fragment and the ability to reduce the joint with closed manipulation. If anatomic alignment can be obtained with closed reduction and the fragment can be stabilized with K-wires, these can be treated as a stable nondisplaced fracture. Often, anatomic reduction requires open exposure. The fragments are often large enough to hold at least one small (1.0 mm) screw and a K-wire or two screws. This provides enough stability to begin early motion and minimizes adhesions to the extensor tendons. When both condyles are involved, initial alignment and stabilization of the articular surface is preferred. Then, the articular surface can be secured to the shaft either with K-wires or plates and screws. Although plates and screws provide good stability, they require more dissection and adhesions to the extensor tendons are likely to occur, often requiring a secondary procedure to remove the hardware and perform a tenolysis.

Technique of ORIF of unicondylar fracture

The procedure can be performed under regional, general, IV sedation, or local with epinephrine without a tourniquet (*Fig. 7.12*). A straight or curvilinear dorsal approach is used from the middle of the proximal phalanx to the middle of the middle phalanx. Skin flaps are elevated to expose the extensor tendon distal to the insertion of the central slip on the middle phalanx. The joint can be exposed by splitting the extensor

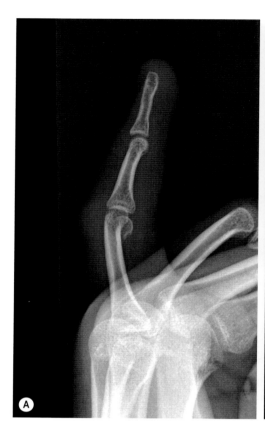
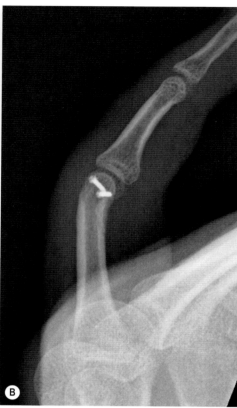

Fig. 7.12 Preoperative lateral radiograph **(A)** of displaced unicondylar fracture. Postoperative lateral **(B)** radiograph in flexion.

tendons (index and small fingers) or to the side of the central slip. Better visualization is obtained through exposure along the side of the central slip on the side with the fracture. The tendon is elevated off the proximal phalanx, taking care to preserve the insertion of the central slip. A capsulotomy is performed, exposing the head of the proximal phalanx. The fragments are reduced under direct visualization and temporarily stabilized with small K-wires. Fluoroscopy is used to confirm alignment and the K-wires are replaced with screws. The capsule can be repositioned, but does not need to be closed with sutures. If the tendons were split, they are repaired with a nonabsorbable suture. The central slip insertion is inspected to confirm it has not been disrupted. The skin is closed, the tourniquet is deflated, and a splint is applied. Rehabilitation begins around the 5th postoperative day with edema control and a figure of eight splint, allowing flexion and blocking the final 10° of extension.

Proximal phalanx shaft and base fractures

Fractures of the shaft of the proximal phalanx can be transverse or oblique. Transverse fractures typically have apex volar angulation and are unstable. Fractures of the base are typically transverse. If not reduced and stabilized, the extensor mechanism will shorten, creating an extensor lag at the PIP joint. Percutaneous fixation has the advantage of stabilizing the fracture and allowing early motion while minimizing

soft tissue injury.[30] Two crossed K-wires typically provide enough stability to allow early motion. The wires can be inserted proximally through the base with one on each side of the metacarpal head or distally, with one entering along the head or neck. Alternatively, the K-wires can be placed through the MCP joint in flexion *(Fig. 7.13)*. The disadvantage is the K-wire is passed through the articular surface, but in cases with significant soft tissue edema, may help prevent MCP joint extension contractures. By 3–4 weeks, the fracture is usually stable enough for removal of the K-wires. Protected motion should occur until complete fracture healing. Radiographic healing lags behind clinical healing, which typically occurs around 6 weeks. ORIF with plates and screws can allow immediate motion, but adherence of the tendon to the hardware can be problematic, often resulting in stiffness and need for secondary procedures.[31]

Oblique or spiral fractures should be evaluated in flexion as well as extension. These often shorten obliquely, resulting in a rotational deformity. Fixation can be accomplished with either K-wires or interfragmentary screws if the length of the fracture is two times the length of the diameter of the bone. ORIF with interfragmentary screws allows enough stability to proceed with early active motion and when anatomically reduced, primary bone healing *(Fig. 7.14)*. Adhesions between the screws and tendons are less when plates are not used, and although removal is sometimes necessary, often the screws can be left in place.

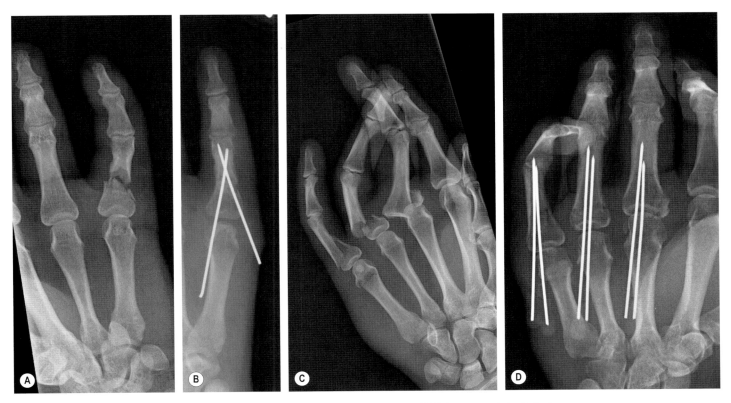

Fig. 7.13 Preoperative and postoperative PA radiograph of proximal phalanx shaft **(A,B)** and base **(C,D)** fractures treated with K-wires.

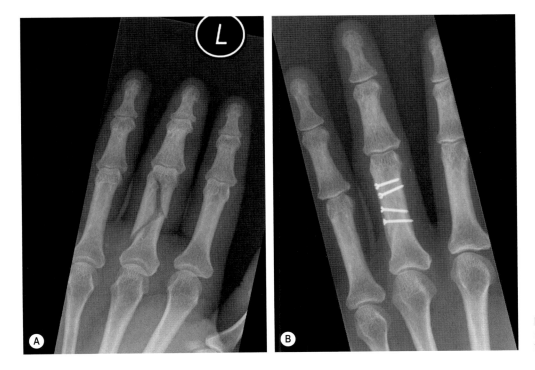

Fig. 7.14 Preoperative **(A)** and postoperative **(B)** radiographs of proximal phalanx fracture treated with interfragmentary screws.

MCP joint fractures and dislocations

Fractures extending into the articular surface of the MCP joint should be reduced anatomically and stabilized, in effort to minimize the development of post-traumatic arthritis.

Dislocations of the MCP joint can occur in any direction, with dorsal being the most common. The border digits (index and small finger) are most commonly involved *(Fig. 7.15)*.[32] The volar plate ruptures from the proximal phalanx and the MCP joint subluxes dorsally, with the proximal phalanx extended in relation to the metacarpal. If the volar plate does not become interposed in the joint, these can be treated with closed reduction. The wrist is flexed to relax the flexor tendons and distal pressure is applied to the base of the proximal phalanx. A snap or pop is often felt, which is the reduction of the joint. Radiographs are obtained to confirm the reduction. The joint is typically stable following reduction, but an extension block splint can be used if instability exists.

When the volar plate becomes interposed in the joint, the dislocation is complex and closed reduction attempts are unsuccessful. Dimpling of the skin is seen over the dislocation. Radiographs will show the proximal phalanx and metacarpal co-linear (as opposed to the convergence seen with simple dislocations). In the index finger, the lumbrical displaces around the radial side and the flexor tendons around the ulnar side. Distal pressure on the proximal phalanx base tightens the lumbrical and flexor tendons around the

metacarpal neck, creating a noose effect and preventing reduction.

In the small finger, the flexor tendons and lumbrical displace radially while the flexor digiti minimi displaces ulnarly, creating the same noose like effect when closed reduction is attempted.

Open reduction through a dorsal or volar approach is necessary.[33] The volar approach is more direct, but the digital nerves are tented beneath the skin and at risk with the skin incision. The A-1 pulley is released, exposing the metacarpal head, and the volar plate is removed from the joint. The flexor tendons are pulled over the metacarpal, allowing reduction. The dorsal approach does not allow direct visualization, but avoids the risk of injuring the digital nerves with the incision. The extensor tendons are split longitudinally. If the volar plate cannot be easily removed from the joint, it can be split longitudinally, allowing each side to be pushed out of the joint. The joint can then be reduced with distal pressure on the proximal phalanx base while pushing the flexor tendons around the metacarpal head. The joint is typically stable following reduction, but extension block splinting can be used if instability exists.

> ### Hints and tips
>
> - For MCP joint dislocations, attempt closed reduction with the wrist maximally flexed; if unsuccessful, proceed to open reduction
> - The volar approach is more direct, but it places the digital nerves at risk during the skin incision as they will be tented beneath the skin
> - The dorsal approach often requires splitting the volar plate to allow complete reduction

Volar dislocations of the MCP joint are rare. Interposed structures can include the dorsal capsule, extensor tendon junctura, collateral ligament or the volar plate.[34,35] When closed reduction is unsuccessful, open reduction is performed through a dorsal approach.

Metacarpal fractures

Metacarpal fractures commonly occur as a result of a direct blow. They can occur through the head, neck, shaft, or base.[36] Fracture configuration is usually transverse, oblique, or spiral. Transverse fractures occur as a result of an axial load with bending and result in apex dorsal deformity. Oblique or spiral patterns occur with torsional stress when an axial load is received. Malrotation of 5° in the metacarpal can result in 1.5 cm of overlap at the fingertips and thus, evaluation of the fingers in flexion is imperative. As the amount of energy increases, the amount of comminution increases and stability decreases, and the incidence of multiple fractures increases.

An open wound over the MCP joint region should be treated as a "fight bite", with irrigation of the wound and inspection of the extensor tendon and joint capsule. Alignment of the fingers is evaluated with the fingers in flexion to check for rotation. Three views of the hand (posterior-anterior, lateral, and oblique) are often adequate for diagnosis of

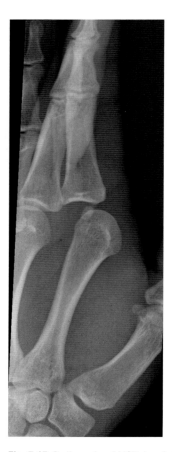

Fig. 7.15 Radiographs of MCP dorsal dislocation.

metacarpal fractures. Additional images include a Brewerton view to improve visualization of the metacarpal heads. This is an A–P view with the phalanges flexed to 45–60° and in contact with the film (the metacarpals are elevated at a 45–60° angle and the beam is directed 15° from ulnar to radial). A 30° pronated oblique view improves visualization of the ring and small finger CMC joints, while a 30° supinated view helps visualize the index and middle finger CMC joints. CT scans can be used when plain radiographs are inconclusive, multiple CMC fracture dislocations are present, or for complex metacarpal head fractures.

Many metacarpal fractures are stable and can be treated nonoperatively. Boxer's fractures (fifth metacarpal neck) are impaction fractures and although there is angulation of the metacarpal neck, are stable. This term is a misnomer as professional boxers rarely sustain this injury; they commonly occur when a firm object, such as a wall, is struck, but the term is commonly used to describe this fracture. The intermetacarpal ligaments stabilize fractures involving the middle and ring metacarpals and often alignment is maintained with minimal shortening.

Metacarpal head fractures

Treatment of fractures involving the metacarpal head involves anatomic reduction and stabilization. A dorsal approach is used and the extensor tendon is split or the sagittal band incised to expose the metacarpal hand and MCP joint. Rigid fixation is preferred when possible, so use of small screws placed through the collateral recess or headless screws are preferred, with the goal of early motion. Severely comminuted fractures are problematic as stiffness and arthritis often result. Hemi arthroplasty, replacing the metacarpal head has been described, but there is no long-term data on outcomes for this procedure.

Metacarpal neck fractures

Metacarpal neck fractures are more common on the ulnar side of the hand (fifth metacarpal), but can occur in any of the fingers. The amount of apex dorsal angulation which is acceptable is debatable and varies between patients depending on vocation and avocations, but increases from radial to ulnar. Acceptable angulation for the index and middle fingers is <15°, with the ring between 20° and 40° and the small finger up to 60°.[37] This deformity will result in loss of prominence of the "knuckle" (metacarpal head) with a proximal prominence along the metacarpal neck and occasionally noticeable prominence in the palm; the flexed metacarpal head. This is unlikely to cause functional limitations. Occasionally, pseudo-clawing will develop secondary to the flexed position of the metacarpal head, resulting in MCP hyperextension and a PIP extension lag.

Treatment is dependent on the existing deformity. Often closed reduction and immobilization provides adequate alignment and can be used for definitive management.[38] Flexing the MCP joint to 90°, which relaxes the deforming intrinsic muscles and simultaneously tightens the collateral ligaments, allows for control of the distal metacarpal fragment. The Jahss maneuver involves flexion of the distal interphalangeal, proximal interphalangeal, and metacarpophalangeal joints followed by dorsally directed pressure over the flexed PIP while applying a volar directed force over the apex of the fracture.[39] This maneuver delivers the three-point fixation needed for fracture immobilization and ensures reduction with appropriate angulation and rotation. After the Jahss maneuver has been performed, the hand needs to be immobilized with the MCP joint flexed and the IP joints extended. A cast or splint is not always successful in maintaining reduction, especially with the swelling associated with the fracture (Fig. 7.16).

Indications for operative treatment include malrotation or unacceptable alignment following closed reduction. Surgical options include closed reduction and percutaneous pinning, IM (intramedullary) wires, and ORIF (open reduction internal fixation). The distal location of metacarpal neck fractures makes stabilization with plates difficult.

The MCP joint is flexed and alignment is evaluated, correcting any malrotation. Percutaneous K-wires can be placed from distal, through the collateral recess or proximal through the metacarpal base. Alternatively, the wires can be placed transverse, stabilizing the fifth metacarpal to the fourth metacarpal, or multiple wires as intramedullary nails. This is completed through an incision proximally near the metacarpal base. After exposing the bone, an awl or similar instrument is used to creating an opening in the bone and wires are placed into the shaft. The reduction is confirmed with fluoroscopy and the wires are advanced across the fracture site and into the bone distally. These wires are typically left out of the bone proximally to allow removal following healing, but can be cut and left within the bone. Depending on stability,

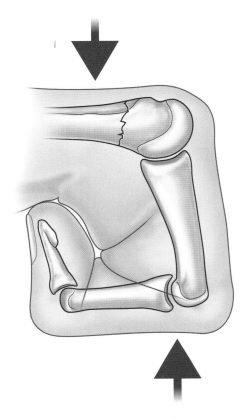

Fig. 7.16 The Jahss maneuver for reduction of a metacarpal neck fracture. The DIP and PIP joints are flexed and dorsal pressure is applied to the PIP joint while counter pressure is applied to the metacarpal shaft proximal to the fracture.

postoperative immobilization is often required for 4–6 weeks, followed by therapy to regain motion.

ORIF is performed when reduction cannot be attained by closed means or when there is a desire to minimize postoperative immobilization. It is completed through a dorsal approach, either splitting the extensor tendons (small or index finger) or along the side. If adequate stability is achieved, the patient can be transitioned to a removable splint and begin active motion when comfortable (usually within the first week).

Metacarpal shaft fractures

Isolated metacarpal shaft fractures are often stable and amenable to nonoperative management. The intermetacarpal ligaments stabilize the distal metacarpal and maintain alignment. Similar to metacarpal neck fractures, the amount of apex dorsal angulation is debated, but increases from radial to ulnar due to increasing mobility at the CMC joint from radial to ulnar. The amount of acceptable angulation is less in the shaft than in the neck, with <10° in the index and middle fingers and approximately 20° in the ring and 30° in the small finger.

Shortening can be noticeable, but typically does not cause a functional problem. Nonoperative treatment includes immobilization for about 4 weeks, with the MCP joints flexed and the IP joints free. Operative indications include open fractures, malrotation and unacceptable angulation *(Fig. 7.17)*. Similar to metacarpal neck fractures, closed reduction and pinning can be completed from distal or proximal, transversely into the adjacent metacarpal[40] or with IM wires.[41]

ORIF can be completed with interfragmentary screws for spiral or oblique fractures or with plates and screws for transverse fractures.[42] Coverage of the plate with periosteum, when possible, will decrease tendon irritation and need for later removal. Early motion should be initiated following ORIF to prevent tendon adhesions.

Severely comminuted fractures, those with segmental bone or soft tissue loss can be treated with external fixation, either temporarily until adequate soft tissue healing for internal fixation, or in some cases definitively.[43-45]

Multiple metacarpal fractures

Multiple metacarpal fractures are often the result of higher energy and result in greater soft tissue disruption. In addition, the stability provided by the transverse intermetacarpal ligament is lost and stabilization is often necessary.

Technique of ORIF of multiple metacarpal fractures

The procedure is completed under regional or general procedure. A dorsal skin incision is outlined. For two metacarpal fractures, the skin incision can be placed between them. The incision can be curved proximally or distally as necessary as the locations of the fractures are often at different in each bone. When three or four fractures are present, more than one incision will be necessary.

The skin incision is completed and dissection is carried to the level of the extensor tendons, taking care to protect sensory branches of the ulnar (fourth and fifth metacarpals) and the radial (second and third metacarpals) nerves. The extensor tendons are retracted and the metacarpal is visualized. There is often hematoma and disruption of the periosteum around the fracture site. A longitudinal incision is completed through the periosteum along the dorsal radial or distal ulnar aspect of the bone, the periosteum is elevated and the fracture is exposed. The adjacent metacarpal is exposed through a periosteal incision, again placed off the central axis of the metacarpal. Beginning with the most radial fractured metacarpal, any interposed tissue is removed from the fracture site. The fracture is reduced and provisionally stabilized (either with a fracture reduction forceps or K-wires), while alignment of the fingers is checked, making sure there is no malrotation.

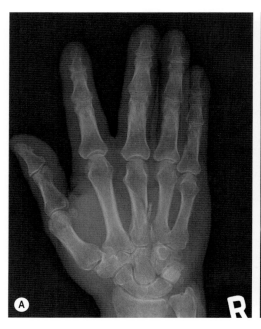
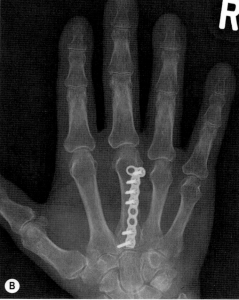

Fig. 7.17 Radiographs of metacarpal shaft fracture treated with ORIF due to malrotation **(A,B)**. (See the preoperative clinical picture in *Fig. 7.3*.)

Interfragmentary screws or plate and screws are applied; fluoroscopy is used to confirm positioning of the hardware and the adjacent metacarpal is addressed. After all fractures are stabilized, the periosteum is closed, creating a layer of tissue between the hardware and the extensor tendons. If the sagittal band was divided distally for exposure, this is repaired and the skin is closed. A splint is applied for comfort and motion can begin as the swelling subsides, typically between 3 and 5 days postoperatively.

CMC dislocations/fracture dislocations

Fractures of the metacarpal base, fracture dislocations of the CMC joint and dislocations involving the CMC joint usually involve the ring and small fingers. Fracture dislocations may involve the capitate and hamate in addition to the metacarpal base.[46,47] These patients will have a prominence along the ulnar side of the hand in the region of the CMC joints. Diagnosis is confirmed in the pronated oblique view, observing the relationship between the carpus and base of the metacarpal. The dorsal aspect should be co-linear and when subluxation is present, the metacarpal will be positioned dorsal to the carpus. CT scan can be used when the diagnosis is not clear on plain radiographs or to define fracture geometry. These injuries are often unstable and require operative treatment. Closed reduction and percutaneous pinning is usually successful when performed within the first several days (*Fig. 7.18*). Delayed presentation usually requires open reduction. Stabilization is obtained using K-wires across the CMC joints. The K-wires are removed at four to six weeks and motion is resumed with protective splinting for comfort. Alternatively, a plate can be applied across the CMC joints with planned removal once soft tissue healing has occurred.

Treatment: thumb

Injuries to the thumb distal and proximal phalanges can be managed similar to the fingers. Metacarpal shaft fractures can tolerate more rotation and angulation due to the greater degree of freedom in three planes (flexion/extension, radial/ulnar deviation, pronation/supination) of the CMC joint. Injuries involving the MCP joint, specifically collateral ligament injuries and those involving the CMC joints require special consideration.

MCP joint injuries

The primary motion of the MCP joint is flexion/extension. The radial condyle of the metacarpal head has a greater height (dorsal/volar dimension), allowing rotation (pronation) with increasing flexion. Stability of this joint is provided by the collateral ligaments, the dorsal capsule and the volar plate, the thenar muscles and the adductor pollicis.

Injuries involving the ulnar collateral ligament are more common than the radial collateral ligament and have been reported to occur at a 10:1 ratio.[48,49] This typically results from forced abduction (radial directed stress), such as falling with an object, such as a ski pole, in the first web space. The dorsal capsule tears along the ulnar aspect of the joint and the proximal phalanx supinates around the intact RCL, creating a prominence of the ulnar aspect of the metacarpal head. Although commonly used to describe this injury, the term "gamekeepers" thumb more accurately defines a chronic injury from repetitive radial directed stress resulting in attenuation of the ligament. This occurred in Scottish gamekeepers while breaking the necks of rabbits between their thumb and index fingers. The term skier's thumb is more accurate and should be used when referring to acute injuries.

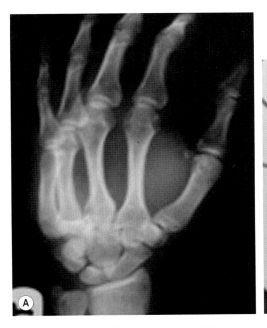
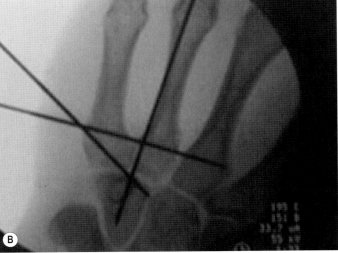

Fig. 7.18 Preoperative **(A)** and Postoperative **(B)** radiographs of CMC 4th and 5th CMC dislocations.

Injuries typically involve disruption of the ligament from the base of the proximal phalanx. This can occur as a bony avulsion or pure ligamentous injury. Larger fractures (those >2 mm), those involving >10% of the articular surface, or those with articular incongruity are best treated with open reduction and stabilization.[49,50]

Isolated ligamentous injuries can be more challenging to diagnose. Avulsion from the proximal phalanx is five times more common than midsubstance tears or avulsion from the metacarpal.[51]

Stener lesion

In 1962, Stener described the injury where the complete ulnar collateral ligament tear retracted proximally and the adductor aponeurosis was interposed between the ligament and the site of avulsion along the base of the proximal phalanx *(Fig. 7.19)*. Without contact between the ligament and bone, healing cannot occur and chronic instability will result.[52] A complete rupture and retraction of the ligament is necessary for the Stener lesion to occur and therefore, it is important to differentiate between partial or complete tears without retraction and those where the ligament has retracted proximal to the adductor aponeurosis. Unfortunately, there is not an absolute clinical criterion for making this diagnosis. The MCP joint is observed for swelling and tenderness along the ulnar side. A palpable mass at the level of the metacarpal neck may be consistent with the retracted UCL. The joint should be tested in both flexion and extension, checking for a definite endpoint and comparing to the opposite thumb. Multiple reports exist in the literature, all using different clinical criteria for diagnosis of a complete tear.[53–56] Stress radiographs may assist in making the diagnosis. In addition, MRI, arthrogram and ultrasound can be used in cases of uncertainty following clinical exam and plain radiographs.

Incomplete tears can be treated with immobilization, allowing the ligament to heal to the bone. When a Stener lesion is present, operative treatment is required. Open ligament repair is the most common procedure performed, but arthroscopic

repositioning of the ligament has been described, placing the ligament deep to the adductor aponeurosis and allowing it to heal to the bone.[57,58] Delayed presentation may make it difficult to repair the ligament primarily and reconstruction may be indicated. With late presentation, radiographs should be evaluated for presence of arthritis and when present, arthrodesis should be considered. Reconstruction techniques produce dynamic (tendon transfers and adductor advancement) and static reconstructions (creation of a static restraint to radial directed stress with a graft).

Dynamic reconstructions typically involve transfer of a tendon to stabilize the MCP joint. Procedures include transfer of the EIP to the extensor mechanism, transfer of the EPB to the ulnar side of the proximal phalanx[59,60] and advancement of the adductor.[61] The adductor is transferred from its insertion on the sesamoid to the proximal phalanx. Static reconstructions involve replacement of the ligament with a graft, such as palmaris longus tendon, through holes created in the metacarpal and proximal phalanx.[49,62]

Primary repair can be completed as long as there is adequate ligament to repair. This can be predictably completed around 6 weeks following the injury. When the procedure is greater than 6 weeks following the injury, the surgeon should be prepared to proceed with reconstruction in the event the ligament is not amenable to primary repair. Surgical treatment should be aimed at anatomic reconstruction of the joint. Repair or reattachment too distal or volar will result in loss of flexion and placement too dorsal may result in persistent instability. With an acute injury, it is often possible to determine the site of avulsion and reattach it to the site of avulsion. The ligament runs from dorsal to volar in a proximal to distal direction. The origin of the proper collateral ligament is 7 mm proximal to the joint and 3 mm from the dorsal cortex. The insertion of the base of the proximal phalanx is located 3 mm distal to the joint and 3 mm from the volar cortex *(Fig. 7.20)*.[63] Reattachment can be completed using suture anchors, a pull out suture exiting the opposite side tied over a button or directly over the bone.

Radial collateral ligament injuries are much less common than their ulnar counterparts. On the radial side of the thumb,

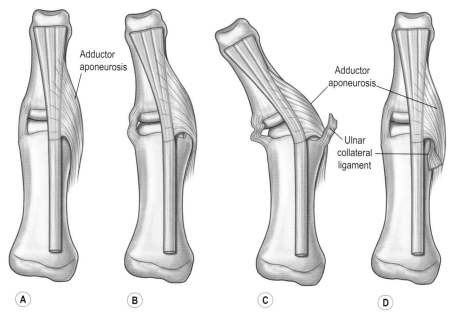

Fig. 7.19 Stener lesion of the MCP joint of the thumb. **(A)** Normal relationship of the adductor aponeurosis. With a radial directed stress **(B)**, the ligament is avulsed from the bone and retracts proximal to the adductor aponeurosis **(C)**. When the joint is reduced, the adductor is interposed between the ligament and bone **(D)**, preventing healing.

the abductor aponeurosis is broad, covering a larger percentage of the joint and there is no interposition of the aponeurosis between the ligament and the bone (Stener lesion). Tear of the RCL typically results from forced adduction on a flexed joint. The dorsal capsule tears along the radial aspect and the proximal phalanx pronates around the intact UCL, creating a prominence of the radial aspect of the metacarpal head. The location of the tear is more variable than the UCL counterpart, with equal frequency between proximal and distal avulsions[48] and mid-substance tears.[64]

Surgical repair of an acute UCL tear

The procedure is performed under regional or general procedure with a tourniquet. The skin incision is outlined in a straight or lazy "S" configuration from the ulnar base of

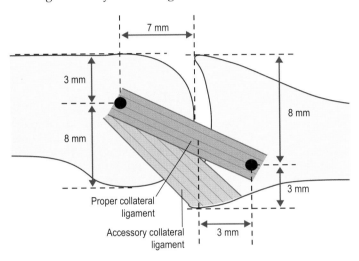

Fig. 7.20 Location of thumb MCP joint UCL on metacarpal and proximal phalanx. The ligament runs from dorsal to volar in a proximal to distal direction. The origin of the proper collateral ligament is 7 mm proximal to the joint and 3 mm from the dorsal cortex. The insertion of the base of the proximal phalanx is located 3 mm distal to the joint and 3 mm from the volar cortex.

the proximal phalanx to the dorsal aspect of the metacarpal head/neck region *(Fig. 7.21)*. After the skin incision is completed, spreading to the level of the adductor aponeurosis is carefully performed. Care should be taken to identify the cutaneous branch of the radial nerve, as injury to this structure can cause a painful neuroma, compromising the final outcome. When a Stener lesion is present, the ligament will be identified proximal to the adductor aponeurosis. The adductor aponeurosis is incised, splitting the fibers until the base of the proximal phalanx can be identified. The ligament is debrided of hematoma and fibrous tissue in preparation for repair. The joint can be opened and irrigated to remove hematoma and the site of repair is identified. When a larger fragment of bone is present, this can be replaced and secured with a screw or K-wires. When the fragment is small, it can be excised and the ligament repaired to the site of avulsion. A suture anchor is placed at the site of avulsion and the ligament is securely reattached to the bone. The adductor aponeurosis is repaired and the skin is closed. If there is a concern about the stability of the repair, a K-wire can be placed across the joint, but this is generally not necessary.

A plaster thumb spica splint is applied, leaving the IP joint free and converted to a short arm cast at 1 week. Motion of the IP joint is encouraged to prevent adhesions of the extensor tendons. At 4 weeks, the cast is removed and a therapy program is instituted to regain motion. A thermoplastic splint is used between exercises and initial motion is directed at restoring flexion and extension with avoidance of radial directed stress. Pinch strengthening is begun at 10 weeks and unrestricted activities are allowed at 12 weeks. Final motion is typically 80% of the noninjured side with grip and pinch strength approximately 90% of the contralateral side.

Reconstruction of chronic UCL tear with tendon graft

This creates a static restraint to radial directed stress and although not the same as the ligament prior to the injury, can

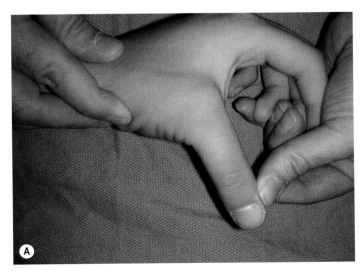

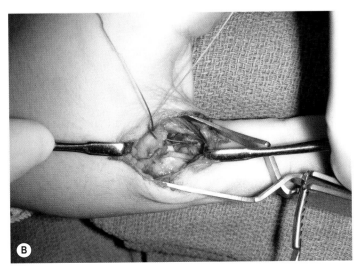

Fig. 7.21 Surgical repair of thumb MCP joint UCL. **(A)** Preoperative clinical photograph illustrating laxity at MCP joint. **(B)** Intraoperative photograph illustrating suture anchor in base of proximal phalanx with suture through the UCL.

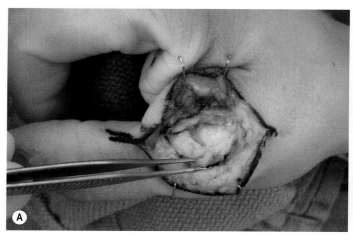
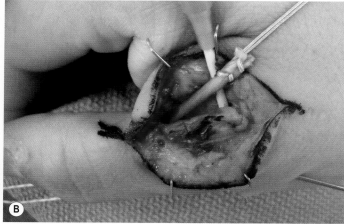

Fig. 7.22 Technique of thumb MCP joint UCL reconstruction with palmaris longus tendon graft. **(A)** intraoperative exposure of the joint following resection of scar and remnants of UCL. **(B)** Tendon graft secured to the proximal phalanx in preparation for securing to metacarpal.

provide a stable thumb MCP joint. The approach to the joint is the same as for acute repairs. After exposing the joint, the remaining collateral ligament is excised. The site of origin and insertion of the graft is identified *(Fig. 7.22)*. A tendon graft is harvested using palmaris longus when present or a strip of FCR in the event the palmaris longus is not present. The graft can be attached either through drill holes or with tenodesis screws (alternatively, the collateral ligament can be left attached to the metacarpal and the graft secured to the native ligament). Two holes are created in the metacarpal head just dorsal to the dorsal volar axis, approximately 8 mm from the joint surface. A bone bridge is left between the two holes and the tendon is placed. The holes must be large enough to allow passage of the tendon and the bone bridge must be of adequate thickness so it does not break following passage of the graft. One hole is created on the base of the proximal phalanx approximately 3 mm from the volar cortex and 3 mm distal to the joint. A suture is placed through each end of the tendon and the graft is pulled through the metacarpal head. Two free Keith needles are placed through the hole in the proximal phalanx, exiting the radial aspect of the base of the proximal phalanx through different sites. The two strands of the tendon are placed in the needle and pulled through bone on the radial side, securing the tendon into the bone. The joint is pinned in slight flexion and ulnar deviation. The sutures are pulled to tighten the tendon graft and the sutures are tied over a button or directly over the bone.

Alternatively, one drill hole can be placed in the metacarpal head and one in the proximal phalanx. The tendon graft can be secured with a biotenodesis screw, anchoring the graft into the bone. The adductor aponeurosis and skin incisions are closed and a thumb spica splint is applied. Postoperative rehabilitation is similar to acute repairs except the joint is immobilized for 6 weeks and pinching is avoided for 3 months. Unrestricted activities are allowed at 4–5 months. Motion tends to be less following reconstructions than acute repairs, but 70% of the flexion extension and 80% grip and pinch strength can often be obtained. The goal of the reconstruction is to produce a stable painless thumb and the slight loss of motion is compensated for at the CMC joint.

Thumb metacarpal fractures

Fractures of the thumb metacarpal are more tolerant of displacement and rotation due to the motion in three planes (flexion/extension, abduction/adduction, pronation/supination). Fractures can occur through the shaft or the base at the metaphyseal-diaphyseal junction. Angulation <20° can be tolerated, but greater than this may result in compensatory MCP joint hyperextension, compromising the function of the thumb. The distal fragment tends to supinate, so closed reduction is performed by applying longitudinal traction, downward pressure of the apex of the thumb, and pronation and extension of the distal fragment. K-wires can be used to stabilize the fracture or alternatively, plates and screws.

Thumb CMC joint injuries

The anatomy of the thumb CMC joint resembles two interlocking saddles (thumb metacarpal and trapezium), which allow motion parallel (abduction and adduction) and perpendicular (pronation and supination). Joint stability is maintained through multiple ligaments, with the anterior oblique, posterior oblique, anterior and posterior intermetacarpal and dorsal radial ligaments being the major stabilizers.[65] Compressive forces are 12 times greater at the CMC joint than the tip of the thumb, so arthritis may develop if incongruence is present at the CMC joint.[66,67]

Isolated dislocations occur much less frequently than CMC fracture dislocations (Bennett and Rolando fractures). When pure dislocations occur, they are dorsal and result from an axial compression of a flexed thumb. There are 16 ligaments which stabilize the thumb CMC joint, with some considered major and other considered minor stabilizers. Although there is disagreement about which structures are torn to allow dislocation, it is likely the anterior oblique (volar beak ligament) and the dorsal radial ligament are disrupted to allow dorsal dislocation of the metacarpal. Partial ligament tears may result in subluxation and may be treated with reduction and immobilization, typically with K-wires. Complete ligament tears result in dorsal dislocation and are unstable. Because these injuries are rare, most reports in the literature are case reports or small series.[68,69] For acute and chronic dislocations, ligament reconstruction with a portion of the FCR, as described by Eaton and Littler[70,71] should provide reasonable results.

Fracture dislocations are much more common. The *Bennett fracture* is a fracture subluxation, which occurs when a flexed metacarpal receives an axial load *(Fig. 7.23)*.[72] The Bennett fragment is maintained due to the attachment of the anterior oblique ligament, while the remainder of the metacarpal subluxes radially, dorsally, and proximally, due to the APL and adductor pollicis muscles. The goals of treatment of this injury are to restore stability to the joint by allowing the displaced

metacarpal to heal to the Bennett fragment and restoration of articular congruity to the base of the thumb. Bennett fractures can be treated with closed reduction and pinning. Indications for ORIF include inability to reduce the fracture by closed means. Some surgeons advocate ORIF when the Bennett fragment involves a significant amount of the joint.[73]

The reduction is performed with longitudinal traction on the thumb, pressure at the metacarpal base, and pronation. It is not necessary to secure the Bennett fragment as long as alignment is maintained and K-wires can be placed in a variety of configurations, most commonly, either through the metacarpal base and into the trapezium or trapezoid, or through the thumb metacarpal and into the index metacarpal. The hand is immobilized in a thumb spica cast, with the

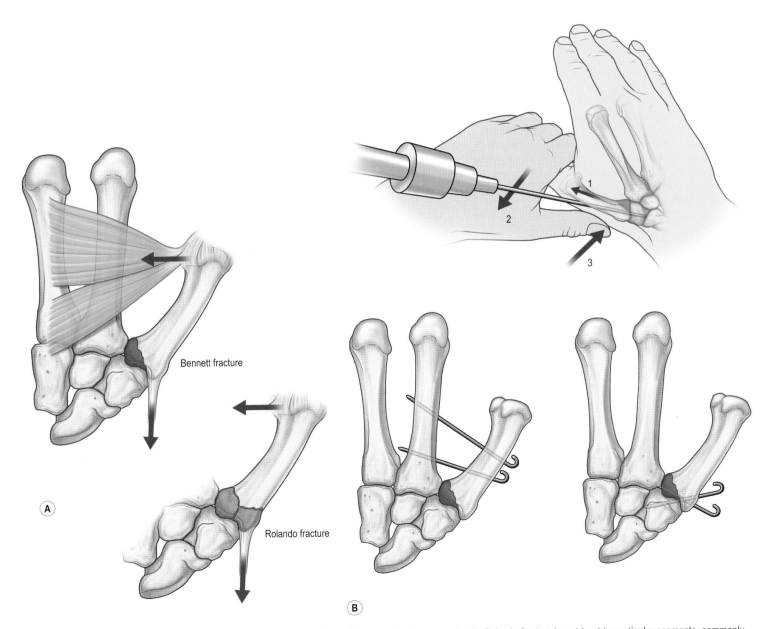

Fig. 7.23 (A) Comparison of Bennett and Rolando fracture (Bennett fracture has one articular segment while Rolando fracture has at least two articular segments, commonly in "Y" or "T" configuration. **(B)** Reduction (distraction, pronation, and dorsal pressure) and pinning of thumb CMC fracture dislocation (Bennett fracture and Rolando fracture).

fingers and IP joint of the thumb free, for 4–5 weeks, followed by protective splinting for an additional 4 weeks.

When ORIF is performed, a Wagner incision is used at the junction of the glabrous and nonglabrous of the skin, extending from the mid-metacarpal to the region of the FCR tendon. The thenar muscles are reflected subperiosteally, and the capsule is incised to expose the joint. Hematoma and is removed from the joint, the fracture is reduced and stabilized with small screws or K-wires. If screw fixation is used, a removable splint and motion can be initiated at one week.

The *Rolando fracture*, as originally described, is a metacarpal base fracture with a "T" or "Y" shaped intra-articular pattern.[74] Currently, the term is used to describe any comminuted intra-articular fracture of the base of the thumb metacarpal. The treatment goals are the same as for the Bennett fracture, but may be more difficult to obtain, as the comminution often makes it difficult to align the articular surface. The true Rolando fracture can be treated with closed reduction, using the same technique as for the Bennett fracture. Stabilization can be completed with K-wires or small screws. Comminuted fractures are more difficult to treat and open reduction can lead to devascularization of the small fracture segments. Bone grafting can be used if there is extensive comminution or a void in the metaphysis, to assist with healing. Stabilization is best accomplished with K-wires from the thumb to index metacarpal or an external fixator. Various designs have been described, including stabilization to the trapezium, or multiple rods securing the thumb to the index metacarpal[75] or in a triangular configuration, securing the thumb and index metacarpals to the radius.[76]

Pediatric fractures

Classification of pediatric fractures has been described in Figure 7.2, Salter–Harris classification of fractures, but fractures of the distal phalanx and the proximal phalanx head deserve special mention. Generally, pediatric fractures are stabilized with smooth K-wires. Effort should be made to minimize the number of passes through the physis and remanipulation of the fracture.

The Seymour fracture is a fracture involving the epiphyseal region of the distal phalanx *(Fig. 7.24)*. This injury appears as an open mallet fracture, with extension of the proximal segment with the attachment of the extensor tendon and flexion of the distal fragment with the FDP attached. There is a transverse laceration of the nail matrix the nail plate superficial to the proximal eponychial fold. The nail matrix can become interposed in the physis. Treatment is irrigation and debridement with reduction of the fracture and repair of the nail matrix. The nail plate is used as a stent on the proximal nail fold to help maintain reduction. A splint of longitudinal K-wire is used to maintain the reduction.[77–79]

Proximal phalanx neck fractures

Fractures of the proximal phalanx neck and occasionally the middle phalanx neck are common in children and result from withdrawal of a finger when caught in a door. These are visualized on a lateral X-ray and are classified according to the amount of displacement *(Fig. 7.25)*.[80–82] The distal fragment can rotate 90°, so the head is directed dorsally and the fracture

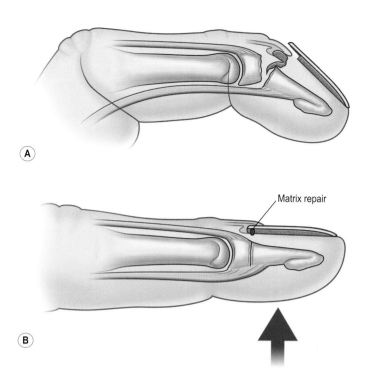

Fig. 7.24 (A) Seymour fracture with nail bed interposed into physis and nail plate dorsal to eponychial fold and **(B)** following repair of nail matrix.

surface is volar. These should be reduced anatomically and stabilized with K-wires. If alignment is not restored, a bony block may occur in the retrocondylar fossa resulting in decreased flexion. If this occurs, an ostectomy of the volar spike can be performed to remove the bony block and restore flexion.

Complications

Many patients with phalangeal fractures have some residual stiffness following treatment. This is not a complication, but a result of the need for tendons to glide along all sides of the proximal and middle phalanx and the adhesions that form between the bone and the tendon.[31]

True complications include infection, loosening of K-wires, malunion, nonunion and compartment syndrome. Infections should be managed with antibiotics. If K-wires have been used, a course of antibiotics will often allow enough healing prior to removal of the implant that the fracture is stable.[83] Malunions can be extra-articular or intra-articular and can occur in any bone in the hand and may cause cosmetic or functional problems. Angular and rotational malunions often cause dysfunction, which must be corrected. Nonunions are uncommon and typically occur with infection, significant bone loss or associated severe soft tissue injuries. They can be atrophic of hypertrophic and are managed with resolution of the infection, providing a stable soft tissue environment and reconstruction with stable fixation and in some instances, bone grafting (atrophic nonunions).

Compartment syndromes are not common in the hand, but may occur with crush injuries. Significant pain following a

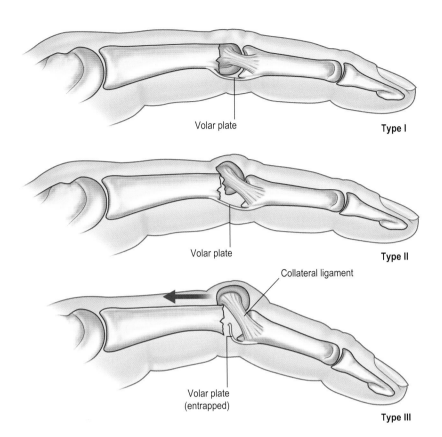

Volar plate

Type I

Volar plate

Type II

Collateral ligament

Volar plate
(entrapped)

Type III

Fig. 7.25 Pediatric proximal phalanx neck fractures. Type I is a stable, nondisplaced fracture. Type II is a fracture with dorsal displacement of the condyles, but contact between the bony surfaces. Type III fractures are defined by dorsal displacement of the condyles with rotation of 90°, so the fracture surface os perpendicular to the dorsal aspect of the proximal phalanx.

crush injury to the hand, which is exacerbated by passive stretching of the digit, should raise the suspicion for compartment syndrome. In the unresponsive patient with significant swelling, compartment pressures can be measured. Pressures >30 mmHg or within 30 mm of diastolic pressure should be treated with urgent fasciotomies, thereby releasing the interosseous, thenar, hypothenar, adductor pollicis and transverse carpal ligament.

Secondary procedures

Secondary procedures can be performed to correct a problem, such as malunion or nonunion or in attempt to improve motion for stiff digits. All wounds should be healed and soft tissues supple before secondary procedures are performed.

Malunion correction

Malunion typically occurs as angular or rotational deformities. Correction of an angular malunion involves an opening or closing wedge osteotomy with internal fixation.[84] Closing wedge osteotomies are easier to perform and are stable, while opening wedge osteotomies often require bone graft. These are best treated at the site of the malunion. Rotational malunions are treated with derotational osteotomies. These can be performed as transverse[85,86] or step cut osteotomies[87–89] and rigid fixation is used to provide stability and early motion *(Fig. 7.26)*. Intraarticular malunions can be corrected with an intra-articular[90] *(Fig. 7.27)* or extra-articular[91] osteotomy. ⊛ FIGS 7.26, 7.27 APPEARS ONLINE ONLY

Nonunion correction

Nonunions are rare in the hand, but can be managed by following principles of nonunion reconstruction in long bones.[92] Any underlying infection should be treated and a good soft tissue envelope should be present prior to reconstruction. Hypertrophic nonunions demonstrate bone formation around the fracture without bridging bone at the nonunion site. These will typically heal if stability and compression are provided at the nonunion site. Atrophic nonunions require bone grafting in addition to internal fixation. Metabolic conditions, such as vitamin D deficiency should be evaluated with blood tests and corrected if necessary, as low vitamin D levels will prevent ossification.

Hardware removal, tenolysis, capsulotomy

Patients with residual stiffness may benefit from secondary procedures to improve motion. When internal fixation with plates and screws has been used for initial treatment of the fracture, adhesions between the plate and the extensor tendons often occur. Removal of the hardware and extensor tenolysis will often improve flexion. Indications include a motivated patient who will be compliant with postoperative therapy program, complete osseous healing and supple soft tissues with passive motion that is greater than active motion. When joints become stiff, the results are much less predictable and outcomes not as good. Results following release of MCP extension contractures are better than PIP flexion or extension contractures.

Bonus content for this chapter can be found online at **http://www.expertconsult.com**

Fig. 7.9 (A) Preoperative and **(B)** postoperative radiographs of patient with middle phalanx base fracture treated with ORIF. **(C)** Clinical photograph in flexion following rehabilitation.

Fig. 7.10 Postoperative radiograph of cerclage wire (and K-wire) used to repair middle phalanx base articular fracture. Radiographically, the wires does not appear secure dorsally because this is secured around the articular cartilage (not seen on radiograph) and can not be placed further distally due to the central slip insertion.

Fig. 7.26 (A–C) Step cut osteotomy for correction of malunion. This can be used in the metacarpal or phalanx. The distal transverse cut is in the direction of malrotation, so the dorsal surface closes as the malrotation is corrected.

Fig. 7.27 Technique for correction of intra-articular malunion of the proximal phalanx head with condylar advancement osteotomy. **(A)** A longitudinal osteotomy is created into the site of the intra-articular malunion, the condyle is advanced and rotated into proper

alignment and secured with screws, leaving the proximal shaft defect to heal secondarily. Clinical example **(B)** preoperative radiograph; **(C)** intraoperative photograph of articular malunion prior to osteotomy. **(D)** Intraoperative photograph following condylar advance osteotomy and fixation. Postoperative PA **(E)** and lateral **(F)** radiographs and clinical example in flexion **(G)**.

Access the complete references list online at **http://www.expertconsult.com**

7. Leinberry C. Mallet finger injuries. *J Hand Surg Am.* 2009;34(9):1715–1717.
   An evidence based review, discussing the literature of operative and nonoperative (splinting) for the treatment of mallet finger injuries.

13. Kiefhaber TR, Stern PJ. Fracture dislocations of the proximal interphalangeal joint. *J Hand Surg Am.* 1998;23(3):368–380.
    This article provides excellent overview of the diagnosis of injuries of the base of the middle phalanx and indications for operative treatment. This article was written prior to hemi-hamate arthroplasty, so this technique is not covered.

20. Williams RM, Kiefhaber TR, Sommerkamp TG, et al. Treatment of unstable dorsal proximal interphalangeal fracture/dislocations using a hemi-hamate autograft. *J Hand Surg Am.* 2003;28(5):856–865.

21. Badia A, Riano F, Ravikoff J, et al. Dynamic intradigital external fixation for proximal interphalangeal joint fracture dislocations. *J Hand Surg Am.* 2005;30(1): 154–160.

31. Page SM, Stern PJ. Complications and range of motion following plate fixation of metacarpal and phalangeal fractures. *J Hand Surg Am.* 1998;23(5):827–832.
    This paper illustrates the challenges associated with plate and screw fixation of fractures in the hand and although often necessary due to open fractures and other conditions, complications, including stiffness, plate prominence, infection and tendon rupture can occur.

56. Heyman P. Injuries to the ulnar collateral ligament of the thumb metacarpophalangeal joint. *J Am Acad Orthop Surg.* 1997;5(4):224–229.

63. Bean CH, Tencer AF, Trumble TE. The effect of thumb metacarpophalangeal ulnar collateral ligament attachment site on joint range of motion: an in vitro study. *J Hand Surg Am.* 1999;24(2):283–287.
    This paper is an excellent study reviewing the precise anatomical location to optimize motion and function following repair/reconstruction of the MCP joint UCL.

77. Al-Qattan MM. Extra-articular transverse fractures of the base of the distal phalanx (Seymour's fracture) in children and adults. *J Hand Surg Br.* 2001;26(3): 201–206.

83. Botte MJ, Davis JL, Rose BA, et al. Complications of smooth pin fixation of fractures and dislocations in the hand and wrist. *Clin Orthop Relat Res.* 1992;(276): 194–201.

84. Freeland AE, Lindley SG. Malunions of the finger metacarpals and phalanges. *Hand Clin.* 2006;22(3): 341–355.
    This paper provides an algorithm for managing malunions in the hand, including the various different osteotomies and concomitant procedures, such as tenolysis and capsulotomy, to improve motion.

90. Teoh LC, Yong FC, Chong KC. Condylar advancement osteotomy for correcting condylar malunion of the finger. *J Hand Surg Br.* 2002;27(1):31–35.

8

Fractures and dislocations of the wrist and distal radius

Kevin C. Chung and Steven C. Haase

SYNOPSIS

- The treatment of scaphoid fractures requires an understanding of the vascular anatomy and judicious treatment based on the fracture pattern in order to assure proper healing.
- The dissociation of the scaphoid and lunate bones breaks the link in the proximal carpal row, causing a predictable pattern of carpal bone misalignment that has major consequences for the management of acute and chronic conditions.
- The dislocation of carpal bones requires a keen eye to determine the instability pattern on wrist radiographs. This is necessary in order to diagnose and treat injury patterns associated with this condition.
- Understanding the treatment of wrist injuries requires the appreciation of carpal bone alignment seen in the AP, oblique, and lateral X-ray views. Subtleties that may provide clues for ligament disruption may not always be easy to discern on the radiograph.
- The treatment of distal radius fractures (DRFs) challenges the surgeon to apply appropriate fixation techniques to not only restore normal radius anatomy, but also to recreate the normal architecture between the radius and the carpal bones, as well as between the radius and the ulna.
- The treatment of DRFs now emphasizes more aggressive surgical treatment in order to restore the anatomy and promote early functional use of the hand.
- Fractures and dislocations of the wrist and distal radius consist of a fascinating array of injury patterns and kinematic complexities that challenge even the most seasoned physician.

Introduction

The wrist is a complex articulation that connects the hand to the forearm. Entire textbooks have been devoted to detailed discussions of the anatomy, physiology, and pathology of this important joint. This chapter will review some of the more common injury patterns seen in the wrist, including fractures of the carpal bones, ligamentous injuries of the wrist, and fractures of the distal radius and ulna.

The epidemiology of wrist fractures has been investigated in detail. Nearly 1.5 million hand and wrist fractures are estimated to occur in the United States, annually.[1] These account for 1.5% of all emergency department visits. Of these, approximately 208 000 are carpal fractures. The scaphoid bone is the carpal bone most commonly fractured; it accounts for 60–85% of carpal fractures.[2] Incidence estimates range from 4.3/10 000 person-years in Norway[3] to 12.1/10 000 person-years in the US military population.[4] The highest incidence is found in the 20–24-year-old age group.[4]

Distal radius fractures are the most common upper extremity fracture; the annual incidence is estimated at 643 000 fractures per year in the United States.[1] When the incidence is examined by age, there are two distinct peaks identified *(Fig. 8.1)*. The greatest "spike" on the chart is in the 5–14-year-old group (55.7/10 000 person-years), and there is an additional peak in the elderly 75–84-year-old group (35.2/10 000 person-years).

Although a common injury, these fractures should never be treated casually. There is significant potential for patient disability if these injuries are not managed with great care and expertise. Khan and Giddins' review of hand and wrist surgery negligence claims in the UK from 1995–2001 revealed that wrist fracture was the most common condition in which negligence was alleged, comprising 48% of claims.[5]

History

The carpal bones are named for their shapes. For example, the scaphoid resembles a boat, whereas the lunate resembles the crescent moon. However, these bones were not described until the 1500s, when Andreas Vesalius first identified the eight carpal bones. Before then, drawings of the hand connected the metacarpals directly to the distal radius, with no mention of wrist anatomy. The names of the carpal bones were not solidified until 1955 when *Nomina Anatomica* established the official

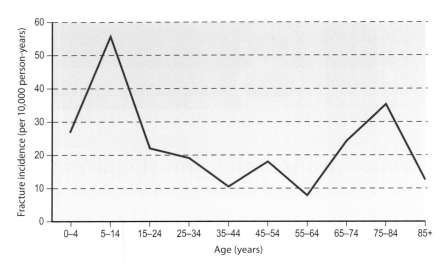

Fig. 8.1 Age-related variation in radius/ulna fracture incidence. (Data from Chung KC, Spilson SV. The frequency and epidemiology of hand and forearm fractures in the United States. J Hand Surg (Am) 2001; 26(5):908–915.)

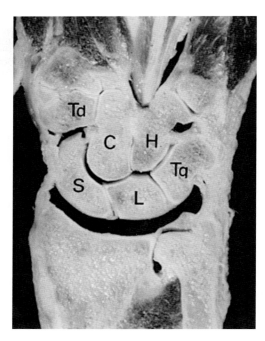

Fig. 8.2 Coronal slice of the carpal bones of the wrist: S, scaphoid; L, lunate; Tq, triquetrum; Td, trapezoid; C, capitate; H, hamate (trapezium and pisiform are not in view).

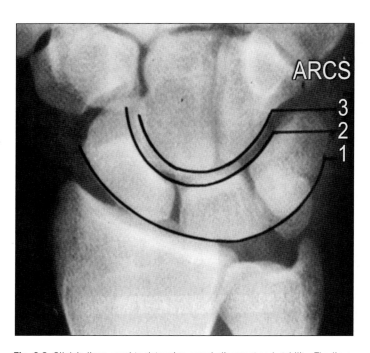

Fig. 8.3 Gilula's lines, used to determine carpal alignment and stability. The lines are defined by (1) the proximal and (2) the distal articular surface of the proximal row of carpal bones, as well as (3) the proximal articular surface of the distal row of carpal bones.

nomenclature for the carpal bones that we use today *(Fig. 8.2)*.[6] Perhaps more useful than nomenclature are the many classification systems that were used to organize the wrist anatomy into discreet packages. The earliest classification separates the wrist joint into two rows, consisting of the distal carpal row and the proximal carpal row. The carpal anatomy is not only distinguishable by rows, but also separated by columnar divisions. Particularly important is the alignment of the carpal bones. Gilula's lines – the arcs formed by (1) the proximal and (2) the distal articular surface of the proximal row of carpal bones, as well as (3) the proximal articular surface of the distal row of carpal bones – are used to determine carpal alignment *(Fig. 8.3)*. Increased joint space or deviation of carpal bones from these lines is indicative of wrist

instability.[7] It is important to note that because of the complex arrangement of the eight bones in the wrist, the pisiform is sometimes considered a sesamoid that is not part of the carpal bones in some classification systems.

The treatment of DRFs is privy to a fascinating 200-year experience. As is often paraphrased from Colles (the Irish surgeon who recognized the common patterns of extra-articular DRFs in the elderly without the assistance of X-rays), even patients treated with simple external anatomic reduction, "have all recovered without the smallest defect or deformity of the limb."[8] Though there is some truth to this 200-year-old statement, the expectations for recovery at that time were quite low because the technology to restore anatomic reduction was unavailable. Nevertheless, it is still often assumed that elderly patients with DRFs will have no functional limitations even with severe malalignments of the distal radius. However in recent years it has been recognized that restoration of the anatomic alignment of the distal radius is *more likely* to achieve better outcomes than less precise anatomic reduction methods. The improvement in internal fixation techniques has been heavily promoted by AO (Arbeitsgemeinschaft fur Osteosynthesefragen or Association for the Study of Internal Fixation, a Swiss organization started in the late 1950s for promoting rigid internal fixation techniques for fractures). These treatment options include the use of K-wires, external fixation, and more recently, a variety of implant technologies that are either placed dorsally or volarly on the radius for even more elegant fragment-specific fixations, where small implants are used to capture fractured columns within the distal radius for assured anatomic reduction. The most important advancement in the treatment of DRFs is the use of volar locking plating techniques, for which low profile plates are placed over the volar distal radius in order to treat a variety of extra-articular and intra-articular fractures regardless of whether the fracture occurs volarly or dorsally.

The high prevalence of DRFs has promoted great interest in restoring earlier functional recovery. Fractures generally occur when an individual falls on the outstretched wrists during slip-and-fall injuries. The younger population experiences a different fracture pattern caused by high energy injuries from motor vehicle accidents or sports trauma, resulting in complex fractures that require a variety of treatment techniques.

Understanding the treatment of the wrist as well as the distal radius, also requires one to be familiar with a variety of eponyms. Although many textbooks discourage the use of eponyms, the eponyms for DRFs display a clear image of predictable injury patterns to convey precise information regarding the type of injury sustained. The major eponyms for distal radius fractures are: dorsal and volar Barton's fractures (a shearing type fracture involving the a volar or dorsal fragment of the articular surface) *(Fig. 8.4A)*; Chauffeur fractures (a fracture involving the radial styloid); Colles fractures (the most common fracture pattern in the elderly in which the fracture fragment is displaced dorsally) *(Fig. 8.4B)*; Galeazzi fractures (a mid-shaft radius fracture associated with distal radioulnar joint disruption) *(Fig. 8.4C)*; and Smith fractures (also called the reverse Colles in which the fracture fragment is displaced volarly). For some cases, these eponyms may help in selecting a treatment modality.[9]

Basic science/disease process

Anatomy

Normal anatomy of the wrist is covered in detail in Volume VI, Section 1, Chapter 1 of this textbook. However, there are a few points that merit emphasis in this chapter with regard to these injuries.

The vascularity of the scaphoid bone bears particular consideration. The scaphoid bone has a single dominant vascular pedicle that enters from the distal pole of the bone. Therefore, the proximal pole relies wholly on the intramedullary blood supply for survival. It is for this reason that proximal pole fractures typically take longer to heal, and have increased incidence of nonunion. Furthermore, in cases of nonunion,

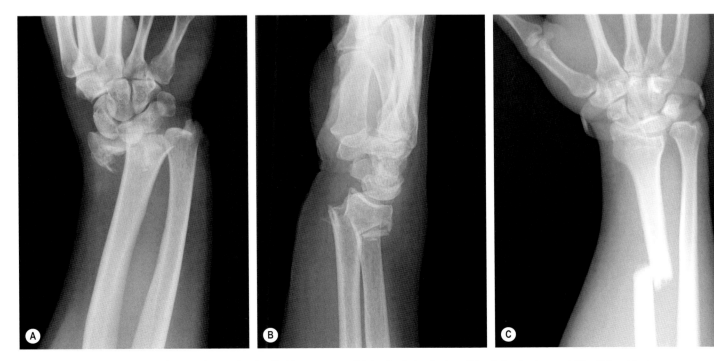

Fig. 8.4 Examples of distal radius fractures that can be classified into eponyms. **(A)** A volar Barton fracture, **(B)** a Colles fracture, and **(C)** a Galeazzi fracture.

the proximal pole is susceptible to avascular necrosis, which further complicates these injuries.[10,11]

The strength of the wrist ligaments helps determine the injury patterns observed. For example, the very strong short radiolunate ligament tends to resist lunate dislocation, retaining the lunate in its fossa on the distal radius in all but the most severe traumas. Instead, the surrounding carpal bones typically dislocate away from the lunate. This perilunate pattern of injury *(Fig. 8.5)* involves: (1) rupture of the scapholunate interosseous ligament; (2) capsular disruption through the space of Poirier, an area of inherent weakness of the volar capsule between the lunate and capitate, and (3) rupture of the lunotriquetral interosseous ligament. If the dislocated carpus rebounds, then the capitate will settle into the lunate fossa, and the lunate rotates volarly, hinged on the short radiolunate ligament.[12,13]

Likewise, the anatomy of the distal radius metaphysis has a direct influence on the types of fractures seen, and the treatment options that are available. Both the diaphysis and the articular surface have heavier cortical bone than is found at the metaphysis. The thinner cortical bone at the metaphysis is vulnerable to fracture, especially in the osteoporotic population. There is a distinct difference within the metaphysis, between the dorsal and volar cortices. The dorsal cortex is much thinner, resulting in extensive comminution in most cases of DRFs from falls on outstretched hands where the force is directed in a volar-to-dorsal direction.

The extensor pollicis longus (EPL) is the tendon most likely to rupture after a DRF. The etiology of this appears to be related to interruption of the tendon's nutritional supply, leading to attritional rupture. This most commonly occurs at

Lister tubercle where there is a natural watershed area of this tendon's intrinsic blood supply. If the extrinsic (diffusion-mediated) nutritional supply is also interrupted by fracture callus, fracture displacement, or swelling from edema or hematoma, rupture of the EPL can occur.[14]

Biomechanics

The biomechanics of the hand and wrist were reviewed in Volume VI, Section 1, Chapter 1, but there are a few points to revisit here.

Disruption of the normal linkages between the bones of the wrist – whether due to ligamentous rupture or fracture – can lead to carpal instability. The concept of carpal instability has evolved rapidly over the past 50 years, as we have learned more about the ways in which the wrist bones move (kinematics) and transfer a load (kinetics). In the modern era, instability has a very specific definition; a wrist is unstable if it is unable to transfer functional loads without sudden changes in stress on the articular cartilage and if it is unable to maintain motion throughout its range without sudden alterations of intercarpal alignment.[15]

Carpal instability has been thoughtfully classified into four major patterns *(Table 8.1)*. Carpal instability dissociative (CID) occurs when there is a disruption within or between the bones of the same carpal row. Carpal instability non-dissociative (CIND) refers to a disruption between the distal radius and the proximal carpal row, or between the proximal and distal carpal rows. When a combination of elements of both CID and CIND exist, it is referred to as carpal instability complex (CIC). Finally, when the instability is an adaptive response to a problem proximal or distal to the wrist itself, it is called carpal instability adaptive (CIA).[16]

Carpal kinematics has perhaps the biggest clinical impact on scaphoid fractures and scapholunate ligament injuries. The proximal carpal row is "pre-tensioned," with the scaphoid subject to a flexion moment, and the triquetrum tending to

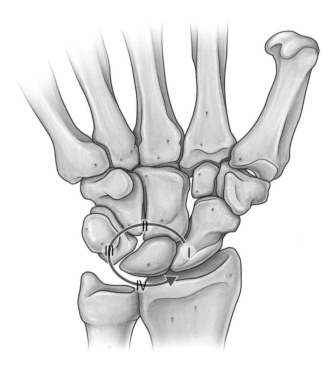

Fig. 8.5 Mayfield's stages of perilunate instability: (I) scapholunate ligament rupture; (II) volar capsule tear at the space of Poirer; (III) lunotriquetral ligament rupture; (IV) lunate dislocation.

Table 8.1 **Patterns of carpal instability**

Pattern	Definition	Example(s)
Carpal instability dissociative (CID)	Disruption within or between bones of the same carpal row	Scapholunate dissociation; Scaphoid nonunion
Carpal instability nondissociative (CIND)	Disruption at the radiocarpal or midcarpal joints, with intact proximal and distal rows	Midcarpal instability
Carpal instability complex (CIC)	Derangement both within and between carpal rows (CID plus CIND)	Perilunate dislocation with ulnar translation
Carpal instability adaptive (CIA)	Instability due to injury proximal or distal to wrist	Distal radius malunion

Source: Data from Gilula LA, Mann FA, Dobyns JH, et al. Wrist: terminology and definitions. J Bone Joint Surg Am 2002;84-A(Suppl 1):1–73.

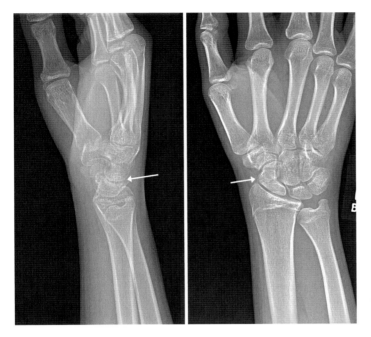

Fig. 8.6 Fracture at the waist of the scaphoid, resulting in a humpback deformity.

follow an extension moment. Any breakage of the connections within this row, whether intracarpal (e.g., scaphoid fracture) or intercarpal (e.g., scapholunate ligament rupture), will result in carpal instability because the disconnected carpal bones rotate in opposite directions. This natural tendency for the components in this row to fall away from each other is in part responsible for the high rate of complications after these types of injury.

Because of the scaphoid's natural tendency to flex when loaded, delayed treatment of comminuted fractures of the scaphoid waist tend to result in the so-called "humpback deformity" *(Fig. 8.6)*. This term describes the shape of the scaphoid as seen on lateral tomograms, reflecting malunion of the bone with an abnormally acute angle between the proximal and distal poles of the scaphoid.[17]

Mechanisms of injury

In elderly osteoporotic patients, wrist injuries are commonly seen after falls from a standing height. Very often, this is an extra-articular fracture with apex volar angulation, the so-called "Colles fracture." With increasing force of injury (e.g. falls from heights, motor vehicle collisions), the chance of associated carpal fracture, intercarpal ligament injury, or triangular fibrocartilage complex injury increases.

Diagnosis/patient presentation

History

A detailed history begins with careful documentation of the circumstances or mechanism of the injury. Patients involved in high-energy falls or collisions should be evaluated for associated injuries by an emergency medicine physician or trauma

specialist. The patient's handedness, occupation, important hobbies or recreational activities, medical and surgical history, and social history should be recorded. It is important to ask about numbness and/or tingling in the hand, because these patients are prone to acute carpal tunnel syndrome which may need to be addressed at the time of operation.

Physical examination

The examination of the patient's upper extremity should be thorough and systematic. Although the focus of this chapter is on the wrist, both the elbow and the hand should be included in the scope of examination, to avoid missing associated injuries. Examination begins with inspection. The signs of acute trauma should be noted: wounds, ecchymosis, bleeding, swelling, etc. Sub-acute or chronic changes may be more subtle and comparison to the patient's contralateral uninjured extremity can be helpful in detecting slight differences in swelling, alignment, and skin characteristics.

Palpation of the extremity can help localize the site of injury. The examining surgeon should be familiar with the topography of the wrist, and be able to identify injury to specific structures by careful, systematic palpation. For instance, focal tenderness just distal to the Lister tubercle could indicate injury to the scapholunate interosseous ligament, whereas pain with palpation of the floor of the anatomic snuffbox may signify a scaphoid waist fracture.

Before assessing the range of motion or performing any provocative testing, it is important to review the radiographs of the extremity to rule out any unstable fractures that might be displaced or otherwise worsened by vigorous physical examination. While assessing the patient's active and passive range of motion, palpation over the joints being moved can yield other useful information about crepitus, clicks, or clunks in the wrist. A complete examination should also include assessment of grip strength, pinch strength, and sensibility. It is particularly important to detect median neuropathy in wrist injury patients, because acute carpal tunnel syndrome may require treatment.[18] Provocative testing of specific intrinsic ligaments of the wrist can be valuable in reaching a diagnosis, but should be conducted with caution when unstable fractures are present to avoid unwanted fracture displacement.

The Watson scaphoid shift test stresses the scapholunate ligament to detect injury or instability *(Fig. 8.7)*. The examiner applies pressure (typically with the thumb) over the distal scaphoid tubercle, while moving the patient's wrist from ulnar to radial deviation.[19] In ulnar deviation the scaphoid is extended, whereas in radial deviation it is flexed. Thus, in the intact wrist, the scaphoid's ligamentous attachments resist subluxation during this maneuver. However, in cases of scapholunate dissociation, the scaphoid may be forced dorsally out of the scaphoid fossa into a painful position for the patient. Upon releasing pressure, a clunk may be heard indicating the self-reduction of the scaphoid back over the dorsal rim of the radius. A painful Watson test in the absence of an obvious clunk may be a sign of scapholunate ligament damage without complete disruption of the ligament.

The lunotriquetral interosseous ligament can be assessed by the Kleinman shear test *(Fig. 8.8)*. The examiner grasps

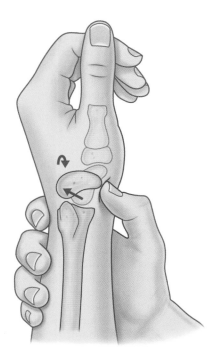

Fig. 8.7 Watson scaphoid shift test.

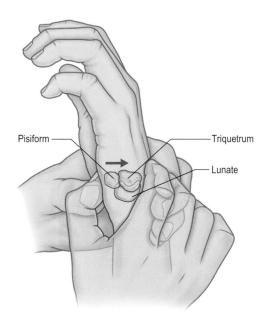

Pisiform — Triquetrum

Lunate

Fig. 8.8 Kleinman shear test.

the patient's wrist in one hand, specifically applying stabilizing pressure over the lunate, which is palpable dorsally just beneath the fourth extensor compartment tendons. With the other hand, the examiner applies dorsally directed pressure over the pisiform, which applies a shear force directed across the lunotriquetral articulation. Laxity can be assessed by further grasping the pisiform/triquetral unit and moving it both palmarly and dorsally in a

"shucking" type maneuver. This latter is referred to as the lunotriquetral ballottement test.[20] Pain and/or instability may indicate injury or disruption of the lunotriquetral ligament.

Diagnostic tests

At a minimum, assessment of wrist injuries should include four radiographs: posteroanterior (PA), oblique, lateral, and PA ulnar deviation. The ulnar deviation view is particularly important in detecting scaphoid injuries. Another helpful view for detecting dynamic instability of the scapholunate ligament is the clenched fist view. When making a tight fist, load is placed across the wrist, and the capitate is driven toward the scapholunate articulation, which will make scapholunate ligament laxity or rupture more evident. To increase the accuracy of the diagnosis, both anteroposterior (AP) and PA stress views should be considered.[21]

Cross-sectional imaging modalities, such as computed tomography (CT) and magnetic resonance imaging (MRI) are also used routinely to investigate wrist injuries. CT is an X-ray-based modality, and as such it is best for assessing complex fracture-dislocation patterns. CT is also better than MRI at determining osseous healing across a fracture site. On the other hand, MRI is the preferred modality for assessing nonosseous structures. MRI technology continues to evolve, and modern machines can detect even very small ligamentous injuries.[22] When the modalities of MRI and arthrography are combined, even small perforations in the interosseous ligaments can be detected.

The indiscriminate use of magnetic resonance imaging (MRI) when one suspects wrist injury is a growing concern. Because the MRI picks up a great amount of detail within the wrist, it is not uncommon to have falsely positive findings relating to potential ligamentous injuries within the wrist. Therefore, the treating physician should have high suspicion of a particular type of wrist injury before ordering an MRI to confirm. This will alleviate false positives and will prevent the unnecessary exposure of the patient to MRI testing. Similarly, when a patient presents with wrist pain that is of short duration without any known trauma, obtaining an MRI is usually not helpful because the likelihood of having a serious injury within the wrist is markedly diminished without an antecedent trauma. In these cases, the MRI may again find certain abnormalities that have no clinical correlation. The use of MRI should be to confirm a clinical suspicion of an occult injury within the wrist when the X-rays do not reveal a distinct pattern for wrist pathology, whereas wrist arthroscopy is done to determine the extent of the injury in order to plan surgical treatments when the options are predicated on the severity of ligament tear or articular cartilage loss. Therefore, the diagnosis of wrist injuries depend on careful history taking, physical examination, and X-rays, followed by confirmation by either MRIs or wrist arthroscopy.

The bones of the wrist are linked by a complex system of intrinsic and extrinsic ligaments *(Fig. 8.9)*. The type of injury sustained in patients presenting with wrist pain may be discerned by soliciting a well defined history. For example, a patient who works with heavy machinery who received a torque-type injury several months ago and continues to have

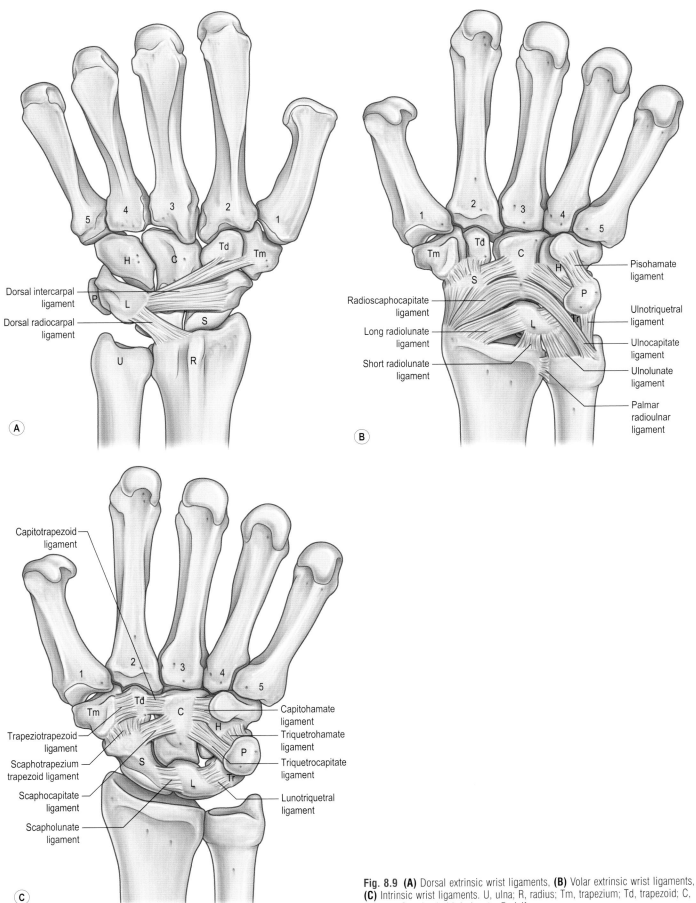

Fig. 8.9 (A) Dorsal extrinsic wrist ligaments, **(B)** Volar extrinsic wrist ligaments, **(C)** Intrinsic wrist ligaments. U, ulna; R, radius; Tm, trapezium; Td, trapezoid; C, capitate; S, schaphoid; L, lunate; P, pisiform.

wrist pain most likely sustained some type of ligamentous injury to the wrist. An X-ray should be able to determine if this ligamentous injury is between the carpal bones, and if it is typical of a dorsal intercalated segment instability (DISI) or volar intercalated segment instability (VISI) deformity *(Fig. 8.10)*. Generally, these injuries are caused by rupture of either the scapholunate or lunotriquetral ligaments. When the X-rays are confirmatory for carpal injuries, the next step is to perform a wrist arthroscopy in order to determine the extent of the injury, whether the injury is treatable, and by what method the injury can be treated after careful consultation with a patient following the arthroscopic findings. Again, obtaining MRIs is quite irrelevant because the predominant confirmatory test is the wrist arthroscopy.

On the other hand, for patients presenting with a vague recollection of wrist injury and with normal carpal alignments as seen on wrist X-rays, physical examination may identify potential tender areas such as pain at the TFCC attachment to the fovea, or potential instability with stressing of the lunotriquetral interval. Only in these situations – when there is a potential inclination for a particular type of injury –

can MRIs be helpful in pinpointing the exact location of the injury. Even in these cases, it is important to note that the confirmatory test will often still be wrist arthroscopy. However, for patients with vague history and inconclusive X-rays, an MRI and arthrogram may detect occult ligamentous injuries. If the MRI of a young, <40 years of age patient is normal, then clinically significant wrist pathologies are eliminated. MRI has an added utility in identifying vascularity in the carpus. Common patterns of scaphoid nonunion particularly with the proximal pole avascular necrosis, or Kienböck's disease with decreased vascularity of the lunate, can be detected quite readily with MRI. Therefore for patients who present with changes in density of a nonunion proximal pole fracture of the scaphoid or sclerotic appearance of the lunate, an MRI can be helpful in defining avascular necrosis of the carpal bones, which needs to be treated with vascularized bone grafting to add more blood supply to these avascular areas.

The use of bone scans has decreased substantially over the years because of the effectiveness of MRIs. Nevertheless, bone scans are still helpful in identifying "hot areas" of the wrist

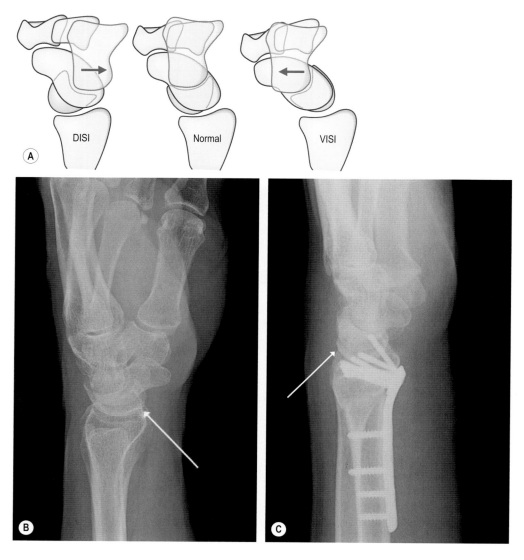

Fig. 8.10 (A) Lunate position in DISI and VISI deformities of the wrist. X-rays of **(B)** DISI and **(C)** VISI deformities.

in difficult cases when the etiology of the patient's wrist pain is uncertain. However, the nonspecific nature of the bone scan limits its usefulness in most settings.

Regarding treatment of DRFs, X-rays are generally sufficient to make a determination about surgical versus nonsurgical treatment. Changes in radial height (normal 12 mm), radial inclination (normal 23°), and volar tilt (average 11°) help define the extent of fracture displacement *(Fig. 8.11)*.[9,23] Additional studies such as CT scans to define the fracture anatomy are not necessary unless X-rays cannot determine the precise intra-articular component of the fracture. In certain situations, the fracture line may extend into the radiocarpal joint and there may be a depressed lunate articular surface that will require the use of CT scans to define the extent of this placement. In general, articular disruptions and incongruity in the distal radius articular surface of about 2 mm is an indication for surgical treatment to avoid potential arthritic changes in the future.

Patient selection

Determining whether a patient will benefit from surgical treatment of a wrist condition requires a great deal of experience in order to anticipate expected outcomes. Of course, situations such as displaced scaphoid fractures or obvious acute scapholunate dissociation (as seen on X-rays), will require surgical treatment to restore the proper anatomy. Hence, unless the patient is infirm or has severe co-morbid conditions that prevent surgical intervention, most cases of acute traumatic injuries such as displaced fractures or ligament tears will require surgical treatment.

Controversy resides around chronic conditions for which surgical treatment may not improve the patient's function. For example, for a patient presenting with incidental finding of scapholunate dissociation on radiographs but has a relatively asymptomatic wrist with minimal pain, scapholunate reconstruction may not be required. Surgical treatment to address scapholunate dissociation should be confined to patients with wrist pain because the outcomes of wrist reconstruction are often associated with decreased wrist motion and recurrence of the deformity. We often inform patients that a good operation for the wrist does not yet exist; therefore, wrist surgical procedures are recommended for intractable pain in chronic conditions or when acute injury is detected.

Patient selection for the treatment of DRFs in the elderly is another controversial area.[24] In the past, many physicians believed that the elderly had low functional demands and that most cases of DRF could be treated with simple casting. However, casting for displaced DRFs predictably results in malunion, especially in the elderly. In the United States, most of the older generation lives independently, and

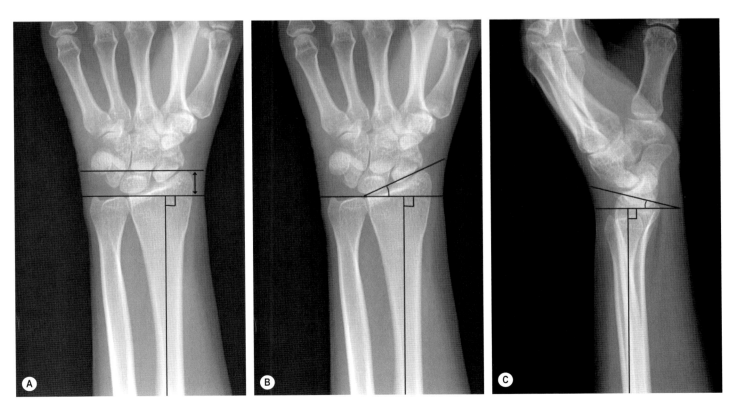

Fig. 8.11 **(A)** Radial height measured as the distance between two lines, the first line perpendicular to the longitudinal axis of the radius and intersecting the distal surface of the ulnar head, and the second line that passes through the distal tip of the radial styloid, **(B)** Radial inclination represented by the angle between the line perpendicular to the longitudinal axis of the radius and a second line connecting the ulnar aspect of the distal radius and the tip of the radial styloid, **(C)** Volar tilt is the angle between the line perpendicular to the longitudinal axis of the radius and a line along the distal articular surface of the radius.

restoration of anatomical alignment of the distal radius will allow them to use their hands much earlier following an injury. This is an important consideration for the elderly because they are much more active and not as infirmed as previous generations. The introduction of excellent fixation techniques including volar-locking plating systems allowed experienced hand surgeons to perform precise anatomic reductions of DRFs to let a patient start moving the wrist as early as within 1 week after injury.[25] The paradigm shift in treating these fractures has resulted in the continued increase in the utilization of internal fixation techniques in the United States. An assessment of Medicare data showed the use of internal fixation techniques increased five-fold, from 3% of fractures treated by internal fixation in 1996 to 16% in 2005.[24] The rate of internal fixation usage continues to grow, although close reduction and cast treatments are still the dominant form of treatment for the elderly in the United States (70% of fractures treated by casting in 2005).[24] It is anticipated that more elderly patients will undergo internal fixation for DRFs in the future, provided that they have no prohibitive risk factors to undergo surgery.

Treatment and surgical techniques

Scaphoid fractures

The scaphoid appears to be in the shape of a cashew nut, and can be divided into three segments: distal pole, waist, and proximal pole. As previously mentioned it has a unique blood supply, receiving the majority of its blood supply dorsally, and a small contribution from the volar side.[26] The blood supply enters from the distal pole of the scaphoid retrograde to the proximal pole. Therefore, any complete transverse fractures of the scaphoid interrupt this tenuous blood supply to the proximal fragment. For distal pole or tubercle type fractures, fracture healing should be rather rapid and unless the fracture is displaced by 1 mm or greater, distal pole fractures will heal with cast immobilization after 6–8 weeks. As the fracture progresses to the waist of the scaphoid, healing can be more difficult. Fractures through the waist can be transverse or oblique. It has been suggested that any fracture that completely traverses through the scaphoid at the waist level is unstable and requires operative fixation. However, this was challenged recently in a paper by Dias and colleagues, which shows comparable outcomes in nondisplaced waist-type fractures when treated with casting as compared to those treated with open reduction and internal fixation (ORIF) with screws.[27] An economic analysis comparing these two techniques based on the societal perspective indicates that for transverse complete fracture of the scaphoid, ORIF with the currently published low complication rate makes it an economically advantageous strategy.[28] ORIF of scaphoid fractures can be challenging because of the need to place a screw within the tight confines of the cashew-shaped scaphoid. Lack of experience leading to injudicious screw placement may result in complications such as distraction of the fracture site, penetration of the screw through the articular surface (as 80% of the scaphoid is covered in cartilage), or other unforeseen events associated with an open approach for the scaphoid. Recently, there is an interest regarding minimally invasive technique to place the screw into the scaphoid using fluoroscopy control with a small incision over the dorsal wrist. Because the placement of the screw is reliant only on fluoroscopy guidance, this lack of direct visualization may occasionally misguide the surgeon, which can result in penetration of the screw through the articular surface. Hence these minimally invasive techniques should only be performed by those who are highly familiar with this procedure.

For proximal scaphoid fractures, the risk of scaphoid nonunion is very high. For these cases (*Fig. 8.12A*), ORIF is preferred through the dorsal approach so that the proximal pole can be fixated rigidly to achieve union.[29] This is done by first locating and marking Lister tubercle, and making an incision that extends distally on the dorsal wrist, ulnar to the tubercle (*Fig. 8.12B*). The incision is made over the third compartment, which allows for the EPL tendon to be identified, and partially released from the third compartment, without completely opening up the third compartment. The wrist capsule is opened longitudinally to expose the wrist joint and to access the scaphoid and the SL joint. Next the wrist is flexed, and a K-wire is passed from the proximal pole of the scaphoid all the way through to the other end. X-rays from several different planes are taken to ensure that the wire is through the axis of the scaphoid. Once this is confirmed, a 0.035 wire is used to fixate the fracture by passing the wire more ulnarly away from the mid-axis of the scaphoid to provisionally fixate the fracture. Another K-wire from the cannulated screw set is passed parallel to the first, but down the mid-axis of the scaphoid to serve as a guide wire for placement of the cannulated screw (*Fig. 8.12C*). This second wire is driven into the trapezium to prevent the wire from coming out once the scaphoid is reamed. A cannulated reamer is guided over the central wire and a drill hole is made along the path of this wire. The reaming should be done by hand and a mini-c-arm is used to continuously check the correct path of the reamer. It is important to maintain the straight trajectory of the reamer to prevent breakage of the guide wire. The second wire prevents rotation of the scaphoid fragments while the screw hole is made. A measuring guide is used to measure the length of the screw (generally 22–24 mm for men; 18–20 mm for women). Note that the wire will overestimate the length of screw needed because the screw itself does not need to pass through the scaphoid entirely. Typically, a 2 mm shorter screw is used, e.g. if the measurement is 22, then a 20 mm screw is chosen. The guide wire should be initially placed just under the articular surface of the distal pole of the scaphoid. Once the measurement is done, the wire is advanced to purchase the trapezium so that the wire will remain in place during the reaming. The cannulated screw is driven in using the K-wire as a guide (*Fig. 8.12D*). The K-wires are then removed, and the incision closed (*Fig. 8.12E*).[29,30] The dorsal approach is preferred for a proximal pole fracture in order to utilize the trailing threads of the screw to purchase and engage the proximal pole for rigid fixation.

Conversely, if casting is used as a treatment for a proximal pole fracture, the patient needs to be immobilized in a thumb spica cast for as long as 6 months for a proximal pole fracture, which can be problematic for the active lifestyle of today.

Scaphoid nonunion

Patients who present with a scaphoid nonunion will require judicious selection of a treatment. It is uncertain what the

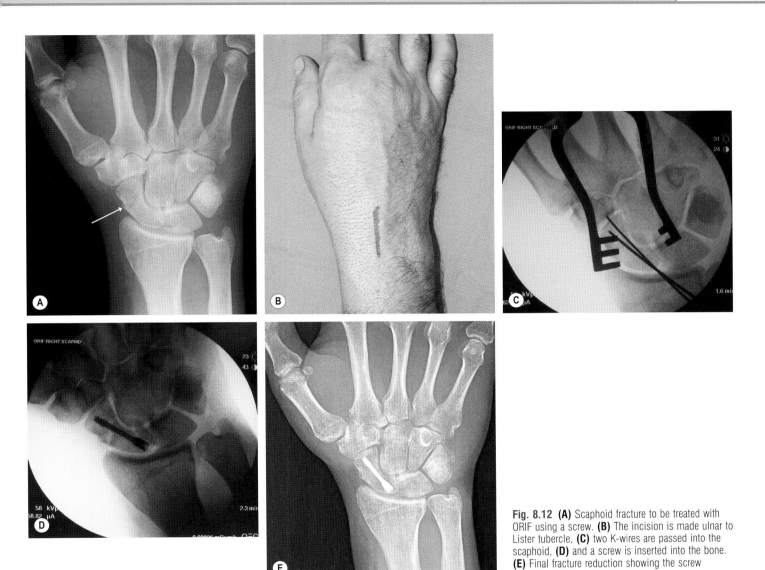

Fig. 8.12 (A) Scaphoid fracture to be treated with ORIF using a screw. **(B)** The incision is made ulnar to Lister tubercle, **(C)** two K-wires are passed into the scaphoid, **(D)** and a screw is inserted into the bone. **(E)** Final fracture reduction showing the screw placement.

natural history of scaphoid nonunion is because only those who are symptomatic are presented for evaluation. To comprehensively analyze this condition, a large cohort of patients with incidental findings of scaphoid nonunion are required to follow their clinical course over time. Unfortunately, many of these patients are asymptomatic and do not realize they have a nonunited scaphoid. In situations where a scaphoid nonunion is found, the patient needs to be counseled appropriately regarding the uncertain risk of developing radioscaphoid arthritis if the nonunion is left untreated. In most cases, patients are followed on a yearly basis to undergo sequential radiographs and to check symptoms in order to determine if wrist deterioration is progressing to a stage that will warrant surgical treatment. As long as the patient is asymptomatic, then the wait-and-see approach is appropriate.

Scaphoid nonunion is not an uncommon occurrence because scaphoid fractures can be missed upon initial examination. Many of those who suffer from a scaphoid nonunion are active young adults who are involved in athletic activities and their fracture is either misdiagnosed as a sprain, or not

diagnosed at all. In many of these situations, the scaphoid assumes a humpback deformity in which the fracture site collapses. This is a very difficult surgical challenge because the fracture must be opened and a structural graft from either the iliac crest or from the distal radius needs be inserted in order to restore the height of the scaphoid. If the malunion is at the waist of the scaphoid, then an osteotomy can be performed and a cortical bone graft can be harvested from the iliac crest to be inserted to fill the fracture site and restore the scaphoid into its typical cashew nut appearance. However, if the nonunion site is more proximal, there is great interest in performing a vascularized bone graft to increase the blood flow to the scaphoid. This bone graft can be taken from either the retrograde vascularized bone graft from the distal radius or a free bone graft from the medial femoral condyle **(Fig. 8.13)**.

Scapholunate ligament injury

Scapholunate (SL) ligament injury is a prevalent wrist injury pattern, given the great amount of stress placed between the

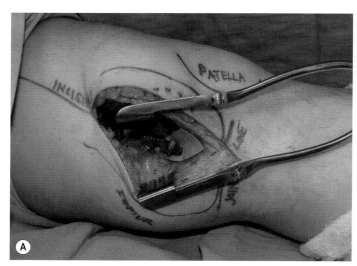
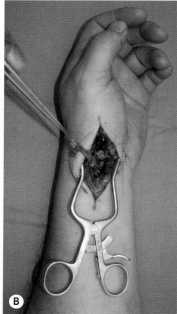
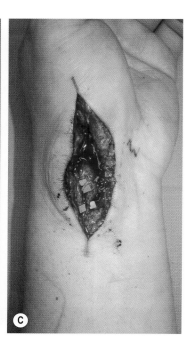

Fig. 8.13 The medial femoral condyle graft **(A)** is taken from the leg **(B)** and grafted into the wrist. **(C)** The increased vascularity will aid in repairing the scaphoid.

scaphoid and lunate during radial and ulnar deviation. Patients present with swelling and pain over the radial dorsal wrist centered between the 2nd and 3rd extensor compartments. In many of these partial acute tears, immobilization of the wrist for 3–4 weeks should allow the SL ligament to heal, with no additional treatment needed. However, for patients who have persistent pain despite 4–6 weeks of immobilization, additional studies may be required. For patients with suspected acute SL ligament tears, there may be widening of the SL interval *(Fig. 8.14)*, which in normal situations is about 2 mm in width. Although acute diastasis caused by a SL ligament tear is uncommon, its presence will certainly give a clear indication of this injury. In most cases, SL diastasis is indicative of a chronic tear in which gradual displacement between the scaphoid and lunate is evident after prolonged stress on the SL interval to result in increased separation of the interval. A more subtle finding is the so-called DISI deformity in which the lunate assumes a dorsally tilted posture and the scaphoid flexes volarly. The SL ligament is a restraint between the scaphoid and lunate, keeping them in a posture that has a 47° angle between the mid-axis of the scaphoid to the lunate *(Fig. 8.15)*. With dorsal tilting of the lunate and volar flexing of the scaphoid, this angle naturally increases and is an indication that the SL ligament is severed.

Treatment for acute SL ligament tear, if diagnosed early, is open repair of the ligament using suture anchors and pinning of the SL interval for 8 weeks to allow the ligament to heal. Generally there should be sufficient remnant ligament between the two bones to allow for the ligament to be repaired with the possible addition of bone anchor sutures. For patients with chronic tears, the treatment becomes much more complex. As the scaphoid assumes a flexed posture, it will impinge on the radial styloid. Constant motion may cause arthritic changes to develop between the scaphoid and the radial styloid that may propagate into the

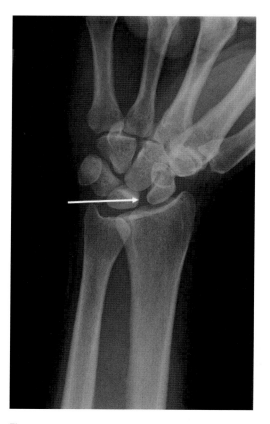

Fig. 8.14 A widened interval between the scaphoid and the lunate as a result of a SL ligament tear.

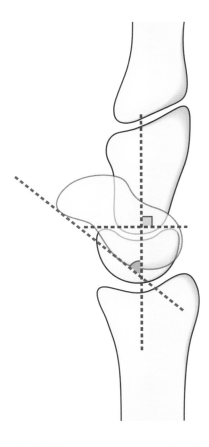

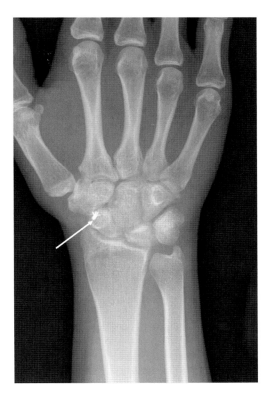

Fig. 8.16 A mini-bone anchor used to anchor the distal pole of the scaphoid to prevent its flexion, which can cause arthritis change at the radial styloid.

Fig. 8.15 The normal angle between the mid-axis of the scaphoid to the lunate is 47°. This angle is maintained by the SL ligament.

entire scaphoid fossa on the radius. In these situations, treatment will depend on the extent of the arthritic change. Arthroscopy is very helpful to determine whether arthritic change has occurred and to gauge the amount of SL diastasis. If there is no arthritic change between the scaphoid and lunate, then it is possible to perform soft tissue reconstruction, which comprises of a multitude of options. Our preference is to perform a dorsal capsulodesis procedure by inserting a mini-bone anchor into the distal pole of the scaphoid *(Fig. 8.16)* to anchor the distal pole to the dorsal wrist capsule, thereby preventing volar flexion of the distal pole of the scaphoid and prevent its impingement on the radial styloid. This procedure is performed if there are still some remnants of ligament left between the scaphoid and lunate. However, when there is no intact SL ligament left, then using a slip of the flexor carpi radialis (FCR) tendon to pass through a drill hole through the scaphoid and repairing it to the lunate can restore SL alignment and prevent abnormal motion between the two bones.[31]

For more advanced conditions, when arthritis has already occurred between the scaphoid and the radius, the scaphoid cannot be salvaged. In these situations, the options are either a proximal row carpectomy *(Fig. 8.17)* or a 4-bone fusion, also known as a 4-corner fusion *(Fig. 8.18)*. Proximal row carpectomy involves removing the scaphoid, lunate, and triquetrum, and then letting the capitate sit on the unaffected lunate fossa on the radius. A 4-bone fusion is done by removing the scaphoid and fusing the lunate, triquetrum, hamate, and

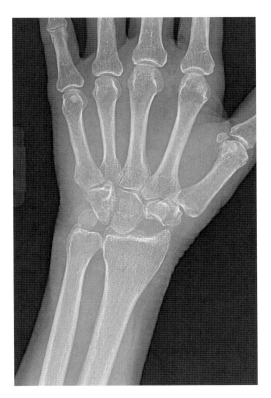

Fig. 8.17 Radiograph after proximal row carpectomy.

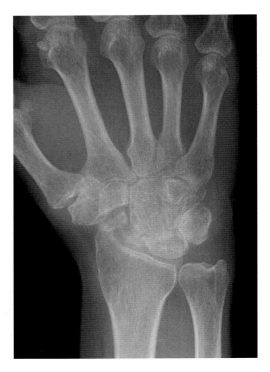

Fig. 8.18 Radiograph after scaphoid excision, 4-bone fusion.

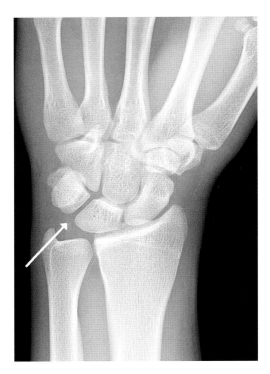

Fig. 8.19 Disruption of Gilula's first-line as a result of an LT ligament injury.

capitate to convert a complex linked joint into a simple joint. Long-term studies have shown the effectiveness of both options but a proximal row carpectomy is much easier to perform, although the articular geometry between the capitate and lunate fossa on the radius is not congruent and radiographic arthritis can occur over time. On the other hand, the 4-bone fusion is much more anatomic because the congruent lunate articular surface on the radius is preserved, but achieving fusion of the four bones can be problematic, and nonunion is certainly a complication that may require additional operative procedures.

Lunotriquetral ligament tear

Lunotriquetral (LT) ligament tears are more subtle than SL ligament tears. This is because unlike SL tears that can be identified by a gap between the scaphoid and lunate, an analogous gap between the lunate and triquetrum is not seen with LT ligament tears. Instead, what is seen in acute cases is a "step," or an unlevel line between the lunate and triquetrum as indicated by a disruption of Gilula's first-line, as seen on a standard PA view radiograph *(Fig. 8.19)*. However, most of these cases are found in chronic situations. The major hint of a potential injury in this area is a VISI deformity pattern in which the lunate tilts volarly. In these chronic situations, patients may go on to develop laxity or weakness of the secondary stabilizers of the LT joint in addition to LT instability. In turn, this may lead to a VISI deformity in which the lunate tilts volarly. Physical examination involves stressing the interval between the lunate and the triquetrum resulting in discomfort in this area. The treatment for the LT ligament is quite similar to that of the SL ligament tear, except that arthritic changes are not seen between the triquetrum and the radius. Patients often complain of a "click" or pain over the ulnar

wrist with this type of ligament injury. If this injury is picked up early, pinning of the LT interval may achieve healing of the ligament. Ligament repair is usually not practical because the ligament is extremely short, which prevents suture repair. Instead a slip of the extensor carpi ulnaris (ECU) tendon is used to pass between the triquetrum and the lunate to recreate the ligament between these two bones. Pins are used to hold this reconstruction in place for at least 8 weeks to achieve a healing of the tendon construct.

Perilunate dislocation

A frequently missed injury is perilunate dislocation *(Fig. 8.20)*. In cases of severe wrist trauma, the ligament injuries around the lunate progress from the radial to the ulnar side. When all of the attachments around the lunate are detached (including the volar radiolunate ligament), the lunate will prolapse into the carpal tunnel through the space of Poirier, which is a weak area in between the volar ligaments. Patients may present with acute carpal tunnel syndrome because of compression of the median nerve by the lunate in the carpal tunnel. The telltale indication is a spilled-cup sign seen on lateral X-rays views *(Fig. 8.21)*, in which the lunate is no longer sitting in its fossa under the capitate but rather is flipped volarly and sits within the carpal tunnel. This is an emergency because the lunate needs to be relocated to prevent its impingement of the median nerve. Reduction of the lunate in the emergency department can be tricky, but with adequate sedation and distraction, pressure can be placed over the volar lip of the lunate to push it under the capitate. However, if the lunate cannot be reduced in this manner, then operative reduction is necessary through both a dorsal and volar incision. The volar incision is similar to a carpal tunnel type incision that extends in a zigzag fashion to the distal wrist. The median nerve and

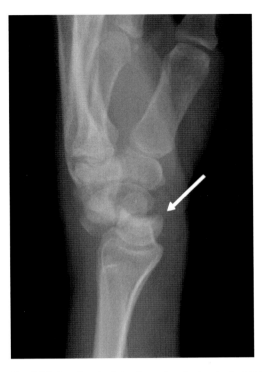

Fig. 8.20 A perilunate dislocation, when the lunate stays in its fossa, whereas the rest of the wrist subluxes dorsally.

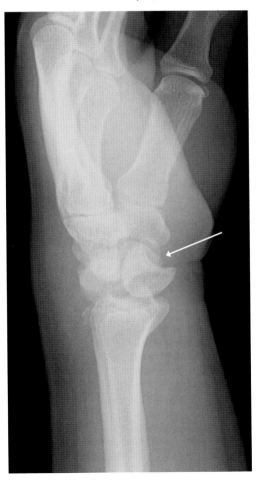

Fig. 8.21 The tell-tale spilled-cup sign, an indication of lunate dislocation.

the flexor tendons are retracted laterally, and the carpal tunnel is decompressed when the lunate is pushed through the opening in the volar wrist capsule to sit under the capitate. The volar capsule rent is closed using 3.0 horizontal mattress Ethibond sutures. A dorsal incision is then made between the third and fourth compartments to expose the wrist to repair the ligament between the scaphoid and the lunate. It is critical that the lunate be perfectly reduced in a neutral position, as confirmed by radiographs. To do this, the lunate is pinned to the scaphoid using a radial pin and to the triquetrum using an ulnar pin. Both pins are cut short under the skin to be removed in about approximately 8 weeks. We prefer to leave the pins under the skin so that the pins cannot be a source of infection, which can be catastrophic if pin-tract infections result in a septic wrist and cause irreparable damage to the wrist joint. The result of lunate reduction and pinning is quite good and interestingly, avascular necrosis is rarely seen after the lunate has been reduced anatomically despite almost complete devascularization of the lunate.

Distal radius fractures

Distal radius injuries are a key component of any hand surgery curriculum. DRFs are the most common fractures of the human skeleton, accounting for 15–20% of all fractures seen by physicians.[32–35] Approximately 80 000 DRFs are suffered by Medicare beneficiaries annually,[36] costing the US healthcare system an estimated US$632 million every year[37] and making DRFs the second most common fracture suffered by the elderly, after hip fractures.[38] As plastic surgery training programs continue to emphasize a comprehensive hand surgery curriculum, the treatment of DRFs is integral to having a rich experience in treating fractures around the wrist.

The essential anatomy of the distal radius can be gleaned from the standard radiograph. The main goal for the treatment of DRFs is to restore anatomic alignment. DRFs can be classified in several ways: displaced or nondisplaced, closed or open, and extra-articular or intra-articular. Open fractures of the distal radius are a surgical emergency because the fracture site needs to be adequately debrided to prevent contaminants from entering into the fracture site. Once the fracture site has been seeded with bacteria, fulminant infection and osteomyelitis are almost impossible to eradicate and will compromise eventual outcomes for these patients. However, other than open fractures, most of these fractures can be treated on an outpatient basis. The exception is closed fractures that are quite displaced and compress the median nerve to cause median nerve symptoms. These fractures typically should be reduced in the emergency department using traction devices to restore at least some alignment of the fracture and to minimize the fracture from impinging the median nerve within the carpal tunnel. If surgery will be delayed for more than a week, reduction of the bony component may prevent soft tissue contractures that will make subsequent reduction of fracture difficult. Our preference is to fix these fractures within a week of injury while the fracture fragments can still be easily manipulated and distracted to restore radial height. The treatments for DRF include closed reduction and casting, K-wire fixation, external fixation, a combination of K-wire fixation and external fixation, and internal fixation.

The introduction of volar-locking plating techniques has revolutionized the treatment of DRFs.[25] Historically, the dorsal approach was preferred to avoid the important neurovascular structures that are found volarly, which made dorsal plating safer and easier. Furthermore, because these fractures tended to displace dorsally, dorsal buttress plating was generally needed. However, dorsal plating is associated with many complications because the dorsal radius is often comminuted, making plating quite complex. Also, because of the close proximity of the dorsal plate to the extensor mechanism, tendon ruptures were common with the dorsal construct.

The modern volar approach is intended to overcome the problems of dorsal plating. The advantage of the volar plating technique is the ability to place the plate under the pronator quadratus, which can shield the plate from injuring the overlying tendons and nerves around the distal radius. In addition, the introduction of locking plates made rigid fixation from the volar side possible irrespective of the amount of comminution over the dorsal surface *(Fig. 8.22)*. Prior plate technology required that the screw purchases both the dorsal and volar cortices of the radius to tighten the plate by friction. This was problematic due to the comminuted dorsal bone, which often left the plate loose. The new locking plate mechanism introduces threads on the plate itself, so there is no need to engage both cortices. By approaching the fracture volarly, the surgeon need only to engage the more intact volar surface of the distal radius. Additionally, the use of distal pegs provides a scaffold to hold the articular surface intact, which adds a novel construct to achieve better anatomic reduction.

Volar plating does have several nuances that one must pay attention to during exposure to prevent unnecessary complications.[25,39] First, the volar incision must be made radial to the FCR to protect the palmar cutaneous branch of the median nerve, which is ulnar to the FCR. Next, instead of incising the pronator quadrates down the middle, the muscle should be elevated as an ulnarly based flap by dividing its insertion on the radius. This makes coverage of the implant easier. To further protect the extensor tendons, the screw length in the distal radius should be 1–2 mm shorter than the depth gauge measurement to prevent screw-tip related injuries to the tendons. Finally, once the plate has been placed on the radius and the fracture reduced, a 30° elevated lateral view should be used to confirm the position of the implant and screw. This will ensure that that the screw has not been inadvertently penetrated into the radiocarpal joint. Adhering to these guidelines will allow for effective plating, with minimal complications.

Ulnar styloid fracture

The ulna is attached to the radius through the triangular fibrocartilage complex that converges at the base of the ulnar styloid. It has been traditionally suggested that any ulnar styloid fracture with a displacement of 2 mm will require open reduction and internal fixation *(Fig. 8.22)*. Our recent prospective study of a large cohort of patients treated with volar locking plates indicates that once anatomic reduction is achieved and there is no instability of the distal radioulnar joint (DRUJ) after DRF fixation, the displaced ulnar styloid fracture does not need to undergo reduction and fixation. The outcomes of those DRFs with corresponding ulnar styloid fractures and those without ulnar styloid fracture are comparable at 1 year follow-up. Therefore, for ulnar styloid fractures, after fixating the DRF, we would stress the DRUJ with the forearm in pronation and supination to determine whether

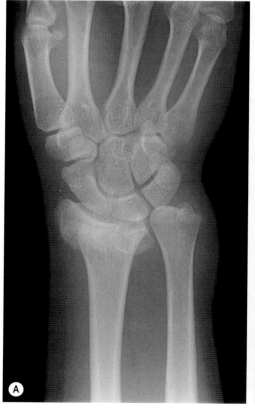
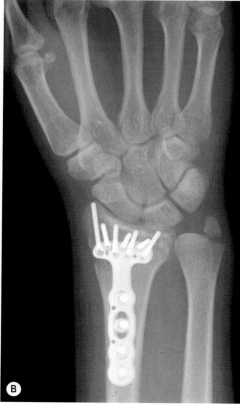

Fig. 8.22 **(A)** A complex distal radius fracture that has been **(B)** reduced using a volar locking plate. Note the displacement of the ulnar styloid fracture, which does not need to be fixated because the distal radioulnar joint is stable with manual testing.

there is instability of the DRUJ. If there is indeed instability, regardless of whether there is ulnar styloid fracture, we would open the ulnar wrist to reattach the TFCC or the large ulnar styloid fracture using a combination of K-wires and/or loop-wires. On the other hand, if there is no instability of the DRUJ after DRF fixation, then the patient can be treated with a standard DRF protocol, which in our protocol is to start active exercises of the wrist 1 week after fixation and to wear a volar wrist splint for the next 4 weeks to allow fracture healing. The patient should maintain finger ROM exercises with an active exercise regimen for the distal radius.

Future directions

Our recent studies of Medicare data show that closed reduction of the distal radius is still the dominant treatment method used for elderly Americans.[24,40] In younger patients, better anatomic reduction leads to better functional outcomes.[41] However, despite the near certainty of fracture malalignment, most elderly patients treated with closed reduction and casting are reported to have satisfactory functional outcomes.[42–47] Somehow the elderly are able to adapt to distal radius deformities. Previous schools of thought held that elderly individuals did not require accurate reduction of the distal fragment to achieve satisfactory functional results.[45,46,48–50] Today's elderly population, however, are more active than any previous generation of elderly individuals. They are continuing to live active, independent lives far longer than their parents or grandparents did. The 2004/2005 National Long-Term Care Survey found that only 19% of Medicare recipients were considered disabled (difficulty performing at least one "Activity of Daily Living"), and that number this is decreasing by approximately 2% per year.[51] This increased activity and independence places more demand on the wrist and may require more accurate fracture fixation to preserve function.[52–55] Because of its better biomechanical properties, volar locking plate systems are being used increasingly in the younger population, and some surgeons have started to apply this technology for the elderly.[56] Although there is some evidence that outcomes in elderly patients are as good as those in young patients,[57] no randomized trials have been performed comparing the current surgical treatments for the elderly. Most of the published series of elderly DRF treatment are hampered by small sample size, inconsistent follow-up times and retrospective study design. Our research group will begin an ambitious study with the participation of 21 leading hand surgery programs in North America to overcome many of the limitations of prior studies.[58] This study will derive evidence-based outcomes data to enhance the quality of care for the US elderly suffering from DRFs.

Acknowledgements

The authors would like to thank Pouya Entezami for help in the preparation of this chapter.

Access the complete reference list online at **http://www.expertconsult.com**

1. Chung KC, Spilson SV. The frequency and epidemiology of hand and forearm fractures in the United States. *J Hand Surg (Am)*. 2001;26(5):908–915.

   ICD-9 codes for hand and forearm fractures were used to extract cases from the 1998 National Hospital Ambulatory Medical Care Survey. Hand and forearm cases accounted for 1.5% of all emergency department cases. Radius and ulna fractures were found to be the most common, accounting for 44% of all hand and forearm fractures, and a majority of fractures (30%) occurred at home.

24. Chung KC, Shauver MJ, Birkmeyer JD. Trends in the United States in the treatment of distal radial fractures in the elderly. *J Bone Joint Surg*. 2009;91(8):1868–1873.

    Medicare data for distal radius fractures over a 10-year time period were analyzed. The rate of internal fixations for treating DRFs for the elderly increased five-fold, from 3% in 1996 to 16% in 2005. Closed treatment still remained the predominant method for treating these fractures (70% of DRF cases in 2005). Differences between specialties were noted: hand surgeons used open reduction techniques more commonly than general orthopedic surgeons.

25. Chung KC, Watt AJ, Kotsis SV, et al. Treatment of unstable distal radial fractures with the volar locking plating system. *J Bone Joint Surg*. 2006;88(12):2687–2694.

    This article presents outcomes of 87 patients with distal radius fractures treated with open reduction and internal fixation using a volar locking plating system. At the 12-month follow-up, the mean pinch strength on the injured side was not significantly different from that on the contralateral side (8.7 compared with 8.9 kg), and the mean flexion of the wrist on the injured side was 86% of that on the contralateral side. These outcomes show that volar locking plates provide effective fixation for the treatment of initially inadequately reduced distal radial fractures.

28. Davis EN, Chung KC, Kotsis SV, et al. A cost/utility analysis of open reduction and internal fixation versus cast immobilization for acute nondisplaced mid-waist scaphoid fractures. *Plast Reconstr Surg*. 2006;117:1223–1235.

    The authors conducted a cost-utility analysis to compare ORIF against cast reduction for acute nondisplaced scaphoid fractures. Utilities were assessed from 50 randomly selected medical students. A time trade-off method was used. This study found that ORIF offers greater quality-adjusted life-years compared with casting, with an increase of 0.21 quality-adjusted life-years for the 25–34-year age group. In addition, because of the lower cost of using ORIF (due to a decrease in lost productivity with this strategy), ORIF is the dominant strategy.

58. Chung KC, Song JW. The WRIST study group. Guide on Organizing a Multicenter Clinical Trial: the WRIST study group. *Plast Reconstr Surg*. 2010;126(2):515–523.

    The authors discuss the stages and importance of organizing a multicenter clinical trial. These types of studies are becoming increasingly important for providing conclusive and useful outcomes research. Guidelines are given beginning with the pre-planning stages, all the way through to the submission of an R01 grant. Performing such studies will help alleviate deficiencies in the current literature on treating fractures of the wrist and distal radius.

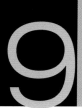

Flexor tendon injury and reconstruction

Jin Bo Tang

SYNOPSIS

■ Tendons transmit forces generated by muscles to move joints or to create action power. Flexor tendon injuries are common, but recovery of satisfactory function, particularly after injuries within the digital sheath, is sometimes difficult. Lacerated flexor tendons should be treated by primary surgical repair whenever possible.

■ The current trend of end-to-end surgical tendon repairs is to use multistrand core sutures (four-strand repairs such as cruciate, double-Tsuge, Strickland, modified Savage, or six-strand repairs such as modified Savage, Tang).

■ In tendon repairs in the digital sheath area, a number of surgeons advocate that the A2 pulley can be released up to two-thirds of its length, and the A4 pulley can be entirely released when necessary and tendon repair is in the proximity of the pulley, given the integrity of the other pulleys. The release may reduce the resistance to tendon motion and the chance of repair ruptures. This technique is somewhat controversial.

■ Postoperatively, early tendon mobilization should always be employed, except in children or in some rare instances; motion protocols vary greatly among different treatment centers.

■ Repair ruptures, adhesion formations, and finger joint stiffness are major complications of primary surgery.

■ Combined use of multistrand core repairs, release of constricting pulley parts, and well-designed postoperative combined passive and active motion protocols – that do not overload, but sufficiently move the tendon – can help minimize adhesions, avoid repair ruptures, and restore optimal function.

■ Secondary surgeries include tenolysis, free tendon grafting, and staged tendon reconstruction. Tenolysis is indicated when restricting adhesions hamper tendon gliding and soft tissues and joint conditions of the hand are favorable. Free tendon grafting is a salvage operation for failed primary repairs, delayed treatment (>1 month) of an acute cut, or lengthy tendon defects. Staged reconstruction is indicated in case of extensive scar formation or multiple failed surgeries. Preservation or reconstruction of major annular pulleys is vital to restoring function of the digits during these secondary surgeries.

■ Closed ruptures of flexor tendons usually require surgical repairs.

■ The success of flexor tendon surgeries is very expertise-dependent. A thorough mastery of anatomy and meticulous surgical technique are requirements for satisfactory restoration of function.

Access the Historical Perspective section online at
http://www.expertconsult.com

Introduction

Tendons are composed of dense connective tissues that transmit forces generated by muscles to move the joints or to create action power. Functionally, the hand is dependent upon the integrity and ample gliding of the tendons. Among all the tendons in the body, those in the hand are most frequently subjected to injuries, due to their length and the varied nature of the activities of the hand. The pursuit of ideal repair techniques has drawn the attention of surgeons ever since hand surgery became a subspecialty. For over a century, flexor tendon repairs have presented challenges to hand surgeons, and aroused enormous enthusiasm of clinicians and investigators.

Difficulties in restoration of function of digital flexor tendons relate chiefly to the intricate anatomy of flexor tendon systems: the coexistence of superficialis and profundus tendons within a tight fibro-osseous tunnel. Frequent peritendinous adhesions jeopardize tendon gliding. Tendons within the synovial sheath (intrasynovial tendons) were once considered to lack the capacity for self-repair; therefore, invasion of adhesions from peritendinous tissues was believed to be a prerequisite in the tendon-healing process.[1-4] As the concepts regarding tendon-healing biology evolved, tendon cells have proved capable of proliferating and of producing collagens to heal the tendons eventually.[5-10] However, the tendon is innately low in cell density and growth factor activity, limiting its early healing strength.

In the early and middle 20th century, secondary tendon grafting dominated the repair of digital flexor tendons. During this period, tendon implants were developed for staged tendon reconstruction. However, as the practice of primary repairs prevailed in recent decades, the number of cases indicated for secondary tendon grafting or staged reconstruction decreased drastically. Primary repair of injured digital flexor tendons was pioneered by Verdan[11] and Kleinert et al.[12] in the 1960s and is the essential approach underlying current practice. Current primary repairs and inception of early tendon motion were based on the recognition of the intrinsic healing capacity of tendons in the 1970s and 1980s by Lundborg, Manske et al., and Gelberman et al.[5–10]

Nevertheless, despite the widespread use of primary repairs, surgical outcome remained unpredictable, and sometimes even disappointing. In the last two decades, major efforts were thus devoted to tackling this problem, with the goal of achieving consistently optimal outcome and minimizing repair ruptures and adhesions. In this regard, a number of multistrand core surgical repairs – such as the techniques of Savage, Strickland, cruciate, Lim-Tsai, or Tang[13–19] – have been developed to replace weaker, conventional two-strand repairs. Subdivisions of zones 1 and 2 of digital flexor tendon systems were proposed by Moiemen and Elliot,[20] and Tang,[21] who offer precise nomenclature when recording the locations of tendon cuts, discussing treatment, and comparing outcome. Surgical procedures to release critical parts of the pulleys have been advocated by Tang[22] and Kwai Ben and Elliot[23] to decompress the tendon and free tendon motion. In the last few years, we witnessed reports in which repair ruptures were completely avoided, with recovery of excellent or good function in most cases.[19,24,25] These recent reports represent remarkable steps towards satisfactory flexor tendon repairs and highlight the promise of predictable tendon repairs *(Box 9.1)*.

Box 9.1 General tips for surgeons of flexor tendon repairs

- Repairing flexor tendons requires meticulous surgery built upon a thorough master of anatomy and biomechanics of the flexor tendon system. Surgeons should know the anatomy in detail, including the length of major pulleys, characteristic changes in the diameter of the sheath, and tendon gliding amplitude
- Primary repairs should be performed by experienced surgeons whenever possible, or if a less experienced surgeon has to be the operator, before surgery the surgeon must review the anatomy of the flexor tendon system, and understand every detail of the requirements of an optimal tendon repair
- The mastery of atraumatic techniques is essential for the operator. The outcome of the repair is very expertise-dependent: repair of tendons by an inexperienced surgeon is a frequent cause of tendon adhesions and poor function, thus should be avoided
- Conventional two-strand repairs are weak; stronger surgical repairs are preferable
- Complete closure of the tendon sheath is not a necessity. Venting of a part of sheath (<2.0 cm), including a critical portion of the pulleys, provides easy access to injured tendons, and decreases resistance to tendon gliding after surgery; this procedure does not lead to loss of digital function when other sheath parts are intact
- Surgeons should emphasize strong suture techniques and decreasing gap formation, which will lead to early active motion exercises and better outcomes

---

Basic science

Anatomy

There are 12 flexor tendons in the hand and forearm regions. They include finger and thumb flexors and wrist flexors. Finger flexor tendons are the flexor digitorum superficialis (FDS) and the flexor digitorum profundus (FDP), and the tendon in the thumb is the flexor pollicis longus (FPL). They originate from muscles at about the midforearm. Except for the index finger, the tendons of the FDP come from a common muscle belly. The tendons of the FDS originate from separate muscle bellies, which allow more independent finger flexion. The FPL tendon arises from the volar aspect of the midportion of the radial shaft and from its adjacent interosseous membrane. Three wrist flexors are flexor carpi radialis (FCR) and ulnaris, and palmaris longus. Palmaris longus is absent in about 15–20% of the normal population. Wrist flexion power is not affected by the absence of this muscle.

Within the carpal tunnel, nine tendons exist – four FDS, four FDP, and one FPL. The relationship of these tendons within the carpal tunnel is fairly constant. The FDS tendons to the ring and middle fingers lie superficially, deeper are the FDS tendon to the index and small fingers, and deeper still are the FDP tendons. The FPL tendon is located deep and radially adjacent to the scaphoid and the trapezium. After emerging from the carpal tunnel, the tendons enter the palm. At about the level of the superficial palmar artery arch, the lumbrical tendons originate from the FDP tendons.

The most intricate portions of the flexor tendons are within the fingers, where the tendons glide within a closed fibroosseous sheath with segmental, semirigid, constrictive dense connective tissue bands present. The digital sheath forms a closed synovial compartment extending from the distal palm to the middle of the distal phalange. Proximally, the synovial sheath ends just proximal to the neck of the metacarpus, forming the proximal reflection of the digital flexor sheath. The FDS tendons lie superficial to the FDP tendons up to the bifurcation of the FDS tendon at the level of the metacarpophalangeal joint (MCP). Then, FDS tendons become two slips coursing laterally and then deeper to the FDP tendons. This FDS bifurcation is in the A2 pulley area. This part of the FDS tendon also serves to constrain the FDP tendon; the FDS segment at bifurcation may be viewed as a structure functioning similarly to a pulley. Deep to the FDP tendon, the FDS slips rejoin to form Camper's chiasm (a fibrous interweaved connection between two FDS slips), and distally insert on the proximal and middle parts of the middle phalanx as two separate slips. The FDP tendon inserts into the volar aspect of the distal phalanx. The FPL tendon is the only tendon inside the flexor sheath of the thumb and inserts at the distal phalanx.

The digital flexor sheath consists of the synovial sheath and interwoven condensed fibrous bands ("pulleys"). The synovial sheath is a thin layer of continuous smooth paratenon covering the inner surface of the fibrous sheath, providing a smooth surface for tendon gliding and nutrition to the tendons. The pulley system of the digital flexor tendon is unique; it consists of annular pulleys (condensed, rigid, and heavier annular bands) and cruciate pulleys (filmy cruciform bands) *(Fig. 9.1)*.[151] There are five annular pulleys (A1–A5),

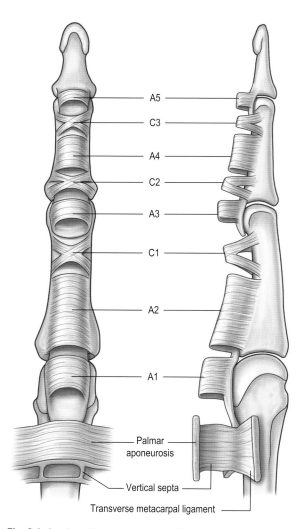

Fig. 9.1 Annular pulleys (condensed, rigid, and heavier annular bands) and cruciate pulleys (filmy cruciform bands) are present in the fingers. There are five annular pulleys **(A1–A5)**, three cruciate pulleys **(C1–C3)**, and one palmar aponeurosis pulley.

three cruciate pulleys (C1– C3), and one palmar aponeurosis pulley.[151,152] The A1, A3, and A5 pulleys originate from the palmar plates of the MCP, proximal (PIP) and distal interphalangeal (DIP) joints, and the A2 and A4 pulleys originate from the middle portion of the proximal and middle phalanges respectively. The broadest annular pulley is the A2 pulley, which covers the proximal two-thirds of the proximal phalanx and encompasses the bifurcation of the FDS tendon at its middle part. The A4 pulley is located at the middle third of the middle phalanx. The A2 and A4 pulleys are the largest among five annular pulleys and have the most important function. The annular pulleys maintain the anatomical paths of tendons close to bones and phalangeal joints, thus optimizing the mechanical efficiency of digital flexion. The more compressible cruciate pulleys allow for digital flexion to occur with condensation of the fibro-osseous sheath at the inner part of flexed fingers. This is called a "concertina effect."

The length of the A2 pulley is about 1.5–1.7 cm in the middle finger of an average adult, and the length of the A4

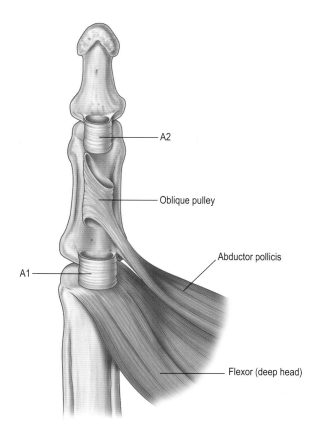

Fig. 9.2 Locations of flexor pulleys of the thumb. There are three pulleys in the thumb: A1, oblique, and A2 pulley, from proximal to distal.

pulley is about 0.5–0.7 cm. The diameter of the flexor sheath is at its narrowest at the level of the A4 pulley and in the middle and distal parts of the A2 pulley. The A2 and A4 pulleys are easily recognizable, because both are remarkably denser and more rigid than their adjacent flexor sheath. The A1 pulley, with a length of about 1.0 cm, is located proximal to the A2 pulley; in some instances, both A1 and A2 pulleys merge to form an especially lengthy pulley complex. The A3 pulley is located palmar to the PIP joint, but it is very short (0.3 cm) and may be difficult to distinguish from the synovial sheath.

In the thumb, there are three pulleys (A1, oblique, and A2) with no cruciate pulleys **(Fig. 9.2)**. The A1 and oblique pulleys are functionally important. The A1 pulley, 0.7–0.9 cm long, is located palmar to the MCP joint. The oblique pulley, 0.9–1.1 cm long, spans the middle and distal parts of the proximal phalanx. The A2 pulley is near the site of insertion of the FPL tendon, and is thin and 0.8–1.0 cm long.

The FDP tendon has two vincula: a fan-like short vinculum and a cord-like long vinculum. The short vinculum is located at the insertion of the FDP tendon **(Fig. 9.3)**. The long vinculum connects the FDP tendon through the short vinculum of the FDS tendon to the floor of the palmar surface of the phalanges. The FDS tendon also has two vincula: one connecting to the proximal phalanx, and another at the insertion of the FDS tendon. Vincula carry blood vessels to the dorsum of these tendons, providing limited nutrition. Tendon insertion sites to bones also carry vessels into tendons over a very short distance.

According to anatomical features, the flexor tendons in the hand and forearm are divided into five zones, which offer the fundamental nomenclature for flexor tendon anatomy and surgical repairs.[153] In the 1990s, the most complex areas – flexor tendons in the digital sheath – were subdivided by Moiemen and Elliot,[20] and by Tang.[21] The zoning is described below, and its relation to the locations of pulleys is shown in *Figures 9.4 and 9.5*:

- Zone 1: from the insertion of the FDS tendon to the terminal insertion of the FDP tendon

- Zone 2: from the proximal reflection of the digital synovial sheath to the FDS insertion
- Zone 3: from the distal margin of the transverse carpal ligament to the digital synovial sheath
- Zone 4: area covered by the transverse carpal ligament
- Zone 5: proximal to the transverse carpal ligament.

In the thumb, zone 1 is distal to the interphalangeal (IP) joint, zone 2 is from the IP joint to the A1 pulley, and zone 3 is the area of the thenar eminence.

The subdivisions of zone 1 by Moiemen and Elliot are:

- 1A: the very distal FDP tendon (usually <1 cm), not possible to insert a core suture
- 1B: from zone 1A to distal margin of the A4 pulley
- 1C: the FDP tendon within the A4 pulley.

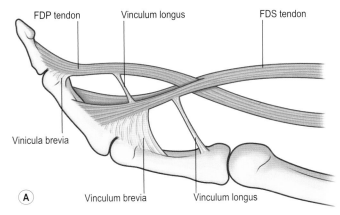

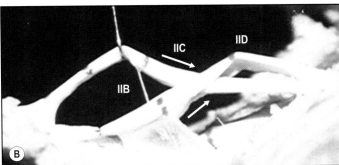

Fig. 9.3 Insertions and relative positions of the flexor digitorum superficialis (FDS) and flexor digitorum profundus (FDP) tendons and vincula. Each of the FDS and FDP tendons has two vincula, one short and one long. The relations of the FDS and FDP tendons are complex in the middle part of the proximal phalanx under the A2 pulley (zone 2C).

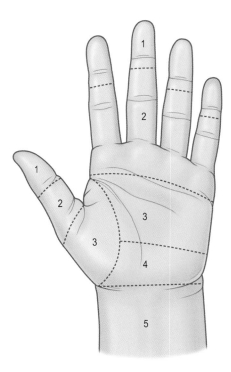

Fig. 9.4 Divisions of the flexor tendons into five zones according to anatomical structures of the flexor tendons, presence of the synovial sheath, and the transverse carpal ligament.

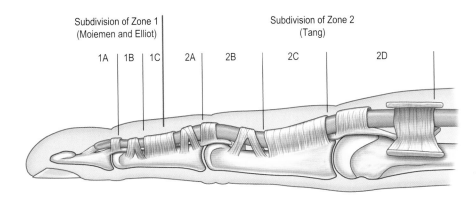

Fig. 9.5 Subdivisions of zones 1 and 2 of flexor tendons in the fingers and their relations to the flexor pulleys.

The subdivisions of zone 2 by Tang are:

- 2A: the area of the FDS tendon insertion
- 2B: from the proximal margin of the FDS insertion to the distal margin of the A2 pulley
- 2C: the area covered by the A2 pulley
- 2D: from the proximal margin of the A2 pulley to the proximal reflection of digital sheath.

Flexor tendon healing

Flexor tendons derive nutrition from both synovial and vascular sources. Flexor tendons outside the synovial sheath are supplied with a segmental vascular network through the paratenon, and the vascular supply plays an important role in the nutrition of these tendons. However, the tendons within the synovial sheath are mostly deprived of a vascular network. Only limited dorsal regions around vincular insertions are vascularized. A series of experiments by Manske et al. showed that intrasynovial flexor tendons are nourished by synovial fluid and that nutrition through vascular supplies is insignificant.[47–50] While the general healing process of the tendon has long been recognized as having early inflammatory, middle collagen production, and late remodeling phases, the healing potential of the intrasynovial flexor tendon has been a subject of intense investigations and debate over several decades.[1–10,52–61]

Before the 1970s, it was widely accepted that the digital flexor tendon lacked intrinsic healing capacity.[1–4] However, in subsequent decades, the intrinsic healing capacity of the tendon came to light in a series of elegant experimental studies. These experiments, by Matthews, Lundborg, Manske, Gelberman, and Mass and others, included observation of the repair process in lacerated flexor tendons within the synovial sheath, investigation of cellular activity in the lacerated tendon within the knee joint, detection of cellular activity, and the ability to produce matrix by in vitro tendon cultures.[5–10,51–61] The work led to the well-supported conclusion that cells in the intrasynovial tendon can proliferate and participate in the healing process, making the tendon itself capable of healing without forming adhesions. This became the scientific basis of early postoperative tendon mobilization.

It is now agreed that intrasynovial flexor tendons can heal through two mechanisms – intrinsic and extrinsic. Intrinsic healing takes place through the proliferation of tenocytes and production of extracellular matrix by intrinsic cells. Growth of tissues or cell seeding from outside the tendon is extrinsic healing. The tendon's intrinsic healing capacity is innately weak; extrinsic healing becomes dominant when intrinsic healing capacity is disabled (such as in the case of severe trauma to the tendon or peritendinous tissues) or under conditions (such as postsurgical immobilization) favoring extrinsic healing. Tendon healing exclusively through the intrinsic healing mechanism occurs only under a few experimental conditions.[7–9] Clinically, the lacerated tendon heals through a combination of both intrinsic and extrinsic mechanisms, whose balance depends upon the condition of the tendon and surrounding tissues. Extrinsic healing may act on the tendon-healing process either by forming adhesions or seeding the extrinsic cells without adhesions to the laceration site. On the other hand, adhesions do not necessarily consist of extrinsic cells. Tenocytes may migrate out of the laceration site for a very limited distance to become part of adhesions. Conceptually, extrinsic healing does not equal adhesion formation. However, it is extrinsic healing in the form of restrictive adhesions that hampers tendon function.

The following five variants (grades) of adhesions are seen clinically: (1) no adhesions; (2) filmy adhesions: formation of visible, filmy, and membranous tissue from tendon to outside tissues; (3) loose adhesions: loose and largely movable; (4) moderately dense adhesions: of limited mobility; and (5) dense adhesions: dense, almost immovable, and invading deep into the tendon.

The first two grades do not affect tendon motion; the third affects motion mildly. Because the fourth and fifth affect motion dramatically, those are the adhesions that surgeons seek to prevent. The density of adhesions relates to the tissues from which they arise. The adhesions arising from bones, periosteum, or major annular pulleys are dense. The density of adhesions can be altered to some extent by tendon motion. Some adhesion fibers can be disrupted as well. Surgeons should do their utmost to preclude or minimize the formation of adhesions which will restrict tendon gliding.

Many strategies have been attempted or suggested to prevent adhesion formation, including medications, use of artificial or biological barriers, and chemical or molecular approaches, with varied results. However, few medications or barriers have become clinically routine. So far, the most effective methods to prevent adhesions in clinic are meticulous surgery and early postoperative motion; the prime cause of adhesions is tendon repair by inexperienced surgeons.

Biomechanics of tendon repair and gliding

Forces generated during normal hand action range from 1 to 35 N, except tip pinch, according to in vivo measurements.[154] Therefore, a surgically repaired tendon should be able to withstand a tension of at least 40 N during motion, with sufficient power to resist gap formation. The repair should be able to withstand cyclic loads under both linear and curvilinear load conditions. Laboratory tests have shown that conventional two-strand core repairs plus running peripheral sutures yield a maximal strength from 20 to 30 N[93]; this is lower than forces generated during normal hand actions and explains why some repairs are disrupted during postoperative motion exercise. Studies showed that failure forces of four-strand repairs are around or beyond 40 N[16,65,94]; six-strand repairs fail with loads over 50–60 N.[13,71,85]

Many factors affect the strength of a surgical repair (Fig. 9.6): (1) the number of suture strands across the repair sites – strength is roughly proportional to the number of core sutures[74–76,81–83,85,94–98]; (2) the tension of repairs – this is most relevant to gap formation and stiffness of repairs[19]; (3) the core suture purchase[84,86,88,94]; (4) the types of tendon–suture junction – locking or grasping[79,88,95,98]; (5) the diameter of suture locks in the tendons – a small-diameter lock diminishes anchor power[80,91]; (6) the suture caliber (diameter)[82,116,117]; (7) the material properties of suture materials[95]; (8) the peripheral sutures[155,156]; (9) the curvature of tendon gliding paths – the repair strength decreases as tendon curvature increases[89,90]; and (10) above all, the holding capacity of a tendon, affected by varying degrees of trauma and posttraumatic tissue softening, plays a vital role in repair strength.

Factors affecting surgical repair strength

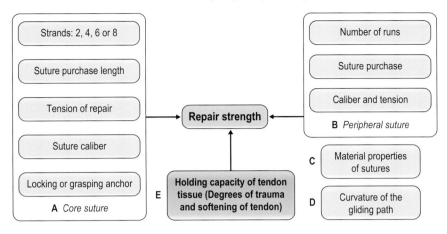

Fig. 9.6 Factors affecting the surgical repair strength of the tendon.

To achieve an optimal surgical repair, the factors outlined above must be considered and incorporated into repair design. A core suture purchase of at least 0.7–1.0 cm is necessary to generate maximal holding power, as recommended by Tang et al.[86,93] and Cao et al.[94] A locking tendon–suture junction is generally better than a grasping junction in terms of holding power. Diameter of the suture locks must reach or exceed 2 mm, according to Xie et al.[91] Tan and Tang recommend a greater core suture purchase (>1.2 cm) and locking repairs for an obliquely cut tendon.[86–88] Barrie et al.[116] and Taras et al.[117] greatly improved repair strength by increasing suture caliber. Clinically, the caliber of suture used in adults is either 3-0 or 4-0; sutures of 2-0 or greater are too large and rigid in the hand.

Tendon–suture junctions in surgical repairs are either grasping or locking; locking junctions vary greatly (*Fig. 9.7*). Grasping repairs are generally weaker than locking repairs. Among locking junctions, cross-locks provide identical strength to circle-locks.[94] Exposed and embedded cross-locks create the same strength.[92] With an identical number of suture strands across the tendon, different locking junctions result in minor differences in strength. Nevertheless, repairs with cross- or circle-locks appear slightly stronger than Kessler-type repairs with Pennington locks. Pennington locks provide a looser junction than cross- or circle-locks.

Peripheral sutures serve to "tidy up" the approximated tendon stumps; they may add strength to repairs as well. Deep-bite peripheral sutures increase repair strength.[155] Increases in suture purchase or complex peripheral sutures, as typified by the Silfverskiöld method,[64] increase overall strength. However, most surgeons choose to insert only simple peripheral stitches. Some surgeons even do not supplement peripheral stitches when multistrand core sutures have been used.[25] In the presence of a strong multistrand core repair, peripheral sutures contribute little in terms of strength. In fact, to simplify repair maneuvers, multistrand core sutures (with or without a few peripheral sutures) may be sufficient.

In addition to surgical factors, tendon curvature affects strength as well. Surgical repair in a tendon under a curvilinear load is weaker than that under a linear load; the repair strength decreases as the curvature increases.[89,90] Mechanically,

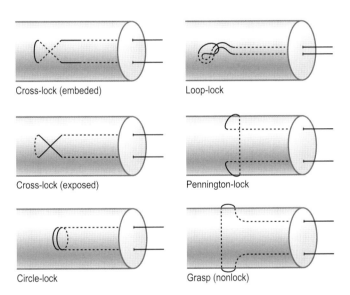

Cross-lock (embeded)

Loop-lock

Cross-lock (exposed)

Pennington-lock

Circle-lock

Grasp (nonlock)

Fig. 9.7 Different tendon–suture junctions in tendon repairs: locking and grasping junctions.

a tendon under linear tension is pulled without being bent, whereas a tendon under curvilinear tension is subjected to both linear pulling and bending forces. Therefore, the repair fails more easily in the flexed finger under curvilinear loads. When the finger moves to approach full flexion, a strongly bent tendon is particularly prone to fail (*Fig. 9.8*).

Annular pulleys are critical to the function of the digital flexor tendons. The pulleys keep the tendons' course close to the phalanges for optimal mechanical efficiency of tendon excursion. Lengthy loss of the sheath and pulleys causes anterior displacement – bowstringing – of the flexor tendon during finger flexion. In fingers, the A2 and A4 pulleys are most critically located and functionally important. Preservation or reconstruction of the two pulleys is necessary in the absence of other pulleys or sheath. Nevertheless, given the presence of other pulleys and sheaths, the loss of any individual pulleys, including the A2 or A4 pulley, appears to result in few detrimental consequences. Both Tang[22] and Tomiano

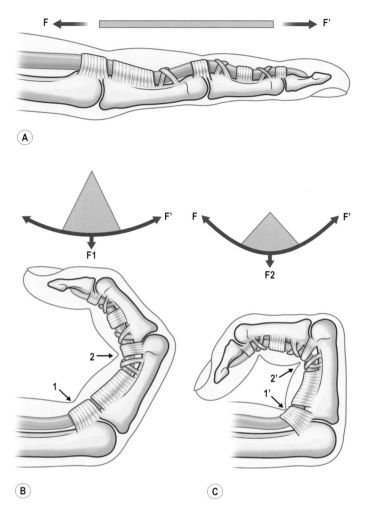

Fig. 9.8 The forces acting on the tendon are different when the tendon is subjected to linear pulling **(A)** or curvilinear tension **(B and C)**. **(A)** The tendon subjected to linear pulling is loaded by only a linear pulling force. **(B and C)** The tendon subjected to a curvilinear tension is loaded by both linear and bending forces. The repaired tendon fails more easily while being linearly pulled and bent. From B to C, as the curvature of the gliding path increases, the bending force on the tendon is increased (F2 > F1). Under greater gliding curvature, the tendon fails with a smaller linear pulling force. From B to C, as the finger flexes progressively, the tendon fails with an increasingly smaller linear tension. **(C)** The tendon is particularly prone to fail when the finger approaches full flexion. The tendon is easier to disrupt in (C) when gliding over joints (1' and 2') with greater curvature than in (B) with smaller curvature.

Flexor tendons in the digits glide in a fairly resistance-free synovial environment. Resistance to tendon motion is increased when the tendons are injured and repaired. The following create resistance to tendon gliding: (1) rough tendon gliding surface; (2) biological reactions of the wound, e.g., subcutaneous and tendon edema; (3) friction caused by exposure of suture materials; (4) increases in tendon bulkiness due to placement of sutures; (5) tight closure of sheath or pulleys that narrows the tendon gliding tunnel; (6) tendon-catching at pulley or sheath edges; (7) postsurgical extensor tethering and joint stiffness that burden the movement of the flexor tendon; and (8) adhesions that restrict tendon gliding.

Following trauma and surgery, tendons undergo inflammation, healing, and edema. The volume of the tendons is increased, which increases the resistance within the narrow sheath tunnel. Subcutaneous edema outside the sheath also impedes tendon motion. These factors affecting the resistance to tendon gliding should be considered in deciding how rigorous the postoperative motion program should be. The safety margin can be enhanced by a strong surgical tendon repair or appropriately decompressing the tendon to avoid repair ruptures.

Biological healing strength is a central issue underlying all tendon repairs. Urbaniak *et al.*,[76] Kubota *et al.*,[77] Aoki *et al.*[78] and Boyer *et al.*[114] have characterized the strengths of the healing flexor tendon using animal models. They found that strength either remained consistent or actually decreased somewhat over the initial few weeks after surgery.[76–78] Decreases in strength, typically those in the second postsurgical week, are thought to be caused by softening of the tendon stumps, which lower the sutures' holding power. Our investigations using a chicken model indicated that the strength of a healing tendon is steady during the initial 4 weeks, followed by a substantial increase (greater than threefold) in the fifth and sixth weeks; thereafter, the tendon heals strongly and is difficult to disrupt. The fifth and sixth weeks after surgery appear crucial to regaining strength. Accelerating healing, aiming to move this critical "strength gain" period to earlier weeks, is a current focus of research into molecular modulation of tendon healing.

Diagnosis/patient presentation

Flexor tendon injuries are open in most cases, resulting from a sharp cut or a crush, but they can also present as closed injuries. Open injuries due to extensive trauma are frequently associated with neurovascular deficits. Closed injuries often relate to forced extension during active flexion of the finger. Flexor tendon rupture can also occur as a result of chronic attrition in rheumatoid disease, Kienbock disease, scaphoid nonunion, or hamate or distal radius fracture.

Careful attention to the patient's history and the mechanism of injury can alert the surgeon to the extent of the tendon trauma and associated injuries. The natural resting posture of the wounded digits is important for evaluation. Complete lacerations of both FDP and FDS tendons are easily diagnosed when the affected fingers are seen in a relatively extended position with loss of active finger flexion at PIP and DIP joints. If the patient can actively flex the DIP joint while the

et al.[111,112] have shown that incision of the A2 pulley up to one-half or two-thirds of its length or of the entire A4 pulley results in no tendon bowstringing and little loss of digital flexion. In *in vivo* settings, incision of the A2 pulley decreases resistance to tendon motion and lessens the chance of repair failure.[109,110] Loss of the A3 pulley alone has few consequences as well, but a lengthy sheath cut adjacent to the A3 pulley, containing C1 or C2, causes tendon bowstringing.[107] Therefore, significant loss of sheath should be avoided to maintain tendon function; however, loss of a small portion (<2 cm in length) of the sheath and pulley, even including a part of the most critically located A2 pulley, has no substantial mechanical consequence.

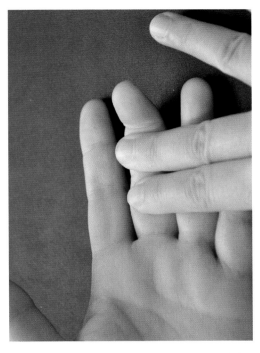

Fig. 9.9 Examination of flexor digitorum profundus (FDP) tendon continuity and function. When the proximal interphalangeal joint flexion is blocked, flexion of the distal interphalangeal joint indicates continuity and function of the FDP tendon.

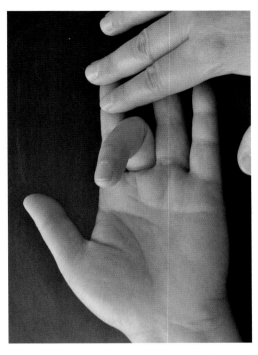

Fig. 9.10 Examination of flexor digitorum superficialis (FDS) tendon continuity and function. If the patient is unable to flex the proximal interphalangeal joint of the examined finger while flexion of the other fingers is blocked, this indicates loss of function of the FDS tendon. Complete flexion of the proximal interphalangeal joint indicates function and continuity of the FDS tendon.

motion of the PIP joint is blocked, no injuries or only partial injuries to the FDP tendon can be diagnosed *(Fig. 9.9)*. To assess the continuity of the FDS tendon, the adjacent fingers are held in full extension by the examiner. If the patient cannot actively flex the PIP joint, the FDS tendon is completely severed *(Fig. 9.10)*. Variations in the FDS tendons in the little finger are frequent. The FDS in 30–35% of the little fingers is connected with the FDS in the ring or middle fingers. Some little fingers (10–15%) are missing an FDS tendon. These patients have limited or no PIP flexion of the little finger during testing. Weakness during resisted finger flexion indicates a possible partial tendon cut. To test the FPL tendon, the thumb MCP joint is stabilized in a neutral position. The patient is asked to flex the IP joint. Loss of active flexion at the joint indicates complete severance of the FPL tendon.

Nerve and vascular function should be assessed routinely because accompanying injuries in the neurovascular bundles in one or both sides of the fingers or median and ulnar nerves at the carpal tunnel or distal forearm are common. Loss of sensation in the finger pulps or loss of function of intrinsic muscles in the hand is indicative of such accompanying injuries; treatment of neurovascular injuries must be included when planning surgical strategies. If fingers or hands are found to be hypovascular or avascular due to vascular lacerations, vascular anastomosis should be a surgical emergency. Otherwise, after wound debridement, either the lacerated flexor tendons can be repaired (when experienced surgeons are readily available) or the skin can be closed to allow for delayed primary repairs within days by experienced surgeons.

Radiographs should always be taken. Associated fractures are not infrequent and require treatment. Computed tomography (CT) scan or magnetic resonance imaging (MRI) is not usually necessary to diagnose open tendon injuries. However, for diagnosis of closed tendon ruptures or suspected ruptures of the primary end-to-end surgical repair, these tools are of particular values. CT or MRI should be prescribed for the cases suspicious of closed tendon ruptures. Ultrasonographic examination may also reveal rupture of the tendons.

Treatment/surgical techniques

Primary and delayed primary repairs

Whenever possible, acutely lacerated flexor tendons in the hand and forearm should be treated primarily or at the delayed primary stage. Primary tendon repair is the end-to-end repair performed immediately after wound cleaning and debridement, usually within 24 hours of trauma. Delayed primary repair is defined as repair performed within 3 or even 4 weeks after tendon lacerations. No clinical investigations actually validated the best time for primary repair. The ideal situation is that of a patient with digital flexor tendon lacerations brought into the clinic soon after injury; surgery begins within a few hours, and an experienced surgeon is readily available. The tendon injured in critical areas (such as zone 2)

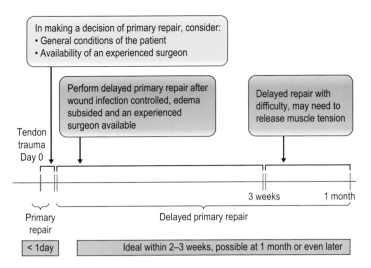

Fig. 9.11 A decision-making flow chart of primary and delayed primary flexor tendon repairs.

Box 9.2 **Primary flexor tendon repairs**

Indications

- Clean-cut tendon injuries
- Tendon cut with limited peritendinous damage, no defects in soft-tissue coverage
- Regional loss of soft-tissue coverage or fractures of phalangeal shafts are borderline indications
- Within several days or at most 3 or 4 weeks after tendon laceration

Contraindications

- Severe wound contamination
- Bony injuries involving joint components or extensive soft-tissue loss
- Destruction of a series of annular pulleys and lengthy tendon defects
- Experienced surgeons are not available

should not be repaired by an inexperienced surgeon. Rather, tendon repair can be delayed until an experienced surgeon is available. My preferred period of deliberate delay is 4–7 days, when the risk of infection can be properly addressed and edema has reduced substantially. Delay of the repair beyond 3–4 weeks may cause myostatic shortening of the muscle–tendon unit; for these late cases, lengthening the tendon within the muscles in the forearm can ease the tension *(Fig. 9.11)*.[157]

Rupture of the repaired flexor tendons after surgery can be re-repaired if the rupture occurs within a few weeks up to a month after surgery; secondary tendon grafts may be the only choice for ruptured cases in the presence of obvious retraction of the tendon end or extensive scarring in the intact FDS tendon when the FDP tendon ruptures.

Indications and contraindications

Primary or delayed primary end-to-end tendon repairs are mainly indicated in clean-cut tendon injuries with limited damage to peritendinous tissues. Neurovascular injury is not a contraindication for primary repairs. Loss of soft-tissue coverage over the tendon and the presence of fractures are borderline indications. Local defects in skin and subcutaneous tissues can be covered by flap transfer. A simple fracture limited to the phalangeal or metacarpal shaft can be securely fixed with screws or miniplates, and then tendons can be repaired. However, serious crush injuries, severe wound contamination, loss of extensive soft tissues, or extensive destruction of pulleys and tendon structures are contraindications for primary tendon repairs. Fractures involving multiple bones, particularly at different levels or not yielding stable internal fixation, are contraindications for primary tendon repairs *(Box 9.2)*.

Surgical techniques

Brachial plexus block is usually sufficient; general anesthesia can also be used when associated injuries are severe. The hand and arm are scrubbed and draped. A tourniquet is placed on the upper arm. The wounds should be thoroughly debrided, devitalized tissues excised, and the wounds washed with antibiotic solution. The position of the fingers or hand is determined by levels of cuts in the tendons in relation to their superficial tissues. The hand is usually held by an assistant, so that it can be adjusted during surgery. Loupe magnification is advised for surgery. The tendons are exposed through zigzag skin incisions on the volar side of the fingers, e.g., Bruner's incision, or a lateral incision. When the wounds are in the palm or forearm, incision by extending the wound opening is often necessary *(Fig. 9.12)*.

Zone 1 injuries

In this area, only the FDP tendon is located. When the tendon laceration is in the distal part of this zone (zone 1A and 1B), because the vincula connect to the proximal tendon to prevent retraction, both the proximal and distal ends can be easily found not far from the skin wound. When cut in zone 1C, the tendon may retract more proximally. For zone 1A injuries, the distal stump is usually too short for direct end-to-end repair. The proximal tendon end can be sutured with Bunnell or modified Becker suture with 3-0 polypropylene, and an osteoperiosteal flap is raised at the base of the distal phalanx *(Fig. 9.13)*. The suture is led through an oblique drill hole, brought out through the nail, and tied over a button above the nail. To avoid passing the suture through the nail, the proximal tendons can be sutured to a fish-mouth opening in the distal tendon stump using reinforced suture repairs or minianchors *(Fig. 9.13)*.[156,157] Another method is to drill a transverse hole through the distal phalanx. After the tendon stump is sutured, the suture is led through the hole and tied to the other end, through an open approach or percutaneously.[158,159] Injuries in zones 1B and 1C usually create tendon stumps of sufficient length for a direct surgical repair, which can be treated by

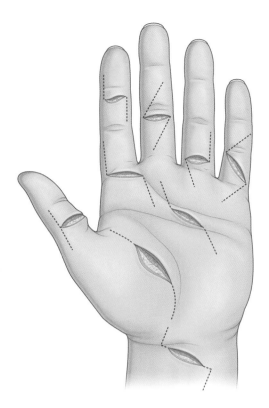

Fig. 9.12 Skin incisions utilized to approach the tendons in the digits and palm.

methods similar to treatment in zone 2. Core tendon sutures, such as the modified Kessler, cruciate, modified Becker, or double Kessler repair, can be placed to the proximal end through a window opening in the proximal sheath. The proximal end is brought underneath the intact sheath between the wound and the proximal opening to approximate the distal end.

Zone 2 injuries

Tendon injuries in this area are often exposed through a Bruner skin incision and a window opening in the synovial sheath, a release, or local excision of a short part of the annular pulleys. If the tendon ends have not retracted far proximally, flexion of the MCP or PIP joint can effectively bring the proximal end into sight. Sometimes the proximal tendon end is found retracted even to the middle of the palm. In this instance, an additional incision is made in the palm to expose the tendons, and the proximal tendon end is pulled distally within the synovial sheath by loosely suturing the tendon to a catheter. The end is brought out of the distal opening in the sheath to approximate the distal end. While the finger is held in slight flexion, a 25-gauge needle is then inserted at the base of the finger through the proximal tendon to hold the tendon temporarily and to release the tension at the surgical suture site.

During surgery, tendons should be handled atraumatically and ragged tendon tissue at the cut ends should be removed with a scalpel. Stronger suture materials are preferred: 3-0 or 4-0 sutures (nylon or coated nylon) are common choices. Basic

requirements of a tendon repair are: (1) sufficient strength; (2) smooth tendon gliding surface, with minimal suture (and knot) exposure; (3) no gapping of the repair site under tension; and (4) easy to perform.

Surgical suture techniques vary among surgeons. Some core suture methods are shown in *Figure 9.14*. The modified Kessler and cruciate techniques are further shown in *Figure 9.15*. The Bunnell method is no longer popular for end-to-end repair. The two-strand modified Kessler method and Tsuge method are among the most widely used over the past 40 years. In the last 20 years, a number of multistrand repair techniques have emerged,[14–19,65–69,] including four-strand repairs such as cruciate, modified Savage, Strickland, and double Kessler; six-strand repairs such as Savage, Lim-Tsai, Tang, M-Tang; and eight-strand Winters–Gelberman methods. I prefer multistrand methods, typically four- or six-strand repair methods when repairing lacerated FDP tendons in zone 2.

In my practice, I have used the double Tsuge method or six-strand methods in the past 20 years. In the last decade, my colleagues and I have started to use modifications of the original methods to repair tendons using fewer looped lines and knots, but maintaining suture strands and repair strength across the repair site identical to those of the original methods *(Fig. 9.16)*. These methods are relatively easy and surgical repair strength is very reliable *(Figs 9.17–9.23)*.

Video 1

Using a needle carrying two separate suture lines, or with remaining pieces of the looped suture line after making the repairs described above, we can make a variety of four-strand Kessler-type repairs by introducing double sutures through one needle passage *(Fig. 9.24)*. These techniques are used in my clinic as well as by my colleagues. We use these methods when repairing flatter tendons in some instances, such as the FDS cut proximal to bifurcation.[72]

Epitendinous stitches smooth the approximation of the tendon ends and resist gapping during tendon movement. Simple running peripheral, locking running peripheral, cross-stitch peripheral, and Halsted horizontal mattress sutures are among those most often used, with the first two more popular *(Fig. 9.25)*. Some surgeons prefer "deep-bite" peripheral stitches to add strength to repairs.[155] An epitendinous suture is usually added after the completion of core sutures, but it can also be added first.[156] Peripheral stitches can be unnecessary given a strong multistrand core suture.[25] Clinically, peripheral repairs vary from complex stitches to none. My preference is to use a simple running peripheral suture with 6-0 nylon after completion of a four- or six-strand core suture repair.

Technically, to make an optimal surgical repair, the length of core suture purchase in each tendon end should be at least 7 mm to 1.0 cm. Surgical repair strength decreases as the length of the suture purchase decreases *(Fig. 9.26)*. In addition, certain tension across repair site is beneficial to resist gapping. In my experience, a certain tension (resulting in about 10% shortening of the encompassed tendon, when the proximal tendon is temporarily fixed during surgery) appears beneficial, because a small amount of baseline tension in the repair would counteract the tension of the locomotor system during resting or active motion. When locking the suture junction in the tendon is incorporated to the core sutures, the locking circles of the suture in the tendon should be of a sufficient diameter (approximately 2 mm). After completing the repair,

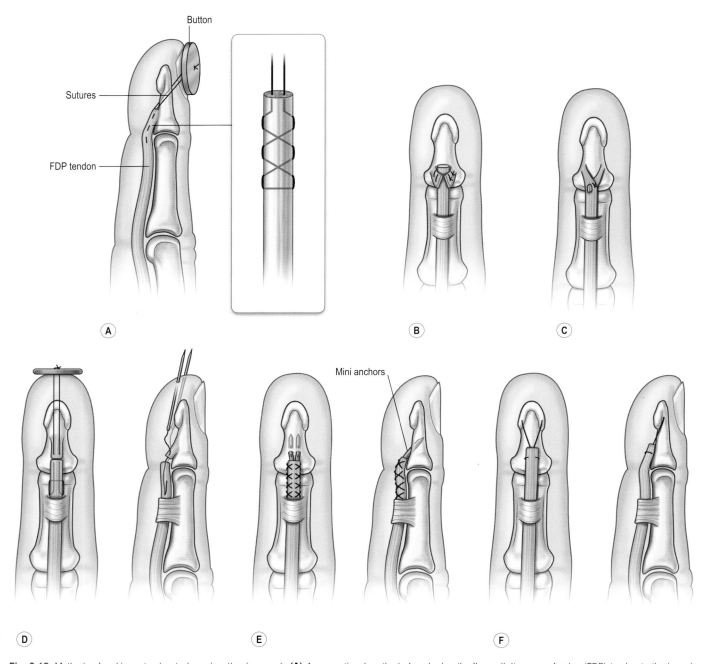

Fig. 9.13 Methods of making a tendon-to-bone junction in zone 1. **(A)** A conventional method of anchoring the flexor digitorum profundus (FDP) tendon to the bone by pull-out sutures through the nail tied over a button. Alternative ways to anchor the distal tendon stump to the bone by: **(B)** directly suturing the stump to residual FDP tendon, **(C)** looping the tendon through the bone, **(D)** pull-out suture over the fingertip, **(E)** minianchors, and **(F)** looping the sutures through a transverse hole in the bone **(F).**

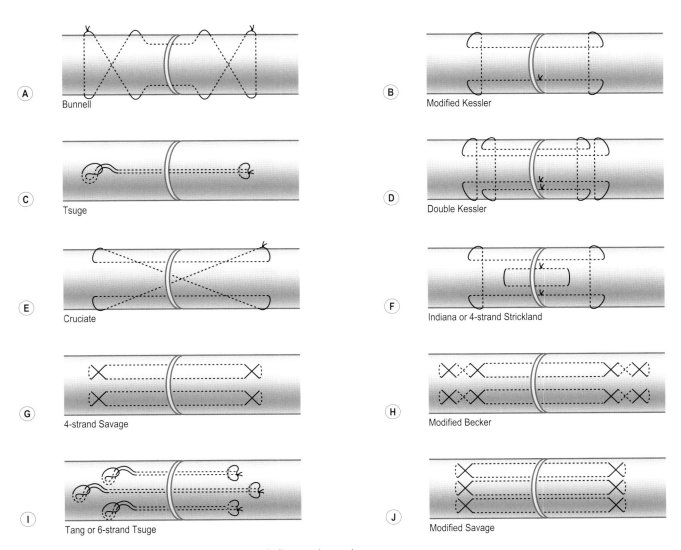

A Bunnell
B Modified Kessler
C Tsuge
D Double Kessler
E Cruciate
F Indiana or 4-strand Strickland
G 4-strand Savage
H Modified Becker
I Tang or 6-strand Tsuge
J Modified Savage

Fig. 9.14 Summary of methods used to make core sutures in flexor tendon repairs.

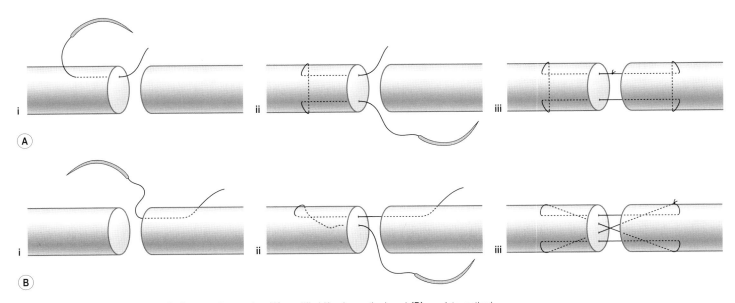

A   i   ii   iii

B   i   ii   iii

Fig. 9.15 Two common techniques in flexor tendon repairs: **(A)** modified Kessler method; and **(B)** cruciate method.

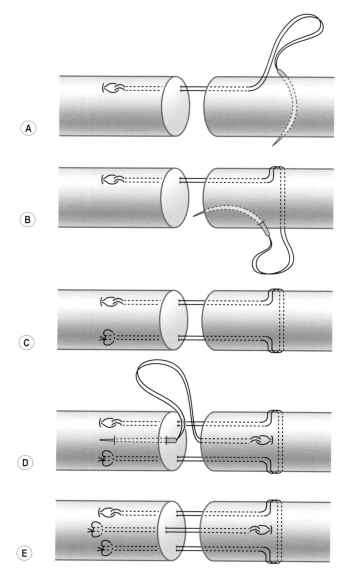

Fig. 9.16 The technique for making a six-strand M-Tang tendon repair. Two separate looped sutures are used to make an M-shaped repair within the tendon. **(A–C)** A U-shaped four-strand repair is completed, which can be used alone for tendon repair. **(D and E)** An additional looped repair is added at the center, to complete the six-strand repair. In tendon cross-sections, three suture groups are placed at points of a triangle to avoid interference to the dorsal center of the tendon where the vascular networks converge. The dorsolateral sutures may act as tension bands to resist gapping of the tendon.

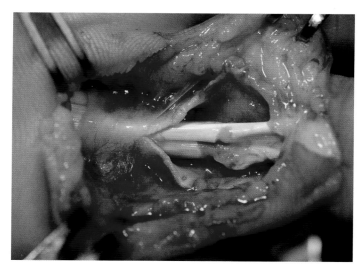

Fig. 9.17 A case with complete laceration of the flexor digitorum profundus tendon and partial flexor digitorum superficialis laceration in zone 2B. The surgery was performed 10 days after injury. The wound was exposed through a Bruner incision, and the distal half of the A2 pulley was incised through the volar midline. A needle is inserted transversely through the sheath and proximal tendon to temporarily fix the proximal tendon to ease tension during repair.

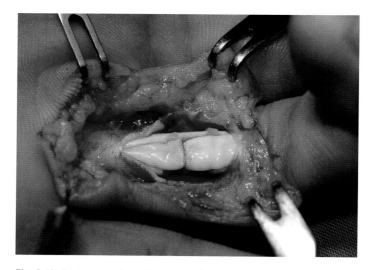

Fig. 9.18 The lacerated flexor digitorum profundus tendon was found through a separate incision in the palm and led underneath the sheath and pulleys to the operation field distal to the A2 pulley, to approximate the distal stump.

the cut tendon ends should align well, and no gapping between the tendon ends should be observed *(Box 9.3)*.

In the past 10 years, novel repair concepts have emerged and novel materials have been used. For example, of potential clinical merit are techniques involving a single passage of the needle carrying double or even triple strands into the tendon[69,160–162]; FiberWire also offers a strong suture material for tendon repairs.[95,163] These methods are effective in enhancing strength with a minimal suture passage in the tendon.

Closure of the synovial sheath is no longer considered essential for tendon repairs after hot debate in the 1980s and

---

Box 9.3 Recommended surgical tendon repairs

- More than two strands as the core repair – four or six strands are recommended
- Certain tension across the repair site – 10% shortening of tendon segment after repair
- Core suture purchase: 7–10 cm
- Locking tendon–suture junctions in core suture
- Diameter of the locks: 2 mm or over
- Suture calibers: 3-0 or 4-0 for core suture
- A variety of nylon sutures, or a FiberWire suture
- A simple running or locking peripheral suture
- No peripheral suture if core repair is very strong
- Avoid extensive exposure of sutures over the tendon surface

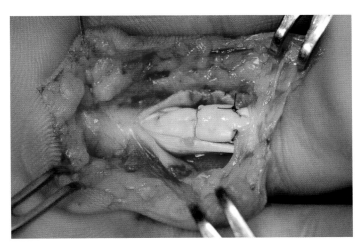

Fig. 9.19 Completion of inserting a four-strand repair using one looped suture line.

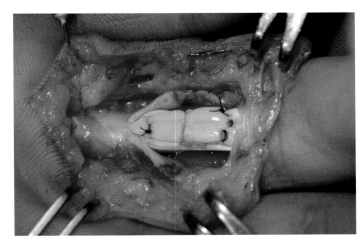

Fig. 9.20 Completion of the six-strand M-Tang repair.

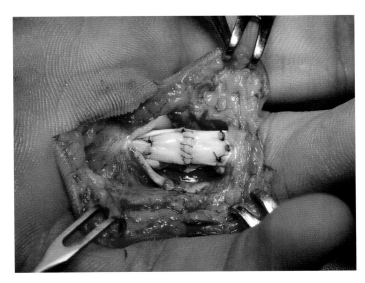

Fig. 9.21 Addition of a simple running peripheral repair.

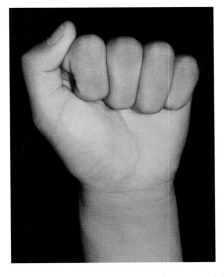

Fig. 9.22 Follow-up at 10 months after surgery: full flexion of the repaired finger, without tendon bowstringing.

Video 1

early 1990s.[164–171] Closure may be attempted in clean-cut injury when sheath defects or abrasions are absent. It is now agreed that avoiding compression or constriction to the edematous tendons by the sheath or annular pulleys after surgery is very important to tendon healing. With major pulleys and a majority of the sheath intact, leaving a part of the synovial sheath open has no significant adverse effect on tendon function and healing. On the other hand, incision of one single annular pulley (A1, A3, or A4) or a critical part (up to two-thirds of its length) of the A2 pulley does not significantly affect tendon gliding when all other pulleys or the synovial sheath are intact. Such a release can in fact be beneficial to tendon healing and gliding: as healing responses and adhesions arise, it releases constrictions on edematous tendons.

Clinically, the A4 or A2 pulley sometimes constitutes an obstacle for the edematous tendon to glide through, which may cause repair rupture during tendon motion exercise. The perceived need for complete preservation of the A4 and A2 pulleys during primary repairs is "borrowed" from the surgery pertaining to secondary tendon reconstructions, and does not hold true when the tendons are cut through a single wound and other sheaths or pulleys are intact. Contrary to the practice of 10 or 20 years ago, releasing the A4 pulley entirely and releasing a part of the A2 has become accepted clinical practice in recent years.[19,23,150,172] In the author's clinic, when the repaired FDP tendons are found tightly entrapped by the A4 pulley after testing during surgery, we completely release the A4 pulley *(Figs 9.27 and 9.28)*. A part of the A2 pulley, either proximal or distal (about one-half to two-thirds the length of the A2 pulley) *(Figs 9.17–9.21)*, is cut when both the FDS and FDP tendons are repaired in the area of or distal to the A2 pulley. When the repair is considerably delayed (3 weeks after injury), the A2 pulley usually collapses or is even embedded within scars. I excise a portion of the A2 pulley to shorten this pulley *(Figs 9.29–9.33)*.

The release usually needs to include a part of the adjacent synovial sheath. The total length of the sheath pulley release

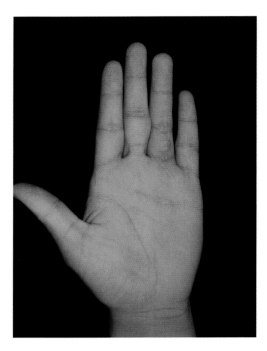

Fig. 9.23 Full extension of the repaired finger.

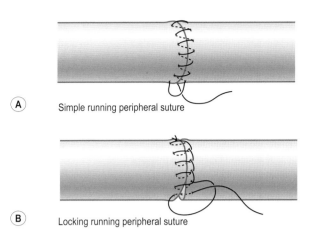

Fig. 9.25 Two simple common methods of peripheral suture. **(A)** Simple running peripheral suture. **(B)** Running locking peripheral suture.

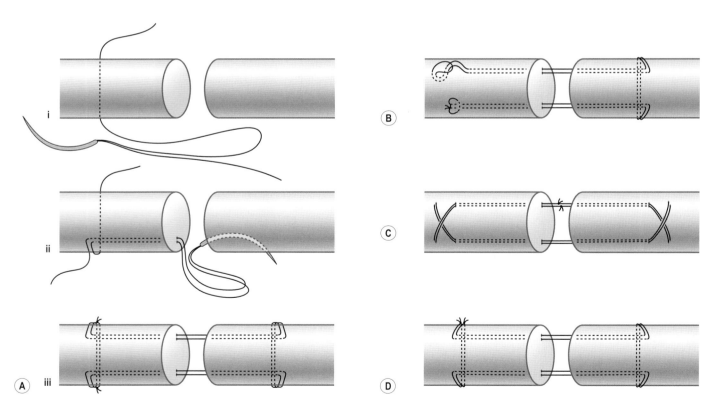

Fig. 9.24 Other designs of four-strand repairs by two separate strands or one looped suture line led by a single needle. These repairs, with fewer needle passages within the tendon, have strengths identical to the double Kessler method. **(A)** A four-strand repair with knots on two lateral sides of the tendon. **(B)** A U-shaped four-strand repair made with one looped suture line. **(C and D)** Two separate strands carried by a single needle to make a four-strand cross-lock repair or a four-strand Kessler repair (knots on one side of the tendon).

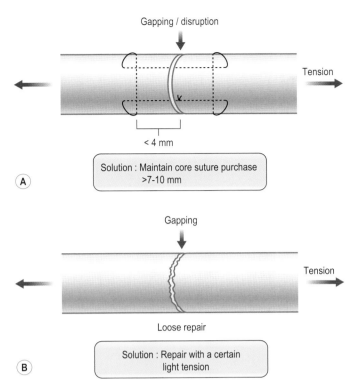

Gapping / disruption

Tension

< 4 mm

(A) Solution : Maintain core suture purchase >7-10 mm

Gapping

Tension

Loose repair

(B) Solution : Repair with a certain light tension

Fig. 9.26 Two bad repairs decrease the strength: **(A)** a repair with insufficient core suture purchase and **(B)** a loose repair. Sufficient core suture purchase and a certain pretension favor resisting gapping and decrease the chance of repair failure during tendon motion after surgery.

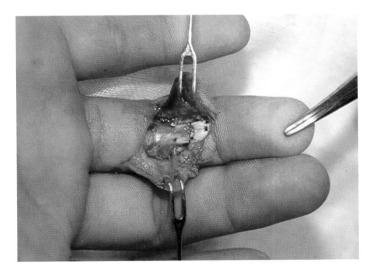

Fig. 9.28 The A4 pulley and a part of its adjacent sheath were vented to allow tendon passage. Other parts of the sheath were not violated. In this case, the flexor digitorum profundus tendon was repaired with a six-strand original Tang repair using three groups of looped sutures.

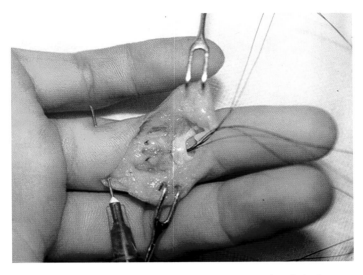

Fig. 9.27 The constricting A4 pulley sometimes presents an obstacle for the passage of the flexor digitorum profundus tendon.

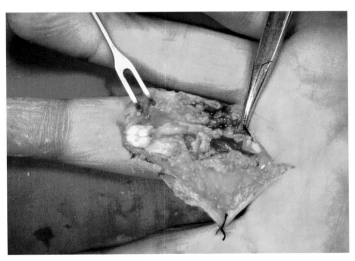

Fig. 9.29 A case of ruptured primary repair referred to the author. We performed direct repair of the ruptured flexor digitorum profundus tendon 3 weeks after the first tendon repair. The flexor tendons and A2 pulleys were found embedded within scars.

Video 1

is about 2 cm in adults, which amply decompresses tendon gliding, but does not lead to functional disturbance. The areas of the release are shown in *Figure 9.34*.

Over the years, release of the pulleys has been achieved differently: (1) incision of the entire or a critical part of the major pulley[19,22,23,150]; (2) excision of a part of the major pulley[19]; (3) omega, Z, or V-Y pulley plasty[173–175]; and (4) sheath enlargement plasty.[176,177] My current pulley release is a simple procedure: incising the A4 or a portion of the A2 pulley, or partially excising the A2 pulley, while obviating complicated sheath- or pulley-plasty surgeries.

Whether or how to repair the FDS tendon when both flexor tendons are injured is a subject of diverse opinions, particularly in the areas covered by the A2 pulley or distal to it. A few reports have discussed it specifically.[21,178,179] Repair of one slip of the FDS is also feasible.[100,108] In the area of the A2 pulley (zone 2C), I prefer to excise the FDS locally in cases with severe peritendinous injuries, when the tendons appear edematous, and in cases with delayed primary repairs. In performing the delayed repair, I find it almost impossible to repair the FDS tendon in zone 2C, because some degree of

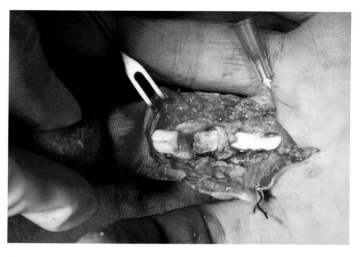

Fig. 9.30 The A2 pulley was partially excised and the intact part of the A2 pulley was released from the scar. The ragged tendon ends were trimmed to fresh tendon surfaces.

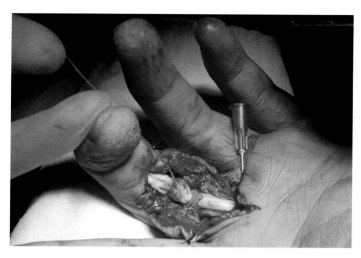

Fig. 9.31 The proximal tendon stump was passed underneath the preserved portion of the A2 pulley. The tendon was repaired with the six-strand M-Tang technique.

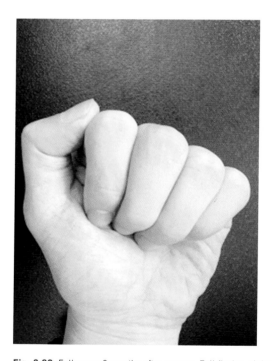

Fig. 9.32 Follow-up 6 months after surgery. Full flexion of the fingers was achieved, without tendon bowstinging during active finger flexion.

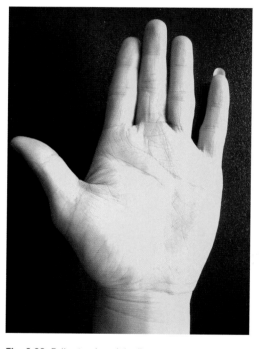

Fig. 9.33 Full extension of the finger, without extension deficits of the finger joints.

collapse or narrowing of the A2 pulley is inevitable, and the tendons are often edematous. In zone 2B, where the FDS tendon is bifurcated into two slips, I use two Tsuge repairs separately in each tendon slip; when the laceration is close to the insertion, I anchor the tendon slips to the phalanx. Treatment of the FDS tendon in zone 2D is straightforward, similar to the FDP tendon, except that the FDS is flatter and four or fewer strands are used.

In deciding surgical options relating to both the FDS and the pulleys, I generally seek to decrease the gliding contents appropriately (by not repairing or excising the FDS tendon) or enlarge the sheath (when both tendons are repaired primarily or only the FDP tendon is repaired at the delayed stage). The underlying idea is that the fibro-osseous digital flexor sheath tunnel is comparable to a tight fascia compartment of extremities; the edematous and healing tendons are easily compromised. Release of compression of the tendon to avoid overloading it during motion can be more vital to the success of treatment than providing it with sufficient surgical strength.

Surgical options currently advised to deal with tendons and pulleys in the most complex areas of finger flexor tendons are summarized in *Table 9.1.*

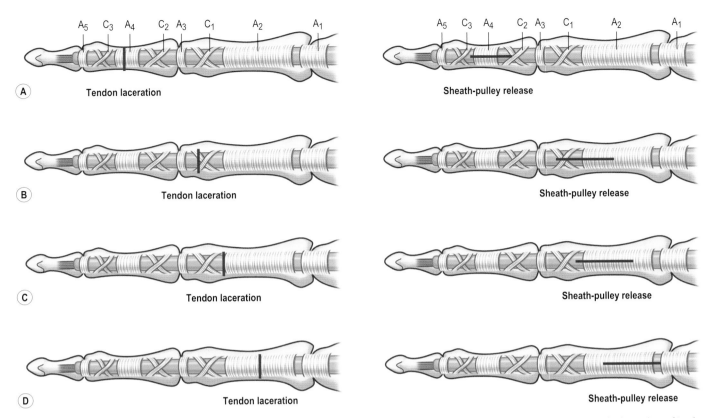

Fig. 9.34 Drawings depicting the length and areas of release of the pulley–sheath complex to decompress the repaired tendons, without bowstringing or loss of tendon function. **(A)** Release of the entire A4 pulley when the flexor digitorum profundus tendon has been cut around the A4 pulley and the tendon cannot pass easily beneath this pulley during surgery. **(B)** Release of a part of the sheath distal to the A2 pulley and the distal half of the A2 pulley, when the tendons are cut slightly distal to the A2 pulley. **(C)** Release of a short part of the sheath distal to the A2 pulley and the distal two-thirds of the A2 pulley when repairing tendons cut at the edge of, or in the distal part of, the A2 pulley. **(D)** Release of the proximal two-thirds of the A2 pulley when repairing a cut in the middle, or proximal part of, the A2 pulley.

Table 9.1 Summary of mechanical basis and surgical options advised to deal with the flexor digitorum superficialis (FDS) tendon and pulleys in zone 2 of the finger

Investigations	Area of FDS Insertion (2A)	Distal to A2 pulley (2B)	Beneath A2 pulley (2C)	Proximal to A2 pulley (2D)
Anatomic				
FDS tendon	Insertion	2 slips, dorsal to FDP, with vincula	Bifurcation	One single band, flattened palmar to FDP
Pulleys	A4, C2, narrow	A3, C1	A2, narrow	A1, PA
Biomechanical				
FDS tendon	No gliding	Not constricting FDP	Constricting FDP, as a moving and second "pulley"	Little constriction
Pulleys	A4 release is feasible[112]	May incise one pulley[107]	Partial release is feasible[22,111,112]	
Clinical options				
FDS tendon		Repair[174,214]	Resection or do not repair[21,23,150] Resect one slip[101]	Repair both tendons when possible
Pulleys	A4 venting[19,23,172]		Partial release[19,23,150,172] Pulley shortening or plasty[100,175]	

FDP, flexor digitorum profundus; PA, palmar aponeurosis.

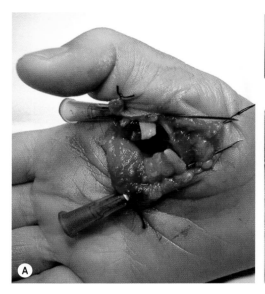

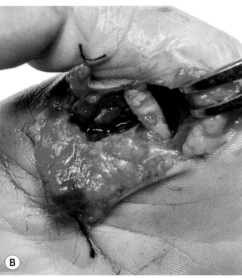

Fig. 9.35 A 9-year-old boy with a complete flexor pollicis longus (FPL) tendon cut. **(A)** The retracted proximal tendon end was found and temporarily fixed with a needle to accommodate tendon repair. **(B)** The FPL tendon was repaired with the six-strand M-Tang technique.

Zone 3, 4, and 5 injuries

The repair techniques for injured flexor tendons proximal to zone 2 are almost identical to those used in zone 2. These zones have a better prognosis because of richer vascularity around the tendon and lack of constricting pulleys over the tendons. Adhesions in these areas are less likely to impede tendon motion. Zone 4 tendon injuries are frequently accompanied by lacerations in the median nerve and arteries. The transverse carpal ligament may be partly opened to facilitate repairs and left partly open after tendon repairs. In most cases zone 5 tendon injuries are presented as multiple tendon lacerations with neurovascular injury. A wrist with transection of a majority of tendons, vessels, and nerves (at least 10 out of 15 of these structures, excluding palmaris longus) is called a "spaghetti" wrist.[179–183] A "spaghetti" wrist was reported to have an adverse effect on the recovery of the independent FDS action but not on the recovery of the digital range of motion.[183] In zone 5, repair of the FDS tendon is preferred, and early postoperative tendon motion is advised,[183–185] This favors independent movement of the superficialis.

FPL injuries

Repair of the injured FPL tendons in the thumb usually follows the same principles and methods of repair of the FDP tendon in fingers. Multistrand repairs are advised, and one or two pulleys can be vented to free tendon motion. Reports have shown that conventional two-strand repairs have a risk of rupture as high as 17%.[25,172] In a recent report from David Elliot's hand center, Giesen *et al.*[25] reported no ruptures and good function after using a six-strand Tang method without peripheral sutures in repairing 50 FPL tendons. In this case series, which reported the best outcomes of FPL tendon repairs thus far, the oblique pulley was vented and the sheath was not closed. The authors found that this six-strand repair was safe for early active mobilization and easier to perform than Kessler core sutures and elaborate Silfverskiöld sutures.

In repairing the FPL tendon, the proximal cut end of the tendon frequently retracts into the thenar muscles. This end can be retrieved with the techniques described for retracted

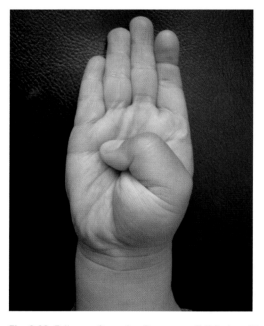

Fig. 9.36 Follow-up 8 months after surgery. Full flexion of the repaired thumb.

FDS and FDP tendons *(Figs 9.35–9.37)*. If the proximal stump of the FPL tendon has retracted proximal to the thenar muscles, a separate incision in the forearm is required to locate the stump. The FPL stump usually lies deep to the FCR tendon and the radial artery.

Injuries in children

Flexor tendon repairs in children have a better prognosis than those in adults.[186–190] As children may be less compliant with instructions to limit movement, the repaired digits are usually immobilized for 3–3.5 weeks after surgery. Either a two-strand or a four-strand repair can be used. In practice, many surgeons use a two-strand repair and achieve good return of function. The outcomes appear unaffected by whether a

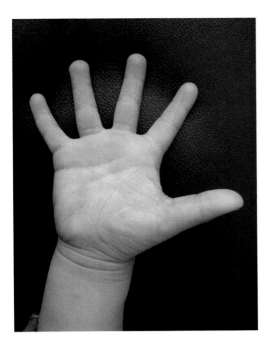

Fig. 9.37 Full extension of the thumb.

commonly in the ring finger. Closed tendon ruptures at the wrist can be associated with fractures in carpal bones.[203] Flexor pulleys are prone to sprains and ruptures during climbing. Rupture of the pulleys occurs in up to 20% of climbers.[204] The A2 pulley of the ring finger is the most often injured. Closed pulley ruptures are treated conservatively or by surgical reconstruction.

Leddy and Packer[200] classified close tendon ruptures into the following types:

I. The FDP tendon is avulsed from the phalanx and retracts into the palm. The vincula of the FDP tendon are disrupted. There is no active flexion of the DIP joint. A tender mass is present in the palm. The tendon should be reinserted within 7–10 days because the sheath collapse may prevent advancing the tendon distally during surgery. Muscle contracture may also prevent tendon advancement.

II. The FDP tendon retracts to the level of the PIP joint. This is the most common type. The sheath is not compromised, and muscle contracture does not develop easily. Repair may be attempted 1 month after injury.

III. A large bone fragment is attached to the FDP tendon. This bone fragment frequently prevents the tendon from retracting proximal to the A4 pulley. Bony fixation using a K-wire or a screw usually suffices.

IV. The FDP tendon avulses from the bony fragment. This type was added by Smith.[200] The avulsed tendon retracts beyond the middle phalanx and even into the palm. In treating type IV injuries, the bony fragment is attached into the distal phalanx first; then the avulsed tendon is advanced. Postoperatively, the DIP joint is immobilized for 4–5 weeks, or a gentle motion regime is prescribed.

Early recognition of closed tendon ruptures is of paramount importance. In cases where there is late diagnosis, primary repair is difficult or even impossible. Chronic cases require free tendon grafting.

two- or four-strand is used or whether the tendon is moved or immobilized early after surgery.[188,189] Navali and Rouhani[188] reported that both a two-strand and four-strand repair achieved good functional return, with no difference in range of active digital motion between the two methods. Elhassan *et al.*[189] reported that early postoperative motion and immobilization did not affect outcomes in children aged 2–14 years with injuries in zones 1 and 2.

Partial tendon lacerations

Laceration through less than 60% of the diameter of the tendon does not necessitate a repair by core sutures. An increased risk of triggering, entrapment, or ruptures is associated with partial laceration over 60%.[191–195] For lacerations less than 60%, the tendon wound can be trimmed to lessen the chance of entrapment by pulley edges and friction against the sheath. Alternatively, the cut portion of the tendon can be repaired with epitendinous stitches to smooth the tendon surface and to strengthen the tendon. Laceration of 60–80% requires at least an epitendinous repair[196–199] and is better repaired using a two-strand core suture through the cut portion. Laceration of 80–90% is treated identically to a complete laceration.

Closed rupture of the flexor tendons and pulleys

Traumatic FDP tendon avulsion from the tendon–bone junction accounts for a major portion of closed rupture cases.[200–203] The injury mechanism is hyperextension of the DIP joint, which subjects the FDP tendon to excessive load. The tendon disrupts at its insertion to the distal phalanx. Athletic injuries can lead to this type of injury. In football, wrestling, or rugby, when one player grabs another's jersey, a finger may be caught and pulled, resulting in disruption of flexor tendons. This injury ("jersey finger") is seen most

Postoperative care

With the exception of a few instances – such as tendon repairs in children, adults who are unable to follow through the protocol, or associated with fractures or particular health conditions – motion of repaired tendons should be initiated from the early postsurgical period. From the 1970s to the 1990s, Kleinert and Duran–Houser protocols were most popular. The protocols have evolved and the methods presently used in many clinics are combined active–passive regimes.

The modified Kleinert method

In the 1960s, Kleinert and associates introduced a controlled active extension–passive flexion motion protocol.[205] The wrist is palmarly flexed with a dorsal protective splint with 30–40° wrist flexion, 50–70° MCP joint flexion, and the IP joints are allowed full extension. Rubber bands are secured to the volar forearm and attached to the tip of the injured finger *(Fig. 9.38)*. Patients are allowed to extend the fingers actively and the fingers are brought back to flexion passively by the tensed

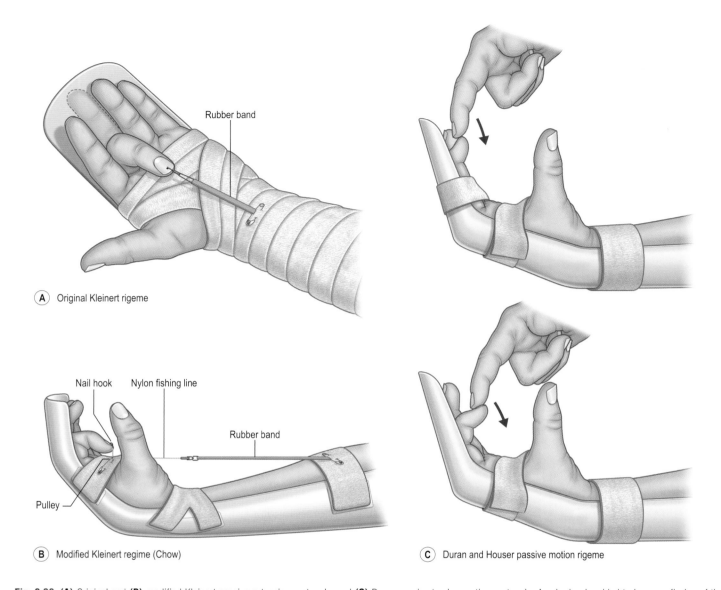

(A) Original Kleinert rigeme

(B) Modified Kleinert regime (Chow)

(C) Duran and Houser passive motion rigeme

Fig. 9.38 (A) Original and **(B)** modified Kleinert passive extension protocols, and **(C)** Duran passive tendon motion protocols. A volar bar is added to increase flexion of the interphalangeal joints in the modified Kleinert protocol.

rubber bands. This method was popularized in the late 1970s and 1980s. Later, rubber band traction was found to lead to flexion contractures of the finger. The original method was largely replaced by its modification with a palmar bar at the level of the MCP joint as a pulley for the rubber bands to create greater flexion of both the PIP and DIP joints **(Fig. 9.38)**.[206,207] In addition, the elastic band is detached at night and the fingers are strapped into extension within the splint to minimize the risk of flexion contractures of the fingers. In recent years, some surgeons have advised to abandon rubber band traction.

Duran–Houser method

This is a controlled passive finger flexion protocol without traction of rubber bands; it was introduced by Duran and Houser in the 1970s.[208] A dorsal splint is applied with the wrist in 20° flexion, the MCP joint in 50° flexion, and the IP joints

are allowed full extension **(Fig. 9.38)**. Within the first 4.5 weeks, the patients perform 10 passive DIP joint extensions with PIP and MCP joint flexions, and 10 passive PIP joint extensions with MCP and DIP joint flexions hourly within the splint **(Fig. 9.38)**. This protocol decreased the frequency of PIP joint contracture seen with Kleinert's rubber band traction.

Strickland and Gettle modified this protocol by adopting a Duran-like protocol for a four-strand tendon repair,[209] later known as the "Indianapolis method." This protocol consists of two splints, the dorsal-blocking splint (used during periods of rest and passive motion, with the wrist at 20–30° of flexion, MCP joints in 50° of flexion, and IP joints in neutral position) and a tenodesis splint (used when performing place and hold exercise). The latter hinged wrist splint permits the wrist position to be varied between flexion and extension. With the tenodesis splint, the patient passively flexes the digits while actively extending the wrist. The patients passively push their fingers into a passive composite fist with the wrist extended and hold for 5 seconds. Then the patients relax the wrist and let it descend into flexion. Patients are instructed to exercise 25 times per waking hour. Four weeks after surgery, active digital flexion and extension are instituted with the dorsal blocking splint still on and the tenodesis splint is discontinued. One week later, active composite fist followed by active extension of the wrist and digits is added to the program. When both flexor tendons are repaired in the digital sheath, differential motion of the two tendons should be practiced. Shifting the finger postures from straight, hook, and fist positions generates differential gliding of the two tendons.

Early active motion

In the late 1980s and early 1990s, protocols containing early active tendon motion components emerged. One requirement is that the tendon repairs be strong enough to tolerate tension during the motion. In 1989, the Belfast surgeons devised an active motion protocol,[210] which was later known as the "Belfast method." Postoperatively, a splint is applied from the elbow to the fingertips with the wrist in midflexion, the MCP joint at slightly less than 90° flexion, and the IP joints straight. The light dressing is removed from the digits and exercises are started 48 hours after surgery. Under supervision, the exercises consist of two passive movements followed by two active movements and are performed at 2-hour intervals. The hand is rested in elevation overnight. During the first week, the PIP joint is actively flexed through about 30° and the DIP joint through 5–10°. In subsequent weeks, the range of active motion is gradually increased. The splint is removed by the sixth week and blocking exercises of the IP joints are initiated when necessary. Variants of the Belfast method have been reported. In one of the variants – the "Billericay regime" – the wrist and the MCP joint are kept in a splint at 30° flexion respectively, and the splint is removed by the fifth week. The patient is instructed to perform 10 repetitions of the active finger flexion exercise hourly.[211]

Author's preferred combined active–passive method (Nantong regime)

After surgery, the hand is protected in a dorsal thermoplastic splint, with the wrist at 20–30° flexion, MCP joint at slight flexion, and the IP joints in extension for the initial 2.5 weeks *(Fig. 9.39)*.[19] We do not encourage patients to move the finger in the initial postoperative days; exercise starts at 3–5 days (in most cases, at 4 or 5 days) after surgery. Patients are instructed to flex the finger actively with gentle force 20–30 times in the morning, noon, evening, and before sleep, up to the range they feel comfortable with (usually from full extension to one-third or one-half of flexion range, and even increasing to two-thirds if achieved with ease). Active flexion over full range is not encouraged, unless it can be achieved very easily. At the beginning of each exercise session, the finger is passively flexed 10 or more times to lessen the overall resistance of finger joints and soft tissues during subsequent active flexion. In this 2.5-week period, full active extension is particularly encouraged, and prevention of extension deficits rather than achieving full range of active flexion is emphasized.

After 2.5 weeks, a new thermoplastic splint is made, and the wrist is splinted at 30° extension *(Fig. 9.39)*. Exercise of finger flexion, both passively and actively, is emphasized in this period. Active motion up to the midrange is required, and can proceed up to two-thirds (or full range). However, digital flexion from the midrange to full range, in particular over the final one-third of the flexion range, is usually achieved passively. In this period, we ensure passive flexion over a full range to prevent joint contracture and active flexion over an increasingly greater range, gradually approaching full flexion range, but discourage active forceful flexion of the finger over the final range where the tendon is subjected to the greatest load and is more vulnerable to rupture. Differential FDS and FDP motion exercise is encouraged throughout the first 5 weeks. From the sixth week, full active finger flexion is encouraged (which can be started earlier when flexion is judged to have less resistance). From 6 to 8 weeks, the splint is removed or used only at night.

The protocols described above represent several distinct categories of exercise. From communications with many hand surgeons and therapists, I have found that hand centers around the globe use variants of these protocols. Motion regimes for zone 4 and 5 repairs are generally not as complex as those described above. There is not yet universal agreement regarding the timing of initiating rehabilitation and frequency of digital flexion–extension motion. Theoretically, tendon adhesions start to develop from 10 days to 2 weeks after surgery. No studies have yet proven the necessity of starting exercise on the first day after surgery. It seems equally reasonable to commence exercise slightly later, though still within 1 week of surgery. Likewise, no studies have identified the optimal frequency of motion in each exercise episode or whether more frequent exercise leads to better results.

Experimental evidence supporting later commencement of tendon motion has been offered by Zhao *et al.*[118] of the Amadio group, and my colleagues Xie *et al.*[119] and Cao *et al.*[122] Digital edema increases resistance to motion, which peaks at 3–5 days.[120–122] Both Zhao *et al.*[118] and Cao *et al.*[122] suggest that motion should be commenced later (5 days after surgery).

Outcomes, prognosis, and complications

Review of outcomes reported over 20 years showed excellent or good active range of finger motion in more than three-fourths of primary tendon repairs.[14,17,19–21,25,210–233] Nevertheless, repair ruptures were documented in a majority of the reports. In the earlier part of this period, the rupture rates ranged from 4 to 10% in the finger flexors and from 3 to 17% in the FPL tendon of thumbs.[14,17,210–230] Adhesions remained the most common complication, preventing satisfactory return of active joint motion. Finger joint stiffness was reported fairly frequently as well. It is worth noting that most of these reports came from the finest hand centers in the world, and each team was supervised by at least one surgeon with expertise in treating tendon injuries. Therefore, the outcomes in a general hospital setting may reflect a lower level of success. Flexor tendon repairs might have been unsuccessful in a larger proportion of patients, with a greater incidence of repair ruptures, adhesion formations, or digital joint contracture.

Nevertheless, the past 20 years have seen impressive improvements in outcomes of flexor tendon repairs. In the

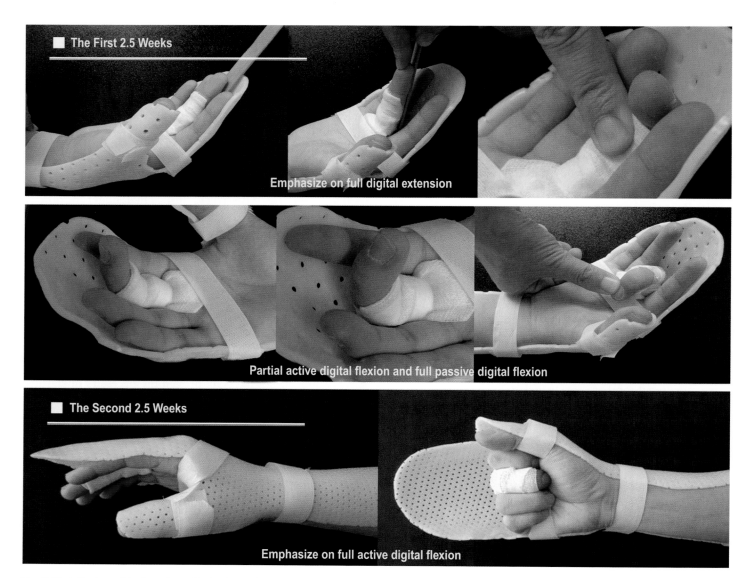

The First 2.5 Weeks

Emphasize on full digital extension

Partial active digital flexion and full passive digital flexion

The Second 2.5 Weeks

Emphasize on full active digital flexion

Fig. 9.39 Author's combined passive–active tendon motion protocol. This protocol is divided into two 2.5-week periods. In the first 2.5 weeks, with wrist in slight flexion, finger extension is emphasized. Only partial active digital flexion is allowed, but full range of passive motion is implemented. In the second 2.5 weeks, with wrist in extension, full active finger flexion is encouraged. This protocol incorporates the concept of synergistic wrist and finger motion. When the wrist is flexed, finger extension is less tensed; when the wrist is extended, finger flexion is less tensed.

late 1980s and early 1990s, Small et al.[210] and Cullen et al.[212] used a two-strand repair and postoperative active motion and had repair ruptures in 6–9% of the repairs, with overall good or excellent results in 78% of digits. Elliot et al.[211] reported a series of 233 patients with complete division of the digital flexor tendons, treated with a two-strand core repair with a controlled active motion regimen. Thirteen (5.8%) fingers and five (16.6%) thumbs suffered tendon ruptures during the mobilization. In the same period, multistrand core repairs were reported by Savage and Risitano,[14] and Tang et al.,[17,214] together with active or active–passive motion therapies.

Trumble et al.[233] used a four-strand Strickland core suture and a running epitendinous suture to repair zone 2 flexor tendon lacerations in 119 digits (103 patients) and examined postoperative therapies in a multicenter prospective randomized trial between 1996 and 2002. They documented significantly greater range of digital motion, smaller digital flexion contractures, and greater patient satisfaction in the active motion group than in the passive motion group. Associated nerve injury, multiple digit injuries, and smoking were factors leading to poorer outcomes. Patients treated by a certified hand therapist had better motion and less severe contractures. Two digits had tendon ruptures in each group. The study supports the combination of multistrand tendon repair and postoperative early active motion therapy in zone 2 primary flexor tendon repairs.

Of note, reports of multistrand core sutures in recent years documented minimal or zero repair ruptures. A stronger surgical repair combined with release of the pulleys offered great safety to the postoperative active motion exercise. After combined use of multistrand repairs and pulley releases, most

Box 9.4 Methods to optimize outcomes

- Master tendon anatomy in detail and use atraumatic techniques throughout surgery
- To expose the tendons, open a window in the synovial sheath, or open the A2 pulley partially or the entire A4 pulley if the repair site overlaps or locates slightly distal to these structures
- May release the distal two-thirds parts of the A2 pulley, where it is the most narrow and most constrictive to the tendons, when the flexor digitorum profundus tendon is cut just distal or under the pulley. A portion of this pulley should be kept intact during surgery
- Adopt a stronger core suture method, with sufficient suture purchase and appropriate locks on tendons
- Add peripheral sutures to smooth the repair and to prevent gap formation
- Properly combine passive and active finger motion into postoperative motion protocols. Fully extend and flex the finger passively, followed by active finger flexion over a certain range. Active motion over the final one-half or one-third is discouraged in the initial weeks to avoid tendon overload (rupture). Postoperatively, apply motion therapy for at least 5–6 weeks
- Passive finger motion before active motion substantially decreases the overall resistance to digital motion, lessening the chance of repair ruptures during active motion
- Surgical tendon repairs are performed by experienced surgeons, and the unit should have established postsurgical rehabilitation guidelines

Table 9.2 Criteria of assessment of functional outcomes of flexor tendon repairs

% return of motion*	Grip strength†	Quality of motion‡	Function grade
Strickland criteria (1980)			
85–100 (>150°)			Excellent
70–84 (125–149°)			Good
50–70 (90–124°)			Fair
0–49 (<90°)			Poor
Moiemen–Elliot criteria (2000) for zone 1 injuries, the distal interphalangeal (DIP) joint only			
85–100 (>62°)			Excellent
70–84 (51–61°)			Good
50–70 (37–50°)			Fair
0–49 (<36°)			Poor
Tang criteria (2007)			
90–100	+	Excellent or good	Excellent +
	–	Poor	Excellent –
70–89	+	Excellent or good	Good +
	–	Poor	Good –
50–69			Fair
30–49			Poor
0–29			Failure

*Percentage return of the normal (contralateral) hand. Strickland and Tang criteria use sum of active range of motion of the DIP and proximal interphalangeal joints. Moiemen–Elliot criteria use motion of the DIP joint only.
†Grip strength is recorded as + when it is greater than that of the contralateral hand (the nondominant hand), or over 70% of that of the contralateral hand (dominant hand). Otherwise, grip strength is considered abnormal and recorded as –.
‡Quality of motion is rated on the basis of direct observation of finger motion by surgeons. It is recorded as "excellent" when all three aspects – motion arc, coordination, and speed – are normal; as "good" when any two are normal; and as "poor" when only one, or none, is normal.
Function is graded as excellent or good when either the grip strength is – or quality of motion is "poor."

cases returned to good to excellent active range of digital motion with zero tendon ruptures (*Box 9.4*).[19,24,25] My own clinical outcomes also indicate that good to excellent return of function can be achieved fairly consistently by means of multistrand tendon repairs, venting of pulleys, and well-designed combined passive and active motion protocols.

Strickland and Glogovac criteria (*Table 9.2*) are most commonly used methods in assessment of outcomes.[15] Moiemen and Elliot criteria (*Table 9.2*),[20] which specifically evaluate the active range of flexion of the DIP joint, are favored by surgeons who record outcomes of zone 1 repair. The total active range of motion (TAM) method proposed by the American Society for Surgery of the Hand is also used, and the Buck–Gramcko method is used often by German-speaking hand societies.[153] Among the less popular methods currently used are White, Tubiana, and tip-to-palm distance methods. I currently use a criterion that implements a more stringent measure of range of active finger motion, as well as grip strength and quality of motion, into the grading system (*Table 9.2*).[19]

Outcomes of flexor tendon repairs are affected by patient age, extent and zones of injuries, timing of the repairs, postoperative exercise, and the expertise of the surgeon. Results of tendon repairs in children are generally better than those in adults. Tendon repairs associated with extended soft-tissue damage or accompanied by phalangeal fractures are likely to have worse outcomes.

Secondary procedures

Secondary tendon repairs are achieved by free tendon grafting, or a staged reconstruction. These procedures are reserved for served tendons that could not be repaired primarily or for lengthy tendon defects. These techniques, developed by the early masters of hand surgery,[38–42,234–244] remain largely unchanged today despite refinements in tendon junction methods, use of novel suture meterials, and widespread adoption of postsurgical rehabilitation in recent decades (*Box 9.5*).[245–249]

Free tendon grafting

Indications and contraindications

Most traumatic lacerations of the digital flexor tendons are now treated with end-to-end tenorraphy primarily. Only some cases require secondary repairs by means of free tendon grafting. Tendon grafting is indicated: (1) when the lacerated tendons are not treated during primary or delayed primary

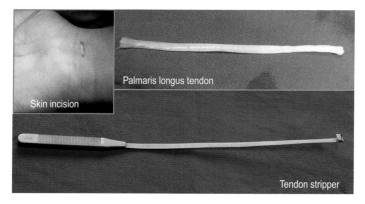

Fig. 9.40 Harvesting a tendon graft through a small skin incision, using a tendon tripper.

stage; (2) when the primary repairs have ruptured and cannot be re-repaired directly; and (3) in the cases not indicative of primary tendon repairs because of severe contamination, infection, lengthy loss of tendon substance, extensive destruction of the pulleys, or accompanying injuries. Patients who have serious scarring in the tendon bed or failed previous efforts at secondary flexor tendon procedures are appropriate for a staged tendon reconstruction, rather than one-stage tendon grafting. Surgeons sometimes need to decide according to intraoperative findings, such as severity of scarring and pulley destruction.

Before surgery is attempted, the soft-tissue wound should be well healed, with supple passive motion of the hand. Physical therapy is prescribed to improve the range of motion of the digits if passive joint motion is limited substantially. Boyes and Stark[42] classified the conditions associated with the cases of tendon grafts and surgical prognosis is worsened by poor hand condition. Lack of passive range of joint motion is contraindicated for one-stage tendon grafting, but may be suitable for staged tendon reconstruction. The timing of tendon grafting is usually 3 months after injury.

Donor tendons

The donors are palmaris longus, plantaris, long toe extensors, or in rare instances the FDS tendon from a normal finger (**Figs 9.40 and 9.41**). The palmaris longus tendon (about 15 cm) from the ipsilateral limb is a frequently used donor and is appropriate for a palm-to-fingertip graft. It can be easily harvested through a short transverse incision over the tendon just proximal to the flexion crease of the wrist. The tendon is divided and grasped with a hemostat, while a tendon stripper is advanced slowly into the proximal forearm. Care must be taken to protect the median nerve trunk lying beheath the tendon and its cutaneous branch of the median nerve.[250] Because this tendon is absent in about 15% of all hands,[251] examination to confirm its presence is essential before surgery. The plantaris tendon is equally satisfactory for a graft, which is obtained by an incision medial to the Achilles tendon and use of a tendon stripper. The length of this tendon (25 cm) is well suited for a long distal forearm-to-fingertip graft.

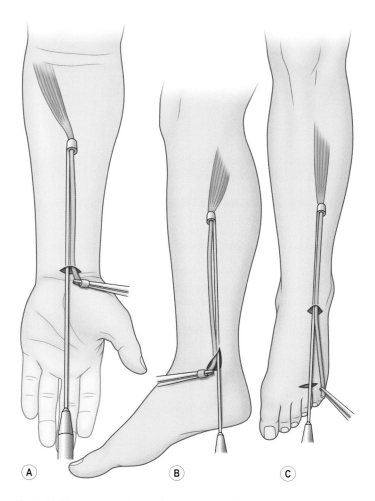

Fig. 9.41 Three common donors of tendon grafts: **(A)** palmaris longus tendon; **(B)** plantaris; and **(C)** toe extensors.

However, this tendon is absent in 7–20% of limbs, and its presence cannot be predicted preoperatively.[252,253] Extensor digitorum longus tendons to the second, third, and fourth toes, the extensor indicis proprius, the extensor digit quinti proprius and the FDS tendon to the fifth finger can be used as well. In my clinic, I use the palmaris longus tendon most frequently and place the proximal junction in the palm.

Operative techniques

The flexor tendon is exposed through a volar Bruner's incision or the midaxial approach.[254–258] Integrity of the major annular pulleys is important to the function of the graft. At least the A2 and A4 pulleys should be preserved. If possible, other annular pulleys such as A1 or A3 and a part of the synovial sheath are preserved to foster better gliding of the grafted tendon. If a series of annular pulleys are found to be destroyed, reconstruction of pulleys is necessary. Most cases requiring reconstruction of multiple pulleys need to proceed to staged tendon reconstruction.

The distal junction of the graft is placed at the fingertip. The common method is to suture the graft directly to the residual FDP stump or bury it under an osteoperiosteal flap in the volar phalanx (*Fig. 9.13*).[258–260] In the latter case, the straight needles are passed through the distal phalangeal drill hole and exit over the proximal portion of the nail. After emerging from the nail surface, the needles are passed through a gauze pad or a sponge, and through the holes of an overlaying button. The sutures are tied over the button to anchor the graft. Additional sutures are used to secure the FDP tendon stump to the graft. Alternative methods are available, as shown in zone 1 repair (*Fig. 9.13*).[156,158,159,244] In children, drill holes at the distal phalanx may damage the open epiphyses; the graft is sutured directly to the stump of the profundus instead. Either at the palm or in the forearm, the proximal junction of the graft is achieved by a Pulvertaft weave suture to the proximal stump of the flexor tendon (*Fig. 9.42*). Placement of the junction at the palm requires only a shorter graft and preserves the function of lumbrical muscles. Care is taken to avoid suturing the tendon to the lumbrical muscle, because this tends to increase the tension in the muscle. Placement of the junction above the wrist allows easy adjustment of the tension of the graft, and the scar may be less severe. In the author's experience, a Pulvertaft weave suture is appropriate for the proximal junction in both areas (*Fig. 9.43*), and the finger is held in slightly greater flexion than in the resting position when the proximal stump is sutured (*Fig. 9.44*).

Postoperatively, the wrist is held in a position of 30–40° flexion, with the MCP joints flexed to 60–70°, and the IP joints at rest in almost full extension. The traditional recommendation is 3 weeks of immobilization within a dorsal splint applied from the fingertip to below the elbow, followed by active exercise of the digits with the protection of a dorsal blocking splint. Some surgeons advocate passive or active finger motion under cautious supervision from a few days after surgery if the graft junctions are strong. Most surgeons still prefer to immobilize the grafted digits for at least 3 weeks to avoid tension on the tendon and to allow some revascularization of the graft. More vigorous exercise can be instituted at 6 weeks after surgery.

The need for tendon graft or reconstruction is controversial when the superficialis tendon is fully functional, but the FDP tendon is cut and has not been repaired directly within 3–4 weeks of trauma.[261–267] There is a risk of losing function if a profundus graft fails. However, such operations are worth the risk in selected cases, such as in young people with a

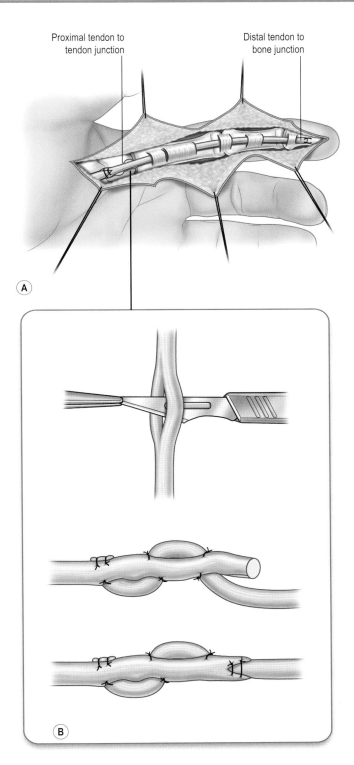

Proximal tendon to tendon junction

Distal tendon to bone junction

(A)

(B)

Fig. 9.42 Skin incision and the method of free tendon grafting to reconstruct the function of digital flexion. As many annular pulleys as possible are preserved. **(A)** The tendon junctions are placed outside the flexor sheath region. To make a proximal junction of the graft with the end of a digital flexor tendon, the Pulvertaft weave technique is commonly used (shown in detail in B). The junction is placed at either palm or distal forearm. The graft is weaved with the digital flexor through holes in the tendons created by a knife **(B, i–iii)**.

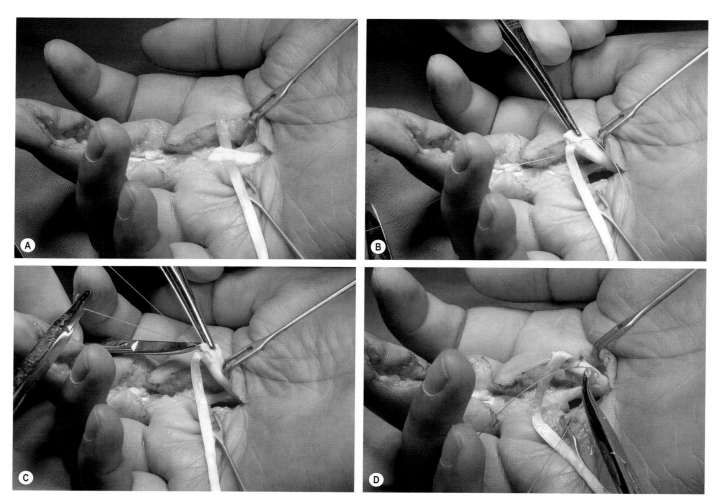

Fig. 9.43 A case of free tendon grafting with a Pulvertaft weave junction of the graft with a digital flexor tendon in the palm. **(A)** The graft was weaved into the digital flexor tendon. **(B and C)** Two sutures were added in either side of the graft and the digital flexor. **(D)** Completion of the weave tendon repair.

reasonable need for active DIP joint flexion. The procedures are similar to those described above. A thinner donor tendon is preferable and the A2 pulley can be shortened, but a series of pulleys are preserved *(Fig. 9.45)*. Alternatively, one slip of the FDS tendon can be removed to favor passage of the graft. During the procedure, while passing the graft through the FDS tendon, injury may occur that results in the formation of adhesions and a loss of finger function. Overall, caution must be exercised with patient selection. Patients with intact superficialis tendon may adapt nicely and require no treatment. Surgeons should fully inform patients about expected gain of function versus risks of this operation.

When the superficialis tendon is intact and the DIP joint is not stable, the DIP joint can be fused or tenodesed in slight flexion. In the presence of a functional FDS tendon, the combination of MCP and PIP joint motion produces approximately 85% of the arc covered by the finger in flexion.

Staged tendon reconstruction

Indications

This operation is indicated in cases with badly scarred digits, as a result of injury or multiple failed attempts to restore

tendon continuity and gliding. The techniques were developed in the middle of the 20th century by Bassett and Carroll,[44] Hunter, Paneva-Holevich, Schneider *et al.*[268–279] This operation consists of procedures in two stages. In the first stage, the tendon and scar from the tendon bed are excised, but the pulleys are preserved or reconstructed. A Dacron-reinforced silicone tendon implant is inserted into the tendon bed to maintain the tunnel and to stimulate the formation of a mesothelium-lined pseudosheath. Following maturation of the sheath, a tendon is grafted in lieu of the implant in the second stage.

Techniques: the first stage

The involved finger is exposed through a volar zigzag incision and the incision is continued to the lumbrical origin level of the palm *(Fig. 9.46)*. The tendons and sheath (pulleys) are usually found embedded within scars. The tendons are excised with a 1-cm stump of the profundus tendon retained at its distal insertion. The critically located annular pulleys are carefully dissected out of scars. All potential useful pulley materials are preserved. When a series of pulleys are damaged, critically located pulleys (A2 and A4) should be reconstructed; this is an important part of the reconstruction. One method is

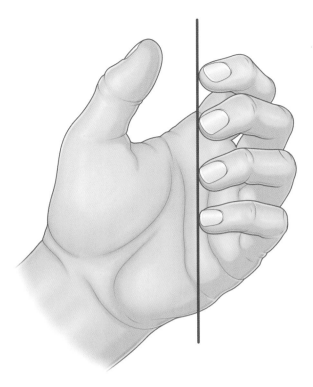

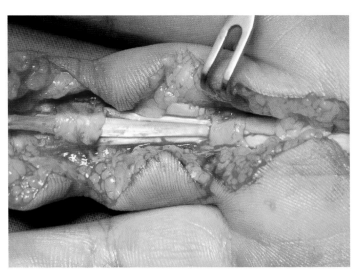

Fig. 9.45 A case of reconstruction of the flexor digitorum profundus tendon in the presence of an intact flexor digitorum superficialis (FDS) tendon. A palmaris longus tendon was harvested as a graft. A series of pulleys (A4, a part of the A2, and A1) were preserved. The thin palmaris longus tendon fits well within the pulleys and intact bifurcating FDS tendon in the finger.

Fig. 9.44 Tension status of the fingers at the time of suturing the proximal tendon junction of a graft. With the wrist in neutral position, the fingers are slightly more flexed than at the resting position, with each finger falling into slightly more flexion than its radial neighboring fingers.

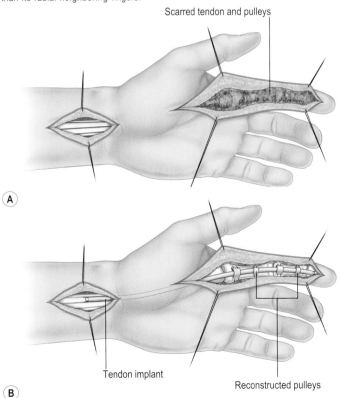

Fig. 9.46 (A) In stage 1 an extensive scar is found after exposure. The scar and the tendon are excised. **(B)** A tendon implant is placed into the scarred tendon bed. The annular pulleys are preserved. The proximal end of the tendon implant is not sutured and is left free.

to use a tendon graft, either a portion of an excised flexor tendon or the palmaris longus tendon, and wrap it around the phalanx twice to obtain sufficient width, but place it deeper than the extensor mechanism in the proximal phalanx or superficial to the extensors in the middle phalanx *(Fig. 9.47)*. Another method is to make use of one rim of a residual pulley, and a tendon graft or a part of the extensor retinaculum is woven back and forth to form a volar part of the residual pulley. A slip of the FDS tendon can be used to make a pulley as well. In the presence of flexion contracture of the finger joint, check-rein extensions of the palmar plate and the accessory collateral ligaments are divided to release the contracture. The profundus tendon is transected at the midpalm.

A set of tendon implants is then tried to determine the appropriate size of the implant, which is judged by the tightness of the digital pulleys and the expected size of the tendon graft in the second stage. In adults, 4-mm implants are often used; these are close in size to the tendon graft. After insertion of the implant underneath the pulleys, the implant should be movable in the tendon bed with minimal resistance. The distal anchor of the implant can be created in several ways *(Fig. 9.48)*. A second incision is made in the distal forearm. The implant is then passed from the proximal palm to the distal forearm using a tendon passer. After the implant is seated, traction is placed on the proximal end of the implant to make sure that it glides freely. A tunnel is created with blunt dissection proximally over the profundus muscle in the proximal forearm. The implant is laid into this tunnel and a space proximal to the implant is ensured for implant migration during exercise.

Postoperatively, the wrist is held with a short arm posterior splint in slight flexion (30°) and the MCP joint in marked

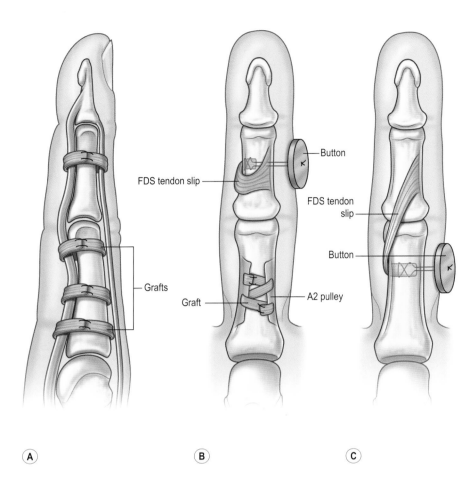

FDS tendon slip

Grafts

Graft

Button

FDS tendon slip

Button

A2 pulley

(A)   (B)   (C)

Fig. 9.47 Methods of flexor pulley reconstruction.
(A) Reconstruction of the A2 and A4 pulleys using flexor tendon grafts passed circumferentially around proximal and middle phalanges. The tendon graft passes deeper to the extensor apparatus at the proximal phalangeal level and superficial to the extensors at the middle phalangeal level.
(B) A tendon graft is weaved through a remnant of the A2 pulley to reconstruct the A2 pulley. **(C)** Use of a slip of flexor digitorum superficialis (FDS) tendon for middle digital pulley reconstruction.

flexion. Passive wrist and digital motion can be started 1 week later. By 8 weeks, full activity is permitted, except powerful grip until 12 weeks. In cases with pulley reconstruction, the fingers must be protected by circumferential taping or orthoplast rings.

The second stage

The second-stage operation is planned approximately 3 months later. A small incision is made adjacent to the distal implant–tendon junction *(Fig. 9.49)*. A portion of the previous incision can be used. After disconnecting the implant from the distal FDP tendon stump, the implant is tagged. A free tendon graft is harvested and inserted into the pseudosheath tunnel. Care is taken not to open the pseudosheath proximal to the DIP joint and to avoid injury to any pulleys. The appropriate motor tendon is then selected. The profundus mass is chosen for grafts to the middle, ring, and small fingers. For index finger reconstruction, the profundus tendon to the index finger is chosen as a motor. For thumb reconstruction, the FPL or one of the FDS muscles is used. The proximal junction can be placed in the palm, but in most cases, it is located in the distal forearm. The tendon graft is attached to one end of the implant. The implant is pulled out through the pseudosheath from one end. The distal tendon junction is secured as previously described for free tendon grafting. Placement of the proximal juncture in the forearm offers the graft a favorable

environment for tendon gliding. Proper tension on the graft is essential for function.

Paneva-Holevich[268] advocated that the FDS tendon should be used proximal to the injury from the same finger as the graft source. This procedure evolved to include placement of a tendon implant together with suturing the proximal FDS to the proximal FDP end at the first stage, and implant removal, grafting the FDS into the finger at the second stage, which yielded favorable results.[269,279]

Postoperatively, the wrist is held in a position identical to that for a tendon graft.

Some surgeons immobilize the hand for 3–4 weeks; others favor an early protected motion program initiated days after surgery. Therapy proceeds carefully through passive and light active motion until at least 6 weeks, when the tensile strength of the tendon and its junctures is sufficiently strong to tolerate more vigorous motion.

Tenolysis

Indications

Tenolysis is indicated when the passive range of digital motion greatly exceeds the range of active flexion several months after direct end-to-end tendon repair or tendon grafting.[234,280,281] Tendon trauma with severe damage to peritendinous tissues

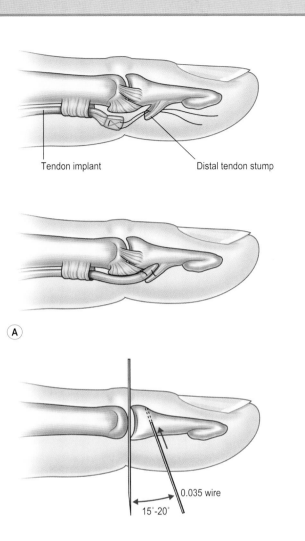

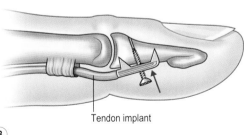

Fig. 9.48 Distal junction of the tendon implant in stage 1. **(A)** The distal junction wire method. A figure-of-eight suture of a monofilament wire (no. 32) is placed in the implant and sutured to the flexor digitorum profundus stump. Additional sutures are supplemented on each side of the implant. **(B)** Screw-plate fixation method. A self-tapping Woodruff screw (2 mm) is used, inserted into a drill hole in the phalanx using a K-wire (0.035-inch (0.1 cm)).

or compound injuries (such as digital or palm replantation) has a greater chance of adhesion formation, thus is more likely to require tenolysis as later surgery.[282] Children can also be candidates for this surgery.[283]

The prerequisites for this operation are: (1) all fractures are healed; (2) wounds have reached equilibrium with soft, pliable skin and subcutaneous tissues, and minimal reactions around the incision scars; and (3) joint contractures must have been corrected and a normal or near-normal passive range of digital

motion achieved. The exact optimal timing of tenolysis remains controversial.[234,284–287] It is reasonable to consider tenolysis if the desired range of motion is not achieved after 3 months of therapy. At least 3 months should have passed since the direct repair or graft to allow necessary healing and revascularization of tendons, so as to avoid endangering tendon strength. To assess the patient's final function reliably, 4–6 months are usually required.[234] However, there is no absolute criteria for how poor the range of motion must be to indicate tenolysis. Surgeons should consider the patient's age, occupational requirements, and functionality of the hand in making a decision. Preoperatively, patients should be informed that intraoperative findings may be incompatible with tenolysis; thus the surgeons need to proceed to the first step of staged reconstruction on finding serious destruction of pulleys or a lengthy lysed tendon segment.

Anesthesia

Active involvement of the patient in assessing tendon mobility and adequacy of release is a key step of surgery. This is achieved by using sedative anesthesia, combined with local anesthesia at the operation area.[234,288] I use 2% lidocaine (without epinephrine) infiltrated locally in the subcutaneous tissues or as a digital nerve block at the metacarpal level. Patients are awakened easily and cooperate dynamically during surgery. Axillary block or general anesthesia is used if the surgeon expects an extensive operation, such as tenolysis in multiple digits, a staged reconstruction procedure, or if the patient is unlikely to tolerate surgery with local anesthesia.

Operative techniques

Through either a Bruner or midlateral incision, dissection proceeds from the unaffected area to the affected area. Tenolysis requires wider surgical exposure. All limiting adhesions are meticulously divided and care is taken to define the borders of the flexor tendons. During dissection, some surgeons advise preservation of the sheath as much as possible, but others prefer to excise the synovial sheath. Regardless, the major pulleys should be maintained, and the synovial sheath embedded within the scar is removed. It is necessary to maintain the A2 and A4 pulleys at a minimum. If possible, the A3 pulley and its adjacent sheath are also preserved. A variety of instruments may aid in dissection of the scarred tendons from inner surfaces of the major pulleys.[288–290] Whenever possible, the FDS and FDP tendons are separated from one another. In some cases with severe adhesions, the FDS tendon has to be resected locally. Dissection is continued until normal tissues are revealed and no scar around the tendon is visible. Adequacy of the release is then checked by active digital flexion of the patient or by a gentle proximal traction on the proximal part of the tendon *(Box 9.6)*. A separate proximal incision in the palm can be created to pull the tendon. The quality of the tendon and integrity of the pulleys are checked. If tendon continuity is maintained only by scar or greater than one-third of the tendon width is lost, the tendon is unlikely to function properly and the case should proceed to staged tendon reconstruction. If the critical pulleys are destroyed, it is appropriate to proceed to pulley reconstruction.

Over the years, many attempts have been made to develop strategies to block or limit adhesion formation.[291–302] Thus far,

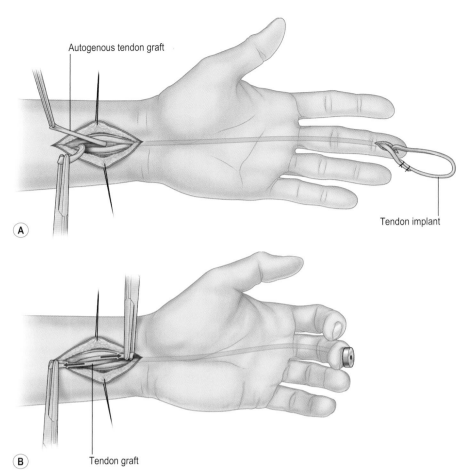

Autogenous tendon graft

Tendon implant

(A)

Tendon graft

(B)

Fig. 9.49 In stage 2, the tendon implant is replaced by a tendon graft. **(A)** The implant is exposed through a small incision at the distal part of the finger. After being disconnected from the flexor digitorum profundus tendon stump, the implant is sutured to the tendon graft. The implant is pulled proximally through the newly formed sheath to lead the grafted tendon. **(B)** The graft has been tunneled in the hand. The distal tendon junction is completed similarly to tendon grafting. The proximal junction of the graft is made.

Box 9.6 Tenolysis: technical pearls

- Local anesthesia is advised, to allow active finger flexion when needed during surgery
- Ensure adequate surgical exposure and start dissection from the border of adhesions
- Strictly preserve the critically located annular pulleys (A2 and A4 as a minimal)
- Check mobility of released tendon to confirm adequacy of surgery before completion
- Postoperative motion is paramount to the success of this procedure
- Rigor of motion regimes is decided according to intraoperative findings of the released tendons. Motion exercise should always be applied and continued for 4–6 weeks

few of these attempts have reliably reduced adhesions clinically and are used routinely. Some surgeons favor the use of steroids.[286] One multicenter clinical trial indicated the benefits of using a hyaluronan gel in reducing adhesions after tenolysis.[303]

Postoperative treatment

Oral analgesics usually alleviate pain during the postoperative period. Transcutaneous placement of local anesthetic catheters may be considered for patients with low pain thresholds or those undergoing extensive operations. Repeated digital nerve block can also be used.[304] Active motion of the fingers can begin on the first day after surgery. Some surgeons advocate waiting for several days or until soft-tissue inflammation and pain subside to start motion.

Postoperative tendon movement is critical to the success of tenolysis and remains the most effective method to prevent recurrence of adhesions.[305–309] The amplitude, frequency, and forces of motion should be decided based on intraoperative findings. The surgeons should directly discuss with the therapists to consolidate a therapy program. A tendon appearing nearly normal in a minimally scarred bed with a strong pulley system is appropriate for a more vigorous motion protocol. When a tendon is of poor quality – with a dense scar, a lysed segment, or a decrease in tendon caliber – or if pulleys have been reconstructed, gentle active motion or delayed initiation of the finger motion is indicated.[234] In this instance, a "place and hold" maneuver after passive digital motion into full flexion is useful to reduce tension and the likelihood of tendon disruption. Passive motion of the fingers is helpful in preventing finger joint contractures and in decreasing the resistance to active finger movement. The motion program is usually continued for 4–6 weeks.

Access the complete references list online at http://www.expertconsult.com

11. Verdan CE. Primary repair of flexor tendons. *J Bone Joint Surg (Am)*. 1960;42:647–657.

14. Savage R, Risitano G. Flexor tendon repair using a "six strand" method of repair and early active mobilization. *J Hand Surg (Br)*. 1989;14:396–399.

19. Tang JB. Indications, methods, postoperative motion and outcome evaluation of primary flexor tendon repairs in zone 2. *J Hand Surg (Eur)*. 2007;32:118–129.

    This article provides a comprehensive and updated review of the current indications for primary tendon repairs in zone 2. The author's techniques of multistrand repairs and rehabilitation are detailed. Most importantly, the author defines the needs, mechanical basis, and areas of releasing the critical parts of the major digital annular pulleys to facilitate tendon repairs. The author highlights the importance of releasing the critical pulley parts and strong surgical repairs in achieving predictable primary flexor tendon repairs in this most difficult area. Subdivision of zone 2 and novel criteria for outcome evaluation are also presented in this article.

25. Giesen T, Sirotakova M, Copsey AJ, et al. Flexor pollicis longus primary repair: further experience with the Tang technique and controlled active mobilisation. *J Hand Surg (Eur)*. 2009;34:758–761.

    This clinical study reported the most up-to-date clinical outcomes of repairs of lacerated flexor pollicis longus (FPL) tendons from a renowned center dealing with flexor tendon injuries. These authors have made a series of reports of their results in treating FPL injuries over the past two decades; this most recent report documents their outcomes in 50 FPL injuries. With a six-strand core tendon repair alone (without peripheral repairs), they achieved good or excellent functional recovery in 80% of thumbs, with zero tendon rupture with an active motion regime. These are the best clinical results of FPL tendon repairs reported thus far. It is worth noting that the authors did not elaborate peripheral sutures in these FPL tendon repairs, and the oblique pulley in the thumb was vented to accommodate tendon repairs.

42. Boyes JH, Stark HH. Flexor-tendon grafts in the fingers and thumb. A study of factors influencing results in 1000 cases. *J Bone Joint Surg (Am)*. 1971;53:1332–1342.

    This classic article reported perhaps the largest case series of free tendon grafting in the fingers and thumbs. The authors analyzed the factors influencing the prognosis for free tendon grafting and showed that the tendon-grafting procedure used can produce clinically acceptable function. However, hand conditions are extremely important. Prognostic factors include conditions of the soft tissues and joints. Extensively scarred tendon bed and joint damage led to the worst prognosis after tendon graft surgeries.

46. Hunter JM, Salisbury RE. Flexor-tendon reconstruction in severely damaged hands. A two-stage procedure using a silicone-Dacron reinforced gliding prosthesis prior to tendon grafting. *J Bone Joint Surg (Am)*. 1971;53:829–852.

150. Elliot D. Primary flexor tendon repair – operative repair, pulley management and rehabilitation. *J Hand Surg (Br)*. 2002;27:507–513.

    This article summarized developments in surgical tendon repair techniques, methods of venting the annular pulleys, and active tendon motion regimes for primary flexor tendon repairs in the hand. Of particular clinical interest, the authors reviewed methods of early active or combined passive–active tendon motion (representing a current trend in digital flexor tendon rehabilitation) and the pulley-venting procedure that the author and his colleagues have been using in their practice.

172. Tang JB. Clinical outcomes associated with flexor tendon repair. *Hand Clin*. 2005;21:199–210.

205. Kleinert HE, Schepel S, Gill T. Flexor tendon injuries. *Surg Clin North Am*. 1981;61:267–286.

234. Strickland JW. Delayed treatment of flexor tendon injuries including grafting. *Hand Clin*. 2005;21:219–243.

    This article provides an update on historical developments of surgical techniques, the author's personal approaches, and current practice of these secondary repair procedures, which are generally considered classic operations. Little has changed over recent decades.

10

Extensor tendon injuries

Kai Megerle and Günter Germann

SYNOPSIS

- A thorough understanding of the complex anatomy is crucial for successful treatment of extensor tendon injuries.
- Injuries are classified into nine anatomic zones. Treatment strategies vary considerably according to the location of the lesion, ranging from splinting to tendon grafting.
- Minimal variations in tendon length may result in considerable alteration in range of motion.
- As in flexor tendon injuries, postoperative care is an essential part of the treatment concept.
- Closed ruptures of the extensor tendon at the level of the distal interphalangeal (DIP) and proximal interphalangeal (PIP) joints are typically treated conservatively.
- Lacerations at the level of the metacarpophalangeal (MP) joint (zone V) are not infrequently caused by human bites and are prone to infection unless thoroughly debrided.
- Ruptures of the sagittal bands may result in subluxation of the extensor tendon at the level of the MP joint.
- The swan-neck deformity is characterized by DIP joint flexion and PIP joint hyperextension. It can be caused by an untreated mallet injury or palmar plate laxity.
- The boutonnière deformity is characterized by hyperextension of the DIP joint and PIP joint flexion. It can be caused by rupture of the central slip of the extensor tendon or palmar subluxation of the lateral bands.
- Complex injuries to the dorsum of the hand can involve skin, tendon, and bone. Adequate debridement is of paramount importance. Before reconstructing tendons, fractures must be stabilized and stable soft-tissue coverage must be provided.

Access the Historical Perspective section online at
http://www.expertconsult.com

Introduction

Injuries to the extensor tendons are frequently underestimated. Several reasons might contribute to this phenomenon, including easy access to the tendons due to the thin soft-tissue envelope, their extrasynovial nature, and limited retraction. However, in contrast to common belief, injuries to the extensor tendon apparatus are often more difficult to treat than those of flexor tendons. First of all, a thorough understanding of the complex interactions between the long extensor tendons and the intrinsic muscles of the hand is necessary to achieve good postoperative results. Second, the extensor apparatus consists of superficial, thin structures that are very close to the underlying bones, which makes them prone to develop severe adhesions. Moreover, their excursion amplitude is limited, so that even subtle lengthening or shortening will result in severe restrictions of range of motion. Postoperative regimes vary considerably in respect to the exact location of the lesion and have to be selected carefully.

However, not only the tendon itself but also the surrounding soft tissues have to be taken into consideration when establishing a treatment concept. Extensor tendons are easily exposed on the dorsum of the fingers and hand even after minor trauma due to the thin tissue envelope. Additional procedures are frequently necessary. Shortcomings in adequate soft-tissue coverage will inevitably result in poor overall results, even if the tendons themselves were addressed properly.

Basic science/disease process

The anatomy of the extensor mechanism is complex and some functional details are still subject to discussion. However, in order to be able to provide the best possible treatment in a given pathologic situation, fundamental knowledge about the functional anatomy of this complex system is paramount.

Anatomy of the extensor tendons

The extensor mechanism consists of extrinsic muscles, which are located on the forearm (extensor communis, extensor indicis, extensor digiti minimi (EDM)), intrinsic muscles, which are located at the level of the metacarpals (interosseous and lumbrical muscles), and fibrous structures.

Extrinsic muscles

All extrinsic tendons pass through the six compartments of the extensor retinaculum on the back of the wrist *(Fig. 10.1)*. The first compartment is attached to the outer rim of the radius and contains the tendons of the abductor pollicis longus (APL) and extensor pollicis brevis (EPB) muscles. In 34% of patients the compartment is further divided by an additional septum, which has implications for the etiology and treatment of de Quervain's disease.[2] The extensor carpi radialis longus (ECRL) and extensor carpi radialis brevis (ECRB) tendons run through the second compartment, which is bordered by Lister's tubercle on the ulnar side. The third compartment crosses the wrist in a diagonal fashion above the second compartment, while Lister's tubercle acts as a pivot point for the extensor pollicis longus (EPL) tendon. While passing through the compartment, the tendon is quite vulnerable to ruptures, e.g., in fractures of the distal radius. The fourth compartment contains both the extensor digitorum communis (EDC) and extensor indicis proprius (EIP) tendons. The EDM and extensor carpi ulnaris (ECU) tendons run through the fifth and sixth extensor compartments, respectively. The ECU not only functions as an extensor for the wrist, but is also part of the triangular fibrocartilage complex (TFCC) and thus a major stabilizer for the distal radioulnar joint.

The two extensor proprii tendons of the index and the little finger are located on the ulnar sides of the corresponding communis tendons and allow for individual movements of the peripheral fingers. On the dorsum of the hand, the EDC tendons are interconnected by the juncturae tendinum which facilitate combined extension of the fingers. Lacerations of the extensor tendons which are located proximal to the juncturae may be masked by the function of these bands. The patterns of the intertendinous connnections are highly variably and have been classified into three types: filamentous, fibrous, and tendinous bands.[3] At the level of the proximal phalanges, the extensor tendons split up into three parts: the central band and two lateral bands *(Fig. 10.2)*. These merge with the intrinsic extensor system to form the complex extensor apparatus of the digits.

The extrinsic extensor tendons themselves have three insertion sites on the phalanges. Proximally, the tendon is fixed at the level of the metacarpal heads to the palmar plate by the sagittal bands. This attachment centers the tendon of the MP joint and prevents hyperextension. The most important insertion is located at the base of the middle phalanx. Distally, the terminal tendon is attached to the distal phalanx. In addition to these three sites, there is a variable degree of attachment of the tendon to the proximal phalanx.

Intrinsic muscles

The intrinsic muscular system of the hand consists of seven interosseous and four lumbrical muscles. The three

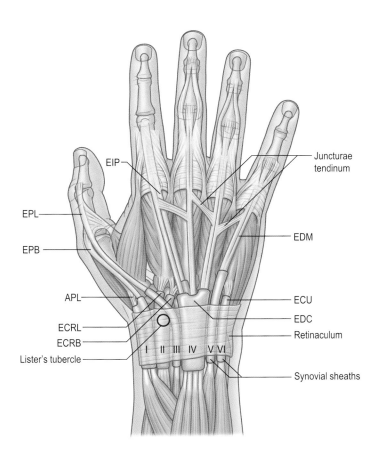

Fig. 10.1 Extensor compartments: I, APL and EPB; II, ECRL and ECRB; III, EPL; IV, EDC and EIP; V, EDM; VI, ECU. EIP, extensor indicis proprius; EPL, extensor pollicis longus; EPB, extensor pollicis brevis; EDM, extensor digiti minimi; APL, abductor pollicis longus; ECU, extensor carpi ulnaris; ECRL, extensor carpi radialis longus; ECRB, extensor carpi radialis brevis; EDC, extensor digitorum communis.

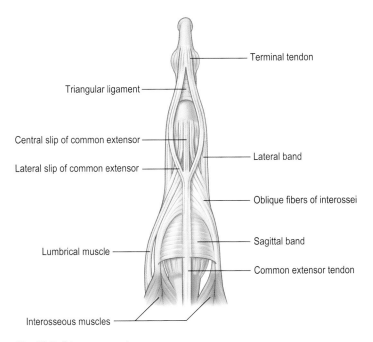

Fig. 10.2 Extensor apparatus.

palmar interosseous muscles arise from the medial sides of the second, fourth, and fifth metacarpal bones and join the extensor apparatus of the digits at the level of the proximal phalanx after crossing palmar to the axis of the MP joint. The four dorsal interosseous muscles originate with two heads each from the adjacent sides of the five metacarpal bones. The first two interosseous muscles approach the index and middle finger from the radial side; the third and fourth approach the middle and ring finger from the ulnar side. They have insertions at the proximal phalanges and the interosseous hood of the extensor apparatus before joining the lateral bands.

The lumbrical muscles are considered some of the most variable muscles of the human body, while the degree of variation increases from the radial to ulnar muscles. In general, they arise from the radial sides of the flexor digitorum profundus tendons at the level of the metacarpals and join the extensor apparatus from the radial side.

With this arrangement, all four digits have three intrinsic muscles contributing to the extensor apparatus, with the missing ulnar interosseous muscle for the little finger being equivalent to the abductor digiti minimi muscle *(Fig. 10.3)*. The thumb also has three short muscles that join the extensor apparatus: the flexor pollicis brevis (FPB) and abductor pollicis brevis (APB) muscles on the radial side and the adductor pollicis (ADP) muscle on the ulnar side.

Functional anatomy

Linked chains

The movement of the fingers is a highly complex mechanism. It is dependent upon a delicate equilibrium between the extrinsic extensor and flexor muscles and the intrinsic muscles. Biomechanically, the finger can be compared to a multiarticular chain comprised of the three phalangeal bones *(Fig. 10.4)*. Landsmeer was able to show that at least three muscles are necessary to control two joints in such a multiarticular chain.[4] For the proximal phalanx, these are the extrinsic extensor and flexor muscles and the diagonal intrinsic system (lumbrical and interosseous muscles). In the middle phalanx there is no diagonal muscle system; instead the third component is made up of the oblique retinacular ligament (Landsmeer's ligament) which has its origin at the flexor pulley and inserts distally into the extensor apparatus. Both of these diagonal systems run palmar to the joint axis proximally and dorsal to the joint axis distally. They play a crucial role in the coordination of extension and flexion movements of the fingers by linking the extrinsic flexor and extensor muscles.

Functions of the intrinsic muscles

It is generally believed that the intrinsic muscles of the hand act as flexors at the MP joints and extensors at the

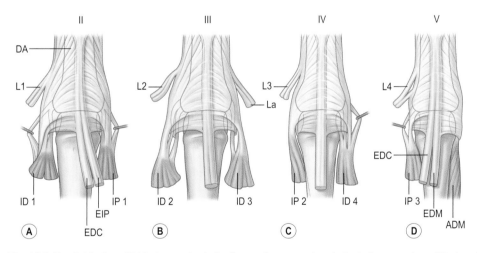

Fig. 10.3 The distribution of intrinsic muscles in the fingers. Roman numbers indicate finger numbers. DA, dorsal aponeurosis; L, lumbrical muscles, numbered from radial to ulnar; La, accessory lumbrical muscle (variation); EDC, extensor digitorum communis; EIP, extensor indicis proprius; EDM, extensor digiti minimi; ADM, abductor digiti minimi; ID, dorsal interosseous muscles; IP, palmar interosseous muscles, numbered from radial to ulnar.

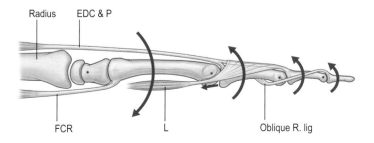

Fig. 10.4 Linked chains. EDC&P, extensor digitorum communis and extensor indicis proprius; FCR, flexor carpi radialis; L, lumbrical muscle; Obliq. R. lig., oblique retinacular ligament (Landsmeer's ligament).

interphalangeal joints. However, this is not always true for the interosseous muscles. They approach the extensor apparatus at a much smaller angle (less steep) than the lumbrical muscles. Due to this little anatomical difference, the function of the interosseous muscles is highly dependent on the position of the interosseous hood and therefore as well of the position of the MP joint. When the MP joints are in extension, the interosseous muscles cover the articular space and the oblique fibers of the interossei are put into tension, which translates into extension of the interphalangeal joints. However, when the MP joints are in flexion, the interosseous muscles slide distally on the proximal phalanx. During contraction of the muscles, the interosseous hood is pulled towards the hand and the flexion movement of the MP joint is enforced. In this position, the interossei lose the extensor function on the distal joints.

The lumbricals join the extrinsic tendon at a much greater angle than the interossei and are therefore not depending in their function on MP joint position. They act as extensors at the proximal and DIP joint in both extension and flexion of the MP joint.

Extrinsic muscle function

It has been shown biomechanically that both the extrinsic flexor and extensor muscles have a component that acts as an extensor on the proximal phalanx. Under physiologic conditions this force is counteracted by the intrinsic muscles. Paralysis of these muscles (as in ulnar nerve palsy) therefore results in hyperextension of the MP joints. Without intrinsic muscle function the long extensors exhaust their potential at the level of the proximal phalanx. Anatomical studies have demonstrated that isolated contraction of the extrinsic extensors results in hyperextended, clawlike position of the MP joints, but not complete finger extension.[3] For complete extension of the interphalangeal joints intrinsic muscle function is therefore mandatory.

Mechanisms of joint extension

The MP joint is extended by the extrinsic extensor tendon. However, there have been debates about how tendon force is transmitted to the joint. The variable direct attachment of the tendon to the proximal phalanx has been shown to have no significant contribution to MP joint extension.[5] It has been postulated that instead the fibrous connections of the extensor tendon to the flexor sheath are the primary transmitters for extension of the joint.

Extension of the PIP joint is mediated by the central slip of the extensor tendon. However, as stated above, intrinsic muscle function is necessary in order to enable the extrinsic extensor tendon to act on the PIP joint. At the level of the PIP joint, the extensor tendon is centered by the transverse retinacular ligaments. Harris and Rutledge have stressed the importance of the correct position and balance between the central slip and the lateral bands in order to maintain normal PIP extension.[5]

Until the late 1940s, extension of the DIP joint was thought only to be mediated by the terminal part of the extensor mechanism. In 1949 Landsmeer defined the function of the oblique retinacular ligament which had been unclear since its

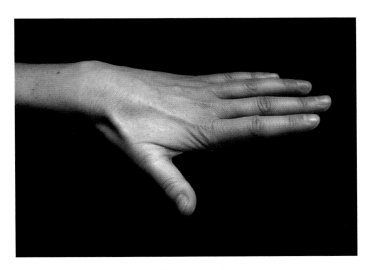

Fig. 10.5 Test of the extensor pollicis longus tendon.

identification in the 1800s.[6] He described the extension of the DIP joint as a combination of the terminal lateral bands and a tenodesis effect mediated by these ligaments. Later these findings were questioned.[5] However, dissection of the ligament results in lack of extension of the DIP joint.

Diagnosis/patient presentation

The diagnosis of extensor tendon injuries is often evident. However, partial lesions can be missed if the remaining tendon is strong enough to create some extension force. As a general rule, open lesions should therefore be surgically explored to identify the extent of the injury and prevent secondary ruptures. The function of the EDC tendon should be assessed by extension of the MP joint of the affected digit against resistance. The EPB tendon inserts into the extensor tendon apparatus of the thumb at varying levels and may be able to extend the IP joint of the thumb. If there is a questionable rupture of the EPL tendon, it should therefore not be tested by extension of the IP joint. Instead, the patient should be asked to lift the thumb off the table, which will be impossible without an intact EPL tendon *(Fig. 10.5)*.

Kleinert and Verdan proposed a system to classify lesions of the extensor tendon apparatus into eight zones according to the level of the lesion.[7] Doyle has added a ninth zone by dividing the forearm into the distal (zone 8) and proximal forearm (zone 9).[8] This classification is presented in *Figure 10.6*.

Patient selection

The repair of simple lacerations of the extensor tendon can be safely performed in the Emergency Room. However, as the lesions are generally underestimated and require sufficient exposure of the tendon, a thorough knowledge of the surgical

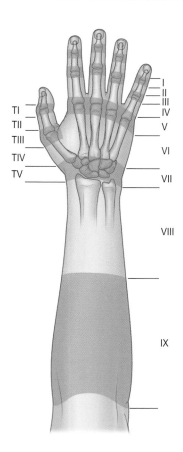

Fig. 10.6 The zones of extensor tendon injuries.

anatomy and treatment regimes is mandatory. Lesions proximal to zone VI should be treated in the operating room. The use of loupe magnification should be considered. The patient should be aware that, despite the often short duration of operations, postoperative treatment protocols can be complicated and may last for several months.

Wide-awake surgery is a concept that is becoming increasingly accepted. In this approach, procedures are performed with no sedation and no tourniquet with the use of tumescent lidocaine and epinephrine. This technique has been proven to be safe and cost-effective.[9–12] Most importantly, however, with the patient able to move the fingers during the operation, the surgeon can verify the success of tenolysis or tendon repair procedures immediately.[13] Not only tendon repairs and tenolysis, but also tendon transfers can be most effectively performed in this approach *(Box 10.1)*.[14]

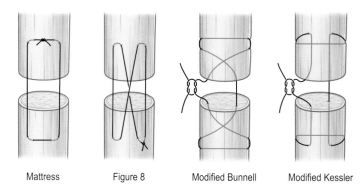

Mattress   Figure 8   Modified Bunnell   Modified Kessler

Fig. 10.7 Different types of core sutures.

Treatment/surgical technique

Suturing techniques

The size of the extensor tendon varies considerably during its course from the distal forearm to its terminal insertion at the distal phalanx. While the tendon is round and thick proximally, it becomes thin and flat more distally. Suturing techniques therefore have to be adapted specifically to the location of the lesion. Whatever technique is chosen, it should provide the best stability with the least shortening possible.

In zones VI and proximally, the extensor tendon resembles a flexor tendon and as such can be repaired with a core suture and an epitendinous running suture. Commonly used suture strengths include 3-0 and 4-0 for core sutures and 5-0 for epitendinous sutures. For neither flexor nor extensor tendons is there any scientific evidence for an advantage of using resorbable or nonresorbable suture materials. *Figure 10.7* gives an overview of common types of core suture. In order to achieve maximum core suture strength, locking stitches should be preferred over grasping stitches in order to prevent suture pull-out and reduce gapping.[15] However, grasping suture techniques have a higher tensile strength and less gap formation in extensor tendon repair than mattress or figure-of-eight stitches.[16] For flexor tendons, it has been shown that at least four core strands should be applied in order to enable early active motion[17] and the same is probably true for extensor tendon repair.

In the more distal zones of injury, locking or grasping core stitches become increasingly difficult due to flattening of the tendon. Newport *et al.* report that grasping stitches in zone IV injuries are strong enough to enable postoperative early active motion.[18] Simple running stitches should be avoided due to the low pull-out strength in favor of more complex locking suture techniques *(Box 10.2)*.

Zone I

The mallet finger

The mallet finger is characterized by persistent flexion of the distal phalanx due to a lesion of the extensor apparatus at the level of the DIP joint. It represents a classic closed injury that is usually treated conservatively, although open injuries may occur as well.

The flat terminal extensor tendon inserts at the base of the distal phalanx where it blends with the joint capsule. Since its excursion is only about 4 mm, even small gaps may result in a considerable lack of extension. It should be kept in mind that the full extension of the distal phalanx is also depended on an intact oblique retinacular ligament.

Mallet fingers can be classified by the degree of osseous involvement. Isolated tendinous ruptures are differentiated from injuries that involve bony avulsions. The latter have been classified into avulsions of small triangular fragments, large fragments that result in palmar subluxation of the phalanx, and epiphyseal detachments in children.

Most surgeons prefer conservative treatment with splints over operative therapy for uncomplicated injuries, although the scientific evidence is limited.[19,20]

Niechajev reviewed 135 patients who had been treated for various types of mallet finger with a minimal follow-up of 12 months.[21] The author concludes that operative treatment should only be performed in cases with subluxation of the distal phalanx or avulsed fragments that are more than one-third of the joint surface and with a diastasis of more than 3 mm. Stern and Kastrup reviewed 123 mallet injuries retrospectively.[22] Thirty-nine patients were treated surgically, resulting in a complication rate of 53%, including infection, nail deformities, joint incongruities, fixation failure, and bony prominence. The authors conclude that splinting is the preferred treatment option in nearly all mallet fingers. Handoll and Vaghela included four trials in a systematic review.[23–27] They concluded that there is insufficient evidence from randomized trials to establish the effectiveness of custom-made or off-the-shelf finger splints, the advantage of surgical treatment over splinting, or even the advantage of splinting over no treatment at all.

The best available evidence therefore supports conservative treatment by splinting for the majority of cases. Conservative treatment usually implies immobilization of the DIP joint in extension while sparing the PIP joint. By extension or slight hyperextension of the joint the two ruptured ends of the tendon are approximated (*Figs 10.8 and 10.9*). The fibrous tissue of the resulting scar is thought to be strong enough to restore extension of the joint. The type of splint is not nearly as important as patient compliance. Prefabricated stack splints have been shown to be equally effective as simple aluminum splints or custom sandwich splints (*Figs 10.10 and 10.11*). Most authors recommend full-time splinting for at least 6–8 weeks followed by a period of 2–6 weeks of splinting at night to enable further shrinking of the immature scar. All patients should be thoroughly instructed to avoid ineffective use of the splints. The splints should only be removed when flexion of the DIP joint by the strong pull of the FDP tendon is

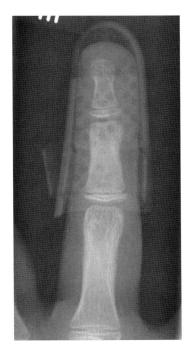

Fig. 10.8 Acute mallet injury, reduced by stack splint: posteroanterior view.

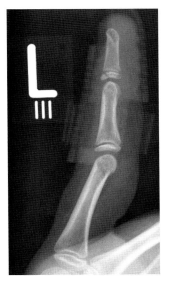

Fig. 10.9 Acute mallet injury, reduced by stack splint: lateral view.

counteracted, e.g., through resting the finger flat on a table. By thorough splinting, a residual lack of extension of 10° or less can be expected.[28]

Surgical treatment for closed injuries should only be considered in fragment sizes greater than one-third of the joint surface. Transfixation of the DIP joint with a Kirschner wire has been suggested for sole treatment of the mallet injury in addition to other surgical interventions.[29,30] To avoid scarring of the finger pulp, Tubiana has suggested an oblique angle when crossing the DIP joint.[31]

When surgical intervention is indicated, the size of the avulsed fragment should be carefully evaluated for direct

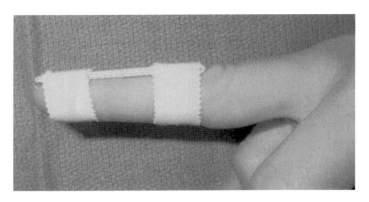

Fig. 10.10 Aluminum splint.

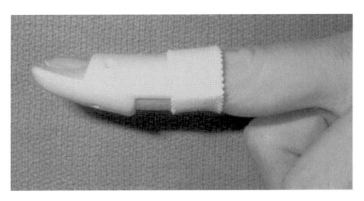

Fig. 10.11 Stack splint.

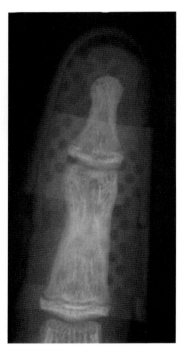

Fig. 10.12 Mallet injury: posteroanterior view.

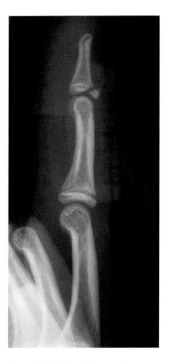

Fig. 10.13 Mallet injury: lateral view. Despite the stack splint, the fragment is not properly reduced.

fixation. This can be very difficult to achieve and may result in further fragmentation of the avulsed bone. In case of a rather small fragment, indirect reduction by extension block pin fixation should be preferred ("doorstop osteosynthesis"). In this technique the distal phalanx is maximally flexed and a 1.0-mm Kirschner wire is advanced into the middle phalanx dorsal to the avulsed fragment at a 45° angle, creating the extension block against which the fragment is reduced. The joint is then extended, reducing the fragment. This position is secured by a second Kirschner wire inserted longitudinally across the DIP joint for transfixation. The wires are cut and a splint is applied for at least 6 weeks **(Figs 10.12–10.15)**.

If the avulsed fragment seems large enough, it may either be pinned directly percutaneously or reduced in an open fashion through a zigzag incision of the distal and middle phalanges. In case of open reduction, screw fixation seems preferable. Alternatively, a pull-out suture may be applied, as described by Doyle.[8]

Open injuries

Most authors agree to operative treatment for open injuries. In some cases, suturing of the skin alone and supporting the joint in extension or slight hyperextension is enough to approximate the ends of the ruptured tendon and allow direct healing. When sutures are needed to approximate the tendon ends, a suture that incorporates both skin and tendon may be superior to individual suturing of the tendon, because further tendon dissection may decrease the blood supply and compromise healing.

Chronic injuries

If tendinous ruptures over the DIP joint are not or insufficiently treated, gapping of the tendon ends will result in the incorporation of fibrous tissue and lack of extension. A swanneck deformity may occur. The approach to these conditions is described below (under secondary procedures).

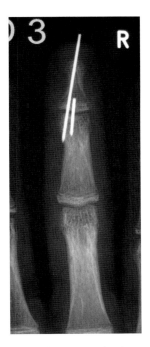

Fig. 10.14 Postoperative doorstop: posteroanterior view.

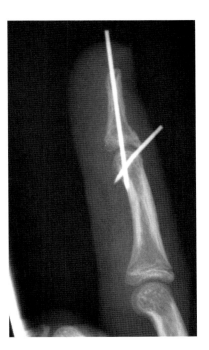

Fig. 10.15 Postoperative doorstop: lateral view 6 weeks after doorstop osteosynthesis.

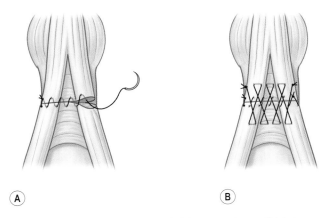

Fig. 10.16 (A, B) Silfverskiöld cross-stitch for sutures in zone II injuries.

Zone II

Injuries to the extensor tendon over the middle phalanx usually result from sharp, direct lacerations or crush injuries. Acute lacerations should be explored to determine the extent of the tendon injury. If less than 50% of the tendon substance are injured, the tendon is considered stable and no further treatment is necessary. If more than half of the tendon is involved, additional suturing is necessary. When evaluating these injuries, phalangeal extension should always be tested against resistance. Doyle recommended a running stitch combined with a Silfverskiöld cross-stitch[8] *(Fig. 10.16)*. Care should be taken to avoid considerable shortening of the tendon which will result in lack of flexion of the DIP joint.

Zone III

Injuries to the extensor tendon at the level of the PIP joint (zone III) occur as both closed and open injuries, ranging from minor strains to complete ruptures or lacerations. Injuries at this level can give rise to the characteristic boutonnière deformity when the proximal phalanx herniates through the central slip defect. However, the deformity will not develop immediately after the injury. Disruption of the tendon first leads to an inability to extend the PIP joint actively while passive extension is possible. Only after the lateral bands migrate palmarly and retraction of the central slip occurs will hyperextension of the DIP joint develop.

Closed injuries

A closed avulsion injury of the central slip may not be immediately evident and extension may be retained by means of the lateral bands. If in doubt, extension of the PIP joint should therefore always be tested against resistance.

The central slip may be restored without surgical intervention by extension splinting. As flexion of the DIP joint stretches the extensor mechanism and facilitates dorsal relocation of the lateral bands, the DIP joint should not be included in immobilization. Instead patients should be encouraged to move the DIP joint actively and passively while wearing the PIP splint *(Fig. 10.17)*. Several authors have proposed pinning the PIP joint in extension by a Kirschner wire.[32–34] Most authors suggest keeping the joint in extension for 5–6 weeks.[33–35]

Surgical treatment has been suggested for avulsion injuries with large bony fragments or unstable transarticular fractures.[31] If the fragment is too small to be pinned directly, it may be excised and the tendon reinserted into the middle fragment with a bone anchor.

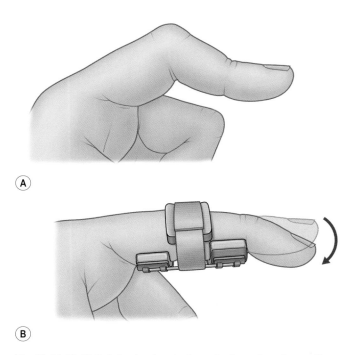

(A)

(B)

Fig. 10.17 (A, B) Splinting for closed extensor tendon ruptures in zone III.

Open lacerations

Open injuries should always be thoroughly explored. Care should be taken specifically to include the lateral bands and the triangular ligament in the inspection. The mechanism of injury is of special importance in open zone III injuries with regard to the extent of injury to both the tendinous structures and the surrounding soft tissues. In clean and sharp lacerations, the wound can be easily enlarged and the injured tendon should be sutured directly or reinserted into the middle phalanx. A Silfverskiöld cross-stitch may be used where appropriate to enforce the suture. In contrast, contaminated defect wounds, e.g., after saw injuries, are a lot more difficult to deal with. If there is considerable loss of tendon, an immediate reconstruction should be attempted. Snow described a retrograde tendinous flap created from the proximal tendon that is flipped over to bridge the defect over the joint *(Fig. 10.18)*.[36] Aiache *et al.* proposed a longitudinal split of the two lateral bands that are joined in the midline to reconstruct the tendinous insertion and to cover the joint *(Fig. 10.19)*.[37] Any loss of covering skin should be replaced immediately as well; options include local random pattern flaps, reversed cross-finger flaps, or flaps from the dorsal metacarpal artery system.

Postoperatively, a Kirschner wire may be used to reinforce splinting of the PIP joint, which should be kept for 4–6 weeks. Tenolyses or joint releases are frequently necessary, but should be delayed until 3–6 months after the injury.

Zone IV

As the extensor becomes very broad over the proximal phalanx, partial lacerations are more commonly observed than complete injuries of the tendons. Therefore extension should be examined against resistance. Surgical inspection is

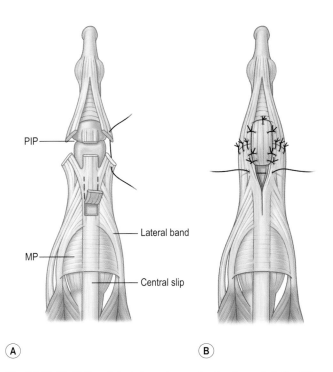

PIP

Lateral band

MP

Central slip

(A)   (B)

Fig. 10.18 (A, B) Snow's technique of reconstructing the central slip. PIP, proximal interphalangeal; MP, metacarpophalangeal.

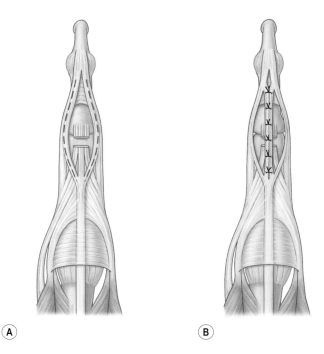

(A)   (B)

Fig. 10.19 (A, B) Reconstruction of the central slip involving splitting of the lateral bands (Aiache's technique).

necessary to assess the exact extent of the injury. Newport *et al.* have demonstrated that modified Kessler sutures do not result in significant shortening of the tendon and allow 30° of flexion in the PIP joint without gapping.[18]

Extensor tendon injuries in zone IV are often associated with fractures of the proximal phalanx.[38] Due to the close relationship between tendon and bone, adhesions frequently occur and tenolysis is often necessary. Some form of a postoperative early active motion regimen is therefore advisable to reduce loss of range of motion. Maintenance of the wrist in an extended position will "unload" the tendon and allow early range of motion of the finger.

Zone V

At the level of the MP joints, the extensor tendon consists of the central extensor tendon and the sagittal bands. Due to the broad width of the extensor apparatus complete lacerations are uncommon. On the other hand, partial lacerations can be easily missed because the remaining tendon may be sufficient to maintain extension function. Surgical exploration is therefore warranted. It should be taken into account that the injury to the tendon may be located more proximally than the skin laceration if the tendon was injured in flexion and the exploration is performed with the digit in extension. If possible, a core suture with an epitendinous running stitch should be performed. In the rare cases of complete lacerations, the tendon will not significantly retract proximally, as it is restrained by the sagittal bands and the juncturae.

Human bite injuries

A common mechanism of injuries to the extensor tendon in zone V is a human bite injury caused by a punch to the opponent's face (fight bites, *Fig. 10.20*). Bite wounds are heavily contaminated and prone to serious infection. As skin damage is often minimal, these injuries are frequently underestimated by the patient and treatment is delayed until infection has developed. Primary inspection is mandatory in fresh injuries, as are X-ray studies to detect avulsed bony fragments or teeth. During exploration, the tendon should be split longitudinally and the MCP joint irrigated with antibiotic solution.[39] Partial lacerations of the tendon often do not require suturing; a number of authors suggest delayed primary treatment after the occurrence of infection has been ruled out.[40]

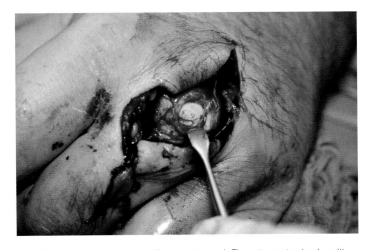

Fig. 10.20 Fight bite in the ring-finger metacarpal. The extensor tendon is split longitudinally.

Sagittal band injuries

The central tendon is centered over the MP joint by the lateral bands which attach to the palmar plate of the joint. Open or closed injuries to the sagittal bands may result in subluxation of the tendon to the unaffected side during flexion. Partial lacerations will not result in subluxation unless two-thirds of the sagittal band is affected.[41] Stable lacerations can be treated by buddy-taping of the affected finger to an adjacent finger for 3 weeks. In case of an unstable tendon, the laceration should be sutured.

Closed ruptures of the sagittal bands are much more common than open injuries and usually occur in the course of a primary disease of the joints such as rheumatoid arthritis. Ishizuki describes two layers of the sagittal bands, a superficial and a deep layer.[42] He postulated that degenerative ruptures affect only the superficial layer, while traumatic ruptures affect both layers. Traumatic and spontaneous ruptures of the sagittal bands may be treated by splinting within 10–14 days.[43,44] In older injuries, direct suturing of the bands should be attempted. Reconstruction of the sagittal bands in chronic subluxation is discussed in the section on secondary surgery, below.

Zone VI

Extensor tendon lesions at the level of the metacarpal bones have a better prognosis than in more distal zones.[38] This is due to several reasons. First, the tendons are very broad and can usually be sutured by a 3-0 core stitch and an epitendinous running suture. Moreover, they are extrasynovial and are not associated with any joints. At the same time, tendon excursion is greater than in more distal locations and imbalances between extensor and flexor systems are less likely to occur. Soft-tissue coverage is better than in distal zones, but still quite thin compared to flexor tendons.

At this level, the function of the extrinsic extensor tendon is to extend the MP joint. Therefore MP joint extension should be tested against resistance. However, the extrinsic tendons are linked by the juncturae tendinum and patients may still be able to extend the joints by means of the adjacent tendons.

Postoperatively, early mobilization with a dynamic splinting regime is indicated to reduce tendon adhesions. Loss of flexion has been reported to be more common than loss of extension.[38]

Zone VII

Injuries to the extensor tendons at the level of the extensor retinaculum are due to either open lacerations that often affect multiple tendons or closed ruptures, most often after distal radius fractures.

In order to repair open lacerations at this level, at least a part of the retinaculum has to be opened. There has been an ongoing debate whether or not to reconstruct the retinaculum over the affected tendon. Some surgeons advocate excising the retinaculum in order to avoid postoperative adhesions. Others suggest reconstructing at least parts of the retinaculum to prevent subluxation or bowstringing of the tendons. Although adhesions between the tendons and the retinaculum seem more likely, Newport *et al.* found no differences between the outcomes of zone VII lesions in comparison to lesions in adjacent zones.[38] The tendon repair itself should be performed with a stable core suture and an epitendinous running stitch. Special attention should also be paid to concomitant injuries of sensory branches of the radial and ulnar nerves. Primary coaptation of the nerve ends should be performed in order to prevent the development of painful and difficult-to-manage neuromas.

As the tendons are arranged very close to each other, injuries of multiple tendons through one laceration occur frequently. Identification of the tendons can be quite difficult, because they tend to retract into the forearm. A thorough knowledge of the surgical anatomy is therefore mandatory. Botte *et al.* described a useful technique of labeling the retrieved tendons by placing sterile labels on hemostats that are clamped to sutures placed in the proximal ends of the tendon.[45]

Ruptures of the EPL tendon are most often associated with fractures of the distal radius or rheumatoid arthritis. Two main causes for EPL ruptures after distal radius fractures have been hypothesized.[46] On the one hand, the tendon may be injured while drilling the holes for palmar plate fixation or by choosing screws that are too long and protrude into the extensor compartments. On the other hand, dislocated dorsal fragments of the fracture may harm the tendon. Because of the degenerative nature of the process, an end-to-end repair of the tendon is usually not possible without unacceptable shortening of the tendon. Instead, reconstruction of the tendon can be performed by EIP to EPL tendon transfers or interposing tendon grafts. Both techniques are discussed in the section on secondary surgery, below.

Zones VIII/IX

Lesions of the extensor tendons at levels VIII and IX include injuries of the musculotendinous junctions and muscle bellies. As in zone VII injuries, the recovery and identification of retracted tendons can be quite challenging. Combined injuries to muscles and/or nerves are possible. Knowledge of the sequence of motor innervation helps to distinguish a motor nerve injury from a tendon injury. The motor branches of the wrist and fingers have been divided into two groups, a proximal superficial group and a distal deep group.[40] The proximal superficial group consists of the ECRL, ECRB, EDC, EDM, and ECU muscles. The entry of nerve fibers into the muscles is near the lateral epicondyle. When exposing the posterior interosseous nerve, the interval between the wrist ECRB and ECRL tendon (proximal to the supinator muscle) and the EDC, EDM, and ECU (distal to the supinator) should be chosen to avoid injury to motor branches. The distal deep group consists of the APL, EPB, EPL, and EIP. They originate in the distal half of the forearm, close to the skeletal plane.

Adequate repair of muscles and tendons can be very difficult in this area. Sutures of muscle fibers alone have virtually no tensile strength. Therefore an effort should be made to suture tendons or fascial layers instead of muscle fibers alone. Nevertheless, these sutures are usually not strong enough for dynamic postoperative treatment protocols and immobilization for 3–4 weeks should be initiated postoperatively.

Postoperative care

As with flexor tendon injuries, the importance of an adequate postoperative treatment cannot be overestimated. Extensor tendon healing itself does not differ very much from flexor tendon healing. However, it has to be considered that the treatment protocol needs to address the powerful antagonist force of the opposing flexor tendons. Initially, static postoperative treatment regimes were considered sufficient for all injuries, as in theory tendon adhesion is limited due to the mostly extrasynovial nature of extensor tendons. In reality however, while prolonged immobilization allows healing of the tendon without disturbances, it still promotes loss of motion due to the formation of adhesions. The problem can be addressed by early active or passive motion which in turn increases the risk of gap formation and ruptures of the sutured tendons. As for flexor tendon injuries, in recent years, dynamic postoperative treatment protocols have been developed that reduce postoperative adhesion formation without jeopardizing the stability of the sutured tendon.

Nevertheless, strict immobilization is the treatment of choice for some indications. Mallet injuries should be treated by full-time static splinting for 8 weeks. The same is true for closed ruptures of the central slip (zone III injuries). Immobilization should also be considered for injuries proximal to the extensor retinaculum (zones VIII and IX) because it may not be possible to achieve adequate tensile strength by suturing fascial layers around the muscle.

Postoperative immobilization of open injuries in zones III–V will inevitably result in severe adhesions, because the tendon is very broad and in close relationship to the adjacent bone in this area. To overcome this problem, Evans described a postoperative treatment protocol that reduces adhesions by limited early active motion ("short arc motion").[47] The regime is based on biomechanical studies that examined the extensor tendon excursions necessary to prevent adhesion formation. Duran et al.[48] found that 3–5 mm of passive tendon glide is sufficient to achieve this goal. Evans[49] compared intraoperative measurements of tendon excursions in zone IV and V with previous measurements of Brand and Hollister,[50] and estimated that 60° of PIP joint flexion translates into 5 mm of tendon glide at Lister's tubercle.

For the protocol, three finger splints are required. The affected digit is immobilized between training sessions in an extension split in 0° extension of the DIP and PIP joints. At every waking hour, the splint is removed and a controlled active motion protocol is followed. First a splint is put on to block flexion of the PIP joint at 30° and flexion of the DIP at 20–25°. After 20 repetitions of active and passive motion within the defined limits, a third splint is put on that stabilizes the PIP joint in 0° extension while sparing the DIP joint. The patient then actively extends and flexes the DIP joint 20 times. During the second and third week of the protocol, flexion of the PIP joint is increased to 40° and 50°. In a retrospective study, Evans reported on significant improvement of clinical results with the dynamic protocol when compared to a group of patients who were immobilized postoperatively.[48]

Dynamic mobilization for injuries in zones V–VII can be achieved by passive extension with a rubber band system combined with active flexion of the affected digit *(Fig. 10.21)*. This protocol has also been termed the "reversed Washington"

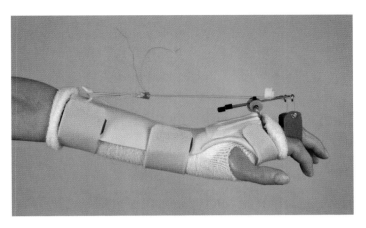

Fig. 10.21 Dynamic extension splint.

or "reversed Kleinert" regimen. The patient is encouraged to perform active flexion and passive extension exercises 10 times every hour for 3 weeks, starting on the second postoperative day. The range of motion for flexion of the MP joint is restricted at 30° in the beginning and gradually increased to 60° until the end of the third week. Active motion is initiated after 3 weeks and the splint is removed after 6 weeks. The load of the tendon is gradually increased over 6 weeks. In a prospective, randomized study, better total active motion was achieved in zone V and VI lesions after 4, 6, and 8 weeks after a dynamic splinting protocol when compared to static splinting.[51]

Early dynamic motion is also superior to immobilization after transfer of the EIP tendon for EPL reconstruction.[52] After performing a Pulvertaft weave, the tendon is more stable and splinting can be discontinued after 3 weeks. However, active extension of the thumb has no advantage over dynamic splinting after transfer of the EIP tendon.[53]

Outcomes, prognosis, and complications

Outcomes

Outcomes vary considerably with the location of the lesion, the extent of concomitant injuries to the bone or surrounding soft tissues, timing of the repair, and adequate postoperative care. Clinical results are most often assessed by total active motion.[54] Hung *et al.* established 270° of total active motion in a digit as a normal value.[55] Some authors have adapted evaluation systems for flexor tendon injuries.[7,56] Alternatively, results can be compared by total lag of extension or flexion, as proposed by Miller in 1942.[57]

Lesions distal to the MP joints lead to less favorable results than more proximal lesions. Newport *et al.* report the results of a retrospective analysis of 101 patients, most of whom were treated with static splinting.[38] Good or excellent results with an average total active motion of 230° were achieved in 64% of patients without an associated injury. However, lesions in zones I through IV resulted in good or excellent results in only 50% of patients. Evans found a total active motion of 147° 6

weeks after repair of lacerations in zone III and an early active motion regimen.[47]

Hung *et al.* reported on 38 patients with an average of 229° of total active motion after postoperative dynamic splinting.[55] Patients with lesions in zones II–IV showed the worst results, with an average of 188° total active motion. For lesions at the level of the MP joint, several studies reported superior results after postoperative dynamic splinting protocols when compared with immobilization, ranging from 237° to 254° of total active motion.[55,58,59]

Complications

The most common complication after extensor tendon injuries is the formation of adhesions between the tendon and surrounding tissues. Under these circumstances, a tenodesis restraint may occur, limiting PIP joint flexion when the MP joint is also flexed. Adhesion formation should be addressed first by hand therapy and splinting of the affected joints in order to improve tendon gliding. If there is not adequate improvement in range of motion after 4–6 months, extensor tendon tenolysis can be considered. A stable skin envelope is a prerequisite before performing any additional procedures. Tenolysis can be elegantly performed utilizing the wide-awake technique with no sedation and no tourniquet with the use of tumescent lidocaine and epinephrine (see patient selection, above).

Tenolysis alone may not be sufficient to achieve an improvement in range of motion. An additional capsulotomy, collateral ligament release, or even flexor tendon tenolysis may be necessary.[60] Creighton and Steichen reported the results of extensor tenolysis after phalangeal and metacarpal fracture repair.[61] Total active range of motion was improved by 31% on average, but only 21% when an additional capsulotomy was necessary.

Secondary procedures

See *Box 10.3*.

The hanging fingertip

Even a minimal increase in tendon length will result in an extensor lag after a mallet injury. In many patients therefore some residual deformity will occur. However, this deformity is rarely of any relevance in terms of long-term prognosis.[62] With the extension lag exceeding 40–50°, however, a considerable number of patients will desire correction. In this case, additional immobilization should be considered for up to 6 months after the injury, especially if there is any doubt about the adequacy of the primary treatment.

If conservative treatment fails, surgical treatment should be discussed with the patient. Due to the delicate equilibrium between the extensor and the flexor tendon system, results are not always satisfactory after secondary surgery. None of the procedures available will invariably provide reliable results. Correction of the deformity may be incomplete, there may be some loss of flexion in the DIP joint, and pain reduction cannot be reliably predicted. Any accompanying arthritis of the joint should be ruled out; in case of cartilaginous deterioration, DIP joint fusion should be considered.

If surgical correction is indicated, a simple combined excision of callus and skin may be the procedure of choice. This dermatotenodesis has also been referred to as the Brooks–Garner procedure. In this procedure, an elliptical wedge of skin and underlying soft tissues, including the scarred extensor tendon, is excised from the dorsum of the involved DIP joint *(Figs 10.22–24)*. The wound edges are closed by en bloc sutures, resulting in a slight hyperextension of the joint. The DIP joint is then transfixed with a Kirschner wire to keep the joint in the desired position for 6 weeks.

Alternatively, a Fowler release (central slip tenotomy) or even a reconstruction of the spiral oblique retinacular ligament may be performed. Both procedures are primarily used to correct swan-neck deformities and require a supple PIP joint. They are therefore discussed in the following section.

The swan-neck deformity

The swan-neck deformity is a classic finger deformity that can be caused by many reasons, including congenital PIP palmar plate laxity and intrinsic tightness. Often it is associated with some form of arthritis; however, it can also result from a mallet injury. A thorough history-taking and physical examination will distinguish the mallet etiology from other causes. In this case, the disrupted extensor tendon results in a concentration of extensor force at the PIP joint *(Fig. 10.25)*. If the palmar plate of the joint is lax, the swan-neck-deformity will occur immediately. However, even if it is not lax to begin with, it will stretch over time due to increased extensor pull. If

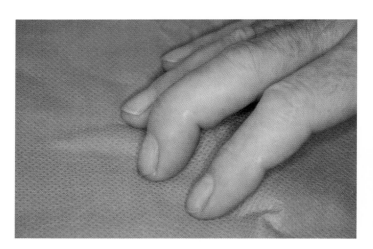

Fig. 10.22 Hanging fingertip.

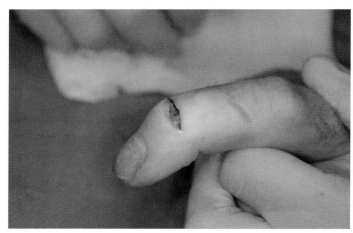

Fig. 10.23 Resection of skin and tendon.

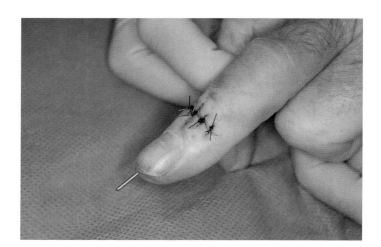

Fig. 10.24 Transfixation of the distal interphalangeal joint.

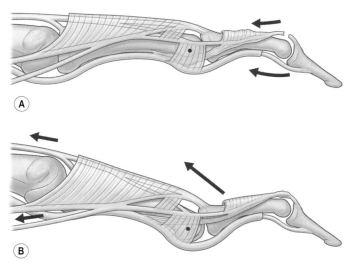

Fig. 10.25 **(A, B)** Pathophysiology of the swan-neck deformity. The deformity persists when the tendon heals with lengthening.

hyperextension of the PIP joint exceeds a critical point, snapping of the joint will occur. This may be often more disconcerting to the patient than the postural deformity.

A tenotomy of the central slip has been used to address the swan-neck deformity in patients with a chronic mallet deformity in which the terminal extensor tendon cannot be repaired.[63] This procedure has also been referred to as the Fowler release. By transection of the central slip, rebalancing of the extensor mechanism should occur in order to increase the extension force on the DIP joint. Grundberg and Reagan reported on a series of 20 patients with an average reduction of PIP joint extension of 10° to less than 2°.[64] A biomechanic study demonstrated the ability to correct an extensor lag of up to 46°.[65] The authors noted that extensor lags greater than 36° may not achieve full correction of the deformity. It should be noted that there is some confusion in the literature about the operation that is referred to as a "Fowler release." Fowler also described a procedure to address the boutonnière deformity by rebalancing the extensor tendon (see below). However, in this operation the extensor tendon is divided distal to the insertion of the central slip and thus even increasing extension forces at the level of the PIP joint.

Alternatively, the extensor tendon may be reconstructed by a tendon graft (spiral oblique retinacular ligament or SORL reconstruction: *Fig. 10.26*). Thompson *et al.* described a procedure using a palmaris tendon to restrain PIP extension and to extend the DIP.[66] In this technically demanding operation, the tendon graft is fixed to the distal phalanx by a pull-out suture. It is then passed between the flexor tendon and the palmar plate of the PIP joint into an osseous tunnel in the proximal phalanx *(Fig. 10.21)*. Although Girot *et al.* reported a 95% success rate to correct PIP hyperextension, experience with this procedure seems to be limited.[67]

Swan-neck deformities which are not primarily related to injuries of the distal extensor tendon should be approached differently. Frequently, these deformities are caused by hyperlax palmar plates at the level of the PIP joint. In these cases, correction of the laxity can be indicated, e.g., by a tenodesis of the flexor digitorum superficialis tendon.

The boutonnière deformity

Acute injury to the central band of the extensor tendon will result in an acute boutonnière deformity as both lateral bands shift palmarly due to the accompanied disruption of the triangular ligament. In the acute phase, the deformity should be easily reducible and may be treated as described above. However, if left untreated, a chronic contracture results from shortening of the oblique retinacular ligament *(Fig. 10.27)*. This condition has long been recognized as one of the most challenging problems in hand surgery.[68]

Preoperative considerations

Any surgical correction of the deformity should only be performed if the PIP joint can be extended passively. This can sometimes be achieved conservatively by a physical therapy program in combination with static and dynamic splinting. In severe cases, an additional operative tenoarthrolysis may be necessary. This procedure can sometimes be combined with

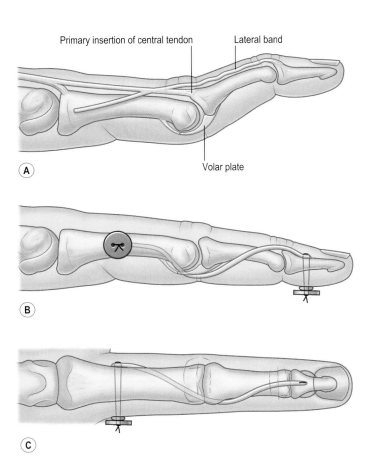

Fig. 10.26 (A–C) Spiral oblique retinacular ligament. A palmaris longus tendon graft is passed between the flexor tendon and the palmar plate and fixed to the distal phalanx by a pull-out suture.

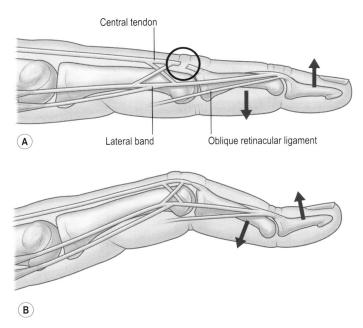

Fig. 10.27 (A, B) Pathophysiology of the boutonnière deformity. Subluxation of the lateral bands results in redistribution of forces and an extensor lag in the proximal interphalangeal joint. Retraction of the oblique retinacular ligament prohibits reduction in chronic deformities.

revision of the extensor tendon from a dorsal approach. However, in severe cases a first-stage palmar approach to release the joint contracture is combined with a staged secondary procedure from dorsally. If combined with a splinting regimen, the tenoarthrolysis may be sufficient to achieve functional improvement, so that further operations can be avoided.

Burton and Melchior have listed several more aspects that should be considered before attempting a surgical correction of the deformity.[69] Patients should be aware that postoperative splinting is an essential part of the treatment strategy and may be necessary for months after surgery. Any attempt to reconstruct the soft tissues around the PIP joint should be avoided if the joint shows any signs of arthritis. In this case, joint fusion or arthroplasty should be considered. The boutonnière deformity does not necessarily compromise the extent of flexion in the PIP joint or grip strength. An increase in extension of the joint should not be traded for a stiff finger or loss of grip strength.

There are two main categories of procedure to address the boutonnière deformity: tenotomy or reconstruction of the extensor tendon by tendon relocation or tendon grafting.

Tenotomy

Tenotomy of the extensor tendon on the middle phalanx is referred as the Dolphin or Fowler procedure.[70,71] It may be the procedure of choice when patients mainly complain about hyperextension of the DIP joint. The incision should be performed just distally to the insertion of the central slip. In Dolphin's description, the tendon is divided more proximally in order to preserve the distal insertions of the oblique retinacular ligament *(Fig. 10.28)*. The lateral bands should be able to slide proximally in order to increase the tone on the PIP joint to allow improved extension and reduce tension on the DIP joint. Postoperatively, the PIP joint should be splinted in extension, allowing free range of motion of the DIP joint. It has been recommended to apply splinting for 6–8 weeks.[69]

Secondary reconstruction of the extensor tendon

If the main patient complaint is the lack of extensor function, secondary reconstruction of the extensor should be considered. This goal can be achieved by either tendon relocation or tendon grafting. Intraoperative transfixation of the PIP joint

with a Kirschner wire has been subject to controversial discussion for any type of reconstruction. In severe flexion contractures of the joint, it may be beneficial.

The central slip can reconstructed as described by Snow *(Fig. 10.18)*. The end of the reconstructed tendon is either sutured to the remaining insertion on the middle phalanx or reinserted directly into the phalanx.

A large number of techniques have been described to reconstruct the central slip using the lateral bands. By relocation of the lateral bands the tension of the terminal tendon on the DIP joint is reduced while increasing the extension force on the PIP joint. Littler and Eaton described the resection of both lateral bands in order to relocate them dorsally and suture them on to the insertion of the central slip, thus combining a tenotomy and tendon relocation *(Fig. 10.29)*.[72] In Matev's technique, the lateral bands are incised at different levels *(Fig. 10.30)*. The distal end of the longer slip is sutured to the proximal end of the other slip, resulting in an increase in length of the terminal tendon in order to reduce tension on the DIP joint. The free slip is then relocated medially to restore the central slip.[73]

In extensive defects of the central slip, the lateral bands may be insufficient for reconstruction. In these cases, free tendon grafts may be indicated. Littler described a figure-of-eight weave through the base of the middle phalanx and the lateral bands.[74] Several other variations of fixation of the graft have been proposed.[30,71,75]

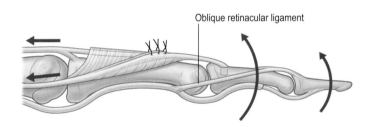

Fig. 10.29 Littler operation. The lateral bands are resected and relocated to the central tendon.

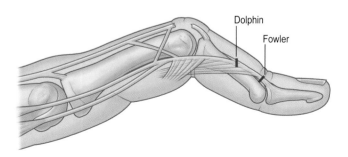

Fig. 10.28 Treatment of the boutonnière deformity by tenotomy as described by Dolphin and Fowler. Dolphin's tenotomy preserves the insertions of the oblique retinacular ligament.

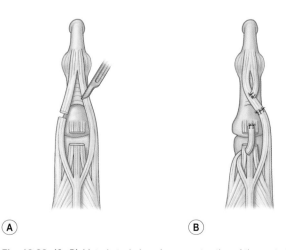

Ⓐ   Ⓑ

Fig. 10.30 (A, B) Matev's technique for reconstruction of the central slip. Both lateral bands are cut at different heights and relocated to reconstruct the central slip.

Delayed sagittal band reconstruction

The function of the sagittal bands is to align the tendon centrally on the MP joint. If the sagittal band is ruptured, the tendon may subluxate to the unaffected side. The lesion most often involves a longitudinal or oblique tear on the radial side of the tendon which leads to an ulnar dislocation at the level of the MP joint.[76] Tendon dislocation rarely occurs in patients not suffering from rheumatoid arthritis. If conservative treatment fails, surgical reconstruction of the sagittal band is indicated. In addition to the reconstruction, a release of the contracted contralateral sagittal band may be necessary in long-standing cases.[41] Several techniques have been described for reconstruction, if direct repair is not possible because of missing soft tissue or severe scarring[76–79] *(Fig. 10.31)*.

Wheeldon described an anchoring of the ulnar-sided junctura tendinum to the radial side of the extensor hood.[79] Elson passed a retrograde tendon slip beneath the deep transverse metacarpal ligament and sutured it to the joint capsule.[80] McCoy and Winsky described another reconstructive procedure that used a proximally based tendon slip.[78] In their "lumbrical loop operation" the tendon was wrapped around the lumbrical muscle and then sutured to itself. Kilgore *et al.*[81] and Carroll *et al.*[77] both described techniques that utilized distally or ulnarly based tendon slips that were passed around the radial collateral ligament and then sutured to themselves. In Watson's technique, a distally based central tendon slip is looped through the deep transverse metacarpal ligament *(Box 10.4)*.[76]

Carroll *et al.* reported the results of three patients who were operated on with their technique in five fingers.[75] No recurrent subluxation was noted. Watson *et al.* found no recurrent subluxation in 21 sagittal band reconstructions in 16 patients after a mean of 16 months.[76]

The missing tendon: tendon transfers versus tendon grafting

In cases of degenerative rupture of an extensor tendon, direct suturing is not usually possible because of an existing gap or extensive degeneration of the tendon ends. In the absence of rheumatoid arthritis, the EPL tendon is most often affected. To reconstruct extensor function two options exist. First, the tendon can be reconstructed with the use of a tendon graft, e.g., derived from the palmaris longus tendon. Second, reconstruction is possible by transfer of another tendon. In case of an EPL rupture, the EIP tendon is most frequently used.

Good results have been reported for both techniques.[82–85] In general, both show similar results.[86] However, each technique has specific advantages and disadvantages. For reconstructions with tendon grafts two weaving sutures are performed, which increases the risk of insufficiencies and ruptures. Harvesting of a tendon graft is necessary, but donor site morbidity should be minimal with the use of a palmaris longus graft. In contrast to tendon transfers no cortical rearrangement and adaption are needed. However, clinical results after tendon grafting are worse in long-standing ruptures because of atrophy and contracture of the affected muscles.[87]

Cortical adaptation is necessary after tendon transfers, but this is usually not a problem even in older patients. The operative technique is usually easier and faster. Because only one

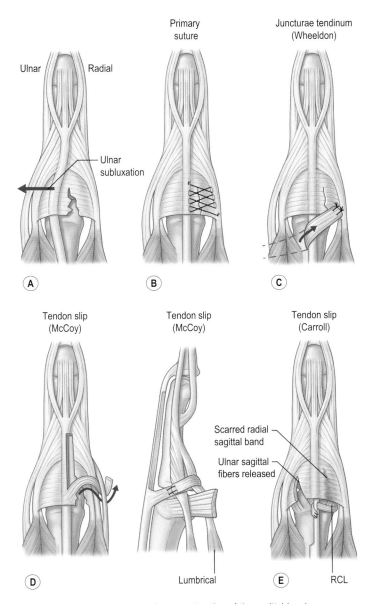

Fig. 10.31 Different techniques for reconstruction of the sagittal band. **(A)** Disruption of the radial sagittal band results in ulnar subluxation of the extensor tendon. **(B)** Primary suturing. **(C)** Wheeldon's technique: the ulnar junctura tendinum is relocated to the deep intercarpal ligament. **(D)** McCoy's technique: the tendon is split distally and wrapped around the lumbricalis muscle. **(E)** Carroll's technique: an ulnarly distal-based slip of the extensor digitorum communis tendon is wrapped around the radial collateral ligament (RCL).

Box 10.4 Clinical tip

Regardless of the preferred technique for sagittal band reconstruction, make sure the tendon is stabilized while maintaining full finger flexion. A dynamic postoperative protocol is advisable.

---

weaving suture is performed, the risk of tendon ruptures may be lower than in tendon transfers. After transfer of the EIP tendon isolated extension of the index finger is maintained in most patients.[88] However, it has to be considered that the strength of isolated index finger extension is weakened.[89,90] This is not a problem for daily life activities, but may be a problem in specific patients, such as musicians.

Soft-tissue management and staged reconstruction in combined injuries

Lesions of the extensor tendons are often complicated by lesions of the bones and joints and by loss of skin. The treatment of these combined defects poses a difficult problem for the treating surgeon. Extensive scarring can be expected and must be taken into consideration when formulating a treatment plan. As in other mutilating injuries, basic reconstructive principles apply. Before attempting reconstruction of the tendons, several requirements must be fulfilled. First of all, radical debridement of all devitalized tissue is mandatory. Before closure, the wound should not contain any contamination or tissue of compromised blood supply in order to prevent infection. Primary radical debridement has been shown to be superior to several serial debridement steps, because of the formation of edema and infected granulation tissue, which is only poorly penetrated by antibiotic treatment.[91–94] Second, osseous structures must be stabilized before turning to soft tissues. This can be achieved by internal or external fixation as appropriate. Third, a stable soft-tissue coverage for tendons and bony structures must be provided. In case of combined lesions of the dorsum of the hand, often pedicled or free tissue transfer is necessary. While the dorsal side of the hand is frequently used as a donor side to harvest soft-tissue flaps for coverage of palmar defects, the opposite is not true. Instead, flaps are usually harvested from adjacent proximal or distal regions on the hand and forearm. The pedicled radial forearm flap is a classic pedicled workhorse flap for coverage of the dorsum of the hand. However, due to sacrifice of the radial artery and the conspicuous donor site, variations of the original technique such as perforator-based flaps or fascial flaps should be considered.[95] Another classic pedicled flap is the posterior interosseous artery flap *(Fig. 10.32–36)*. With the advancement of microsurgical techniques, free tissue transfers are now more frequently performed.[96]

The timing of combined reconstructive procedures has been subject to discussions. Traditionally, these injuries have been addressed by multistage procedures.[97] However, since

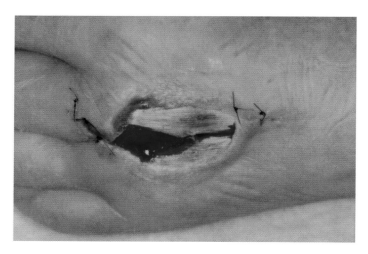

Fig. 10.32 Postinfectious defect of the dorsum of the hand with exposed extensor tendons.

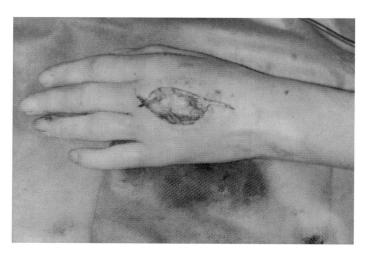

Fig. 10.33 Defect after debridement of the extensor tendons. The metacarpal bones are exposed.

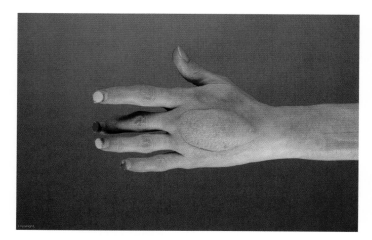

Fig. 10.34 Soft-tissue reconstruction by a posterior interosseus artery flap. The missing tendons have been reconstructed by transfer of the extensor indicis tendon.

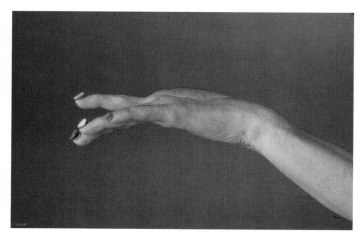

Fig. 10.35 Recovery of extensor function.

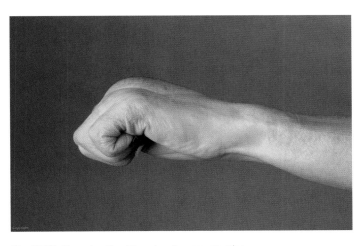

Fig. 10.36 Flexor function 12 weeks after reconstruction.

Godina's classic work on the value of early debridement and free tissue transfer for lower-extremity defects, today probably most surgeons apply the same principles in upper-extremity reconstruction with the aim of achieving soft-tissue coverage within 72 hours.[98] Several authors have reported excellent results after one-stage procedures for defects involving the dorsum of the hand with the use of emergency free flaps.[99–101] Reconstruction of missing tendons is usually performed at the time of soft-tissue coverage by primary grafting or tendon transfers. Because the creation of a secondary tendon sheath is not necessary, staged reconstruction of extensor tendons utilizing silicone rods is rare.[102–104] Adams reported on six patients who were treated by two-staged reconstructions of complex defects of the extensor tendon at the level of the PIP joint.[104] Active extension of the PIP joint could be achieved in all patients with an average extensor lag of 15°. In contrast, Quaba *et al.* presented good clinical results in nine patients with complex defects in zones VI and VII who received soft-tissue coverage only without reconstruction of tendon defects.[105]

Conclusion

Extensor tendon injuries are frequently underestimated. However, even slight disturbances in the delicate balance between the flexor and the extensor tendon systems will result in significant loss of finger function. Therefore, a clear understanding of the pertinent anatomy is essential to achieve good treatment results. Acute injuries require early diagnosis and treatment, which should always take the surrounding soft-tissue structures into consideration. Chronic injuries and subsequent finger deformities such as swan-neck and boutonnière deformities are very difficult to correct and require a thorough analysis of the underlying tendon imbalance. As is true for other tendon injuries, good results cannot be achieved without the choice of the right postoperative treatment protocol.

Access the complete references list online at **http://www.expertconsult.com**

5. Harris CJ, Rutledge GLJ. The functional anatomy of the extensor mechanism of the finger. *J Bone Joint Surg Am.* 1972;54:713–726.

6. Landsmeer JM. The anatomy of the dorsal aponeurosis of the human finger and its functional significance. *Anat Rec.* 1949;104:31–44.

    Classic description of the function of the oblique retinacular ligaments which is the anatomical foundation for numerous reconstructive procedures of the distal extensor tendon.

16. Newport ML, Williams CD. Biomechanical characteristics of extensor tendon suture techniques. *J Hand Surg Am.* 1992;17:1117–1123.

23. Handoll HH, Vaghela MV. Interventions for treating mallet finger injuries. *Cochrane Database Syst Rev.* 2004;CD004574.

36. Snow JW. Use of a retrograde tendon flap in repairing a severed extensor in the pip joint area. *Plast Reconstr Surg.* 1973;51:555–558.

    Although only 6 cases in 3 years are reported, this is the classic description of one of the most commonly used techniques to reconstruct defects of the central slip.

47. Evans RB. Early active short arc motion for the repaired central slip. *J Hand Surg Am.* 1994;19:991–997.

    Based on several anatomical studies, Evans introduces a new early active motion protocol for extensor tendon injuries in zones III and IV. Sixty-four digits in 55 patients were investigated. Patients who were treated by early active motion demonstrated better functional results than those who were treated by immobilization.

48. Duran RJ, Houser RG, Stover MG. Management of flexor tendon lacerations in Zone 2 using controlled passive motion postoperatively. In: Hunter JM, Schneider LH, Mackin EJ, et al, eds. *Rehabilitation of the Hand.* St. Louis: CV Mosby; 1978:217–224.

51. Mowlavi A, Burns M, Brown RE. Dynamic versus static splinting of simple zone V and zone VI extensor tendon repairs: a prospective, randomized, controlled study. *Plast Reconstr Surg.* 2005;115:482–487.

63. Bowers WH, Hurst LC. Chronic mallet finger: The use of Fowler's central slip release. *J Hand Surg Am.* 1978;3:373–376.

70. Dolphin JA. Extensor tenotomy for chronic boutonnière deformity of the finger; report of two cases. *J Bone Joint Surg Am.* 1965;47:161–164.

    Description of the classic technique to address the problem of the boutonnière deformity.

72. Littler JW, Eaton RG. Redistribution of forces in the correction of boutonnière deformity. *J Bone Joint Surg Am.* 1967;49:1267–1274.

    Littler and Eaton describe the pathophysiology of the boutonnière deformity and the results of 8 patients who were treated by detachment and proximal reinsertion of the lateral bands.

11

Replantation and revascularization

William W. Dzwierzynski

SYNOPSIS

- Replantation should be considered for all amputated parts; the only absolute contraindication to replantation is preserving life over limb.
- A string sign or ribbon sign in the digital vessels suggests the digit is not suitable for replantation.
- Skeletal shortening should be considered. Bone shortening facilitates a primary nerve and vessel repair.
- Rigid bone fixation is desired for early mobilization. Interosseous wires offer an excellent option for rigid fixation.
- Revascularization of wrist and more proximal amputations should be performed before 12 hours of cold ischemia or a maximum 6 hours of warm ischemia. If ischemia time is over 4 hours, consideration should be given to temporary arterial shunting prior to bone fixation.
- Pharmacological management of replantation and revascularization remains controversial. Our current protocol includes heparin irrigation at a dilution of 100 units/ml during surgery and a heparin bolus of 50–100 units/kg before release of microvascular clamps.
- The psychological implications of amputation and replantation must be considered. The hand plays a significant role in a patient's identity and psyche.

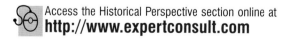

Access the Historical Perspective section online at
http://www.expertconsult.com

Introduction

Restoring life has always been a dream. From the mythological resurrection of the phoenix to the rising of Lazarus from the dead, returning life to the dead remains a miracle. Replantation restores life to the lifeless extremity: a miracle of modern surgery.

Basic science/disease process

Pathophysiology of ischemia and reperfusion

Tissue tolerance to ischemia varies significantly. In normal ambient temperature, irreversible changes can occur in muscle with only 2 hours of ischemia; skin properly cooled and stored in a nutrient media can be viable for over a month.[4] Ischemia causes tissue hypoxia and the conversion from aerobic to anaerobic metabolism. Adenosine triphosphate (ATP) is produced by glycolysis which leads to the buildup of lactic acid in the tissue and the resultant reduction of intercellular pH.[5] As the supply of ATP is diminished, intracellular Na^+ and Ca^{2+} concentrations are increased. Chemical mediators and enzymes are triggered by ischemia, resulting in the production of phospholipase A_2 and lysozymes. If continued beyond the critical point these processes lead to eventual cell necrosis.

Revascularization is essential before these processes become irreversible, but revascularization can lead to its own problems. Reperfusion injury can cause problems as severe as the initial ischemic insult. When ischemic tissue is suddenly reperfused, reactive oxygen species (ROS) are produced. These include superoxide (O^-_2), hydrogen peroxide (H_2O_2), and hydroxyl radical (OH^-).[6] The ROS react with the cell membranes, especially in the endothelial cells. They cause direct cell damage and produce inflammatory mediators, complement activation, and leukocyte adhesion. This cascade increases vascular permeability and can cause cell death despite revascularization. Reperfusion-generated mediators may have systemic effects when vessels are unclamped and the inflammatory mediators are released to the circulation. This can lead to a decreased level of consciousness, jaundice, cardiac arrhythmia, metabolic acidosis, myoglobinuria, and multifailure organ system.[7] Methods to prevent or reduce ischemia–reperfusion injury include hypothermia, interarterial flushing, ischemic preconditioning, antithrombotic agents, free-radical scavengers, and leukocyte inhibitors.[4,5] While many of these techniques show promise experimentally or in elective free flap surgery, pretreatment is not an option in traumatic replantation and revascularization. Aside from expedient revascularization the only current useful techniques are cooling of the amputated part, interarterial flushing, and antithrombotic agents. In major limb replantation, once arterial flow is established, the vein should be allowed to bleed to eliminate ROS, prior to establishing flow to the systemic circulation.

Diagnosis/patient presentation

Transportation

The most critical factors in replantation and revascularization surgery is management of the patient and the amputated part. Proper handling of the amputation is essential to revascularization and replantation success. The first responders must be educated in the proper transportation of the injured part. This includes proper cooling of the amputated part and stabilization of the patient. The part is wrapped in moist saline gauze and placed in a waterproof plastic bag. The plastic bag is placed in a container of ice *(Fig. 11.1)*. The part should not come into direct contact with the ice. Freezing the severed extremity can cause direct irreversible damage to the microvascular system. Timely, efficient transportation of the patient and the amputated part to the replantation center is critical for survival and function. Because of the rapid irreversible changes that occur in muscle, this is essential in major limb amputations. Muscle undergoes irreversible damage with ischemia times greater than 6–9 hours. Digits tolerate longer periods of ischemia. Successful replantation can be achieved even after prolonged ischemia. VanderWilde *et al.* reported a successful hand replantation after 54 hours of cold ischemia.[8] Wei *et al.* reported a series of three successful digital replants with 84, 86, and 94 hours of cold ischemia.[9] All patients had satisfactory functional results and no vascular compromise. Lin *et al.* reviewed their experience with 31 replantations (two thumb, 21 finger, and two hand amputations), all with over 24 hours of either cold or warm ischemia. The overall success rate was 64%. Only one of the hands was successfully replanted; 15 of the 23 digits were salvaged.[10]

Replantation center

Digital and major limb replantation can be performed in any hospital with a microscope or even a pair of high-powered surgical loupes. A replantation center, usually a trauma center, offers a dedicated team to serve the patient better. The replantation center should include an emergency room and paramedic system familiar with the transportation of the injured patient and the amputated part *(Table 11.1)*. This often includes a medical air transportation system to facilitate rapid transportation from the accident scene. At the replantation center, the operating room should be large enough to allow two independent surgical teams to operate, one on the patient and the second on the amputated part *(Fig. 11.2)*. The replantation center should have a minimum of two sets of microsurgical instruments and two microscopes if possible. Chung *et al.* reviewed the database from the Agency for Healthcare Policy and Research, evaluating 304 cases of finger replantation. Over 906 hospitals were represented in the database but only 15% performed a finger replantation in the year reviewed; 60% of these hospitals performed only one replant. Only 2%

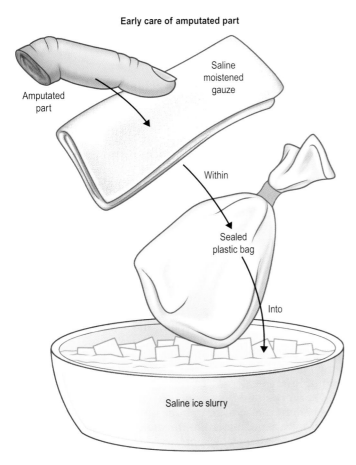

Early care of amputated part

Amputated part

Saline moistened gauze

Within

Sealed plastic bag

Into

Saline ice slurry

Fig. 11.1 The amputated part should be wrapped in moist gauze placed in a plastic bag which is chilled in an ice-water mixture. Direct contact of the part with the ice must be avoided.

Table 11.1 Replantation center criteria

1. An efficient ground and air transportation system to transfer the patient from the injury site or referring hospital to the replant center
2. Experienced microsurgical teams, able to work in shifts
3. A well-prepared emergency room staff to stabilize and quickly evaluate the patient with physical examination, X-rays, and laboratory tests
4. Experienced anesthetists, operating room, and microsurgical staff available 24 hours/day, 7 days/week
5. Proper microscopes, instruments, and sutures
6. A carefully trained nursing staff for postoperative care and monitoring
7. Physical and occupational therapists trained in postreplantation rehabilitation
8. Psychologists and social workers to help the patient cope with his or her injuries and continue an active and useful life

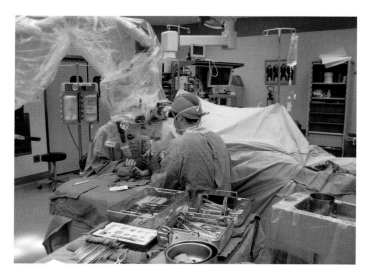

Fig. 11.2 Replantation operation room set-up. The pressure pump is situated at the patient's head. The fluid cooler/warmer (far right) is used for icing the amputated part.

Table 11.2 Indications for replantation
Strong indications
• Multiple digital amputations
• Thumb amputations
• Whole hand
• Transmetacarpal and partial hand amputations
• Any amputated part in a child
• Single digit amputation distal to flexor digitorum superficialis insertion
Relative indications
• Sharp injuries at elbow or proximal forearm
• Humeral-level amputations

of the hospitals in the database performed 10 or more cases. He postulated that replantations should be best performed at high-volume centers.[11] Chen and Narayan reviewed the economic trends of upper extremity replantations over a 10-year period and found an increasing tendency for these surgeries to be performed at large teaching institutions.[12] A survey of members of the American Society of Surgery of the Hand found that only 56% of its members perform replantation surgery, despite 94% of the responders describing their microsurgical training as good or excellent.[13]

Patient selection

Indications and contraindications

Needless to say, the critical patient selection criterion for replantation is a patient with an amputation. The amputated part must be both available and in satisfactory condition for the replantation *(Table 11.2)*. Digits recovered from the stomach of an attacking animal or extracted from industrial grinders generally do not meet this criterion. Outside these obvious examples, replantation should at least be considered for all amputated parts. This includes not only amputation of the upper extremity but the lower extremity or any other body part. Accepted indications for replantations in the upper extremities are thumb amputations, multidigit amputations and amputations in children.[14] Replantation of parts otherwise not generally thought to be replantable are often indicated in the child. Often adult patients with single-digit amputations, especially the index finger, are generally not considered candidates for replantation.[15] Replantation of a single digit is generally indicated in children. This is partly due to improved healing in children but also because of the future potential of the child. A replanted digit may allow a child to follow her dream as a great musician or athlete, whereas an amputation revision may preclude this possibility. Lower-extremity and upper arm replantations may also be

indicated in a child. The child possesses improved nerve regeneration that may allow improved function for amputations at these levels.

Thumb amputations also deserve special emphasis. It is our opposable thumb which separates us from other species. While thumb reconstruction can be achieved with methods such as pollicization or toe transfer, these reconstructions have a significant donor site cost. Thumb replantation should be considered even if the digit may be shorter or if arthrodesis is necessary due to joint trauma. The thumb primarily functions as a post for opposition. Whereas lack of motion in a replanted finger decreases the usefulness and function of the hand, decreased motion in a thumb is generally well accepted, and a stiff thumb still contributes to the overall function of the hand.

Patients who have lost multiple digits also deserve an extra consideration in replantation. Where a single digit loss may be well tolerated, patients who have lost multiple digits have a significantly greater disability. Salvaging one or two fingers in a mutilated hand may preserve essential function of the hand. In multiple-digit amputations consideration should also be made for "spare-parts surgery." If an amputation is through the metacarpophalangeal (MCP) joint of the long finger and more proximal on the index finger, replantation of the index finger to the long finger ray, preserving the joint, may increase the patient's overall function. Replantation above the elbow is advocated for preservation of elbow function but generally distal function in the hand is poor.[16] Fingertip replantations, once considered nonindicated, are now seen as an excellent level of replantation. Replantation of a digit distal to the flexor digitorum superficialis (FDS) insertion generally has excellent function because only one flexor tendon requires repair, and should be strongly considered.

The only absolute contraindication to replantation is preserving life over limb. A patient with life-threatening injuries or multiple medical problems who cannot withstand prolonged surgery should not undergo replantation. An uncooperative patient is also a contraindication for replantation.[14] In a patient with acute major life-threatening injuries, an amputated hand or digit may be kept in cold storage and the patient reassessed in 24 hours. If the patient is stable enough to undergo surgery, delayed replantation may be considered.

There are several relative contraindications to digital replantation[17] *(Table 11.3)*. These contraindications are related

Table 11.3 Relative contraindications to replantation
• Concomitant life-threatening injury
• Systemic illness (e.g., small-vessel disease)
• Poor anesthesia risk
• Mentally unstable patients
• Single finger proximal to flexor digitorum superficialis insertion in adults
• Multiple segmental injuries in the amputated part
• Severe crushing or avulsion of the tissues
• Extreme contamination
• Prior surgery or trauma to the amputated part
• Prolonged warm ischemia time
• Ribbon sign, red line sign
• Most index finger amputations

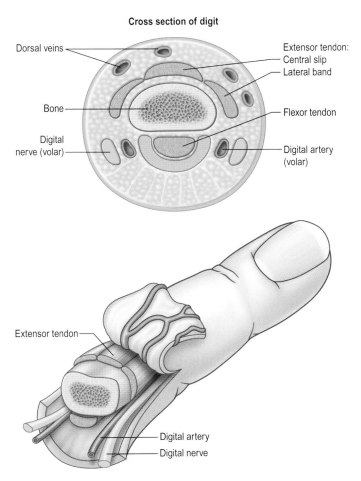

Cross section of digit

Fig. 11.3 **(A, B)** A mid-lateral exposure of the amputated part offers greater access to the neurovascular structures.

more to microvascular success and hand function as compared to an amputation revision. All patients must be evaluated individually to determine if they are a candidate for digital replantation. While age is not an absolute contraindication for replantation, older patients carry a greater risk of arteriosclerosis of the vessel, joint stiffness, and generally decreased function secondary to less recovery of sensation. Okada *et al.* reviewed eight replantations in patients over 65 years old. Function of these digits was generally classified as poor, although all patients were satisfied with their results. Expectations in the elderly patient may be less than those of a younger patient.[18]

Treatment/surgical technique

Operative sequence

Replantation surgery is an exacting and strenuous operation. It should proceed in an organized and deliberate fashion. When replantation is considered feasible, the amputated part is brought to the operating room and explored to identify the neurovascular structures. This may even be performed while the patient is still in the emergency room being evaluated and stabilized.

If two surgical teams are available (at least for a short time during this surgery) both the amputated part and the patient can undergo simultaneous surgery. If there is any delay in getting the patient to the operating room, the amputated part is brought to the operating room first. Using loupe magnification, all structures are examined. The blood vessels and nerves are usually examined at high magnification with the operating microscope before committing to perform a replantation. Under the operating microscope, the part is examined for suitability of replantation. Tissue loss is evaluated, along with the level of amputation. Multiple levels of injury may be found which were not apparent during the emergency room examination. The neurovascular structures should be evaluated for evidence of avulsion injuries. A string sign or ribbon sign means the digit is not suitable for replantation. These signs are indicated by a red streaking of blood along the path of the artery, usually implying an avulsion injury. The artery and nerves should be identified and tagged with a 7-0

polypropylene suture or microclips. If the digital vessels cannot be readily identified through the traumatic wound, the digital vessels can be exposed through a midaxial incision *(Fig. 11.3)*. Dorsal veins are identified and tagged in a similar fashion. The location of the veins is more variable, and they may not be readily visible. Two or three veins should be identified. Preliminary bone fixation and methods of tendon repair are considered at this time. The digital core tendon suture may be placed while the part is on the back table. The distal aspect of the bony fixation can also be secured, whether this is with K-wires, interosseous wires, or a mini fixation plate.

Once the patient is under anesthesia, the proximal level of the injury is explored. Replantation surgery is usually performed under general anesthesia. Regional anesthesia may be considered for a cooperative patient. Regional anesthesia offers the added benefit of decreased postoperative pain and possible vasodilatation. A Foley catheter is inserted and proper body warming is assured by utilizing a warming blanket and warming the operating room. All pressure points should be well padded to avoid pressure injuries; this includes the occiput to avoid scalp alopecia.

The sequence of the repair in digital replantation varies among surgeons, with some advocating arterial repair after bony fixation and flexor tendon repair while others advocate

Video 1

repair of the dorsal structures, including the extensor tendon, dorsal veins, and skin prior to repairing any volar structures.[17] The author favors repairing the volar structures first, and then proceeding to the dorsal structures. Repair of the extensor tendon prior to releasing the tourniquet is advantageous in those cases where visualizing the vein is difficult and better seen when the digit is revascularized.

Bone fixation

The time spent in achieving secure digital fixation is well worth the additional effort required in this fixation *(Fig. 11.4)*. Adequate fixation of the replanted digit is essential not only for short-term healing but also for long-term function. Rigid fixation of the bony fracture can reduce pain, allow early mobilization of the hand, and improve long-term function. Conventional thinking suggests that time is of the essence and bony fixation should be rapid in order to get to the ultimate goal of the microvascular repair. This logic ignores the fact that the final outcome of the replantation lies in the ultimate function of the hand. Function is linked to motion, and motion is optimized by early mobilization. Rigid bone fixation is desired for early mobilization. Skeletal shortening should be considered in all replantations; this can allow more secure bone fixation and lessen the need for vessel and nerve grafting.[14] In a thumb, shortening of the digit should be performed judiciously.[19]

A variety of methods are available for bone fixation. The simplest method is K-wire fixation. K-wires are universally available and can be easily and rapidly inserted. The simplest fixation is a longitudinally placed K-wire. While easily performed, longitudinal K-wires have many disadvantages. K-wires do not offer rigid fixation, longitudinal K-wires do not control against rotation and, almost by necessity, must go through the joint. Longitudinal K-wires are best utilized in distal replants and revascularizations where other fixation methods may not be technically feasible.

Cross K-wires offer more advantages than longitudinal K-wire fixation, most notably the control of rotation. Cross K-wires can be difficult for the novice to perform in simple fracture fixation and devascularization injuries, but complete amputation simplifies the process of cross K-wire placement. While the amputated digit is on the back table, the K-wires can be inserted in a retrograde fashion. The neurovascular structures need to be meticulously protected and the amputated part securely held to avoid spinning the part uncontrollably.

Kirschner wires offer control of rotational deformity but greater care must be taken with early digital motion. Cross K-wires give an acceptable result although early rigid fixation is not achieved. Late digital stiffness and fracture malunion may occur. Kirschner wires should be reserved for cases where rapid fixation is necessary and in children.[19]

Interosseous (I-O) wires offer an excellent option for rigid fixation in amputations. I-O wires can be technically demanding to perform, but offer the advantage of rigid fixation and the ability to correct for any rotational deformity prior to final tightening of the wires. Three sets of wires, two longitudinal and one radial ulnar, give as much rigidity as a fixation plate. The exposure granted by the amputation allows easier access to the bone for I-O wire placement. The ends of the wires should be turned in to the fracture site to add additional strength to the configuration and to avoid impingement on the tendons.[20] Ninety-ninety-wire bone fixation has a low nonunion rate and provides secure compression of the fractures.[17,19,21–23]

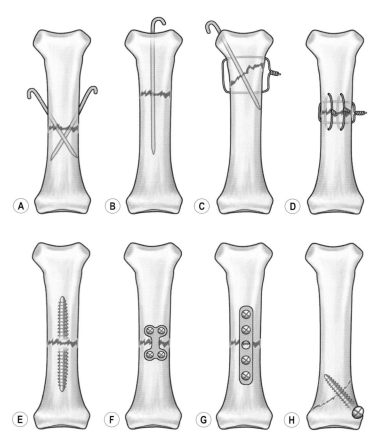

Fig. 11.4 Techniques of bony fixation include: **(A)** crossed K-wires; **(B)** single longitudinal K-wire; **(C)** I-O wire and K-wire; **(D)** 90-90 I-O wires; **(E)** intermedullary fixation; **(F)** compression plate; **(G)** H-plate; and **(H)** lag screw.

Hints and tips

Interosseous wire fixation is a quick and secure method of bony fixation for digital replantations. While the amputated part is on the back table two tunnels, one radial to ulnar and one dorsal to volar, are made with a 21-gauge needle. The 21-gauge needle allows a 26-gauge wire to pass through the tunnel easily.

Plate fixation offers secure fixation for fractures. Standard miniplates, while offering secure fixation and compression, have the disadvantage of requiring significant periosteal stripping and more extensive soft-tissue exposure. Small "H" plates offer similar fixation strength with less exposure and periosteal stripping. One disadvantage of plates is the lack of adjustability. If distinct registration points are not present on the bone, improper fixation can lead to rotational deformities. The increased dissection and periosteal stripping may lead to increased scarring and tendon adhesions. Generally plate fixation is more time-consuming than other methods of fixation. A low-profile H-plate may allow less dissection; however, this application is technically demanding and angulation and malunions can occur.[19]

Tendon repair

Secure tendon repair is necessary for early-motion protocols. Inexperienced surgeons may desire to fix the tendons quickly in order to move on to the revascularization of the fingers. In properly cooled digital amputations, ischemia time can be safely prolonged without any deleterious effects on success rates and overall function. The extra 20–30 minutes required to obtain a good tendon repair is time far better spent to avoid tendon rupture, protracted therapy and tenolysis surgery. We prefer to use a modified Kessler repair along with an epitendinous suture. The Kessler repair is easy and relatively quick to perform. The use of a looped 4-0 braided polyethylene fiber suture allows a strong four-strand repair without significant bulk. The epitendinous repair is essential for proper tendon excursion. This additional suture supplies increased strength, facilitates tendon glidin, and allows proper tendon tensioning of the core suture. The pulleys should always be preserved. The distal core suture may be first performed and then the tendon is glided under the pulley for the final repair.

The distal core tendon suture is usually performed on the back table. To repair the tendon the distal phalanx is flexed to expose and relax the tendon. The proximal tendon is identified and secured with a 25-gauge needle to the underlying tissue to prevent retraction. Utilizing a 6-0 polypropylene suture, the epitendinous repair is started on the dorsal aspect of the tendon, with a locked, running suture. After completion of the dorsal epitendinous repair, the core suture repair is woven through the proximal portion of the tendon. The knot is tied in the substance of the tendon. Use of this technique may prevent tendon bunching. Finally, the volar epitendinous repair is performed with a running locking stitch, utilizing the remaining portion of the 6-0 polypropylene suture. This four-strand repair is strong enough to initiate early active motion protocols.

Hints and tips

In tendon repair, performing the back wall of the epitendinous suture first allows better approximation of the core suture. The tendon is held securely with a 25-gauge needle to the soft tissue, and then a running locking 6-0 polypropylene suture is used for the back wall. The core suture is placed without any tendon "bunching." The running polypropylene suture is then continued on the volar aspect of the tendon.

Controversy exists among surgeons as to whether both and FDS and flexor digitorum profundus (FDP) tendons should be repaired in zone 2 replantations.[24] Waikakul et al., in their series of 1018 replantations, found patients who had a sharp guillotine zone 2 amputation had good to acceptable results in terms of range of motion with repair of both tendons. In crush, degloving, or avulsion injuries, repairing only the FDP tendon or both tendons gave poor results. Repairing the FDP stump to the proximal superficialis tendon gave the best result, which was statistically significant.[25] Ross et al. prospected and evaluated tendon function after replantation using a modified Kessler repair with 4-0 polyester suture. The average total active motion was 129°. Patients with zone 1 and 5 injuries had a significantly better active range of motion. Replantation after avulsion injury resulted in lower range of motion compared to sharp injuries. When they evaluated patients who had one tendon repaired versus those with a repair of both tendons, the average motion for fingers with both tendons repaired was 136° compared to 111° for fingers with only the FDP tendon repaired. This was statistically significant. Of all factors in the surgeon's control, the most important was initiating early therapy. Early therapy increased both active and passive range of motion and did not significantly increase the incidence of tendon rupture.[24]

Artery repair

A patent arterial repair is essential to successful replantation. The red line sign, or ribbon sign, is an indication of torsion or stretch of the vessel and suggests a relative contraindication to replantation.[26] Arteries should be debrided to beyond the zone of injury. The lumen of the artery should be explored to make certain there are no intimal flaps which can cause thrombosis. The arteries should be examined and cut back, as necessary, prior to inflation of the tourniquet. The vessel is flushed with a dilute heparin solution at a concentration of 100 units/mL. The heparinized saline solution can be placed in a pressure bag to assure a constant, accurate irrigation pressure (Fig. 11.5). Manual irrigation with a standard 3-cc syringe may produce excessive irrigation pressure. Yan et al. found that irrigation pressures under 80 mmHg are as effective as higher pressures at removing clots and did not damage the vessel endothelium.[27] After irrigation, the vascular clamp is released to visualize the arterial flow. If the artery does not have a strong pulsatile flow, the vessel is cut back and irrigated until pulsatile flow is obtained. It is preferable to repair both digital arteries, if possible. Zumiotti et al. found that when two arteries and more than one vein were anastomosed, the success rate was highest.[28] In the index finger, long finger, and thumb, the ulnar digital artery is usually larger and should be preferentially repaired. In the small finger, the radial digital artery is usually of larger diameter. There is usually no difference in size in the ring finger vessels. Adequate exposure to the blood vessels is essential. Skin hooks attached to rubber bands may facilitate artery exposure. If this is not adequate, additional incisions should be made to aid exposure. In the proximal and middle phalanx, zigzag incisions are preferable, while in distal replantations a mid-axial incision is preferred.[14]

If after proper debridement the gap precludes primary repair, a vein graft should be used. Theoretically an increased potential of thrombosis exists when vein grafts are used since there are two microvascular anastomoses. However, clinical studies do not support an increased incidence of thrombosis. When vein grafts are utilized, venous discrepancies may be managed by a variety of techniques, including fish mouth incisions, sleeve anastomosis, or end-to-side coupling or step-down vein grafts.[29] Vein grafts are usually harvested from the palmar side of the thenar eminence of the hand or from the distal volar forearm or the dorsal foot (Fig. 11.6).[30] For arterial reconstruction in the finger, the author prefers the dorsal foot veins because they are thicker-walled and better match the

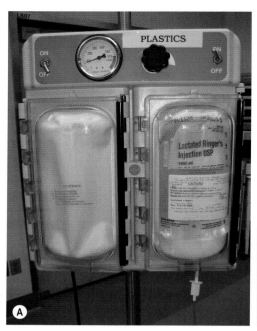
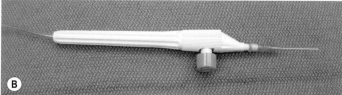

Fig. 11.5 (A) Pressure bag irrigation with pharmacy-prepared heparin irrigation solution. **(B)** Irrigation hand control.

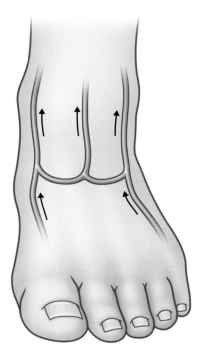

Dorsal venous arch of foot

Fig. 11.6 The dorsum of the foot provides a source of potential vein grafts. The branching pattern allows revascularization of several vessels.

digital artery. For more proximal amputations the greater or lesser saphenous veins can be harvested.

Lee *et al.* prospectively followed 75 finger replantations with Doppler examinations for 60 days postoperatively. In 37% of successful replantations Doppler signals, which were initially present, were not heard on postoperative day 15. This rate was five times greater for crush injuries than for guillotine amputation. Their replantation center now routinely administers anticoagulants for 2 weeks in all replantations, regardless of the degree of tissue damage. They postulate that by continuing anticoagulation, reduced morbidity such as cold intolerance and sensory abnormalities may be achieved.[31]

Vein repair

Repair of the veins is one of the most crucial steps in replantation. The number of veins repaired correlates well with success in digital replantation.[32,33] In a devascularized extremity or digit, a small skin bridge of only a few millimeters can allow adequate venous outflow. In a complete amputation, the vein repair is critical. Dorsal veins can be found by identifying bruising or small hematomas just under the skin *(Fig. 11.7)*. The veins are usually repaired after repair of one or both of the digital arteries. If ischemia time is prolonged, the vein can be repaired after the first digital artery and then the hand supinated to repair a second digital artery. Veins grafts to bridge segments of venous loss are used as required. Additional length on dorsal veins may be achieved by dividing the interconnecting branches between the veins. At least one vein should be repaired prior to release of the arterial clamp. If a vein could not be identified on the initial exploration of the amputated part, release of the arterial clamp will allow visualization of the dorsal veins as they fill with blood; but the resulting bleeding may obscure the clean microvascular field.

A functional venous anastomoses is important to overall success rate in replantation; however, the more distal the amputation, the less this factor comes into play. Distal amputations can be successfully replanted even without a venous anastomosis as long as some method of venous egress is assured.[34–38] In a series of 120 replantations distal to the FDS

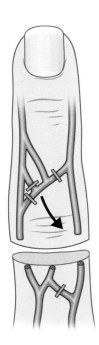

Fig. 11.7 Ligation of branches of the dorsal subcutaneous veins can provide additional length for primary venous repair.

insertion a 91.7% success rate was achieved when two veins were repaired. This success rate dropped to 84.4% when only one vein was repaired, but with no vein anastomosis, a 40% success rate was still achieved.[39] Various methods of venous outflow other than direct vein coaptation have been described. These include use of leeches (Hirudo medicinal), arterial venous anastomoses, nail plate removal, heparin rubs, subcutaneous heparin instillation, nail ablation, and dermal implantation.[34,35,39–41]

Nerve repair

Sensibility in the replanted finger is an important factor in final functional outcome. Sensibility is even more important than range of motion.[14] Primary repair of the nerve can be performed in most clean guillotine-type injuries. Bone shortening facilitates a primary nerve repair.[42] Patient factors influencing nerve recovery are age, level of injury, and mechanism of injury. Surgeon-controllable factors include digital blood flow and postoperative sensory re-education. Repair of more than one artery improves nerve recovery.[43] If there is any question of the quality of the nerve it should be debrided to identify a good fascicular pattern. Nerve grafts or conduits can be used for small nerve defects. Conduits may be constructed utilizing a variety of materials, including segments of vein, collagen, silicone, Gore-Tex®, polyester, and polyglycolide.[44] Conduits are best limited to defects of less than 2 cm in length.[45] Some conduits are extremely rigid and may impede motion if placed over a joint or are at risk for erosion of overlying skin. Conduits are best used for sensory nerve defects; for motor nerves standard nerve grafts are preferred. Nerve grafts can be harvested from a variety of donor sites. In the upper extremity these include the posterior interosseous or median antebrachial cutaneous nerves. The sural

nerve is the standard donor graft in the lower extremity. The fascicles of the sural nerve match the digital nerve topology well. After successful nerve repair, replanted fingers typically achieve protective sensation with a two-point discrimination under 15 mm. The majority will achieve static two-point discrimination less than 12 mm.[46]

Skin closure

Skin closure should be performed with special precautions not to constrict arterial inflow or, more importantly, venous outflow. Tight closures may compromise success in replantation. If there is any concern a skin graft should be utilized. A small graft over the mid-lateral incision covering the vascular pedicle is far safer than a tight closure. If there is a deficit of skin and an arterial defect requiring a vein graft, consideration should be given to using a venous flowthrough flap (vascularized by the digital artery).[47] The flap is harvested from the distal ipsilateral volar forearm. A vein of sufficient size is identified and a skin flap slightly larger than the skin defect is designed, centered over the vein. The flap should not extend more than 1.5 cm from the vein. The vein is reversed and used to bridge the arterial defect and the skin island covers the skin defect.

Special circumstances

Thumb replantation

Thumb replantation and revascularization deserve special consideration *(Fig. 11.8)*. Technical considerations in thumb replantation include the liberal use of vein grafting. The ulnar digital artery of the thumb is usually of larger caliber and is preferentially repaired. The ulnar digital artery of the thumb however is difficult to access under the microscope. Even with the use of a lead hand, exposure is a challenge. It is the rare revascularization where a direct arterial repair is possible. The use of an interpositional vein graft from the radial artery to the snuff box simplifies revascularization in thumb replantation[17,19] *(Fig. 11.9)*. An 8–10-cm vein graft is harvested, usually from the dorsal foot or saphenous vein. The graft is reversed and irrigated. The distal anastomosis of the vein graft is performed on the back table before bone and tendon fixation. Performing the anastomosis on the back table allow easy positioning of the amputated thumb. The distal aspect of bone fixation should be performed prior to the distal revascularization. Care should be taken when doing the proximal bone fixation, as the vein graft can easily become wrapped up in the power equipment. In the thumb pulp sizable palmar veins can usually be identified superficial to the arteries and these should be identified.[48]

Rosson *et al.* compared the functional outcome of thumb replantation versus great toe transplantation. In 384 thumb amputations over a 20-year period, an 85% success rate was obtained in thumb replantations. Complications occurred in 29% of cases. The average replant patient underwent four additional operations. Patients achieved 30% diminished protective sensation and light touch as compared to the normal contralateral thumb. In great toe to thumb transplantations the surgical success rate was 93%, but 43% of patients had complications. The motion in the interphalangeal joint was

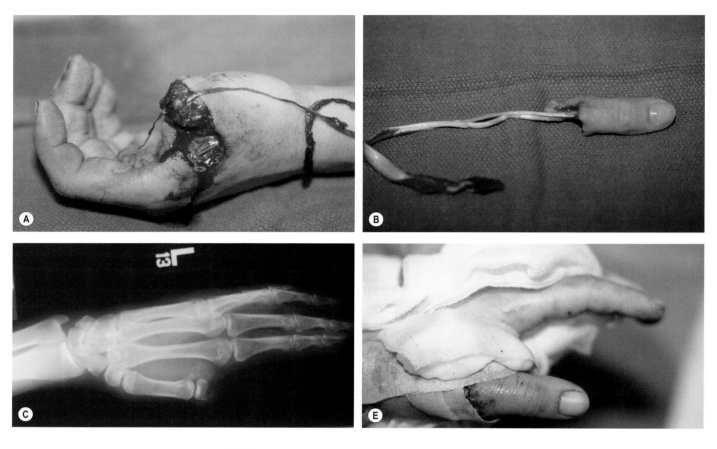

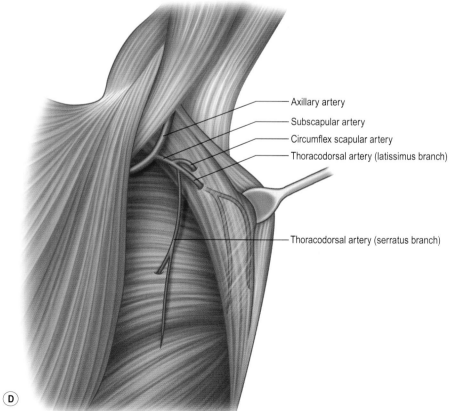

Axillary artery
Subscapular artery
Circumflex scapular artery
Thoracodorsal artery (latissimus branch)

Thoracodorsal artery (serratus branch)

Fig. 11.8 (A) A 22-year-old college student with a thumb avulsion amputation. The arteries were avulsed at the level of the interphalangeal joint. The digital nerves were avulsed in the carpal tunnel. **(B)** The amputated thumb with avulsion of the flexors and extensor tendons from the muscle origin. **(C)** Radiograph of hand. **(D)** The subscapular arterial tree provides an accessible source for a stepdown arterial graft. **(E)** Early postoperative photo of successful revascularization. The patient developed protective sensation and useful opposition function of the thumb.

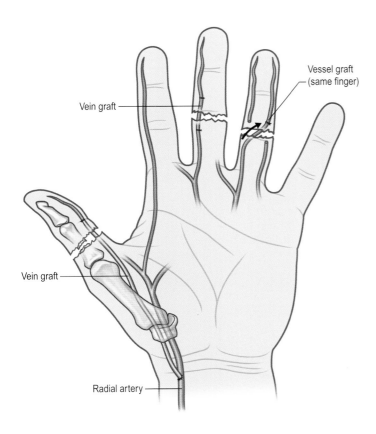

Fig. 11.9 If a primary anastomosis cannot be performed, the gap can be bridged with a reversed vein graft or transposition from an adjacent proper digital artery.

better in toe transplants than in the replanted thumb; sensation was comparable in both groups.[49]

Multiple digits

Multiple digit replantations are a significant surgical challenge and it should be performed in a replantation center with significant experience in this type of surgery *(Fig. 11.10)*. The time commitment is considerable: 3–4 hours should be allowed for each amputated finger. In most centers this will average 4 hours per finger. There may be a time-saving benefit from performing all the bony and tendon work first, then bringing in the microscope to do the microvascular repairs. Although total surgical time may be reduced, the warm ischemia time for each digit is increased. As many digits as possible are replanted. The finger with the best chance of function is repaired first. An exception to this rule is the index finger. If the index finger is stiff or has decreased sensation, the patient often avoids use of this finger.[19] Replantation of the distal amputation of the ring and little finger is strongly advocated because of their need for full length in order to get optimal hand closure and good grip function, especially when torque needs to be applied.[14]

A functional hand can be achieved with an opposable thumb, a satisfactory first webspace, a stable wrist, and at least two fingers. Heterotrophic replantation can maximize hand function. If the thumb and index finger are amputated and the distal thumb is not replantable, replantation of the index finger to the thumb position, a microvascular

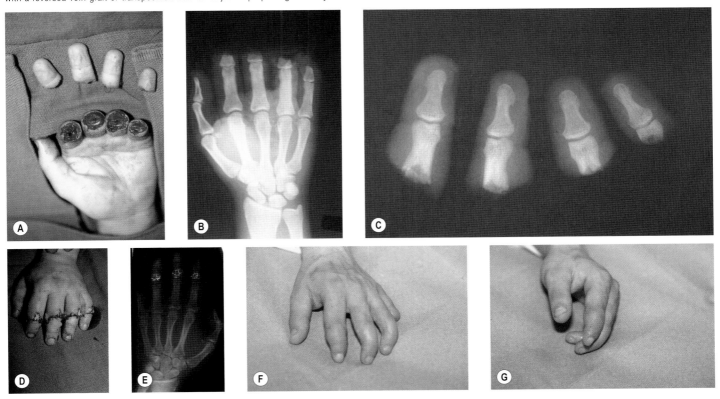

Fig. 11.10 **(A)** Four-finger amputation in a 26-year-old smoker. **(B)** Radiographs demonstrate amputation distal to the flexor digitorum superficialis insertion. **(C)** Radiographs of the amputated digits. **(D)** Immediately postoperative, after four-finger replantation. Small skin grafts were harvested to cover dorsal veins. **(E)** Radiographs demonstrate secure fixation with 90-90 I-O wire technique. **(F)** Six months postoperatively. The replantation was lost on the small finger despite salvage attempts. **(G)** Excellent function of the hand was achieved despite minimum motion at the distal interphalangeal joints.

pollicization, should be performed.[50] Forty to 50% of hand function is accounted for by the thumb. Restoration of at least two fingers is most important in achieving hook grasp, power grasp, and precision handling.[51] The value of the ulnar digits to hand function, especially power grip, is underappreciated. Priority should be given to restoration of the ulnar digits after salvage of the thumb.

A functional MCP joint is a significant priority for determining digital reconstruction. Digits with injuries through the MCP joint should be considered for heterotrophic transfer to another ray with a functional MCP joint. "Spare-parts surgery" should be considered in any multidigit amputation. If a digit is nonreplantable, skin can be harvested for use as a skin graft. Tendon, nerves, and vessels can also be used for grafts.

Proximal amputations

Amputations at the level of the palm and proximal forearm offer unique challenges and opportunities. The functional deficit of amputations at this level is devastating and replantation and revascularization offer the opportunity for meaningful function of the hand. At this level, the vessels are larger and the procedure is technically easier. Because of the presence of muscle in the amputated part, timing of revascularization is critical. Revascularization of wrist and more proximal amputations should be performed before 12 hours of cold ischemia or 6 hours of warm ischemia at the very maximum.[3] With proximal forearm revascularization it is necessary both to preserve muscle viability and prevent myoglobinuria. For injuries at the level of the distal forearm and hand, preservation of the intrinsic muscles is important to hand function but unlikely to result in myoglobinuria if critical ischemia time is exceeded. The risk of reperfusion injury is low due to their small mass; if function of the muscle is to be preserved revascularization should be expediently performed *(Fig. 11.11)*. If the injury is at the level of the palmar arch or distal, an arterial graft or reversed "Y" vein graft, usually from the dorsal foot, can be harvested to revascularize multiple common digital arteries *(Fig. 11.12)*.

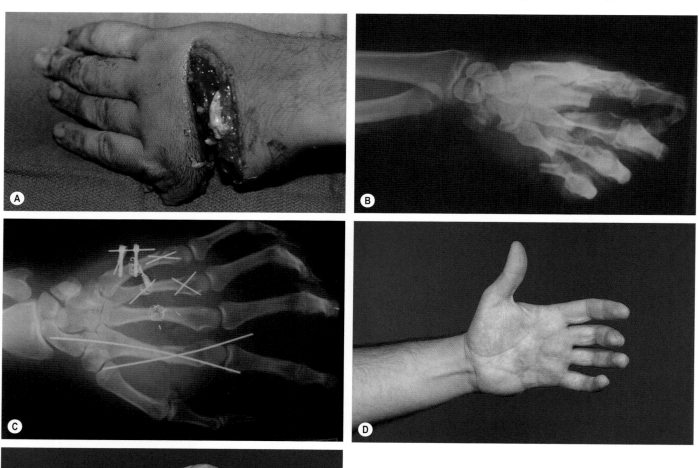

Fig. 11.11 (A) Miter saw injury in a 26-year-old carpenter; all fingers were avascular. **(B)** Preoperative radiograph. **(C)** Radiograph demonstrating fixation with I-O wires and crossed K-wires. **(D)** Postoperative extension. **(E)** Postoperative flexion.

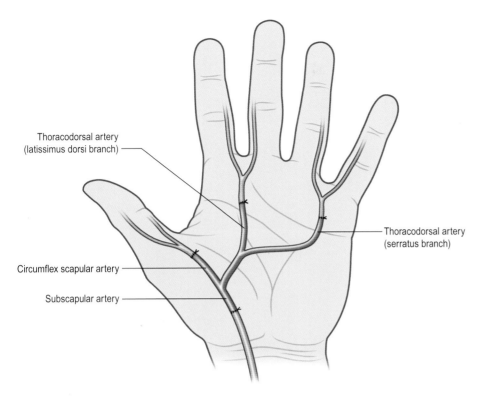

Fig. 11.12 Branches of the subscapular artery are utilized for revascularization of multiple distal vessels.

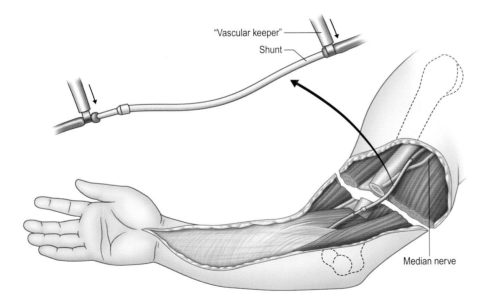

Fig. 11.13 Silicone temporary vascular stent is used in major limb replantation prior to bone fixation if ischemia time is prolonged.

Injuries in the distal forearm and wrist have excellent functional results after replantation and every effort should be made to salvage these injuries.[52] Bone fixation should be performed first in these injuries. Shortening of the bones at this level provides quicker fixation and decreased need for vein and nerve grafts, and yields almost no functional loss. If ischemia time is over 4 hours, consideration should be given to temporary arterial shunting prior to bone fixation. A carotid shunt or an intervascular catheter is used *(Fig. 11.13)*. Only one artery and one vein is required to revascularize the extremity successfully. After opening the arterial clamp, bleeding from multiple distal veins will require ligation or clamping with microvascular clamps. The risk of exsanguination with arterial and venous shunts is significant. Considerable bleeding can occur and the patient should have matched blood available. If shunting is utilized, the vein should be allowed to drain prior to connecting it to the proximal circulation.[53]

In patients with a multiple-level mangled extremity, the goal of treatment is to restore prehension and sensibility. A sensate partial hand is quite often better than a prosthesis[16] *(Fig. 11.14)*. However patients with crush or avulsion injuries may be poor candidates for replantation. Adequate debridement is the critical first step in reconstruction.[54] Vein grafts

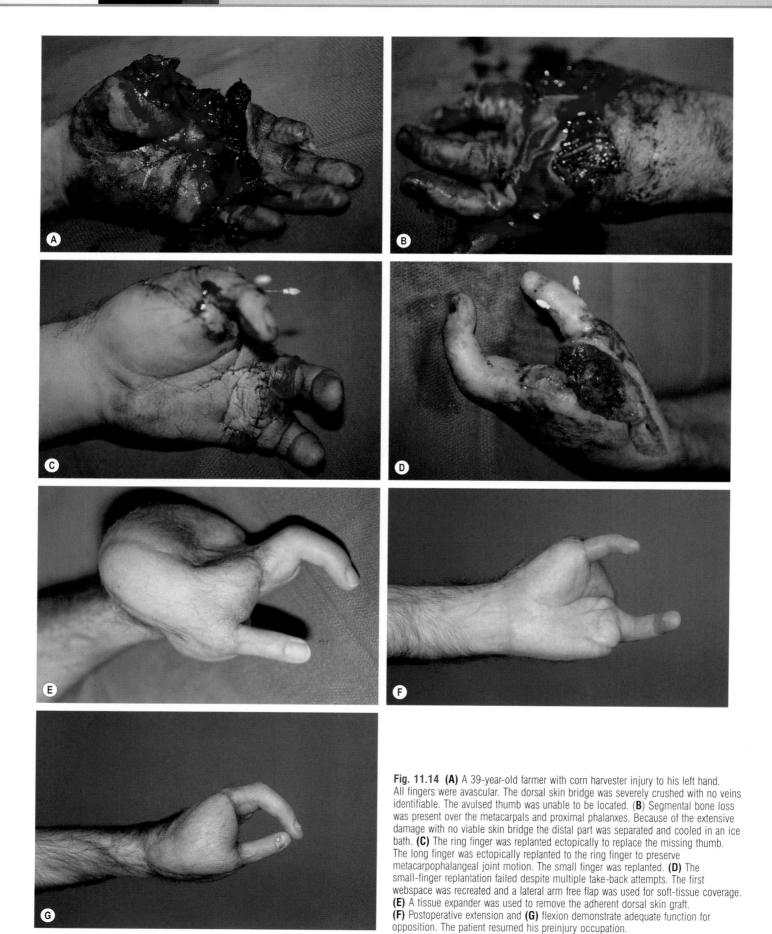

Fig. 11.14 (A) A 39-year-old farmer with corn harvester injury to his left hand. All fingers were avascular. The dorsal skin bridge was severely crushed with no veins identifiable. The avulsed thumb was unable to be located. **(B)** Segmental bone loss was present over the metacarpals and proximal phalanxes. Because of the extensive damage with no viable skin bridge the distal part was separated and cooled in an ice bath. **(C)** The ring finger was replanted ectopically to replace the missing thumb. The long finger was ectopically replanted to the ring finger to preserve metacarpophalangeal joint motion. The small finger was replanted. **(D)** The small-finger replantation failed despite multiple take-back attempts. The first webspace was recreated and a lateral arm free flap was used for soft-tissue coverage. **(E)** A tissue expander was used to remove the adherent dorsal skin graft. **(F)** Postoperative extension and **(G)** flexion demonstrate adequate function for opposition. The patient resumed his preinjury occupation.

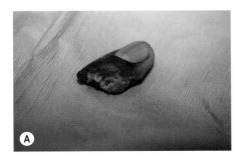 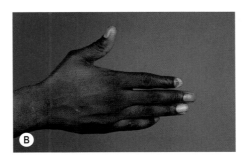 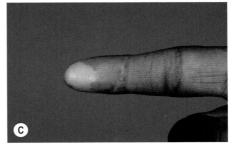

Fig. 11.15 (A) Single-digit amputation of the index finger at the level of the distal interphalangeal joint. The patient desired replantation. The surgery was performed as an outpatient, with the patient discharged home on oral aspirin. **(B)** Postoperative view of the hand. **(C)** Volar view of replanted finger.

should be liberally used to avoid injured segments of artery and vein.[29] With major limb replantation, fasciotomies are usually required. Godina emphasized that, upon completion of aggressive debridement, the wound should resemble a tumor resection.[55] Nonviable tissue with bacterial contamination is associated with loss of salvaged limb. The sequence of repairs for forearm replantation is bony fixation followed by arterial and venous repair. The vena comitantes should be repaired primarily; if this is not successful, then dorsal or antecubital veins are utilized. Nerves should be repaired after the arteries with the possible exception of the ulnar nerve, which lies deep to the ulnar artery.[54]

Amputations at the proximal forearm present a difficult clinical decision process. Functional results are generally much worse at this level than in more distal amputations. Because of the loss of muscle tissue, poor motor nerve recovery, loss of intrinsic function and postoperative scarring, results after replantation at this level are disappointing.

Amputations proximal to the elbow should be considered, if only to salvage a functional elbow joint. Recovery of distal function is poor. The greater muscle mass in a proximal limb amputation is more susceptible to ischemia time. Metabolic breakdown products from the muscles entering the systemic circulation after revascularization can result in reperfusion syndrome. Death may occur in patients with above-elbow replants who develop reperfusion syndrome.[56] A functional elbow and below-elbow prosthesis may offer the patient the best reconstructive results, but many patients are reluctant to undergo a revision amputation after a successful replantation despite having poor function.

Distal amputations

Replantation distal to the distal interphalangeal (DIP) joint was once considered as folly. Patients with amputation revisions at this level generally did very well functionally *(Fig. 11.15)*. Recent experience with distal replantations now shows both excellent success and functional and aesthetic results with replantations. These distal anastomoses can challenge the surgeon's microvascular skills *(Fig. 11.16)*. In distal crush injuries it is often difficult to get the proper size match of the distal artery. Transfer of a digital artery from an adjacent digit may be utilized, especially in children where the size match is critical.[57] A step-down arterial graft should be utilized if a vein graft is required and the reversed vein segment has too great of a size mismatch. A method of temporary intravascular stenting using 4-0–6-0

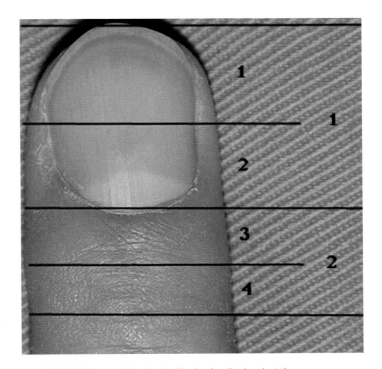

Fig. 11.16 Ishikawa and Tamai classification for distal replantation.

(0.199–0.07 mm) nylon monofilament stents for very-small-vessel anastomoses has been advocated for distal fingertip amputations; 11-0 or 12-0 sutures are placed in the vessel around the stent, which is removed prior to the last two sutures being placed. Vessels as small as 0.15 mm have been anastomosed using this technique. Microvascular survival of 85% has been reported.[58]

While arteries in very distal replants can be difficult to repair, veins may be a nightmare. The surgeon should be familiar with the venous anatomy of the digits and the thumb. Repairing volar veins may be preferable in these distal injuries, since they are easier to dissect than the dorsal veins, which lie in a dense fibrous tissue.[59] Occasionally suitable veins for repair are not available; a successful outcome can still be obtained in these cases if there is an effective means of ensuring temporary venous outflow while the collateral circulation develops. The primary method of temporary venous outflow is medicinal leeches. Leeches effectively remove congested blood and detach when engorged. Additionally, they inject hirudin, a potent anticoagulant which results in bleeding long after the leech detaches.

The leech is applied to the congested part and allowed to attach. If the arterial blood supply is poor, which usually implies that the diagnosis of venous congestion is wrong, the leech may detach prematurely and attempt to wander to another site. The patient's dressing should be fabricated to allow the leech to attach only to the congested part. Leeches feed usually for 10–40 minutes, after which they detach or should be removed. Absorbent dressing is utilized to avoid further constriction from the continued oozing, which may last for up to 6 hours. A new leech is applied if the finger appears congested again, usually no sooner than 4 hours.

Leech therapy is slowly weaned at approximately 5 days. At this point venous circulation should be re-established. *Aeromonas* species bacteria in the leech gut are essential for digestion of blood.[34] *Aeromonas hydrophila* is not normally a pathogen, but precautions should be utilized. Prophylactic antibiotics to cover *Aeromonas* should be considered. These are mainly third-generation cephalosporins or aminoglycosides. Leeches may not always be available and other methods of venous outflow can be utilized. Removing the distal nail plate and mechanical rubbing of the sterile matrix followed by application of a dressing with a 1000 unit/mL heparin solution may achieve active oozing in the congested finger. This technique is repeated hourly until congestion is improved.[35,59] Another option is the injection of heparin subcutaneously. In this technique, a fish mouth incision is made in the distal digit to allow venous outflow. A solution of 1000 units of heparin in 0.1 mL saline is injected subcutaneously into the tip of the congested replanted finger. Heparin subcutaneous injections are reported to be more cost-effective than medical leeches and simpler to administer, and heparin action can last for over 6 hours.[36]

Another technique which can be considered is subcutaneously pocketing the distal replantation. This technique was initially described using a subdermal pocket on the chest wall.[37] To prevent the awkward immobilization of a chest flap, the subdermal pocket has been described on the palm.[60] The pulp of the finger is de-epithelialized; a subdermal pocket is made in the palm or thenar crease. The finger is secured in a flexed position attached to the palm for 7 days. After 7 days the patient is brought to the operating room and the finger is detached.[61]

With distal phalanx amputation, replantation can achieve over a 90% success rate when venous anastomosis is performed. Even without venous anastomosis, success rates over 75% can be achieved.[38,41,43,44,62,63] Given these success rates, distal fingertip amputation is justifiable and these fingers should be aggressively replanted.[64] The aesthetic and psychological benefit of distal fingertip replantation should not be ignored.

Ring avulsion injuries

Ring avulsions are some of the most difficult injuries to treat. The classification scheme popularized by Urbaniak *et al.*[65] and modified by Kay *et al.*[66] is commonly used *(Table 11.4)*. Injuries of class 2 and above require microvascular repair; class 3 ring avulsions are the most challenging, due to their degloving, avulsion, and amputation *(Fig. 11.17)*. Under the operating microscope a mid-lateral incision is made on the ulnar

Table 11.4 Ring avulsion injuries classification

I	Circulation adequate
II	Circulation inadequate, no skeletal injury
	a Arterial circulation inadequate only
	v Venous circulation inadequate only
	av Arterial and venous circulation inadequate
III	Circulation inadequate, skeletal injury
	a Arterial circulation inadequate only
	v Venous circulation inadequate only
	av Arterial and venous circulation inadequate
IV	Complete amputation

aspect of the amputated digit. Nonviable tissue should be debrided. Damaged arteries should be bypassed. Inadequate debridement leads to poor outcome. Vein grafts are almost universally required due to the significant extent of the vascular damage. Because of difficulty in arterial size matching, a second step-down vein graft can be harvested; alternatively, an arterial pedicle from the adjacent digit may be used.[67,68]

A minimum of two veins should be repaired. Vein grafts should be utilized if needed. If the amputation occurs at the DIP joint, primary arthrodesis of the joint should be considered. Following replantation at this level, motion at the DIP joint is poor and fusion may permit bony shortening, which may aid in nerve repair and skin closure. The skin should not be pulled taut in order to close the skin defect or to attempt to get a primary skin closure. Skin grafts should be utilized to avoid a tight closure. A venous flap should be considered for coverage of the skin defect. A retrospective review of venous flaps used for ring avulsion injuries showed 100% survival of all flaps and fingers. The venous flaps produced a supple skin envelope and made subsequent surgeries such as tenolysis or capsulotomy easier to perform. Venous flaps should be vascularized only by the arterial inflow, as flaps vascularized with venous outflow have had poor survival rates.[47]

Survival rates for ring avulsion injuries requiring revascularization range from 60% to 81%.[67] The factor most significantly associated with revascularization failure is repair of fewer than two veins. Cigarette smoking and level of bone injury have not been found to affect survival. The most commonly occurring complications are flexion contracture, cold intolerance, and malunion. A majority of patients can expect two-point discrimination greater than 8 mm.[68] In patients with ring avulsion injuries, finger reconstruction generally gives a better result than amputation, although in patients with ring avulsion amputation proximal to the insertion of the flexor superficialis tendon, amputation or ray amputation should be considered, since these patients are likely to have poor hand function.[69]

Hints and tips

In type III and IV ring avulsion injuries, fusion of the distal interphalangeal (DIP) joint can allow easier bony fixation and sufficient shortening to allow primary approximation of the dorsal veins, skin, and nerves. Range of motion of the DIP joint is generally poor even after attempts to preserve the joint.

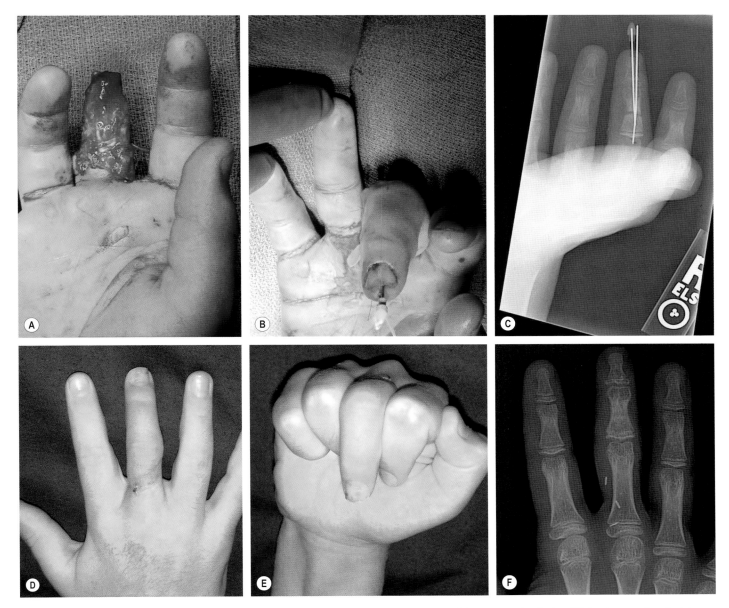

Fig. 11.17 (A) Child with a type IV ring avulsion injury. **(B)** Immediately postoperative after replantation. **(C)** Crossed K-wire fixation. **(D)** Fourteen months after injury, extension of finger. **(E)** Flexion of fingers. **(F)** Radiographs demonstrate bone union but premature closure of growth plate. (Courtesy of James R. Sanger, MD.)

Ectopic transplantation secondary at replantation

Godina *et al.* performed the first ectopic replantation in 1983 when they transferred an amputated hand to the axilla after a contaminated multilevel farm injury.[70] Sixty-five days later the hand was successfully replanted to the forearm. This technique has subsequently been utilized for a variety of amputated parts, including fingers, thumbs, ears, penises, and scalps.[71–76] The recipient sites best used are the thoracodorsal, the deep inferior epigastric, the superficial inferior epigastric, the radial and the dorsalis pedal vessels. These vascular pedicles are familiar to most microsurgeons. The choice of recipient vessel for ectopic replant depends on the length of the expected pedicle as well as donor site morbidity *(Fig. 11.18)*. Adequate surgical debridement is essential prior to

replantation of the digit. Often a staged local or free flap is needed for soft-tissue coverage prior to second-stage transplantation. The ectopic site must be outside the zone of injury.

Complications were significant in all series of ectopic replantations.[72] These occurred mostly after the second stage of transplantation. Nazerani and Motamedi[76] reported a series of 24 staged distal finger ectopic replantations, initially transplanting the digit to the ipsilateral groin, anastomosing an artery and a vein. After 8–12 weeks, the finger was transferred to the hand as a pedicle groin flap. A success rate of 75% was achieved by this method with few complications. This technique may be of clinical use in thumb amputation where there is need for flap coverage along with salvage of bony length and the cosmetic appearance of the thumb.

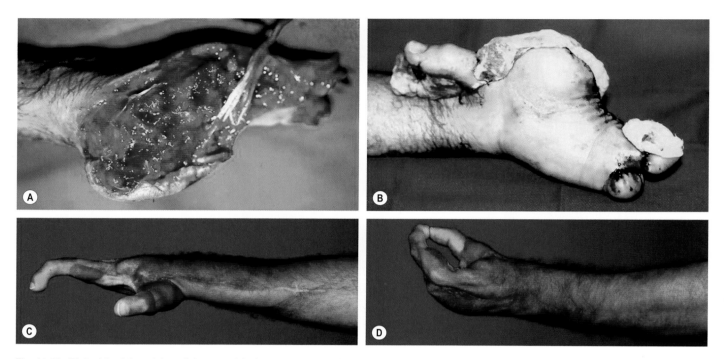

Fig. 11.18 (A) Avulsion injury of the radial aspect of the forearm and wrist. **(B)** Thumb ectopically transplanted to the wrist via the radial artery. **(C)** Thumb replantation after staged reconstruction with second toe second metatarsophalangeal joint and dorsalis pedis free flap. **(D)** Opposition of the thumb and toe transfer. (Courtesy of N. John Yousif, MD.)

Pediatric replantation

In children, less stringent criteria for replantation and revascularization are generally employed. Replantation should be considered for all amputated parts, including amputations of the lower extremity. Success rate in replantation is generally lower in children than in adults, but this may be due to the fact that surgeons are more aggressive in salvaging and attempting to replant parts in children. Clean guillotine amputations generally have the greatest success; however, crush and avulsion injuries from bicycle and mechanical sports equipment with spokes or chains are the most common form of injury in children. The operative procedure in children is similar to that in adults, and the sequence of the procedure is identical. Surgery may be more challenging because of the size of the vessels and a greater tendency for spasm in the pediatric age group.[57] Replantation of multiple digits should begin with the thumb, then with the most ulnar amputated digits. An opposable thumb and two ulnar digits provide essential power grip. In finger replantation, K-wire fixation is preferred over plate fixation to avoid growth disturbances.[77] The replanted part can be expected to grow to 90% compared to normal unless there is significant damage directly to the growth plate.[78]

Recovery of nerve and muscle function is generally better in pediatric patients. After a mutilating hand injury, children tend to rebound more quickly from both functional and psychological aspects. However, parents add a level of complexity to the care of the child, often because of guilt issues. Family psychological counseling may be beneficial. A long-term follow-up of 14 children with digital replantation shows an 88% success rate. Satisfactory sensory recovery was obtained

in all fingers. The growth rate of the digit was 86% compared to the contralateral, noninjured extremity. Twelve of the 14 cases were judged to have excellent results.[79]

Postoperative care

Anticoagulation

Pharmacological management of replantation and revascularization remains a controversial topic. Platelet aggregation is the most prevalent underlying cause of arterial thrombosis. Venous thrombosis is generally caused by fibrin clotting. The risk of thrombosis is highest in the first 2 postoperative days, with 80% of thromboses being seen in this time period. Various schemes of pharmacological management have been utilized. No consensus exists on the use of anticoagulation therapy after microsurgery. The most commonly utilized agents are heparin, low-molecular-weight dextran, and aspirin, but little evidence is available on the efficacy of any of these regimens. A survey of microsurgeons showed that 90% used anticoagulation in free flap and microvascular surgery.[80]

Heparin has been used for over 50 years. Heparin binds to antithrombin III, enhancing its antiprotease activity. Various factors, including thrombin and factor Xa, are rendered inactive.[81] Heparin also has a vasodilatory effect. Heparin can be administered systemically by intravenous methods, by subcutaneous injection, or by direct irrigation. When given intravenously or subcutaneously, heparin needs to be monitored by measuring activated partial thromboplastin time levels. Side-effects of heparin include hematoma formation and heparin-induced thrombocytopenia. Low-molecular-weight heparin (LMWH) is a derivative of standard unfractionated heparin with the same activity against factor X but weaker antithrombotic factor II activity. LMWH is as effective as heparin in its antithrombogenic effects but has fewer adverse reactions. The advantage of LMWH is that there is no need for monitoring and it can be used on an outpatient basis. Chen *et al.* examined topical effects of LMWH compared to unfractionated heparin in a crush injury model and found the thrombosis rates were significantly reduced with both treatments.[82]

Dextran 40 is a group of polysaccharides synthesized by *Leuconostoc mesenteroides* streptococcus. The exact mechanism by which Dextran 40 works is unclear. The antithrombotic effect of dextran is thought to be due to binding to erythrocytes, platelets, and the vascular endothelium. It is mostly thought to interfere with the formation of fibrin clot and to prevent the aggregation of red thrombi. This effect is thought to be significantly greater than any effect on platelets. Dextran has a low risk of postoperative bleeding and hematoma formation. It has some rare, but serious, consequences, including that of pulmonary edema due to fluid overload.[83]

The use of Dextran 40 has been shown to be beneficial in animal studies. There has been no trial to date that demonstrates any significant beneficial effect in humans with the use of dextran. There is no generally accepted regimen for the administration of dextran. Jallali in his review on the use of dextran advocates initiation of Dextran 40 at a rate of 0.4 cc/kg per hour for 2 days, then reducing the rate to 0.2 cc/kg per hour on day 3 and 4, and weaning on day 5.[83] Ridha *et al.*[84] surveyed the practice of 161 microsurgeons and found 45% routinely used dextran postoperatively with 17% combining it with aspirin or heparin. Forty percent of surgeons using dextran used it for less than 72 hours; 52% used it for 5 days. Eight percent used it for greater than 5 days. There was no difference of survival in the patients who used dextran versus those who did not use dextran. A single institutional study from Memorial Sloan Kettering compiled data from 505 free flap surgeries. One group treated by surgeons who routinely used only aspirin was compared to a group treated by a surgeon who routinely used low-molecular-weight dextran. There was no significant difference between the two groups in regard to microvascular thrombosis, flap loss, hematoma, or bleeding.[85] Disa *et al.*[86] prospectively analyzed 100 consecutive patients undergoing microvascular free flap surgery. All patients were randomized into one of three anticoagulation groups, which included low-molecular-weight dextran (20 cc/h for 48 hours), low-molecular-weight dextran (20 cc/h for 120 hours), or aspirin (325 mg for 120 hours). There were no total flap losses, three flaps were re-explored, and systemic complications were greatest at 51% in patients with 120 hours of dextran, 29% in patients who had 48 hours of dextran, and only 7% in patients receiving aspirin. Based on this prospective study, the surgeons at this institution eliminated the use of dextran for microvascular surgery at their institution.[86]

Aspirin (acetylsalicylic acid) inhibits platelets enzyme cyclooxygenase and impedes arachidonic acid breakdown through thromboxane and prostacyclin. Preoperative aspirin has been shown to decrease microvascular thrombosis formation; however, the administration is very time-dependent. Rat studies suggest aspirin needs to be given 10 hours before surgery.[80]

Many animal studies have suggested that anticoagulation may be useful, especially in the crush or avascular injury, yet prospective studies in human are limited. Khouri and the International Microvascular Research Group prospectively studied the use of anticoagulation in microvascular surgery. This was a 6-month study of 23 free flap surgeons analyzing data for 493 free flaps. While the study was prospective in nature, it was not randomized, and all of the surgeons performed their standard anticoagulation therapy, including the use of heparin, aspirin, and Dextran 40. This study was on elective free flap surgeries and not replantation. They found the overall rate of thrombosis was 9.9% with a 60% salvage rate after re-exploration of thrombosed vessels. There was no increased risk of thrombosis in young or old patients, smokers, or diabetics. The use of intraoperative anticoagulation therapy did not reduce the risk of thrombosis. They concluded that only subcutaneous heparin given postoperatively may have decreased the rate for thrombosis, but the use of heparin irrigation intraluminally had no beneficial effect on preventing thrombosis.[87]

Conrad and Adams reviewed the use of anticoagulation in microsurgery. They conceded that most of the better studies have been performed in animals and very few studies with a high level of evidence have been performed in humans. Irrespective of these limitations, they recommended in replantation surgery using a loading dose of aspirin, 1.4 mg/kg (100 mg aspirin in a 70-kg adult) followed by aspirin 1.4 mg/kg/day for 2 days. They advocate the use of heparin irrigation at a dilution of 100 units/mL during surgery and a heparin bolus of 50–100 units/kg before release of a microvascular clamp.[88]

Continuous brachial plexus blockade may be beneficial in preventing microvascular thrombosis and for early continuous pain relief. Sixteen patients were evaluated after replantation or revascularization surgery. One group received continuous brachial plexus blockade; the second received conventional management. The group undergoing conventional treatment had two microvascular thromboses, which were explored and salvaged. Pain control was adequate in both groups, although those in the conventional anesthesia group required more intravenous pain medication.[89]

For revascularizations and sharp guillotine-type injuries, the author uses heparin irrigation intraoperatively (100 units/mL) and aspirin. Aspirin 325 mg is given in the recovery room and daily for 1 month. In patients with crush or avulsion injuries, LMWH at a deep-vein thrombosis prophylaxis dose is utilized. The first dose is given in the operating room, and it is continued for 2 weeks postoperatively. The patient and family are instructed on home injection prior to discharge. The LMWH regimen is based on animal studies on the efficacy of heparins in crush injuries.[90] The advantage of the LMWH regime is that patients can be discharged home while still on therapy.

Postoperative monitoring

Careful postoperative monitoring is essential in replantation surgery. Eighty percent of vascular occlusions occur within the first 48 hours after surgery. The salvage rate in a failing replantation explored early ranges from 66% to 80%.[91] A dedicated replantation team is essential for monitoring the patient.

Table 11.5 Circulation

	Normal circulation	Venous occlusion	Arterial occlusion
Color	Pink	Blue/purple hue, cyanotic	Pale, mottled
Capillary refill time	1–2 seconds	Increased, <1 second	Decreased, >2 seconds
Temperature	Warm	Warm-cool	Cold
Turgor	Full	Distended, swollen	Hollow
Dermal bleeding	Bright red blood	Dark red or bluish Bleeds briskly	Minimal bleeding only serum

The best monitor is a conscientious nursing staff. When the patient arrives on the floor, the physician should examine the replant with the nurse, judging its color, capillary refill, and turgor. The finger is examined every hour by the nursing staff. If there is any change from the baseline level, the physician should be notified *(Table 11.5)*. Proper handoff between nursing shifts is essential: at the bedside the clinical parameters are assessed with both nursing teams at each shift change. Venous occlusion is more insidious and harder to assess than acute arterial thrombosis. Venous occlusion will eventually lead to arterial thrombosis. If there is any doubt regarding the clinical assessment of the digit, the pulp of the finger can be pricked with a 25-gauge needle. If the blood is blue, has brisk bleeding, delayed bleeding or serous fluid exudate; exploration of the digit should be performed.

Technology cannot replace a dedicated, experienced nurse, but can aid in the postoperative assessment of viability. The most commonly used devices are pulse oximetry, ultrasonic Doppler, digital thermometry, and the laser Doppler.[91] Each of these devices can help identify an early vascular occlusion, but each has its shortcomings. While temperature measurements are inexpensive, variations such as room temperature can affect the accuracy. Laser Dopplers have a high sensitivity and specificity. When compared to thermometry, the sensitivity of the Doppler is 93% while that of thermometry is 84%. Specificity is 94% with the laser Doppler and 86% with thermometry.[92]

Hints and tips

The best monitor of the replanted digit is a well-trained nursing staff. The surgeon should examine the replantation with the nursing staff and ask to be called at any change in appearance. Shift change handoffs should be made at the bedside, so that all care members know the physical appearance of the replantation.

Postoperative therapy

Therapy after mutilating hand injuries is essential to regaining function. During the first few days after surgery the therapist fabricates splints, and initiates gentle range of motion to the nonaffected joints. At postoperative days 5–7, a formal therapy program is initiated; this includes dressing changes, passive splint formation, and instruction regarding activities of daily living. Blood vessel and nerve repairs are protected for 3–4 weeks. Tendon therapy initially involves immobilization to prevent injury, but early active and passive mobilization can be initiated if there is rigid bone fixation and a solid multistrand tendon repair. After 6–8 weeks, the therapy program is increased to include strengthening and full range-of-motion programs. Sensory re-education is initiated after any nerve injuries. Desensitization programs start using fabric textures and progress to vibratory sensory re-education.[93,94] Patients who started therapy before day 14 postoperatively have better eventual motion than those who start therapy later.[24]

Psychosocial aspects of replantation

The surgeon treating a patient with an amputation must not only treat the amputation, but the whole patient, and at times the family. The psychological implications of amputation and replantation must be considered when caring for these patients. The hand has a significant role in a patient's identity and psyche. The hands are an individual's second most visually prominent structure, second only to the face. Most individuals view their hands far more than they view their own faces. The hands are not only a source of contact with the world, but a means of communication and an instrument of sexuality. Injury or disfigurement to the hands is a source of tremendous psychological difficulty. The psychological consequences of amputation may not correlate with the degree of injury.[95] The consequences of a distal single-digit injury in one patient may be more severe than that of a major limb amputation in another individual. Despite common misconceptions, the presence or absence of worker's compensation or litigation does not seem to correlate with the patient's psychological reaction after injury.[96]

The psychological response to amputation may take various forms, including anxiety, depression, anger, guilt, fear, frustration, and sadness. All of these emotions are normal after an injury, but their prolonged manifestation may be pathological and lead to full acute stress disorder and posttraumatic stress disorder (PTSD). PTSD symptoms may include flashbacks, nightmares, sleep disturbances, avoidance, and detachment.

The physician should convey hope but also give the patient realistic expectations prior to surgery. Patients need to be reassured that everything possible will be done to make them whole again.

Nightmares and flashbacks are commonly seen after traumatic injuries. Flashbacks are an almost universal component of the traumatic hand injury. These can be replay flashbacks where an individual replays the entire traumatic event, or an appraisal flashback where the patient sees a snapshot of the injured hand. Patients may also have projection flashbacks where the injury is seen as more severe than it actually is. The type and persistence of flashbacks are strong prognostic factors in predicting PTSD and the eventual return to work and function. Psychological care of the patient with a traumatic hand amputation begins immediately in the emergency room. The patient is asked two questions: how did this accident occur, and what do you perceive was responsible for the injury? Whether patients take responsibility for the injury or attribute it to something out of their control is an important prognostic sign. Patients who see the accident as under their control, e.g., I knew I should not have removed the blade guard, do significantly better than those who believe they lack control, e.g., the machine intermittently malfunctions.

Patients are also asked how the injury appears to them and their emotional reaction. Finally they are asked about flashbacks. After discharge from the hospital, patients should be followed up with psychological treatment. Patients who are experiencing signs of PTSD are begun on a course of desensitization and systematic exposure training. Grunert et al.[96] were able to achieve over 90% return to work with a graded return-to-work exposure program in patients with PTSD.

Children with traumatic injuries are a special challenge to the surgeon. Rusch et al. found that 98% of children with traumatic injuries had symptoms of PTSD, depression, or anxiety 1 month after injury. Twelve months after injury, 21% still met the criteria for PTSD.[97]

Outcome, prognosis, and complications

Outcome after replantation and revascularization surgery can be measured in many ways. The simplest of these is survival of the replanted part. Overall survival can be expected in over 90% of digits. The largest single-institution study found a success rate of 92.9%.[25] Several factors are associated with worse prognosis. The most significant of these is mechanism of injury. Crush and avulsion injuries have a poorer anastomotic success rate than clean amputations. The anastomotic success after a clean amputation approaches 100%.[25,98,99]

Other factors associated with poorer success rate include the total number of anastomosed vessels but not necessarily the number of anastomosed arteries or veins independently. The more vessels anastomosed (whether arteries or veins) improved survival. Even in very distal replantation where anastomosis of a vein is not possible, a high success rate of over 60% can still be possible.[28] A positive correlation exists between the number of vessels anastomosed and the mechanism of injury; crush injuries generally reduce the number of anastomosed vessels and veins.[33] The use of vein grafts is not associated with a poorer outcome. Cigarette smoking leads to a poorer outcome, but alcohol consumption does not affect survival.

Another indicator of outcome is objective measurement of hand function. Standard measurements include range of motion, grip strength, and sensation. These measurements can be compared to noninjured hands or to hands with amputations. Long-term follow-up of 59 successfully replanted digits showed that average active range of motion was 44–56% of the normal contralateral hand. Grip strength was 67% of the contralateral hand. Only three digits had normal two-point discrimination. Over one-half achieve 10 mm or less two-point discrimination.[100]

The best measurement of outcome is the use and function of the hand. A variety of tests are available to judge outcome, including the short-form 36 (SF36), upper extremity functional test (UEFT), and the Disability of the Arm, Shoulders and Hand (DASH). Outcome assessment after major upper extremity replantation is difficult.[101,102] Outcome of replantation can be compared to amputation, the normal hand, or other surgical reconstructions.[58] Various scales have been devised to try to assess and predict functional recovery after mutilating hand injuries and replantations; these include the Tamai scale, the Chen scale (Table 11.6), and the Campbell hand injury severity scale (HISS).[56,103–106] The HISS performed at the time of injury can be predictive in assessing return to work and functional recovery of the patient. The more proximal level of injury and the more injured fingers predicted poorer functional outcome.[107] Despite results of functional outcome, patient satisfaction after replantation is high; long-term follow-up in successfully replanted digits shows good satisfaction by a majority of the patients.

Replantation distal to the FDS insertion offers excellent functional results. Hattori et al. compared the functional results of single fingertip amputations versus replantation in regard to symptoms of pain, paresthesias, cold intolerance, and DASH scores. Grip strength did not differ between the amputation group and the replantation group. Range of motion of the proximal interphalangeal joint was better in the replantation group. Replantation patients had significantly improved DASH scores. Ninety-six percent of patients obtained protective sensation. Less than 10% of replantation patients complained of pain, while 60% of patients with amputation complained of pain and half of these patients rarely or never use their affected fingers for activities of daily living. All patients with successful replantations were highly or very satisfied. Only 60% of patients in the amputation group were highly or very satisfied.[98] Patients with primary amputation revisions have a higher incidence of painful and uncomfortable sensation in their amputation stumps. Patients with replanted index and middle fingers have improved use and function of these fingers compared with patients with amputation revision. When cost was compared, a successful

Table 11.6 Chen classification of functional results after replantation/revascularisation

Grade	Return to work	AROM (%)	Sensation	Cold intolerance	Grip strength (five-grade scale)
I	Same profession	>60	Normal	–	4–5
II	Other profession	40–60	Satisfactory	–	3–4
III	Not returned to work	30–40	Protective	Yes	Slight
IV	The limb survived, but is functionally severely disabled				

AROM, active range of motion.

replantation cost 20% more than unsuccessful replantation and 300 times more than primary amputation revision.[107] The level of injury had a significant influence on the final function, with the worse function in amputations in flexor tendon zone II. In this area, repairing the profundus stump to the superficialis had improved outcome.[25]

The surgical success rate for major limb replantation ranges from 36% to 100% depending on the level of amputation, etiology of amputation, and age of the patient.[100] Using the Carroll Quantitative Test of Upper Extremity Function, the Louisville group compared the outcomes of replantation to prosthesis in adults with amputations proximal to the wrist. In injuries between the wrist and elbow, good to excellent outcomes were achieved in 50% of replantation patients. No patients in the prosthetic group had good or excellent function.[108] Better outcomes were seen in younger patients and those with more distal injuries. Outcome for amputations proximal to the elbow was significantly worse in both groups.

Replantation, even after significant mangling injuries, is still worthwhile. Avulsion amputations in the forearm were evaluated based on the patient's overall satisfaction, recovery of motion, and ability to perform daily activities: 100% success rate of replantation was achieved. Postoperative function was rated as excellent to good in 40%, but poor in 30% of patients.[109]

Amputation at the transmetacarpal level is a bridge between the digital amputation and major limb replantation. A review of 10 patients with transmetacarpal-level replantations showed 90% salvage of the replanted hands. Intrinsic muscle function was weak or absent in all patients. Only one patient was able to resume his prior occupation. Despite this fact, all patients were satisfied with their replantation.[110]

Complications

The most significant complication after replantation and revascularization is anastomotic failure. Re-exploration to correct arterial insufficiency can be successful in over 50% of patients with a failing replantation.[106,111] Close observation of the patient postoperatively for signs of thrombosis and urgent re-exploration of the vessel is the essential first step in successful re-exploration. In the patient's room, the dressing should be removed and if skin sutures appear to be constricting venous outflow, they should also be removed. The patient is given a bolus of intravenous heparin and the operating room is readied. The anastomosis is opened and clots are atraumatically evacuated. The use of a Fogarty catheter is considered; however a catheter can cause significant intimal

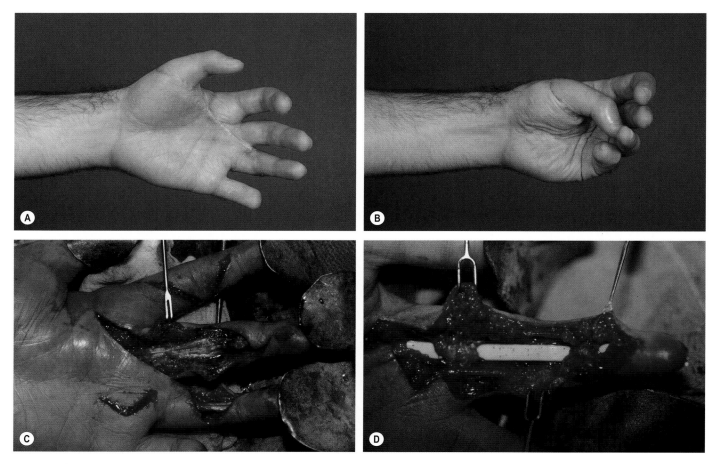

Fig. 11.19 (A and B) A 24-year-old status post five-finger amputation and replantation with stiff fingers. **(C)** Exploration at time of tenolysis shows severe scarring and attenuation of the digital pulleys. **(D)** Hunter rod inserted, and A2 and A4 pulley reconstruction.

damage. If white thrombus or intimal injury is present, a vein graft should be utilized. Intravascular tissue plasminogen activator is considered; however, there is very limited clinical data and outcome of its effectiveness. After establishing flow, prophylactic therapy with aspirin or heparin should be strongly considered.[85,112]

Cold intolerance is common in varying degrees in almost all replanted digits; it may resolve in 1–2 years or may be permanent.[100] Eighty-one adults from Norway were evaluated for cold sensitivity after successful replantation or revascularization. Twenty percent were severely or extremely cold-hypersensitive. Cold-hypersensitivity is significantly higher in replantations as compared to revascularizations.[113] Only 40% of children with replanted digits reported cold intolerance.[50]

Secondary procedures

The incidence of secondary procedures after digital replantation ranges from 15% to 80%.[110,111,114] Most series report an approximate 50% rate of reoperative surgery. Procedures include those performed immediately, mostly related to vascular anastomosis and skin closure, and late secondary procedures relating mainly to bony nonunion, or tendon adhesions. Yu et al. reviewed a series of 102 secondary procedures in 55 patients with injuries in 79 digits. Ninety-two percent of the early procedures were for soft-tissue coverage and 67% of later procedures were for tendon function. Significant factors related to the need for secondary surgeries are avulsion or degloving injuries, and proximal replantations in zones 3–5.[115] In digital replantations proximal to the superficialis insertion, a high rate of secondary procedures can be expected. Many of these secondary surgeries have a poor outcome.[116] Tenolysis after finger replantation and revascularization is one of the most challenging operations of all tendon surgeries. Although technically demanding, the results of tenolysis can be rewarding (*Fig. 11.19*). Tenolysis in these digits may produce a modest total improvement in motion, but this functional improvement can be substantial. The risk of tendon rupture in these patients is significantly greater.[117,118]

Revascularization and replantation remains one of the most challenging procedures in hand surgery. The surgeon must have a meticulous plan and exacting surgical technique. The postoperative management may be as complicated as the surgical procedure itself. Yet the rewards of a successful replantation for the patient and the surgeon are immeasurable.

Access the complete references list online at **http://www.expertconsult.com**

3. Buncke Jr HJ. Microvascular hand surgery transplants and replants over the past 25 years. *J Hand Surg [Am]*. 2000;25:415–428.

   The pioneer of US microsurgery discusses the history of microsurgery and replantation. Tips and techniques from a lifetime of experience are included.

11. Chung KC, Kowalski CP, Walters MR. Finger replantation in the United States: rates and resource use from the 1996 Healthcare Cost and Utilization Project. *J Hand Surg*. 2000;25A:1038–1042.

    The database from the Agency for Health care Policy and Research was reviewed to obtain data on the frequency and cost of digital replantation. Only 60% of the 906 hospitals performed any replantation. Only 2% of hospitals performed 10 or more cases of replantation.

25. Waikakul S, Sakkarnkosol S, Vanadurongwan V, et al. Results of 1018 digital replantations in 552 patients. *Injury, Int J Care Injured*. 2000;31:33–40.

    The largest series of digital replantation published from Bangkok, Thailand with at least 2-year follow-up. A 92.9% success rate in digits. Risk factors and outcome are discussed.

33. Chaivanichsiri P, Rattanasrithong P. Type of injury and number of anastomosed vessels: Impact on digital replantation. *Microsurg*. 2006;26:151–154.

    A retrospective review of 130 digital replantions was performed. The type of injury and the number of vessel anastomoses were the most significant predictors of successful outcome. *Crush injuries had significantly worse outcome than sharp injuries. In distal replantations, an arterial repair even without repair of a vein can achieve a high success rate.*

38. Zhang X, Wen S, Wang B, et al. Reconstruction of circulation in the fingertip without vein repair in zone 1 replantation. *J Hand Surg*. 2008;33A:1597–1601.

49. Rosson GD, Buncke GM, Buncke HJ. Great toe transplant versus thumb replant for isolated thumb amputation: critical analysis of functional outcome. *Microsurgery*. 2008:598–600.

59. Li J, Guo Z, Zhu Q, et al. Finger replantation: determinants of survival. *Plast Reconstr Surg*. 2008;122:833–839.

    A retrospective review of 211 finger amputations was performed over a 16-year period. An 81.5% success rate was achieved. Injury mechanism, platelet count, smoking, and the use of vein grafting were found to be the main predictors for the survival of the replanted fingertip.

69. Sanmartin M, Fernandes F, Lajoie AS, et al. Analysis of prognostic factors in ring avulsion injuries. *J Hand Surg*. 2004;29a:1028–1037.

81. Levin LS, Cooper EO. Clinical use of anticoagulants following replantation. *J Hand Surg*. 2008;33A: 1437–1439.

91. Bakri K, Moran SL. Monitoring for upper extremity free flaps and replantations. *J Hand Surg*. 2008;33A: 1905–1908.

12

Reconstructive surgery of the mutilated hand

William C. Pederson and Randolph Sherman

 Access the Historical Perspective section online at
http://www.expertconsult.com

Introduction

Management of the mangled upper extremity is complex, demands special skills and expertise, and is facilitated by a team approach with participation of all those dedicated to upper extremity surgery. When adequate facilities, equipment, and surgical expertise are not available to manage the patient's degree of injury, the patient should be transferred with the extremity splinted. If the limb is ischemic, or if part of the limb is amputated, the extremity should be cooled. The ischemic limb should be carefully covered in ice, with a protective barrier to prevent frostbite injury. The amputated part should be wrapped in a saline-soaked gauze, placed on ice, and sent with the patient. The ideal temperature is +4°C. Dry ice or alcohol should not be used to aid in cooling during transport of the part as this can cause actual freezing of the tissues.

Resuscitation of the patient is a priority over addressing the extremity injury. However, in the event of a coexisting life-threatening injury, the extremity injury must not be neglected. Assessment of vascularity, realignment, and splinting are not time-consuming and should be done as soon as possible. Provisional revascularization through shunting may be an option to restore circulation to the extremity quickly while the trauma team simultaneously addresses the coexisting injuries. Consent of the patient should initially be obtained for wide debridement of the wound; internal versus external fixation; repair or reconstruction as indicated of nerves, vessels, tendons, and muscles; use of vein grafts for arterial and venous reconstruction; possible donor sites for flap coverage; and primary amputation. The selected treatment is based on the intraoperative findings.

The initial treatment includes meticulous debridement, wound irrigation, wound culture, antibiotic administration, and tetanus prophylaxis. Copious irrigation of the wound coupled with debridement is important because it removes foreign bodies and decreases the bacterial load. High-pressure and/or pulsed lavage of the soft tissues is to be avoided in these types of injuries, as it may force debris and bacteria into the tissues and has a tendency to force fluid into the tissues, potentially creating more edema in the postoperative period. The cultures most predictive of later infecting organisms are the postirrigation cultures. Antibiotics will help reduce infection and should be administered in the emergency department and continued intravenously for at least 72 hours. Antibiotic coverage should be effective against both Gram-positive and Gram-negative organisms. The authors currently prefer to use a first-generation cephalosporin and an aminoglycoside in combination. In cases of soil contamination, as in farm injuries, coverage against anaerobic organisms should always be added. High-dose penicillin provides excellent anaerobic coverage. The possibility of gas gangrene should also be considered in these cases. The antibiotic regimen

Key points

- Thorough debridement is essential in the management of these patients to decrease risk of infection and scarring
- In cases of arterial insufficiency, provisional revascularization via a shunt or temporary vein graft should be considered
- Adequate skeletal stabilization should be performed early and preferentially is done with internal fixation to allow definitive repairs of neurovascular structures and soft-tissue coverage
- Definitive vascular reconstruction is usually delayed until after skeletal stabilization is achieved
- Musculotendinous reconstruction should be done early if possible, to the point of performing early tendon transfers
- Nerve repair is also best performed early, to allow proper alignment of nerves and to avoid having to dissect the nerve out of scar at a secondary procedure
- Proper management of the soft-tissue envelope is essential to allow all of the other structures to be repaired as noted above. Proper flap selection allows early rehabilitation and facilitates secondary surgery when necessary
- Postoperative management revolves around proper planning at the first stage of reconstruction. Every surgery should be performed with an eye to what will need to be done in the future

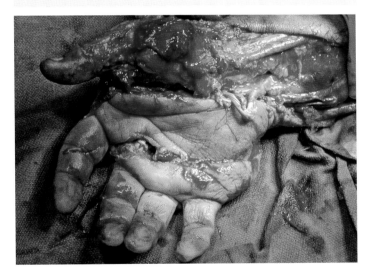

Fig. 12.1 A 43-year-old patient who suffered a crush injury to his hand when an airplane fell on it while under repair. This hand will require extensive debridement to delineate which tissues are viable and which are not.

should subsequently be modified depending on the culture results. Tetanus prophylaxis should be administered in accordance with the status of previous immunization.

Debridement

Radical debridement with elimination of all nonviable tissue is the crucial step in the management of these injuries. This is performed under tourniquet control to provide the best visualization of the extent of injury and to prevent iatrogenic injury to intact structures. Once nerves and vessels are identified, the tourniquet may be released to assess the viability of the remaining tissue better *(Fig. 12.1)*.

Skin and subcutaneous tissues are sharply debrided to bleeding edges. Muscle is debrided until bright red blood is seen. Color and twitch are used to assess muscle tissue; however, these characteristics are not totally reliable in determining viability. If the muscle does not bleed, it is dead and should be debrided. Small bone fragments devoid of soft-tissue attachments are avascular and should be discarded unless they constitute part of an articular surface. Contused or contaminated nerves are left in continuity. Superficial dissection above the epineurium can be carefully done to remove foreign material if it is present. Cut nerves are debrided to healthy-appearing fascicles. At the time of reconstruction, this is done under microscopic visualization because a primary repair or nerve graft will fail if the entirety of the injured segment is not resected.

The wound is copiously irrigated. Tissue margins are re-evaluated, and further debridement is performed as necessary. Hemostasis should be done cautiously. Do not cauterize vessels that may be needed for arterial or venous reconstruction. Side branches may be controlled with small sutures or vascular clips. Arterial debridement is performed for cut or thrombosed vessels. Definitive debridement of arteries that are to be reconstructed is done with the tourniquet released. At the completion of debridement, assess and record what structures remain intact and what the functional losses are. Some of the remaining intact muscles may be suitable for immediate tendon transfer to replace important functional losses.

Provisional revascularization

When the extremity is amputated or ischemic and the delay to surgery or anticipated length of time for debridement and definitive skeletal stabilization exceeds 6 hours, provisional revascularization can be done with use of a shunt, such as a Javid, Ishihara, or comparable segment of plastic tubing *(Fig. 12.2)*. While different shunts are available, their use is similar. Whichever shunt is chosen (primarily by what might be available for use by the vascular surgeons), it is generally flushed with heparinized saline and then clamped. The concentration of this is usually 100 units heparin per cc saline. The shunt is then carefully slipped into the ends of the vessels to be shunted (artery to artery). The shunt is either held in place with moist umbilical tapes placed around the vessels and clamped tight with a piece of red rubber catheter *(Fig. 12.2)*, or some shunts come with a special clamp which goes around the artery and holds it flush on the shunt. While generally utilized for only short periods of time (i.e., minutes to a few hours), these types of shunt have recently been utilized to great effect in the conflict in the Middle East for up to 8 hours on major arteries, without systemic heparinization. In this application, however, their use should only be necessary for the time it will take to perform an initial debridement and bony fixation. Another option is rapidly to perform reversed vein grafting between the arterial ends to re-establish arterial inflow. After definitive skeletal stabilization, the length of the vein graft can be adjusted and the anastomosis revised.

Skeletal stabilization

Definitive stable internal fixation should be done immediately when possible to allow therapeutic access to the extremity for

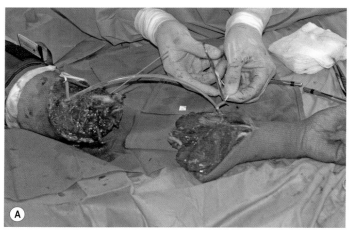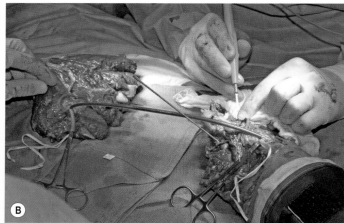

Fig. 12.2 (A) A 24-year-old patient after mid-forearm amputation. Shunt placed from radial artery to radial artery to perfuse limb while debridement and bony fixation are performed. **(B)** View of shunt perfusing limb while debridement is performed.

wound care and early joint range of motion when applicable. In general, the use of external fixation is to be avoided. These devices carry the risk of neurovascular injury during pin placement, restrict circumferential access to the extremity, and may limit rehabilitation. They may be useful as a temporary solution for severely contaminated wounds with extensive soft-tissue injury, however. External fixation should not be used for the reason of avoiding exposed hardware. Potentially exposed hardware should be addressed with appropriate soft-tissue coverage.

Diaphyseal fractures of the arm and forearm are usually amenable to plate fixation. If the fracture is segmental or comminuted over a large segment, a flexible interlocking intramedullary nail can be used. Fractures should be reduced anatomically with respect to rotational alignment. One must carefully check pronation and supination prior to final fixation to avoid placing the hand in a poor position. Comminuted bone fragments without soft-tissue attachments should be removed. Shortening of the humerus up to 5 cm and of the radius and ulna up to 4 cm is acceptable. Indications for shortening include significant comminution over a segment with bone and soft-tissue loss. Bony shortening has the advantage of allowing primary repair of vessels and, more importantly, of nerves.

Complex diaphyseal fractures include Galeazzi fractures (radial diaphyseal fracture with disruption of the distal radioulnar joint), Monteggia fractures (proximal ulna fractures with radial head dislocation or radial head or neck fracture), and Essex–Lopresti injuries (radial head fracture with associated rupture of the interosseous membrane to the level of the wrist). These fractures must be restored to anatomic length to restore joint congruity and alignment.

Diaphyseal fractures of the hand are fixed with Kirschner wires, with attention to maintaining rotational alignment. Shortening of the metacarpals or phalanges between 5 and 6 mm may be necessary in replantation. For other injuries, length can be restored or maintained with internal or external fixation and primary or delayed bone grafting. In general, initial use of plate fixation is not recommended in the hand, particularly in the phalanges. This requires more stripping of the periosteum and later has an adverse effect on functional outcome because of potential tendon adhesions around the plate.

In contrast to lower-extremity injuries, primary bone grafting is acceptable and recommended in the upper extremity. Primary iliac crest bone graft or bone allograft may be used for defects up to 4 cm. For larger defects, vascularized bone grafts, in particular a vascularized segment of free fibula, should be considered. With massive bone loss, creation of a one-bone forearm can be considered as a salvage procedure when other options are not available. The results of this procedure in trauma are inferior to those in limb salvage surgeries for tumor reconstruction.

Intra-articular fractures should be anatomically reduced. Stable fixation is imperative to allow early range of motion. Fixation can be done with plates, screws, K-wires, or tension band wiring as dictated by the fracture pattern and location. Articular fragments free of soft-tissue attachments should be preserved to reconstruct the joint surface. Primary bone grafting should be done to address bone defects, to enhance the stability of the fixation, and to promote bone healing. When the joint surface cannot be reconstructed owing to severe comminution or bone loss, other reconstructive options are available. At the shoulder and elbow, a primary allograft or a prosthesis can be used. At the wrist joint, primary fusion should be the first treatment option. If wrist motion is critical to the patient, vascularized free fibula, retaining the proximal articular cartilage, can be used to reconstruct the joint surface. Prosthetic devices for total wrist arthroplasty are poor at present, and historically do not do well in posttraumatic wrists regardless.

In summary, the goal of skeletal stabilization is to achieve stable anatomic fixation to allow early range of motion and rehabilitation. Soft-tissue stripping of bone is limited to only that which is necessary for fixation. Comminuted fragments with attached soft tissue are retained. Bone defects are treated primarily whenever possible. The potential of exposed hardware should not limit the choice of fixation. Exposed bone, hardware, or joints are addressed with appropriate soft-tissue coverage, whether it be pedicled or free.

Vascular reconstruction

Definitive revascularization is done once skeletal stabilization is completed. Lacerated vessels are resected to

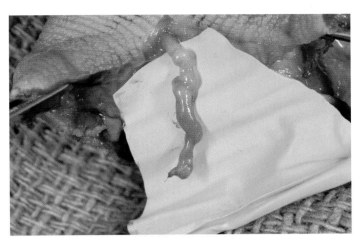

Fig. 12.3 "Ribbon" sign in an avulsed finger. Note corkscrewing of vessel which indicates severe avulsion damage to the adventitial layer.

healthy-appearing vessel wall both proximally and distally. Contusion along the adventitia suggests injury within the intimal layer as well. A "ribbon sign" (convoluted or tortuous course of the digital vessels) indicates injury to the media layer of the vessel and requires resection of the length of the involved area and reversed vein grafting *(Fig. 12.3)*. Inflow is assessed, and if it is not adequate, the vessel should be resected more proximally until pulsatile flow is achieved.

When possible, primary repair is preferred. However, it is better to resect appropriately and to use a reversed vein graft than to perform a primary repair under tension. Reversed vein grafts are available from several sites. The most commonly used for long segments in the upper extremity is the saphenous vein. For reconstruction in the hand, local grafts from the dorsal or volar forearm can be used.

Reconstruction of the superficial palmar arch and its multiple common digital arteries may be difficult. Branched vein grafts from the dorsum of the foot and use of the subscapular artery and its branches have been described for this. The descending branch of the lateral femoral circumflex artery may also be utilized as a smaller arterial graft to make use of its branches to reconstruct the arch. The conventional method is to harvest two Y vein segments from the volar forearm and to perform end-to-end or end-to-side anastomoses as necessary. Vein grafts should be routinely used to reconstruct venous outflow if primary repair cannot be achieved. There is a minimal role for artificial grafts for vascular reconstruction in the upper extremity distal to the axillary artery, particularly in contaminated wounds.

When the need for coverage and vascular repair present themselves simultaneously, one can consider "flow-through" free flaps both to bridge the arterial defect and to obtain coverage at the same time. The radial forearm free flap is very useful in this regard, as the radial artery offers an excellent choice for a long bypass.[1] Due to trauma to the forearm, however, this may not be an appropriate choice of flap. In this case, the anterolateral thigh flap with its long segment of the descending branch of the lateral femoral circumflex can be utilized.[2,3] Small venous free flaps with arterialized segments of vein can be utilized to great utility for revascularization of fingers in the face of a soft-tissue loss volarly.[4,5]

Musculotendinous reconstruction

Primary tendon repair is preferred when permitted by the injury. There is often a crush or avulsion component to the injury which may preclude primary repair. In these cases, treatment options include primary or delayed reconstruction with tendon grafts or Silastic tendon rods. Immediate reconstruction is favored with the use of available donor tendons (palmaris, plantaris, local tendons that cannot be reconstructed, and toe extensors).

In flexor tendon injuries in the hand, priority is usually given to reconstruction of the profundus tendons. If there is trauma to the distal interphalangeal joint requiring fusion, priority is rather given to the superficialis tendon. The lesser-priority tendon can be used for reconstruction of the other when necessary. It can be used as a donor tendon for other sites or for pulley reconstruction as necessary. One should pay close attention to the status of the pulleys in the fingers, and the A2 and A4 should be reconstructed with portions of tendon grafts when necessary.

Functional reconstruction of muscle deficits and tendon injuries should be done immediately whenever possible. Unrecoverable muscle function can be treated with tendon transfer, and it is preferable to perform this as a primary procedure. However, this can also be performed at a later stage of reconstruction. Delayed transfers are generally more difficult because they have to be performed through a scarred tissue bed, and this requires additional surgical procedures and further delays the patient's rehabilitation and recovery. When no donor tendons are available for transfer, muscle function can be restored with functional free muscle transfer. The gracilis is the most commonly used muscle for functional reconstruction and can actually provide both coverage and restoration of muscle function to the fingers. Again, this can be done either primarily or at a later stage of reconstruction; however primary reconstruction is favored as available nerves and vessels are easier to locate and one is not operating through a scarred bed of tissue. This procedure will be discussed in more detail below and in Chapter 35.

Nerves

Nerves may have internal derangement without loss of anatomic continuity and they can be partially or completely disrupted. Severe contusion to the nerve with internal hemorrhage without actual division may mitigate against functional return; however contused or attenuated nerves are usually left intact. If lacerated, the nerve ends should be debrided serially under magnification until healthy-appearing fascicles appear. The resection should not be compromised in order to preserve length, as nerve regeneration will not occur through scarred nerve tissue, and nerves repaired under tension also do not regenerate well.

Mobilizing the proximal and distal stumps to achieve primary repair is not recommended because this results in devascularization of large segments of the nerve. Mobilization can be done over a 1–2-cm distance to allow repair, but to avoid repair under tension, nerve grafting is preferable. If a staged repair is planned, nerve ends are tagged with 6-0 polypropylene suture for later identification. Primary nerve grafting is recommended, however, as the orientation is much

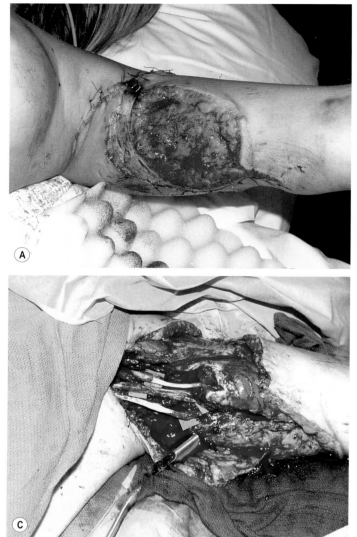

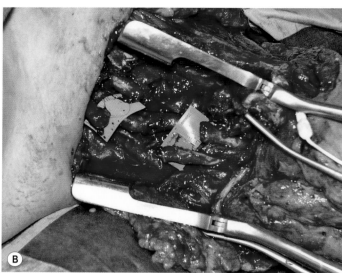

Fig. 12.4 (A) View of upper arm in patient suffering avulsion injury and global nerve palsy in the hand. **(B)** Close-up view of nerves. Median and ulnar nerve over background in front and radial behind. **(C)** Nerves after debridement to healthy fascicles and sural nerve grafting.

clearer at the time of injury rather than later and dissecting a nerve out of a scarred bed is technically challenging *(Fig. 12.4)*. Common donor nerves include the sural or saphenous nerves, sensory branch of the radial nerve (if lacerated from the injury), medial or lateral antebrachial cutaneous nerves, and the posterior interosseous nerve. In multiple nerve injuries, primary nerve transfers can be performed.[6] These include transfer of the anterior interosseous nerve (distal to the branch to the flexor pollicis longus) to the motor branch of the ulnar nerve and transfer of the sensory branch of the radial nerve to the digital nerves of the thumb and index finger.[7] When a nerve defect is greater than 15 cm, an end-to-side neurorrhaphy of the distal stump of the injured nerve to a neighboring intact major nerve can be done, although functional outcomes of this procedure are generally poor.

Skin and soft-tissue reconstruction

Appropriate soft-tissue coverage is of paramount importance for coverage of bone, joint, tendons, neurovascular structures, and hardware. The selection of coverage should provide a

gliding surface for mobile structures and enhance vascularity in the injured area.

Extensive skin and soft-tissue loss is one of the major problems in the mangled upper extremity. Isolated skin loss may be managed by split-thickness skin grafting (if not over a bony prominence, hardware, or exposed tendons). Local random skin flaps have limited utility even in superficial soft-tissue defects owing to their restricted mobility, precarious blood supply, and frequent involvement in the injury.

Soft-tissue loss can be managed in a variety of ways. A simple approach is to leave the wound open and let it heal by secondary intention with granulation tissue. However, exposed tissues sensitive to desiccation, such as nerves and tendons, will become necrotic, scarring will be promoted, and function will be compromised. Local muscle flaps are usually not suitable because of their proximity to the zone of injury, the limited amount of coverage that they provide, and the resulting functional deficit. Two-stage distant pedicled flap procedures are avoided when possible; immobilization of the reconstructed area will lead to stiffness and swelling. If this means of coverage is required, the most common sources are the pedicled groin flap, cross-arm flap, thoracoacromial flap, and abdominal flap. In mangling injuries, the need for extensive coverage, reliable vascularity of the flap, and early mobilization usually necessitates use of axial flaps (local or regional), one-stage distant pedicled flaps, or free flaps. The type of coverage depends on the site and extent of the defect. This is particularly important for bone, tendon, nerve, and hardware coverage, as well as for facilitation of future reconstructive procedures in planning a staged reconstruction. As discussed above, one should think one or two steps ahead in terms of what reconstructive procedures are potentially going to be performed later under or though the chosen flap.

Fasciocutaneous flaps or cutaneous flaps with subcutaneous tissue are recommended when tendons are exposed as this tissue facilitates tendon gliding. However, many fasciocutaneous flaps over time do not have a good cosmetic appearance (color match can be poor and they can be too bulky). The primary fasciocutaneous flaps used with acceptable cosmetic appearance include the radial forearm flap, as either a free or rotational flap; the lateral arm flap; and the groin flap. These can all be utilized as free flaps, but the groin flap is generally utilized today as a pedicled flap due to the small size and short available vascular pedicle. An alternative to the fasciocutaneous flap is a fascial flap. Donors for this include the temporoparietal fascia, the parascapular fascia, and the radial forearm fascia. The free fascial flap is placed on the defect and then covered with an unmeshed split-thickness skin graft. It has been our experience, though, that it can be difficult to elevate a fascial flap later for tenolysis or other procedures.

Muscle flaps are used when a moderate to large soft-tissue defect is present. Although muscle flaps may be harvested with a skin component, harvesting of muscle alone is preferred. This is then covered with a split-thickness skin graft. In the arm and elbow, the latissimus dorsi can be used as a one-stage distal pedicled rotational flap. Most other reconstructions are done with a free muscle transfer using the gracilis, rectus abdominis, latissimus dorsi, or serratus anterior. When a functional deficit is present, consideration should be given to use of a functional free muscle transfer to provide both functional restoration and soft-tissue coverage. The gracilis is most commonly used for this transfer in the forearm, as noted above.

Postoperative management

In the immediate postoperative period, the extremity is splinted in an appropriate position to prevent capsuloligamentous shortening and tension on repaired structures. Elevation is necessary to reduce edema and help control pain. The patient's pain and anxiety should be adequately controlled. The ambient temperature should be at least 25°C and adjusted to the patient's body temperature. Hydration should be sufficient to maintain urine output between 80 and 100 mL/h. Anticoagulant therapy is used by many surgeons. However, the authors are selective in using heparin; aspirin is used daily for 4–6 days after surgery. Appropriate antibiotic therapy is continued in the postoperative period and later modified as necessary according to culture results.

Extremity and flap monitoring is critical. Early recognition of arterial hypoperfusion or venous congestion will occur only in a well-monitored environment with trained nursing

staff. If there is a question about tissue viability, the dressings are released and the entirety of the revascularized tissue is exposed for further assessment of perfusion, congestion, temperature, turgor, and color with Doppler examination. Release of the dressings alone may be sufficient to alter the vascular issue. If viability is still in question after 30 minutes, immediate re-exploration and further assessment may prevent failure of the revascularized tissue, whether it be the extremity or a free flap.

Early and motivated rehabilitation of the extremity is an important factor in achieving a successful outcome. Early motion reduces edema, adhesions, and scarring. It prevents muscle atrophy and facilitates healing of the soft tissues by remodeling of collagen fibers. The details of the rehabilitation program are determined by the existing injuries and the reconstruction procedure.

Basic science/disease process

Upper extremity function and facial appearance and expression are the two central defining features of our humanity. Movement of the hand through space along with precise grasp, pinch, and positioning allows us to perform the most rudimentary to the most highly complex tasks to actualize the entire range of our wishes, dreams, and ambitions. Man without hands is akin to a plane without wings. Nearly all tasks combine positioning of the hand with shoulder, elbow, and wrist motion followed by intricate manipulation of finger joint position with both intrinsic and extrinsic muscle force modulation.

Injuries to any part of the upper extremity, no matter how minor, may immediately compromise and chronically debilitate the user's ability to perform. Witness the enormously negative impact of work-related injuries on our economy. Productivity is reduced, medical costs are escalated, and the work environment is disrupted, not to mention the enormous personal and family suffering caused by pain and loss of function. Some have estimated the cost to our economy from upper extremity trauma to run in the hundreds of billions of dollars. In light of the significantly problematic consequences that result from extensive upper extremity injuries, it is paramount that early diagnosis and, more important, strategically sound treatment be instituted from the outset.

Extensive skin and soft-tissue trauma along with composite injuries involving multiple structures must be managed actively, there being few circumstances in the hand in which open wound management and healing by secondary intention play a role. Maximum preservation of motion and sensibility should be ever present in the mind of the reconstructive surgeon from the moment of first evaluation, with prompt wound closure given high priority.

The term "mangled" is commonly used to describe the hand and upper extremity after major trauma. Gregory *et al.* used the term "mangled" to describe a severe injury to at least three of the four organ and tissue systems of skin, bone, vessel, and nerve.[8] According to the *Oxford English Dictionary*, to mangle is "to reduce by cutting, tearing or crushing to a more or less unrecognizable condition." Each of these definitions implies a severe, high-energy injury that involves multiple anatomic structures, usually over an extended topography.

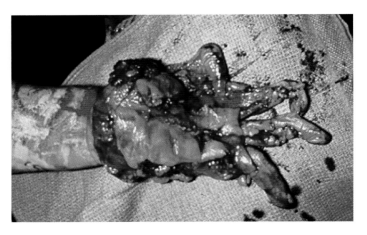

Fig. 12.5 View of hand after it was trapped in a 9-ton press. This is the definition of mangled; it was also unfortunately unsalvageable.

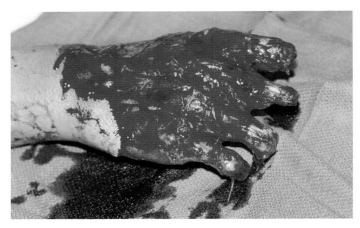

Fig. 12.6 Hand of a 25-year-old male with avulsion injury of entire skin of hand and distal portions of phalanges. This is a devastating injury and will require a number of procedures for adequate reconstruction.

Mangling injuries are produced by high-energy forces. High-power equipment – agricultural (corn picker, grain auger), industrial (punch press, power saw), or household (lawn mower, snow blower) – may cause such an injury *(Fig. 12.5)*. In addition, gunshot wounds, explosives, and motor vehicle accidents (especially with the arm of the patient being outside the car window) account for many cases. The injury may have a combination of sharp, crushing, avulsive, and thermal components. The wound may be severely contaminated, depending on the location and mechanism of injury.

Types of injury

Amputation involves complete severing of a part from the body. This is common in the upper extremities, and ranges from fingertip amputation (an extremely common injury and one of the most common ones seen in emergency departments) to amputation of the entire upper extremity at the shoulder. While fingertip amputations may be managed in any number of ways (most by benign neglect) with excellent outcomes, management of major limb amputations can lead to significant functional and cosmetic deformity and present significant local and systemic problems in management. Replantation of amputated parts requires microsurgical skills and may necessitate other procedures to lead to final restoration of function.

Crush injuries may and may not lead to amputation, but involve significantly more damage to the involved structures than straightforward and sharp amputations. These injuries often lead to major loss of bony and soft-tissue structures and have much poorer results both in terms of survival (if replantation is required) and function. Familiarity with various options for bony and soft-tissue reconstruction, as well as nerve and musculotendinous reconstruction, is often required.

Avulsion injuries primarily involve the soft tissues of the upper extremity. The etiology of these injuries is often due to industrial accidents in roller press machines which both cause bone dislocations in the hand and can lead to loss of the entire soft-tissue envelope to the hand *(Fig. 12.6)*. These injuries predictably lead to severe scarring and often poor function despite the type of reconstruction performed. Early motion is essential for reasonable outcomes in these injuries.

Roller injuries occur when the hand is caught between two rollers whose function is usually to compress sheets of metal. This can result in an array of injuries, including degloving of the skin of the hand, fractures, and potentially crushing of all the tissues of the hand and forearm. These are devastating injuries and call on the entire armamentarium of the surgeon to manage the bony fractures, dislocations, and coverage and functional issues from soft-tissue damage *(Fig. 12.7)*.

Careful evaluation of both the patient and the injury, formulation of a treatment plan, meticulous operative treatment by an experienced team, and early, motivated rehabilitation reduce the morbidity associated with these injuries.

Diagnosis/patient presentation

Evaluation of the patient in the emergency room

Evaluation of the patient with a high-energy injury includes a thorough trauma workup, beginning with the basics of airway, breathing, and circulation. Whereas the mangled extremity is often the most apparent injury, careful evaluation of the entire patient for potential life-threatening or other associated injuries is critical to formulation of a treatment plan.

The patient's history focuses on the time and mechanism of injury and any associated chemical, electrical, or thermal components of the injury. The mechanism of and the time from injury, which is especially crucial when ischemia is present, are the most important factors in determining the zone of injury and predicting the ability to salvage the extremity. A medical history is taken to determine the patient's ability to tolerate a prolonged anesthetic with the potential for significant blood loss, fluid shifts, and release of metabolic byproducts after revascularization of ischemic tissue. Medical conditions such as diabetes, hypertension, vasculitis, or other inflammatory diseases, and smoking history can adversely affect outcome and should be considered in developing a treatment plan. Similarly, the occupational history and social history are important in determining postoperative

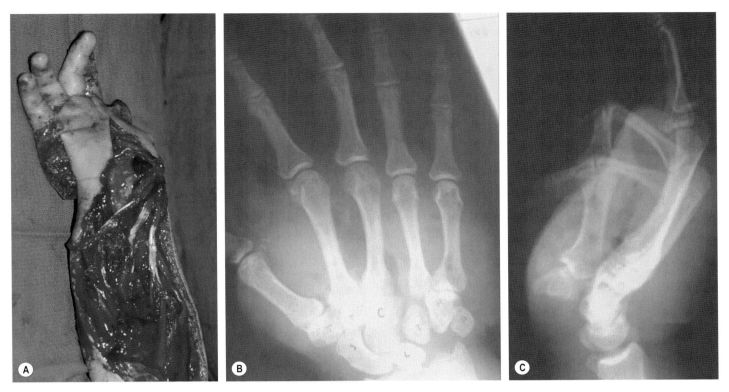

Fig. 12.7 (A) A 27-year-old male with a roller press injury. Note avulsion of muscles and position of hand. **(B)** Anteroposterior X-ray of hand and wrist. Patient has a longitudinal dislocation between the third and fourth rays (a "perihamate peripisiform" injury) which is typical of crushing injuries to the hand. **(C)** Lateral X-ray of the hand and wrist. Note the carpometacarpal dislocation of the thumb in this view, also fairly typical of crushing injuries to the hand.

compliance and in addressing the reconstructive goals. The presence of one or several adverse factors is not an absolute contraindication to salvage of an extremity or to microvascular repair and/or reconstruction. However, these factors should be considered in selecting the type of reconstruction to be used and in better predicting outcome.

Examination of the mangled extremity should be systematic and address vascular status, skeletal stability, motor and sensory function, and soft-tissue loss. The vascular status is evaluated by assessment of peripheral pulses, color, temperature, and capillary refill time in the distal extremity. Pulse oximetry is generally readily available in the emergency department and is helpful in assessing ischemia in the fingers. Doppler examination and angiography can also be used. Arteriographic exam in the mangled extremity may simply delay revascularization, however, and should be utilized very selectively. Skeletal injury is assessed clinically by the presence of deformity, crepitance, or bone tenderness. Radiographs should be taken of the entire extremity – particularly to evaluate the joints above and below the level of injury. A motor and sensory examination should be documented. The examiner should be aware that motor or sensory loss can result from muscle, tendon, or nerve injury as well as from ischemia. The ultimate assessment of the mangled extremity occurs in the operating room, however, after the debridement of nonviable tissue.

In the case of limb-threatening ischemia in a mangling injury, evaluation of the status of the vessels is generally performed in the operating room without the delay necessary for an arteriogram. An intraoperative angiogram may aid in determining the level and extent of arterial injuries, however. Radiographs taken in the operating room are usually of better quality than those taken in the emergency department because the extremity can be positioned without causing the patient discomfort. Traction radiographs allow better delineation of the fracture pattern and number of fragments, especially in evaluating intra-articular fractures about the wrist and elbow. Photographic documentation of the injury should be done throughout the course of treatment from initial evaluation to conclusion of treatment.[9]

Emergency room to operating room – making a plan

Planning in patient management starts when the patient is first seen in the emergency room. As a general rule, however, multiple examinations of the extremity by multiple physicians (emergency physician, intern, resident, fellow) are to be avoided. In the unanesthetized patient this is painful and leads to further anxiety which can lead to vasospasm and further problems. The quality of circulation in the extremity must be assessed, and a rough idea of the soft-tissue deficit should be obtained in a single examination. X-ray studies done in the emergency room of the extremity (and of the distal portion in cases of amputation) also can give an idea of what might be necessary in terms of bony fixation. Consent must be obtained for whatever might be necessary to include bony fixation, revascularization (including potential vascular graft donor sites), and coverage. While an emergency free flap is rarely indicated, the patient should be informed of potential soft-tissue flap donor sites as well. The patient and family should also be informed of the need for further surgery, including second looks/washouts which should be performed in the first several days.

Planning for reconstruction

In deciding how best to treat the mangled extremity, a variety of factors are considered. They can be broadly classified as patient and extremity factors. Pertinent patient factors include the general condition, age, handedness, occupation, functional requirements, and socioeconomic background of the patient. Associated injuries resulting in cardiopulmonary or hemodynamic compromise as well as pre-existing medical problems will mitigate against a lengthy salvage procedure, especially in a patient of advanced age. Conditions adversely affecting the blood vessels, such as diabetes mellitus, vasculitis, or smoking, will increase the risk of anastomotic failure and should be taken into consideration. Psychiatric disorders may be a contraindication to reconstruction because of possible repeated suicide attempts or anticipated noncompliance with the rehabilitation program. A morose patient may be temporarily incompetent to participate in determining treatment. Because time is a critical factor in treatment, it may be better to err in attempting to salvage an extremity than to perform a primary amputation.

Important extremity factors include the time since the injury, the severity of the injury, and the previous functional status of the extremity. Warm ischemia time longer than 6 hours results in progressively irreversible changes in cellular structure of muscle. Even if vascularity is re-established, tissue necrosis will not be avoided. Systemic risks of revascularizing a limb with prolonged ischemia must also be considered and addressed. These include acidosis, hyperkalemia, and rhabdomyolysis. In amputations of digits, where no muscle is present, the delay until reperfusion with use of cold ischemia may be extended to 20 hours. Finally, the previous condition of the extremity is considered. A history of major trauma, neurologic disease, or congenital deformity resulting in impaired function may not justify a salvage attempt.

The multitude of factors and the complex interrelations among them make reaching a decision a difficult task, even for experienced surgeons. Specialized scoring systems have been developed on the basis of lower-extremity injuries. These may offer valuable guidelines for evaluating the lower extremity but cannot be applied well to the upper extremity.[10] Each case is unique, however, and the final decision should be an individualized one based on assessment of the patient and extremity parameters as well as sound judgment. The patient's knowledge of the potential risks and benefits of surgery and the possibility of early or later amputation is important.

A third factor which is rarely discussed is the surgeon factor. The skill and experience of the surgeon managing the patient are extremely important in determining the outcome.[11] While the experienced surgeon is more likely to have a more favorable outcome, reasonable results can be obtained by others if they follow basic principles and stick to what they are comfortable doing. The surgeon who only occasionally performs microsurgical tissue transfer may better serve the patient by performing a pedicled flap for initial coverage than attempting an esoteric and complex microsurgical procedure. It is always better to perform an initial reconstruction using a technique with which you are familiar rather than attempting to perform a procedure that has a high potential for failure. In any case, it is preferable to refer a patient with a complex extremity injury to a center which routinely deals with these problems rather than attempt reconstruction if one is not familiar with these types of problems.

The most important factor in planning reconstruction of a mangled extremity is in fact to have a plan and to know what you are going to need to do next. While the merits of early reconstruction and primary versus delayed reconstruction will be discussed below, the surgeon must have a plan and be ready to alter this depending on the findings at surgery and potential problems as they arise. Reconstructive surgeons must always think at least one or two steps ahead of where they are today in order to maximize their reconstructive efforts. Anticipation of what will need to be done in the future is the primary determinant of what needs to be accomplished today. If one decides to delay bone grafting but proceed with soft-tissue coverage (which is often applicable) the soft-tissue reconstruction should be done in such a manner to make the secondary bony reconstruction both feasible and easy. If there is a large bony defect which may potentially require vascularized bone grafting, the soft-tissue flap should be performed in such a manner as to facilitate performance of the vascularized fibula transfer later. This may mean that a pedicled soft-tissue flap is a superior choice to a free flap (to save recipient vessels for the later bone transfer), but if this type of coverage is not feasible, then the anastomosis for the soft-tissue transfer should be performed in a location and to a vessel which will not make a second microsurgical bone transfer technically more challenging than it already is. The same philosophy applies when one anticipates later toe transfer(s) for thumb or digital reconstruction. Another example is the potential need for later tenolysis or tendon grafting under a soft-tissue flap which is placed at the initial surgery. There is no question that it is much easier to reoperate through a soft-tissue flap than it is under a muscle flap. Muscle flaps scar rather severely underneath when placed on a wound, while soft-tissue flaps do not. Tendons also glide much easier under a fascia or fatty tissue flap than they do under a muscle flap, thus it is preferable to cover exposed tendons (or wounds with gaps in tendons) with some type of fascial or fasciocutaneous flap.

Timing of reconstruction

Definitive reconstruction of the mangled extremity may be undertaken either early or late. In both reconstructive plans, the initial treatment includes aggressive debridement, skeletal stabilization, revascularization, and soft-tissue coverage. Early soft-tissue coverage is of paramount importance to limb salvage. This improves the vascularity to the traumatized area, limits exposure to hospital pathogens, and reduces the risk of infection. Coverage is technically easier to perform early; with delay, edema obscures tissue planes, vessels become friable, and vascular grafts may be needed to perform microanastomoses out the zone of injury.[12]

Reconstruction of bone, tendons, and nerves can be performed either early or late. Early reconstruction implies repair or reconstruction of all injured structures during the initial phase of treatment, up to 10 days from the initial injury. Delayed reconstruction implies staged repair of bone, tendon, nerve, and soft tissue at different periods in the course of treatment. The choice of reconstructive approach depends on the characteristics of the injury and the preference and expertise of the treating surgeon.

Early reconstruction (single-stage)

This approach requires debridement of the wound followed by reconstruction of all structures: bone, tendon, and nerve. This is done ideally within 24–72 hours. Primary corticocancellous bone graft or vascularized bone grafts, nerve grafts, tendon transfers, tendon grafting, and free functional muscle transfer are performed at the time of soft-tissue coverage. Reconstruction can be delayed up to 10 days in the event of a severely contaminated wound, which requires several debridements to reduce the contaminant load.

Primary reconstruction of all structures is technically easier to perform when the tissue bed is fresh rather than later through a scarred soft-tissue bed. It decreases the number of subsequent procedures, total hospitalization time, and cost. Also, rehabilitation can begin earlier. The development of adhesions is decreased, and the functional outcome is improved.[13,14] This type of reconstruction by its nature, however, usually mandates experience and skill with microsurgical repair (nerves) and tissue transfer (for complex and composite tissue loss). If one lacks experience in this type of reconstruction, it is usually best to get primary soft-tissue coverage by whatever means is best and delay the reconstruction of the other structures until a stable soft-tissue bed is obtained.

Delayed reconstruction (multiple stage)

In the past, delayed staged reconstruction was the primary method of treatment of severe injuries with multiple structural defects. In this treatment plan, vascularity is established, and the soft-tissue injuries are treated with serial debridements performed at 24–72-hour intervals. Appropriate wound coverage is performed when the wound is clean and all necrotic tissue has been debrided. This should be within the first 10 days from injury, regardless of the technique chosen, however. Bone, tendon, and nerve reconstruction is delayed until "soft-tissue equilibrium" is achieved. This is when the tissues have healed and are free of infection, edema has resolved, scar tissue has matured, and the joints are supple and have achieved their maximum passive range of motion. Delayed reconstruction is a good option when the patient's comorbidities or a severely contaminated or infected wound prevent early definitive treatment.

Salvage versus amputation

The surgeon may be confronted with the decision to attempt salvage or to amputate a mangled, nonviable upper extremity. The appropriate decision is difficult because recovery of function in a salvaged extremity may be limited or absent. Thus, multiple reconstructive procedures with associated morbidity, prolonged hospitalization, disability time, psychological distress, and financial demands may be too expensive a price to pay for the end result of a useless and painful limb. In contrast to prostheses for the leg, prostheses for the hand and forearm offer limited restoration of function, however. Even with the most advanced prosthetic devices available today, there is no sensory feedback from the prosthesis, and for most purposes, this makes a prosthesis less functional than a sensate yet injured hand. Thus, most mangled upper extremities should be considered for salvage. Nevertheless, serious associated injuries or diseases, ischemia time longer than 6 hours, and parts that are severely crushed, avulsed, contaminated, or injured at multiple levels constitute unfavorable conditions for a replantation or revascularization attempt. In this setting, amputation is not a failure but rather a step toward stabilization of the patient and rehabilitation of the extremity.

Spare-parts utilization

In some instances in severe injury to the upper extremity, there may be uninjured tissues, which, while not salvageable in their native position, may be utilized for coverage and/or reconstruction of the defect. This is certainly the case in multiple digital amputations when the thumb is severely damaged and another finger can be placed in the thumb position to reconstruct this important function (Fig. 12.8). Likewise, the tissue from an amputated finger or forearm can be utilized for coverage of another defect, or even an amputation stump, to salvage length and preclude the necessity for another flap. One should remember to salvage whatever may be useable for reconstruction from parts not deemed suitable for replantation, and this can include skin (grafts or flaps), bone graft, joints (vascularized or not), nerves, and tendons.

Treatment/surgical technique

Options for bony reconstruction

Mangling injuries to the hand and upper extremity usually involve the bone structure as well as the soft tissue. This can range from dislocations to significant bone loss. Each of these must be managed primarily to allow stabilization for vascular and soft-tissue repairs. Dislocations are generally managed with relocation and pinning with Kirschner wires, which usually require 6–8 weeks in place to allow for healing of ligamentous structures. Crushing and roller press injuries commonly lead to longitudinal dislocations in the metacarpal and carpal bones, most frequently between the third and fourth rays (axial loading dislocations or "meat cleaver" injuries). One may also see the thumb ray dislocated with the trapezium on the radial side of the hand. Ligament repair is rarely possible in these injuries, and the bony injury can be missed due to the fact that the soft-tissue issues are often quite dramatic (Fig. 12.7B and C). Management of these injuries is appropriate reduction of the dislocations and/or fractures and pinning (Fig. 12.9). Immobilization is needed for 6–8 weeks. Other wrist dislocations are usually managed in a similar manner.

Fractures of the hand are often best managed with simple K-wire fixation, as this is a rapid and reliable technique. Taking a great deal of time to perform plate fixation in the case of severe injuries in the hand is often counterproductive, especially if the distal extremity is ischemic. This type of fixation usually will not allow early motion, but this is frequently difficult to do in any case in mangling injuries. On the other

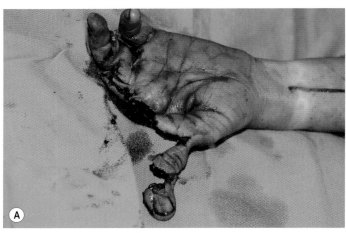

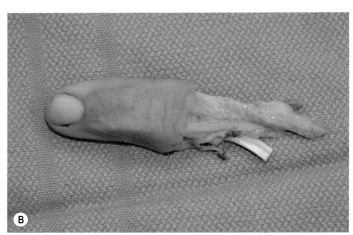

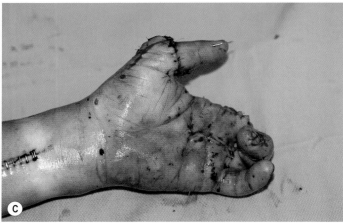

Fig. 12.8 (A) Hand of a 38-year-old male after saw injury with amputation of index and middle fingers with mangling injury to thumb. Thumb is not replantable. **(B)** View of index finger after debridement and identification of structures for replantation. **(C)** Hand after replantation of index finger in thumb position.

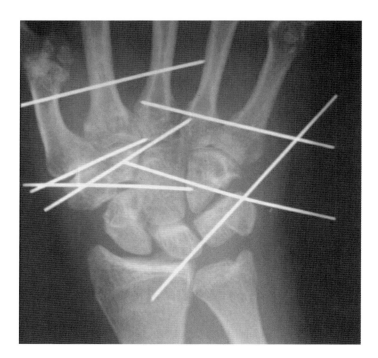

Fig. 12.9 X-ray of patient shown in *Figure 12.7* after reduction and pinning of dislocations using Kirschner wires.

hand, fractures of the radius and ulna are best managed by internal plate fixation. This can be performed relatively rapidly, and gives very stable fixation. We prefer to utilize stainless steel locking plate fixation, and ideally there should be three screws placed on either side of the fracture. The state of the soft tissues should not be a deterrent to plate fixation, as providing good soft-tissue coverage (with an appropriate flap) should be part of the initial plan. The bone must be thoroughly debrided and contaminated fragments with no blood supply should be discarded, however. In the case of severe contamination, a second washout at 48–72 hours should be planned with elevation of the soft tissues, further debridement, and irrigation.

Bone loss may or may not present a problem. Small segments may not preclude healing, but large segments may need reconstruction. Bones should still usually be placed in proper relationship with internal fixation whenever possible, and, as noted above, with the ends in anatomic alignment around the gap. In heavily contaminated wounds, primary bone grafting (with nonvascularized grafts) is not indicated, as the bone graft could be lost to infection. Soft-tissue coverage should be obtained first and the gap dealt with by either standard bone graft (if the defect is less than 6 cm) or vascularized bone grafting (usually a free fibula transfer in the upper extremity). In cases where a significant amount of bone has been lost in both bones of the forearm, an external fixator may be required until adequate soft-tissue reconstruction can be performed and internal bony stabilization applied.

Options for vascular reconstruction

Ideally, primary repair of vascular injury will be possible, but if there is any doubt about potential injury to the ends of the vessels, one should rapidly perform a bypass graft. For most purposes in the upper extremity, this will involve the use of vein grafts. Artificial conduits smaller than 6 mm (primarily expanded polytetrafluoroethylene or Gore-Tex®) have extremely poor patency rates, and are not indicated for bypass grafting. That leaves primarily venous grafts and in some instances arterial grafts. For long segments in the upper arm or forearm, the preferred vein graft is the saphenous from the medial thigh or lower leg *(Fig. 12.10)*. The lesser saphenous,

located on the posterior lateral portion of the ankle and running up the midline of the calf, presents another option if the saphenous is absent or severely varicose. Arm veins (the basilica or cephalic) can be utilized for bypass in the arm, but in the face of severe injury, these may not be available and in fact may be needed for venous outflow (particularly in the face of replantation).

For reconstruction of injuries distal to the wrist, small vein grafts from the volar forearm or dorsal foot may be used. The use of arterial grafts in reconstruction of the ulnar artery and arch has some advocates, and donor sites for this include the subscapular–thoracodorsal axis from the axilla and the descending branch of the lateral femoral circumflex artery in the lateral thigh.[2] Both of these give a reasonable size match for the vessels of the arch, and may offer multiple side branches to anastomose to the common digital vessels as they come off the reconstructed arch. In cases of traumatic injury with ischemic distal tissue, however, the time it takes to

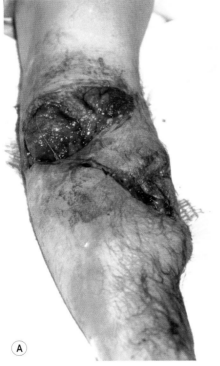

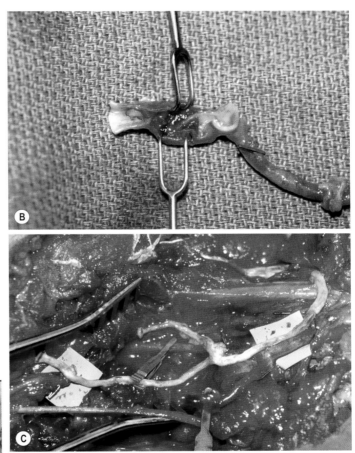

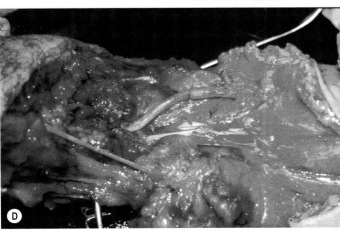

Fig. 12.10 (A) Arm of patient after vehicle roll-over with crush-avulsion injury. There were no palpable pulses in the wrist and the hand was cool. **(B)** View of brachial artery after excision. Note severe intimal avulsion injury in mid-portion. **(C)** Portion of saphenous vein harvested for revascularization. Note branch taken with graft, which is to be utilized for anastomosis to free muscle transfer for coverage. **(D)** Vein graft distended with blood after removal of vascular clamps.

dissect these arterial grafts out (as compared to subcutaneous veins) is probably not worth it. To date, we are not aware that there is any proven benefit to utilizing arterial grafts over venous grafts.

Another option in the face of a moderately large wound with the need for arterial bypass grafting is the use of "flow-through" flaps. As noted above, several flaps are available for this, and the radial forearm free flap, anterolateral thigh, temporoparietal fascia,[15] and omentum have all been utilized as arterial flow-through free flaps. One can also utilize arterialized venous flaps, which have a great deal of utility in digital revascularization to cover small volar defects and provide arterial inflow at the same time,[5] while larger flaps based on the saphenous vein with large skin paddles have been successfully utilized.[16] Another option in the case of large segments of amputated tissue is to provide both coverage and salvage of length utilizing all or a portion of the amputated tissue as a flow-through flap. The use of all of these flaps for both coverage and bypass is unusual, but the surgeon dealing with severe extremity injuries should be familiar with the options.

Nerve reconstruction

The ideal time for nerve reconstruction is usually at the time of injury, because it is easiest to determine level of damage (by observing bruising of the nerve), and dissection and orientation of the nerve are obvious prior to the onset of scarring. Nonetheless, the goal should be repair of nerve damage at the time of initial treatment with the caveat that nerve repairs and/or grafts should be surrounded with well-vascularized tissue. This may require the use of vascularized flap transfer to maximize nerve recovery; however a flap may be needed regardless. Nerve repairs and nerve grafts should not be done if there is inadequate soft tissue surrounding the repair and should certainly not be placed under skin grafts.

Primary repair of damaged nerves is the ideal, but if this cannot be achieved, the nerve should be grafted. Small gaps of smaller sensory nerves may be treated with any of the number of "tubes" available[17]; however their utility in larger nerves and in longer gaps remains unproven.[18,19] The recently approved nerve allograft has shown some possible application in nerve gaps, but the results in larger nerves have not proven to be the equal of autologous nerve grafts.[20] Autologous nerve grafts remain the gold standard, and a number of donor sites are available. The most commonly utilized is the sural nerve running from the posterior knee to the lateral ankle, but other peripheral sensory nerves can be utilized as well. These include the saphenous nerve, the medial and lateral antebrachial cutaneous nerve, the radial sensory branch, and the medial brachial cutaneous nerve. These secondary sources of nerve graft are all limited by their diameter and available length compared to the sural. When nerves are grafted, an attempt must be made to line up similar areas of fascicular bundles on the nerves to maximize functional recovery.

As noted above, nerve transfers may be the best option when multiple nerves have been injured.[6,7] The reader is referred to Chapters 32 and 33 for more information on these subjects.

Muscle and tendon repair and reconstruction

As with other structures, primary repair of muscles and tendons is desirable. Tendons and tendon repair will also require good, vascular soft-tissue coverage in order both to survive and have maximal function. Flexor tendons in the hand and fingers should be repaired with a four-strand core suture technique whenever possible, with the addition of an epitenon stitch of fine monofilament suture to aid in gliding.[21] In the case of injury to both the flexor digitorum superficialis and profundus tendons in the finger, one may opt simply to repair only the profundus, particularly if the cut ends are untidy. If the ends cannot be brought together, one must consider either primary tendon grafting or the possibility of tendon transfer to provide the missing function if it is essential. Primary tendon grafting should not be performed in a bad wound bed, as the odds of success are small. In these cases, one might also consider placing Silastic tendon rods along the course of the tendon requiring reconstruction. Grafts can then be placed in the tracts of the rods. This scenario would most commonly accompany flap coverage, however, and in general cutaneous flaps are a much better bed than muscle for placing tendon grafts. Direct injury to muscles can often be sutured, but with severe injury the damaged muscle will often require debridement. Loss of function from removing muscle can be reconstructed with tendon transfers on occasion but may require free innervated muscle transfer to repair the loss.

Soft-tissue reconstruction

The approach to wounds of the upper extremity should follow the usual parameters of soft-tissue reconstruction, the so-called reconstructive ladder. In complex wounds, however, this concept is being replaced by that of the "reconstructive elevator," which proposes bypassing simple reconstructions and providing the best functional coverage available (despite the fact that a wound might "get by" with a skin graft). Many wounds nonetheless can be covered with a split-thickness skin graft or with regional flaps, particularly in the hand. The ultimate morbidity of any local or regional flap must be considered, however, especially in relation to later hand function. Because the hand is highly visible, the cosmetic aspect of certain local and regional flaps must be considered as well. Although certain wounds may be adequately covered with a flap from the same extremity, one should consider what offers the best coverage in terms of the overall reconstruction.[22] This will often lead to use of a free flap for many hand and upper-limb wounds. The selection of flap coverage for a clean wound allows use of composite tissue in many cases.[23–25] Whereas many smaller wounds in the upper extremity are amenable to small local or regional flaps, this discussion centers on the use of major axial-based pedicle or free flaps for the management of larger wounds.

Wounds should be definitively closed as soon as the wound bed is clean. This applies equally to flap coverage as well as simple primary closure. As discussed above, wound debridement is essential to provide control of tissue necrosis and infection. If the status of the tissue is in doubt, serial debridements should be performed to avoid removal of viable tissue and yet assure a well-vascularized wound with minimal bacterial contamination. In patients with vital structures exposed, it is often best to place a muscle flap (usually a free muscle flap), with the plan to return to the operating room every 48 hours. The flap is not definitively sutured down, and is lifted at each subsequent procedure and debridement and irrigation are carried out. Once the muscle flap starts becoming adherent to the underlying tissue and there is a decrease in cloudy fluid under the flap, it is ready for definite insetting and coverage with a skin graft *(Fig. 12.11)*. Vacuum-assisted wound closure provides an excellent temporizing measure between debridements,[26,27] and may be utilized in the upper part of the arm to optimize a wound bed prior to skin grafting. This wound management technique has the advantage of removing edema and exudate from the wound and tends to decrease swelling in our experience. It should be utilized with caution in the hand, however, as extended use can lead to increased scar (in the form of granulation tissue) and additional stiffness. When utilized for a relatively short period of time, however, it can be advantageous.

Types of flaps – cutaneous versus muscle

Wounds of the hand and upper extremity can be covered by either cutaneous flaps or muscle flaps. Myocutaneous flaps are not utilized as much today as in the past, because surprisingly they are not generally as cosmetic as a simple muscle flap covered with a split-thickness skin graft. Muscle flaps have always been thought of as superior for coverage of untidy and/or infected wounds[24]; however fasciocutaneous flaps (at least with inclusion of the well-vascularized fascia) are equally applicable to these wounds in terms of the ability to manage infection.[25] For hand coverage, we prefer cutaneous flaps whenever possible, as it is usually easier to reoperate through skin and subcutaneous fat than muscle. While the muscle has the advantage that it atrophies over time, there tends to be a fairly severe amount of scarring under a muscle flap, which makes it more difficult to raise for secondary procedures and mitigates against tendon gliding. Thus, in general, we prefer to utilize any of the number of fasciocutaneous flaps when covering the hand. In severe injuries and in

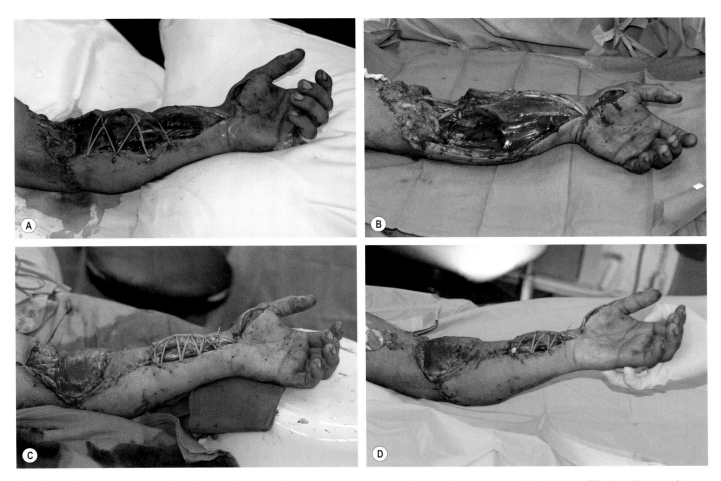

Fig. 12.11 (A) Forearm of young patient 48 hours after replantation at proximal forearm level. Note necrotic-appearing muscle in forearm. **(B)** View of forearm after debridement. Note exposed vein bypass grafts. **(C)** Patient at same surgery after placement of rectus abdominis muscle free flap to cover vessels and bone. **(D)** View of forearm at time of re-exploration 48 hours after last debridement and flap cover.

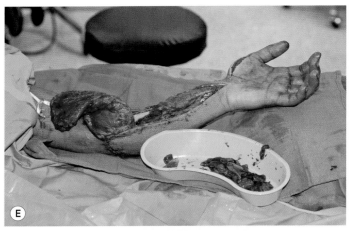

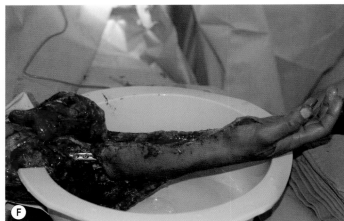

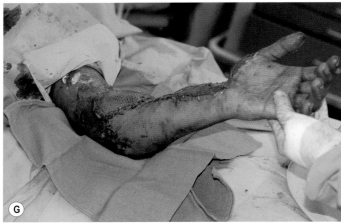

Fig. 12.11, cont'd (E) Nonviable muscle debrided at this surgery. Note rectus muscle flap flipped back to allow debridement and washout and nonviable muscle in basin. **(F)** Forearm at third washout, 6 days after injury. There was no further muscle necrosis noted on this exploration, and the muscle flap was becoming adherent to the underlying tissues. **(G)** Forearm at fourth washout, 9 days after injury. The wounds were very clean and the muscle flap was sutured down and a split-thickness skin graft was placed. This patient never developed evidence of sepsis and no infection developed in either the soft tissues or bone, despite severe contamination at the time of injury.

the face of a large dead space needing to be filled, however, muscle is probably superior. While the hand and upper extremity afford a large number of local and regional flaps, this chapter will deal primarily with larger flaps and emphasize free tissue transfer for coverage of the hand.

Pedicled flaps – the groin flap

The pedicled groin flap remains one of the workhorses for hand coverage. It provides a very large portion of soft tissue which can cover many large defects in the hand and forearm. This flap was the first axial pattern flap described, and was the first flap transferred microsurgically. Its use as a free flap has been supplanted by many flaps with better vasculature, but it should be a part of the armamentarium of every hand surgeon. The blood supply is based on the superficial circumflex iliac vessels, which exit the femoral vessels in the groin and run approximately 2 cm below and parallel to the inguinal ligament *(Fig. 12.12)*. This artery can be located with a pencil Doppler and can be mapped out roughly to the level of the anterior superior iliac spine (ASIS). This flap can (and should be) taken out beyond the ASIS to allow the proximal portion to be tubed to allow some shoulder and elbow motion. It can be radically defatted, especially the more distal portion (which will be placed on the hand), and contours very well on the hand. It can be utilized for coverage of the dorsal hand, forearm, and first webspace, and has great

utility as a first step prior to toe transfer for thumb or digital reconstruction.

The flap is first marked out with the vessel in the center axis of the flap (which we prefer to locate with a Doppler) *(Fig. 12.13)*. Dissection proceeds from lateral to medial. Care should be taken to avoid leaving a great deal of the fat from the iliac area on the deep surface of the flap, as this will have to be removed regardless. The landmark to look for as dissection proceeds medially is the sartorius, as the artery pierces the fascia of the sartorius at its medial edge. We prefer to incise the fascia at the lateral edge of the muscle and stop the dissection short of the space medial to the muscle, which obviates damage to the vascular pedicle. Once the flap has been dissected up, the donor site is closed. The edges of the donor site should not be undermined, as this simply makes the wound larger. Closure is facilitated by bending the hip and placing a pillow under the knee. Once the donor site is closed, the proximal portion of the flap is usually sewn into a tube. The distal flap to be placed on the hand is defatted centripetally, avoiding defatting the central portion too much to avoid damage to the pedicle. Once this is done, the flap is sewn in place in the defect on the hand *(Fig. 12.14)*. Closure of the donor site and tubing of the flap prior to inset as described above greatly facilitates this operation.

We have not seen patients pull the flap off the hand once they are fully awake, but it is prudent either to strap the arm down to the torso or put a very large suture between the wrist and the body until the patient is fully awake and on the ward. If the arm is strapped, this should be removed once the patient is awake and lucid as it can lead to swelling and congestion in the hand. In the postoperative period, the patient is instructed how to move the shoulder and elbow through available range based on the tubed portion of the pedicle. The flap can usually safely be divided at around 3 weeks, but this is dependent on how well the flap is healed on the hand. If

healing has been delayed or there has been a partial dehiscence, division may need to be delayed. The flap can also be "delayed" prior to division, which is accomplished by either making a small incision in the tubed portion and dividing all the deep tissues (i.e., the pedicle) or conversely by incising the tube circumferentially to interrupt the subdermal plexus. Once this has been done, the flap can usually be safely divided in 5–7 days.

At the time of division, the donor site is closed and the flap is gently inset on the hand. Some advocate leaving the tubed portion dangling on the hand to allow for potential demarcation of the flap into viable and nonviable portions. Our experience has been that if the flap is well healed on the hand, the flap can usually be safely trimmed and inset. The patient is begun on a rigorous physical therapy program to regain

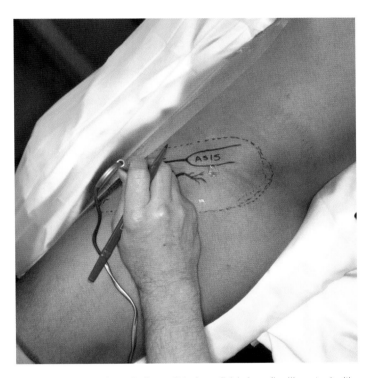

Fig. 12.12 Anatomy of groin flap and superficial inferior epigastric artery (SIEA) flap. Note that the superficial circumflex iliac artery runs approximately 2 cm (or two fingerbreadths) below the inguinal ligament. These two flaps can provide coverage of very large wounds of the hand.

Fig. 12.13 Locating the groin flap pedicle (superficial circumflex iliac artery) with a pencil Doppler.

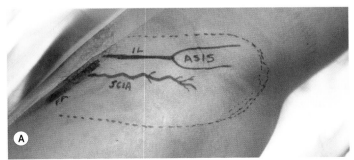

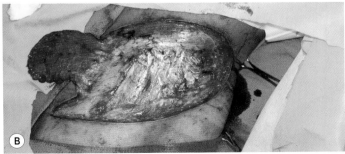

Fig. 12.14 (A) Markings on groin of patient for pedicled groin flap. Patient had failed replantation of thumb and flap is to prepare for later toe transfer for thumb reconstruction. **(B)** Flap elevated. Note size of donor defect after elevation. Be aware that undermining these edges simply makes this defect more difficult to close.

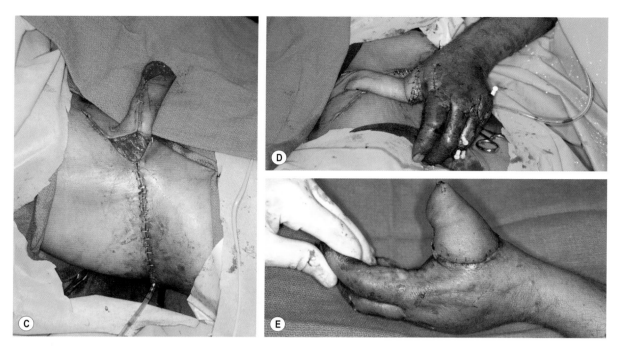

Fig. 12.14, cont'd (C) Donor site has been closed primarily and flap has been tubed. **(D)** Flap after placement on hand. **(E)**. Final view after 3½ weeks at time of division and insetting of flap.

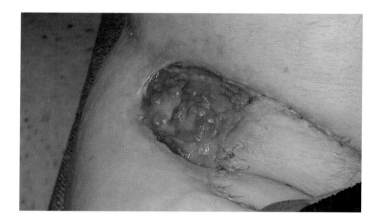

Fig. 12.15 Patient who suffered infection and dehiscence of groin flap donor site after 3 weeks of wound care, prior to placement of split-thickness skin graft. This can be avoided by treating the wound carefully in the postoperative period and avoiding leaving it open.

shoulder and elbow motion, as well as motion in the hand. The pedicled groin flap can usually be contoured (defatted) adequately when first placed on the hand, but on occasion will require secondary procedures to inset and decrease the bulk later. The primary advantage of the pedicled groin flap is that it does not require microsurgical expertise, while the primary disadvantage of this flap is that the hand is placed in a dependent position and may lead to stiffness in the shoulder. One caveat concerning the donor site is that if this area becomes infected, is it unwise to remove all the sutures. This will lead to a gigantic wound which can be quite difficult to

manage *(Fig. 12.15)*. It is much better to treat this by removing a few sutures and irrigating the area under the sutures daily, which will rid the area of infection without the morbidity of a massive open wound on the hip.

Free flaps – fasciocutaneous flaps

The radial forearm flap

This flap offers almost ideal characteristics for hand reconstruction.[1] Its primary application is as a pedicled flap, based on reversed flow through the distal radial artery and venae comitantes.[28] It may be elevated on a proximal vascular pedicle to cover wounds in the forearm or about the elbow. Nonetheless, it may be used as a free flap in certain instances and affords excellent hand coverage. This flap can be raised anywhere along the course of the radial artery, and a skin island from very small to quite large may be taken *(Fig. 12.16)*. The radial artery provides a large-caliber vessel for anastomosis and may be used for revascularization of the distal limb if necessary as a "flow-through" free flap. The venous drainage is through the dual concomitant veins of the radial artery; larger flaps can be drained by cutaneous veins. There has been some controversy as to the primary venous drainage of these flaps, but the venae comitantes offer reliable drainage even in the absence of superficial veins. This flap may be innervated by anastomosis of the lateral antebrachial cutaneous nerve, part of which is invariably in the flap. The quality of sensation in such reinnervated flaps is not great, but it may be useful. If the patient has a palmaris longus tendon, it may be taken in the flap as well and offers an excellent option for tendon reconstruction, especially on the dorsal hand. Because the tendon is taken with its surrounding tissue, it has excellent

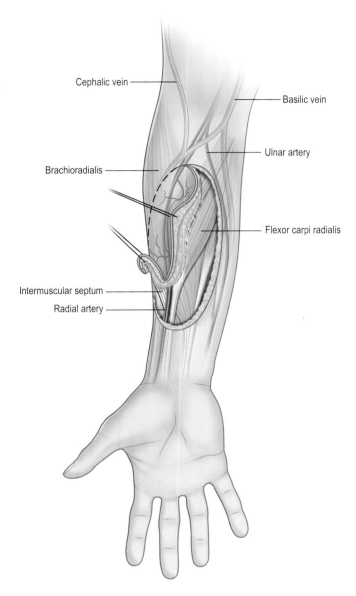

Cephalic vein

Basilic vein

Ulnar artery

Brachioradialis

Flexor carpi radialis

Intermuscular septum

Radial artery

Fig. 12.16 Anatomy of radial forearm flap on forearm. This flap can be taken anywhere over the radial artery in the forearm, and can include skin, fascia, tendon, and bone.

gliding when transferred as part of the flap. A portion of the volar radius may be harvested with the flap as well and is particularly useful in reconstruction of missing segments of metacarpal[29,30] *(Fig. 12.17)*. The radial artery can be taken with the fascia only, which offers a thin flap that is particularly useful in reconstruction of the palm.

The advantages of this flap as a free flap are its thinness, its reliability (based on the radial artery), and the multitude of other tissues that may be harvested with it. The main disadvantage of this flap is the resulting donor site, which must usually be covered with a skin graft. The donor site is usually aesthetically unpleasing but causes few functional problems. Another relative contraindication to this flap is the loss of the radial artery, but studies have shown that significant

problems are unusual. Cold sensitivity is seen but may be related to other factors. Whereas the radial forearm flap is an excellent free flap, it can usually be used as a distally pedicled island flap for hand reconstruction *(Fig. 12.18)*. If this flap is not available for some reason as a pedicled flap, a skin flap is usually selected from another area, and a radial forearm flap is not taken from the contralateral uninjured arm.

Lateral arm free flap

This fasciocutaneous flap from the lateral distal upper arm is based on the posterior radial collateral artery, a branch of the profundus brachii.[31] This vessel runs with the radial nerve in the spiral groove and comes to lie in the posterior intermuscular septum between the brachialis and lateral head of the triceps *(Fig. 12.19)*. It gives arterial supply to the skin overlying the septum as well as the underlying humerus *(Fig. 12.20)*. Distal to the intermuscular septum, the posterior radial collateral artery has a rich system of anastomoses with vessels in the proximal lateral forearm, which will allow extension of the flap on to the proximal forearm. This flap can also be based distally for coverage of small to moderate defects of the elbow *(Fig. 12.21)*. The pedicle for this flap is relatively short (5–7 cm), and the proximal artery has a small diameter (1.5–2 mm) compared with the flaps previously discussed. The length of the pedicle is limited by the fact that it exits the spiral groove with the radial nerve, and damage to this nerve must be avoided in the dissection. Acland and Shatford, in unpublished video demonstrations, have demonstrated a safe and effective method to lengthen the pedicle significantly through an alternative proximal dissection. The skin paddle can be based directly over the intermuscular septum for a smaller flap or extended distally for a larger one.

Donor sites up to 7 cm in width can be closed primarily, but larger ones require a skin graft.[32] When closed primarily, the donor site can be cosmetic, but the scar will widen significantly in some patients. The posterior cutaneous nerve to the arm may be taken to innervate the flap; the posterior cutaneous nerve to the forearm may be used as a flow-through vascularized nerve graft.[33] A portion of the lateral humerus can be taken with the flap for bone reconstruction, based on its vascular supply from the overlying pedicle.[34] The lateral arm flap is purported to be a "thin" flap, but because of the tissue in the intermuscular septum, it is a bit bulky when placed on a flat recipient site (i.e., the back of the hand). This problem can be avoided by using the fascia only, which also decreases donor site problems.[32,35] The primary advantages of this flap are that it can be taken from the ipsilateral arm (of injury) *(Fig. 12.22)*, it avoids the sacrifice of a major vessel, it has the potential to serve as a multicomponent composite transplant, and the donor site can often be closed primarily. The primary disadvantages of the lateral arm free flap are its somewhat limited size, the short and small-diameter pedicle, the resultant contour deformity in the arm, and forearm dysesthesias. It is useful in coverage of small defects of the hand and works well in the first webspace *(Fig. 12.23)*. In thin patients, it can be used to cover a degloving injury of the thumb with the added benefit of reinnervation through the cutaneous nerve. It has served nicely as a composite osteocutaneous flap to reconstruct multicomponent defects about the antecubital fossa and elbow.

Text continued on page 272

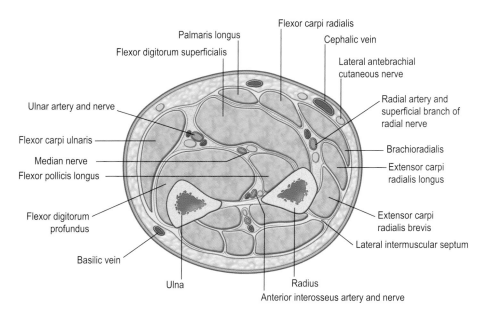

Palmaris longus

Flexor digitorum superficialis

Flexor carpi radialis

Cephalic vein

Lateral antebrachial cutaneous nerve

Ulnar artery and nerve

Flexor carpi ulnaris

Median nerve

Flexor pollicis longus

Flexor digitorum profundus

Basilic vein

Ulna

Radius

Anterior interosseus artery and nerve

Radial artery and superficial branch of radial nerve

Brachioradialis

Extensor carpi radialis longus

Extensor carpi radialis brevis

Lateral intermuscular septum

Fig. 12.17 Cross-section anatomy of the forearm. The radial forearm flap is based on the radial artery as it runs between the flexor carpi radialis muscle and the brachioradialis muscle. Muscle and/or bone may be harvested with this flap.

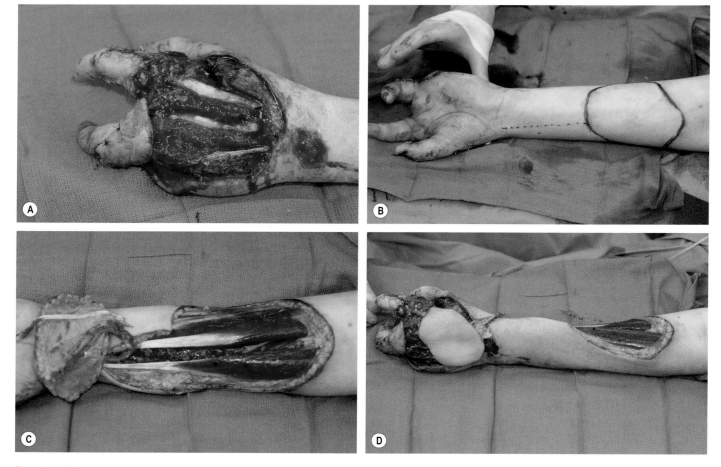

Fig. 12.18 (A) Degloving injury in 13-year-old boy after automobile roll-over injury. **(B)** Outline of distally based pedicled radial forearm flap for coverage of wound. **(C)** Flap elevated. Note that the palmaris longus tendon has been harvested in the flap for extensor tendon reconstruction. **(D)** Flap placed on hand. Note that flap and pedicle will be placed through a subcutaneous tunnel to reach the dorsal hand.

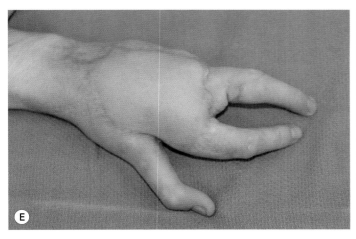

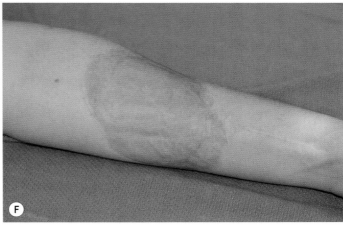

Fig. 12.18, cont'd (E) Healed flap on dorsal hand. Note color and texture match of flap with hand. **(F)** Donor site on volar forearm after healing of split-thickness skin graft.

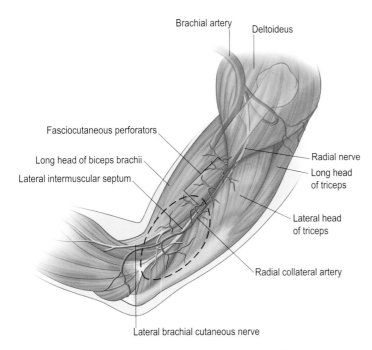

Fig. 12.19 Anatomical depiction of anatomy of lateral arm free flap.

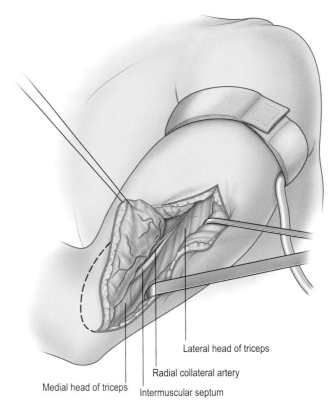

Fig. 12.20 Dissection of lateral arm free flap.

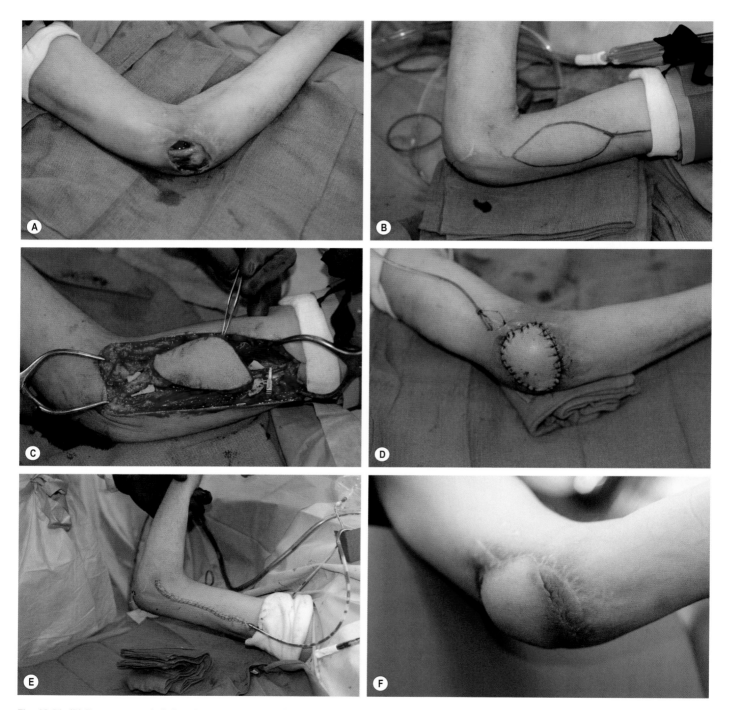

Fig. 12.21 (B) Recurrent wound of elbow in paraplegic patient. **(B)** Markings for distally pedicled lateral arm flap for coverage. Note that distal extent of recurrent radial artery has been located with a pencil Doppler and marked. **(C)** Flap after elevation. Note distal pedicle at elbow. Vascular clamp is on proximal vessel; note excellent perfusion of flap without evidence of venous congestion. **(D)** Flap sutured in place. **(E)** Donor site closed primarily. **(F).** Flap healed at 3 months with good coverage.

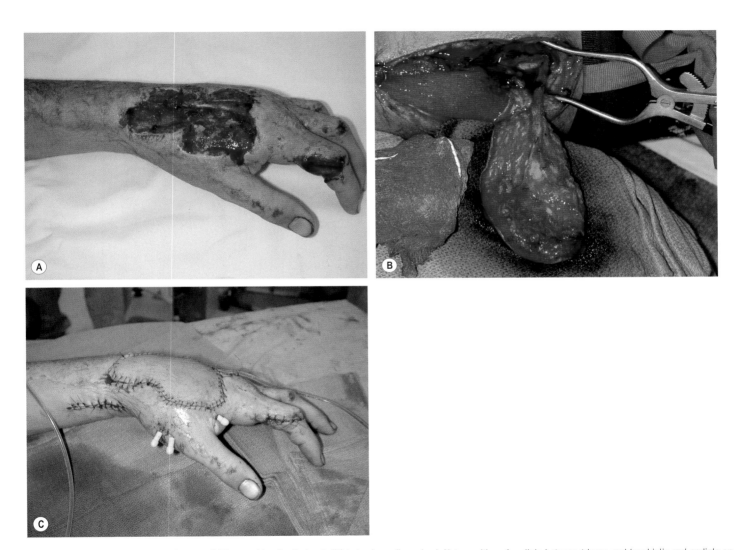

Fig. 12.22 (A) Avulsion injury on dorsum of 24-year-old patient's hand. **(B)** Lateral arm flap raised. Note position of pedicle between triceps and brachialis and pedicle on deep surface of fascia of flap. **(C)** Free flap after being inset on hand. Anastomosis was to radial artery in anatomic snuffbox.

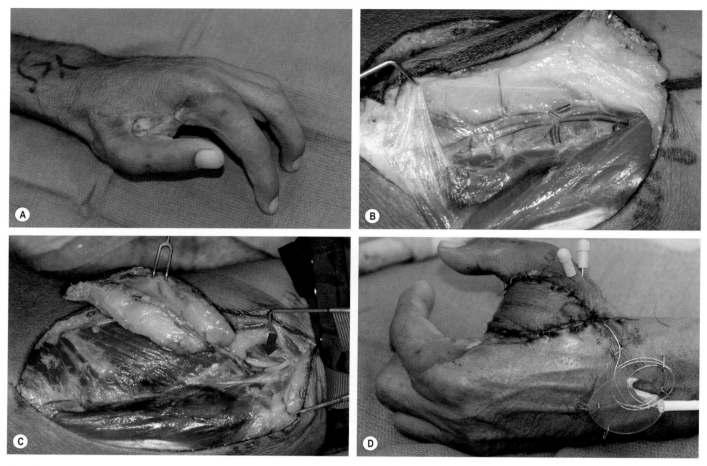

Fig. 12.23 (A) Patient with severe first webspace contracture after crush injury. **(B)** Flap being raised from posteriorly. Underside of flap showing pedicle at base of septum; note triceps muscle posterior to flap. **(C).** Flap raised on its pedicle. Arrow points to radial nerve in septum. **(D)** Flap after suturing in place.

Scapular flap

The scapular and parascapular flaps offer a versatile large skin flap for coverage of defects in the upper extremity.[36] The vascular supply is based on the circumflex scapular vessels that branch from the subscapular system.[37] The pedicle for this flap is long (4–6 cm) because the subscapular vessels can be taken if necessary, and this provides vessels of large diameter at the takeoff from the axillary artery. The vessels lie in the fascia with branches to the overlying skin. There are two primary branches, giving rise to the transverse scapular flap, which is sited transversely across the back, and the parascapular flap, which is sited obliquely down the back *(Fig. 12.24)*. Based on this vascular supply, a large skin flap can be designed that will cover most defects of the forearm and arm.[38] Although a number of cutaneous nerves enter the skin, there is not a dominant nerve to this area, and thus this flap has poor potential for innervations. Branches from the primary pedicle feed the lateral surface of the scapula, and a portion of this bone can be taken to repair bone defects. This bone is flat, however, and its primary indication is reconstruction of smaller defects in the hand. Donor sites in the 8-cm range can usually be closed primarily, but this is usually limited to the parascapular design of the flap.

The primary advantages of this flap are the length and diameter of its pedicle along with its potential large size. The primary disadvantage of this flap is the need for turning the patient to harvest it. The scapular flap is an excellent choice for coverage of large wounds of the forearm and can be used in place of a pedicled groin flap for hand coverage *(Fig. 12.25)*. It can be combined with the latissimus dorsi and serratus anterior muscle flaps on a single pedicle to provide a huge amount of tissue and for coverage of different surfaces of the hand and arm.[38] Fascia alone can be harvested if back skin and subcutaneous tissue are deemed too bulky for an effective transfer.

Temporoparietal fascia flap

The temporoparietal fascia offers a flap of specialized tissue that has great utility in reconstruction of the hand.[15] This flap is supplied by the superficial temporal artery and vein and has a pedicle in the 2–3-cm range, which is about 1.5–2.5 mm in diameter[39] *(Fig. 12.26)*. The temporal fascia lies on the temporal region of the skull, beginning on the zygoma and running superiorly. There is a larger superficial layer as well as a deep temporal fascial layer, and both may be taken with this flap. The use of both layers of fascia has been promoted

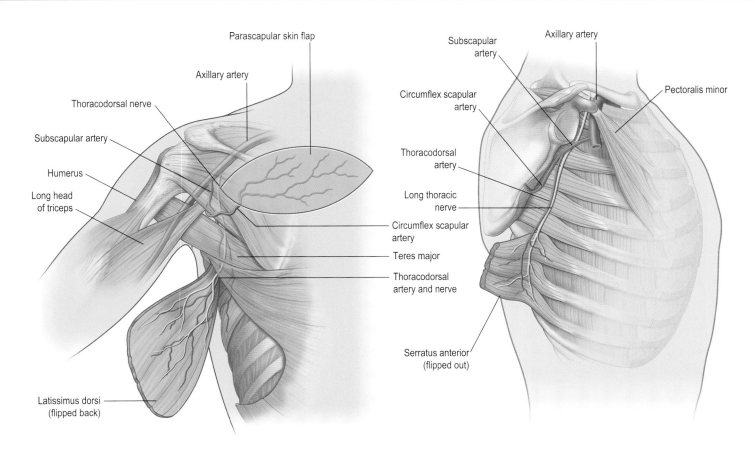

Fig. 12.24 Anatomy of the thoracodorsal/subscapular vascular tree with the flaps (scapular/parascapular/latissimus/serratus anterior) that can be raised on this pedicle.

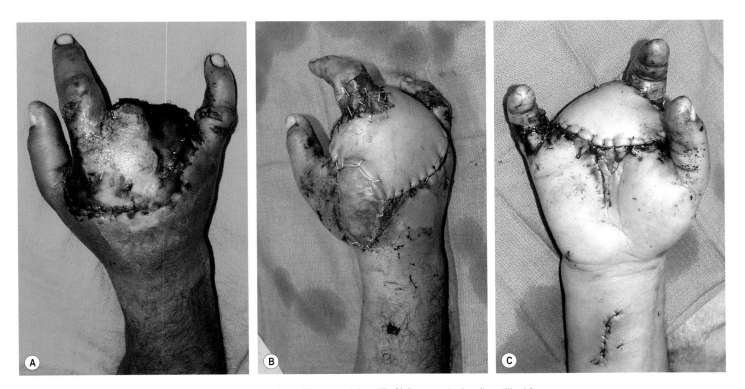

Fig. 12.25 **(A)** Patient with amputation and degloving of dorsal hand from rope injury. **(B, C)** Parascapular free flap utilized for coverage.

for wrapping adherent tendons on the dorsum of the hand after tenolysis in a scarred bed. The deep fascia can provide tissue for reconstruction of small tendons on the dorsal hand as well. A flap of moderate dimensions may be taken, in the 8–10-cm range. The potential for harvesting vascularized bone with this flap exists, but the thin, outer table bone available has little indication in the hand. Although the donor scar is one of the best in terms of cosmesis, the problem of alopecia exists because the superficial fascia must be dissected from just beneath the hair follicles of the scalp.

The primary advantages of this flap include the potential to provide a gliding surface and a donor site that is one of the best in terms of cosmesis. The primary disadvantage of this flap is that it is thin and must be covered with a skin graft. The frontal branch of the facial nerve can be injured in its dissection. Temporoparietal fascia offers nice coverage for defects of the fingers and hand, but the size of the flap is limited.[40] This tissue does seem to improve the gliding ability of tendons, particularly on the dorsum. When covered with a split-thickness skin graft, the temporoparietal fascia flap offers the thinnest coverage available (excluding other fascial flaps) *(Fig. 12.27)*.

Anterolateral thigh flap

The anterolateral thigh flap is a more recently popularized flap which has application in reconstruction of wounds in the hand. It is based on the descending branch of the lateral

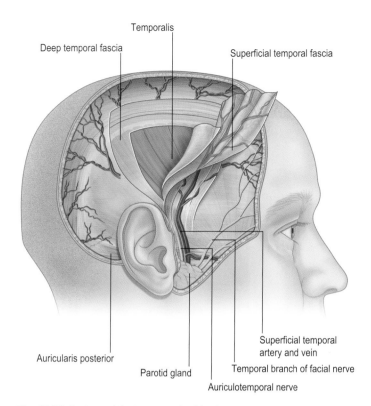

Fig. 12.26 Anatomy of the temporoparietal fascia.

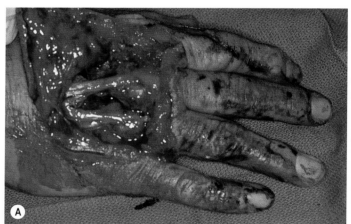

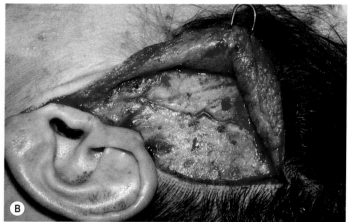

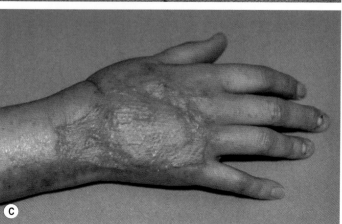

Fig. 12.27 (A) Degloving injury of dorsal hand. **(B)** View of temporal vessels within temporal fascia on side of head. Temporal artery is tortuous, vein is anterior and straighter. **(C)** Healed dorsal hand after flap covered with meshed split-thickness skin graft.

femoral circumflex artery in the thigh, and can be taken with a large skin paddle, fascia, and potentially muscle *(Fig. 12.28)*. This flap was originally thought to be a septal perforator type of flap, but it is well recognized now that most of these flaps are supplied by intramuscular perforators through the vastus lateralis muscle.[41] Donor sites in the 6–7-cm width range can be closed primarily, but larger flaps will require a skin graft for the donor site. This flap can supply a large amount of tissue for coverage, and the fascia may be useful in reconstruction of tendons (i.e., the distal triceps tendon). It can also be utilized to revascularize the distal extremity as a flow-through flap via the descending branch which also supplies the flap.[42] When placed on the hand, the flap can be radically thinned to avoid excessive bulk.[3]

The flap is designed by marking a line from the anterosuperior iliac spine to the lateral border of the patella. This should roughly follow the septum between the rectus femoris and the vastus lateralis. The primary perforators are located roughly halfway down this line. While some design the flap without identifying the perforators,[43] we prefer to utilize a pencil Doppler to locate the primary perforators along the medial border of the vastus lateralis. Once the central axis of the flap is laid out, the dissection begins by raising the medial aspect of the flap. This is raised over to the intermuscular septum between the rectus femoris and vastus lateralis, which is inspected to see if there are any perforators present. The dissection then proceeds from medial to laterally over the vastus, and great care must be taken to lift the flap very carefully and identify and preserve any and all perforators coming through the muscle and fascia lata into the skin paddle. Once these perforators are identified, the lateral edge of the flap can be incised and the remainder of the flap lifted. The perforators are then carefully dissected out of the muscle down to the level of the descending branch of the lateral femoral circumflex vessels. Once these are dissected out, the flap pedicle can be ligated and the flap moved.

The primary indication for the anterolateral thigh flap is in large defects of the forearm and/or hand *(Fig. 12.29)*. As noted above, it can be utilized for distal revascularization as well. The donor site is generally well tolerated, even if it has to be grafted.[44] The primary disadvantage of this flap is that it tends to be bulky, particularly in obese patients.

Free flaps – muscle flaps

Latissimus dorsi

The latissimus dorsi muscle is a large muscle of the back and shoulder, and its vascular supply for free transfer is based on the subscapular–thoracodorsal system[45,46] *(Fig. 12.24)*. The pedicle is lengthy (8–11 cm) and has a relatively large diameter proximally (up to 6 mm). This is the largest single muscle available for transfer, and its area of coverage can be expanded by including a portion of the serratus anterior muscle by its nourishing branch that arises from the thoracodorsal artery.[47] It can be used as an innervated muscle because of the single thoracodorsal nerve,[48] but the latissimus is generally used in the upper limb for coverage of large, degloving-type wounds *(Fig. 12.30)*.

The advantages of this muscle are that it has a totally reliable vascular supply and is very large. Its primary disadvantage is that the patient must be turned in the lateral decubitus position for harvest of the muscle. If the contralateral muscle is taken, the patient can be turned on the side and the injured arm can be prepared simultaneously with muscle harvest (assuming that appropriate surgical assistance is available). It can be taken as a musculocutaneous flap or harvested with the entire subscapular axis to include up to two muscles (latissimus and a portion of the serratus anterior), a fasciocutaneous paddle, and vascularized bone; but for most indications in the upper extremity, the muscle only is taken and covered with a split-thickness skin graft. The donor site is easily closed, but seroma formation is a common sequela of this donor site. The functional morbidity from the loss of muscle is minimal in most patients, but its use should be avoided in patients who must adduct the arm strongly (crutch-walkers and paraplegics).

Rectus abdominis

The rectus abdominis is a muscle widely used in microsurgery, primarily today as the transverse rectus abdominis

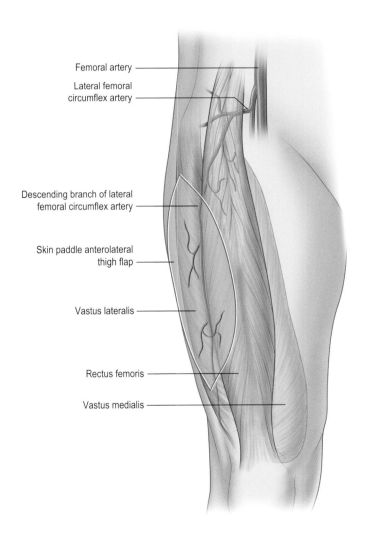

Fig. 12.28 Anatomy of descending branch of lateral femoral circumflex artery and anterolateral thigh flap. This flap offers one of the largest cutaneous free flaps available, and can be taken with vascularized muscle and/or fascia.

Labels on figure:
- Femoral artery
- Lateral femoral circumflex artery
- Descending branch of lateral femoral circumflex artery
- Skin paddle anterolateral thigh flap
- Vastus lateralis
- Rectus femoris
- Vastus medialis

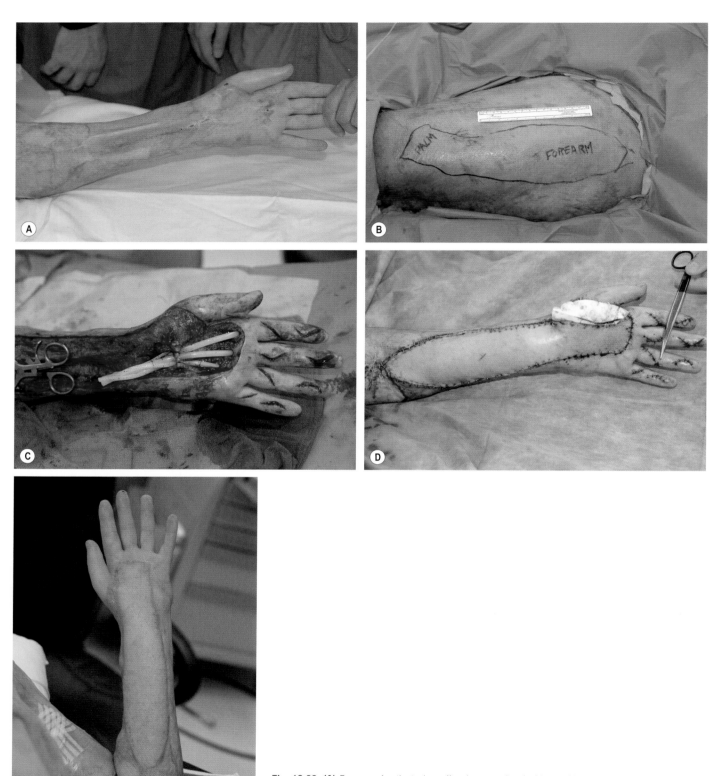

Fig. 12.29 **(A)** Forearm of patient who suffered severe electrical burn with loss of all volar musculature. Plan is for coverage with free anterolateral thigh flap and placement of tendon rods followed by innervated muscle transfer and tendon grafting. **(B)** Markings on leg for flap. Hip is to the right and knee to the left in this view. **(C)** Forearm and hand after placement of tendon rods and pulley reconstruction. **(D)** View after vascular anastomosis and insetting of flap. **(E)** Hand and forearm after 3 months prior to innervated gracilis transfer.

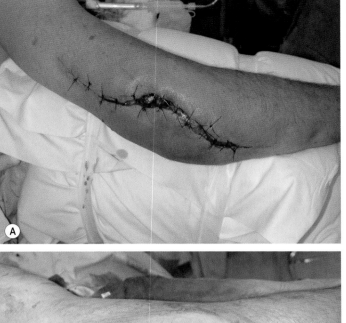

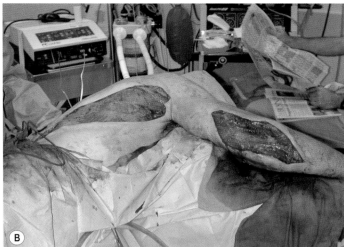

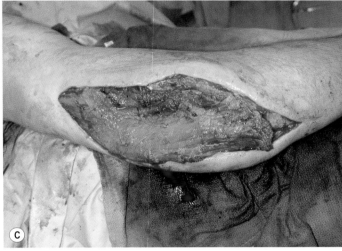

Fig. 12.30 (A) View of patient's elbow with wound breakdown after total elbow replacement for traumatic fracture/dislocation. **(B)** Patient after wound debridement, and pedicled latissimus dorsi for coverage. **(C)** Close-up of muscle in wound. Note that there is plenty of length to reach beyond the elbow proper.

muscle flap and perforator variants for breast reconstruction. This muscle is on the anterior abdominal wall and runs from the medial lower ribs to the pubis. It lies in a sheath composed anteriorly of continuations of the external and internal oblique muscle layers. The posterior sheath is a continuation of the transversus abdominis but is quite thin in the lower abdomen (below the linea semicircularis). It is a fairly large muscle and has a reliable vascular pedicle based on the deep inferior epigastric system. The pedicle is fairly long (5–7 cm) and the diameter fairly large (2.5–3 mm).

The rectus abdominis muscle will cover most defects of the hand and/or forearm,[49,50] and it will cover large defects of the forearm if most of the muscle is harvested and placed "barber pole" fashion around the arm.[51] The advantages of this muscle are that it has a reliable vascular pedicle and may be taken with the patient supine. The disadvantage of this muscle is that a hernia can result from its harvest if fascia is taken (for a myocutaneous flap) or if the anterior sheath is weak. For coverage of the upper extremity, this muscle is usually harvested without a skin paddle and covered with a split-thickness skin graft. The muscle can actually be harvested as a pedicled flap and placed on the forearm in rare situations where microsurgery might be difficult or pose other problems *(Fig. 12.31)*.

Serratus anterior

This muscle is useful for coverage of smaller hand defects.[47,52] It consists of nine slips of muscle that connect from ribs at the anterior axillary line to the tip of the scapula. The lower slips are vascularized by a branch coming off the thoracodorsal artery; the upper slips are vascularized by a branch of the lateral thoracic artery. The lower three slips may be taken individually or together as a free muscle flap based on the thoracodorsal pedicle. This dissection is tedious because branches of the long thoracic nerve may be intertwined with the vessels, and damage to the nerve supplying the remaining slips of muscle can lead to winging of the scapula.[53] The branch to the serratus is usually taken with the proximal thoracodorsal vessels, both for lengthening the pedicle and because of the larger diameter of the proximal vessel. This can give a lengthy pedicle (15–17 cm) with a large diameter (3–6 mm) *(Fig. 12.24)*.

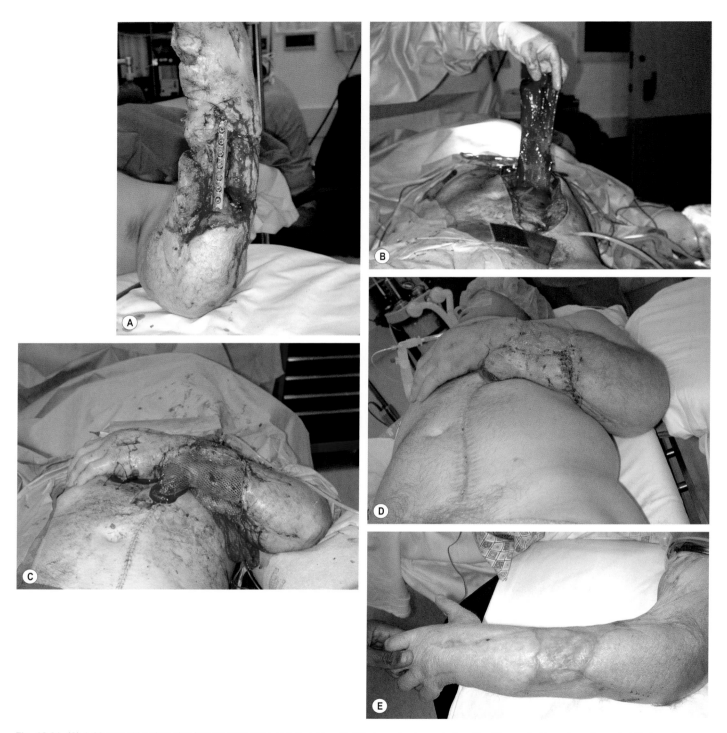

Fig. 12.31 (A) A 33-year-old patient after forearm amputation and coverage with latissimus dorsi muscle flap. Hand is supplied by vein grafts, as is latissimus flap. **(B)** View of rectus abdominis muscle being raised proximally as a pedicled flap. **(C)** Flap after insetting on arm. **(D)** Flap healed at 4 weeks. **(E)** View of flap at 3 months after division.

The primary advantage of this muscle is its small size and lengthy vascular pedicle. The disadvantages of this muscle are the potential for long thoracic nerve injury and the decubitus position necessary for harvest. This flap can be used for coverage of the dorsal or palmar hand and first webspace. It has the potential for innervation through a branch of the long thoracic nerve, but this application would be limited in the upper extremity.

Postoperative care

In the immediate postoperative period, the extremity is splinted in an appropriate position to prevent capsuloligamentous shortening and tension on repaired structures. Elevation is necessary to reduce edema and help control pain. The patient's pain and anxiety should be adequately controlled. The ambient temperature should be at least 25°C and adjusted to the patient's body temperature. Hydration should be sufficient to maintain urine output between 80 and 100 mL/h. Anticoagulant therapy is used by many surgeons. However, the authors are selective in using either heparin or dextran[54]; aspirin is used daily for 4–6 days after surgery. Appropriate antibiotic therapy is continued and later modified according to the culture results.

Flap monitoring is critical. Early recognition of arterial hypoperfusion or venous congestion will occur only in a well-monitored environment, with trained nursing staff. If there is a question about tissue viability, the dressings are released and the entirety of the revascularized tissue is exposed for further assessment of perfusion, congestion, temperature, turgor, and color and Doppler examination. Release of the dressings alone may be sufficient. If viability is still in question after 30 minutes, immediate re-exploration and further assessment may prevent failure of the revascularized tissue.

Early and motivated rehabilitation of the extremity is an important factor in achieving a successful outcome. Early motion reduces edema, adhesions, and scarring. It prevents muscle atrophy and facilitates healing of the soft tissues by remodeling of collagen fibers. The details of the rehabilitation program are determined by the existing injuries and the reconstruction procedure.

Outcomes, prognosis, and complications

Reconstruction of complex hand injuries remains a challenge. The ultimate desired outcome is "normal" function of the hand and upper limb, but this can rarely be obtained. Actual outcome studies in terms of the management of these injuries are very limited, however. Based on the few studies available, the primary determinants of the quality of eventual function are the severity of nerve injury and the need for emergency fasciotomy (which may lead to functional muscle loss).[55] Likewise, it is not surprising that outcomes have been shown to be better in younger patients, both from their ability to recover function and to adapt.[56] del Pinal has suggested that the initial goal in reconstruction of mutilating hand injuries should be the "acceptable hand," which he defines as a hand with three fingers, near-normal length, near-normal sensation, and a functional thumb.[11] This would seem to be a reasonable approach in these severe injuries; however it is not always obtainable.

There are many complications that can arise in the management of these injuries, with the early problems centering around infection. As noted above, this can be largely mitigated by early and thorough debridement, with return to the operating room frequently in the early period to reassess the wound and to perform more debridement of nonviable tissues as necessary.[57,58] Appropriate antibiotic coverage is helpful, but is not a substitute for debridement. While the principle of "early" coverage in the first days after injury was proposed by Godina and has been the gold standard for nearly 25 years,[13] recent experience with the management of war wounds in the conflicts in the Middle East has proven that wounds can be safely and properly managed in a delayed fashion. These studies have shown that early debridement, followed by wound management with negative-pressure therapy, can temporize and decrease the infection rate in heavily contaminated wounds. The results of management of patients in this fashion are equivalent to that with early coverage in most instances.[59–61] These patients also suffer from the complications (or more properly labeled "sequelae") found in any injury to the hand or upper extremity, including tendon adhesions, poor nerve recovery, and bony problems (malunion and/or nonunion). These are managed by the surgeon in standard fashion, but particular problems will be addressed below.

Free fibula transfer

Most bone defects in the upper extremity can be managed with standard bone grafts; however, long defects (>6 cm) and those associated with recurrent nonunions may be candidates for microvascular bone transfer.[62] Whereas several flaps are available that can include a portion of vascularized bone (iliac crest, scapula, lateral arm, radial forearm, dorsalis pedis), the fibula osseocutaneous flap offers the best piece of bone for reconstruction of significant defects of the long bones of the upper extremity.[63,64] Smaller defects, such as those in the hand, can be managed by one of the previously discussed flaps with inclusion of a segment of bone. Larger defects of the radius, ulna, or humerus will usually require a piece of bone such as the fibula.[65,66] (Fig. 12.32). The vascular supply of the free fibula is based on the peroneal vessels of the leg. These vessels run along the deep surface of the fibula from just below the tibioperoneal trunk to the level of the ankle. Whereas the peroneal vessels provide an endosteal nutrient artery to the medullary canal of the fibula, they also provide rich periosteal blood supply to the cortical surface. The proximal portion of the fibula can be taken for reconstruction of the radiocarpal joint, but this segment of bone gets its primary blood supply from a branch of the anterior tibial artery,[65] which must be taken to ensure viability of this segment. The proximal portion can be taken with the vascularized epiphysis in children to promote later growth,[67] and this application will be discussed further in Chapter 30.

A portion of the skin overlying the fibula can be taken with the bone, and thus compound defects can be managed with this flap. The perforators to the skin run around the posterior

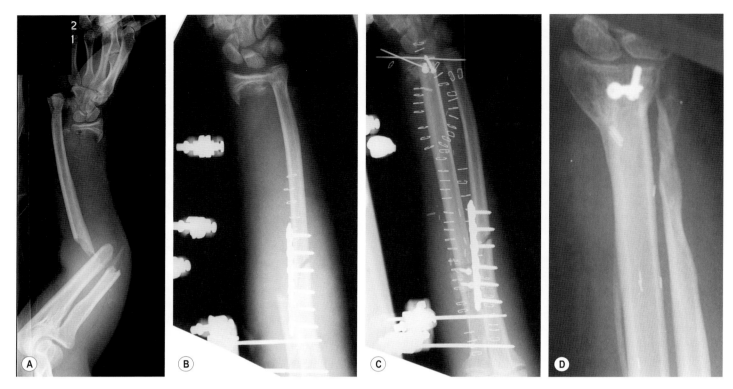

Fig. 12.32 (A) X-ray of forearm of 15-year-old male after automobile accident with loss of majority of radius through open fracture. **(B)** X-ray view of arm after external fixation to align bones. **(C)** X-ray after vascularized free fibula transfer to reconstruct defect of radius. **(D)** View of X-ray at 6 months. Note interface between fibula and distal radial remnant (patient developed osteomyelitis of distal ulna and required long-term intravenous antibiotics, but functionally had no problems from this).

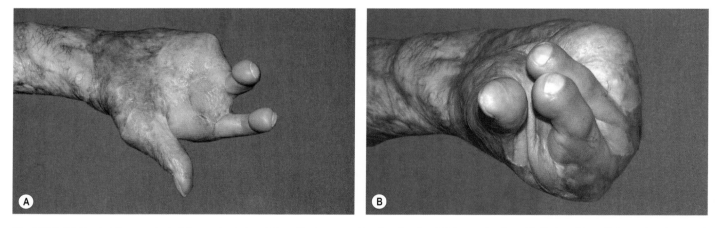

Fig. 12.33 (A) Hand of fireman who lost fingers due to burn injury after two second-toe transfers for digital reconstruction. **(B)** Flexion of toes. Note good motion at native metacarpophalangeal joints but rather poor motion of interphalangeal joints of toes.

aspect of the bone, and thus it is best to include a cuff of muscle along the posterior surface of the bone if a skin paddle is to be included. If a skin paddle is taken, most donor sites will require a skin graft on the overlying muscles. The primary advantage of this donor site is the large amount of bone that can be taken. In adults, a total of up to 24–26 cm of bone may be harvested. The fibular head should be left in place at the knee level, and 6 cm of the distal fibula should remain to avoid problems with the ankle. In children, a screw should be placed across the distal fibular–tibial joint to avoid proximal migration of the fibula. The disadvantages of this donor site are few; the pedicle is relatively short (2–4 cm) and there is

some morbidity from harvesting, but this usually does not present functional problems.

Digital reconstruction with toe transfer

Microvascular toe transfer represents one of the pinnacles of reconstructive surgery. The ability to replace in kind a missing digit with a mobile, sensate toe offers the best type of reconstruction available. Although this is a complex microsurgical procedure that should not be undertaken without experience,[68] it remains the benchmark for thumb and most digital reconstructions *(Fig. 12.33)*. There are a number of variations of toe transfer, and almost any tissue needed for digital reconstruction can be transferred. These range from pulp-only transfers to double second- and third-toe transfers to reconstruct the metacarpal hand.[69,70] All great- and second-toe transfers ideally have their vascular basis on the dorsalis pedis – first dorsal metatarsal system. This anatomy is highly variable, however, and a thorough knowledge of this is the basis for safe harvesting of these flaps. The venous drainage is based on dorsal superficial veins of the foot; the deep system that accompanies the arterial supply is usually very small.[71] The flaps can be innervated by the proper plantar digital nerves to the toe as well as by the deep peroneal nerve that accompanies the dorsalis pedis – dorsal metatarsal vessels. The details of all the complexities of digital reconstruction with toe transfer are beyond the scope of this chapter, but the reader is referred to several excellent review articles on this subject.[69–71] Toe transfer for thumb reconstruction is discussed in detail in Chapter 14.

Innervated muscle transfer

In the case of loss of functional muscle in the forearm, the options for reconstruction of this function are either tendon transfer or innervated microvascular muscle transfer. Although many losses can be adequately reconstructed with standard tendon transfers, patients with significant loss of muscle substance (such as those with Volkmann ischemic contracture) may benefit from reconstruction of function with a microvascular muscle transfer.[72] The muscles available for this include the gracilis, latissimus dorsi, and rectus femoris. The latissimus dorsi can be used in the forearm as a free functional transfer,[73] but it is not ideal. It is better suited as a replacement for elbow flexion when biceps function is lost. In this case, a pedicle transfer is perfectly adequate. The rectus femoris has been used for this in the past, but again, it is not the optimal muscle due to its short excursion. The gracilis muscle, on the other hand, is nearly ideal for reconstruction of the muscles of the forearm. It has adequate excursion to provide finger flexion or extension, it is of appropriate size (both length and width), and it has an excellent neurovascular pedicle. The reader is referred to Chapter 35 for the details of this procedure.

 Access the complete references list online at **http://www.expertconsult.com**

11. del Pinal F. Severe mutilating injuries to the hand: guidelines for organizing the chaos. *J Plast Reconstr Aesthet Surg*. 2007;60:816–827.

    This paper by a well-known European hand and microsurgeon is an excellent overview of the management of severe hand trauma from the standpoint of making the most of what is available. Professor del Pinal espouses the principle of the goal of an "acceptable" hand as an outcome in severe trauma.

13. Godina M. Early microsurgical reconstruction of complex trauma of the extremities. *Plast Reconstr Surg*. 1986;78:285–292.

    This is the classic paper by Godina on early coverage of severe trauma with free flaps, in which he proves the rationale for early coverage.

14. Gupta A, Shatford RA, Wolff TW, et al. Treatment of the severely injured upper extremity. *J Bone Joint Surg Am*. 2000;81(A):1628–1651.

    This paper from an AAOS instructional course lecture gives a very organized and well-structured overview of the subject from the orthopedic standpoint.

55. Topel I, Pfister K, Moser A, et al. Clinical outcome and quality of life after upper extremity arterial trauma. *Ann Vasc Surg*. 2009;23:317–323.

    This paper from Germany looked at 33 patients with arterial trauma with DASH scores at the time of final follow-up. Not surprisingly, they found that nerve and orthopedic trauma had more long-term impact than vascular injury (apart from those patients with muscle damage from ischemia.)

59. Kumar AR, Grewal NS, Chung TL, et al. Lessons from the modern battlefield: successful upper extremity injury reconstruction in the subacute period. *J Trauma*. 2009;67:752–757.

    This recent paper dealing with injuries in US soldiers from the Middle East wars notes that successful flap reconstruction can be performed in a delayed fashion (contradicting the long-held notions of Godina). Average time to flap reconstruction was 31 days, with a 4% flap loss rate and 8% infection rate, which are both very acceptable.

13

Thumb reconstruction: Nonmicrosurgical techniques

Nicholas B. Vedder and Jeffrey B. Friedrich

SYNOPSIS

- Thumb reconstruction should aim to restore the cardinal thumb actions: mobility, stability, sensibility, length, and appearance.
- Level of thumb loss is divided into thirds: distal (tip to interphalangeal joint), middle (interphalangeal joint to metacarpal neck), and proximal (metacarpal neck to carpometacarpal joint).
- Distal third reconstruction typically requires only soft-tissue restoration.
- Numerous options exist for middle-third reconstruction, including increasing thumb ray length (metacarpal lengthening, osteoplastic reconstruction) and increasing relative length (phalangization).
- Proximal third reconstruction is best accomplished with pollicization or on-top plasty (pollicization of a damaged index finger). However, microsurgical reconstruction (discussed in another chapter) is preferred at this level.

 Access the Historical Perspective section online at
http://www.expertconsult.com

Introduction

- When thumb loss occurs due to trauma, replantation is the best method of reconstruction for many patients. When replantation is not possible, thumb reconstruction is warranted.
- The level of thumb amputation guides the type of reconstruction. Determination of level of loss is based on physical examination and radiographs.
- Any thumb reconstruction method requires input and acceptance by the patient. The reconstruction should be tailored to the patient's personal and professional needs. Because significant rehabilitation may be required, the patient must be a willing participant in both the reconstruction and rehabilitation.
- Functional compensation following distal-third thumb loss is easily achieved, therefore, reconstruction at this

level is chiefly soft tissue alone. Techniques such as the neurovascular advancement (Moberg) flap and the cross-finger flap remain reliable methods for reconstruction at this level.
- For losses in the middle third of the thumb, restoration of length is a priority. This can be done via absolute length restoration with metacarpal lengthening or osteoplastic reconstruction, or via relative length restoration using phalangization of the thumb.
- Proximal third thumb losses are best treated with microsurgical reconstruction. However, in some cases this may not be possible. In these situations, transfer of another finger can provide an excellent thumb replacement. A normal finger (typically the index) can be pollicized to become a thumb. A damaged index finger can also be transferred (on-top plasty) to become a stable post for opposition, pinch, and grip.
- Hand rehabilitation after reconstruction is absolutely necessary, especially following middle- and proximal-third reconstructions. Rehabilitation can last months, but allows the patient to regain motion and strength. For some procedures, such as neurovascular island flaps and digit transfer, sensory re-education is an important part of the rehabilitation.
- This chapter will provide a comprehensive description of nonmicrosurgical thumb reconstruction, including reconstruction decision-making, technical approaches, and postreconstruction management.

Basic science/disease process

By far, the most common "disease process" necessitating thumb reconstruction is traumatic injury. The majority of these patients are working-age males. Within the larger trauma classification, thumb injury can be the result of a variety of different mechanisms. These include sharp cut, avulsion, and crush. There are some mechanisms that have characteristics of more than one injury type. This phenomenon is best illustrated by saw and lawnmower injuries, which have both cutting and crushing components, resulting in a larger zone of injury.

Other insults that can result in thumb loss requiring reconstruction are infections and neoplasms. Because tumors are less acute than trauma or infections, thumb reconstruction planning can be more deliberate, and can even be performed at the time of tumor extirpation.[10]

Diagnosis/patient presentation

The diagnosis of thumb trauma is relatively straightforward, as there will be, in most cases, open wounds. It is important to obtain history regarding the mechanism and other details of the traumatic insult, time from injury to presentation, handedness, occupation, pertinent social issues such as tobacco use, and pertinent medical problems (including problems that can compromise peripheral circulation and/or wound healing). If feasible, replantation of the amputated thumb will generally yield a thumb that is superior in appearance and function to any other type of thumb reconstruction. However, this is sometimes not possible, in which case, other reconstruction methods are employed.

Evaluation of the traumatically injured thumb requires complete evaluation of all tissues of the thumb including integumentary, neural, vascular, and musculoskeletal. The wound(s) on the thumb should be carefully inspected. The integrity of the sensory nerves supplying the thumb is assessed. Assessing any compromise in the circulation to the thumb is crucial, as is assessing the feasibility of arterial and venous reconstruction. Finally, assessment of the integrity of the thumb tendons and skeletal structures is performed. Radiographs are a necessity in evaluating thumb skeletal structure.

Evaluation of the thumb following infection is similar to that following trauma. All tissues must be assessed, making particular note of the cutaneous defect requiring reconstruction.

Evaluation of a thumb affected by a tumor will be guided by the tumor itself. Specifically, tumor type and grade will determine the extent of extirpation that will need to be determined prior to reconstruction. This will also determine which procedures will be needed either intraoperatively (sentinel lymph node biopsy, lymphadenectomy) or perioperatively (radiation, chemotherapy).

Patient selection

Because there are many ways to reconstruct a deficient thumb, patients must be educated about the various options so that they may make an informed decision as to which type of reconstruction will serve them best in both the personal and professional settings.

Many thumb injuries occur in the workplace, and these patients will be affected by the injury because their work involves significant hand use. In these patients especially, it is essential to work toward a thumb that has adequate length

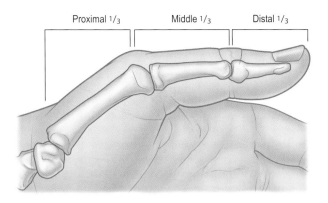

Fig. 13.1 Thumb loss classification, divided into thirds. Distal third is from thumb tip to interphalangeal joint. Middle third is interphalangeal joint to metacarpal neck. Proximal third is metacarpal neck to carpometacarpal joint.

for both gripping and pinching, is stable during activities, has reasonable motion, and, importantly, is sensate in order to give tactile feedback during these actions and to prevent recurrent ulceration or injury. That said, adequate length, stability, motion, and sensibility are the end-goals for any patient requiring thumb reconstruction, regardless of profession or vocation.[11]

In addition to patient input regarding reconstructive methods, the patient must also commit to the reconstructive process. Most of the reconstructive options will result in edema, stiffness, and pain in the near term; therefore, adherence to a supervised hand therapy program is critical to reconstruction success.

As with any type of reconstructive surgery, medical optimization prior to procedure(s) allows superior outcomes. This includes, but is not limited to, tobacco cessation, cardiopulmonary stabilization, and good diabetes control. If the thumb is being reconstructed following cancer extirpation, the physician must ensure adequate local disease control prior to reconstruction, and coordination of the patient's reconstruction with any systemic adjuvant therapies that will be required. Similarly, in patients for whom a thumb is deficient due to infection, infection control prior to reconstruction is paramount.

The most important factor in patient selection is the amount and nature of tissue loss that must be reconstructed. The level of amputation is the easiest way to classify thumb deficiencies, and is listed in thirds[12] (**Fig. 13.1**). The distal third extends from the interphalangeal joint to the thumb tip. The middle third is the portion between interphalangeal joint and the metacarpal neck, and the proximal third is from metacarpal neck to the carpometacarpal joint. Each amputation level presents unique challenges for patient and physician, and each level can be reconstructed with multiple modalities.

Treatment/surgical technique

Distal third

Thumb distal-third amputations rarely, if ever, require restoration of length, as a thumb amputated through the interphalangeal joint remains very functional.[12] Therefore, the chief goals of thumb tip reconstruction are soft-tissue coverage of bone and length preservation. When there is no bone exposed at the tip of the thumb, closure can be achieved with either healing by secondary intention or skin grafting. Secondary healing of tip amputations has been shown to result in a stable scar and good two-point discrimination, and is therefore a relatively easy (and usually the preferred) method of achieving coverage.[13] Secondary healing by wound contracture has the advantage of bringing stable, sensate skin together to close the defect, as opposed to skin grafts, which remain insensate. Defects up to 1.5 cm in diameter with no bone exposure can be effectively treated with dressing changes. Daily dressing changes with petroleum or bismuth-impregnated gauze are relatively easy for patients. Larger defects with a stable base, however, require skin grafting. Full-thickness grafts are usually preferred, as they are more durable and stable, especially in the contact areas subject to pressure and shear. Small full- or split-thickness skin grafts can be harvested from the hypothenar eminence or the volar wrist crease. Larger skin grafts, however, are best harvested from the groin crease.

When phalangeal bone is exposed at the thumb tip, vascularized coverage is required to preserve length, and there are several flaps that can accomplish these goals. The main criteria for flap selection are defect size and location of soft-tissue loss, specifically if it is volar, dorsal, or at the tip. The V-Y advancement flap described by Atasoy *et al.* provides good coverage of the tip of the distal phalanx when only a very small amount of bone is exposed[14] (*Fig. 13.2*). The technique involves incising the volar pulp of the thumb in a V shape. Scissors are then used to spread the subcutaneous tissue carefully. The subcutaneous attachments deep to the flap, which provide the neurovascular supply to the flap, are left intact. The flap is then advanced distally to close the defect and the proximal aspect of the V is closed side to side, thereby creating the Y shape of the final scar. In practice, there is limited application for this flap due to the limited advancement that is possible without devascularizing the flap.

The neurovascular volar advancement flap, which goes by the eponym of the Moberg flap, is well suited to cover volar and tip defects of the thumb.[11] It is often described as an advancement flap, but in reality, the amount of advancement achieved with the conventional rectangular Moberg flap is limited. Instead, the elevation of the flap allows flexion of the

interphalangeal joint of the thumb, thereby allowing the flap to appear to "advance" distally (*Fig. 13.3*). To elevate the flap, one incises the mid-lateral lines on either side of the thumb, down to the base of the proximal phalanx. The flap is then elevated from the deeper tissues, directly off the flexor retinaculum, with sharp dissection. The flap includes both neurovascular bundles and all of the subcutaneous tissue down to the flexor tendon sheath. The interphalangeal joint is flexed, and the flap is inset at the tip. If necessary, a Kirschner wire can be placed across the interphalangeal joint to stabilize it, though this is seldom required. This flap can easily cover a defect of 1–2 cm^2 (*Fig. 13.4*). A variation of the Moberg flap is an island flap in which flap is incised transversely across the proximal base, and the only remaining attachments are the two neurovascular bundles. Unlike the conventional Moberg flap, this method will allow a small amount of actual advancement, thereby covering more distal defects. The proximal gap at the base of the flap will then require a small skin graft.

The cross-finger flap from the index finger is an excellent reconstructive technique for larger volar and tip defects of the thumb, up to 2–3 cm^2.[15] The tissue transferred is reliable and durable.[16] The chief disadvantages to this technique are thumb coaptation to the index finger for 2–3 weeks, and the need for a skin graft on the index donor site. A radially based rectangular flap is marked on the dorsum of the index proximal phalanx that extends from the ulnar to the radial mid-lateral lines (*Fig. 13.5*). The flap is incised and elevated from ulnar to radial in the plane between the subcutaneous tissues and the extensor mechanism. It is critically important to leave the paratenon on the extensor to allow skin grafting. Upon reaching the radial aspect of the flap, one must release Cleland's ligaments along the length of the base of the flap to prevent kinking at the flap "hinge." The flap is then sutured to the thumb – this may require some trial and error to find the best flap orientation (*Fig. 13.6*). A full-thickness skin graft is then sutured to the dorsum of the index finger. A bulky thumb

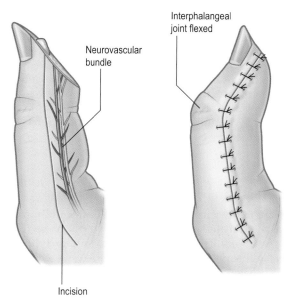

Neurovascular bundle

Interphalangeal joint flexed

Incision

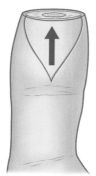 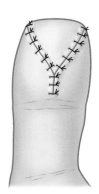

Fig. 13.2 Thumb tip closure via volar V-Y advancement flap. The flap is perfused by small vessels traversing the subcutaneous tissues immediately deep to the flap.

Fig. 13.3 Moberg thumb volar advancement flap. It is a sensate flap by virtue of the digital nerves remaining in the flap, and is perfused by the digital vessels.

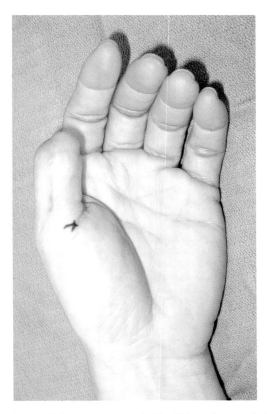

Fig. 13.4 Thumb reconstructed with a Moberg flap for a distal amputation. Note the flexed posture of the interphalangeal joint.

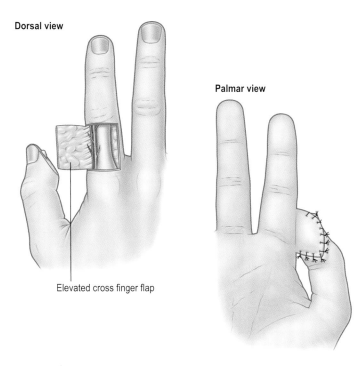

Dorsal view

Palmar view

Elevated cross finger flap

Fig. 13.5 Diagrammatic representation of the cross-finger flap to the thumb. The flap is elevated from the dorsum of the index finger proximal phalanx and inset to the thumb volar defect. Once elevated, Cleland's ligament of the index radial neurovascular bundle can restrain and kink the flap, therefore release of this ligament allows greater flap freedom.

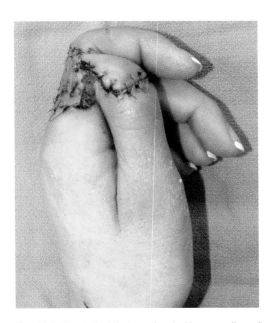

Fig. 13.6 Thumb tip defect resurfaced with a cross-finger flap from the index finger.

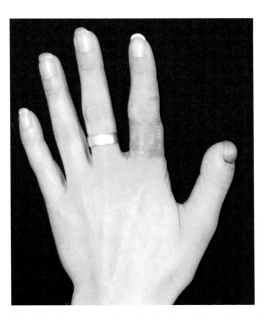

Fig. 13.7 Reconstructed thumb following division of the cross-finger flap seen in *Figure 13.6*.

splint is applied. At 2 or 3 weeks, the flap is divided and the inset to the thumb is completed *(Fig. 13.7)*. After division, aggressive range-of-motion therapy for both the thumb and index finger should begin.

The neurovascular island flap attributed to Littler is a valuable tool in thumb reconstruction.[17] It is rarely used as a primary coverage flap, although it is certainly possible to use it in that manner. Rather, its most common use is for the restoration of sensation to the thumb pulp following reconstruction.[17,18] The flap is based on the ulnar neurovascular bundle of either the middle or ring finger *(Fig. 13.8)*. The ulnar side of the digit is chosen because its loss will have

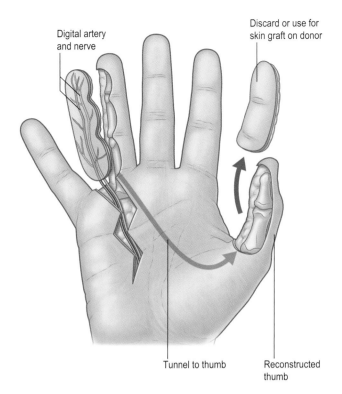

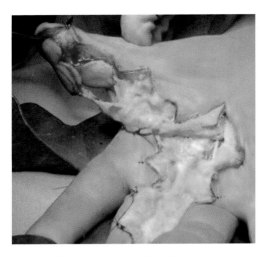

Fig. 13.9 Neurovascular island flap following dissection.

Fig. 13.8 Depiction of neurovascular island flap taken from ulnar side of ring finger. The flap will then be tunneled through the palm to the thumb to provide sensate reconstruction of volar thumb.

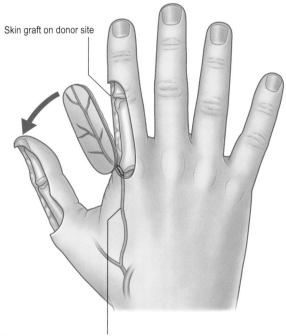

Fig. 13.10 Diagram of dorsal metacarpal artery flap ("kite flap") from index-finger dorsum. It is important to include subcutaneous fat and interosseous muscle fascia with the pedicle.

minimal effect on grip and pinch activities. The dimensions of the flap needed are marked on the ulnar pulp of the chosen donor finger. Often, the flap will require harvesting of skin over the distal and middle phalanges of the donor finger. The flap is incised, and a mid-lateral incision proceeding from the proximal aspect of the flap is made. The flap is elevated from distal to proximal, and the entire ulnar neurovascular bundle is elevated in continuity with the flap. It is critical to raise the neurovascular bundle with a fairly thick cuff of surrounding fatty tissue containing the vasa vasorum of the artery, as that is the only source of venous outflow for the flap. Failure to do this will result in flap congestion. One must dissect fairly proximally in the palm to allow adequate transposition to the thumb, and the other branch of the common digital artery (i.e., the radial digital artery to the ring or small finger) must be divided. The common digital nerve can be split along the fascicles to allow adequate flap mobility. The flap can then be transposed to the thumb either via subcutaneous tunnel, or a connecting incision from the donor site to the thumb can be made *(Fig. 13.9)*. The flap is then inset into the volar defect of the thumb. The donor site is grafted with full-thickness skin. In addition to postoperative restoration of motion, patients must work with a hand therapist on sensory re-education of the thumb.

The proximally based first dorsal metacarpal artery (FDMA) flap is an excellent tool to achieve thumb coverage, although it is better suited for dorsal thumb defects than palmar defects.[19,20] Its harvest causes virtually no donor site functional loss. The FDMA is found using a conventional Doppler

device, beginning proximally with the radial artery at the anatomic snuffbox. The radial artery then branches into the princeps pollicis artery radially and the FDMA ulnarly. At approximately the metacarpal head level, the artery then becomes difficult to trace further distal. The flap is then centered over the FDMA *(Fig. 13.10)*. The flap is incised and dissected from distal to proximal, leaving paratenon over the extensor mechanism for later skin grafting. To ensure inclusion of the FDMA with the flap, it is reasonable to incise the thin fascia over the first dorsal interosseous muscle and include it with the flap. Once the flap is elevated and the

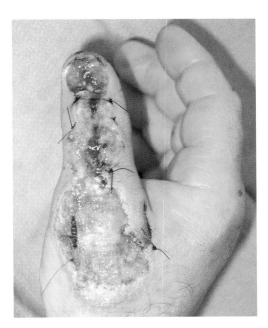

Fig. 13.11 Dorsal-thumb defect following avulsion injury. The extensor pollicis longus tendon was exposed and required reinsertion into the distal phalanx with a suture anchor.

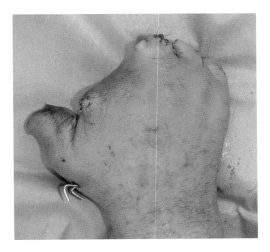

Fig. 13.13 Severe wood chipper injury that later resulted in a first webspace contracture that prevented radial and palmar thumb abduction.

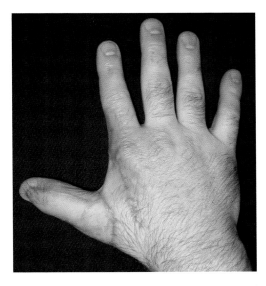

Fig. 13.12 Dorsal-thumb defect from *Figure 13.11* resurfaced with a dorsal metacarpal artery flap. Note the ability of the flap to reach the thumb tip.

BOX 13.1 Clinical pearl: distal-third reconstruction

Loss of the distal third of the thumb is minimal in terms of functional loss.[12] Therefore, the chief priority is soft-tissue coverage. The choice of soft-tissue reconstruction is determined by the location of loss. Volar defects can be reconstructed with secondary healing (wound contraction), full-thickness skin grafts, Moberg flaps, cross-finger flaps, and neurovascular island flaps, while dorsal defects may be dealt with using skin grafts or first dorsal metacarpal artery flaps.

---

proximal vascular leash fully mobilized, it can then be tunneled to the thumb in the subcutaneous plane, or a connecting incision can be made *(Figs 13.11 and 13.12)*. The donor defect is then closed with a skin graft. It is critical to raise the vascular pedicle of the FDMA flap with a fairly thick pedicle of surrounding fatty tissue containing the venae comitantes of the artery, as that is the only source of venous outflow for the flap *(Box 13.1)*.

Middle third

Loss in the middle third of the thumb is more functionally limiting than that of the distal third. Therefore, the priorities are both soft-tissue coverage and functional restoration. Commonly, the soft-tissue coverage of amputations at this level will have been achieved acutely by revision amputation in which the skeletal components are shortened to allow primary closure. Reconstruction then occurs weeks or months after the initial insult.

Phalangization is a set of reconstruction techniques that increases the effective, rather than the absolute, length of the thumb. The chief component of phalangization is first webspace deepening.[12] The webspace can be injured or not injured during the initial injury to the thumb. Webspace deepening allows better thumb excursion, specifically both palmar and radial abduction, thereby improving the thumb's oppositional function. First webspaces with mild or moderate tightness can be deepened with skin grafts or local tissue rearrangement (commonly Z-plasties). The main assessment of the webspace is whether the contracture is broad or is a discrete linear band. If it is broad, then scar contracture incision, followed by skin grafting, is warranted, whereas if the contracture is linear, Z-plasties are the preferred treatment. Full-thickness skin grafts are usually used for the first web, although a thick split-thickness skin graft can be used *(Figs 13.13 and 13.14)*. A single Z-plasty can be used for a linear scar band, although two combined Z-plasties are uniquely suited to this anatomic area. The four-flap Z-plasty (which is essentially two superimposed Z-plasties) *(Fig. 13.15)* and the double-opposing Z-plasty ("jumping man" flap) *(Fig. 13.16)* have been commonly used for the first web. In both cases, the scar band itself is the middle limb of both z's, and the triangular flaps then are mobilized from the dorsal and volar sides of the scar contracture. When using either skin graft or Z-plasty for the first webspace, the adductor muscle is often tight due to scarring. A portion of it can be released to allow further thumb abduction prior to skin closure.

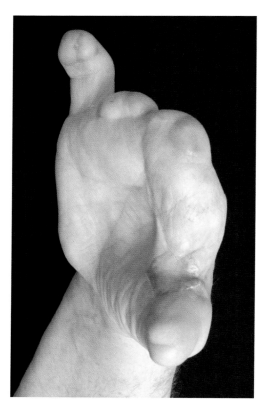

Fig. 13.14 First webspace from *Figure 13.13* that has been deepened with a full-thickness skin graft. Note improved thumb abduction.

More significant first webspace contractures can require transposition of vascularized tissue into the space, rather than the less-complex local tissue rearrangement. The dorsal hand flap can accomplish this task in a straightforward fashion. This flap is proximally based on the dorsum of the hand and is vascularized by the metacarpal artery system *(Fig. 13.17)*. Unlike the FDMA flap, it is not an island flap, and can include more than one metacarpal artery. The flap's distal extent is at the level of the metacarpal heads and is elevated in the plane between subcutaneous tissue and extensor tendon paratenon. The flap is then transposed radially into the first webspace, following release of all constraining structures in the space. The donor site is then skin-grafted.

If the dorsal hand skin has been injured, or if a larger amount of vascularized tissue is required to resurface both the first web and the thumb itself, then regional flaps will be necessary. The radial forearm flap and the posterior interosseous artery flap are good choices. The utility of the radial forearm flap has been repeatedly demonstrated in a variety of hand reconstruction settings, including the thumb. The major drawback to use of a reverse-flow radial forearm flap is that its use may compromise future thumb reconstruction. Specifically, if a microvascular toe transfer is being considered for thumb reconstruction, the radial artery is the preferred recipient vessel, and the transposition of a pedicled radial forearm flap will make that later microvascular transfer difficult, if not impossible. It is, however, possible to harvest a radial artery perforator flap, leaving the radial artery intact.[21,22]

The radial forearm flap is extremity versatile, and can be harvested as a fascia-alone flap, fasciocutaneous flap, or a suprafascial skin flap. For thumb reconstruction, the use of the fascia-alone flap with skin grafts applied directly to the flap allows maintenance of the normal contour of the thumb[23] *(Figs 13.18 and 13.19)*. An Allen's test is always performed to ensure the digits will remain perfused by the ulnar artery. The pivot point of the flap pedicle is approximately at the radial styloid, although it can be more proximal than this. The flap

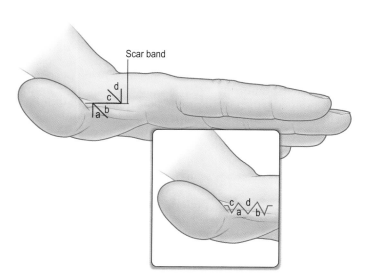

Fig. 13.15 Depiction of four-flap Z-plasty used for deepening of the first webspace and/or releasing a first webspace contracture.

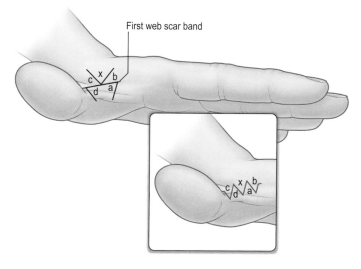

Fig. 13.16 Diagram of the double-opposing Z-plasty (known as the "jumping man" flap). This Z-plasty and the four-flap Z-plasty provide similar substantial amounts of first webspace release.

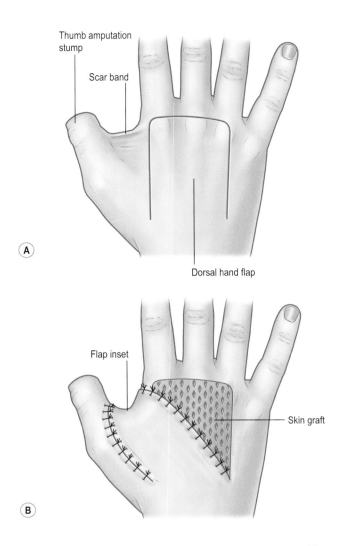

Fig. 13.17 **(A, B)** Diagram of the dorsal hand flap. This flap can provide a substantial amount of coverage for first webspace deepening.

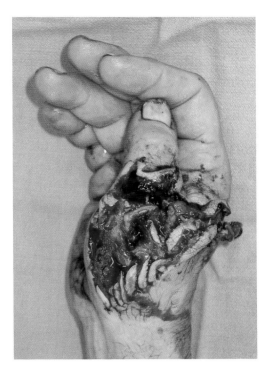

Fig. 13.18 Severe dorsal thumb injury from a router. The fractures were stabilized, and the extensor pollicis longus tendon was reconstructed with a transferred extensor indicis proprius tendon.

should then be drawn on the forearm such that the pivot point is midway between the distal end of the thumb or first web defect and the proximal end of the radial forearm flap. The flap is elevated on the radial and ulnar sides. Upon reaching the ulnar edge of the brachioradialis muscle on the radial side of the flap, and the radial edge of the flexor carpi radialis tendon on the ulnar side of the flap, dissection then proceeds directly down toward the radius. The dissection then proceeds under the deep aspect of the radial vascular bundle. Prior to dividing the proximal end of the radial artery, a microvascular clamp can be placed on the artery just proximal to the flap, and the tourniquet released. After several seconds, if both the flap and all the digits are well perfused, the proximal radial artery can then be divided. The flap is then transposed distally to the first webspace and/or thumb. Depending on the type of flap used, the donor site is primarily closed (fascia-alone flap) or skin-grafted (fasciocutaneous or suprafascial). Because venous outflow from the reverse radial artery flap is retrograde through the venae comitantes against the venous valves, venous congestion can occur. It is imperative to include the venae comitantes and surrounding fatty tissue

with the arterial pedicle when raising the flap. Performing an antegrade venous microvascular anastomosis to a vein in the hand can reduce venous congestion and flap swelling.

The vascular supply to the posterior interosseous artery flap is both an advantage and a disadvantage: the flap is perfused by reverse flow-through in the posterior interosseous artery via anastomotic connections with the anterior interosseous artery just proximal to the distal radioulnar joint.[24] This allows preservation of the radial and ulnar arteries to the hand, but the vascular supply can be compromised if the zone of injury is anywhere near the wrist. The posterior interosseous artery is found with a Doppler and the flap centered over it. The vessel is along a line drawn between the lateral epicondyle of the elbow and the ulnar head. The pedicle of the flap runs in the diminutive septum between the extensor carpi ulnaris and extensor digiti minimi (quinti) tendons. Dissection is performed from distal to proximal so as first to locate the anastomotic connection with the anterior interosseous artery and then include the posterior interosseous artery with the flap as one dissects proximally. Once fully dissected, the flap is transposed to the first webspace, and the donor site is skin-grafted. Another disadvantage of the flap is the appearance of the donor site, which is on the easily visible dorsal forearm.

Metacarpal lengthening allows increase in the absolute length of the thumb ray. This is usually performed for more proximal losses in the middle third of the thumb, and was popularized by Matev.[8,9] Matev reported that the only absolute contraindication to the procedure is less than 3 cm of remaining thumb metacarpal.[25] One should note that this reconstruction technique requires a long period of time with external fixation, and multiple outpatient visits, therefore

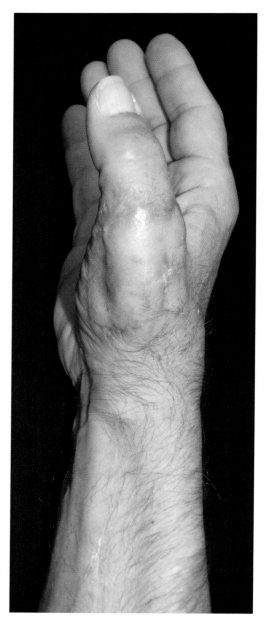

Fig. 13.19 Thumb from *Figure 13.18* satisfactorily reconstructed with a pedicled radial forearm fascia flap. The flap was skin-grafted and the donor site closed primarily as no skin was harvested from the forearm.

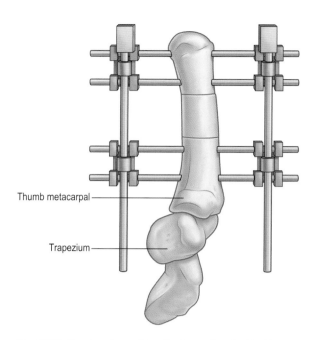

Fig. 13.20 Thumb metacarpal lengthening as described by Matev.

patient acceptance of the technique should be established prior to reconstruction. The pins for the distraction device are placed distally and proximally prior to osteotomy *(Fig. 13.20)*. Through a dorsal incision over the metacarpal, the distraction device is applied first, and the bone is then cut at the diaphysis and the skin closed. Distraction is initiated at 1 mm/day until the desired length is achieved. While some patients, especially children, will spontaneously ossify the bony gap of the metacarpal, most patients will require bone grafting at a second surgery. This bone can be harvested from the iliac crest, or with small defects, from the distal radius. While the bone graft is consolidating, the original frame may be left in place, or one may change to internal fixation. In Matev's experience, a number of patients had first-webspace creep due to the

distraction drawing the first web skin distally.[25] If this occurs, one of the first web-deepening techniques described previously may be used.

Osteoplastic thumb reconstruction allows restoration of good thumb length, and, when combined with a neurovascular island flap, can result in fairly good thumb pulp sensation. While not absolute prerequisites, the osteoplastic thumb reconstruction method works best when there is intact and functioning thenar musculature and a working thumb carpometacarpal joint. It is generally accepted that osteoplastic thumb reconstruction is performed in three stages: (1) skeletal reconstruction with iliac crest bone graft wrapped with a flap (typically a groin flap); (2) groin flap division and serial thinning; and (3) pulp reconstruction with a neurovascular island flap.

The groin flap is a versatile and reliable flap.[26] It is an axial flap, perfused by the superficial circumflex iliac artery, which runs parallel to and 2 cm below the inguinal ligament. The flap is centered over this line. It is incised and elevated from lateral to medial just superficial to the muscle fascia. Upon reaching the lateral border of the sartorius, the sartorius muscle fascia is incised and elevated with the flap to prevent kinking of the pedicle. Typically, dissection to the medial border of the sartorius is sufficient length for a thumb groin flap. The proximal end of the flap is tubed upon itself. At this point, an iliac crest tricortical bone graft may be harvested from the lateral aspect of the groin flap incision. An oscillating saw allows rapid and neat harvest of the bone graft. The bone graft is then fixed to the distal end of the thumb stump (either proximal phalanx base or distal metacarpal). Fixation can be provided in a variety of ways; however, plate and screw fixation allows early motion *(Fig. 13.21)*. Following bone graft fixation, the groin flap is then wrapped around the graft and inset to the thumb. The groin flap is usually divided 2–3 weeks after inset. Several stages of flap thinning are usually required *(Fig. 13.22)*. At approximately 3–6 months after

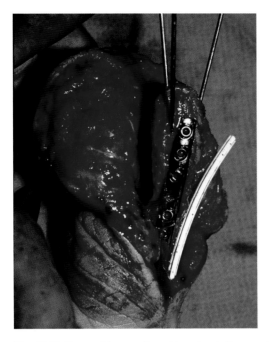

Fig. 13.21 Iliac crest bone graft used for osteoplastic reconstruction of a thumb. The fixation of the bone graft is in progress, and will be covered by a groin flap.

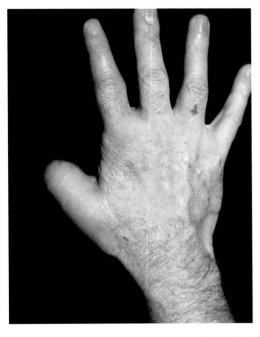

Fig. 13.22 Osteoplastic reconstruction from *Figure 13.21* following thinning of the groin flap.

skeletal and soft-tissue reconstruction, sensibility is supplied by transfer of the neurovascular island flap. The chief disadvantages of the osteoplastic reconstruction technique for the thumb are possible bone graft resorption, the multiple stages required, and the bulky appearance of the reconstructed thumb.

Quite often, thumb amputations do not happen in isolation – there is often damage to other finger(s), especially the index finger. In the ultimate example of "spare-parts" surgery, the

---

BOX 13.2 Clinical pearl: middle-third reconstruction

For thumb losses in the middle third, length restoration becomes a primary goal. This is done by extending either the absolute length or the relative length of the thumb:

1. Relative length ("phalangization"): restoring or deepening the first webspace. This may be accomplished as follows:
   (a) Small webspace deepening: either skin grafting or Z-plasties. If the patient has a linear scar band, Z-plasties; skin grafting is required for broader scar contractures
   (b) Large webspace deepening: vascularized tissue imported from another location, achieved by the dorsal hand flap, radial forearm flap, or posterior interosseous artery flap
2. Absolute length: several techniques can increase absolute length of the thumb:
   (a) Metacarpal lengthening
   (b) Osteoplastic reconstruction: bone graft wrapped with a flap, most commonly the groin flap
   (c) On-top plasty: transposition of a damaged index finger on to the remaining thumb ray

---

damaged/amputated index finger stump can be transferred on to the thumb amputation stump. This is an excellent reconstructive option for patients with a middle-third amputation of the thumb, especially at the proximal end of that zone.[12,27] The index transfer procedure has been variably referred to as "pollicization" and "on-top plasty." On-top plasty is probably more accurate as pollicization is most often used to denote transfer of a normally functioning index to the thumb. On-top plasty does not necessarily need to be accomplished with the index stump – the middle- or ring-finger stump may instead be used.

On-top plasty may be accomplished with a variety of skin incisions; however "racket"-type incisions at the base of the index and the end of the thumb stump are usually made. Perhaps the most important part of the surgery is the dissection of the dorsal veins. At least one vein must be preserved, but when possible, it is recommended that the majority of the dorsal vein arcade be taken with the digit. Volarly, both neurovascular bundles to the index are carefully dissected. Either before or after index dissection, the thumb is prepared for receipt of the transferred digit. This consists of soft-tissue elevation and metacarpal exposure for bone fixation. Internal fixation is preferred because it does not need to be removed, and early motion can be performed. At this time, a microvascular clamp is placed on the ulnar digital artery to the index, and the tourniquet released. If the index stump is perfused, then the ulnar digital artery is divided. Alternatively, the radial digital artery to the middle finger can be divided, and the common digital artery taken with the index. The ulnar digital nerve will need to be separated from the common digital nerve to allow transposition. As this is a damaged index stump, the flexor and extensor mechanisms are not usually transferred (in contrast to pollicization), and can be divided. The second metacarpal is cut at the appropriate length for the thumb reconstruction. The remainder of the second metacarpal (down to proximal metaphyseal flare) is removed to allow a full first-webspace. Fixation of the index metacarpal neck to the thumb metacarpal shaft or base is then performed. In order to gain webspace closure and ensure an adequately deep webspace, a dorsal hand flap may need to be transferred to the webspace (*Box 13.2*).

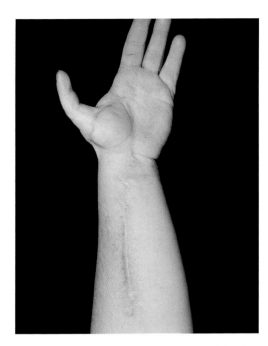

Fig. 13.23 Completed index-finger pollicization following traumatic thumb loss at the base of the thumb ray.

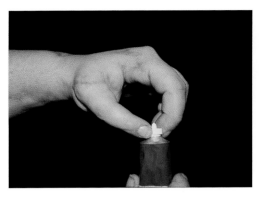

Fig. 13.24 Pollicization from **Figure 13.23** demonstrating good opposition of the pollicized finger and good tip pinch.

Proximal third

Loss of the thumb at the level of the proximal third is a challenge for reconstruction, as this is essentially total thumb loss. While the divisions between middle-third and proximal-third loss are somewhat arbitrary, one chief difference is that loss at the proximal third can include loss of some or the entire cuff of thenar musculature. This muscle loss then precludes use of previously mentioned techniques such as osteoplastic reconstruction, distraction osteogenesis, and perhaps on-top plasty. Because of the paucity of local reconstruction options, microvascular techniques play a primary role in thumb reconstruction at this level. This primarily is performed with various types of toe transfer, and these techniques are detailed in a separate chapter.

There are some instances of proximal-third loss in which on-top plasty may be appropriate. As stated, if some or all of the thenar musculature is missing, mobility of the transferred index will be limited, and may need to be augmented by an opposition transfer at a later time. In the adult, this opposition transfer can be accomplished with either the ring-finger flexor digitorum superficialis tendon, or the extensor indicis proprius tendon. The technique of on-top plasty is performed the same way as discussed in the section on middle-third loss.

Short of microvascular techniques, index-finger pollicization is the only other viable technique for proximal-third thumb reconstruction *(Figs 13.23 and 13.24)*. The procedure's utility in children with thumb hypoplasia or aplasia is undisputed. Its use in adults is also fairly reliable, although it may be more difficult for adults than children to adapt to the new finger position. In Brunelli and Brunelli's description of pollicization in adults, this group highlights one of the chief differences in pollicization between children and adults: in children, the thenar musculature and the adductor pollicis are

entirely missing, whereas in adults, there may be at least a remnant.[28] This then slightly changes what is done with the index palmar interosseous (becomes the adductor pollicis) and the dorsal interosseous (becomes the thenar muscles). In children, these muscles are transferred with the index, whereas in adults, the muscles themselves are eliminated and their tendons sutured to the thenar and adductor remnants.

A variety of skin incision patterns can be used. Once the skin is incised, the dorsal veins are carefully dissected. Vein preservation is critically important, and is often the most tedious portion of the pollicization surgery. Next, the neurovascular bundles to the index are dissected. The palmar and dorsal interosseous tendons are divided from the muscles. The flexor and extensor tendons are dissected after opening the first and second annular pulleys. The thumb is then prepared by dissection of the soft tissue and exposure of the metacarpal remnant. The thenar and adductor pollicis muscles or their remnants are also prepared. At this point, the tourniquet is released. There are two possibilities for the ulnar digital artery of the index finger: it can be divided if the radial digital artery adequately perfuses the finger, or the radial digital artery to the middle finger can be divided and the common digital artery to the second webspace can be taken with the index finger. The second metacarpal is then cut at the neck. The remainder of the second metacarpal down to the metaphyseal flare is removed to open the new webspace. The index is transferred and rotated.

In general, the pulp of the new thumb should be facing the ring finger when bony fixation is completed *(Fig. 13.25)*. The tendon of the first dorsal interosseous muscle is sutured to the thenar muscle remnant (opponens pollicis if possible) and the tendon of the palmar interosseous muscle is sutured to the adductor pollicis muscle or its remnant. Some authors recommend no shortening of the extrinsic extensor and flexor tendons is done, whereas others advocate tendon plication.[12,28] The metacarpophalangeal joint is pinned for 6 weeks in slight flexion to counteract the tendency of the index metacarpophalangeal joint to hyperextend. The skin is then closed. If any of the skin closure appears tight, one should have a low threshold for placement of skin grafts to complete the closure. As with on-top plasty, the thenar musculature may be later found to be inadequate for functional opposition, and in these cases, opposition transfer (ring-finger flexor digitorum

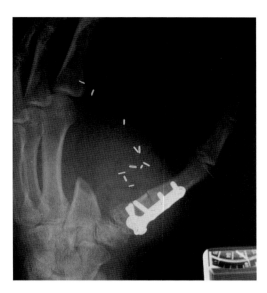

Fig. 13.25 Pollicization from *Figures 13.23* and *13.24* demonstrating fixation of the index metacarpal to the thumb metacarpal remnant.

---

superficialis or extensor indicis proprius) can be performed at a later time *(Box 13.3)*.

Prosthetics

Prosthetics for thumb loss are a viable option for patients who do not wish to undergo reconstruction. In general, prosthetics are aesthetic in nature, which is to say they have minimal or no function. Pillet has the largest experience with upper extremity prosthetics, and his aesthetic results are impressive.[29] There are scattered reports of osseointegrated digital and thumb prosthetics, which would render them slightly more functional and durable.[30] In general, there must be at least a remnant of thumb proximal phalanx for an aesthetic prosthetic to remain on the thumb.[12] Otherwise, a hand-based extension may be required for prosthesis stabilization.

Postoperative care

Immobilization is the cornerstone of any hand postoperative care, and the thumb is no exception. Generally, distal-third thumb reconstruction is soft tissue alone, therefore,

immobilization in a postoperative plaster splint is only done for approximately a week. After that, the thumb can be supported with a removable splint, and normal showering and hand-washing can begin. Sutures are removed at 2 weeks postoperatively.

More proximal reconstructions can involve skeletal reconstruction, in addition to soft tissue. Plate and screw fixation allows early mobilization, typically initiated at 1–2 weeks postoperatively. Kirschner wire fixation can be slightly less rigid; however, at least some passive gliding exercises can still be initiated at 2 weeks. Again, removable splinting allows hand-washing and bathing.

At approximately 6 weeks, bony consolidation will have proceeded to the point that some resistive exercises can be started (provided that on radiographs the fixation has remained stable and there is at least some evidence of consolidation). It is also at this point that scar modification techniques can usually begin in earnest.

Outcomes, prognosis, and complications

Unfortunately, there is a scarcity of well-controlled outcomes studies related to the various types of thumb reconstruction. There are, however, a number of large retrospective series for each of the above-listed reconstruction methods that, in general, demonstrate good results.[11,14–16,19,25,27]

There are five goals when reconstructing a thumb: restoration of (1) functional length; (2) stability; (3) mobility (especially opposition); (4) sensibility; and (5) aesthetic appearance. The treating physician should help the patient choose the technique that will allow restoration of (hopefully) all five of these aspects to the thumb. If all five are restored, then the prognosis for a functional thumb and a satisfied patient is good. If all five cannot be restored, then, at the least, restoration of a stable thumb with adequate length will allow some grip and pinch activities.

Secondary procedures

First-webspace deepening is frequently required after thumb trauma and possibly after prior reconstructive procedures. This can be done with skin grafts or local tissue rearrangement, as discussed previously. Other scar contractures that are functionally limiting or aesthetically unpleasing can be treated with a variety of releases and transpositions, including Z-plasties and Y-V plasties.

Tendon adhesions are also common after thumb reconstruction. The primary method of treatment of this problem is early and aggressive hand therapy to minimize their impact. If therapy cannot overcome the adhesions, then flexor and/or extensor tenolysis may be required. Following tenolysis, therapy should resume within 24–48 hours.

As mentioned in the section on metacarpal lengthening, bone grafting is often required. Nonunions in the hand are rare but may require later bone grafting. Malunions of the thumb ray are extremely well tolerated and compensated;

however, severe malunions may require osteotomy and fixation.

Joint contractures in the nonthumb digits can be particularly detrimental, especially the proximal interphalangeal joint. However, in the thumb, these are less an issue, and in fact can help with thumb stability. If there is a severe flexion contracture of the metacarpophalangeal joint, this may need joint release.

Distal-third thumb loss may result in painful neuromas that require later excision. However, this can largely be mitigated by traction neurectomy of the digital nerve(s) at the time of initial reconstruction.

Access the complete references list online at **http://www.expertconsult.com**

1. Littler JW. On making a thumb: one hundred years of surgical effort. *J Hand Surg*. 1976;1:35-51.

   Authored by one of the pioneers of hand surgery, this manuscript is a detailed and richly illustrated history of thumb reconstruction up to 1976. Many of the techniques described in this article remain common today. These include digit transfer, toe transfer, osteoplastic reconstruction, and phalangization.

12. Muzaffar AR, Chao JJ, Friedrich JB, et al. Posttraumatic thumb reconstruction. *Plast Reconstr Surg*. 2005;116:103e-122e.

    The authors present a comprehensive review of the classification of thumb loss in thirds, as well as reconstructive options for each level of amputation. This article includes both microsurgical and nonmicrosurgical reconstructive techniques. The focus of the article is reconstruction of the traumatically injured thumb, but the principles contained within are applicable to other thumb loss etiologies.

25. Matev I. Thumb metacarpal lengthening. *Techniques hand upper extremity surg*. 2003;7:157-163.

    This paper by Dr. Matev describes his experience with thumb metacarpal lengthening over a 40-year period. It is both a historical reference as well as an excellent technical guide to the procedure. While most of his patients required bone grafting following distraction, he describes situations in which the gap spontaneously ossified. Finally, Dr. Matev addresses other considerations such as the effects of distraction on the first webspace and the thumb carpometacarpal joint.

27. Bravo CJ, Horton T, Moran SL, et al. Traumatized index finger pollicization for thumb reconstruction. *J Hand Surg*. 2008;33:257-262.

    This article is one of a very few that analyze the on-top plasty (pollicization of a damaged index finger). The authors review 7 patients who underwent this reconstruction method, including pinch strength and sensibility. They find that, in general, this is a sound method of thumb reconstruction, and most patients reported favorably on their postoperative funcationality. The article also includes a valuable list of technical points necessary to accomplish the procedure.

28. Brunelli GA, Brunelli GR. Reconstruction of traumatic absence of the thumb in the adult by pollicization. *Hand Clin*. 1992;8:41-55.

    This is a technique manuscript describing index finger pollicization which can be used for proximal third thumb loss. The authors present in detail the steps required to accomplish pollicization. Additionally, they address important considerations including management of the dorsal and palmar interosseous muscles of the index finger, as well as management of the transferred metacarpophalangeal joint. They also briefly describe pollicization of other digits if the index finger is unavailable.

14

Thumb and finger reconstruction: Microsurgical techniques

Fu Chan Wei and Wee Leon Lam

SYNOPSIS

- Microsurgical toe-to-hand transplantation has allowed the possibility of replacing "like for like" tissues, achieving good functional and aesthetic results with acceptable donor site morbidity.

- Early consideration of toe-to-hand procedures at the initial debridement ensures careful preservation of all viable neurovascular bundles, flexor and extensor tendons, mobile joints, and skin in order to maintain or achieve maximal functional results with minimal dissection of the foot.

- Retrograde dissection of the vascular pedicle facilitates toe harvest and alleviates concerns regarding any variations in the vascular anatomy of the donor vessels.

- Amputated thumbs can be successfully reconstructed with various modifications of the great toe, including whole great toe, trimmed great toe, great-toe wrap-around flaps, and the second toe.

- Amputated fingers can also be successfully reconstructed with various configurations from lesser toes, achieving results comparable to that of the thumb.

- The "metacarpal hand" refers to a hand with amputations of all fingers proximal to a critical functional level with or without accompanying thumb amputations. Toe-to-hand transplantations can help restore maximal hand function to this once permanently crippling condition, even for bilateral defects.

- Our large series of over 1700 cases allows continual pioneering of new concepts, refinements of existing techniques, improved classification systems, and strategic management algorithms that will enable easier mastery of toe-to-hand transplantations.

 Access the Historical Perspective section online at
http://www.expertconsult.com

Introduction

The first toe-to-thumb procedures were performed by Yang[1,2] in 1966 and Cobbett[3] in 1967. These were among the first

free tissue transfers to be attempted and probably reflects the central role of the hand, and the obvious logic in using toes to replace missing digits. The human hand functions through a combination of different prehension patterns, adequate motor strength, and sensory feedback. Such a unique combination requires the presence of mobile joints, specialized glabrous skin composition with a rich sensory input especially in the fingertips, with accompanying splintage from healthy nails. Following digital amputations, the replacement of "like for like" tissues that restores these exacting demands is only achievable by a successful replantation.[4-6] In cases of failed replantations, toe-to-hand transplantations remain the next best option with a superior result than the use of prosthesis or other nonmicrosurgical techniques to achieve functioning digits with acceptable sensibility and appearance.[7-13]

To date, toe transplantation for thumbs has been established as the gold standard in replacing mutilated or unreplantable thumbs.[14-17] The use of toes to replace missing fingers, however, has been somewhat less acknowledged and controversial, partly due to the perceived insignificance of finger loss and overall discomfort with the technical challenge involved, resulting in a general reluctance to carry out a "big operation" for a "small injury." In certain select patient groups, however, especially those with demanding functional[18] or aesthetic concerns,[19] replacing single fingers with composite tissues offers satisfactory results, even when carried out solely for cosmetic and psychological reasons.[20-22] In certain occupations, e.g., musicians, these operations provide the only hope of continual meaningful employment. When multiple fingers are amputated, the resultant disability is comparable to the loss of the thumb and drastically alters the appearance of the hand.[8,23-26] The "metacarpal hand" is a devastating injury with amputations of all fingers proximal to a functional level with or without accompanying thumb amputations.[12,27,28] Toe-to-hand transplantations remain the only useful option for this condition to restore functional usefulness, especially in bilateral defects.[29,30]

The growing literature, especially in the area of toe-to-hand transplantations for finger amputations, reflects the

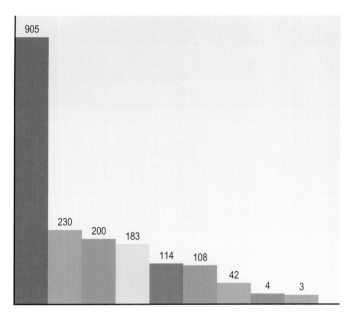

905

230

200

183

114

108

42

4

3

Total: 1789 operations, 1992 toes transferred
From Jan. 1985 to Dec. 2009

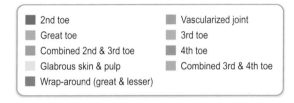

■ 2nd toe   ■ Vascularized joint
■ Great toe   ■ 3rd toe
■ Combined 2nd & 3rd toe   ■ 4th toe
■ Glabrous skin & pulp   ■ Combined 3rd & 4th toe
■ Wrap-around (great & lesser)

Fig. 14.1 Number of cases performed at Chang Gung University Medical College Hospital from 1985 to 2009.

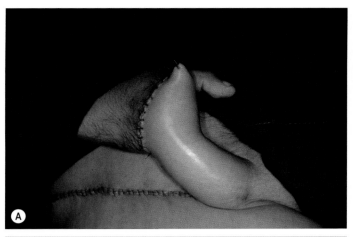

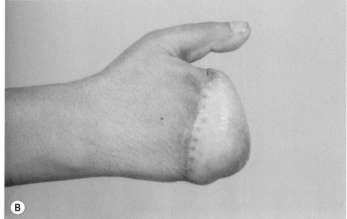

Fig. 14.2 (A, B) Coverage of an injured hand with a pedicled groin flap before toe transplantation.

increasing acceptance among surgeons for this procedure and also a relentless pursuit to achieve excellence in outcomes[31–38] and improved donor site morbidity[39–41] through continuous innovation. The reconstructive surgeon wishing to replace missing thumbs or fingers with toes now has a wide range of options for selection in order to achieve optimum results. This chapter outlines the current experience of toe-to-hand transplantations, drawing from our experience of more than 1700 cases over a 30-year period at Chang Gung University Medical College Hospital *(Fig. 14.1)*.

Diagnosis/patient presentation

The initial management of the potential toe-to-hand transplantation patient is similar to any other trauma or patient requiring digital replantation, with resuscitation and management of concomitant life-threatening injuries if necessary, and appropriate preservation of the amputated digits. Initial assessment of the injured hand allows pre-emptive discussion of toe-to-hand transplantation with the patient, especially when the possibility of a successful replantation is in doubt, such as in severely avulsed, crushed, or multiple amputations. In particular, patients whose occupation requires a

high-demand use of their hands or those with special needs and hobbies requiring a fine degree of dexterity and 10 fingers, e.g., musicians or athletes, should be given all information available concerning different reconstructive options. If there is significant soft-tissue damage, or anticipated soft-tissue lack following debridement, additional cover with the use of pedicled groin flaps should be considered at the time of the initial operation and discussed with the patient *(Fig. 14.2)*.

The initial operation

Anticipation of either primary or secondary toe-to-hand operations ensures careful preservation of all viable structures at the initial debridement or following failed replantation.[49,50] Excessive shortening of structures in order to achieve direct wound closure or the use of local flaps should be avoided[10] with the use of a pedicled groin flap instead; with the following advantages: (1) donor site on the foot can be primarily closed without the need to harvest large amount of skin with the toes; (2) skin grafts in the hand can be avoided, thus improving the appearance of the toe transplantation; and (3) an adequate webspace can be created with the excess skin available. Although some reports have suggested other methods of additional soft-tissue harvest with the toe transplantation, either as a single-stage microvascular procedure with combined free flaps,[51] or the use of native foot tissue,[31,52] we recommend a groin flap for the majority of cases as it is quick and simple to perform and leaves an almost negligible donor scar.

As the use of intraosseous wires is an effective method of osteosynthesis[53] and only requires 0.5 cm of bone for wire placement, as much remnant bone should be preserved as possible. In transjoint amputations, any intact articular cartilage and accompanying ligaments should be preserved to facilitate joint reconstruction with disarticulated toe joints.[54] Amputations at the level of the thumb metacarpals can be augmented with the use of bone blocks, thus avoiding the need for a transmetatarsal osteotomy in great-toe harvest, as preservation of the metatarsophalangeal joint is important for foot function and appearance.[12,55]

Avulsed or shredded extensor and flexor tendons should be debrided but never sacrificed for the sole purpose of obtaining wound closure. In fingers, preserving the native intrinsic extensor apparatus as far as possible, especially over the proximal interphalangeal joint, allows preservation of the arrangement of the intrinsic and extrinsic extensor systems[56] following reconstruction. Similarly, preserving the insertion of the flexor digitorum superficialis, wherever possible, has proved useful in achieving better functional results.[50,57]

Excessive shortening and the use of cauterization of arterial and venous ends are to be avoided in order to minimize intimal damage and preserve length, avoiding more extensive foot dissection and the need for vein grafts which prolong the operation and increase complications.[58] The same applies to nerves. Traditional teaching of the "pull and cut" method for prevention of neuromas in amputated stumps is to be avoided, as sensory recovery is much faster when nerve length is preserved and neurrorhaphy performed nearer to the transferred toe.[59] All neurovascular bundles should be tagged carefully with 10/0 sutures to ensure easier identification at the subsequent reconstruction.

Patient selection

Patient factors

Careful patient selection is the key to success. Age is not a contraindication, although the demands of hand function decrease with advanced age. Furthermore, the higher risks of thrombosis[60] as well as lessened sensory recovery[61] have to be carefully discussed with the elderly patient. Ideal patients are well motivated and clear about their needs and goals with good overall health. Decision-making for each patient is individualized not simply for the injury status but also to take into account the hand dominance and occupation as well as socioeconomic status.

Primary versus secondary reconstruction

Although secondary toe-to-hand procedures may appear to be the logical choice to ensure better wound control and definition of the zone of injury, a primary reconstruction (before the wounds are closed or have healed) allows a one-stage procedure, earlier rehabilitation, and subsequent return to

work, as advocated by several authors.[20,62–64] In our study of 26 primary cases versus 96 secondary cases, there was no significant difference in terms of vascular re-exploration rates, recipient site complications, or requirement for secondary revision.[64] In a well-informed and motivated patient without extensive soft-tissue loss or other significant injuries of the ipsilateral upper limb, primary toe-to-hand transplantation offers the ideal method of replacing digit loss. On the other hand, the procedure is best delayed in patients who are unsure about their decisions and who also communicate their reluctance to undergo further rehabilitation.

Injury factors

Decision-making for the thumb

The functional thumb depends on adequate length, sensibility, mobility, and stability. Microvascular toe-to-thumb transplantations allow these four objectives to be achieved in a single stage with a superior aesthetic result. The function of the thumb decreases by 50% once the amputation level is proximal to the proximal interphalangeal joint and reaches 100% once it crosses the metacarpophalangeal joint.[65] Amputations distal to the interphalangeal joint are generally well tolerated but, in certain patients, the additional length, stability, and sensibility from a transplanted distal toe transfer should always be offered as an option.[59,66]

Various classifications and reconstructive algorithms exist for thumb defects,[67–69] although the underlying principles relate mainly to the types of tissue and the length of thumb missing.[70] Toe-to-thumb transplantations can be successfully reconstructed with various modifications of the great toe, including whole great toe,[66] trimmed great toe,[71] great-toe wrap-around flaps,[72] pulp flaps,[73] and the second toe.[29,52] The decision to use which toe or its variation should be individualised not only to the thumb defect and the patient's needs, but also with careful consideration to the donor site. In general, thumb reconstruction using the great toe or its variants provides a better functional and aesthetic outcome than use of the lesser toes, although augmentation procedures for second toes to improve bulk have been described.[52] If the great toe is used, at least 1 cm of the proximal phalanx should be preserved in the foot to ensure better push-off and preservation of foot appearance; the great toe is therefore an ideal option for thumb amputation levels distal to the mid-metacarpal shaft. In more proximal amputations, a transmetatarsal transfer of the second toe or additional methods like preliminary distraction lengthening of the existing metacarpal or interpositional bone grafting between the transferred toe and the metacarpal without sacrificing the metatarsophalangeal joint of the great toe are preferred.[12,30,59]

Decision-making for fingers

Classification of finger defects is similar to the thumb and pertains to the type of tissue and length of finger missing, with the additional consideration of which finger is involved and whether there is single or multiple amputations. The definition of proximal or distal amputations is determined by its relation to the insertion of the flexor digitorum superficialis tendon.[49,59,74] Toe transplantation to more distal finger amputations can be achieved by a wide variety of options, including the use of vascularized nail grafts,[75–77] pulp flaps,[78] wrap-around flaps,[33] and partial second toe,[19] depending on what tissues are missing. These operations are rewarding due to the restoration of high-density pulp sensation, fine pinch, and cosmetic appeal of the nail.[74,75,79] A partial second-toe flap includes either only the distal interphalangeal joint or both the proximal and distal interphalangeal joints, and is indicated in amputations distal to the flexor digitorum superficialis insertion.[18,74,80,81] In contrast, a whole second-toe flap is indicated in carefully selected patients with more proximal amputations[59]; the ideal level, however, is distal to the middle of the proximal phalanx as reconstructions for more proximal amputations usually result in a slightly shorter finger.[82]

Decision-making for patients with multiple finger amputations are largely guided by the specific occupational and cosmetic needs of the patient. In general, two adjacent fingers should be reconstructed wherever possible to allow a stable tripod pinch or hook grip.[12,26,81] Preferential reconstruction of the radial two fingers should be recommended for patients who require fine pinch and the ulnar two digits for manual workers who require a strong grip.[24,83]

Decision-making for the metacarpal hand

The term "metacarpal hand" refers to a hand injury with multiple finger amputations at the level of the metacarpophalangeal joint, or immediately proximal or distal to it. Delitala was perhaps the first to coin this term[84] and, since then, various classification systems have been proposed,[85–88] with varying levels of clinical usefulness. A classification system based on reconstructive options and different stages of injury has proved useful in our experience[12,55,84] *(Tables 14.1 and 14.2)*. This takes into account the level of finger amputations and relative involvement of the thumb, and provides guidelines for the reconstructive technique as well as prediction of the functional outcome after reconstruction. Further subclassified into two types for these purposes, type I refers to an injury with four-finger proximal amputations without thumb or only distal-thumb involvement (no thumb reconstruction necessary). In type IA injuries, where the amputation level is distal to the metacarpophalangeal joint, the focus is on the selection of two separate toes or combined second and third, or third and fourth toe transplantations *(Fig. 14.3)*. To ensure that the different digits curve around an object more evenly in grasp prehension, the length of the remaining amputation stumps should not be longer than that of a normal little finger when considering a combined second- and third-toe transfer.[83] For type IB injuries, where the amputation level is through the joints with intact articular surfaces, combined second and third toes are harvested as composite joint transfers. More proximal injuries (IC) where the amputation level is proximal to the metacarpophalangeal joints require the harvest of combined second and third toes as transmetatarsal transfers. Reconstruction of two adjacent fingers allows for a stable tripod pinch, although reconstruction of all four fingers is possible in certain selected patients *(Fig. 14.4)*.[12]

Type II injuries refer similarly to four-finger proximal amputations but with various levels of thumb involvement. The reconstruction of fingers with toe transplantations follows a similar decision-making process as for type I defects, but reconstruction of the thumb is determined by the presence or absence of a functional thenar musculature. If the thenar muscle is intact or possesses adequate function (types IIa and IIb), a one-stage procedure to reconstruct the thumb and two adjacent fingers is recommended. If the thenar muscle presents with missing or inadequate function (IIC), the thumb reconstruction should be delayed until after the finger reconstructions and the thumb position first determined by the aid of a prosthetic thumb while the fingers assume its final positions *(Fig. 14.5)*. This is to allow proper length and positioning of the reconstructed thumb in a suitably adducted and opposed posture at the second stage to facilitate an effective tripod pinch prehension. Tendon transfers for opposition transfers can also be carried out at the time of the second stage, if necessary.[89]

Table 14.1 Metacarpal hand classification for type I defects		
Subtype	**Thumb amputation levels**	**Finger amputation levels**
IA	Amputation distal to the interphalangeal joint	Distal to the level of metacarpophalangeal joint
IB		At the level of the metacarpophalangeal joint
IC		Proximal to the level of the metacarpophalangeal joint

Table 14.2 Metacarpal hand type II defects and proposed reconstruction algorithm			
Subtype	**Thumb amputation level**	**Reconstructive options**	**Stage**
IIA	Distal to the metacarpal neck	Whole or trimmed great toe	Simultaneous
IIB	Proximal to the metacarpal neck with adequate thenar muscle function	Whole or trimmed great toe ± lengthening or bone augmentation Transmetatarsal second-toe transfer	Simultaneous
IIC	Any level with inadequate thenar musculature	Same as in IIA or IIB Opponenplasty	Staged
IID	Any level with damaged carpometacarpal joint	Same as in IIA or IIB Immobile thumb post	Staged

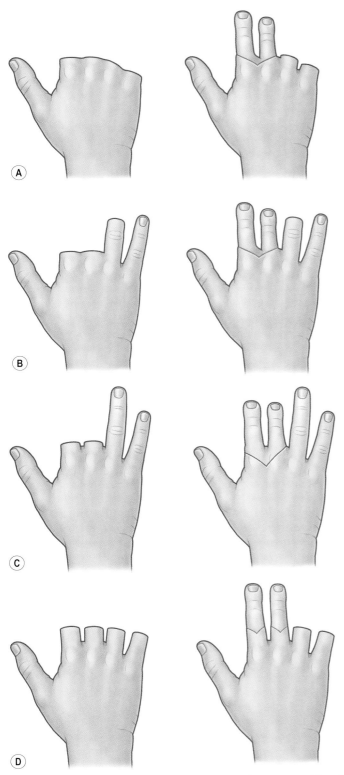

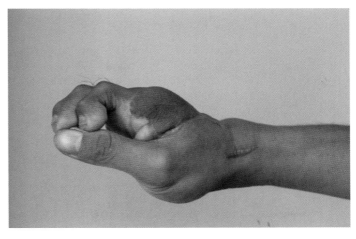

Fig. 14.4 The reconstructed tripod pinch of a type I metacarpal hand, showing stability of grip and good opposition with the thumb.

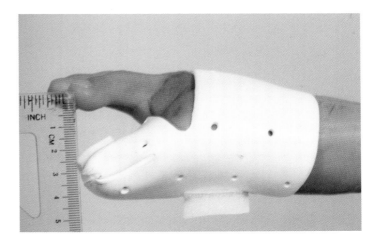

Fig. 14.5 Use of a prosthetic thumb for a type IIC metacarpal hand after combined second- and third-toe transplantation for middle- and ring-finger reconstruction. This is useful for determining the exact position of the future transplanted thumb and for planning additional procedures (e.g., opponenplasties).

Fig. 14.3 Indications for combined second- and third-toe harvest versus bilateral toe harvest. A combined second- and third-toe transplantation is preferred for: **(A)** amputations proximal to the webspace (indicative of a level at or proximal to the metacarpophalangeal joints); or **(B)** when the remaining fingers are at the level of, or shorter than, the little finger. Using this technique when the remaining finger is longer than the little finger will produce a hand with gross unequal finger lengths and an uneven digital arcade **(C)**. **(D)** Bilateral second toes are best suited when the webspaces are preserved, indicative of amputations distal to the metacarpophalangeal joints with adequate bone for osteosynthesis.

Decision-making in bilateral metacarpal hand injuries requires a careful balance of the severity of injury (type I or II), the patient's needs, and acceptable level of donor morbidity. Type II injuries are much more difficult than type I, requiring up to but not exceeding five donor toes to achieve a functional level of prehension.[30] In general, the use of a great toe, usually from the left or nondominant foot, is sacrificed for dominant thumb reconstruction together with a combined two-toe reconstruction from the opposite foot to achieve a tripod pinch. In the nondominant hand, single-digit pulp-to-pulp pinch is considered adequate with the use of a lesser toe for thumb reconstruction.[30] Although the option of sacrificing both great toes or more lesser toes for hand reconstruction may seem attractive, we have found that the donor morbidity reaches a level that is incompatible with activities of daily

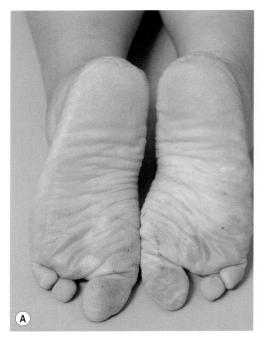
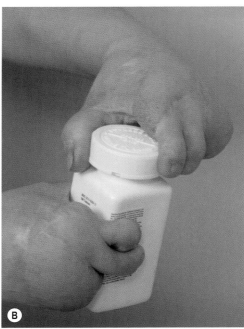

Fig. 14.6 (A, B) Appearance of bilateral metacarpal hands and donor sites after toe-to-hand transplantations. Up to a total of five toes can be harvested for the most severe defects of bilateral type II metacarpal hands requiring reconstruction of opposing digits in both hands.

living. In instances where multiple toes are needed, the patient needs to participate fully in the decision-making with regard to the foot morbidity, especially in certain populations where patients are far less tolerant of sacrificing their toes to reconstruct their hands *(Fig. 14.6)*.[29]

Treatment/surgical technique

Despite the many configurations and combinations of toe-to-hand transplantations available, a few important principles exist for all cases which, when adhered to, allow easier dissection, reduced foot morbidity, and improved overall functional and aesthetic outcomes.

General principles in vascular dissection

Dissection of the vascular pedicle remains a source of confusion and frustration for surgeons wishing to embark on toe-to-hand transplantations. Adopting a retrograde dissection method of the arterial pedicle alleviates concerns regarding vascular anatomy and greatly facilitates easier dissection.[90,91] Begin by dissecting the pedicle in the web space and identifying the dominant blood supply to the toes, having a working knowledge of the three types of arterial supply. The first dorsal metatarsal artery (FDMA) is usually dominant (70%) and identified by its dorsal relation to the intermetatarsal ligament *(Fig. 14.7)*.[59,92] Once this is confirmed, it permits early ligation of the plantar system which greatly facilitates further dissection. In the 20% of cases where a first plantar metatarsal arterial (FPMA) system is dominant, as identified by its plantar relations to the transverse metatarsal ligament *(Fig. 14.7)*, the FDMA is then ligated and the plantar dissection continued together with the harvest of the digital nerves. The

length of the arterial pedicle harvested should be able to reach the chosen recipient artery. However, in a dominant FPMA system dissection should be limited to the nonweight-bearing zones, with the use of vein grafts if necessary to increase pedicle length. In cases where both the FDMA and FPMA appear equally dominant (10%: *Fig. 14.7*), the dorsal system is always selected due to its easier harvest and less donor morbidity. Following toe harvests, at least 20 minutes should be allowed for observation of adequate perfusion before detaching the flap. The venous drainage system is usually identified after the arterial system, and follows a lazy "S" incision on the dorsum of the foot. One sizeable vein is usually enough from the plexus of veins located in an intermediate layer and drained by the great saphenous vein; they should not be confused with the superficial dermal veins.

Hints and tips

- To facilitate easier dissection and alleviate concerns regarding vascular anatomy, start in the webspace and then trace the arterial pedicle in a retrograde fashion. In 80% of cases, the first dorsal metatarsal artery can be used as the arterial pedicle
- To improve the profile at the toe–digit junction and prevent a bulbous appearance, create four equal mobile flaps through a cruciate incision, and interpose these with the V-shaped flaps of the transplanted toe

General principles in recipient preparation

A two-team approach greatly reduces the overall operating time, surgeon fatigue, and risks of anesthesia.[49] Proper preparation of the recipient site allows a smooth transition from flap

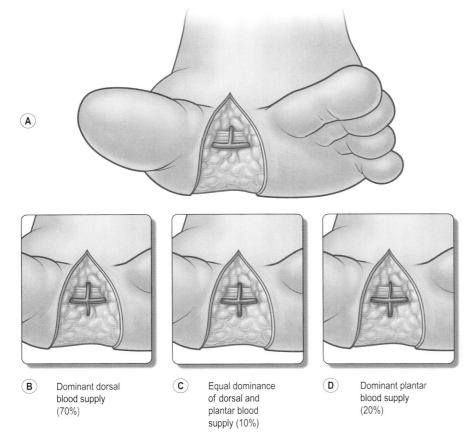

Fig. 14.7 (A) Retrograde dissection of the arterial pedicle begins in the first webspace and allows early confirmation of a dominant dorsal or plantar system. **(B)** In 70% of cases, a dominant first dorsal metatarsal artery is present, whereas in 20% of cases, a dominant first plantar metatarsal artery is present **(C)**. In 10% of cases, both systems are equally dominant, in which case the dorsal system is selected **(D).**

(B) Dominant dorsal blood supply (70%)

(C) Equal dominance of dorsal and plantar blood supply (10%)

(D) Dominant plantar blood supply (20%)

harvest to inset without any delays. Preservation of all viable lengths of bone, joints, neurovascular bundles, and tendons should have been performed at the initial operation by a surgeon who has working knowledge of toe-to-hand transplantations.[50] A cruciate incision allows the creation of four equal triangular flaps for smooth interdigitation with the V-shaped flap of the transplanted toe and prevents the ugly "cobra" appearance that features prominently at the toe–digit junction *(Fig. 14.8)*. Following preliminary inset, excess fatty tissues are trimmed by skeletonizing the neurovascular bundles of the recipient flaps. All these maneuvers allow the creation of a finger or thumb with a more natural-looking appearance.

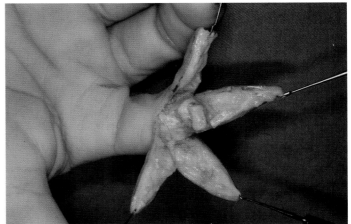

Fig. 14.8 A cruciate incision at the recipient site allows the creation of four equal triangular flaps and prevents a bulbous appearance at the subsequent toe-to-finger junction.

Hints and tips

To reduce foot morbidity and avoid the use of skin grafts, pay careful attention to the placement of incisions on the foot. Webspace incisions should not cross the midline on to the territory of the contralateral toes, and all proximal incisions should converge to a V proximal to the osteotomy sites. In addition, scars should be kept away from all weight-bearing sites.

General guidelines in donor closure

Careful placement of incision lines in the donor foot minimizes weight-bearing pain and scar tenderness and permits earlier mobility. V-shaped flaps are sited proximal to the

osteotomy site whereas distally, the incisions are situated midway between the webspaces to permit tension-free closure, even with combined second–third or third–fourth-toe transplantations. Incisions on weight-bearing areas as well as extensive foot dissection should be avoided. Skin grafts are generally discouraged due to difficulties in replacing glabrous skin, wound breakdown due to repeated pressure from weight-bearing and footwear, and also because it prevents early ambulation. When skin grafts are required, for example, after pulp flap, webspace flap, and wrap-around flap harvests, they should be carried out meticulously with strict prevention of ambulation until the grafts are healed.

General principles in flap inset

Intraosseous wires provide a stable method of bone fixation, achieving a union rate of 98.5%.[53] They are also advantageous for the following reasons: a shorter segment of recipient bone is required for osteosynthesis; the semirigid fixation allows early postoperative correction if the transplanted toe is found to be malaligned or malrotated *(Fig. 14.9)*.

Hints and tips

To preserve maximum bone length in the amputation stump, use parallel intraosseous wires as the preferred method of osteosynthesis, as this requires only 0.5 cm of available bone, achieves a good union rate, and allows postoperative correction of any malalignment or malrotation.

Careful attention to tendon repairs increases range of motion and also corrects the natural tendency of the toe to claw. The extensor tendons are always reconstructed first. Preserving the extensor tendon apparatus over the proximal interphalangeal joint, wherever possible, allows the intact intrinsic system of the hand to work synergistically with the reconstructed extrinsic system. Release of the extensor digitorum longus attachment from the metacarpophalangeal joint capsule, suturing of the extensor digitorum brevis to the dorsal expansion or to the interosseous musculotendinous structure, and a tight extensor repair in full extension are different ways of overcoming the naturally flexed position of the toe.[34] In addition, a K-wire is also inserted at the end of the procedure, transfixing the distal interphalangeal joint and the proximal interphalangeal joint in full extension. The flexor tendon repair is carried out against the tension of the extensor repair to restore a normal digital cascade. In proximal amputations, the flexor tendon of the transplanted toe

should be pulled through proximally into zone III for repair to prevent an increased risk of tendon adhesions in "no man's land" (zone II).

Hints and tips

- To achieve the best functional outcome of the reconstructed tendons, preserve all extensor apparatus as far as possible to allow synergistic action of the native intrinsic system with the reconstructed extrinsic system. To correct the natural tendency of the toe to claw, perform a tight extensor tendon repair and insert a K-wire insertion with the distal and proximal interphalangeal joints in extension for 6 weeks followed by splinting for up to a year
- To achieve maximal stability of the interphalangeal joint following a trimmed great-toe harvest, ensure that the perijoint flap consisting of the periosteum, medial collateral ligament, and joint capsule is redraped and closed in a tight manner around the trimmed interphalangeal joint of the great toe

Nerve repair is carried out next. The proper digital nerves are selected for end-to-end anastomosis with recipient digital nerves that have been trimmed back to reveal healthy nerve stumps. If additional dorsal recipient nerves are available, these can be sutured to any harvested branches of the superficial and deep peroneal nerves. Following nerve repair, the skin flaps are closed temporarily to allow for final skin adjustments if necessary. Care must be taken to prevent a tight closure which may eventually compress the pedicles. If in doubt, a skin graft should be used rather than try to force primary closure. A single arterial anastomosis is then performed and perfusion of the toe checked before the venous anastomosis. If it is judged to be inadequate, the entire pedicle should be assessed for any kinking, twisting, or compression with further stripping of the adventitia if necessary. If required, further shortening or a vein graft should be used to ensure healthy inflow.

Hints and tips

To ensure maximal success and reduce vascular complications, harvest the combined second- and third-toe flap with the first dorsal metatarsal artery as the dominant pedicle, and the second and third common digital artery as a backup in case of inadequate perfusion. To reduce donor site morbidity, close the donor site primarily in all cases. It is not necessary to reconstruct the transmetatarsal arch even when disturbed, for example, in transmetatarsal osteotomies, as this does not affect gait and walking ability in the long term.

In a combined second- and third-toe transplantation, two anastomoses should be prepared as a higher rate of arterial spasm and re-exploration rates of up to 20%[93] have been found when using a single dominant artery; the second anastomosis using the second and third common plantar artery should be carried out when the perfusion to the third toe is uncertain. Once perfusion is established, the hand is then

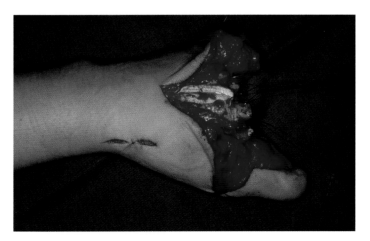

Fig. 14.9 A prepared recipient site with interosseous wires inserted, ready for inset of the toe flap.

turned around and the venous outflow checked for healthy back bleeding. Venous anastomosis is carried out through a separate incision on the dorsum of the hand. A recipient vein of suitable calibre is selected and mobilized from the adjacent fingers if necessary. The skin incisions are then loosely closed definitively over small Silastic drains placed in the dorsum of the hand and fingers, and finally the K-wire is inserted across the distal and proximal interphalangeal joints in full extension. The hand is then wrapped in a noncircumferential, noncompressive dressing with the transplanted toe largely exposed to monitor perfusion.

Specific operations

Trimmed great toe

Harvest of the trimmed great toe begins with measurements taken and compared at three locations on the normal contralateral thumb and the great toe to reconstruct a new thumb with matching proportions: the nail eponychium, the interphalangeal joint, and the middle of the proximal phalanx *(Fig. 14.10)*. The size discrepancies are marked on the medial aspect of the great toe as an area of tissue to be excised, with an excess of 2–3 mm on each side and tapering of both the proximal and distal ends to facilitate closure.

Elevation of the trimmed great toe begins in the first web-space to identify the dominant blood supply and carry out retrograde dissection, as previously described. Following identification of the flexor and extensor tendons and also after careful preservation of the deep peroneal nerves, the trimming of the great toe is commenced. The marked area of redundancy is excised with incisions down to and superficial to the medial collateral ligament of the interphalangeal joint. The next step is removal of bony excess. To facilitate access to the phalanges, a plantar-based perijoint flap composed of periosteum, joint capsule, and medial collateral ligament is raised. About 4–6 mm of the joint prominence and 2–4 mm of the phalanges are removed with an oscillating saw and the

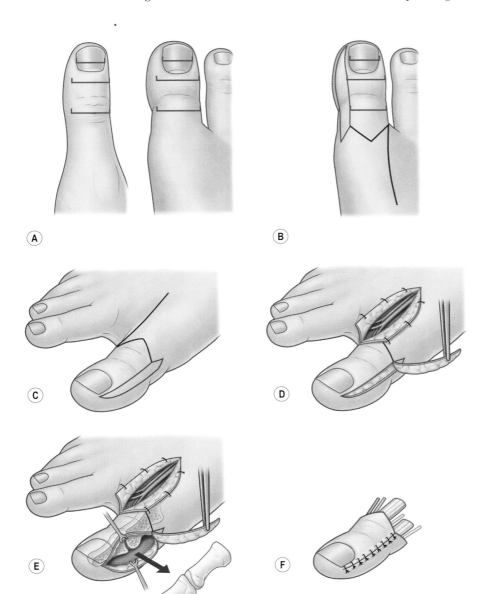

Fig. 14.10 Trimmed great-toe harvest technique. **(A)** Markings of the thumb are made at three positions on the thumb and transposed to the toe: nail eponychium, widest point (interphalangeal joint), and middle of proximal phalanx. **(B, C)** The discrepancies are marked on the medial side as an area to be excised. **(D)** The skin flap is elevated superficial to the collateral ligament and joint capsule. **(E)** The perijoint flap is created by raising the periosteum, medial collateral ligament, and joint capsule as a single flap, exposing the phalanges. The medial joint prominence and 2–4 mm of the proximal and distal phalanges are removed by an oscillating saw. **(F)** Following tight redraping of the perijoint flap, the skin is closed to create a toe of smaller circumference, ready for transfer.

remaining bones smoothed with a burr. The perijoint flap is then redraped with the excess tissue excised and sutured in a tight manner to ensure the stability of the joint. Finally, the medial skin incisions are approximated and the overall appearance checked before carrying out the transverse osteotomy at the level of the proximal phalanx and the flap islanded, ready for inset *(Fig. 14.10)*.

Second toe: total and partial

Video 2

The decision for total or partial second-toe harvest is determined by the level of finger amputation (see definition above). For either, the skin markings encirculate the base of the second toe and cross the midpoints of the first and third webspaces, finally converging as a V proximally and extending at least 5–10 mm beyond the osteotomy site *(Fig. 14.11)*. The toe harvest commences by identifying the dominant arterial supply in a retrograde fashion and one sizeable vein, as previously described. Both the extensor digitorum longus and brevis tendons are identified and traced proximally for adequate length. Branches of the peroneal nerves are usually not harvested in preference of the plantar digital nerves. The dissection is then continued on the plantar aspect of the foot, similarly with a V extending from the base of the toe and further extension with avoidance of any weight-bearing areas. The flexor sheaths are opened and the flexor tendons pulled out and cut at a proximal level to ensure adequate length. The plantar nerves are traced proximally to the bifurcation of the common digital nerves and internal neurolyses carried out if necessary to obtain adequate length before dividing them.

The removal of excess fibrofatty tissues by skeletonization of each neurovascular components is routinely carried out, as this greatly facilitates wound closure and improves the aesthetic appearance of the transplanted toe. This is especially so for partial toe transfers, due to the relative lack of space for flap inset at the level of the middle phalanx.

The bone length required for a complete second-toe transfer is achieved by an osteotomy at the proximal phalanx, the metatarsal shaft, or via a metatarsophalangeal joint disarticulation. In a partial toe transfer, the neurovascular bundles are freed distal to the osteotomy sites at the middle or proximal phalanges or the disarticulated joint. Metatarsophalangeal joint disarticulation is usually necessary to permit direct skin closure, even following partial toe transfers.

Wrap-around flaps: great and second toes

The great-toe wrap-around flap was originally used in conjunction with a nonvascularized iliac bone graft for reconstructing thumb loss distal to the metacarpophalangeal joint,[72] although reconstructions at more proximal levels have been described.[94] The use of these flaps can be extended to the replacement of skin and nail loss in the thumb and ring avulsion finger injuries with an intact skeleton, tendon, and proximal interphalangeal joints. Reconstruction of the latter is better achieved with a second-toe wrap-around flap which provides an excellent contour and nail match and also avoids using the great toe as a donor.[33]

Harvest of the great-toe wrap-around flap follows similar principles as per the trimmed great-toe technique, as

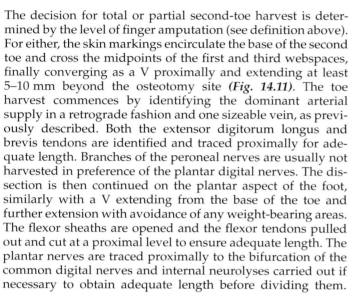

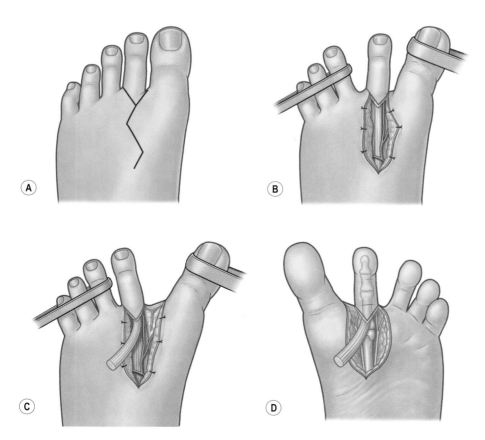

Fig. 14.11 Second-toe harvest technique. **(A, B)** A dorsal S incision is made on the dorsum of the foot to expose the donor veins, extensor mechanism, and arterial pedicle, although dissection begins in the first webspace to allow a retrograde dissection **(C)**. Plantar dissection begins with a midline incision, avoiding the weight-bearing areas of the foot, to expose the digital nerves and to harvest the flexor tendon **(D)**.

previously described. Preoperative markings are made with measurements taken from the contralateral thumb and transposed on to the great toe *(Fig. 14.10A)*. The flap utilizes the dorsal, lateral, and plantar skin, leaving behind a cuff of skin and subcutaneous tissue on the medial aspect for donor closure. Disarticulating the remaining interphalangeal joint and closing the medial skin flap over the proximal phalanx is preferred rather than using a cross-toe flap from the second toe. The second-toe wrap-around flap begins in exactly the same manner as the partial or complete second-toe flap (see above). The flap is then carefully degloved from the underlying skeleton, except for the distal phalanx, which is always included in the flap to maintain distal stability and prevent bone resorption. Careful consideration is also given to the placement of scars during flap harvest for their subsequent positioning on the "trailing" edges of the fingers. Disarticulation at the metatarsophalangeal joint in the remnant toe provides a donor defect amenable to primary closure and improved appearance.

Pulp flaps

The size of the defect is outlined and marked on the selected toe *(Fig. 14.12)*. The lateral aspect of the great toe is preferred for its richer nerve supply, more abundant tissues, and therefore increased likelihood of primary closure.[59] Principles for flap harvest are similar to those previously described, but important considerations are keys to achieving success: (1) identifying and including both the branches of the deep peroneal nerve and digital nerve proper to provide the best sensory outcome; (2) dissection and inclusion of the proper digital artery by tracing its origin from the first dorsal or plantar metatarsal artery in the first webspace; (3) skeletonizing the neurovascular bundle to allow tunneling of the vessels during flap inset.

First-web neurosensory flap

This is a useful flap due to its rich sensory innervation, pliability, and size, with dimensions of 14 × 7 cm achievable[95] for resurfacing of bigger defects in one or multiple fingers,

and the potential to replace glabrous skin for palm defects.[94,96,97] After outlining the defect in the first webspace, the vein is first identified, as previously described. The location of the intermetatarsal ligament is identified next as this structure points to the first dorsal or plantar metatarsal artery and the distal communicating artery that supplies this flap. Once the dominant blood supply is confirmed, retrograde dissection continues in a straightforward manner, continuing with either the dorsal or plantar approach. Branches of the proper digital arteries must be traced and included if the flap dimensions extend to the pulps of the great or second toes. Likewise, in this situation, the proper digital nerves are harvested in conjunction with the deep peroneal nerve branches to provide adequate sensation. The donor defect is readily reconstructed with a split-thickness skin graft and tie-over dressings. Careful attention to detail and strict nonweight-bearing reduce the incidence of wound-healing complications and the need for prolonged foot care *(Fig. 14.13)*.

Combined second- and third-toe transplantation

Combined second- and third-toe transplantations carry the advantages of only needing potentially one set of micovascular anastomosis, less operative time, and confining donor morbidity to one foot.[83] Its popularity has been limited, however, by the length of digits achievable following reconstruction and probably concerns regarding the donor morbidity, especially in certain populations.[29] If carried out carefully, however, this procedure is extremely useful in replacing two adjacent finger amputations at a level proximal to the webspace, especially when the other remaining fingers are shorter than the little finger. It is especially useful in the metacarpal hand deformity to provide tripod pinch function, hook grip capability, and lateral stability.

Skin incisions in the first and third webspaces should not cross the midline, and converge to a V 1 cm proximal to the level of osteotomy. In proximal phalanx amputations with at least 5 mm of bone remaining, the toe is disarticulated from the metatarsophalangeal joint and then subsequently shortened to the required length and osteosynthesized to the finger skeleton. Through metacarpophalangeal joint amputations are reconstructed with the corresponding metatarsophalangeal joints of the toes with their joint capsules intact. Even more proximal amputations require harvest of the respective metatarsals *(Fig. 14.14)*.

Retrograde dissection of the dominant arterial supply is performed in the first webspace, as previously described. The second and third plantar arteries should be dissected and preserved as a backup in case a second set of anastomosis is required. The common digital nerve to the second and third toe, together with their respective proper digital nerves, is also isolated and preserved for transfer during the plantar dissection. Direct closure of the donor site in a tension-free manner should be achievable without the need for a skin graft. In cases where the metatarsals have been osteotomized, our present unit policy is not to replace the foot defect with a bone graft as previous analysis of our patients has demonstrated no difference in walking and gait performance.[59]

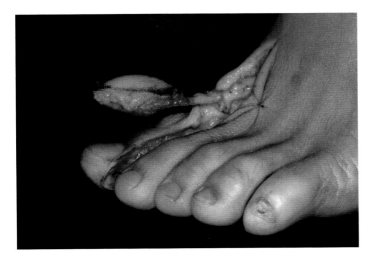

Fig. 14.12 Pulp flap harvested from the great toe.

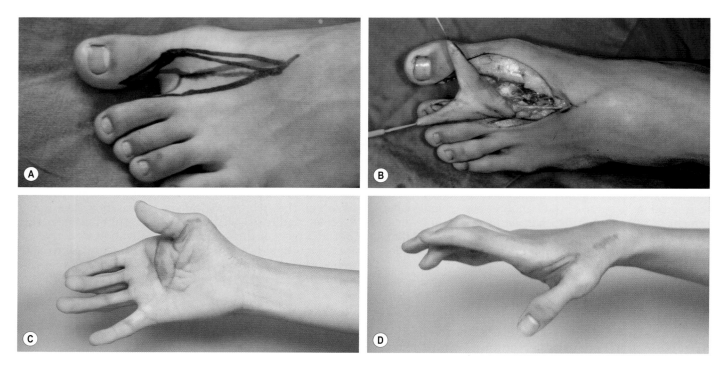

Fig. 14.13 (A–D) First-web neurosensory flap harvest from the left foot for reconstruction of the first webspace of the right hand.

Postoperative care

Immediate postoperative period

The immediate postoperative care is critical to ensure the success of the microsurgical procedure. Patients ideally can be kept for close monitoring of the flap in a microsurgical intensive care unit for a minimum of 5 days. If this facility is not available, they should be kept in a warm room and nursed by experienced staff who are trained in the routine monitoring of free flaps. Although both internal devices like implantable Doppler[98] and external devices like infrared temperature assessment and pulse oximetry may be useful modalities,[99] the most reliable method of flap monitoring is still clinical observation. At the first sign of vascular compromise, rapid action should be taken to avoid further flap deterioration.[100] Beside flap monitoring, all patients are carefully monitored to ensure they are warm, well hydrated, and painfree. The hand is kept slightly elevated above the level of the heart but not any higher than that. Nonconstricting or nonbulk dressings should be used as this prevents clot formation which could induce vasospasm during dressing change and also prevents early mobilization. A routine intraoperative bolus of dextran is given, followed by continuous infusion over the next few 5 days. In addition, a 2-week course of oral aspirin is also administered to reduce the incidence of platelet aggregation.

Motor rehabilitation

Toe-to-hand transplantations require a close collaboration between surgeons, nurses, physiotherapists, occupational therapists, and prosthetists to provide the necessary

postoperative rehabilitation program and maximize the functional outcome. Individual patient motivation and employment needs also have to be considered. A five-stage rehabilitation program[59] ensures that these objectives are met:

1. Protective stage (days 1–3): The objectives of this stage are to establish an interaction between the patient and the hand therapist and to support the patient through the initial first few difficult days while the patient recovers from the surgery.

2. Early mobilization stage (day 4 to 4 weeks): This stage aims to maintain a balance between achieving bone union through immobilization of the osteosynthesis site and prevention of joint stiffness. The hand, and especially the transplanted toe, receives careful passive mobilization of the joints distal to the bony union site from day 4 to 2 weeks after withdrawal of the K-wire, followed by passive mobilization of the joint proximal to this site. At week 4, the dressings should be reduced to light, tubular adhesives that conform to the fingers, allowing maximal joint movements. During this period, correction of any malalignment or malrotation can also be carried out by the use of a splint in between exercises.

3. Active motion stage (5–6 weeks): In this stage, patients are encouraged to perform active mobilization and also scar management under guidance. A dynamic or blocking splint, such as those popularized for traditional flexor tendon repair, is used until the sixth week. Strict nonweight-bearing on the reconstructed digits should be advised until at least the end of this period to permit full tendon healing.

4. Activities of daily living training stage (7–8 weeks): Close liaisons between the occupational and physiotherapists allow integration of activities of daily living for the

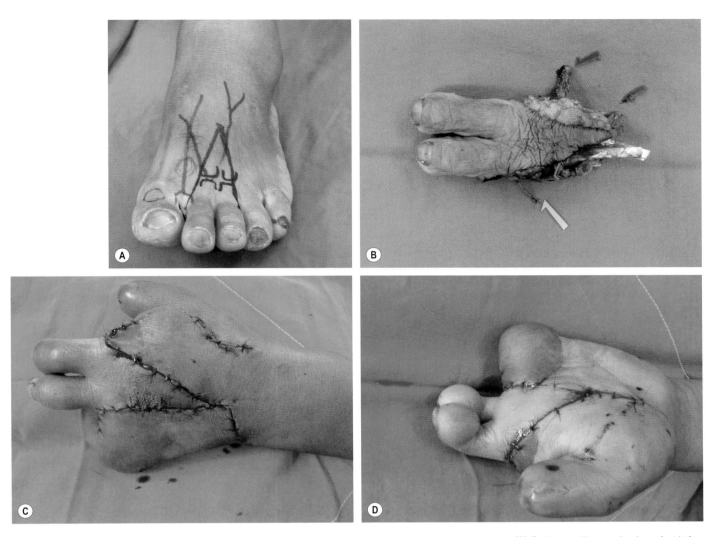

Fig. 14.14 Combined second- and third-toe harvest as a transmetatarsal transfer for reconstruction of a metacarpal hand. **(A)** Surface markings on the donor foot before harvest showing the position of the first dorsal metatarsal artery and a suitable vein. **(B)** Harvested toe with artery, veins, nerves, and tendons. **(C, D)** Reconstructed hand following inset showing primary closure of all wounds without tension.

reconstructed hand(s). Patient confidence is slowly restored as the patient engages once again in normal household activities. In addition to strengthening forearm muscles, this stage is also vital for sensory re-education in improving proprioception, dexterity, and object identification (see below).

5. Prevocational training (8 weeks onwards): The success of the operation can only be determined by the continual use of the reconstructed digit(s) in the long term, with one of the most important determinants being useful employment. Before discharging the patient back into the community, the individual occupational context has to be assessed to see if the patient can return to the original job, find a new job, or whether retraining or new training is required. Pediatric patients may require longer-term follow-up for future occupational advice. The use of a night splint to keep the fingers in full extension for up to a year reduces any recurrences of clawing.

Sensory rehabilitation

The finger and thumb pulps are unique in that they contain a higher density of sensory nerve endings than other body areas, packed within a relatively small area of skin that is tightly adhered to the underlying bone via fibrous septa.[101] Although toe transfers allow the replacement of this specialized glabrous skin, targeted sensory rehabilitation plays an important role in producing an optimal functional result. Several studies have demonstrated the importance of sensory re-education in maximizing both subjective and objective sensory recovery following nerve repair in digits[61,102–104]; this is of even greater importance in toe-to-hand transplantations due to the fewer number of sensory endings in the toe as compared to the fingertip.[105] Two types of sensory re-education program are used in our unit: early and delayed.

Early re-education focuses on improving the local adaptation to the submodalities of light touch, pinprick, and pressure with correct localization, as according to Dellon.[61] Static and moving two-point discrimination tests are usually chosen to measure local sensory recovery[63,80,97,106] following early re-education, although our unit has shown that there is very little correlation between this method of assessment and sensory threshold testing using the Semmes–Weinstein monofilament kit.[107] These results suggest that subjective recovery of functional sensibility may not always reflect the actual recovery of nerve function at the microscopic level. In fact, from our earlier study, the actual number of Meissner corpuscles was found to be decreased after transplantation, even though good functional sensibility was restored,[108] stressing again the importance of delayed sensory education which emphasized the retraining of central cortical functions like concentration, memory, and relearning.

Delayed sensory re-education consists of touching objects, both blinded and nonblinded, to appreciate further the differences in texture, size, shape, and consistency from different surfaces. The significant improvement that can be seen following this re-education can probably be explained by the increased cortical reorganization caused by increased neural activity in the postcentral gyrus that compensates effectively for the decreased local neural activity.[109–111]

Outcomes, prognosis, and complications

Outcomes and prognosis

The microsurgical success of toe-to-hand transplantations compares favourably to that of other free tissue transfers, with failure rates generally not exceeding 5% in most series in adult and pediatric populations.[47,112–114] In our series of 1734 procedures in 1553 patients carried out over a 20-year period (1985–2004) at Chang Gung University Medical College Hospital, a success rate of 97% was achieved *(Fig. 14.1)*. Success in toe-to-hand transplantations, however, is much more than simply achieving survival of the toe flap, and must be a cumulative outcome in terms of a mobile, painfree, and stable digit with good sensory feedback and aesthetic appearance.

Range of motion

In terms of range of motion, an average of 25° and 29° following thumb reconstruction using the great toe should be achievable at the metacarpophalangeal joint and interphalangeal joint respectively.[113] The trimmed great-toe technique generally results in an anticipated reduction of movement at the interphalangeal joint of 18°, although this did not seem to affect pulp-to-pulp pinch prehension.[71] In toe-to-finger transplantations, an average total range of motion of 50–60° is usually achievable for the proximal and distal interphalangeal joints.[54,115] If a metatarsophalangeal joint has been transferred to reconstruct the metacarpophalangeal joint, the expected range of movement should average 50°, or 52° if a composite joint reconstruction has been carried out via a metatarsophalangeal joint disarticulation during harvest.[12,83]

Strength assessment

In general, an average of more than 75–80% approximation to the opposite thumb has been reported for both grip and pinch strength following thumb reconstruction, in many instances exceeding the strength of its counterpart.[21,113,116] Independent strength assessment in finger reconstructions is more difficult to measure and is often dependent on an intact thumb function to produce a stable tripod or pulp-to-pulp pinch. The reconstructed finger is also often shorter and may not be accurately assessed using conventional methods of assessment like the traditional dynamometer or pinch meter. These instruments may need to be specially modified to conform to the length and profile of transplanted toes. Furthermore, restoring the prehensile patterns of the hand may be a much more valid measure of outcome and has been achieved in most series, especially following reconstructions for multiple-finger amputations and the metacarpal hand deformity.[8,25,74,117,118] In addition, from our series of toe transfers for isolated finger amputations, we have also found restoring the digital arcade and storage function of the hand to be useful both functionally and psychologically.[22,119]

Appearance and sensory outcomes

A major advantage of toe-to-hand transplantations is the replacement of tissue that bears a near-normal resemblance of what was lost. Both Chung and Wei[116] and Poppen *et al.*[113] found a much higher use of the reconstructed hand following toe-to-thumb transplantation as compared to its use before thumb reconstruction. With improved sensory recovery comes an enhanced appreciation of the reconstructed digits and also a better overall integration into the body. These improvements are largely dependent on a comprehensive sensory re-education program as described. Performing the toe-to-hand transplantation surgery within a month of the injury has also been shown to lead to better sensory results.[111] Overall, the average recovered two-point discrimination should not expect to exceed approximately 7–8 mm.[45,69,97,108]

Donor site outcome evaluation

Foot morbidity is completely acceptable after isolated harvest of the second toe[32,33,82] *(Fig. 14.15)*. In contrast, foot deformity appears to be more evident following great-toe harvest or combined second and third toe.[120,121] Despite increased dynamic and static loading on the first metatarsal head and heel, this very seldom translates into significant complaints regarding gait or appearance[59] *(Fig. 14.15)*. Previous advocation of the use of nonvascularized bone blocks to replace harvested metatarsals is no longer routine in our practice as we have found that the great toe and heel provide adequate compensation for avoidance of any problems with walking or takeoff. All precautions should be taken to ensure additional potential complications such as skin necrosis, hypertrophic scarring, or painful neuroma[122] are minimized. The potential donor defect should always be discussed in detail with the needs of each patient individualized with regard to lifestyle, hobbies, and concerns regarding appearance.

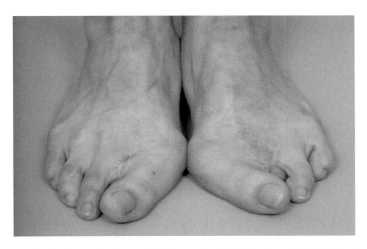

Fig. 14.15 Donor site after combined second- and third-toe harvest in the left foot and second-toe harvest in the right foot.

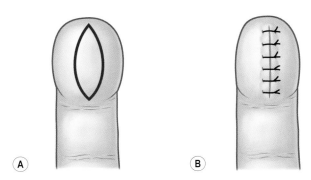

Fig. 14.16 **(A, B)** Pulp plasty technique.

Complications

The most common complication in the immediate postoperative period is vascular compromise due to vasospasm or arterial thrombosis. Emergency re-exploration of the anastomosis is warranted following failed bedside measures such as release of sutures, topical application of lidocaine, and fluid optimization. Additional anastomoses using another arterial pedicle may be required in certain cases, for example, combined toe units. Venous compromise is much less common and is usually due to preventable and correctable causes. Despite careful preoperative planning and early recognition of problems, around 3–5% still end up failing, possibly due to irreparable damage or inherent problems with the suitability of the vessels.[123,124] Once the cause of the problem is identified, a repeat toe transfer may be indicated with the use of an interim groin flap.[125] Other complications, including skin flap necrosis or wound-healing problems with resultant exposed structures, must be remedied as soon as possible to prevent desiccation of tendons or neurovascular bundles, which result in further complications from the injury. Longer-term complications may be directly related to the original injury or indirectly as a result of suboptimal reconstruction, often correctable by secondary procedures.

Secondary procedures

Despite meticulous planning and prevention of unfavorable results, secondary procedures are still required in a percentage of cases (14–20%) to improve the functional and aesthetic outcome of the hand and foot following toe-to-hand transplantations.[38,126,127] Revision procedures for functional improvement such as tenolysis, arthrodesis, and webspace deepening usually yield good results.[38] Flexor tenolysis is one of the most common secondary procedures described for most series and may be related to the methods of bone osteosynthesis or the severity of the original injury requiring a period of immobilization.[38,128]

Revision procedures for aesthetic improvement are usually minor, and aim to increase resemblance of the toe to the finger or thumb.[34,36,129] The most common procedure is a pulp plasty carried out under local anesthesia to reduce the bulbous appearance of the toe, although other procedures including scar revision and flap thinning may be required (*Fig. 14.16*).

Access the complete references list online at **http://www.expertconsult.com**

12. Wei FC, el-Gammal TA, Lin CH, et al. Metacarpal hand: classification and guidelines for microsurgical reconstruction with toe transfers. *Plast Reconstr Surg.* 1997;99:122–128.

   Metacarpal hand refers to the hand that has lost its prehensile ability through amputation of all fingers with or without amputation of the thumb. Functional restoration can be achieved by a wide variety of microvascular toe transfer techniques. When deciding which procedure should be used, careful consideration must be given to the level of amputation of the fingers as well as the functional status of the remaining thumb. In this article, a classification is proposed for the various patterns of the metacarpal hand along with guidelines for selection of the proper toe transfer procedure.

22. Demirkan F, Wei FC, Jeng SF, et al. Toe transplantation for isolated index finger amputations distal to the proximal interphalangeal joint. *Plast Reconstr Surg.* 1999;103:499–507.

30. Wei FC, Lutz BS, Cheng SL, et al. Reconstruction of bilateral metacarpal hands with multiple-toe transplantations. *Plast Reconstr Surg.* 1999;104: 1698–1704.

36. Wei FC, Yim KK. Pulp plasty after toe-to-hand transplantation. *Plast Reconstr Surg.* 1995;96: 661–666.

50. Wei FC. Tissue preservation in hand injury: the first step to toe-to-hand transplantation. *Plast Reconstr Surg.* 1998;102:2497–2501.

This article gives useful guidelines in the initial management of amputated digits, especially if a pre-emptive view of future toe-to-hand transplantation is to be considered and discussed with patients. The main recommendations outlined in this editorial emphasize tissue preservation, facilitating future toe-to-hand transplantation in terms of reconstructive options, functional and aesthetic outcomes in the hand, and donor site morbidity in the foot. Although tissue conservation is the main goal at this stage of treatment, this should not be at the expense of tissue viability. If in doubt about management issues, advice should be sought from the reconstructive microsurgery unit.

70. Wei FC, Chen HC, Chuang CC, et al. Microsurgical thumb reconstruction with toe transfer: selection of various techniques. *Plast Reconstr Surg.* 1994;93:345–351; discussion 52–57.

    This review looked at the established method of thumb reconstruction using different options. Selection of technique requires balancing the patient's functional needs, appearance of the reconstructed thumb, and donor site cosmesis. Based on their experience with 103 toe-to-thumb transfers performed over the previous 9 years, this paper attempts to provide guidelines for appropriate selection among the four most commonly employed toe transfer techniques (second toe, total great toe, great toe wrap-around, trimmed great toe) so that both optimal results and patient acceptance can be achieved.

83. Wei FC, Colony LH, Chen HC, et al. Combined second and third toe transfer. *Plast Reconstr Surg.* 1989;84:651–661.

    This study reported a 4-year experience with 26 consecutive combined second- and third-toe transfers to replace missing adjacent fingers in order to delineate the indications and technical considerations and to emphasize prevention of donor site complications. The surgical technique is described in detail. Combined second- and third-toe transfer is reserved for adjacent finger amputations proximal to the digital webspace with remaining fingers no longer than the small finger. Radial amputations are replaced with contralateral combined toe units, while ipsilateral toes are more ideal for ulnar amputations. When properly applied in selected patients, this single-stage microsurgical procedure can restore prehensile function, improve the appearance of the hand with multiple digital amputations, and preserve near-normal donor foot function.

92. Wei FC, Silverman RT, Hsu WM. Retrograde dissection of the vascular pedicle in toe harvest. *Plast Reconstr Surg.* 1995;96:1211–1214.

    A retrograde approach to dissection of the vascular pedicle in toe-to-hand transfer is presented, along with a simplified view of the vascular anatomy of the first webspace. This paper described the several advantages of this approach. First, the dominant vascular supply to the toe is elucidated early in the procedure, allowing for less unnecessary dissection of an inadequate pedicle. This also eliminates the need for preoperative arteriography. Furthermore, in cases where a lengthy pedicle is not required, retrograde dissection dispenses with harvest of a proximal vessel, which will not be needed for the transfer, thus minimizing donor morbidity.

107. Lin CH, Lin YT, Sassu P, et al. Functional assessment of the reconstructed fingertips after free toe pulp transfer. *Plast Reconstr Surg.* 2007;120:1315–1321.

109. Wei FC, Ma HS. Delayed sensory reeducation after toe-to-hand transfer. *Microsurgery.* 1995;16:583–585.

15

Benign and malignant tumors of the hand

Justin M. Sacks, Kodi K. Azari, Scott Oates, and David W. Chang

SYNOPSIS

▪ Benign and malignant tumors of the hand arise from distinct tissue
  types.
▪ The majority of these tumors are benign.
▪ Accurate assessment, diagnosis, and treatment will optimize
  clinical outcomes.
▪ Reconstructive procedures of the hand and upper extremity should
  be performed only after the diagnosis is confirmed and appropriate
  surgical margins are achieved.

Introduction

- Most tumors of the hand are benign, recognized early,
  and treated by excision.
- Ninety-five percent of hand tumors that do not involve
  the skin are benign.
- Malignant tumors of the hand can be divided into two
  categories: primary and metastatic. Primary tumors can
  arise from the skin (e.g., melanoma, basal and squamous
  cell carcinoma), soft tissues (e.g., sarcoma), or bone (e.g.,
  osteosarcoma). Metastatic disease originates most
  commonly from cancers of the breast, kidney, thyroid,
  lung, and colon.
- Appropriate evaluation, diagnosis, and treatment for
  tumors of the hand are required for optimal patient care.
  A careful history and physical examination will rapidly
  focus the investigation of a suspicious mass found in the
  hand.
- Magnetic resonance imaging (MRI) has become the "gold
  standard" to evaluate soft-tissue masses for malignancy.
  Computed tomography (CT) is preferred for osseous
  lesions.
- Incisional or excisional biopsy is required for definitive
  diagnosis in many cases.

- Surgical incisions must be planned carefully with
  definitive surgery in mind, utilizing a longitudinal
  incision in line with or parallel to a potential limb salvage
  procedure.
- Reconstructive procedures, in the setting of a neoplasm of
  the hand, are performed only after the final pathological
  diagnosis and clear resection margins are established.
- An understanding of both oncologic and reconstructive
  principles is required in order to achieve an optimal
  clinical outcome.

Basic science/disease process

Tumors of the hand can arise from the skin, adipose tissue,
synovium, tendons, cartilage, bones, muscles, fibrous tissue,
nerves, and blood vessels. The majority of hand tumors are
benign, most are recognized early, and the prognosis is typically good.[1,2] Malignant tumors also occur in the hand and
can be divided into two categories: primary and metastatic.
In addition, premalignant lesions such as actinic keratoses
and atypical nevi can occur on the hands.

   In this chapter, benign and malignant tumors are classified
and discussed by their tissues of origin. Understanding the
origin of hand lesions will assist in accurate diagnosis and
appropriate therapeutic interventions.[3]

   The management of hand tumors requires the hand surgeon
to function as both oncologic surgeon and reconstructive
surgeon. A complete understanding of both oncologic and
reconstructive principles is therefore required to achieve an
optimal outcome. The role of the oncologic surgeon is to eradicate the tumor completely, which can compromise both aesthetics and function. In contrast, the role of the reconstructive
surgeon is to optimize hand function. Balancing these sometimes competing goals can be challenging.[4]

   An effective strategy to evaluate, diagnose, and treat
tumors of the hand and associated upper extremity is required
for optimal patient care. A careful analysis of the history and

physical examination will rapidly focus the investigation of a newly evident hand lesion. The use of radiography (X-rays), CT, and MRI will strengthen the apparent diagnosis.[5] However, incisional or excisional biopsy will, in most instances, be the final determinant of diagnosis.

Diagnosis/patient presentation

History

A thorough history and physical examination remain the foundation of proper initial diagnosis. Questions concerning the history of the tumor are solicited. These include duration, changes in size or color, associated pain, and occurrence of ulceration. Pain can signify a malignancy or a mass that has encroached on neurologic structures. The sensitivity of the mass to cold or heat needs to be clarified, as the former typifies a subungual glomus tumor.[6]

Inquiring about risk factors for tumors of the hand will strengthen eventual diagnostic conclusions. The patient should be questioned about a history of cutaneous malignancies, extensive sun exposure or sunburns as a child, chemical and ionizing radiation exposure, and trauma or infections. The patient should also be questioned about rheumatologic conditions, such as gout, psoriasis, and rheumatoid arthritis.

The age of the patient needs to be considered when evaluating a mass in the hand. Certain masses are specific to certain age groups. For instance, bone cysts are typically seen in adolescents and young adults, whereas metastatic tumors in the hand are rare under the age of 50 years.[7]

Questions about previous biopsies or excisions will complete a thorough historical evaluation of the patient with a hand tumor. Pathology reports for previous biopsies or excisions will need to be obtained and reviewed. Prior operative reports will help clarify the diagnosis and optimize future surgical interventions in instances in which the current pathology is unknown.

Physical examination

The physical examination of the hand involves a complete examination of the skin, tendons, muscles, ligaments, bones, and neurovascular structures. An evaluation of the regional lymph nodes for adenopathy is the cornerstone for assessing the malignant potential of a hand mass. For example, adenopathy can be observed in epithelioid or clear cell sarcomas.[8,9]

An inspection of the lesion begins in the examination room. An adequate light source is essential to visualize the lesion's characteristics. Color and texture changes are noted, and an examination for ulcerations, erythema, and edema is performed. Transillumination of the mass can be helpful in distinguishing between solid and cystic etiologies. The lesion is palpated, and the mass size is appreciated along with its shape and contour. The mobility of the mass is assessed to determine whether it is fixed to underlying anatomic structures. Having the patient flex and extend the fingers and wrist will further delineate whether the lesion is associated with tendons or deeper structures within the joints. A complete vascular examination with palpation of pulses is required. If pulses are not palpable, Doppler ultrasonography can be used to define the vascular status of the hand and upper extremity. Allen's test is mandatory. Neurologic testing of fine and gross motor and sensory function is also performed.

When benign lesions are to be followed clinically, photographic documentation is an essential tool to judge the rate of growth over time. Photographs are also recommended for patients with multiple and subtle lesions.

Laboratory studies

Laboratory studies are helpful in determining the etiology of some hand tumors. A hematology profile can determine an infectious etiology. Serum calcium, phosphorus, and alkaline phosphatase levels are often increased in patients with metastatic tumors, and alkaline phosphatase is also increased in patients with osteosarcoma. An erythrocyte sedimentation rate assesses for inflammation; the rate is often increased in Ewing's sarcoma, lymphoma, and myeloma. An extremely elevated prostate-specific antigen level is specific for metastatic prostate cancer. In male patients older than 50 years with evidence of blastic hand lesions on X-rays, a serum prostate-specific antigen test should be performed. Although these laboratory findings are not specific for hand tumors, they can help focus the search for a diagnosis.

Imaging

Multiple radiologic modalities are available for imaging benign and malignant hand lesions and masses. Radiographs are not essential for most skin lesions. However, radiographs are required for very large skin lesions and for those apparently fixed to underlying anatomic structures based upon physical examination.

The plain X-ray is one of the most important studies for evaluating lesions and masses of the hand. X-rays are easily obtained and can evaluate a mass from multiple angles. The size of the mass can be inferred from X-rays. In the hand, a mass >3 cm in diameter should be considered potentially malignant. The architecture of the mass as it relates to the cortex of the associated bone can be determined rapidly by X-ray. Sharp cortical margins indicate a benign process, while a "moth-eaten" or destroyed cortex indicates a malignant process. Erosions and periosteal elevation on X-rays can signify a potential malignancy or an infectious process. Soft-tissue calcifications may signify a malignancy *(Fig. 15.1)*. Rounded calcifications with central lucencies can portend a vascular etiology.

Ultrasonography can be helpful in assessing soft-tissue masses. This technique is noninvasive and inexpensive. Ultrasonography can determine if a tumor is solid or cystic and differentiate between a discrete mass and diffuse edema. In many instances, ultrasonography can be used to guide needle biopsy.

Scintigraphy or bone scanning is beneficial in screening for skeletal masses. This technique is sensitive in isolating abnormalities, but the findings are not very specific for malignancy. For example, there is intense uptake with osteoid osteoma, a benign bone tumor. Bone scans are very helpful when searching for sources of metastasis in the workup of hand and upper extremity primary malignancies.

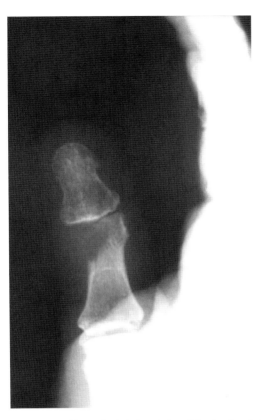

Fig. 15.1 In this proximal phalanx lesion of the thumb a destroyed cortex potentially indicates a malignant process.

CT is extremely useful for the assessment of bones and cortical destruction. CT scans have markedly greater bony resolution than standard radiographs. If bone involvement by the mass is equivocal on X-rays, CT is the next appropriate radiographic modality. CT also distinguishes calcification patterns from ossification and is superior in assessing periosteal versus endosteal reactions.

MRI is superior to CT for the evaluation of soft-tissue masses. MRI is better able to assess the intra- and extraosseous extent of soft-tissue masses. It has become the gold standard to evaluate soft-tissue masses for malignancy.[10] The MRI study should include T1-weighted, fat-suppressed T2-weighted, and short tau inversion recovery images. The contrast agent gadolinium can further enhance the visualization of soft-tissue tumors. An MRI study obtained with various views can clearly delineate the extent of soft-tissue involvement prior to operative intervention. A drawback of MRI is that it cannot reliably distinguish between benign and malignant processes. In addition, for MRI of hand masses, a dedicated hand coil is required.

The next logical progression in the workup of a skin, soft-tissue, or bony lesion is a biopsy. The accuracy of pathologic assessment is dependent on the type of specimen obtained. A frozen-section analysis can be performed to assess the adequacy of the tissue sample. However, the accuracy of frozen-section diagnosis is only 80%, whereas permanent-section diagnosis is accurate 96% of the time. The accuracy of core needle biopsy is intermediate between the two, at 83–93%.[2]

A biopsy can be closed or open. In a closed biopsy, a needle or trephine is used to obtain samples. Closed biopsy is useful for metastatic workup. However, tissue samples from closed biopsy are often inadequate for initial diagnosis.[11]

Open biopsies can take many forms: the type of open biopsy performed is determined by the patient's history, physical findings, and imaging findings. For all open biopsies, longitudinal incisions should be in line with or parallel to incisions that would be used in a later limb salvage procedure if the tumor proves to be malignant. If a tourniquet is used, the upper extremity must not be exsanguinated because doing so may cause spread of malignant cells into the lymphatics. Proper hemostasis should be maintained, and adjacent anatomic compartments should not be violated unless a radical excision is required. An important tenet is to biopsy all infections and culture all masses.[3,12] Chronic infections can masquerade as malignancies, and masses can result from subclinical infections.

In an incisional biopsy, only a piece of the lesion is removed. A longitudinal incision is made; if soft-tissue masses invade adjacent compartments, muscle fibers are split longitudinally. A piece of the lesion is then excised for pathological diagnosis.

An excisional biopsy removes the entire lesion and is potentially a single-stage cure for a benign lesion. Excisional biopsy is limited to lesions ≤1 cm.

Enneking developed a method for musculoskeletal tumor dissection based on the histologic grade, location, and extent of the mass. An intralesional dissection is through the plane of the tumor, whereas a marginal dissection is through the tumor "reactive zone." A wide dissection involves removal of the mass plus a margin of normal tissue but remains within a single compartment.[12] A wide dissection is performed when there is a suspicion of malignancy. A radical dissection involves extracompartmental resection.

Patient selection

All patients with a lesion or a mass of the hand must be appropriately evaluated. A history and physical examination are critical to determining what further workup is needed. Once the process needed to investigate the lesion or mass is determined, it is then the physician's responsibility to determine the appropriate diagnosis and plan the treatment.

Treatment/surgical treatment by tissue of origin

Skin tumors

Neoplasms of the skin can be benign, premalignant, or malignant. In addition, there are masses such as sebaceous cysts and cutaneous horns that can masquerade as tumors but are not true neoplasms and thus are considered pseudotumors.[13] For the majority of benign neoplasms or tumors, an excisional biopsy will completely eradicate the mass. For malignant skin neoplasms, such as melanoma, complete excision with clear margins does not always correlate with complete eradication

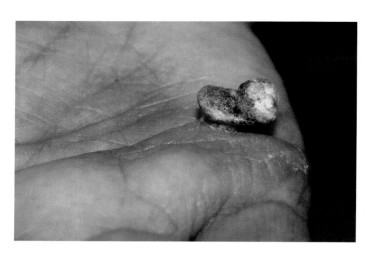

Fig. 15.2 Cutaneous horn. The lesion typically presents on the palmar surface of the hand. This lesion represents the typical keratin horn.

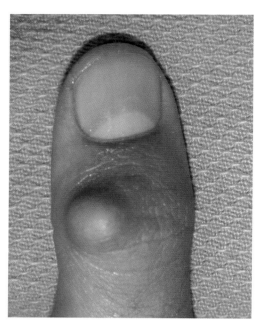

Fig. 15.3 Epidermal inclusion cyst. These masses, which originate from an invagination of epithelium, can follow trauma, injection, or an incision. The epithelium is internalized, resulting in subcutaneous keratin deposition.

of the skin tumor because of the potential for metastatic spread.[1]

Cutaneous horn

A cutaneous horn is an exophytic lesion that originates from the skin and is composed of keratotic material *(Fig. 15.2)*.[13] Cutaneous horns are located on sun-exposed areas of the body such as the dorsum of the hands and forearms. These unsightly lesions can interfere with function. They can occur in association with a variety of tumors, including epidermal inclusion cysts, epidermal nevi, fibromas, and pyogenic granulomas. In addition, cutaneous horns can be associated with both premalignant and malignant neoplasms such as actinic keratoses and squamous cell carcinomas. In fact, 10% of cutaneous horns are found in association with squamous cell carcinoma.

Cutaneous horns are treated by excisional biopsy with 1–2-mm margins. Incisional biopsy is not recommended for this lesion because of the potential for sampling errors.[2]

Epidermal inclusion cyst

Epidermal inclusion cysts are the third most common hand tumors *(Fig. 15.3)*. These masses, which originate from an invagination of epithelium, can follow a trauma, injection, or incision.[2,14] The epithelium is internalized, resulting in subcutaneous keratin deposition. Epithelial cysts are typically painless and most commonly occur in the digits.

Treatment of an epidermal inclusion cyst involves a complete marginal excision of the cyst and its wall. The risk of recurrence of this lesion following complete excisional biopsy is extremely low.

Sebaceous cyst

A sebaceous cyst is another lesion originating from the skin and is similar in appearance to an epidermal inclusion cyst *(Fig. 15.4)*. Sebaceous cysts arise from an obstructed apocrine gland, which produces sebum as opposed to keratin.[2] When they occur in the hand, sebaceous cysts are found on the dorsal aspect. Palmar skin does not contain sebaceous glands,

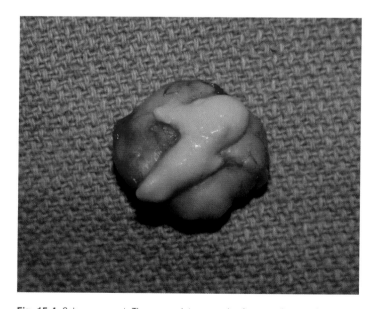

Fig. 15.4 Sebaceous cyst. These pseudotumors arise from an obstructed apocrine gland, which produces sebum as opposed to keratin.

so sebaceous cysts do not appear there. Treatment is similar to that of an inclusion cyst, and the risk of recurrence is low.

Verruca vulgaris

The human papillomavirus causes verruca vulgaris or common warts *(Fig. 15.5)*. Types 1–4, 7, and 10 have been implicated in the etiology of skin lesions involving keratinized epithelium. Verruca vulgaris presents as a rough raised

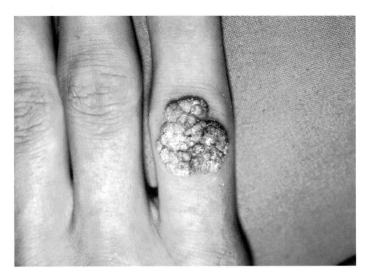

Fig. 15.5 Verruca vulgaris. This lesion presents as a rough raised surface commonly on the dorsum of the hand.

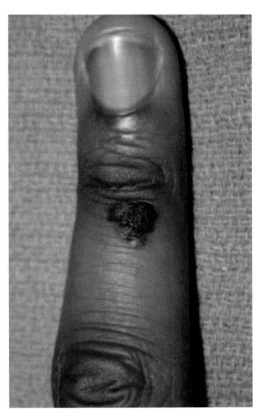

Fig. 15.6 Nevus. A benign proliferation of melanocytes, either acquired or congenital.

surface anywhere on the hand and is 20 times more common than the verruca plana or flat wart, which is found commonly on the dorsum of the hand. Verrucae vulgaris are often found at sites of trauma in the periungual region (such as from habitual nail biting). The typical course of these benign neoplasms is self-limited, with spontaneous resolution in 1–2 years. However, there have been reports of malignant transformation of verrucae vulgaris, most commonly when they occur on the mucosa.[15]

Treatment is instituted if the lesions become cosmetically unacceptable or if they interfere with hand function. The first-line therapy is topical agents such as salicylic acid, which results in cure rates of 70–80%. Cryotherapy is considered the second-line therapy for lesions unresponsive to topical agents and offers cure rates of 60–80%. Third-line treatments include immunomodulatory agents, lasers such as carbon dioxide and pulse dye, and photodynamic therapy. It is critical to be highly suspicious of lesions that do not respond to therapy, as they may be malignant. Excision is therefore recommended for treatment-refractory verrucae or to rule out malignancy.

Nevi

A melanocytic nevus or benign pigmented nevus is a benign proliferation of melanocytes *(Fig. 15.6)*. Nevi can be either acquired or congenital. The acquired form typically begins to appear 6 months after birth, and acquired nevi increase in both number and size throughout childhood and adolescence. Congenital nevi require surveillance because of the potential for malignant transformation. Nevi are classified by size as small (<1.5 cm), medium (1.5 cm to <20 cm), and large or giant (>20 cm). The lifetime risk for malignant transformation of giant congenital nevi is 10%.[16]

Common acquired nevi are defined by their anatomic location within the epidermis and dermis. Junctional nevi are found at the dermal–epidermal junction. These lesions transform into compound nevi when their growth extends into the dermis. Nevi found completely within the dermis are termed intradermal nevi. Acral nevi are typically found on the palmar or plantar surfaces. Longitudinal melanonychia refers to

streaking of the nail secondary to melanin deposits in the nail plate; these lesions can result from acral nevi involving the nail matrix.

Nevi of the hand and upper extremity should be evaluated for any clinically suspicious changes. These include asymmetry, border irregularities, color changes, diameter >6 mm, or elevation of the lesion. A useful mnemonic for these changes is "ABCDE." When there is any doubt about diagnosis, excisional biopsy is recommended.[17]

Keratoacanthoma

Keratoacanthoma is thought to be derived from the epithelium of hair follicles *(Fig. 15.7)*. This skin lesion closely resembles squamous cell carcinoma. However, keratoacanthoma growth is more rapid and central necrosis is more dominant. These lesions are typically found on hair-bearing regions. A keratoacanthoma begins as a small red papule and progresses to a large ulcerated mass. This mass is "volcano"-shaped, with a large central crater. The natural course of the lesion involves regression after a latent phase of 6 months to several years.[18]

Excisional biopsy is necessary to rule out a malignant neoplasm, most commonly squamous cell carcinoma. Treatment can include curettage if a benign nature is considered likely. Because the natural history of these lesions is to involute, classically they have been treated conservatively. However, poor cosmetic outcomes can result from this approach.

Muir–Torre syndrome is an autosomal-dominant disorder associated with multiple keratoacanthomas. This clinical entity is also associated with visceral malignancy, and the

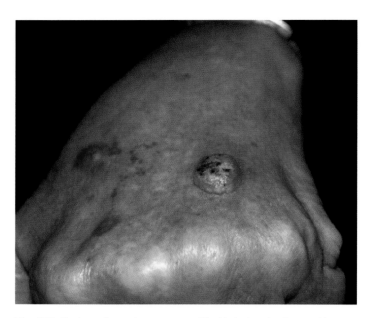

Fig. 15.7 Keratoacanthoma. In appearance, this skin lesion closely resembles squamous cell carcinoma. The lesion begins as a red papule progressing to a large ulcerated mass.

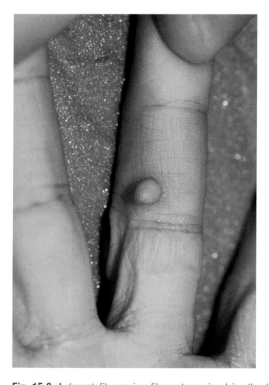

Fig. 15.8 A dermatofibroma is a fibrous tumor involving the dermis. These lesions form in young adulthood and are found more typically in females.

workup of patients with multiple keratoacanthomas should include colonoscopy and CT.[19,20]

Dermatofibroma

A dermatofibroma is a fibrous tumor involving the dermis *(Fig. 15.8)*. This neoplasm contains fibroblasts, collagen, and

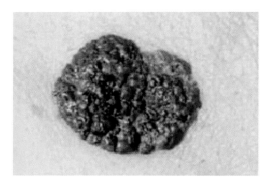

Fig. 15.9 Seborrheic keratosis. A benign neoplasm originating from keratinocytes, common in middle-aged and older patients and distributed widely over the body.

histiocytes. The clinical presentation is that of a firm, solitary mass of varying color. Dermatofibromas usually form in young adulthood and are found more typically in females. Excisional biopsy is performed to rule out a malignant lesion such as a sarcoma, squamous cell carcinoma, or melanoma.[21]

The malignant form of this lesion is a dermatofibrosarcoma protuberans, which is occasionally found in the hand.[22] While the metastatic potential is low, there is a potential for recurrence after excision. A wide excision with 3-cm margins is recommended and should include underlying fascia and muscle. The likelihood of local control associated with this procedure exceeds 90%, with the probability of regional or distant metastases being less than or equal to 5%. Adjuvant radiotherapy is indicated in the event that a patient has unresectable macroscopic disease.[23]

Seborrheic keratosis

A seborrheic keratosis is a benign neoplasm that originates from keratinocytes *(Fig. 15.9)*. Seborrheic keratoses are very common, typically present in middle-aged and older patients, and can be distributed widely over the body. Initially, they appear as a hyperpigmented lesion but later coalesce into a characteristic waxy, "stuck-on" appearance. The clinical conundrum with these lesions is that, although they are benign in nature, they may mimic melanoma. These lesions require a biopsy to rule out a malignancy. If a malignancy is not suspected, these lesions can be treated with cryotherapy, curettage, or excision.

Actinic keratosis

Actinic keratoses are premalignant lesions and in fact are the most common precancerous skin condition *(Fig. 15.10)*. An actinic keratosis presents as a rough, scaly, erythematous plaque found in an area of chronic sun exposure. The lesion is commonly tender to palpation. Histologically, this lesion shows dysplastic keratinocytes confined to the lower third of the epidermis. Actinic keratoses are the direct result of chronic sun exposure and are more common in fair-skinned persons. The potential for malignant conversion to squamous cell carcinoma ranges from 0.25% to 1.00% per year. Regression can be spontaneous if sun exposure after diagnosis is limited.

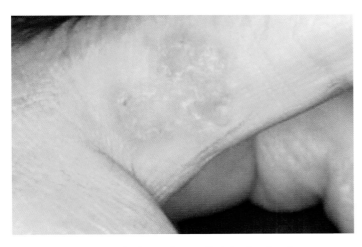

Fig. 15.10 Actinic keratosis. A premalignant skin lesion found on the upper extremity. It presents as a rough, scaly, and erythematous plaque found in areas of chronic sun exposure.

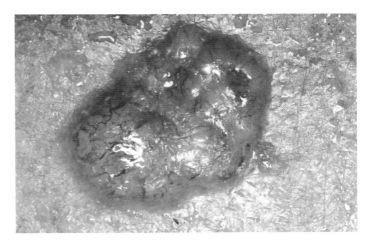

Fig. 15.11 Basal cell carcinoma. These lesions are malignant neoplasms of the basal epithelium forming insidiously but rarely metastasizing.

Treatment ranges from continued clinical observation to ablation. Cryotherapy can be used for isolated lesions. For more dispersed lesions, topical 5-fluorouracil, dermabrasion, and cutaneous peels such as trichloroacetic acid peel can be used. Newer reports have shown positive benefits using photodynamic therapy with porphyrin derivatives acting as a photosensitizer. Cure rates with this new modality have been reported as similar to those with topical 5-fluorouracil.[24]

Basal cell carcinoma

Basal cell carcinoma is the second most common skin malignancy on the hand and is the most common form of skin cancer *(Fig. 15.11)*. Basal cell carcinomas are malignant neoplasms of the basal epithelium. Five major types of basal cell carcinoma exist: fibroepithelioma, morpheaform, nodulo-ulcerative, pigmented, and superficial. The nodulo-ulcerative is the most common form, and the morpheaform variant is the most aggressive form of the tumor. The lesions form insidiously and rarely metastasize.[1,2,25]

Basal cell carcinomas present in sun-damaged areas. The middle to older age group is commonly afflicted. Clinically, the lesion is observed as ulcerated skin with pearly elevated edges. Treatment consists of excisional biopsy with 2-mm margins. The key is surgical resection until only normal tissue remains. Regular follow-up is indicated to identify recurrences and new lesions. Since there is a low likelihood of metastasis, no further workup is required.

Squamous cell carcinoma

Squamous cell carcinoma is the most common malignant tumor in the hand *(Fig. 15.12)*.[26] The tumor typically presents in late middle age or later. Usually, squamous cell carcinoma is found on the dorsum of the hand secondary to chronic sun exposure. Squamous cell carcinomas are pink or skin-colored and can present as firm hyperkeratotic lesions. Since there is a potential for malignant spread, it is critical to evaluate lymph node status by physical examination.

Etiologies of squamous cell carcinoma, in addition to sun exposure, include a history of therapeutic radiation, chronic

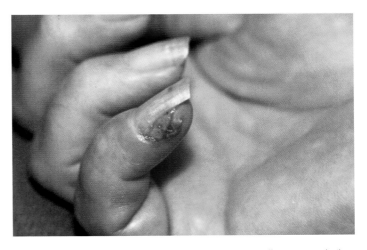

Fig. 15.12 Squamous cell carcinoma. The most common malignant tumor in the hand, typically found on the dorsum of the hand secondary to chronic sun exposure. It is critical to evaluate lymph node status upon physical exam.

inflammation, chronic sinus sites secondary to osteomyelitis, and immunosuppression. A Marjolin's ulcer is a squamous cell carcinoma present in a chronic burn ulcer. It is important to beware of nonresponsive subungual lesions mimicking fungal infections. It is essential to biopsy all chronic infections to rule out malignancy.

Treatment of squamous cell carcinomas ranges from electrodesiccation and curettage for low-risk tumors to excisional biopsy for high-risk lesions. Excision with 5-mm margins of normal tissue results in complete clearance of 95% of tumors.[27] Other studies have shown that wide local excision with 4-mm margins has a clearance rate of 96% and that 6-mm margins clear 99% of tumors. Metastasis is found within the first 5 years in 5% of patients with squamous cell carcinoma. This is in contrast to basal cell carcinoma, which typically does not metastasize. Long-term follow-up after treatment of these lesions is therefore critical to assess for recurrence or metastatic spread.

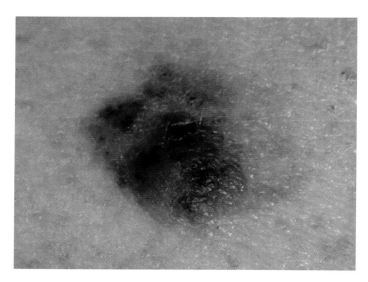

Fig. 15.13 Melanoma. A highly malignant tumor of melanocytes, melanoma may arise from atypical moles. One-half of these tumors develops *de novo* and is unrelated to pre-existing nevus.

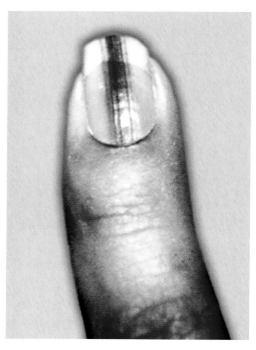

Fig. 15.14 Subungal melanoma. These lesions must be differentiated from hematoma and onychomycosis. Evaluation of lymph node basins must be determined clinically and pathologically in lesions of intermediate thickness.

Melanoma

Melanoma is a highly malignant tumor of melanocytes *(Fig. 15.13)*. Although melanomas represent only 5% of all skin cancers, they are responsible for 75% of the deaths from skin cancer.[2,28] Based on these percentages, the prompt, accurate diagnosis and treatment of these tumors are critical for the well-being of all patients who present with a suspicious skin lesion on the upper extremity. The typical presentation of melanoma is a pigmented mass with appearance changes (ABCDE; see above). Melanomas may arise from atypical moles, but half of these tumors develop *de novo* and are unrelated to a pre-existing nevus *(Fig. 15.14)*.[1] Acral lentiginous melanoma is a variant that occurs on the palmar, plantar, and nail plate surfaces.[29]

Diagnosis is established by incisional or excisional biopsy. Determination of the depth of invasion is a critical component of pathologic analysis. The Breslow system, which is most commonly used, reports the depth of invasion in millimeters and correlates with rates of lymphatic spread and distant metastasis. The Clark system reports invasion based on anatomic levels.

Treatment of melanoma *in situ* is excision with a 0.5-cm tissue margin. For invasive lesions <1.0 mm thick, a 1-cm margin is used. For lesions that are 1–4 mm thick, a 2-cm margin is used; and for lesions >4 mm thick, a 2–4-cm margin is used. The risk of metastasis is only 2% for thin (<1 mm) lesions but higher for lesions that are 1–4 mm thick (addressed below). It is important to examine clinically the lymph nodes that drain melanomas.

Lymphatic metastases from melanoma are believed to occur in an orderly, anatomic progression. The first node to which a melanoma metastasizes is considered the sentinel lymph node (SLN) and can be predicted by the lymphatic drainage pattern of the skin area where the tumor is located. By performing a biopsy of the SLN in patients with intermediate-thickness melanomas, the potential for metastasis to other nodes can be predicted. The SLN is identified at the time of tumor resection by lymphoscintigraphy and the use of dye.[30] Technetium-99m is given the morning of the operation, with surgery being performed 4 hours later after Lymphazurin blue is injected intradermally around the lesion. Next, the "hot" lymph node is searched for using a radioactive sensor and by visualizing the path of the blue dye. This lymph node, the SLN, is then sent for frozen-section pathologic assessment. If the SLN is positive, a full dissection of the draining lymph node basin(s) is performed. Consideration should then be given to adjuvant chemotherapy. No further treatment is given if the SLN is negative.

For thick melanomas (>4 mm), the risk of nodal metastasis is high (60–80%). Any clinically identified positive nodes are resected along with the primary lesion. If the clinical node examination is negative, SLN biopsy is not routinely indicated because this group will probably not benefit from locoregional disease control.

Subungual melanomas may masquerade as a subungual hematoma or onychomycosis. Typically, treatment of subungual melanoma is an amputation at the distal interphalangeal joint.[29]

Synovial lesions

Ganglion cysts

Ganglion cysts are the most common soft-tissue tumors of the hand and upper extremity *(Fig. 15.15)*. Ganglion cysts are mucin-filled structures associated with joint capsules, tendons, or tendon sheaths. The etiology of these cystic structures is

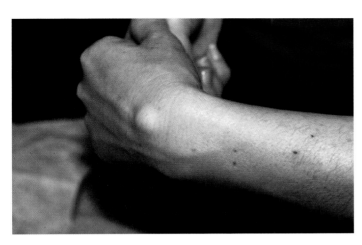

Fig. 15.15 Ganglion cysts. The cyst is a mucinous-filled structure associated with joint capsules, tendons, and tendon sheaths. The etiology of these cystic structures is presumed to be secondary to synovial herniation and trauma.

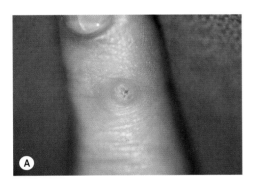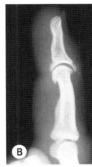

Fig. 15.16 Mucous cyst. **(A)** Ganglions found on the dorsal proximal interphalangeal joint associated with osteoarthritis are termed mucous cysts. **(B)** Excision of the cyst along with excision of osteophytes must be performed to treat this clinical entity completely.

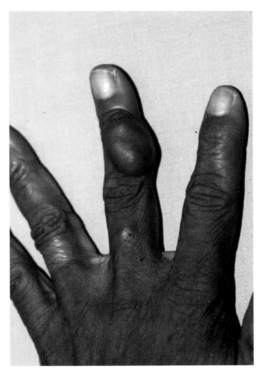

Fig. 15.17 Giant cell tumor (pigmented villonodular synovitis). A benign tumor containing multinucleated giant cells and xanthoma cells found in synovial fluid-producing sites such as joints, capsular ligaments, and tendon sheaths.

presumed to be secondary to synovial herniation and trauma but remains unclear.[31]

In the hand, ganglion cysts typically occur in the dorsal carpal region (60–70%) and originate from the scapholunate interosseus ligament. The volar carpal region is the next most commonly involved region, with 20% of ganglion cysts originating from the scapho-trapezio-trapezoid ligament. Ganglion cysts are also found on the volar retinaculum (10–20%). Ganglion cysts found on the dorsal proximal interphalangeal joint associated with osteoarthritis are termed mucous cysts *(Fig. 15.16)*. These are treated by excision of the cyst along with associated osteophytes. If atypical presentations occur or if clinical examination does not clarify a potential ganglion cyst, then ultrasonography or MRI can be helpful in determining a diagnosis.

A key point in the treatment of ganglion cysts is to clarify their benign nature for the patient. Patients often seek reassurance when confronted with this lesion. The natural course of volar retinaculum ganglion lesions is spontaneous resolution in almost two-thirds of patients. Aspiration of these masses results in complete resolution in the same proportion of patients. Aspiration of volar and dorsal ganglions in other

locations with fenestration techniques has improved results. However, recurrence is still observed.[31]

The definitive management of ganglion cysts is surgical excision with a cuff of retinaculum. For larger ganglions in the volar and dorsal regions of the hand, removal of the ganglion with its stalk and a portion of the cuff of the joint capsule is required. The capsule is not repaired so as not to limit motion. Arthroscopic removal of ganglion cysts in the dorsal region of the wrist is currently being performed. Success rates have been favorable, although long-term follow-up data are currently lacking.

Giant cell tumor (pigmented villonodular synovitis)

Giant cell tumors are the second most common soft-tissue masses in the hand *(Fig. 15.17)*. A giant cell tumor is a benign tumor containing multinucleated giant cells and xanthoma cells. Giant cell tumors are found in synovial fluid-producing sites such as joints, capsular ligaments, and tendon sheaths.[32,33] They are slow-growing and can have a mass effect on adjacent structures, at times indenting cortical bone. They are firm, nodular, and nontender. Most commonly, they are found over the volar aspect of the hand.

The treatment for this tumor is careful, complete excision. When dissecting these tumors out of the hand, the surgeon must beware of nerve displacement. The main problem with these masses is the potential for recurrence; the recurrence rate has been reported to be 5–50%. A malignant form of this tumor has been described but is extremely rare.

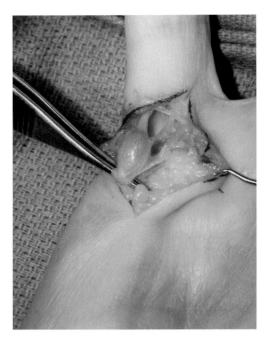

Fig. 15.18 Schwannoma/neurilemmoma. This soft-tissue mass arises from Schwann cells and is typically found on the volar surface of the hand and forearm.

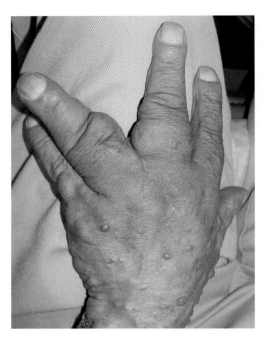

Fig. 15.19 Neurofibroma, a benign slow-growing tumor arising within nerve fascicles. When encountered in groups, von Recklinghausen's disease or neurofibromatosis should be considered as a diagnosis.

Nerve tumors

Schwannoma/neurilemoma

Schwannomas, the most common benign nerve tumors of the hand, arise from Schwann cells *(Fig. 15.18)*. The presentation of schwannoma is one of a slow-growing, well-circumscribed, eccentric, and essentially painless mass.[34] However, there may be a neurologic deficit or pain if the lesion is in the distribution of motor or sensory nerves. Schwannomas are mobile transversely, not longitudinally. They are typically found on the volar surface of the hand and forearm in the fourth to sixth decades of life.

The treatment for schwannoma is to "shell it out" from surrounding intact nerve fascicles, under magnification. The risk of a postoperative neurologic deficit is 4%. There are very rare reports of malignant transformation.

Neurofibroma

Neurofibromas are benign, slow-growing tumors arising within nerve fascicles *(Fig. 15.19)*.

The lesions appear histologically as diffuse growths of Schwann cells, fibrous tissue, and axons. When groups of these lesions are encountered, von Recklinghausen's disease or neurofibromatosis should be considered as a diagnosis.

The treatment for neurofibromas is excision; however, this is likely to require segmental nerve resection and nerve grafting based on the anatomy of the tumor in that normal nerve fascicles are incorporated into the tumor.

Malignant transformation of neurofibroma is possible, and rapid enlargement may indicate malignant transformation.[2]

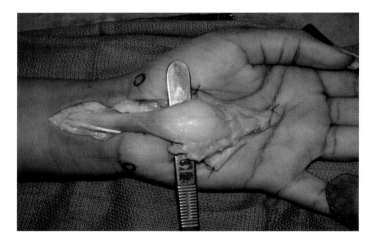

Fig. 15.20 Lipofibromatous hamartoma. This mass is a fibrofatty infiltration of the nerves, most commonly found in the median nerve. In a child who presents with carpal tunnel syndrome, this should be considered part of the differential diagnosis.

In patients with neurofibromatosis, malignant degeneration into plexiform neurofibromas can occur. A pseudoarthrosis, which is a rare condition frequently associated with neurofibromatosis, can occur in the upper extremity. This appears as "sucked candy" on radiographs.

Lipofibromatous hamartoma

Lipofibromatous hamartoma represents a fibrofatty infiltration of the nerves *(Fig. 15.20)*. This tumor is most commonly found in the median nerve. In a child who presents with

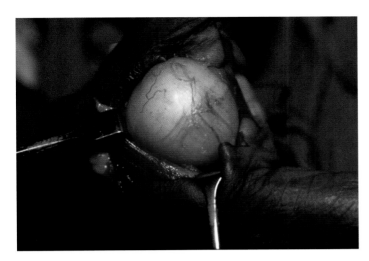

Fig. 15.21 Lipoma. This lesion is a benign tumor composed of adipose tissue. Commonly they are located subcutaneously or intramuscularly in the upper extremity.

carpal tunnel syndrome, lipofibromatous hamartoma should be considered part of the differential diagnosis.[35] Exploration of the mass reveals fusiform swelling of the nerve without invasion into perineural tissue.

Interfascicular resection is not possible and in fact is contraindicated for the treatment of this lesion. Instead, simple decompression is recommended. Gradual deterioration of nerve function can occur; only then should resection and nerve grafting be considered.

Fat tumor: lipoma

A lipoma is a benign tumor composed of adipose tissue *(Fig. 15.21)*. Lipomas can be located subcutaneously or intramuscularly. If present in the carpal tunnel or Guyon's canal, lipoma can lead to nerve compression. Lipomas typically have a long-standing history with very slow growth. Physical examination and history will invariably lead to the diagnosis. If imaging is warranted, X-rays will reveal lucent soft-tissue shadows, and MRI will show a signal intensity consistent with adipose tissue.

The treatment of lipoma is simple excisional biopsy consisting of a marginal resection. The well-defined margins of the tumor make excision not technically challenging. The primary indication for excision is size increase and mass effect (nerve compression).

The malignant form of this mass, liposarcoma, has rarely been reported in the hand. However, liposarcoma can be confused with a lipoma if encountered.

Fibrous tissue lesions

Benign lesions

The majority of the lesions of fibrous tissue found in the hand are benign. These include simple scars, hypertrophic scars, and keloid tissue. Hypertrophic scars are confined within the original wound margins, whereas keloids grow beyond these margins. Both exhibit increased cellularity and vascularity. Other benign fibrous tumors found in the hand include juvenile aponeurotic fibroma, desmoid tumors, fibrous histiocytoma, and Dupuytren's disease. The last of these constitutes fibrosis of the palmar fascia that leads to subsequent contractures of the fingers involving the metacarpophalangeal, proximal interphalangeal, and distal interphalangeal joints.

Sarcomas

Malignant fibrous histiocytoma is the most common soft-tissue sarcoma in adults *(Fig. 15.22)*.[35,36] It develops in the sixth to eighth decades of life. This tumor presents as a painless enlarging mass that is most common in the forearm. Treatment is wide excision or amputation. Neoadjuvant therapy can be administered to reduce tumor bulk and avoid amputation of the limb. A metastatic workup is required, with the most common site of metastasis being the lungs.

Synovial sarcoma is among the more common sarcomas in the hand and wrist. This malignant soft-tissue tumor occurs near tendons and joints and may invade bone. Its most common presentation in the upper extremity is that of a firm, indolent, painless mass on the dorsum of the hand.[8] It typically presents in young adults to middle-aged patients. Synovial sarcoma is a very aggressive tumor. Treatment is wide or radical surgical excision. Nodal status must be evaluated because of the high rates (50%) of metastasis from this mass. Adjuvant radiotherapy or chemotherapy is recommended.

Epithelioid sarcoma is the most common malignant soft-tissue tumor of the upper extremity *(Fig. 15.23)*. It most commonly appears on the hand and forearm in adolescents and young adults as a firm, slow-growing mass.[8] Epithelioid sarcoma can affect the digits and palm with proximal spread along tendon sheaths. It can be misdiagnosed as a wart or an ulcer. Treatment of epithelioid sarcoma is wide or radical excision. Nodal status needs to be evaluated as metastasis is typically to regional lymph nodes.

Chemotherapy and limb salvage surgery with reconstruction has become the standard treatment for sarcomas of the extremities, including the hand. Local flaps are often inadequate for repairing extensive defects resulting from tumor resection. Such defects may require free tissue transfer. The use of free flaps in reconstructing oncologic defects has enabled reconstructive surgeons to affect a paradigm shift in limb salvage. Complex free flap reconstructions are now routinely being used to preserve limbs that, due to locally advanced disease, would have been previously amputated. This has redefined the surgical management of sarcomas of the extremities. This shift toward limb preservation has prompted surgeons to re-evaluate the indications for amputation and thus improved patients' quality of life. In addition, tremendous advances in the multidisciplinary management of sarcoma have been made. Neoadjuvant chemotherapy and radiotherapy are now used to reduce tumor size to enable neurovascular-sparing resections that preserve limb function.

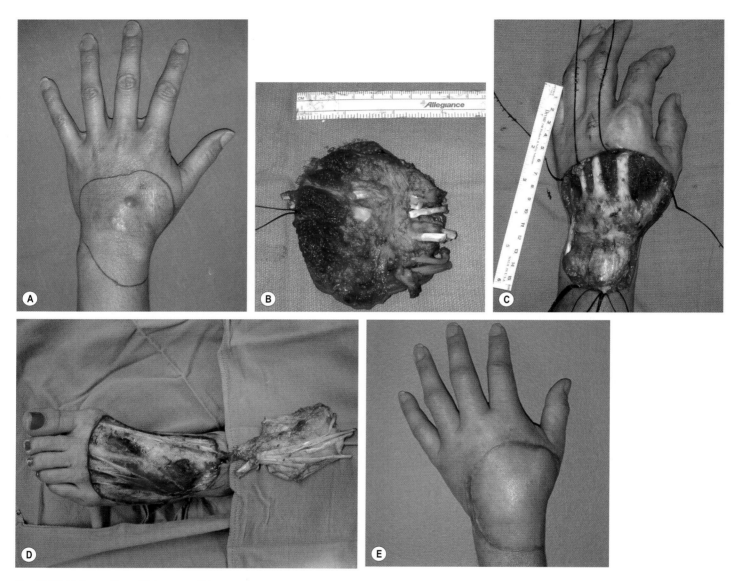

Fig. 15.22 Malignant fibrous histiocytoma. This sarcoma presents as a painless enlarging mass commonly found on the upper extremity. Treatment for this tumor is wide excision with mandatory metastatic evaluation. **(A)** Dorsal hand lesion. **(B)** Specimen revealing composite resection involving extensor tendons. **(C)** Wide local excision with proximal and distal extensor tendons tagged for reconstruction. **(D)** Dorsalis pedis flap elevation, including dorsal foot extensors. **(E)** Postoperative flap.

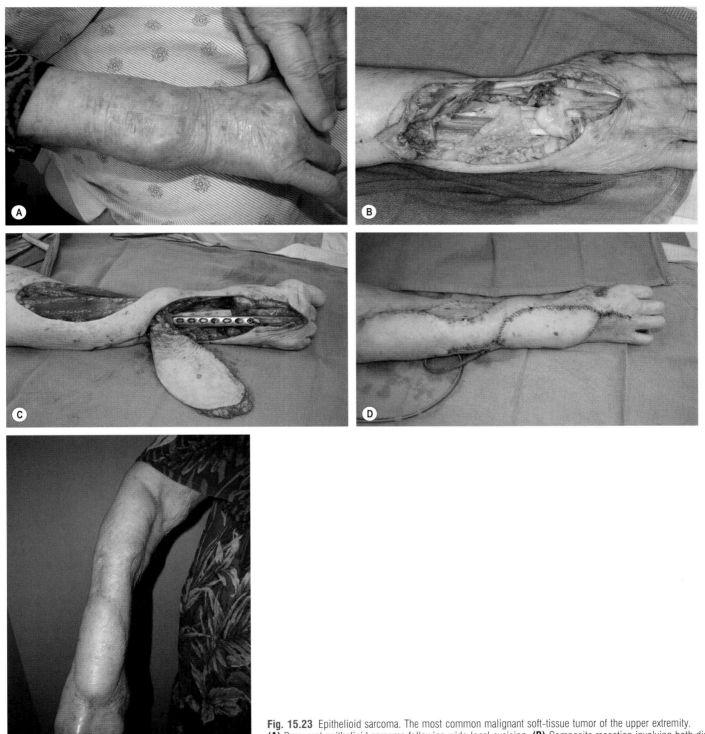

Fig. 15.23 Epithelioid sarcoma. The most common malignant soft-tissue tumor of the upper extremity. **(A)** Recurrent epithelioid sarcoma following wide local excision. **(B)** Composite resection involving both distal radius and ulna. **(C)** Bone allograft with internal fixation. Soft-tissue coverage supplied by a reverse radial forearm flap. **(D)** Intraoperative flap inset. **(E)** Postoperative result.

Vascular lesions

Hemangioma

Hemangiomas are benign capillary malformations. They can present as superficial, cutaneous lesions; as deep, cavernous lesions; or as a mixture of the two forms *(Fig. 15.24)*. Hemangiomas typically are not present at birth but appear in the first month of life. They are characterized by a rapid growth phase during the first year. The rate of involution is 50% by 5 years of age and 70% by 7 years of age.[37]

Treatment is typically observation, as most will involute. However, laser therapy, systemic steroids, intralesional steroids, and interferon have all been shown to have beneficial effects. When hemangiomas become symptomatic in adults, they require a marginal resection. Even after resection, these lesions can recur.

Infantile hemangiomas can be associated with Kasabach–Merritt syndrome *(Fig. 15.25)*. This aggressive hemangioendothelioma leads to a consumptive coagulopathy secondary to platelet trapping. High-dose steroids and vincristine have been used to treat this syndrome.[38]

Maffucci's syndrome is a condition characterized by multiple hemangiomas and enchondromas.[39] The digits in patients with this condition are short and angulated. There is a risk of malignant transformation of the enchondromas and hemangiomas into chondrosarcomas and angiosarcomas.

Vascular malformations

Vascular malformations are typically present at birth, in contrast to hemangiomas, and represent malformed vascular channels. Malformations are described by their location as capillary, venous, lymphatic, or mixed venous–lymphatic malformations *(Fig. 15.26)*. These are considered "low-flow" tumors. Treatment can be observation, laser therapy, sclerosing agents, or excision.[40]

"High-flow" vascular malformations have arterial or arteriovenous components. These masses represent a "time bomb" with the potential for rapid expansion. Treatment of these tumors involves preoperative embolization followed by excision.

Other vascular malformations seen in the hand are aneurysms and pseudoaneurysms *(Fig. 15.27)*. The former can originate from the radial, ulnar, or digital artery. Aneurysms involve all three layers of the vessel wall – the intima, the media and adventitia. In contrast, pseudoaneurysms represent a defect in the arterial wall contained by fibrous tissue.

Glomus tumor

A glomus tumor is a benign tumor of the neuromyoarterial apparatus, which is responsible for controlling circulation to the skin. Glomus tumors frequently present subungually *(Fig. 15.28)*. The classic triad of symptoms is cold hypersensitivity, intermittent severe pain, and point tenderness.[6,41]

Diagnostic workup for a suspected glomus tumor should include radiography and MRI. Radiographs reveal a "scalloped" osteolytic defect. MRI will commonly reveal a high-signal-intensity lesion. Excisional biopsy is curative.

Pyogenic granuloma

Pyogenic granuloma is a rapidly progressing vascular lesion *(Fig. 15.29)*. Pyogenic granulomas of the hands are commonly

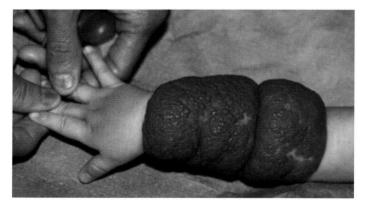

Fig. 15.24 Hemangiomas present as: (1) superficial in the cutaneous form; (2) deep, which represents cavernous lesions; or (3) a mixture of both. Not present at birth, they are characterized by a rapid growth phase during the first year. Expected involution is 50% by 5 years of age and 70% by 7 years of age, respectively.

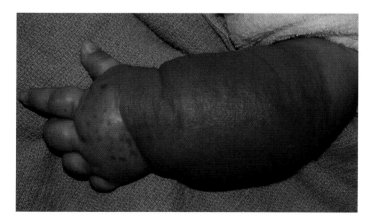

Fig. 15.25 Kassabach–Merritt syndrome. This aggressive hemangioendothelioma leads to a consumptive coagulopathy secondary to platelet trapping.

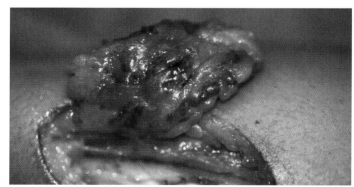

Fig. 15.26 Vascular malformations, p at birth, in contrast to hemangiomas, and representing malformed vascular channels. Treatment can be observation, laser therapy, sclerosing agents, or excision.

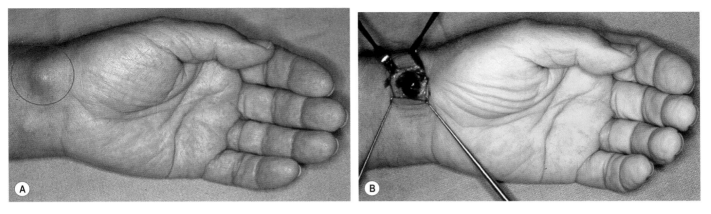

Fig. 15.27 Pseudoaneurysm. This represents a defect in the arterial wall contained by fibrous tissue as opposed to an aneurysm, which involves all three-vessel wall layers (intimae, media, and adventitia). **(A)** Radial artery psuedoaneurysm. **(B)** Radial artery pseudoaneurysm exposed.

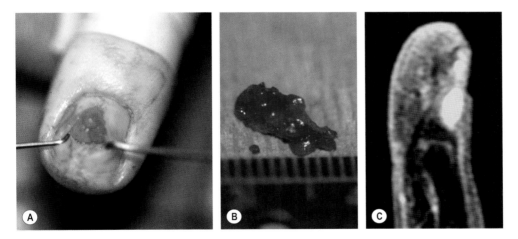

Fig. 15.28 Glomus tumor. A benign tumor of the neuromyoarterial apparatus responsible for controlling skin circulation presenting in a subungal location. **(A)** Glomus tumor *in situ*. **(B)** Glomus tumor excised. **(C)**. Magnetic resonance imaging scan of glomus tumor distal phalanx.

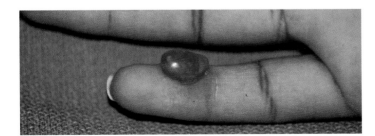

Fig. 15.29 Pyogenic granuloma. Rapidly progressing benign vascular lesion commonly found in the finger. Etiology is unknown.

found on the fingers. The lesion begins as a solitary "red" nodule and progresses to a chronically inflamed vascular lesion. The exact etiology is unknown.[40] Current beliefs are that the lesion begins with trauma followed by a subsequent subclinical infection. Treatment modalities range from excision with 1-mm margins, to curettage, to topical silver nitrate; however, all are associated with some incidence of recurrence.

Muscle lesions

Myositis ossificans

In myositis ossificans, benign ossification occurs in muscles and other soft tissues *(Fig. 15.30)*. The etiology can be traumatic. In the upper extremity, the deltoid and brachialis muscles are involved most frequently. Over time, the volume of heterotopic bone will diminish.

Leiomyoma

Leiomyoma is a benign, smooth-muscle neoplasm *(Fig. 15.31)*. Leiomyomas are rare in the hand. Treatment is excisional biopsy. If a lesion is clinically suspicious, biopsy is necessary to differentiate leiomyoma from leiomyosarcoma.[21]

Rhabdomyosarcoma

Rhabdomyosarcoma is a malignant tumor of muscle stem cells. Presentation is typically before 15 years of age. In the hand, rhabdomyosarcoma presents as a slowly developing, deep, painless mass. Rhabdomyosarcomas have been observed in the thenar eminence and between the metacarpals.

The treatment for rhabdomyosarcoma is wide resection or amputation. Regional lymph node dissection is usually necessary. Adjuvant radiotherapy and chemotherapy are recommended.[36]

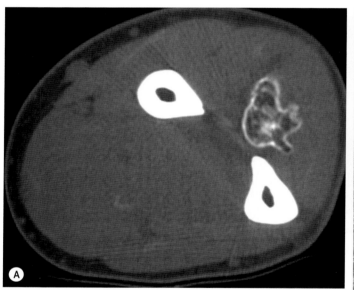

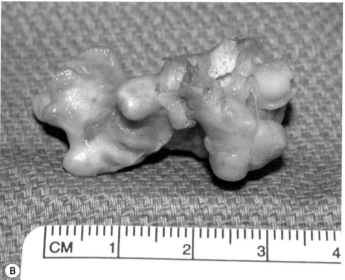

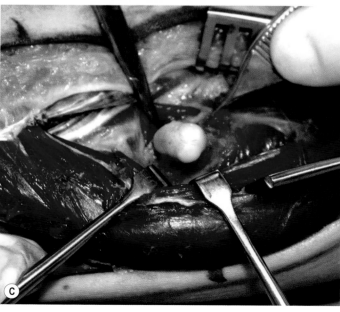

Fig. 15.30 Myositis ossificans. Extraskeletal ossification seen here in the upper extremity. **(A)** Computed tomographic scan showing extraskeletal lesion in distal upper extremity. **(B)** *In situ* lesion. **(C)** Excised specimen.

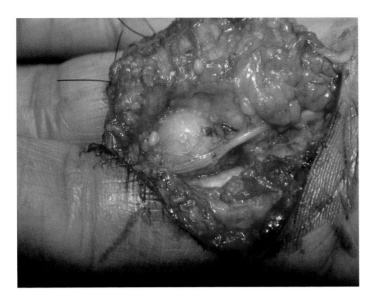

Fig. 15.31 Leiomyoma. A benign smooth-muscle neoplasm seen here on the velar aspect of the hand in close proximity to neurovascular structures.

Cartilage and bone tumors

Enchondroma

Enchondroma is the most common primary tumor in the bones of the hand. Essentially, it is a benign cartilage lesion within the bone. The tumor most commonly presents in the fourth decade of life. Typically, it arises in a proximal phalanx or metacarpal. The common clinical presentation is pain and edema secondary to pathologic fracture. The diagnosis is strengthened by radiographic patterns showing a radiolucent lesion with cortical thinning and "popcorn" calcification *(Fig. 15.32)*.[42,43]

Treatment can begin with observation. However, solitary lesions have a potential for malignant transformation to chondrosarcoma (<5% risk).[43] A healing fracture resembles a chondrosarcoma, so it is important to follow up these lesions radiographically. If a pathologic fracture occurs, it is recommended that the fracture be treated first, followed by curettage of the tumor. A bone graft or allograft is placed into the bone cavity.

Ollier's disease is a nonhereditary condition characterized by multiple enchondromas.[43] The tumors occur mainly unilaterally. Pain is uncommon unless there is a fracture. There is a 30–50% risk of malignant transformation, so it is critical to follow patients with Ollier's disease closely.

Osteoid osteoma

Osteoid osteoma represents a benign bone-forming lesion typically affecting the distal radius, carpus, and phalanges *(Fig. 15.33)*. These bone tumors rarely form in the hand (<1%). They present during the first two decades of life, and patients may complain of persistent pain relieved only by nonsteroidal anti-inflammatory agents. Radiographs reveal sclerosis around a central lucency.[44,45] Treatment can be either curettage or resection. There is a potential for recurrence if a lesion is incompletely removed.

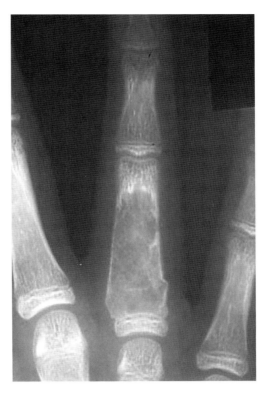

Fig. 15.32 Enchondroma. A benign cartilage lesion within the bone presenting here in the proximal phalanx.

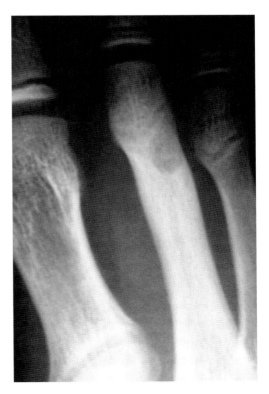

Fig. 15.33 Osteoid osteoma. A benign bone-forming lesion found here in the phalanges. Radiographs reveal sclerosis around a central lucency.

Osteochondroma

Osteochondroma represents the most common benign bone tumor *(Fig. 15.34)*. It develops during adolescence and enlarges during puberty. Osteochondroma is a benign bone prominence with a cartilage cap. Osteochondroma can present in the hand as multiple enchondromas or as an asymptomatic hard lump, which can cause a growth deformity (e.g., short deformed ulna or radius displacement). Osteochondroma can also cause a mechanical block to flexion from the angular growth disturbance.[42]

The treatment of this lesion is observation initially, with excision if there is pain or deformity. Bone grafting is performed for the correction of angular deformity. There is a 10–25% chance of malignant degeneration when multiple osteochondromas are present.

Solitary unicameral bone cyst

Solitary unicameral bone cysts are rare in the hand and usually present in the forearm. The cyst usually becomes clinically evident because of a pathologic fracture causing pain and edema. Radiographs show radiolucency in the affected metaphysis with a thin cortical wall *(Fig. 15.35)*. Treatment is curettage and bone graft.

Aneurysmal bone cyst

Aneurysmal bone cyst is a benign vascular tumor of bone, rare in the hand and usually found in the forearm *(Fig. 15.36)*.

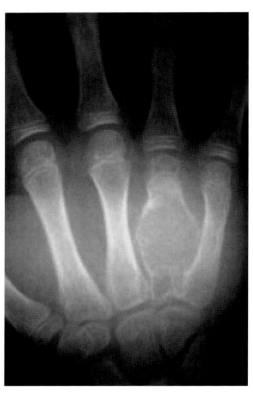

Fig. 15.36 Aneurysmal bone cyst. A benign vascular tumor of bone seen here in the metacarpal bone. Radiographs reveal a large radiolucency with a "blown-out" cortex.

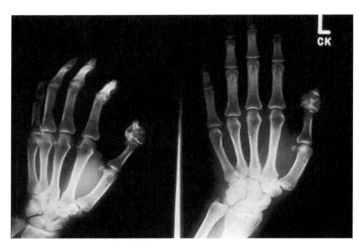

Fig. 15.34 Osteochondroma. The most common benign bone tumor. Seen here in the distal phalanx of the thumb, it is a benign bone prominence with cartilage cap.

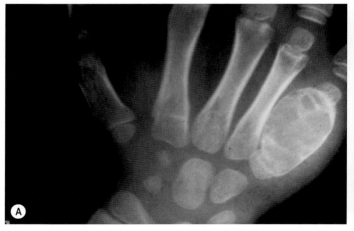

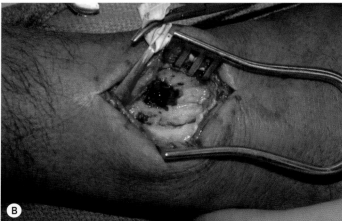

Fig. 15.35 (A, B) Solitary unicameral bone cyst: a benign cyst of the bone usually presenting in the forearm. This lesion, seen here in the small-finger metacarpal, shows radiolucency in the metaphysis with a thin cortical wall.

Growth is rapid and can be locally invasive. Radiographs reveal a large radiolucency with a "blown-out" cortex. Treatment of this mass is curettage and bone or strut grafting. Amputation has been used for destructive distal phalanx lesions. There is a high recurrence rate (60%) following curettage. Ray section will treat recurrences.[46]

Giant cell tumor of bone

Giant cell tumor of the bone is a distinct entity from a giant cell tumor of the tendon (*Fig. 15.37*). The tumor may present with joint pain and swelling. Pathological fracture is commonly seen as the presenting diagnosis in up to 10% of the affected population.[47] The neoplasm is multicentric, with a potential for metastatic spread, most often to the lungs (<2% of cases). The tumor appears in the distal radius up to 10% of the time, with other sites more commonly the proximal tibia and distal femur.[47] Metastatic workup is appropriate for this tumor secondary to the potential for metastatic spread.

Surgical treatment can include extended curettage, wide excision, or amputation.[48,49] Recurrence rates for extended curettage are significant.[50] However, when extended curettage is performed the cavity can be packed with either cancellous bone graft or methylmethacrylate cement.[50] In cases of wide local excision reconstruction where the bone is made unstable, such as the distal radius, reconstruction is required typically with an autograft or allograft.

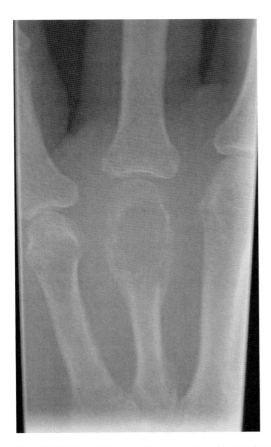

Fig. 15.37 Giant cell tumor of bone. A multicentric neoplasm with a potential for metastatic spread. Treatment of this mass is wide excision or amputation.

Reconstruction of the distal radius is performed to optimize the function of the wrist, specifically the radiocarpal joint. Surgical reconstruction can be performed with either an arthroplasty or arthrodesis involving the use of nonvascularized (tibia, fibula, iliac crest, or distal part of ulna) or vascularized (fibula and distal portion of the ulna) bones.[51–54] Reconstruction with vascularized and nonvascularized fibular grafting has been shown to give the patient improved function over arthrodesis.[51,55] However, distal radius resection managed with a radiocarpal arthrodesis through use of an intercalary bone graft stabilized with a long plate also has shown proven functional benefits.[56]

Healing complications related to the use of a bone allograft or autograft may involve malunion and nonunion of bone. In addition the graft can fracture, necessitating further surgical intervention.[52] In reference to distal radius reconstruction potential subluxation of the carpus, and degenerative osteoarthritis can lead to limited wrist movement and pain. Donor site complications related to autograft harvest involving the fibula, such as ankle instability, pain, footdrop, and paresthesia, might develop.[57]

Osteosarcoma

Osteosarcoma is the most common primary malignant bone-forming tumor. Presentation is a firm, rapidly enlarging, painful mass. Although rarely found in the hand, osteosarcoma can occur in the metacarpals and proximal phalanges.

Treatment starts with incisional biopsy. Local and systemic staging is then performed. This is followed by wide excision, or possibly finger or ray amputation for osteosarcoma in the hand. Neoadjuvant chemotherapy and postoperative adjuvant chemotherapy are recommended for high-grade lesions of the hand.[58–60]

Chondrosarcoma

Chondrosarcoma is a malignant cartilaginous tumor and the most common primary malignant tumor of the hand, although this site is rare. This mass presents typically in patients >40 years old. In the metacarpals and proximal phalanges, chondrosarcoma is firm, insidious, and painful. Radiographically, the presence of lytic lesions with cortical destruction and soft-tissue destruction differentiates chondrosarcoma from enchondroma.[42,61]

Treatment for hand tumors is incisional biopsy to establish the diagnosis and then wide excision or ray amputation. Local and systemic staging is critical.

Staging and treatment of musculoskeletal sarcomas

A sarcoma, as previously discussed, is described as a malignant neoplasm arising from transformed connective tissue cells originating from embryonic mesoderm.[62] These cells can include adipose tissue, bone, cartilage, muscle, and bone. Commonly they can present as an asymptomatic mass originating in an extremity. However, this neoplasm can occur anywhere in the body such as the trunk, retroperitoneum, or the head and neck.[62]

Table 15.1 Enneking's classification system of musculoskeletal sarcomas

Stage	Grade	Site	Metastases
IA	G1	T1	M0
IB	G2	T2	M0
IIA	G1	T1	M0
IIB	G2	T2	M0
IIIA	G1–G2	T1	M1
IIIB	G1–G2	T2	M1

Grade:G1, low; G2, high.
Site: T1, intracompartmental; T2, extracompartmental.
Metastases: M0, no regional or distant metastases; M1, regional or distant metastases.

Enneking *et al.* developed a classification system for the staging of musculoskeletal tumors.[63] This three-stage classification system is based on grade (G), site (T), and metastasis (M), using histological, radiologic, and clinical criteria. Grade 0 refers to benign lesions, G1 to low-grade, and G2 to high-grade lesions. Low or G1 lesions have a low risk of metastases (<25%). They are well differentiated, and have fewer mitoses and moderate cellular atypia. G2 lesions, high-grade lesions, are characterized by an increased rate of metastasis.[3] T0 represents a benign intracapsular and intracompartmental lesion, whereas T1 is an intracapsular and T2 an intracompartmental lesion. M0 represents no regional or distant metastasis and M1 represents regional and distant metastasis. Stage I represents a low-grade lesion without metastasis, stage II represents a high-grade lesion without metastasis, and stage III represents a metastatic lesion regardless of tumor grade *(Table 15.1)*. The Enneking classification correlates the tumor stage with the recommended excision margins depending on whether it is a benign or malignant mass. Based on the stage, the appropriate surgical margin is chosen to obtain appropriate local control.

Four types of surgical margin are typically described when removing tumors of the hand. An intralesional resection is through the plane of the tumor, leaving gross or macroscopic tumor behind. A marginal resection is performed through the tumor pseudocapsule or "reactive zone," potentially leaving "satellite" or "skip" lesions. A wide resection plane involves removal of the mass with normal tissue but remains within the relative tissue compartment. This resection can potentially leave "skip" lesion. Finally, a radical resection of tumor involves removing the entire intracompartment and extracompartment of involved and uninvolved tissue. An example of this would be a soft-tissue sarcoma of the hand requiring a radiocarpal disarticulation.

Oncological treatment for upper extremity sarcoma emphasizes limb salvage as an alternative to amputation and is determined mainly by the stage of the disease.[3] Treatment options for musculoskeletal sarcomas include chemotherapy, radiation therapy, and surgery. Since neither radiation nor chemotherapy alone or in combination has been shown to attain long-term local control of disease, surgical ablation is a critical step in the management of these neoplasms.[62,64] A

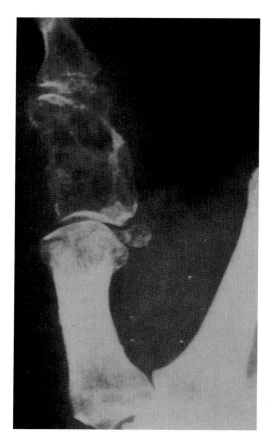

Fig. 15.38 Metastasis. Sources of metastatic spread to the upper extremity most commonly are from primary breast, kidney, thyroid, lung, or colon cancer. The distal phalanx, as seen here, is the most common site.

multidisciplinary team involving the medical and surgical oncologist along with an integrated hand surgeon adept at reconstructive surgery best handles the overall treatment of a sarcoma of the upper extremity.

Metastases

In the hand, metastases from tumors at other sites are rare. However, the most common sources of metastatic spread to the hand are primary breast, kidney, thyroid, lung, and colon cancers. The distal phalanges are the most common site of metastasis in the hand *(Fig. 15.38)*.[7] The symptoms and signs reported are pain, edema, and erythema. Radiography can reveal destructive lytic lesions. The diagnosis is confirmed by incisional biopsy.

Treatment of metastatic lesions in the hand begins by identifying the primary tumor. Once a primary tumor is identified, a systematic workup is undertaken that takes into consideration other metastatic lesions in the body. Treatment of hand lesions may include local radiotherapy for tumors that are radiosensitive, such as metastases from breast, prostate, and thyroid cancers. A digit or ray amputation can be performed to reduce the tumor load or effect a cure. However, metastasis to the hand is an ominous sign. Life expectancy in these patients is usually <6 months.[1,7]

Postoperative care

For most lesions of the hand, simple excision and closure will suffice for treatment. In these instances, a sterile bulky dressing with or without a splint will be required. For larger soft-tissue resections with concomitant reconstruction, appropriate volar or dorsal splinting is required. The patient is instructed to elevate the extremity for the first several days to alleviate postoperative swelling. If bone reconstruction is performed, appropriate postoperative radiographs must be obtained during the first week to determine if there is displacement of fixated structures.

The success of upper extremity reconstruction is quantified by limb function, sensation, cosmesis, and stable wound coverage. Appropriate postoperative splinting and aggressive rehabilitation to maximize long-term upper extremity function are critical to complete postoperative care.[65] The role of the upper extremity reconstructive surgeon is critical as the team-leader to obtain optimal clinical outcomes.

Outcomes, prognosis, and complications

Tumors of the hand are typically recognized early. They may originate from any cell type, and most are benign. Malignancy is uncommon but must be ruled out. A careful history and physical examination followed by an appropriate diagnostic workup will typically lead the hand surgeon to the correct diagnosis. When the tumor type remains in question, excisional biopsy will very often lead to both diagnosis and cure. The critical element when dealing with tumors of the hand is to follow a careful surgical plan that preserves function as much as possible while simultaneously removing the neoplastic process completely.

Access the complete references list online at **http://www.expertconsult.com**

1. Plate AM, Steiner G, Posner MA. Malignant tumors of the hand and wrist. *J Am Acad Orthop Surg.* 2006;14:680–692.

   Malignant tumors in the hand and wrist compose a wide variety of lesions involving skin, soft tissues, and bone. Squamous cell carcinomas are described as the most common, followed by basal cell carcinomas and malignant melanomas. Other soft-tissue malignancies are defined as less common and can present diagnostic problems. These lesions often remain clinically indolent for some time prior to diagnosis. Delay in diagnosis of these tumors can have morbid and fatal consequences. Bone malignancies involve both primary lesions, with chondrosarcomas being the most common, and metastatic lesions. Treatment of malignant tumors in the hand and wrist requires special considerations because of the critical function role in the upper extremity. It is critical for upper extremity surgeons to be familiar with the wide clinical array of these tumors, the appropriate evaluation necessary to arrive at a precise diagnosis, and the treatment plan that will achieve the most favorable outcomes, oftentimes requiring a multidisciplinary approach.

2. Chakrabarti I, Watson JD, Dorrance H. Skin tumours of the hand. A 10-year review. *J Hand Surg Br.* 1993;18:484–486.

   This was a retrospective study performed over 10 years. The incidence, histological type, and clinical progression of skin tumors of the hand that were referred to a regional plastic surgery unit were evaluated. Eighty-five patients were studied with 98 malignant or premalignant lesions identified. The majority of skin lesions were squamous cell carcinoma. Recurrence after excision was seen in lesions greater than 1.5 cm in diameter. The overall incidence of squamous cell carcinoma of the hand was seen to be five cases per million per year. Other skin lesions and tumors were noted to be rare.

4. Upton J, Kocher MS, Wolfort FG. Reconstruction following resection of malignancies of the upper extremity. *Surg Oncol Clin North Am.* 1996;5:847–892.

   A multidisciplinary approach using utilizing diagnosis, staging, adjuvant therapy, surgical resection, and reconstruction is described as the standard of care for upper extremity neoplasms. The reconstructive surgeon's involvement with preoperative planning is crucial for optimal functional and aesthetic outcome. Varied techniques currently available for both salvage and restoration of function, including local soft-tissue flaps, regional pedicled and vascular island flaps, and free tissue transfers, bone autografts, and allografts, were described. This article reviews both new and well-established reconstructive options after resection of upper extremity malignancies in children and adults.

7. Kerin R. The hand in metastatic disease. *J Hand Surg Am.* 1987;12:77–83.

8. Murray PM. Soft tissue sarcoma of the upper extremity. *Hand Clin.* 2004;20:325–333, vii.

   Soft-tissue sarcomas of the upper extremities are rare. It is critical for the physician to review the characteristics of these tumors and understand their biology. These lesions typically are misdiagnosed and treatment is often delayed. The most common soft-tissue sarcomas of the upper extremity are the epithelioid sarcoma, synovial cell sarcoma, and malignant fibrous histiocytoma. Limb salvage surgery is the standard of care for soft-tissue sarcomas in order to preserve upper extremity function. Following wide tumor resection, adjuvant therapies such as chemotherapy, external beam radiation therapy, and brachytherapy may lessen local recurrence rates, but their effect on overall survival remains unclear.

12. Enneking WF, Spanier SS, Goodman MA. A system for the surgical staging of musculoskeletal sarcoma. 1980. *Clin Orthop Relat Res.* 2003;415:4–18.

A surgical staging system for musculoskeletal sarcomas is presented which stratifies bone and soft-tissue lesions of varied histological type and by the grade of biologic activity, anatomic setting, and the presence of metastasis. Three stages – I, low grade; II, high grade; and III, presence of metastases – were subdivided by whether the lesion is anatomically confined within surgical compartments or beyond such compartments. Operative margins are defined as intralesional, marginal, wide, and radical relating to the surgical margin of the lesions, its reactive zone, and anatomic compartment. The system defines prognostically significant progressive stages of risk with their surgical implications and probability of survival.

31. Thornburg LE. Ganglions of the hand and wrist. *J Am Acad Orthop Surg*. 1999;7:231–238.
42. O'Connor MI, Bancroft LW. Benign and malignant cartilage tumors of the hand. *Hand Clin*. 2004;20:317–323, vi.
58. Daecke W, Bielack S, Martini AK, et al. Osteosarcoma of the hand and forearm: experience of the Cooperative Osteosarcoma Study Group. *Ann Surg Oncol*. 2005;12:322–331.
65. Saint-Cyr M, Langstein HN. Reconstruction of the hand and upper extremity after tumor resection. *J Surg Oncol*. 2006;94:490–503.

16

Infections of the hand

Sean M. Bidic and Tim Schaub

SYNOPSIS

- A thorough understanding of underlying anatomy and pathophysiology of hand infections along with the advent of antibiotics has all but eliminated mortality from most hand infections.
- The potential for considerable morbidity from hand infections may be lessened with the correct diagnosis of type and location of infection to allow effective and fastidious treatment.
- Effective and appropriate treatment of severe soft-tissue infections is based on prompt and correct diagnosis, early initiation of appropriate empiric broad-spectrum antibiotics, early aggressive surgical intervention, and pathogen identification with proper de-escalation of antimicrobial therapy.
- Infections that do not appear improved within 24–48 hours of intervention should have the treatment plan reassessed.
- Early and aggressive range-of-motion therapy should begin as soon as swelling, pain, and erythema allow.

 Access the Historical Perspective section online at
http://www.expertconsult.com

Introduction

One of the greatest impacts on the outcomes of hand infection treatment was the discovery of penicillin by Alexander Fleming in 1929. The advent of antibiotics for the treatment of infections decreased morbidity of hand infections considerably, and decreased mortality to almost zero.[1] Unfortunately, bacteria demonstrated resistance to penicillin *in vitro* as early as 1941, and by 1942 resistant bacterial strains were identified in patients. By the mid-1950s, nearly three-quarters of all staphylococcal species isolated from patients in large hospitals were highly resistant to penicillin.[1] Fortunately, alternative antibiotics were being discovered and developed, and continue to be researched today.[2]

The treatment of hand infections is based on a thorough understanding of underlying anatomy and physiology. The availability of antibiotics has changed these infections from one of potential mortality to one of almost certain cure, but they are not a substitute for appropriately indicated and performed surgical drainage.[2]

Basic science/disease process

Hand and wrist infections are frequently encountered in emergency departments. Paronychias-eponychias (35%), felons (15%), cellulitis (35%), and tenosynovitis (10%) are the most common types encountered. Inception of the infection occurs 60% of the time by direct inoculation of organisms through a variety of traumatic breaks in the protective skin layer: human bites (25–30%), drug abuse (10–15%), and animal bites (5–10%). How severe the infection becomes is largely dependent on the immune status of the host, the viability of the surrounding tissue, the location of the inoculation, and the virulence of the organism or organisms.[5]

Particular groups of patients with weakened immunity, such as those with acquired immunodeficiency syndrome (AIDS),[6–8] intravenous drug abusers,[9–11] diabetics,[12,13] those with chronic corticosteroid use, and alcoholics,[12] are all more susceptible to infections. Infections in these populations can be more challenging to diagnose for several reasons:

- Infections are often caused by diverse organisms, including those not usually considered to be pathogenic in otherwise healthy patients.
- Infection of the soft tissues may occur as a part of a more systemic infection.
- The degree and type of immune deficiency can attenuate the clinical presentation and findings.[14]

The likelihood of infection can also be heightened by local-tissue ischemia from traumatic injuries disrupting blood flow, and foreign bodies. The principles for adequate prevention of infection in traumatic injuries, in addition to appropriate antibiotic administration, include copious wound irrigation, adequate surgical debridement of devitalized tissue, and stable fixation of fractures, as required.[15]

Diagnosis/patient presentation

The initial evaluation of any patient should include a thorough history and physical examination. Determining a patient's age, handedness, and occupation can often lead to clues as to the etiology and risk factors for infection. The traditional OPQRST questions (onset, provocation factors, quality, radiation, severity, and temporal onset) can lead to important clues to the chronicity, severity, and depth of the infection. Previous injuries can also reveal critical elements in determining a diagnosis. In a careful review of systemic diseases, determine if there is a history of heart, lung, liver, or kidney problems. Also review the past medical history for contributing factors, such as diabetes, cancer, human immunodeficiency virus status, steroid use, and other immune-compromising diagnoses. In the past surgical history, previous hand and upper extremity surgeries may explain confusing physical exam findings, reveal a history of a transplant requiring immunosuppressive medications, or determine the presence of chronic conditions. A brief review of immunization history will help determine if the tetanus status is known and if a dose should be given at the time of evaluation. The patient's social history may also reveal clues as well as help determine a patient's in-hospital care. It may also reveal risk factors for methicillin-resistant *Staphylococcus aureus* (MRSA) infections *(Table 16.1)*.

When performing a physical examination, it is critical to examine the entire upper extremity. This will allow for identification of lymphangitic spreading, lymphadenopathy, and any concurrent infection sites. A systematic method of examination should be performed every time so as to minimize the chance of missing a clinical finding. Signs indicative of infections are many, including the traditional swelling (tumor), erythema (rubor), warmth (calor), and pain (dolor). More severe infections will often herald the Kanavel signs of flexor tenosynovitis (see below), signs of compartment syndrome, palpable crepitus, and skin necrosis. These signs and symptoms are imperative to recognize and require prompt, if not emergent, surgical treatment.

Imaging modalities can be helpful in the assessment of upper extremity infections. They can reveal subcutaneous emphysema, identify foreign bodies, rule out osteomyelitis, and serve as a baseline for future studies. Importantly, however, most hand infections are diagnosed by clinical determination.

Hints and tips

The treatment plan for all hand infections should follow the four following principles:

1. Infections should be treated with rest, elevation, and immobilization
2. Infected tissue requires debridement and all closed-space infections must be adequately drained
3. Appropriate type and amount of antibiotics for the given clinical situation must be administered
4. As soon as pain, swelling, and erythema subside enough to allow it, hand therapy needs to begin

---

If the hand does not improve within 24–48 hours, then the treatment plan needs to be reassessed.[18] Prompt and correct diagnosis of type and location of infection is crucial, as is the timely instigation of the appropriate intervention in order to prevent the potential disastrous consequences of the inflammation and scarring that can follow these types of infections.[16,17]

The most common bacteria encountered in hand infections are *Staphylococcus aureus*, *Streptococcus* and Gram-negative species.[18] The principal organism in 50–80% of infections is *Staphylococcus*. Gram-positive organisms are usually responsible for industrial and home-acquired injuries. Intravenous drug use, bite injuries, severe farm injuries, and those found in diabetics are usually polymicrobial and can include Gram-positive, Gram-negative, and anaerobic species. Human bite infections usually have alpha-hemolytic *Streptococcus* and *Staphylococcus aureus*, although *Eikenella corrodens* is isolated in one-third of victims. Animal bite and scratch wounds will commonly harbor *Pasteurella multocida*. Chronic indolent infections are suggestive of fungal or atypical mycobacterial infections.[16,18,19]

Infections should be routinely sent for aerobic and anaerobic cultures and Gram stain to direct therapy. The history of the infection can help direct other cultures and stains. The Ziehl–Neelsen stain illuminates acid-fast bacilli for the diagnosis of *Mycobacterium tuberculosis*. All *Mycobacterium* and *Nocardia* species are potentially acid-fast, so a positive smear is not pathognomonic for tuberculosis. Also, these organisms are fastidious, so false negatives are common. Multiple tissue samples grown with cultures under specific temperature conditions and cultures at 28–32°C in Lowenstein–Jensen medium for 3–6 weeks are necessary for atypical mycobacteria.[16,19] Fungal infections can be diagnosed with potassium hydroxide

---

Table 16.1 Risk factors for community-associated methicillin-resistant *Staphylococcus aureus* (MRSA) skin and soft-tissue infections

Persons at risk for skin and soft-tissue infections caused by community-associated MRSA

- Household contacts of a patient who has proven community-associated MRSA infection
- Children
- Day care center contacts of hospitalized patients who have MRSA infections
- Men who have sex with men
- Soldiers
- Incarcerated persons
- Athletes, particularly those involved in contact sports
- Native Americans
- Pacific Islanders
- Persons with a previous community-associated MRSA infection
- Intravenous drug users

(Reproduced from Napolitano LM. Severe soft tissue infections. Infect Dis Clin North Am 2009;23:571–591.)

Table 16.2 **Classification of severe skin and soft-tissue infections by the US Food and Drug Administration**

Uncomplicated
Superficial infections, such as: • Simple abscesses   • Impetiginous lesions   • Furuncles   • Cellulitis   • Can be treated by surgical incision alone
Complicated
Deep soft tissue, requires significant surgical intervention   • Infected ulcers   • Infected burns   • Major abscesses   • Significant underlying disease state that complicates response to treatment
(Reproduced from Napolitano LM. Severe soft tissue infections. Infect Dis Clin North Am 2009;23:571–591.)

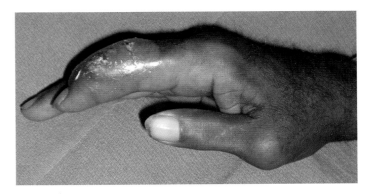

Fig. 16.1 Gout tophus involving the index finger.

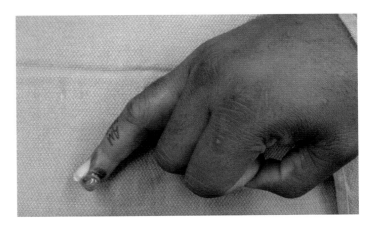

Fig. 16.2 Pyogenic granuloma on the fingertip.

preparations from skin scrapings from the periphery of lesions.[20] Tzanck smears may be useful in diagnosing herpes simplex virus infections.[21] Antibiotic therapy should only be delayed as long as necessary to obtain cultures and Gram stains.[16]

Classification of infections

Several methods of classifying infections have been proposed. The most common divides infections into complicated and uncomplicated and was developed by the US Food and Drug Administration (FDA) for pharmaceutical companies to categorize skin and soft-tissue infections (SSTI) during clinical trials *(Table 16.2)*. The Infectious Disease Society of America developed practice guidelines for the diagnosis and management of SSTIs, but they do not utilize the FDA categorization. The guidelines are described in reference to the specific disease entity, the mechanism of injury, or host factors.

Mimicks of infection

It is important to be able to distinguish infectious and noninfectious forms of inflammation in the upper extremity. The treatments are obviously different, and applying the wrong treatment can lead to morbidity, even mortality.

Gout

Gout, the most common of the crystalline deposition diseases, is also the most likely to be misdiagnosed as an infection in the upper limb *(Fig. 16.1)*. Gout can be a primary metabolic disease or may present as a secondary manifestation of another primary disease process, such as myeloproliferative or renal disease.[22] In acute cases of gout the hand may have swelling, erythema, pain with motion and, occasionally, fever, especially if secondarily infected. It is not typical, but the hand and upper extremity may be the initial presenting ground for the diagnosis of gout. The diagnosis is made by aspiration or procurement of the crystals from the

tissue. The treatment is dependent on severity, and may include splinting, oral anti-inflammatory medications, colchicine, and in select cases, surgical extirpation of tophaceous material.

Pseudogout

Pseudogout (calcium pyrophosphate deposition disease) is often seen with aging, and most frequently involves the wrist. Although uncommon, the acute inflammatory reaction seen in the wrist can be mistaken for an acute infection. The diagnosis is made by joint aspiration and evaluation of the synovial fluid for crystals using a polarizing microscope.

Pyogenic granuloma

Pyogenic granuloma is a proliferative tissue in the hand that consists of inflammatory cells and exuberant granulation tissue. It is reddish, friable, and bleeds easily *(Fig. 16.2)*. It is usually found following a penetrating injury that fails to heal. It may be treated with silver nitrate or surgical excision for larger lesions.

Pyoderma gangrenosum

This is a rare skin lesion that starts as a small, painful ulcer. The central region becomes necrotic and spreads in a centrifugal pattern with increasing peripheral creep. The lesion is associated with an underlying systemic disease process, most commonly ulcerative colitis, but may also be seen with Crohn's disease, carcinoid syndrome, polyarteritis nodosa, rheumatoid arthritis, and diabetes mellitus. The lesions are treated conservatively with local wound care. Surgical excision is contraindicated as it can lead to additional problems. The lesion has a very characteristic appearance *(Fig. 16.3)*.

Brown recluse spider bite

Brown recluse spiders (genus *Loxosceles*), endemic to the Midwest and southeastern US, are identified by the violin-shaped pattern on the back of their cephalothorax. The initial bite is usually trivial-appearing; however, the area of injury may progress to a varying degree, from simple pruritus to full-thickness tissue necrosis. A severe systemic reaction, known as loxoscelism, is a rare life-threatening systemic symptom that can occur after a brown recluse spider envenomation and may include pyoderma gangrenosum, intravascular hemolysis, renal failure, pulmonary edema, and systemic toxicity. Because the initial injury is not usually witnessed, one should have a high index of suspicion with a history of working around warm, dark, dry environments. Most brown recluse spider bites can be treated with rest, ice, compression and elevation and will heal without further treatment. The true benefit of adjunctive therapy, such as dapsone, hyperbaric oxygen, and electric shock therapy, have also been called into question.[23,24]

Granuloma annulare

Granuloma annulare is an idiopathic illness that is self-limited and usually resolves within 2 years. It most commonly presents on the hands and feet. The differential diagnosis includes primary dermatoses and chronic infections, such as tuberculosis, secondary syphilis, and sarcoidosis.

Rheumatoid arthritis

Rheumatoid arthritis can cause an intense inflammatory reaction that is easily mistaken for an acute infection, particularly in a patient not yet diagnosed with the disease. More likely, however, is secondary infection of an inflamed rheumatoid

focus. Joint aspiration is the best method to differentiate the two.

Types of infection

Cellulitis

Cellulitis is characterized by a spreading diffuse hyperemia and edema of skin and subcutaneous tissue with infiltration of leukocytes. It is often accompanied by acute lymphangitis. Cases of cellulitis associated with abscesses, carbuncles, or furuncles are most often caused by *Staphylococcus aureus*. Diffuse cellulitis, or cellulitis without a defined entry point, is most commonly seen with streptococcal infections. Other questions to include in the history should center on recent physical activities or traumas, water and travel exposures, and bites by insects, animals, and humans.[25] Treatment for uncomplicated cases of cellulitis include a first-generation cephalosporin, unless it is common in the community to have resistance to these agents. For penicillin-allergic patients, clindamycin or vancomycin is a good choice. If a lack of clinical response is noted, resistant strains, unusual organisms, or a deeper infection should be suspected. In those patients who are becoming increasingly ill, toxic shock syndrome, myonecrosis, or necrotizing fasciitis should be considered.[20]

Paronychia

The significance of nail loss or deformity can be both aesthetic and functional. It is, therefore, important for those treating hand conditions to understand the anatomy and physiology of the fingertip and its relationship to the nail in order to provide optimum care[26] *(Fig. 16.4)*.

The paronychium is the fold on each lateral side of the nail where the nail forms a curve into the fingertip. The junction of the nail bed and the skin of the finger occurs in this area. An infection along this fold or under the edge of the nail is known as a paronychia. Paronychial infections can be either acute or chronic. Acute infections are usually associated with some form of trauma, either direct or indirect. Acute paronychia is the most common form of hand infection, comprising 30% of all septic hand infections. Paronychia is a result of

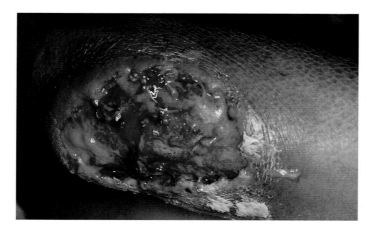

Fig. 16.3 Pyoderma gangrenosum of the elbow. (Courtesy of Yale Residents' Slide Collection. Reproduced from Bolognia JB, Jorizzo JJ, Rapini RP. Dermatology, 2nd edition. Elsevier, 2007.)

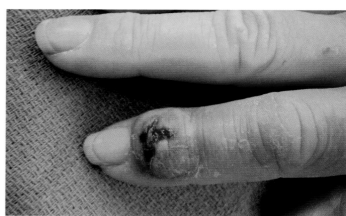

Fig. 16.4 Acute paronychia.

bacterial inoculation of the space between the nail fold and the nail and any violation of the nail vest, which serves as a waterproof nail sealant, can provide a portal of entry for bacteria. Meat handlers and haircutters are particularly prone to this type of infection. The index finger and thumb are most commonly involved, and the diagnosis has been associated commonly with nail biting and manicures. Most acute cases of paronychia are caused by staphylococcal infections. The infection usually starts on one paronychium, but with time can progress to the eponychial fold and then to the opposite paronychium ("runaround" infection). When the infection involves one lateral nail fold and the eponychium, it is termed an eponychia. Purulence buildup can eventually result in elevation of the nail off the nail matrix.

Reiter's syndrome, psoriasis, and herpetic whitlow can all present with symptoms similar to an acute paronychia. Reiter's and psoriasis can usually be ruled out on history alone. Herpetic whitlow usually has a prodrome of pain prior to advent of a single or multiple vesicles in a honeycomb pattern along the nail fold. This diagnosis should be suspected in patients with recurrent acute paronychial infections. Diagnosis can be confirmed by viral culture or Tzanck smear. Herpetic whitlow should not be treated with incision and drainage, but rather with topical or systemic antivirals.

In the early stages of this infection, warm soaks with systemic oral antibiotic and rest of the affected hand can be effective. In the presence of superficial abscess, the thin layer over the abscess can be unroofed without anesthesia. The most superficial portion of the abscess should be the site of drainage. If the infection is more extensive, such as a runaround abscess, surgical decompression should occur under digital tourniquet and digital block. If the infection affects the finger deep to the nail, that portion of the nail should be removed. When the entire nail is involved, the entire nail plate should be removed as pressure necrosis can result in damage to the germinal matrix and temporary or permanent loss of nail growth.[27]

Chronic paronychia can result from long-standing acute infection and is also common in patients with diabetes mellitus or hands exposed to prolonged moisture. The infection has generally been present for at least 6 weeks to be considered chronic. Certain systemic drugs are also associated with chronic paronychia, such as protease inhibitors, retinoids, cetuximab (Erbitux) and an antiepidermal growth factor receptor antibody used against solid tumors. The infectious agent in chronic paronychia is often *Candida albicans*. The presentation of chronic paronychia is similar to acute paronychia with erythema, swelling, and tenderness of the nail fold. There may also be retraction of the eponychial fold, and pus may form along the paronychium. One or more nails may be affected, and the nail plate usually becomes thickened and discolored with distinct transverse ridges.

Chronic paronychia is most commonly treated by eponychial marsupialization. This is performed under digital tourniquet and block. A symmetric crescent-shaped area of the eponychium is excised starting about 1 mm proximal to the distal eponychial fold and extending proximally for 3–5 mm. The tissue is removed down to the level of the germinal matrix, but the matrix should not be removed. The wound is left open to heal by secondary intention. If a nail deformity is seen, it may be beneficial to remove the nail as this is reported to improve the cure rate and prevent recurrence.[28]

Felon

A felon is a distinct infection affecting only the pulp of the fingertip. It is a subcutaneous abscess of the closed spaces created by the multiple vertical fibrous septa. The natural history of felons usually starts with penetrating trauma to the distal finger *(Fig. 16.5)*.

After inoculation of the bacteria, an abscess forms, and the subsequent inflammation of the noncompliant pulp spaces results in increased pressure and subsequent vascular congestion and impairment. If left untreated, tissue necrosis then follows and secondary infections of surrounding structures can occur, such as decompression into the flexor tendon sheath, distal phalangeal osteomyelitis, or rupture of the overlying skin. The characteristic findings of this diagnosis are the rapid onset of swelling and throbbing pain. The swelling does not extend proximal to the distal interphalangeal joint crease unless surrounding structures are involved, as in long-standing cases. *S. aureus* is the most common organism associated with felons, although other organisms are being encountered with increased frequency, especially in immuno-compromised patients.

The longitudinal palmar incision described by Kilgore[21] is a method of felon drainage that leaves a thin, fine, and painless scar. It also preserves the integrity of the palmar pad and minimizes the risk to the digital nerves and vessels. It is the preferred method when a sinus tract is present. The incision extends to 3 mm distal to the distal interphalangeal joint flexion crease proximally, and to the extent of the underlying phalanx distally. The blade extends through the dermis, and the underlying soft tissue is dissected bluntly with a small hemostat. The necrotic tissue can be excised and the underlying abscess irrigated and drained.

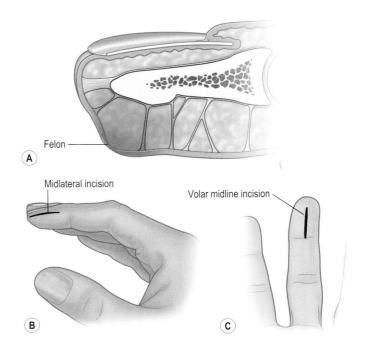

Fig. 16.5 Anatomy of a felon and options for felon incisions.

The wound is irrigated and packed with a sterile gauze. The affected digit should be elevated for at least 48 hours, at which time the gauze is removed and the wound evaluated for continued infection. Some form of soaking is recommended, either dilute povidone-iodine or saline, until the wound closes. The wound is kept open with wick drainage for 2–5 days. Following surgical drainage, antibiotics covering suspected bacteria should be given. If the patient has suspected osteomyelitis and is being hospitalized, intravenous antibiotic therapy is recommended with coverage of *S. aureus*. Outpatient treatment should utilize a course of oral antibiotic therapy. All patients should have early finger range of motion.

Deep space infections of the hand

The intricate anatomy of the hand provides for several potential spaces that can develop localized collections of pus. These spaces include the dorsal subaponeurotic space, the webspaces, hypothenar and thenar spaces, the midpalmar or subtendinous space, and the space of Parona *(Fig. 16.6)*. The most clinically important are the thenar and midpalmar space. These infections account for as much as 15% of all hand infections. *S. aureus* is the most common pathogen. Patients routinely require surgical drainage.

The dorsal subaponeurotic space is a potential space volar to the digital extensor tendons and dorsal to the metacarpal periosteum and fascia of the interosseous muscles. Infections in this region are usually due to penetrating injuries or extension from other parts of the hand *(Fig. 16.6)*. Typical presenting symptoms of dorsal subaponeurotic space infections include swelling and pain with finger extension.

The webspace, or interdigital space, infection can occur in the second, third, and fourth webspaces. It occurs in these webspaces most often in manual laborers, originating in the calluses on the palm. Wshen infections occur in the webspace and the purulence communicates between the palmar fascia and the dorsal subcutaneous webspace, a "collar-button" abscess forms *(Fig. 16.7)*. Treatment is aimed at proper

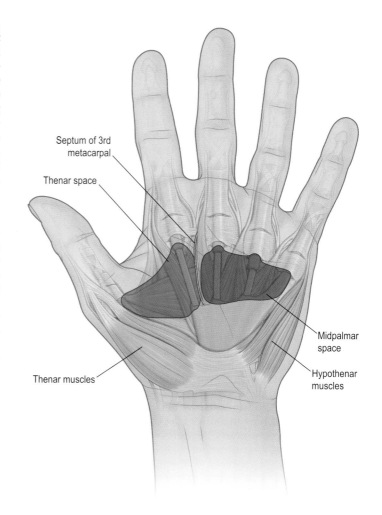

Fig. 16.6 Deep spaces of the hand.

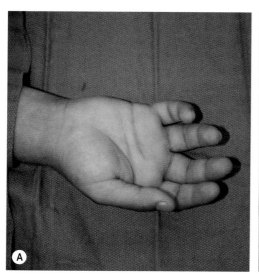 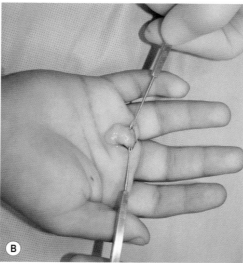

Fig. 16.7 Deep spaces of the hand. **(A)** Collar button abscess – note the abduction of adjacent digits. **(B)** Collar button abscess after incision.

drainage of both the palmar and dorsal fluid collections, and opening the connection between the two.

The signs and symptoms of a thenar space infection include a remarkable amount of swelling and exquisite tenderness. The swelling may extend to the dorsum via a "pantaloon" infection where the purulence extends from deep to the index finger flexors dorsally over the adductor pollicis and first dorsal interosseous muscles. It is imperative to make sure both areas are evaluated when performing drainage of this area.

The midpalmar space is encompassed radially by the midpalmar septum, ulnarly by the hypothenar septum, running from the palmar periosteum of the fifth metacarpal to the palmar fascia, and lies volar to the fascia of the second and third palmar interosseous muscles and dorsal to the long, ring, and small fingers' tendons. The typical distinguishing feature of this type of infections is the loss in concavity of the normal palm.

The space of Parona is a deep potential space in the distal forearm formed between the flexor digitorum profundus tendons and the pronator quadratus muscle. It is in continuity with the radial, ulnar, and midpalmar spaces. Those with a space of Parona infection have swelling, tenderness, and sometimes fluctuance of the distal forearm. The flexion of the fingers may be painful and difficult.

Pyogenic flexor tenosynovitis

The synovial sheaths of the flexor tendons provide fluid-filled gliding planes in a closed compartment that allows excursion of the flexor tendons. The synovial sheath extends from the midpalmar crease at the level of the A1 pulley to just proximal to the distal interphalangeal joint. The thumb flexor tendon sheath is in continuity with the radial bursa of the palm, and the small-finger sheath is continuous with the ulnar palmar bursa. The two bursae communicate in nearly 80% of humans. This communication explains why a horseshoe abscess occurs, where flexor tenosynovitis of the flexor pollicis longus can result in an infection of the ulnar bursa, and vice versa.

Prior to the advent of antibiotics, the diagnosis of flexor tenosynovitis was a life-threatening event. Today, it is still a source of significant morbidity, but rarely mortality. The four cardinal signs of flexor tenosynovitis, as described by Kanavel,[3] include: (1) fusiform swelling of the finger; (2) partially flexed posture of the digit; (3) tenderness over the entire flexor tendon sheath; and (4) disproportionate pain on passive extension. The last sign is the one most consistently present, and the one seen earliest in the infection process. Early infections may respond to conservative management with heat, elevation, rest, and antibiotics. However, the majority of infections will appear later or more severely, and require operative intervention. Infection of the tendon sheath leads to tendon necrosis and may lead to proximal propagation if not treated early. The most common organisms identified are S. aureus and Streptococcus species.

The goal of treatment is to drain the deep space while protecting the superficial structures. The space is packed with a gauze wick. The patient should remain on intravenous antibiotics postoperatively. The first dressing change should be within 12 hours of the operation. The patient can then be treated with sink hydrotherapy or dilute povidone-iodine soaks three times a day, and the hand should be elevated and splinted. If there is no improvement within 48 hours of drainage, the patient should be taken back for repeat debridement and irrigation (Fig. 16.8).

Flexor tenosynovitis

1. This is a surgical emergency: watch for Kanaval's signs (two visual signs – swollen, flexed digit – and two signs by palpation – tender tendon sheath and painful passive extension of digit).
2. Open tendon sheath proximally and distally; use Brunner incision proximal to A1 pulley and Brunner encompassing distal interphalangeal crease.
3. Culture for appropriate antibiotic coverage.
4. Irrigate tendon sheath copiously.
5. Leave in angiocath proximally for continuous irrigation (Fig. 16.9).

Septic arthritis

The three major routes of infection in septic arthritis are direct penetration, extension from contiguous infection, or hematogenous spread (Fig. 16.10). The misdiagnosis or delayed diagnosis of septic arthritis can lead to considerable articular cartilage destruction.

The most prevalent causative organisms are Staphylococcus aureus and Streptococcus organisms. In young children, consider Haemophilus influenzae and, in young adults, Gonococcus may be the etiology of monoarticular nontraumatic septic arthritis.

The diagnosis of septic arthritis can be subtle in the absence of obvious penetrating trauma. Fluctuance or fullness may be appreciated in affected joints, along with pain with active and passive motion. The joint is usually held in a position that allows the most volume in the joint capsule. A thorough examination must include visualizing the skin, the elbow, and axilla for lymphadenopathy, and any other affected joints. Laboratory findings often show an elevated erythrocyte sedimentation rate and C-reactive protein, but white blood cell count is normal in at least half of patients. Joint aspiration should be performed when possible. Gram stains may or may not show organisms. Aspiration of digital and midcarpal joints can be difficult to perform, but the radiocarpal joint is relatively easy and useful to confirm the diagnosis in this region.

The metacarpophalangeal joint may be approached through a dorsal midline longitudinal incision. The extensor hood is split in the midline and the joint is exposed beneath. The joint is then debrided of all infected synovium and purulence. The articular surface should be examined for signs of injury. The wound is then packed and left open to be addressed with dressing changes. The wound may also be addressed with a closed irrigation system in which a 14–18-gauge catheter is inserted into one side of the wound and a drain is established on the other side (e.g., Penrose drain). The wound is then closed over catheter and drain, and the wound continuously irrigated for 48 hours. The wound is then reassessed at that time and the drain and catheter removed.

Proximal interphalangeal joint septic arthritis should be approached through a midaxial inicision to avoid disruption of the central slip. The incision is made from the proximal

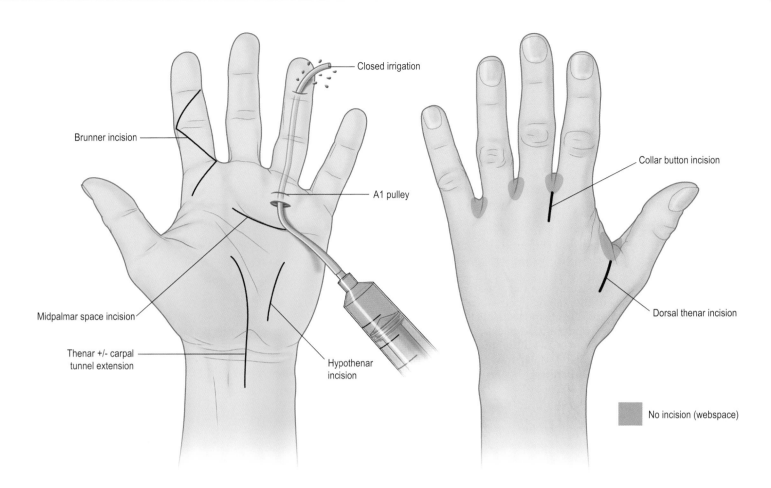

Fig. 16.8 Hand incisions.

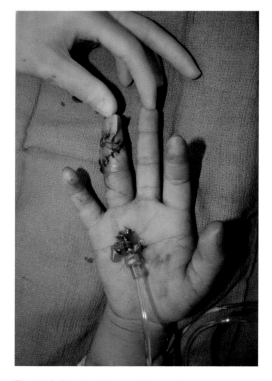

Fig. 16.9 Closed catheter irrigation for flexor tenosynovitis – typical setup.

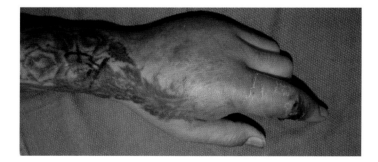

Fig. 16.10 Septic arthritis of index-finger proximal interphalangeal joint from fight bite.

extent of the digit longitudinally to just proximal to the distal interphalangeal joint. The transverse retinacular ligament is incised to expose the collateral ligament complex. The accessory collateral ligament is then incised, followed by capsulectomy. The infected synovium is debrided, the articular surface evaluated, and the wound left open to heal by secondary intention or closed irrigation by an 18-gauge catheter irrigation system for 48–72 hours. The latter requires suturing over the catheter and placing a drain at the other end of the incision. It is critical to begin motion once the catheters are removed.

Distal interphalangeal joint septic arthritis should be addressed through a dorsal H or Y incision. The skin flaps are elevated over the terminal tendon. The terminal tendon is then retracted to one side and the arthrotomy performed. An alternative approach is through a midaxial incision, perhaps as an extension of the proximal interphalangeal joint if both are affected or in flexor tenosynovitis. In this approach, it is necessary to excise the collateral ligament to gain access to the joint. The wound is left open with a surgical wick to heal by secondary intention.

Hints and tips

- This is a surgical emergency. Inaction can cause rapid erosion of cartilage, often after bite or penetration injury over joint
- Access joint via dorsal incision
- Culture wound for appropriate antibiotic coverage
- Irrigate joint copiously
- Leave wound open and begin early range of motion

Osteomyelitis

Osteomyelitis is a pyogenic infection of bone with the potential of affecting any bone in the body. Open fractures are the leading cause of osteomyelitis in the hand. Other routes of infection include through other traumatic injuries, spread from adjacent infected tissues, or by seeding from hematogenous spread. The periosteum serves as a protective barrier to infection; however, in traumatic injury this cortex is often damaged, allowing easy infection of the bone. Infected bony sequestrums do not respond well to nonsurgical methods of treatment due to lack of local delivery of antibiotics. Similarly, implanted hardware has no intrinsic blood supply, and infective bacteria often are able to form a protective layer over the inorganic surface, termed a biofilm.

The rate of infection in open fractures range from 1 to 11%, with increasing incidence with increasing severity of injury. *Staphylococcus aureus* and *Streptococcus* are the most common inciting organisms in immunocompetent hosts. Where there is failure of resolution of soft-tissue infections following standard treatment or persistence of a nonhealing wound, this should alert the treating physician to the possibility of osteomyelitis.

Radiologic evidence of osteomyelitis is difficult to detect on plain radiographs prior to 2–3 weeks after onset. The typical signs are metaphyseal rarefaction, osteopenia, osteosclerosis, and periosteal reaction or elevation. These same signs are seen with healing fractures, making the diagnosis difficult on X-ray alone. When a sequestrum and involucrum are seen, this indicates an advanced and chronic infection. Technetium bone scans and indium-labeled white blood cell scans can allow early diagnosis and are accurate.

Early diagnosis and treatment are needed for optimal outcome in patients with osteomyelitis, which requires both surgical and medical management. Eradication of the infection often requires debridement of necrotic soft tissue with decompression and curettage of necrotic bone, followed by repeat debridement and cultures when clinical improvement is absent in the first 72 hours. These wounds should not be closed. It is far better to plan a bone and soft-tissue reconstruction once the infection is under control than to have inadequate debridement or fail an attempted primary closure. In those patients with osteomyelitis of the distal phalanx, particularly when associated with septic arthritis, amputation may be the best option.[29] In instances where bone loss is created after debridement, the bone space can be maintained with an external fixator and the space filled with delayed bone grafting once complete wound healing has been achieved.

Necrotizing fasciitis

Necrotizing fasciitis is a group of rapidly progressive, potentially fatal infections that can involve one or more soft-tissue components: skin, fat, fascia, and muscle *(Fig. 16.11)*. The optimal outcome for patients with this type of SSTI relies on the following, as described by Napolitano[29]:

- Early diagnosis and differentiation of necrotizing versus nonnecrotizing SSTI
- Early initiation of appropriate empiric broad-spectrum antimicrobial therapy with consideration of risk factors for specific pathogens and mandatory coverage for MRSA
- Source control (early, aggressive surgical intervention) of early SSTI
- Pathogen identification and appropriate de-escalation of antimicrobial therapy.

Differentiating nonnecrotizing from necrotizing infections is crucial to achieving adequate surgical therapy. The classic signs of necrotizing fasciitis include skin necrosis, bullae, subcutaneous air, crepitus, and a systolic blood pressure <90 mmHg. Unfortunately, studies have indicated that less than 50% of patients presenting with necrotizing fasciitis have these signs. A white blood cell count of $15\,400 \times 10^9/L$ or serum sodium less than 135 mEq/L was found to assist reliably in differentiating necrotizing from necrotizing soft-tissue infections. Clostridial myonecrosis is a similar, and even more serious, infection of skeletal muscle.

The microbiology of necrotizing fasciitis has typically been infection with group A streptococcus,, More recently, 15–80% of necrotizing fasciitis cases involve community-acquired MRSA, and the incidence appears to be rising. In any patient suspected of having necrotizing fasciitis, anti-MRSA empiric antibiotics should be started immediately.

Critical to control and eradication of this infection is early aggressive surgical intervention for drainage of abscesses and debridement of necrotizing soft-tissue infections. Also known as source control, this aggressive debridement should be performed in conjunction with early initiation of appropriate empiric broad-spectrum antimicrobial therapy with consideration of risk factors for specific pathogens and MRSA

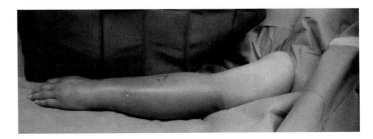

Fig. 16.11 Necrotizing fasciitis.

coverage. Once identified, the antimicrobial therapy should be de-escalated to cover the pathogen's or pathogens' sensitivities. Appropriate critical care management should be instituted, including fluid resuscitation, organ support, and nutritional support.

Hints and tips

- Necrotizing faciitis is a surgical emergency. Watch for progressive infection advancing proximally in an immunocompromised patient (e.g., diabetic) with subcutaneous crepitus and severe pain
- Open subcutaneously to infection demarcation line. One will often find murky clear fluid
- Debride all nonviable tissue – if it doesn't bleed, it should be gone
- Culture wound for appropriate antibiotic coverage
- Monitor progress and repeat debridements as needed
- Reconstruction (e.g., skin grafts) to be performed only after infection has been eradicated and appropriate antibiotic course provided

---

Herpetic whitlow

Herpetic whitlow is a superficial infection with herpes simplex virus type 1 or 2. Herpetic whitlow is often clinically confused with true felons, but should follow a very different algorithm *(Fig. 16.12)*. The infection is an occupational hazard of those who commonly are exposed to orotracheal or genital secretions. A painfully cytolytic infection usually occurs 2–14 days after exposure, and matures over the subsequent 2 weeks. Vesicles will form, coalesce, and unroof, forming characteristic ulcers.

The natural course of the infection is usually self-limited with resolution after 10–14 days. The lesions are no longer contagious once they are epithelialized. The infection then maintains a latent state in the nervous ganglia, and recurrences can be induced by certain stressors, such as physiologic

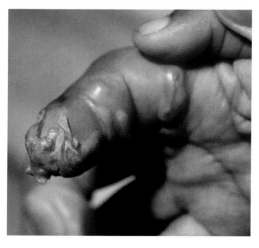

Fig. 16.12 Herpetic whitlow. (Courtesy of Yale Residents' Slide Collection. Reproduced from Bolognia JB, Jorizzo JJ, Rapini RP. Dermatology, 2nd edition. Elsevier, 2007.)

or psychological stress, fever, sun exposure, and other infections. There is often a prodrome of pain and tingling prior to eruption. The diagnosis is usually based on clinical history and exam, but may be confirmed by culturing the vesicular fluid, Tzanck smear, or a rise in serum antibody titiers.

The treatment of herpetic whitlow is based on not mistaking it for a felon or paronychia. The unnecessary incision of this lesion can lead to a superinfection. Acyclovir has been recommended for treatment of those with a prodrome, decreases the clinical course in protracted cases, induces remission in patients with AIDS, and may be used to prevent recurrences in otherwise healthy patients.

Mycobacterial infections

More than 75% of atypical mycobacterial infections involve the hand. The most frequently identified of these organisms is *Mycobacterium marinum*. The source of these infections typically comes from a penetrating injury from contaminated fish tanks, swimming pools, boats, or injuries from fish spines, fins, or bites. The infections are categorized as cutaneous (verrucal), subcutaneous (granulomatous), or deep (involving bone, bursal synovium, joint, and/or tendon).

The typical physical exam findings are few and none are pathognomonic. Patients will frequently present with abundant tenosynovitis or joint synovitis. Many cases are initially misdiagnosed, causing delay in appropriate therapy. Systemic symptoms do not usually occur and white blood cell count and erythrocyte sedimentation rate are usually normal. Biopsy of the affected areas usually shows granulomas and cultures must be incubated in Lowenstein–Jensen medium at 30°C for up to 8 weeks.

For the verrucal form, the infection is usually self-limited. If the lesion has been picked at or biopsied without postoperative prophylaxis, the infection can become subcutaneous. This granulomatous infection must then be treated with debridement followed by 2–6 months of antibiotic administration. Deeper lesions will need synovectomy, tenosynovectomy, or incision, drainage and debridement of bone or joint, with antibiotic administration for 4–24 months.

With hand tenosynovitis, it is necessary to remove the synovium of the flexor completely while preserving the annular pulleys. Minocycline is the drug of choice for this type of infection.

The presentation for *M. tuberculosis* is a long history of progressive, painful swelling and decreased hand function. It may take over a year for symptoms to appear after infection, and it can sometimes take years to have a proper diagnosis. Many patients never present with the constitutional symptoms of pulmonary tuberculosis, and over time the infection causes significant bony and soft-tissue destruction. Purified protein derivate is unreliable for diagnosing the disease, but is often positive. Diagnosis is usually made by biopsy of the lesion with acid-fast stain and culture.

Treatment of *M. tuberculosis* of the upper extremity should involve the help of infectious disease colleagues. A trial of chemotherapy alone before surgical debridement is recommended by some. When required, the surgical debridement is usually extensive. The osseous destruction from dactylitis will often recoup itself; however, when affecting the carpus, a carpectomy and/or wrist fusion is necessary. With tenosynovitis, the typical "rice bodies" are seen and debridement of the entire synovium is recommended. Fortunately, the cure rate for these infections is reportedly 80–100%.

The second most common atypical mycobacterial species seen in the upper extremity is *Mycobacterium avium* complex. It is the most common opportunistic infection seen in AIDS patients; infections often require multiple debridements and combination chemotherapy to help eradicate the infection.

Noncholera *Vibrio* infections

Vibrio vulnificus is an aggressive and destructive infection that can cause upper extremity necrotizing fasciitis. It is often seen following fish handling or consuming raw seafood. The infection causes rapidly progressive skin and deep-tissue necrosis. These infections will continue to produce significant soft-tissue destruction in the presence of appropriate antibiotics. Treatment should be early and aggressive with extensive surgical excision of all infected, necrotic tissue.

Fungal infections

Fungal infections of the upper extremity can be roughly categorized into three major groups: cutaneous, subcutaneous, and deep or systemic. The cutaneous infections are caused by dermatophytes. They rely on keratin as a substrate for food and invade cornified tissue such as hair, skin, and nails. Subcutaneous infections originate from low-virulence organisms that enter the tissue through traumatic implantation. Deep or systemic infections, usually caused by dimorphic fungi, usually originate as naturally found soil saprophytes but produce disease in animals when a sufficient number of spores are implanted traumatically or inhaled from the air. The cutaneous and subcutaneous forms are the most common and relatively benign. The deep or disseminated mycotic infections are rare, but are usually a much more serious clinical entity, with potential for significant morbidity or mortality. Patients who are immunocompromised are particularly vulnerable to fungal infections.

Bites

Bite wounds are a common injury that is all too often mistaken to be harmless by both bite victims and treating physicians. They require, however, special attention as the mouths of humans, dogs, cats, and other animals contain flora that may not be sensitive to the standard antimicrobial therapy. Like a needle, the sharp pointed teeth of some animals can puncture and inoculate deep into tissues bacteria living in their mouth.[30]

Animal bites

Ninety percent of animal bites in humans are by dogs. Five percent are from cats. More than 50% of dog bite injuries involve children who are less than 12 years old and half of these wounds are of the hand and forearm. Approximately a dozen people die yearly from dog bites; one-third of these are infants less than 12 months old. Only bees and venomous snakes cause more fatalities.[30] Patients presenting in the first 8 hours after injury are usually more concerned with crush injury, care of the disfigurement caused by the attack, and the need for rabies or tetanus therapy. The wounds are typically contaminated with multiple strains of aerobic and anaerobic bacteria. "Treated wounds" will become infected between 2 and 30% of the time. Patients presenting longer than 8 hours after injury usually have an established infection from the bite. Puncture wounds become infected more often than avulsions and can lead to abscess formation. Bites close to bones or joints may cause septic arthritis, osteomyelitis, tenosynovitis, or abscesses in potential spaces. Punctures over or near a joint, especially in the hands, should be treated aggressively with antibiotics and elevation because of a high incidence of osteomyelitis and septic arthritis.

Dog bite wounds are considered predominantly from the dog's oral flora. Multiple strains of the genus *Pasteurella* have been identified, as well as many others. Wounds inflicted by cats are usually scratches or tiny punctures on the extremities and have a high likelihood of becoming infected. Rattlesnake bite wounds should cover for fecal flora, as the snake's prey often defecate while being consumed.

Infected wounds should be cultured for aerobic and anaerobic bacteria and a Gram stain obtained. Small tears and infected puncture wounds should be cultured with a min-itipped swab, such as a nasopharyngeal swab. The wound should be irrigated and any devitalized or necrotic tissue should be debrided. It is important to obtain radiographs to determine if a fracture is present and if any tooth foreign bodies were left behind. It will also provide a baseline for future concerns of osteomyelitis. Primary wound closure is not indicated, except in fresh, uninfected facial wounds. Wound edges can be approximated, when possible, by adhesive strips. Antimicrobial prophylaxis for initial presentation of hand bite wounds is recommended and should cover *P. multocida, Staphylococcus aureus*, and anaerobes.

If the patient presents early after a bite and only mild to moderate signs of infection are present, amoxicillin/clavulanic acid, 875/125 mg bid or 500/125 tid with food, will cover most bite pathogens. There has been no alternative established for penicillin-allergic patients. If hospitalization is required, intravenous ampicillin/sulbactam or cefoxitin is recommended.

Human bites

Human bite wounds have a much higher rate of infection than do animal bite wounds. Occlusional human bites can affect any part of the body, but most often involve the distal phalanx of the long or index fingers of the dominant hand. Bites to the hand are more frequently infected and more seriously than bites to other areas. Infections sustained from human bite wounds should have appropriate surgical drainage and debridement, admission to the hospital, and administration of intravenous antibiotics. A Gram stain with aerobic and anaerobic cultures should be obtained with all infected wounds prior to any therapy.

Clenched-fist injuries are a specific subtype of human bite wounds that deserve special attention. These are traumatic injuries that occur when the patient strikes another in the mouth with a clenched fist. This occurs most commonly over the third and fourth metacarpophalangeal joints of the dominant hand, but may also occur over the proximal interphalangeal joints (*Fig. 16.13*). These injuries often present delayed, and therefore have a high rate of complications.

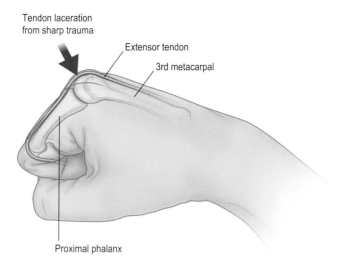

Tendon laceration
from sharp trauma

Extensor tendon

3rd metacarpal

Proximal phalanx

Fig. 16.13 Clenched-fist injury.

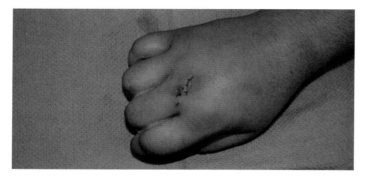

Fig. 16.14 Fight bite injury.

In this clenched-fist injury *(Fig. 16.14)*, as the patient punched his opponent, the opponent's tooth passed through the skin, subcutaneous tissue, tendon, subtendinous space, and joint capsule and into the articular surface of the metacarpal head. Because this occurred with the hand in the clenched position, this is the only hand position in which the pathway of the tooth can be seen. Typically, the hand is examined, and operated on, with the hand laying flat. It is important to remember that, in this position, the pathway of the tooth is no longer collinear.

Debridement and copious irrigation are usually required for treatment of infections resulting from fight bites. In patients hospitalized for clenched-fist injuries, deep structure involvement occurs in 75% of patients. In one study, joint capsule violation occurred in 67.8%, tendon involvement in 20.3%, articular bone indentations in 16.5%, and free articular cartilage fragments in 5.8%. The conclusion of this study of 191 patients with 194 skin lacerations was that all patients with clenched-fist lacerations or puncture wounds over joint

should be surgically debrided and explored for damage to deep structures, including the joint, at the time they first seek medical care.[31] Empirical antibiotics should include either cefoxitin or ampicillin/sulbactam or a carbapenem until culture results are known. Failure of first-generation cephalosporins and penicillinase-resistant penicillin, as a monotherapy, has been reported and is most often due to *Eikenella corrodens*.

Hardware infections

Hardware infection can be of two varieties, external and internal. Pin track infections from external fixators and Kirschner wire placement occur anywhere from 1% for major infections (requiring removal of one or more of the pins before infection can be resolved) to 33–80% for minor infections (benign, easily treatable with antibiotics and notable for prolonged drainage, crusting, swelling, and erythema).[27,29,32,33] The optimal method for pin care has not been established; however, there may be a role for burying pins when able and requiring longer than 8 weeks for placement.[33]

Fortunately, the incidence of internal hardware infection is rare. Careful patient selection, appropriate preparation, and proper technique should lead to very low infection rates.[34] Procedures lasting over 2 hours, those involving bone, and those involving hardware placement should utilize prophylactic antibiotics. Other elective, clean hand surgery procedures have not been proven to require routine prophylactic antibiotics.[5,34]

Patient selection

The care of a patient with a hand infection requires not only knowledge of anatomy, but also an understanding of types of infection, as well as experience to know the spectrum of presentations from simple cellulitis to necrotizing fasciitis and mimickers of infection. Signs of infection can be subtle to overt, and providing the wrong treatment can lead to severe morbidity, or even mortality.

Outcomes, prognosis, and complications

The outcome and prognosis of hand infections are usually related to the amount of delay in treatment, and the appropriateness of the treatment modality. Those infections that are neglected or inadequately treated can go on to cause more extensive damage, resulting in a poorer prognosis, and subsequent outcome. Early, aggressive, comprehensive therapy is essential to infection eradication.

Access the complete references list online at **http://www.expertconsult.com**

3. Kanavel AB. An anatomical and clinical study of acute phlegmons of the hand. *Surg Gynecol Obstet*. 1905;1:221–259.

    In this timeless and clinically important work, Kanavel defined the five fascial spaces of the hand (dorsal subcutaneous, dorsal subaponeurotic, middle palmar, thenar, and hypothenar) and the patterns of communication between these fascial spaces. He also noted that, as purulence accumulates and pressure increases in these tight spaces, the purulence spreads in defined and predictable patterns. As such, Kanavel was able to develop the surgical techniques that form the foundation for modern treatment of hand infections. Many of these incisions are still in use today.

10. Summanen P, Talan D, Stron C, et al. Bacteriology of skin and soft-tissue infections: comparison of infections in intravenous drug users and individuals with no history of intravenous drug use. *Clin Infect Dis*. 1995;20(Suppl 2):S279–S282.

    In this study of bacteriology of cutaneous or subcutaneous abscesses (86 specimens) from intravenous drug users compared to those of patients with no history of intravenous drug use (74 specimens), the researchers found that intravenous drug abusers have more upper extremity infections than nonintravenous drug abusers. More importantly, the type of infections each sees is often different. This study showed that intravenous drug abusers are more likely to have mixed infections with aerobe/ anaerobe infections containing oral flora. Staphylococcus aureus and Streptococcus milleri were the most commonly isolated aerobes. In nonintravenous drug abusers, Staphylococcus aureus was the most common isolate.

15. Gosselin RA, Roberts I, Gillespie WJ. Antibiotics for preventing infection in open limb fractures. *Cochrane Database of Systematic Reviews*. 2004, Issue 1. Art. No.: CD003764.

    Most studies in this Cochrane review lacked sufficient power; however, a meta-analysis supported the effectiveness of antibiotics active against Gram-positive organisms in reducing the incidence of early infection when the antibiotic was given before or at the time of initial treatment of an open limb fracture, at least in the short term. It was clear from all articles reviewed that antibiotic therapy was to be utilized only as an adjunct to, and not a replacement for, comprehensive open fracture management protocol (e.g., surgical debridement, stabilization, wound coverage). In subgroup analysis of finger fractures, it was found that prophylactic antibiotics may not reduce the incidence of early infection, but the difference was not significant.

25. Napolitano LM. Severe Soft Tissue Infections. *Infect Dis Clin North Am*. 2009;23:571–591.

    This is an excellent review of how to approach soft-tissue infections. The article summarizes the best evidence available on how to identify and treat the spectrum of soft-tissue infections, from simple to severe. It also gives an up-to-date literature review of treatment modalities, and algorithms for managing those patients presenting with MRSA (both community-acquired and hospital-acquired) and methicillin-sensitive Staphylococcus aureus infections. The article also reviews the epidemiology of the infections, and risk stratification for the development of severe soft-tissue infections.

    Houshian S, Seyedipour S, Wedderkopp N. Epidemiology of bacterial hand infections. *Int J Infect Dis*. 2006;10:315–319.

    This study is a retrospective review of patients who presented with hand infections at a single institution in Denmark over an eight year period with hand infections. They had 418 patients between 1992 and 2001. 44% of the patients had an infection with Staph aureus, followed by 11.7% having mixed flora infections. They also noted that gram negative organisms were commonly isolated from diabetics and intravenous drug abusers.

17

Management of Dupuytren's disease

Andrew J. Watt and Caroline Leclercq

SYNOPSIS

- Dupuytren's disease is a benign fibromatosis of the palmar and digital fascia characterized by nodular thickening and subsequent contracture.
- Successful treatment requires a detailed understanding of the normal palmar and digital fascial structures and their corollary diseased states.
- Operative indications are based on the degree of contracture and the resultant functional disability of the hand.
- Palmar fasciectomy remains the mainstay of surgical treatment.
- Evolving treatments include percutaneous (needle) aponeurotomy and collagenase injection.
- Despite appropriate management, recurrence and disease progression remain the primary obstacles to treatment.

 Access the Historical Perspective section online at
http://www.expertconsult.com

Introduction

Dupuytren's disease is a progressive disease of the palmar and digital fascial structures characterized by nodular thickening and subsequent contracture. Deformity of the hand occurs primarily at the metacarpophalangeal (MCP) and proximal interphalangeal (PIP) joint level, resulting in functional limitations. This disease process is quite familiar to hand surgeons and presents a challenge in terms of both treatment and prognosis.

Epidemiology

Dupuytren's disease belongs to the overarching category of benign superficial fibromatoses and, as such, is closely related to Peyronie's disease (penile fibromatosis) and Ledderhose's disease (plantar fibromatosis). Historically, Dupuytren's disease has been successively referred to as a Nordic, Caucasian, Anglo-Saxon, and finally a Viking disease.[1-4] Although most prevalent in populations with a strong northern European ancestry, Dupuytren's disease affects populations throughout the world. Critical evaluations of the migrations that have occurred throughout history, particularly those originating in northern Europe, suggest that the disease likely originated among Celtic and Germanic tribes around 1200 BC and dispersed throughout Europe with the great migrations beginning around 200 BC.[5] Few populations are spared at least anecdotal cases of Dupuytren's disease; however, the incidence remains highest among individuals of northern European ancestry, with overall estimates ranging from 2% to 42% depending on the population being studied.[6] Men are six times more likely to develop Dupuytren's disease than are women and typically exhibit an onset in the fifth decade of life, in comparison to onset within the sixth decade for women.[7] Population studies support an autosomal-dominant inheritance pattern with variable penetrance.[6]

Associations with repetitive trauma, alcohol abuse, hepatic disease, diabetes mellitus, smoking, chronic obstructive pulmonary disease, human immunodeficiency virus, malignancy (paraneoplastic manifestation), and epilepsy have been proposed.[8-10] These associations are often weak and most likely represent factors that may increase the penetrance or exacerbate an underlying genetic predisposition.

Palmar and digital fascia

Dupuytren's disease is ultimately manifest as the transformation of the normal palmar and digital fascial structures to thickened diseased cords through the deposition of type I and type III collagen and the contractile forces generated by myofibroblasts. An intimate understanding of both the native and pathologic anatomy is paramount in assessing and appropriately treating patients with Dupuytren's disease.

Palmar fascia

The palmar fascia provides a flexible yet firm framework for the soft tissues of the palm, tethering the skin to the underlying musculoskeletal structures. Classic descriptions of the anatomy of the palmar fascia provided by Legueu, Juvara, and Testut have withstood the test of time.[11,12] The palmar fascia consists of two distinct layers: the deep fascia and the superficial fascia or palmar aponeurosis. The deep fascia covers the interosseous muscles and is not involved in Dupuytren's disease. The superficial fascia, in contrast, is affected by the pathologic progression of Dupuytren's disease.

The palmar aponeurosis is a triangular-shaped fascial structure consisting of longitudinal, transverse and vertical fibers with its apex in continuity with the palmaris longus tendon *(Fig. 17.1)*. Although these structures are in continuity, the palmar aponeurosis is histologically distinct from the palmaris longus and is invariably present even in patients with an absent palmaris.

The longitudinal fibers course superficial to the flexor retinaculum, forming pretendinous bands. These bands travel distally and insert into the deep surface of the dermis at the distal palmar crease, contribute to the retrovascular fascial structures, and bifurcate around the flexor tendon sheath to insert on the radial and ulnar sides of the MCP joint.[13]

The transverse fibers are characterized by two distinct bands, one proximal and one distal. The proximal transverse fibers, located at the level of the distal palmar crease, course deep to the longitudinal pretendinous bands and are not typically affected by Dupuytren's disease.[14] Radially, these fibers form the proximal commissural ligament of the first webspace. The distal transverse fibers, alternately referred to as the natatory ligament, course superficial to the longitudinal pretendinous bands and are affected by Dupuytren's disease. The natatory ligament extends from the radial border of the index finger to the ulnar border of the small finger. Ulnarly, the natatory ligament divides to envelop the abductor digiti minimi (ADM) and the ulnar neurovascular bundle. Radially, the natatory ligament is continuous with the distal commissural ligament of Grapow within the first webspace.

The vertical fibers of Legueu and Juvara connect the superficial palmar aponeurosis to the deep fascia. These fibers form a series of eight vertical septa on the radial and ulnar sides of the flexor digital apparatus. These septa divide longitudinal compartments containing the flexor tendons from those containing the lumbricals and digital neurovascular bundles.[11,15] Additional vertical fibers connect the superficial palmar fascia to the overlying dermis, providing resistance to shear forces within the palm.[13]

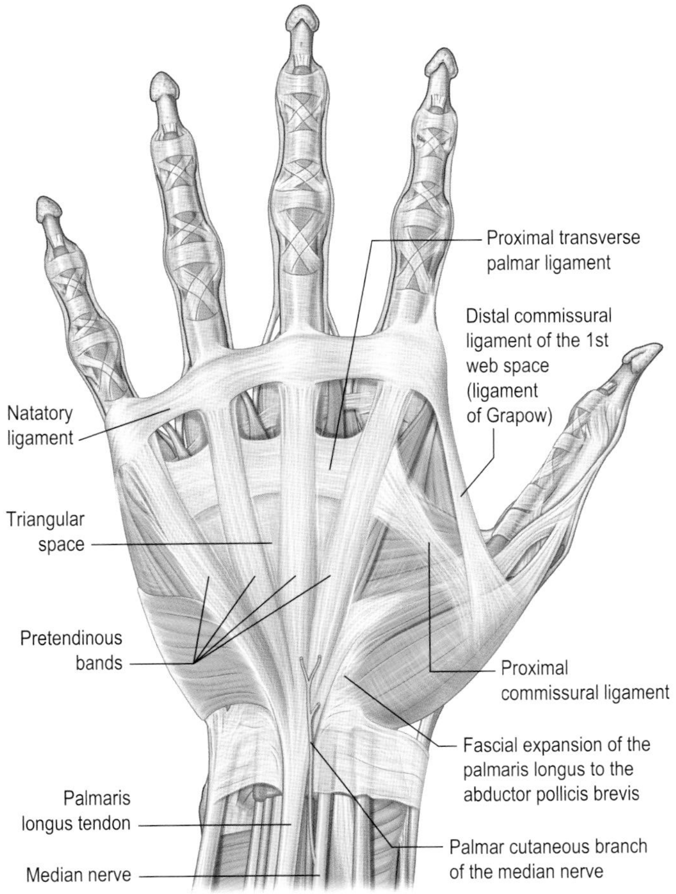

Digital fascia

The palmar and digital fascia is contiguous with a complex digital–palmar junction in which intermediate and deep fibers of the longitudinal bands bifurcate, contributing to the formation of digital retrovascular bands. Anatomic studies have revealed more variability in the anatomy of the digital fascia in comparison with the relatively constant palmar fascial anatomy; however, relative agreement exists over the basic structure. The finger is invested by an elliptical fascial covering consisting of volar and dorsal fascial sheets that lie superficial to the flexor and extensor mechanisms respectively. These sheets unite along the radial and ulnar aspects of the finger. The volar and dorsal aspects of the finger are separated by a series of lateral structures that envelope the neurovascular structures of the finger.[16] These lateral structures include Cleland's ligaments, Grayson's ligaments, and transverse retinacular ligaments. Cleland's ligaments consist of a series of dorsal fiber bundles that arise proximal and distal to the interphalangeal joint, fanning laterally to insert in the skin. These fiber bundles do not form a contiguous sheet and run within several planes dorsal to the neurovascular bundle. Grayson's ligaments are more distinct, arising from the volar surface of the flexor tendon sheath, fanning laterally to insert into the skin, volar to the neurovascular bundle. The transverse retinacular ligaments originate from the volar capsule of the PIP joint and course dorsally to insert into the lateral margin of the extensor mechanism[17] *(Fig. 17.2)*.

First webspace

The radial longitudinal fibers of the superficial palmar aponeurosis extend distally into the thumb, inserting into the dermis

Natatory ligament

Triangular space

Pretendinous bands

Palmaris longus tendon

Median nerve

Proximal transverse palmar ligament

Distal commissural ligament of the 1st web space (ligament of Grapow)

Proximal commissural ligament

Fascial expansion of the palmaris longus to the abductor pollicis brevis

Palmar cutaneous branch of the median nerve

Fig. 17.1 Anatomy of the palmar fascia. (Redrawn from Tubiana R, Leclercq C, Hurst L, et al. (eds) Dupuytren's Disease. London: Martin Dunitz, 2000, p. 22.)

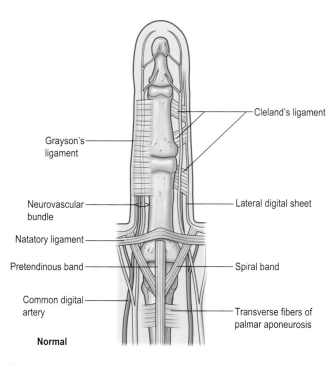

Fig. 17.2 Normal fascial anatomy of the digit.

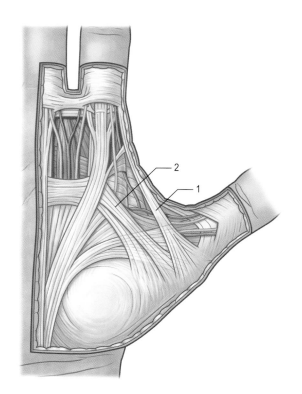

Fig. 17.3 Normal fascial anatomy of the first webspace. 1, Distal commissural ligament (ligament of Grapow). 2, Proximal commissural ligament.

at the level of the MCP joint. Additional fibers insert into the intermuscular septum between the adductor pollicis and the first dorsal interosseous muscles while additional fibers insert into the flexor tendon sheath of the index finger.

The natatory ligament is contiguous radially with the distal commissural ligament within the first webspace. The proximal transverse fibers are contiguous with the proximal commissural ligament *(Fig. 17.3)*.

Basic science and disease process

Basic science

Although Dupuytren's disease has been formally recognized and clinically treated for over two centuries, the etiology and pathogenesis of Dupuytren's disease remained a matter of both speculation and incidental correlation. It has been only over the past 30 years that surgeons and scientists have begun to unravel the cellular mechanisms that contribute to the development of the disease.

Histopathologic studies have provided the foundation of scientists' nascent understanding of Dupuytren's disease. Initial studies have demonstrated not only involvement of the palmar aponeurosis but also absence of adipose tissue, a paucity of sweat glands, and increased vascularity within the affected palm.[23] Histologically, nodular rests of myofibroblasts surrounded by dense collagen characterize affected tissue. Molecular analysis reveals a preponderance of type III collagen, which is not typically observed in mature palmar fascia, and increased concentrations of prostaglandins as

well as several subtypes of transforming growth factor-β (TGF-β).[24,25] DNA microarray analysis comparing diseased and control palmar fascia has revealed a host of gene expression changes, including both up- and downregulation of expression. These include genes previously implicated in the pathogenesis of Dupuytren's disease, including fibronectin, tenascin C, TGF-β, collagen III, IV, and VI, as well as novel genes, including musculoaponeurotic fibrosarcoma oncogene homolog B (MafB).[26] Although the intricate interrelationship between these gene expression patterns remains a field for future inquiry, this knowledge has provided potential clinical targets for pharmacologic intervention in halting or potentially preventing Dupuytren's disease.

In 1959, Luck described the pathogenesis of Dupuytren's contracture in pathologic terms consisting of proliferative, involutional, and residual phases. This description has provided a framework within which molecular advances may be analyzed as well as a foundation for clinicians' understanding of disease progression. The proliferative phase is characterized by nodule formation within the palmar fascia and biochemically by increased fibrinolytic activity. At this stage, fibroblasts differentiate into myofibroblasts and comprise the majority of nodular architecture. Myofibroblasts are fibroblastic in origin; however, they contain an actin microfilamentous structure analogous to smooth-muscle cells. These actin microfilaments are arranged in bundles oriented along the long axis of the cell and communicate with the extracellular matrix fibronectin, thereby allowing transmission of intracellular contractile forces to the extracellular tissues. Marked nodular thickening and signs of early joint contracture characterize the involutional phase. Throughout the involutional phase, type III collagen is synthesized and the myofibroblasts reorient along the lines of tension within the palm. Type III collagen deposition continues and is gradually replaced with type I collagen throughout the residual phase. Myofibroblasts have largely disappeared by the residual phase, resulting in a relatively hypocellular amalgam of type I and type III collagen.[27–29]

The inciting event resulting in myofibroblast proliferation remains unknown. Authors have suggested multiple hypotheses, including trauma, focal ischemia, and a host of growth factor and cytokine aberrations. Murrell *et al.* hypothesize that ischemia within the palmar fascia results in the generation of free radicals that damage the surrounding tissue. This damage incites repair with the deposition of collagen and the proliferation of myofibroblasts, and leads to further ischemia and disease progression.[30] Mechanical stress has been shown to upregulate myofibroblast differentiation and supports the traumatic theory.[31] Myofibroblast proliferation is also stimulated by a number of growth factors and cytokines, including TGF-β_2 and inhibited by platelet-derived growth factor (PDGF), basic fibroblastic growth factor, interleukin-1α, and interleukin-1β.[32] Actin expression may also play a pivotal role in the progression of Dupuytren's disease and is increased by TGF-β_2 and degreased by PDGF-BB.[33] The expression of androgen receptors within Dupuytren's nodules has also raised the question of hormonal influence on disease development and progression. Myofibroblasts from Dupuytren's patients stimulated with 5α-dihydrotestosterone demonstrated higher rates of proliferation than myofibroblasts from control subjects, suggesting that androgens may play a role in disease progression. This theory gains support from the male predominance of the disease. Ultimately, none of these theories and biomolecular interrelationships is mutually exclusive and Dupuytren's disease may very well represent the culmination of a host of environmental and cellular events in a genetically prone individual.

Disease process

The net effect of these cellular and pathologic mechanisms is the transformation of normal palmar and digital fascial structures into fibrotic diseased cords. Each normal anatomic structure within the palmar and digital fascial system maintains a pathologic correlate. Diseased components may be further subdivided into palmar, palmodigital, digital, first webspace, and hypothenar cords *(Table 17.1)*.

Within the palm, involved pretendinous bands become pretendinous cords. These cords course distally and insert into the deep surface of the dermis at the distal palmar crease, resulting in pitting of the palmar skin. They are also continuous with the retrovascular fascial structures and contribute to formation of the spiral cord.[13] The remaining fibers contribute to the formation of the central cord within the finger itself. The pretendinous cord is the primary contributor to MCP flexion contracture and is located superficially, leaving the deeper neurovascular structures undisturbed. Dissection within the palm, proximal to the distal flexor crease, is therefore relatively safe with respect to neurovascular bundles. The vertical fibers of McGrouther and the septa of Legueu and Juvara also become involved and may result in painful triggering with extension of the finger following full flexion *(Fig. 17.4)*.

Table 17.1 Fascial anatomy of Dupuytren's disease

Diseased structure	Anatomic origin	Clinical significance
Palmar cords		
Pretendinous cord	Pretendinous band	MCP joint flexion contracture
Vertical cord	Vertical fibers of McGrouther or septa of Legueu and Juvara	Causes painful triggering
Palmodigital cords		
Spiral cord	Pretendinous band, spiral band, lateral digital sheet, Grayson's ligament	Displaces the neurovascular bundle medially and superficially (spiral nerve)
Natatory cord	Natatory ligament (distal fibers)	Webspace adduction contracture
Digital cords		
Central cord	Pretendinous cord (digital extension)	PIP joint flexion contracture
Retrovascular cord	Retrovascular band of thomine	PIP and DIP joint flexion contracture; prevents full correction of PIP joint contracture
Lateral cord	Lateral digital sheet (often closely associated with pretendinous and natatory cord)	PIP and DIP joint flexion contracture; displaces neurovascular bundle medially
Abductor digiti minimi cord	Abductor digiti minimi tendon	PIP joint flexion contracture
Thumb and first webspace cords		
Proximal commissural cord	Proximal commissural ligament	First-web adduction contracture
Distal commissural cord	Distal commissural ligament	First-web adduction contracture
Thumb pretendinous cord	Pretendinous band	MCP joint flexion contracture

MCP, metacarpophalangeal; PIP, proximal interphalangeal; DIP, distal interphalangeal.

Two key cords are located within the palmodigital region. The spiral cord forms from the diseased confluence of the pretendinous band, spiral band, lateral digital sheet, and Grayson's ligament. The spiral cord wraps around the neurovascular bundle, displacing the digital nerve and artery medially, superficially, and proximally, placing them at risk for injury during skin incision and dissection *(Fig. 17.5)*. The spiral cord not only displaces the neurovascular bundle, but also results in significant PIP joint contracture.[34] The natatory ligament,

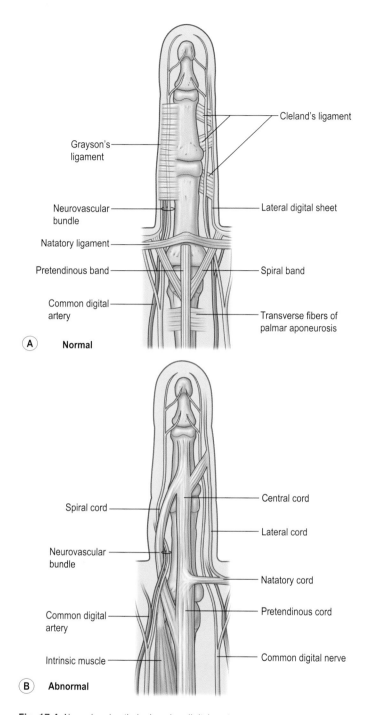

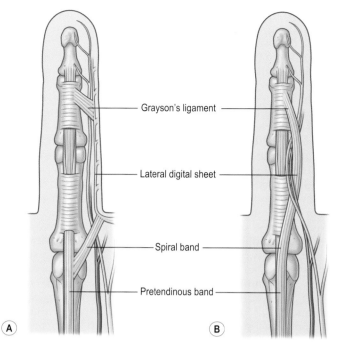

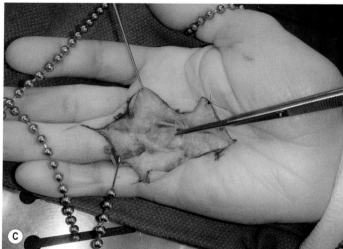

Fig. 17.5 Spiral cord. **(A)** Normal fascial palmodigital fascial structures contributing to the formation of the spiral cord. 1, Pretendinous band. 2, Spiral band. 3, Lateral digital sheet. 4, Grayson's ligament. **(B)** Spiral cord. **(C)** Spiral cord: note displacement of the ulnar neurovascular bundle radially.

Fig. 17.4 Normal and pathologic palmodigital anatomy.

which traverses the palm transversely at the level of the metacarpal heads, is transformed into the natatory cord. The natatory cord results in webspace adduction contracture.

Within the finger, involved pretendinous bands become central cords. These cords are contiguous proximally with the pretendinous cords of the palm and insert laterally on the radial and ulnar side of the PIP joint and on the flexor tendon sheath of the middle phalanx. The central cord acts in concert with the spiral cord, contributing to PIP joint contracture. Additionally, the retrovascular band of Thomine becomes the

retrovascular cord, which contributes to PIP and distal interphalangeal (DIP) joint contracture. The lateral digital sheet may also become involved in disease progression as the lateral cord, contributing to the spiral cord and resulting in PIP and DIP joint contracture.[35]

The first webspace may also be involved in Dupuytren's disease. The proximal and distal commissural ligaments, which represent the radial extension of the proximal transverse fibers of the palmar aponeurosis and the natatory ligament, respectively, become the proximal and distal commissural cords. These cords contribute to first-webspace adduction contracture. A thumb pretendinous band, analogous to the longitudinal pretendinous fascial structures of the

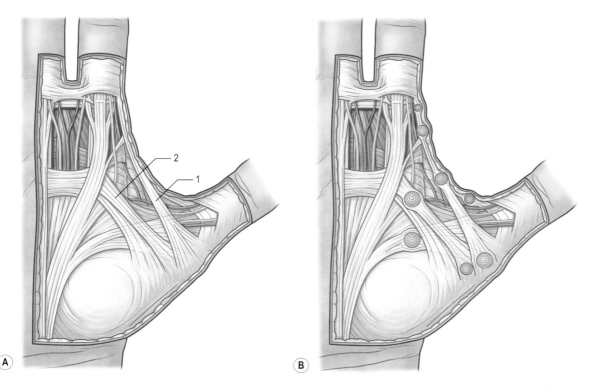

Fig. 17.6 Normal and pathologic anatomy of the first webspace. **(A)** Normal anatomy. **(B)** Pathologic anatomy. 1, Distal commissural ligament (ligament of Grapow). 2, Proximal commissural ligament.

fingers, evolves into a pretendinous cord and results in MCP joint contracture *(Fig. 17.6)*.

In addition to the palmar and palmodigital cords analogous to those of the index, long, and ring fingers, the small finger has a unique ADM cord. This cord represents pathologic involvement of the fascia associated with the ADM tendon and results in an abduction contracture of the small finger.

Diagnosis/patient presentation

Clinical presentation

Patients with Dupuytren's disease present throughout the spectrum of disease progression, and diagnosis is made based upon history and clinical examination. The characteristic progression from nodule to fibrotic cord with contracture of the affected palm and digits is pathognomonic for Dupuytren's disease. Onset is typically insidious with progressive contracture and disability developing over the course of years. The earliest signs of disease consist of pitting or dimpling of the palm with distortion of the distal palmar crease resulting from connections between the dermis and longitudinal fibers of the palmar aponeurosis[13] *(Fig. 17.7)*. Distortion of the skin creases can appear as a deepening of the crease or widening of the crease (Hugh Johnson sign).[36] These skin changes are typically the first signs of the disease, preceding the development of nodules. Nodules develop within the palm and are the palpable manifestation of myofibroblast proliferation. These nodules are most commonly located within the ulnar aspect of the palm overlying the ring-finger ray at the level of the distal palmar crease and at the PIP joint level within the finger. Nodules may develop anywhere within the finger, palm, and,

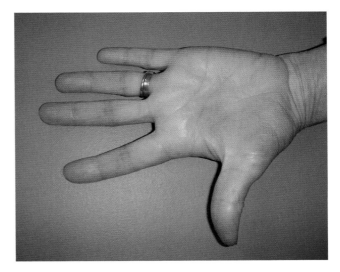

Fig. 17.7 Early Dupuytren's disease: note the nodule formation within the ring ray at the level of the distal palmar crease.

rarely, as proximal as the wrist. The nodules are typically painless; however, some patients note discomfort, particularly with grip, and a sensation of tension within the palm.

Disease progression is characterized by the development of longitudinal cords, most commonly in the ulnar aspect of the palm and extending distally into the fingers. The overlying skin is typically undisturbed in the proximal palm and increasingly adherent to the underlying cord distally *(Fig. 17.8)*. The ring finger is most commonly affected, followed in prevalence by the small finger, thumb, middle, and index fingers. A soft palpable fullness immediately adjacent to the

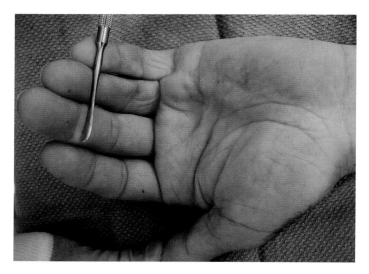

Fig. 17.8 Palmar and palmodigital disease.

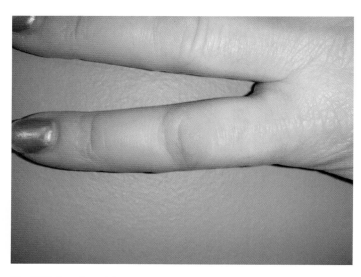

Fig. 17.9 Garrod's nodules.

cord at the level of the MCP joint may indicate displacement of the neurovascular bundle by a pathologic spiral cord (Short–Watson sign).[34]

The distal course of the cord varies. The cord may terminate in the dermis at the distal palmar crease, laterally on each side of the MCP joint, or continue distally as the central digital cord. The digital cord typically terminates just distal to the PIP joint, either centrally or laterally. A large volar nodule located at the level of the proximal phalanx often becomes intimately associated with the dermis of the overlying skin. These relationships are discernible with palpation of the cords or clinical examination. Cords are unusual distal to the middle phalanx. When present, they often lie along the radial and ulnar aspects of the finger, crossing the DIP joint. Nodules and cords strictly isolated to the finger in the absence of palmar involvement are rare but may occur.

The net effect of myofibroblast activity within palmar nodules and the deposition of collagen as pathologic cords is progressive joint contracture. The MCP joint is typically involved first, followed, in more severe cases, by PIP joint contracture. Initially, joint contracture presents as limitation in hyperextension at the MCP joint and progresses to a permanent lack of extension. MCP and PIP joint contracture result in progressive disability of the hand. Common complaints include impairment in hand shaking, fitting of gloves, difficulty placing the affected hand in a pocket, and impairment in grasping large objects. The DIP joint is typically unaffected by Dupuytren's disease; however, deformities of both flexion and extension may occur. Flexion deformity results from involvement of the lateral and retrovascular cord. DIP hyperextension, in contrast, is compensatory in the setting of PIP flexion contracture, and results from imbalance of the flexor and extensor mechanisms.

Patients may also present with Garrod's nodules, or knuckle pads located dorsally over the PIP joints *(Fig. 17.9)*. Garrod's nodules suggest a higher likelihood of bilateral hand involvement; however, their presence does not suggest stage or severity of disease, nor do they result in any functional limitation themselves.[37] Knuckle pads have been reported in

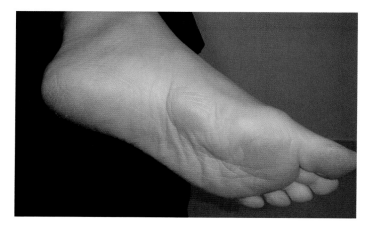

Fig. 17.10 Plantar fibromatosis.

15% of patients with Dupuytren's disease and may occur in isolation.[38,39] Knuckle pads suggest a higher likelihood of concomitant fibromatoses, including Peyronie's (penile fibromatosis) and Ledderhose's disease (plantar fibromatosis). Peyronie's disease affects the tunica albuginea of the corpora cavernosa of the penis and is present in 1–3% of patients with Dupuytren's disease.[40,41] Fibrosis develops as a well-circumscribed plaque, usually on the dorsum of the penis. The disease is generally painless; however, discomfort may occur with erection.[42] Plantar fibromatosis is present in 5–20% of patients with Dupuytren's disease, presenting as a nodular thickening within the nonweight-bearing (arch) portion of the sole of the foot[43] *(Fig. 17.10)*. These lesions are typically asymptomatic; however, they may produce discomfort or even severe pain with ambulation in a select number of cases.[44,45] Contracture of the toes does not develop. Additional presentations of Dupuytren's disease include triggering secondary to involvement of the vertical palmar septa, and an isolated tender palmar nodule whose discomfort will typically dissipate with time.

Several other lesions have been reported in association with Dupuytren's disease; however, no clear relationship has been established. Matev reported involvement of the auricular concha.[46] Allen reported the presence of nodules within the tensor fascia lata in patients with Dupuytren's disease, and Hueston has described involvement of the Achilles tendon.[44,47]

Differential diagnosis

Differential diagnosis of Dupuytren's disease includes camptodactyly, traumatic scar contracture, burn scar contracture, Volkmann's ischemic contracture, intrinsic joint ankylosis, locked trigger finger, and spastic digital contracture. Callosity, foreign body, desmoid fibroma, nodular fasciitis, and fibrosarcoma should also be considered in the differential for a primarily nodular palm. The classic history of nodule appearance with insidious progression to cord formation and joint contracture is pathognomonic for Dupuytren's disease. Diagnosis is further bolstered in the setting of a family history or in the presence of knuckle pads, Peyronie's disease, or Ledderhose's disease. No radiographic imaging or tissue diagnosis is required to confirm a diagnosis of Dupuytren's disease.

Patient selection

The primary objective of treatment in patients with Dupuytren's disease is correction of deformity, thereby reducing disability and restoring hand function. It therefore follows that the degree of joint contracture, and, more importantly, the extent of functional disability, are the primary indications for intervention. Commonly accepted surgical indications include greater than 30° of MCP joint contracture and any degree of PIP joint contracture, as these degrees of joint contracture are functionally limiting. The urgency of operative intervention is also related to the degree of joint involvement and, more critically, to the joint involved. Surgical intervention for MCP joint contracture is not urgent as the collateral ligaments are taut in MCP joint flexion. This position is protective with respect to joint motion. Surgical intervention may therefore be delayed without compromising functional outcome. In contrast, PIP joint contracture necessitates expeditious operative attention. Longstanding PIP joint contracture results in shortening of the collateral ligaments and precipitates articular changes with loss of subchondral bone resulting in a recalcitrant flexion contracture of the joint. In an effort to preserve functional PIP joint motion, surgery is indicated with any degree of contracture.

Additional operative indications include a functionally limiting first-webspace adduction contracture, small-finger abduction contracture, unremitting tenosynovitis secondary to a palmar nodule overlying the A-1 pulley, and palmar contracture resulting in maceration of the distal palmar crease.

Few contraindications to surgery exist beyond those considerations that would preclude regional or general anesthesia. Poor operative candidates include those patients with longstanding PIP joint contracture and documented underlying articular changes. These patients may require PIP arthroplasty, musculotendinous lengthening, joint fusion, or even amputation in more severe cases. Special consideration must be given to patients with a history of complex regional pain syndrome (CRPS). These patients should receive preoperative neuropathic medication therapy and operation should be performed under regional anesthesia. Relative contraindications also include conditions in which the micro- or macrovascular circulation may be impaired, including tobacco abuse, peripheral vascular occlusive disease, and diabetes mellitus. Anticoagulants should be held in the preoperative period in order to minimize the risk of palmar hematoma. Antiplatelet agents, including aspirin and clopidogrel, should be discontinued 7–9 days prior to operative intervention, while warfarin should be held 3–5 days prior to surgery so as to allow for normalization of the patient's international normalized ratio.

Treatment

Treatment of Dupuytren's disease may be subdivided into modality therapy, injection, and surgical intervention. Although promising interventional treatments, including enzymatic lysis of diseased tissue with collagenase and percutaneous needle aponeurotomy, are emerging, treatment remains primarily surgical, and results for all interventions are tempered by high rates of disease recurrence and progression.

Modality therapy

A host of nonoperative treatments have been explored for the treatment of Dupuytren's disease. This array of therapies underscores both a physician and patient desire to develop nonoperative alternatives to palmar fasciectomy as well as the general ineffectiveness of these modalities. Extension splinting may prevent contracture; however, the splint must be worn continuously and is incompatible with functional use of the hand. Intermittent splinting has not demonstrated effectiveness in preventing the progression of Dupuytren's disease. Ultrasound therapy has been reported to soften palmar nodules but has not been effective in the treatment of cords or contracture.[48] External-beam radiation therapy has been advocated for the treatment of Dupuytren's disease; however, this therapy presents significant risk for the treatment of a benign condition and has not proven effective.[49–51] Additional therapies, including the use of dimethyl sulfoxide, vitamin E, methylhydrazine, allopurinol, colchicine, and interferon-γ, have been investigated without beneficial results.[52–56]

Injection treatment

Injection therapy has demonstrated greater promise than topical and modality therapies. Authors have investigated both the use of corticosteroid injection as well as enzymatic fasciotomy with a host of degradative enzymes, including trypsin and, most recently, clostridial collagenase.

Steroids have demonstrated a restrictive effect on the formation of fibrous tissue and scar. The use of corticosteroids as a postoperative adjunct was first reported in 1952.[57] The efficacy of steroid therapy remains a subject of debate with reports ranging from no efficacy to complete resolution of palmar nodules.[52,58,59] Corticosteroid injections maintain complications, including dermal atrophy, skin depigmentation, and flexor tendon rupture. In general, corticosteroid injection may have a role in the treatment of a symptomatic palmar nodule; however, no efficacy in the treatment of Dupuytren's cords or joint contracture has been established.

The concept of targeting abnormal collagen deposition via enzymatic degradation followed by manual rupture is not novel. Reports of attempted enzymatic fasciotomy appear as early as 1907 and ,over the past century, greater refinement in the activity and specificity of the enzyme injected has occurred.[60] In 1965, Bassot reported his technique of "exerèse pharmodynamique," utilizing a mixture of trypsin, alphachymotrypsin, hyaluronidase, thiomucase, and lidocaine. Bassot reported correction of severe contracture in 34 patients.[61] In 1971, Hueston reported his experience with a simplified formula consisting of trypsin, hyaluronidase, and xylocaine, achieving favorable initial results.[62] McCarthy reported his experience with enzymatic fasciotomy in 14 patients, noting recurrence of initial contracture in 75% of patients at an average of 2–3-year follow-up. He concluded that there was a similar rate of recurrence with both enzymatic fasciotomy and surgery.[63] This technique subsequently fell into disfavor given concerns for neurovascular injury and tendon rupture with the use of nonspecific degradative enzymes.

Collagenase emerged as a candidate for enzymatic fasciotomy in 1996 and offers a potential advantage over nonspecific degradative enzymes by specifically targeting collagen. *In vitro* biomechanical testing has demonstrated a 93% decrease in the tensile modulus of Dupuytren's cords injected with a 3600-unit dose of collagenase.[64] Initial human studies focused on dose–response, collagenase pharmacokinetics, and immunologic response. Complications of treatment in phase II trials included pain with injection and manipulation, edema, ecchymosis, lymphadenopathy, and skin tears. The phase II trial showed an initial response to injection results in reduction of joint contracture to within 0–5° of normal in 90% of patients.[65,66]

A recently completed prospective, randomized, doubleblinded, placebo-controlled, multicenter phase III clinical trial further evaluated the efficacy of clostridial collagenase in the treatment of Dupuytren's disease. Results were reported in terms of a primary endpoint consisting of reduction in contracture to 0–5° of full extension within 30 days following injection. Overall 64% of patients met this primary endpoint with an improvement of range of motion from 44° to 81°. When subdivided according to the joint treated, 76% of MCP contractures and 40% of PIP contractures met the primary endpoint, with less severe contractures more reliably exhibiting correction. Complications were primarily limited to localized skin reactions, peripheral edema, and injection site pain; however, 2 out of 308 patients experienced flexor tendon rupture.[67]

Injection in enzymatic fasciotomy is performed with 0.58 mg clostridial collagenase diluted in 0.25 mL (MCP joint) or 0.20 mL (PIP joint) of sterile diluent. The cord is located by manual palpation and injection is performed at three points along the length of the cord via a single puncture with a 25-gauge needle. Care is taken to inject within the mid-substance of the cord as lateral injection may result in neurovascular injury, while deep injection results in intratendinous injection *(Fig. 17.11)*. Patients return to clinic on postinjection day 1 for manual manipulation *(Fig. 17.12)*.

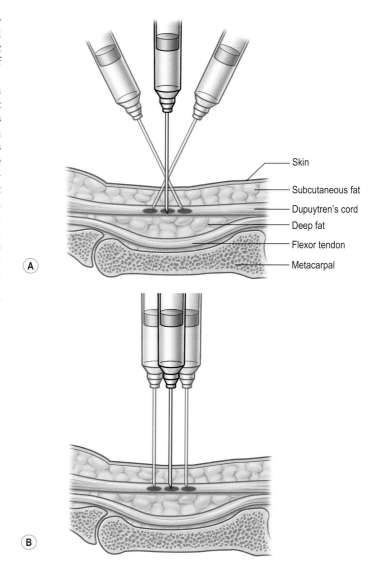

Fig. 17.11 Collagenase injection technique.

Night extension splinting is performed for 4 months following injection. A 1-month interval is allowed before repeat injection is attempted. Long-term disease recurrence rates as well as the clinical role of collagenase injection are yet to be established.

Surgical treatment

Surgical treatment of Dupuytren's disease consists of both fasciotomy and fasciectomy. Fasciotomy involves division of the diseased cords without excision and may be performed via an open technique or percutaneously. Fasciectomy involves excision of the diseased cords. Fasciectomy varies in the treatment of the skin as well as the extent of surgical dissection *(Table 17.2)*.

Percutaneous fasciotomy (needle aponeurotomy)

Percutaneous fasciotomy represents the least invasive operative modality for the treatment of Dupuytren's disease and

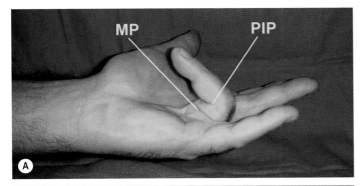

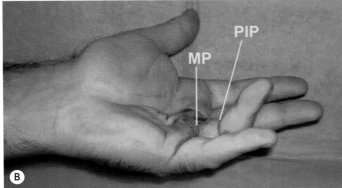

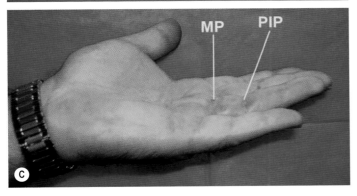

Fig. 17.12 Collagenase treatment of Dupuytren's disease. **(A)** Metacarpophalangeal and proximal interphalangeal joint contractures prior to collagenase injection. **(B)** Manipulation following collagenase injection: note ecchymosis-associated edema. **(C)** Correction of metacarpophalangeal and proximal interphalangeal joint contractures 1 month following treatment with collagenase.

Table 17.2 Surgical options for the treatment of Dupuytren's disease

Surgical technique	Description
Fasciotomy	Division of diseased cords without excision
Local fasciectomy	Removal of segment of diseased cord
Regional fasciectomy	Removal of all diseased fascia as well as local region of grossly normal tissue
Radical fasciectomy	Removal of the entire palmar and digital fascia
Open-palm technique (McCash)	Division of the palmar aponeurosis without closure of the skin deficit created
Dermatofasciectomy	Removal of the diseased fascia as well as the overlying skin. Closure typically obtained with the use of a full-thickness skin graft

---

BOX 17.1 Clinical pearl: percutaneous (needle) aponeurotomy

Percutaneous aponeurotomy involves division of Dupuytren's cords with a beveled needle under local anesthetic. Successful release requires detailed knowledge of the pathologic anatomy, meticulous technique, and a reliance on sensory feedback.

1. Extension of the involved finger by an assistant places traction on the cords within the finger and palm
2. Only distinctly palpable cords should be addressed percutaneously
3. The bevel of the needle is used to scrape and progressively weaken the involved cord in a longitudinal fashion
4. Work on several areas of the same cord prior to rupturing or dividing the cord in order to maintain tension
5. Avoid transverse movements as these present the greatest risk of neurovascular injury

---

was first described by de Seze and Debeyre in 1957.[68] The original technique described direct injection of corticosteroid into the affected cord followed by division of the cord via scoring with a 15-gauge needle and manual manipulation.[69] This technique has been modified and further refined by Foucher and its clinical utility is expanding as practitioners become more accustomed to the technique and comfortable with the pathologic anatomy *(Box 17.1)*. Using local anesthetic and a forearm tourniquet, a 19-gauge needle is used to score and divide the involved cords *(Fig. 17.13)*. No corticosteroid is utilized to weaken the cord structure and division is carried out in a distal to proximal manner to avoid disappearance of the digital cord following proximal division. Cords are divided at two or more levels and a separate fasciotomy is used to free the skin in the setting of palmar pitting.[70]

Percutaneous fasciotomy is best suited for isolated palmar cords with moderate flexion at the MCP joint level. Distal fasciotomies, including treatment of PIP contractures and spiral cords, are being performed by practitioners familiar with the percutaneous technique and anatomy with increasing clinical efficacy and success. Diffuse infiltrating cords, nodules, postsurgical recurrence, longstanding PIP flexion contracture, and deep lateral cords are poor indications for percutaneous treatment and carry a higher risk of complications. Published results demonstrate the technique to be relatively safe but limited by recurrence. In a multicenter trial in which 3736 percutaneous aponeurotomies were performed, 70% correction was reported in 93% of patients with stage I disease (less than 45° of flexion at the MCP and PIP), 78% of patients with stage II disease (45–90° of flexion at the MCP and PIP), 71% of patients with stage III disease (90–135° of flexion at the MCP and PIP), and 57% of patients with stage IV disease. Complications included two flexor tendon ruptures and two nerve transections requiring operative repair.[71] Immediate failure of therapy is reported at 15–19%.[70] Long-term recurrence rates have not been established; however, a survey of midterm results indicates a high level of recurrent contracture.[72]

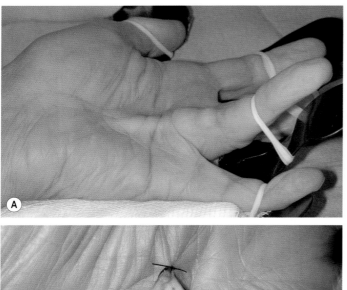
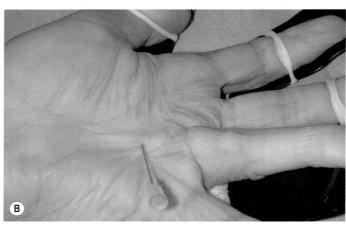
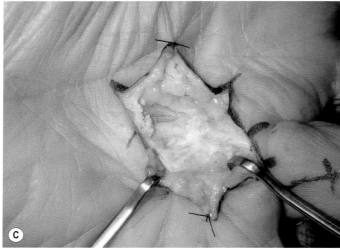

Fig. 17.13 Percutaneous (needle) aponeurotomy. **(A)** Preprocedure. Note 60° metacarpophalangeal flexion contracture. **(B)** Postprocedure, demonstrating correction of metacapophalangeal flexion contracture with percutaneous technique. Note residual digital disease. **(C)** Open dissection. Note transection of cord which has been completed percutaneously. The proximity of the radial neurovascular bundle is well visualized. The palm was opened to address digital disease.

Open fasciotomy

First described by Dupuytren, open fasciotomy consists of division of the diseased cord under direct vision.[73] A limited longitudinal incision is made over the affected cord. The cord is visualized, isolated, and divided transversely. The resultant defect may be closed directly, rearranged with a Z-plasty incorporating the cord and skin, or closed with a skin graft.[74–77] Open fasciotomy techniques reliably provide for correction, particularly in the setting of isolated MCP contractures; however, recurrence sufficient to warrant reoperation is reported in 43% of patients.[78]

Fasciotomy is a simple and safe technique when performed within the palm. Its primary utility remains in elderly patients with an isolated palmar cord in whom substantive health problems preclude a more extensive procedure. Use of fasciotomy within the finger presents some risk of neurovascular injury.

Local fasciectomy

Local or limited fasciectomy is a technique designed to remove a portion of the diseased aponeurosis, disrupting continuity of the diseased tissue. This procedure is a compromise between removal all of the diseased aponeurosis via extensive palmar and digital dissection and fasciotomy. Theoretically,

local fasciectomy limits the risk of complications associated with dissection, including palmar hematoma and neurovascular injury, while addressing the possibility of local recurrence by creating discontinuity of the diseased tissue.

A longitudinal or Z-plasty incision is performed over the involved cord analogous to that performed in an open fasciotomy. The cord is isolated and divided with resection of 1–2 cm of the cord itself. Residual diseased aponeurosis is left behind. The role of local fasciectomy is limited and overlaps with that of fasciotomy.

Regional (partial) fasciectomy

Until recent developments with needle aponeurotomy and enzymatic treatment, regional fasciectomy has provided the mainstay of operative treatment in Dupuytren's disease. Regional fasciectomy consists of excision of all macroscopically abnormal fibrous tissues within the palm and finger. Successful operative intervention requires an intimate understanding of the normal palmar and digital fascial anatomy as well as the pathologic correlates. This technique limits palmar dissection while disrupting the continuity of the aponeurotic tissue and limiting focal recurrence. By leaving residual aponeurosis, the possibility of disease progression remains. This technique is performed under regional or general anesthesia with a brachial tourniquet placed sufficiently high as to allow access to the medial arm should a skin graft be required. The arm is abducted, supinated on a hand table. A lead or Tupper hand is a valuable adjunct to allow the surgeon to work with minimal assistance. Loupe magnification is invaluable in allowing fine dissection of the common and digital neurovascular bundles.

Digital and palmar disease may be approached through a variety of incisions either separately or conjunction (*Fig. 17.14*). The skin incision should provide adequate exposure for dissection of the disease tissues and the neurovascular bundles in the palm and fingers, preserve vascularized skin flaps to avoid skin necrosis, allow skin lengthening along the longitudinal axis of the finger, and avoid scar contractures. Although some surgeons advocate transverse palmar incisions, longitudinal incisions are more useful for digital exposure and may be extended into the palm for exposure of the aponeurosis. Longitudinal incisions with Z-plasties at the flexion creases or a zigzag Brunner-type incision both provide excellent exposure. Closure with Y to V tissue rearrangement provides for additional length and is particularly useful in patients with significant contracture in which a relative deficiency of skin exists upon correction of the contracture. Contracture of the first webspace is best approached through a T-incision combined with Z-plasties to prevent scar contracture. Transverse incisions within the palm allow for excellent palmar exposure and present no risk of flexion contracture; however, this approach typically requires relatively extensive undermining and does not lend itself to facile proximal or distal extension. When the skin is markedly adherent to the underlying diseased aponeurosis, the incision should pass through the center of this region to avoid extensive devascularization.

Following skin incision, dermal flaps are developed sharply with preservation of the subcutaneous tissue. A scalpel is used to sweep the skin/subcutaneous flaps sharply off the cord in the palm region. Proximal to the distal palmar crease, the digital neurovascular structures are safely deep to the cord itself, and are therefore protected. With the cord skeletonized, the digital nerves and arteries may be identified proximally and traced distally. All abnormal tissue is excised, including the involved vertical fibers of Legueu and Juvara. The proximal transverse metacarpal ligament is preserved as it is not affected by Dupuytren's disease. The aponeurosis may be in intimate association with the underlying flexor tendon sheath and pulley system; however, a natural plane of dissection exists and the sheath is preserved. Once the palmar aponeurosis and pretendinous cords have been disrupted, the MCP joints will extend without constraint, allowing for more facile dissection within the finger (video clip).

Distal to the proximal transverse metacarpal ligament, the diseased tissue becomes increasingly adherent to the overlying dermis, necessitating sharp dissection. From this point distal, the dissection is focused on the neurovascular structures, and excision of diseased tissue is performed only after the nerve and artery have been identified and protected. Of particular note, the common digital arteries lie superficial to the common digital nerves within the palm, while the proper digital arteries lie deep to the digital nerves within the finger. The digital nerves bifurcate more proximally than the arteries, crossing over the digital arteries at the level of the metacarpal heads.

The termination of the pretendinous cords is variable, and each termination should be dissected separately and divided. Once the pretendinous cord has been divided, MCP extension is typically full. The natatory ligament, which crosses the tendons and neurovascular bundles superficially, is excised, thereby allowing release of any adduction contracture.

At the digital–palmar junctions, multiple anatomic components converge. The pretendinous cord, spiral cord, lateral digital sheet, and Grayson's ligament may coalesce to form a spiral band, displacing the neurovascular bundle medially, superficially, and proximally. Meticulous care is exercised in order to avoid damage to a displaced neurovascular bundle resulting from the presence of a spiral cord. Removal of diseased tissue within the finger is the most delicate portion of the operation. The path of the neurovascular bundles, altered by an assortment of fibrous cords, is unpredictable. The digital artery may, on occasion, be separated from its companion nerve by a sheet of fibrous tissue. To navigate this anatomy successfully and to avoid injury to the digital neurovascular structures, the digital artery and nerve should be identified distally within uninvolved tissue and traced proximally (*Box 17.2*).

Retrovascular cords are notoriously occult, and failure to recognize this structure often results in residual PIP contracture. DIP joint hyperextension is infrequent and is often associated with severe PIP contracture. Release of the PIP contracture typically corrects the distal deformity. Residual DIP hyperextension may require oblique tenotomy of the lateral bands of the extensor apparatus. Release of the lateral bands is performed over the middle phalanx through a dorsal incision. The bands are allowed to slide distally, restoring DIP flexion.

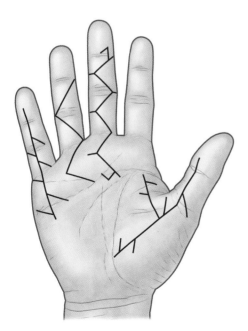

Fig. 17.14 Surgical incisions for regional fasciectomy. Thumb illustrates T- with Z-plasties at the flexion creases, long finger illustrates Y to V advancement, ring finger illustrates traditional Brunner incision, and small finger illustrates axial incision with Z-plasties at the flexion creases.

Fasciectomy within the small finger and first webspace require special attention due to the unique pathologic anatomy in these regions of the palm. The small finger is often severely involved in the disease process and dissection is particularly difficult given the diminutive size of the ulnar digital artery and nerve. Fascia surrounding the ADM and its retrovascular correlate are routinely affected. This structure originates from the muscular fascia of the ADM immediately superficial to the ADM tendon and is frequently mistaken for the ADM tendon itself. The cord is usually deep and ulnar to the neurovascular bundle; however, the bundle may spiral dorsal to or through the cord. The dorsal ulnar sensory nerve may also be displaced volarly and should be identified prior to division of the ADM cord.

Although radial-sided palmar involvement in Dupuytren's disease is rare, a marked first-webspace adduction contracture and thumb MCP contractures may be quite functionally limiting. Contracture of the first webspace is best approached through a T-incision combined with Z-plasties to prevent scar contracture or a four-flap Z-plasty.[79] The neurovascular bundles should be carefully identified and preserved. The ulnar bundle is reliably found at the base of the thumb. The radial bundle, in contrast, may be quite difficult to localize as it is covered with decussating fibers at the level of the MCP joint, and should be identified more proximally within the thenar eminence. The proximal and distal commissural cords

should be excised. In longstanding contractures of the first webspace, the dorsal structures may become contracted secondary to positional deformity rather than involvement of the Dupuytren's disease process, and may require release.

Several additional techniques may be required when complete range of motion cannot be restored with fasciectomy alone. These procedures should be employed judiciously with consideration given to the fact that a finger with mild residual PIP deformity is more functional than a stiff finger with full extension. Residual deformity may be attributed to shortening of the flexor tendon sheath, capsular contracture of the PIP joint, or articular changes within the PIP joint. The latter is not amenable to further correction with manipulation of the soft tissue alone and requires arthodesis or arthroplasty to address residual deformity. Shortening of the tendon sheath is addressed by making one or two transverse incisions within the sheath at the level of the PIP joint to allow for lengthening. The pulley system should be preserved. PIP joint contracture presents a more formidable challenge. Complete capsulectomy should be avoided in favor of a limited artholysis, which involves selective division of the volar plate check rein ligaments.[80,81] Check rein division should be performed just proximal to the arterial branch for the vinculum longum, which is preserved[82] **(Fig. 17.15)**. Once full passive extension is achieved, the integrity of the central slip should be assessed. If the central slip is deficient, the PIP joint should be immobilized postoperatively in static extension for 3 weeks. Alternatively, gentle passive manipulation under anesthesia may be performed.[83] This method does not allow for dramatic correction, but minimizes trauma and potential complications of recurrent PIP joint capsular contracture.

Radical fasciectomy

Radical fasciectomy involves extensive dissection of the palm and digital fascial structures in an effort to remove both normal and diseased palmar and digital fascia. This procedure has been proposed and advocated by several surgeons with the theoretic advantage of eliminating the risk of disease progression and recurrence.[84] This theoretic advantage has not been borne out in practice.[85,86] The procedure has been plagued by significant postoperative complications, including

---

BOX 17.2 Clinical pearl: dissection of a spiral cord

Safe dissection of the neurovascular bundle which has been displaced proximally, medially, and superficially by a spiral cord is the most technically demanding component of an open fasciotomy. Several key techniques will ensure clinical success:

1. Identify the involved neurovascular bundle proximally within the normal tissue of the palm (outside the zone of disease)
2. Identify the involved neurovascular bundle distally within the normal tissue of the finger (outside the zone of disease)
3. Dissect from proximal to distal between these two "known" regions
4. Division of the cord proximally may assist in distal dissection
5. Avoid undue traction on the neurovascular bundle

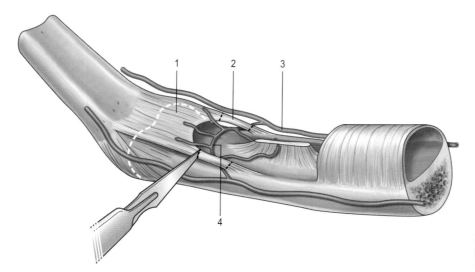

Fig. 17.15 Technique of check rein release. 1, Volar plate. 2, Check rein ligament. 3, Collateral artery. 4, Transverse arterial branch. (Redrawn after Tubiana R. The Hand. Philadelphia: WB Saunders, 1999, p. 463.)

hematoma and skin necrosis, and has largely been abandoned in favor of regional excision.

Dermatofasciectomy

Dermatofasciectomy involves excision not only of the involved facial structures of the palm and fingers, but the overlying skin as well. This practice has its foundation in the histopathological studies of Meyerding *et al.* that demonstrated pathologic changes in the palmar fascia, thinning of the subcutaneous tissue, and a reduction in the number of dermal sweat glands.[23] The dermis is often thought to represent a repository for active disease and the nidus for disease recurrence. Although this relationship has never been definitively established, dermatofasciectomy retains a role primarily in the treatment of recurrent disease or in cases with extensive cutaneous involvement. Excised skin is allowed to heal secondarily (open-palm technique of McCash) or replaced with a full-thickness skin graft obtained from the groin or medial arm.[87] The open-palm technique alleviates the risk of hematoma; however, it is complicated by prolonged healing times and scar contracture. This technique is advocated only for small lesions within the palm. Skin grafts provide a viable alternative to the open-palm technique; however, no skin graft can adequately replace the glabrous skin of the palm. Skin grafts have, however, bee demonstrated to prevent local recurrence in several studies.[88–93] A single series of 103 patients published by Logan and colleagues noted only nine histologically confirmed recurrences in patients treated with dermatofasciectomy.[93] Dermatofasciectomy is most clearly indicated in cases of recurrent disease and in patients with early-onset primary disease with significant skin involvement.

Postoperative care

Postoperative therapy in Dupuytren's disease couples early motion to maintain joint mobility with extension splinting to reduce the risk of early contracture. The interrelationship between these two opposing regimens is dictated by the procedure performed.

Patients undergoing enzymatic or percutaneous fasciotomy are placed in a soft, bulky dressing postoperatively in order to provide mild compression and for comfort. This dressing is removed 1–3 days after the procedure and patients are encouraged to use their hand normally as tolerated by level of comfort. Hand therapy is rarely required in order to facilitate mobilization and extension night splinting is encouraged for 3–4 months following contracture release.

Patients undergoing fasciectomy typically have more discomfort and postoperative stiffness compared with those undergoing percutaneous techniques. A volar splint with the MCP and PIP joints placed in maximal extension is placed, leaving unoperated fingers free. The fingertips should be visible to allow for assessment of perfusion. In the absence of a skin graft, this splint is taken down and physical therapy for active and passive range of motion is begun at 3–5 days after surgery. The suture lines are dressed daily with antibiotic-impregnated gauze and sutures are left in place for 14 days. Skin grafts are held in place with tie-over bolsters consisting of antibiotic gauze and this dressing is taken down after 5 days. In these patients range of motion is delayed until postoperative day 7 to allow for sufficient revascularization of the graft.

Hand therapy is generally required in patients with severe MCP and any degree of PIP joint contracture and should be initiated as early as possible as allowed by postoperative pain and edema. Therapy first targets recovery of full finger flexion, followed by progressive restoration of finger extension. If articular interventions are performed, including check rein release, early dynamic splinting should be instituted. If central slip tenodesis was performed, immobilization must be continued for 3 weeks prior to the initiation of dynamic splinting.

Outcomes, prognosis, and complications

Percutaneous interventions in Dupuytren's disease seek to minimize wound complications and recovery. Complications arise as a consequence of the blind nature of these techniques. The short-term efficacy and complications of enzymatic fasciotomy have been well quantified in the recent phase III evaluation of clostridial collagenase. Edema (73%), bruising (51%), and injection site pain (32%) were the most commonly reported complications. Patients also noted discomfort with manual manipulation. No systemic side-effects or type IV hypersensitivity reactions were noted. Serious complications included two tendon ruptures and one case of CRPS in 308 patients. Overall 64% of patients met the primary endpoint of correction of contracture to within 0–5° of full extension within 30 days of injection with an improvement of range of motion from 44° to 81°. When subdivided according to the joint treated, 76% of MCP contractures and 40% of PIP contractures met the primary endpoint with less severe contractures more reliably exhibiting correction.[67] Although clostridial collagenase can effectively correct flexion contractures resulting from Dupuytren's disease with a reasonable margin of safety, long-term studies of recurrence and disease progression have not yet been completed. This lack of long-term data remains a primary barrier to widespread use of this technique.

Percutaneous (needle) aponeurotomy has been more widely employed and data regarding efficacy and prognosis have been established. In a multicenter trial in which 3736 percutaneous aponeurotomies were performed, 70% correction was reported in 93% of patients with stage I disease (less than 45° of flexion at the MCP and PIP), 78% of patients with stage II disease (45–90° of flexion at the MCP and PIP), 71% of patients with stage III disease (90–135° of flexion at the MCP and PIP), and 57% of patients with stage IV disease. Immediate failure to correct the underlying contracture is reported in 15–19% of patients.[71,94] Two large series have evaluated complications in percutaneous fasciectomy. The first evaluated complications in 138 patients undergoing needle fasciotomy. Complications were reported as skin ruptures (16%), nerve transections (2%), and infections (2%).[71] A larger multicenter study evaluating 799 patients undergoing 3736 percutaneous aponeurotomies reported complications including cutaneous rupture (2%), flexor tendon rupture (0.8%), and nerve transections (0.8%). Long-term data regarding recurrence and progression are sparse; however, Foucher *et al.*

report a recurrence rate of 58% of patients undergoing needle aponeurotomy with a reoperation rate of 24% at 3.2 years.[70]

Complications in the surgical treatment of Dupuytren's disease may be categorized as perioperative, early postoperative, and late postoperative complications. Operative complications most commonly involve damage to the neurovascular bundle. Experienced surgeons have reported rates of arterial and nerve injury less than 0.4% and 2.3% respectively.[95] Damage to the neurovascular bundle may be avoided by maintaining a high suspicion for a spiral nerve in all patients and particularly in those patients with PIP joint contracture. Dissection between the distal palmar crease and proximal digital crease should be specifically directed at identifying and preserving the neurovascular bundle. Nerve or vascular injury should be recognized and repaired immediately should it occur. The surgeon should be particularly vigilant during reoperation for recurrent contracture as a single digital artery may supply the digit. Digital ischemia is addressed intraoperatively by: (1) minimizing compression from skin closure and dressings; (2) infiltrating agents (papaverine, lidocaine) to decrease vasospasm; (3) decreasing extension of the digit to prevent unaccustomed stretch on the digital vessels; and (4) microsurgical exploration and repair as necessary *(Box 17.3)*.

Early postoperative complications include infection, hematoma, skin necrosis, and postoperative flare reaction. Postoperative wound infection typically occurs in 1–4% of patients, but has been reported to be as high as 9.5%.[96] Infections are likely attributable to bacterial overgrowth within the macerated distal palmar crease as well as to tenuous blood supply to the palmar flaps. Another common complication of palmar dissection is postoperative hematoma, which often results in palmar skin necrosis if not identified and evacuated. The reported incidence in populations undergoing a variety of surgical techniques is 2%; however, the risk with radical fasciectomy is significantly higher.[96] The risk of palmar hematoma may be minimized by obtaining hemostasis with the tourniquet deflated, prior to application of the final dressing, and by minimizing palmar dissection. Some authors advocate application of a pressure dressing; however, this intervention is unnecessary if meticulous operative hemostasis is obtained. The incidence of palmar hematoma may also be reduced with the use of the open-palm technique of McCash.[87,95] Postoperative flare reaction may also occur. Flare reaction consists of significant pain, swelling, and joint stiffness, characteristically occurring in the third to fourth week following surgery. Flare reaction is significantly more common in women and its incidence is further increased with concomitant procedures, including carpal tunnel release.[96,97] For this reason multiple procedures should not be performed at time of operation for Dupuytren's disease. This syndrome may be a precursor of CRPS, and the incidence is minimized with operation under regional anesthesia.

Late postoperative complications include CRPS, scar contracture disease recurrence, and disease progression. CRPS refers to a syndrome characterized by pain, allodynia, and hyperalgesia disproportionate to the extent of inciting injury accompanied by evidence of vasomotor instability. The reported incidence of CRPS in patients undergoing fasciectomy for Dupuytren's disease ranges between 4.5 and 40%, and varies on the choice of anesthetic. Regional analgesia provides the lowest postoperative incidence, with comparable results achieved with intravenous regional anesthesia accompanied by clonidine. The highest reported incidence occurs with general anesthesia.[98] For this reason, infraclavicular or axillary block should be considered the anesthetic method of choice when operating for Dupuytren's disease. Scar contracture occurs with longitudinal digital incisions. The risk of contracture is minimized by careful incisional planning, the use of Z-plasties at the flexion creases, or Brunner's incisions. Prolonged postoperative stiffness is reported in 10% of patients. The most common complication of Dupuytren's disease is recurrence. Recurrence is distinct from disease progression and is defined as the reappearance of Dupuytren's disease, nodules or cords, in a region previously cleared of abnormal fascia via operative excision. The incidence of recurrence varies with technique and ranges between 32 and 40% with open techniques, and is reported to be as high as 58% with percutaneous fasciotomy of the diseased cords.[99,100] In general, recurrence may be minimized with appropriate digital dissection coupled with more extensive palmar dissection. The benefits of more extensive dissection must, however, be weighed against higher incidence of wound complications. Interestingly, most severe recurrences develop early, whereas later recurrences typically remain discrete, resulting in little or no functional disability.[101] Recurrence does not invariably require additional surgery. Rodrigo and colleagues found that only 15% of patients required re-excision following disease recurrence.[78]

BOX 17.3 Clinical pearl: treatment of arterial insufficiency in Dupuytren's contracture release

Arterial insufficiency is a known surgical complication in the treatment of Dupuytren's disease. Ischemia may result from direct trauma to the digital artery as a consequence of dissection or, more commonly, as a result of traction and vasospasm as a previously contracted finger is straightened. The surgeon should have a methodical approach to the treatment of arterial insufficiency.

1. Flex the finger to alleviate traction on the digital artery
2. Warm the finger with warm irrigant solution
3. Apply topical papavarine (30 mg/mL) to facilitate smooth-muscle relaxation (lidocaine may be used alternatively or in addition to papavarine)
4. Be patient. Allow the relaxation, warming, and antivasospasm interventions time to work. The artery may require up to 10 minutes for the restoration of perfusion
5. If arterial insufficiency persists beyond 10 minutes, explore the digital artery throughout the extent of dissection. Repair of a partial or complete laceration should be performed under the operating microscope. A vein graft may be necessary if undue tension is present

---

Secondary procedures

Disease recurrence and progression are common in Dupuytren's disease and, consequently, operation for disease recurrence is the most common secondary procedure performed.

Severely contracted, functionally limiting fingers may require ray amputation; however, several alternatives to amputation exist and have gained an integral role in the treatment of recalcitrant disease. These procedures include skeletal traction, wedge osteotomy, total volar tenoarthrolysis, and PIP arthrodesis.

Skeletal traction

Severe PIP joint contractures may be addressed with the application of a dorsally based external distraction device. Described by Messina in 1989, the continuous elongation technique involves application of progressive continuous extension via an adjustable external device.[102] Full extension is typically achieved over the course of 2–4 weeks. This technique allows for ready access to the palm and a regional or dermatofasciectomy is performed concomitant with removal of the distraction device.

Biochemical studies have demonstrated an increase in the enzymatic activity of fibroblasts and increased collagen deposition in response to skeletal traction.[103] If left unaddressed, this stimulus results in disease progression, and, therefore, distraction alone is contraindicated unless coupled with subsequent fasciectomy. This technique is a useful addition to the surgeon's repertoire in addressing advanced Dupuytren's disease and may provide salvage in settings under which amputation might be considered.

Wedge osteotomy

Wedge osteotomy provides for a more functional range of motion in recalcitrant PIP contractures with residual flexion deformity despite attempts at surgical release. The operation consists of removal of a dorsal wedge from the proximal phalanx placing the PIP joint into a position in which the existing range of motion is functionally useful. Although advocated by some, wedge osteotomy maintains a very limited role in the treatment of advanced Dupuytren's disease.[104]

Total volar tenoarthrolysis

Analogous to wedge osteotomy, total volar tenoarthrolysis redistributes the existing PIP range of motion to within a more functional range. Via a lateral digital approach, the volar plate and flexor digitorum superficialis and profundus are sectioned. This leaves the extensors and intrinsics as the only active determinants of digital motion. The finger passively falls into flexion due to the contracture of the palmar fascia.[105,106]

PIP arthrodesis

Arthrodesis is indicated in patients with severe PIP joint contracture that has proven recalcitrant to surgical correction. Underlying articular or degenerative change, pain upon restoration of motion, and immobility in a nonfunctional position are clear indications favoring PIP arthrodesis. MCP arthrodesis should be avoided as articular change does not occur with prolonged contracture at this joint and fusion at the MCP joint level is functionally limiting.

Amputation

Although commonly employed in the past in cases of severe primary contracture and recurrent, severe secondary contracture, amputation is now a relatively rare treatment of Dupuytren's disease. Skeletal traction has emerged as a useful adjunct in treating patients who might otherwise be considered candidates for amputation. Clear indications for amputation exist, including multiply recurrent contractures and in severely contracted fingers with nerve or vascular lesions. Ray amputation is preferable for the index, long, and ring fingers. Amputation at the MCP joint level is indicated to address small-finger contracture. Thumb amputation is contraindicated regardless of the severity of contracture. Dorsal skin should be preserved and may be useful in resurfacing the palm.

Conclusion

The management of Dupuytren's disease remains a challenging problem for hand surgeons. Operative results are tempered by relatively high rates of disease recurrence and each subsequent operation affords a narrower margin for functional improvement and higher risk to the neurovascular structures of the hand. Bench and clinical research continue to identify and evaluate new clinical targets and novel therapeutic interventions. The opportunity to modify the underlying disease process via pharmacotherapeutics and interventional treatments offers the greatest promise for functional preservation and disease prevention.

 Access the complete references list online at **http://www.expertconsult.com**

21. Dupuytren G. *Leçons orales de clinique chirurgicale faites a l'Hôtel-Dieu de Paris*. Paris: Baillière; 1832.

27. Luck JV. Dupuytren's Contracture. A New Concept of the Pathogenesis Correlated with the Surgical Management. *J Bone Joint Surg (Am)*. 1959;40:635–664.
   In this seminal manuscript, Luck provides a detailed description of the histopathologic anatomy and disease progression in Dupuytren's disease. Luck's proliferative, involutional, and residual phases provide a framework within which molecular advances may be analyzed and a foundation for clinicians' understanding of disease progression.

33. Shaw RB, Chong AK, Zhang A, et al. Dupuytren's Disease: History, Diagnosis, and Treatment. *Plast Reconstr Surg*. 2007;120:44e–54e.

35. McFarlane RM. Patterns of Diseased Fascia in the Fingers in Dupuytren's Contracture. *Plast Reconstr Surg*. 1974;54:31–44.
   In this manuscript, McFarlane details the normal and pathologic disease correlates in the progression of Dupuytren's disease. A detailed description of the formation of the spiral cord has provided the foundation for all subsequent manuscripts. The detailed illustrations are useful and frequently reproduced.

67. Hurst LC, Badalamente MA, Hentz VR et al. Injectable Collagenase *Clostridium histolyticum* for Dupuytren's Contracture. *N Engl J Med.* 2009;361:968–979.

This manuscript describes a multicenter, randomized, double-blind, placebo-controlled trial of clostridial collagenase injection in the treatment of Dupuytren's disease. A total of 64% of patients met the primary endpoint of correction to within 0–5(of full extension. When subdivided according to the joint treated, 76% of MCP contractures and 40% of PIP contractures met the primary endpoint, with less severe contractures more reliably exhibiting correction. This study provides the first large-scale assessment of the efficacy, safety, and reliability of clostridial collagenase injection therapy.

78. Rodrigo JJ, Niebauer JJ, Brown RL, et al. Treatment of Dupuytren's Contracture: Long-term Results After Fasciotomy and Fascial Excision. *J Bone Joint Surg (Am).* 1976;58:380–387.

Rodrigo's manuscript provides the first and largest assessment of the clinical outcomes following fascial excision in Dupuytren's disease. This manuscript established the commonly quoted 32% recurrence rate and established that only a portion of recurrences (15%) require reoperation.

84. McIndoe A, Beare RL. The Surgical Management of Dupuytren's Contracture. *Am J Surg.* 1958;95:197–203.

88. Tonkin MA, Burke FD, Varian JP. The Proximal Interphalangeal Joint in Dupuytren's Disease. *J Hand Surg (Br).* 1985;10:358–364.

95. Bulstrode NW, Jemec C, Smith PJ. The Complications of Dupuytren's Contracture Surgery. *J Hand Surg (Am).* 2005;30:1021–1025.

100. Foucher G, Medina J, Navarro R. Percutaneous Needle Aponeurectomy: Complications and Results. *J Hand Surg (Br).* 2003;28:427–431.

Foucher provides a detailed description of the technique of needle aponeurotomy, including operative indications, patient selection, and technical considerations. A review of the complications and outcomes provides the reader with a detailed understanding of the evolving role of percutaneous aponeurotomy in the treatment of Dupuytren's disease.

18

Occupational hand disorders

Steven J. McCabe

SYNOPSIS

- Upper extremity problems that are attributed to the workplace require experience, a knowledge base, and skill set that set them aside from non occupational injuries.
- To evaluate causation requires a careful history and physical examination as well as knowledge of the disease process and literature.
- The Workers' Compensation environment creates external forces on the provider and patient that can adversely affect patient management and recovery.
- Management of work related upper extremity disorders should include nonsurgical care when it is known to be efficacious.
- Return to meaningful employment and high quality of life are the desired outcomes.

Introduction

There are several reasons why upper extremity problems relating to work activities are considered as a distinct entity. Some upper extremity problems are closely identified with work activity and hence could correctly be called occupational injuries. High pressure injection injuries and vibration induced problems are closely identified with a certain occupational activity. In addition to these problems that are closely identified with specific work, there are upper extremity problems that seem to occur in greater than expected numbers, i.e., their incidence rate may be higher, in certain working populations. Although tendon entrapments are often seen in the nonworking population their occurrence is often attributed to work activity. The surgeon is often called upon to determine causation or if the upper extremity problem is related to the work activity. Second, illness related to the work place requires considerations for management not needed in problems unrelated to work. Documentation and justification of attribution to the workplace, guiding the return to some form

of modified work and full duty work are examples of issues in management that are more profound in the work related injury. Finally, the outcomes of treatment in upper extremity problems related to the workplace are qualitatively and quantitatively different than similar problems not related to the workplace. Return to previous work is an outcome of interest unto itself. The surgeon will be involved in determining the return to regular or modified work activities, the completion of active medical care, and the assignment of a permanent impairment rating.

Hints and tips

- Some upper extremity problems are closely associated with work activity.
- Work related upper extremity disorders require management considerations that are different than nonwork related problems.
- Return to full activity at work is one important outcome goal.

Causation

Physicians and surgeons are often called on to judge whether a specific work activity could cause the upper extremity problem of a patient. To do this, the surgeon must bring to bear all the evidence that is available from the history of injury, the time course of events since the injury, the physical examination, information from diagnostic tests, as well as knowledge of the upper extremity problem diagnosed in the patient.

Patient history

Initial events

The history must be detailed and thorough. It is important to consider the sequence of events, the history of injury, the behavior of the patient, co-workers, and medical providers at the time of the injury. Often a careful history will reveal features of the injury that were previously unclear such as the nature of a crushing injury or the lack thereof. A severe injury will usually demand an immediate response and care. When a patient was able to complete vigorous work for the remainder of the day following an injury and reported the injury some days later, many severe injuries can be excluded. Similarly a review of the original medical records is often informative. The description of the emergency room doctor or first examining physician provides contemporaneous information on the severity of injury. Severe swelling, bruising, or radiographic evidence of soft tissue swelling or fracture at the time of the injury will all document the nature of the original injury. Similarly a lack of physical findings at the time of the injury may be important for lingering symptomatic problems. The initial behavior of the patient and documentation of the injury before the initiation of the Workers' Compensation system of care and the influence of society will be informative for future management. For an observed traumatic event, immediate contemporaneous actions and information are the result of the injury whereas later behavior is a result of the injury, and the influence of a number of other societal factors that have to be considered.

The course of illness

Through education and experience, surgeons understand the expected course of an illness and can detect when there is variation from this. When the course of illness varies to some large degree it is sometimes possible to determine that the symptoms and physical findings of a current evaluation could not be consistent with an injury that is described in the history and verified by review of initial medical records. In other words, knowledge of the natural course of an injury can be used to make strong statements about the lack of causation.

Physical examination

A detailed perceptive history and physical examination are required for careful evaluation of a work related injury. The surgeon must use all of her senses to gather information. Open ended questions, active listening, and fact checking are all important. Classic techniques such as repetition to check important physical findings, distraction, and use of a tool box of physical examination skills specific to the situation must be developed and practiced. Adequate time must be devoted to obtain accurate impressions and information.

Knowledge of the disease process and its causation

The concept of causation has evolved as our understanding of illness has changed. The concepts of Hill have stood the test of time as guidelines to evaluate associations as possibly causative however it is clear there are no single or combination of characteristics of an association that can prove causation. The concept of causation requires in depth knowledge of the content of the research to measure associations as well as their context and characteristics. It is difficult to suggest associations are causative from observational data alone. Therefore for many illnesses of the upper extremity related to the workplace there will always be some uncertainty as to the accuracy of their attribution. This problem is magnified when considering an individual patient.

The role of force and repetition

In 1991, Gerr and associates reported that: "Sufficient evidence is available at this time to conclude that several well-defined soft-tissue disorders of the upper extremities are etiologically related to occupational factors. These disorders include tendinitis of the hand and wrist, CTS, and hand-arm vibration syndrome. Force, repetition, and vibration have been established as risk factors in the etiology of these disorders."[1] These conditions are discussed further below.

Szabo has well advised against the use of *"cumulative trauma disorder"* or *"repetitive strain injury"* as diagnostic labels, suggesting the term *"work-related musculoskeletal disorders"* to describe an amorphous category of upper extremity problems, often characterized by pain, with no clear diagnosis or anatomic basis for symptoms, and clinical course that is not easy to understand given the traditional concepts of illness and injury.[2] It is plausible that highly repetitive activity of high enough force can lead to symptoms and disorders of the upper extremity but it seems most appropriate to consider these as attributes leading to potential causation rather than a diagnosis of an illness. Upper extremity pathology with a clear clinical diagnosis such as carpal tunnel syndrome or de Quervain's tendonitis should be managed according to the standards available for the problem. A new diagnostic category is not required and confuses the management of the patient. Upper extremity problems without a clear diagnosis should be dealt with as such. A pseudo-diagnostic label will not help the patient recover from an illness.

Although the concept of causation is philosophical, practically, the best evidence that can be gathered would be the results of a randomized experiment where the causative agent is randomly distributed to two otherwise equivalent groups. Unfortunately, it is typically not possible to randomize the exposure to work activities. Failing this, it is important to understand this uncertainty and try to understand the consequences and minimize the negative impacts of this uncertainty.

What is the purpose of this attention being delivered to determine if the upper extremity problems are related to work and why is it the surgeon's responsibility to arbitrate this decision?

1. To provide the best management, the surgeon should have an accurate evaluation of the patient's illness, which includes the pathology located in the upper extremity, how that is experienced by the patient, and the external factors that can influence the management and recovery.

2. It is important to the patient. In a work-related disorder the financial benefits of the Workers' Compensation

system may be the only source of financial security for the patient.

3. An accurate and definitive decision about work attribution may be the best way to avoid the negative effects that accompany the Workers' Compensation system of insurance coverage. A rapid and accurate decision either affirmative or negative will reduce the potential for conflict and will be in the patients' best interest.

4. The surgeon is in the best position to gather and weigh all the evidence that is available.

5. It is important to be truthful.

Clinical care in illness related to the workplace

Injuries at the workplace can be broadly divided into acute traumatic injuries and those without a single identifiable traumatic incident.

When a worker suffers a verifiable traumatic injury at the workplace that is directly observed and an injury is present under any reproducible and acceptable method of its presence, the attribution to work is not an issue. Efforts are provided at the best management and rehabilitation of the injured worker.

Millender et al. has divided the more chronic occupational injuries of the musculoskeletal system into four categories that provide a useful framework for discussion *(Table 18.1).*[3]

In category one, most patients are highly motivated and when the appropriate treatment is provided for the patient, the upper extremity problem resolves. The patient can resume work and there are no lingering effects.

In category two, some difficulties may arise as permanent impairment is possible. When the patient is left with permanent impairment the easiest resolution is for the injured worker, upon recovery, to return to the same regular duty work that pre-dated the injury. If this is not possible, then a modified job with the same employer may be possible. Failing this, the worker may have to consider new work with a new employer, or retirement. This can be a difficult decision that requires coordination with a case manager or rehabilitation

counselor. There are some patients with conditions usually well treated either nonsurgically or surgically by the hand surgeon, who do not seem to have the capacity to recover to the extent that would let them return to their original job. This group of people may be difficult to identify before treatment begins but eventually they can be identified by a recovery that falls below the threshold that allows them to return to their pre-injury job. This group of patients is difficult for the hand surgeon to manage, and care should be taken to avoid a repetitious exposure to invasive treatments and repeated surgeries that never quite reach the expected result.

In category three, the patients may have pain that is out of proportion to their physical injury. They can be angry and frustrated at the lack of improvement, despite adequate medical care. Patients may have definite upper extremity pathology but this is difficult to improve to a degree that will be satisfactory to the patient. Surgeons will immediately recognize this group of patients, as features of the history and physical examination will be identified as falling outside the expected norms for the conditions being cared for. This embellishment of symptoms and physical findings may represent frustration on the part of the patient, an attempt to make the surgeon realize the depth of their problem, or conscious magnification of symptoms and findings. Unfortunately, this is a group of patients that is difficult for the surgeon to manage. An honest approach will result in anger on the part of the patient, but management that deals with the upper extremity problem as an isolated independent part of the patient will not succeed.

In category four, the diagnosis of the upper extremity problem is unclear. Many of these patients will have vague diagnoses and may have had surgical procedures. They may have previous experience with other Workers' Compensation injuries and may have seen other hand surgeons. For example the patient may present with a problem whose existence is controversial, its pathology unproven, its treatment ill-defined, and its outcome uncertain. The patient may be in conflict with their employer and may be terminated from employment. When the worker has this type of an upper extremity disorder, there may be conflict at every aspect of the patient's interaction with the surgeon and healthcare system. The role of the hand surgeon is to take a careful history, perform a physical examination, recommend the appropriate diagnostic tests and provide honest recommendations for further management. Going for a surgical "Hail Mary" will be a disappointing misadventure.

At each step of care, the surgeon must be aware of the play of internal and external forces that promote and limit recovery. The structure of the Workers' Compensation system can create perverse incentives the surgeon must be perceptive about and must guard against. The surgeon may have perceived or real pressures to do things that are uncomfortable from an ethical standpoint. For example the surgeon may be pressured to return the injured worker back to the workplace early after surgery on limited work such as "one hand duty." Workers with pain in one extremity from a workplace injury or recent surgery may be required to go to the workplace and answer the phone or even perform useless or demeaning tasks or simply sit in a room or lie on a stretcher. This so-called presenteeism is a warping of societal norms that has occurred to circumvent the negative impact of workers compensation protections. The physician wants to do the best for the patient

Table 18.1 Chronic occupational injuries of the musculoskeletal system	
Category 1	Diagnosis is easily established, good methods are available for treating the condition, and the prognosis for returning to work is good.
Category 2	Diagnosis is established, but neither nonsurgical nor surgical treatment is always successful in returning the patient to the original job.
Category 3	The condition combines definite physical problems and additional nonmedical issues.
Category 4	Diagnosis is unclear

Reproduced from: Millender LH, Louis DS, Simmons BP, eds. Occupational Disorders of the Upper Extremity. New York: Churchill Livingstone; 1992.

but feels those decisions are beyond the scope of their influence. The presence of "one hand work" creates the aura of reasonableness creating a plausible justification for the surgeon to agree to this. An alternative perspective is that the early return to the workplace is important in the recovery of the injured worker.

The patient may feel trapped in a closed system. The patient can be suspicious of the compensation system and lose the sense of control of their healthcare. Attempts to recover this control can be self-destructive and misunderstood.

An awareness of these forces will help the surgeon provide the best care for the patient and prevent a fatalistic approach by both. A clear focus should be on providing the best possible care for the upper extremity problem with perception of and attention applied to the other concerns of the patient.

Tendinopathy

Medial and lateral epicondylitis

van Rijn and associates have reviewed the literature evaluating the associations between lateral and medial epicondylitis and work related factors such as force, repetition, posture and psychological issues.[4] They report that handling tools of weight >1 kg; repetitive movements >2 h/day; low job control, and low social support, are associated with lateral epicondylitis. Handling tools >5 kg two times, at a minimum of 2 h/day, or tools >20 kg at least 10 times per day; high-hand grip forces for >1 h/day; repetitive movements for >2 h/day and working with vibrating tools, are associated with medial epicondylitis. The clinical management of these conditions have recently been reviewed by Rineer and Ruch.[5]

Lateral epicondylitis

Lateral epicondylitis, tennis elbow, presents with well localized lateral elbow pain that is exacerbated by certain activities such as gripping. The diagnosis is made by history and physical examination. Physical examination will show point tenderness directly over the lateral epicondyle. Pain will be increased with resisted wrist extension, especially in elbow extension.

The management of lateral epicondylitis has gradually shifted to less intervention as it has become disseminated that this condition will resolve over time. Treatment is therefore used to temporize symptoms.

Splinting, counter force bracing, NSAIDs, physical therapy, steroid injection, or simple observation without intervention have all shown to result in satisfactory results for a majority of patients. In addition, new modalities are being evaluated continuously.

Surgical treatment is reserved for long time failures. A variety of surgical techniques that typically include debridement or tenotomy of the extensor carpi radialis brevis origin are used with reported good success.

Tendinopathy at the wrist and hand

In a review of data collected in 1988 Tanaka et al.[6] reported that the period prevalence for tendonopathies, including tendonitis, synovitis, tenosynovitis, de Quervain's, or epicondylitis, ganglion cyst, or trigger digit was 0.46% of the population

working within the previous year. Of these, 28% were thought to be work related. The authors found bending and twisting of the wrist at work and female gender were associated with reporting these disorders.

De Quervain's tenosynovitis

Tenosynovitis of the first dorsal compartment is the signature work related tendinopathy *(Fig. 18.1)*. Interestingly, this condition is commonly seen in new mothers and in the worker. Nevertheless the presence of this condition in the nonworkers' compensation population is supportive evidence of its existence and sheds credibility on its genesis and that of other tendonopathies. It is clear that with repetitive activity, perhaps one that has recent initiation that a painful condition can develop where a tendon traverses a synovial lined tunnel. It is therefore plausible that any of the common sites for tenosynovitis could be related to activity.

Symptoms of de Quervain's are typically well localized to the radial side of the wrist. The Finkelstein's test is a sensitive test for this problem and point tenderness is a specific test. The diagnosis is made by history and physical examination. Occasionally there will be a small ganglion overlying the first compartment.

Nonsurgical treatment, including oral non-steroidal anti-inflammatory medication, steroid injections, splinting and therapy are often used to treat de Quervain's tenosynovitis. A recent review by Ilyas, of nonsurgical treatment, pointed out the lack of randomized trials for this common condition.[7] Nevertheless, one randomized trial of injection of triamcinolone versus placebo showed benefit from the active drug.[8]

The anatomy of the first dorsal compartment, specifically the presence of a septum between the extensor pollicis brevis and abductor pollicis longus is an interesting finding more prevalent in de Quervain's tenosynovitis requiring surgical treatment than in cadaveric dissection. This anatomic feature has direct surgical importance as each tendon must be identified and released during surgery (see *Fig. 18.1*).

Surgery is performed using local anesthesia. A longitudinally oriented zigzag incision is made directly over the first dorsal compartment. The subcutaneous tissue is gently spread to avoid injury to small branches of the radial nerve and the

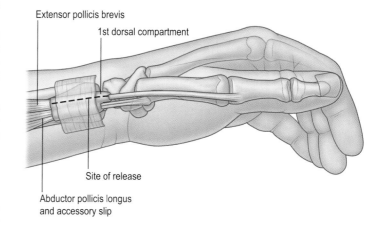

Extensor pollicis brevis

1st dorsal compartment

Site of release

Abductor pollicis longus and accessory slip

Fig. 18.1 De Quervain's tenosynovitis. Tendons of first dorsal compartment and planned release on dorsal half of sheath.

medial antebrachial cutaneous nerve of the forearm. The first dorsal compartment is identified and opened dorsal to the midline. After complete release, each tendon is identified making sure the extensor pollicis brevis is released. If it is not identified, it will lie in a separate tunnel on the dorsal margin of the open first compartment. This is easily released from within the first dorsal compartment. The tourniquet is released before wound closure and a short thumb spica splint is worn until suture removal about 10–14 days later.

Trigger finger

Trigger digit is one of the most common disorders of the hand. A comprehensive review with extensive references has been published by Moore.[9] A case–control study found associations of trigger digit with female gender (OR 7.57, 95% CI 5.07–11.31); diabetes (OR 3.72, CI 2.43–5.70); obesity (OR 1.49, CI 1.02–2.19); occupation as a homemaker (OR 2.44, 95% CI 1.62–3.69); seamstress (OR 4.8, CI 1.3–21.6); and secretary (OR 2.74, CI 1.38–5.52). It is not clear from the abstract if gender was controlled for in these calculations although it would seem to be difficult to accomplish.[10] A study in a meat packing plant found a person-year incidence rate of 12.4% for workers using tools and 2.6% for those without tool use. The authors believe high worker turnover may cause an underestimation of the rate in the workplace.[11]

The diagnosis of trigger digit is relatively straightforward and relies on history and physical examination. Triggering will usually be demonstrable in the office. Two situations often occur that require further discussion. The patient who presents with no active triggering and work attribution should be managed without invasive intervention. These patients may have triggering in the morning or heightened sensitivity to symptoms. I recommend initial management with a night time splint and re-evaluation of these patients. This will give the surgeon the opportunity to spend more time with the patient and determine if they have extraneous problems that could interfere with obtaining a good result. Patients who present with triggering and the presence of a flexion contracture of the PIP joint can present a challenge. The surgeon must point this out before treatment starts and combine treatment of the trigger digit with splinting and mobilization of the PIP joint *(Fig. 18.2)*.

Treatment for trigger digit includes rest, splinting, steroid injection, and open or percutaneous surgery. Splinting can be used at any joint and is primarily used at night. This is particularly valuable if the finger is locked upon waking in the am as night time splinting can prevent this problem. Steroid injection is the mainstay of initial management for trigger digit. A Cochrane review supports the use of steroid as an efficacious treatment.[12] Kerrigan and Stanwix used decision analysis and showed that management with one or two injections prior to surgery minimizes the cost of management.[13]

To inject the A1 pulley, I mix 0.25 cc of Triamcinolone 10 with 0.25 cc of 1% plain lidocaine. I have the patient's hand resting palm up on the examining table with the fingers pointed to my left. This allows me to position my hand over the patient's wrist and angle the needle in a slight proximal to distal direction. I push the needle through the skin and identify its position in the tendon by gentle passive flexion and extension of the digit with my left hand. Using gentle pressure on the syringe the needle is slowly withdrawn

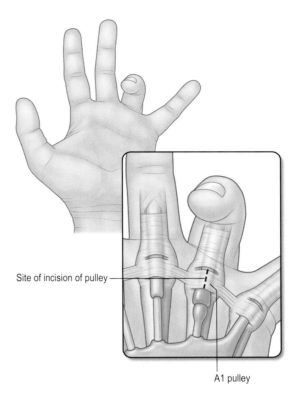

Site of incision of pulley

A1 pulley

Fig. 18.2 Trigger digit. Location of A1 pulley and planned incision on radial side of the pulley.

until there is a drop in resistance to injection. The needle tip is then between the tendon and the sheath or more likely directly on the surface of the pulley system. The 0.5 cc is then injected.

Surgical treatment is performed using local anesthetic. The A1 pulley is released under direct vision and unrestricted motion of the digit is demonstrated in the operating room. Percutaneous release of trigger digit has been reported in the literature and can be performed in the office with lower cost than traditional surgery. One randomized trial found a high success rate in both treatment groups without serious complications.[14] Like many other surgical procedures, the choice of procedure will depend on surgeon training and experience and the wishes of the informed patient. The proximity of the digital nerves to the A1 pulley in the index and the thumb must be considered.

Nerve compression

The work attribution of nerve compression has a well documented history and is still the object of intense research effort. As research designs are improved the relationship of carpal tunnel syndrome to keyboard use for example has become less certain. A recent review of the literature reveals the association between keyboard use and CTS has been based on epidemiologic studies with significant flaws.[15] In fact, Atroshi et al. recently reported a study where use of a keyboard was found to be protective of CTS.[16] It is clear from the literature there is an inverse relationship between the specificity of the diagnosis of a disorder and the prevalence of the disorder. In other words, as the diagnostic criteria become more specific, i.e., other noncarpal tunnel syndrome causes of symptoms are ruled out, the prevalence of CTS is reduced. The incidence rate of CTS when it is diagnosed with high specificity is quite low even in the population of patients using a keyboard suggesting that this is unlikely to be a major work related condition in keyboard users.

In addition to the studies cited above, a recent review of CTS and its epidemiologic associations suggested occupational factors play a minor and debatable role in the etiology of CTS. In spite of some objections to the development of a scorecard based on the characteristics of an association defined by Hill this review is a comprehensive review and thought provoking discussion of the potential causation of work attributed CTS.[17]

Even if work-attributed CTS is an upper extremity problem defined administratively and not by causative mechanism or pathology, it has been found the attribution to the workplace results in inferior outcomes compared to nonwork related surgical care for CTS.[18] Manktelow and colleagues, in reviewing a large population of CTS patients, found that residual symptoms after release of the carpal tunnel are common.[19]

For CTS that has been attributed to the workplace, I recommend the patient proceed with a course of nonoperative treatment before surgery is considered. Nonsurgical treatment is efficacious and the improvement after splinting and or injection is a good diagnostic test of the ability of the patient to obtain improvement from further intervention. If the diagnosis is correct, then any improvement following efficacious nonsurgical treatment will be a good indicator that the patient has at least some potential for improvement.[20] If absolutely no benefit is achieved from nonsurgical care, then the surgeon should confirm the diagnosis as much as possible and recommend a thorough course of nonsurgical treatment. Further detailed information on nerve compression syndromes can be found in Chapter 24.

Vascular disorders

In some occupations, the heel of the hand is used as a hammer to push objects into place. Some commonly recognized activities are "hammering" a board into place or putting on a hub cap. The ulnar artery and ulnar nerve pass through Guyon's canal and are susceptible to injury in the hypothenar area. Thrombosis, pseudoaneurysm formation, embolic phenomena, and nerve symptoms are possible.

The history is usually highly suggestive of ulnar artery or nerve problems. Examination of the fingers may show signs of emboli and the Allen's test may show occlusion of the ulnar artery. The history will likely be specific if a pseudoaneurysm is present and it will usually be obvious on physical examination

Treatment of the so-called hypothenar hammer syndrome is based on the presence of symptoms. The presence of an ulnar artery occlusion on the Allen's test without symptoms or peripheral signs does not necessitate surgical intervention. If there are compression symptoms and findings related to the ulnar nerve in Guyon's canal or evidence of ischemia or emboli, then imaging is indicated. Magnetic resonance imaging (MRI) will define localized vascular pathology as well as masses within of deep to Guyon's canal. Surgery will

usually be indicated in the presence of neurologic or vascular symptoms.

Surgery for hypothenar hammer syndrome will start with release of the ulnar artery and nerve from the wrist crease to distal to Guyon's canal. The motor branch of the ulnar nerve should be identified and followed deep into the palm. For ulnar arterial lesions, the area of obstruction is resected and the flow in the hand is evaluated. Resection of the artery alone has been reported to increase flow to the hand by way of a regional sympathetic effect. Treatment of choice is to perform an interposition vein graft with a short saphenous vein or a forearm vein. Further detailed information on hand ischemia syndromes can be found in Chapter 22.

Hand–arm vibration syndrome (HAVS)

The relationship of vibration to upper extremity pathology has been the subject of extensive literature and regulatory interest. For the upper extremity surgeon, there are criteria that score the vascular and neurologic components of vibration injury.

The classification scheme that was produced at a workshop in Stockholm bears its name as the Stockholm Workshop Scale (*Table 18.2*) and is divided into neurologic symptoms and vascular symptoms.[21]

Although there is clear experimental evidence that vibration can cause injury to tissues, many of the symptoms of vibration induced injury can be caused by other means. For example the vascular symptoms of vibration injury can also be caused by smoking, something that is highly prevalent in some populations. The relationship of vibration to vascular disorders is also potentially confounded not only by smoking

Table 18.2 **Stockholm workshop scale**		
Neurologic symptoms		
0 SN		Exposed to vibration but no symptoms
1 SN		Intermittent numbness, with or without tingling
2 SN		Intermittent or persistent numbness, reduced sensory perception
3 SN		Intermittent or persistent numbness, reduced tactile discrimination and/or manipulative dexterity
Vascular symptoms		
0	–	No attacks
1	Mild	Occasional attacks affecting only the tips of one or more fingers
2	Moderate	Occasional attacks affecting distal and middle (rarely also proximal) phalanges of one or more fingers
3	Severe	Frequent attacks affecting all phalanges of most fingers
4	Very severe	As in stage 3, with trophic skin changes in the fingertips

Reproduced from: McGeoch KL, Lawson IJ, Burke F, et al. Diagnostic criteria and staging of hand-arm vibration syndrome in the United Kingdom. Ind Health 2005;43:527–534.[21]

but also other problems such as peripheral vascular disease of other etiologies. The neurologic symptoms of vibration injury are typical of peripheral nerve compression so there is often confusion between a diagnosis of CTS and vibration induced injury. The relationship between vibration injury and nerve compression is not clearly elucidated. For patients with nerve compression symptoms however it seems prudent to limit exposure to future vibration.

Patient management

When a working patient has a vascular complaint or a history of numbness or tingling, the surgeon should enquire about vibration in the workplace as well as other potential causative mechanisms for the symptoms including a cardiovascular history, a smoking history, and a family history. Similarly, a detailed history related to nerve symptoms may be helpful. If the worker has been exposed to vibration, it is important to create a temporal history of the time and degree of exposure over their entire work history.

The physical examination will evaluate the upper extremity for evidence of vascular and neurologic findings. This will include measuring the blood pressure in each arm, listening to the heart and for bruits along the major vessels, palpating pulses at various levels, performing an Allen's test, and evaluating the fingertips for color, trophic changes, and temperature. The examination of the peripheral nervous system includes measuring sensory and motor function, and evaluation for sites of nerve compression.

Additional evaluations will often include electrodiagnostic testing and noninvasive vascular testing. Angiograms are not indicated unless there is evidence of a structural problem that may require surgical planning.

Patients presenting with vascular or neurologic symptoms should be advised to avoid exposure to vibration. This advice does not implicate vibration as a cause of their symptoms but seems prudent, given the experimental evidence of the potential for vibration to cause injury.

Management of the patient further depends on the accurate diagnosis and management of other pathology such as CTS.

Return to work

Keeping the injured worker in the workplace or reintegration of the injured worker into the workplace, is a vital outcome of management of occupational illness of the upper extremity. When an injury forces a patient to leave the workforce, even temporarily, the surgeon should be aware of several possible points of view. (1) The injury or illness may be more severe causing symptoms that make work impossible. This can have implications in the application of more invasive treatment at an earlier stage of management. (2) The patients work activities may be more physical, requiring more intense use of the upper extremities, something that will influence their potential for return. (3) The financial stakes for the employer become higher, as salary replacement and a history of lost time injury may be important. (4) When the injured worker is unable to work, a set of emotional circumstances is potentially set into play that can possibly make it difficult for the worker to return to work.

In trying to return the patient to work, the first consideration is whether the patient has the ability to work in any capacity. The second consideration is whether the change in ability to work is either permanent or temporary. For temporary changes in the ability to work, restricted duty work is often available if the employee has a work related injury. This may take the form of one-hand work if the injury is limited to one extremity and the patient's general condition allows safe return. For a patient who has a temporary inability to work in any capacity the surgeon will need to follow the patient closely and communicate with the workplace about return to work when the medical situation allows. If the patient has an injury or illness that permanently prevents unrestricted work the surgeon will play an important role in returning the patient to gainful employment. The first step is to determine the permanent restrictions that will be recommended to the patient to keep him/her safe in the workplace. For practical purposes, this is done when the patient has reached their level of maximum medical improvement. Further active medical management would not be expected to increase the patient's status. At this time, the patient can have an impairment rating calculated to facilitate compensation for the permanent effects of the injury. The second step is to return the patient to the workforce. Given a permanent impairment the first choice of return to the workplace is the previous employer and return to the pre-injury work. If this is not possible due to the restrictions, then return to the previous employer in a modified work capacity is often the easiest plan. This may not be possible and the injured worker may be required to search for a new job, limited by the restrictions that have been imposed to ensure safety. It is obvious each step of the process can have a big influence on the patients return to the workplace and the ability to find future employment.

Measuring impairment

In measuring permanent impairment, the surgeon is providing a basis for financial compensation of the patient for the permanent effects of an injury in the workplace. This measurement is often performed by hand therapists. This measurement is indicated at the time when no further diagnostic testing or interventions are planned for the patient. It is meant to be a tally of the permanent effects of an injury after all steps have been taken to minimize them. Often, when the surgeon perceives the patient has reached this stage of maximum medical improvement, the evaluation of permanent impairment and the decision about permanent work restrictions will be accomplished simultaneously. If this is straightforward and without conflict, this can be done by the surgeon at the time of a final visit. If there is conflict, or if the return to work restrictions are complicated, a hand therapist may be of assistance.

In some situations of work-related upper extremity illness, the patient may have prolonged symptoms and an inability to work, despite maximum care, the determination that the patient is at maximum medical improvement, the assignment of permanent restrictions, and the determination of an impairment rating can allow the patient to move on with their life and provide a stopping point for further nonbeneficial interactions with the surgeon.

The most recent version of the *Guides to the Evaluation of Permanent Impairment*, 6th edn., put forward by The American Medical Association has a fundamental change in the evaluation of permanent impairment, shifting to the ICF model, 'The International Classification of Functioning, Disability and Health.'[22] This is outlined in the first chapter, "Conceptual Foundations and Philosophy."

"In this edition there is a paradigm shift, which adopts a contemporary model of disablement: it is simplified, functionally based, and internally consistent to the fullest extent possible."

"The vision … is articulated in terms of five specific new axioms":

1. The terminology and conceptual framework of the ICF are adopted
2. Diagnosis and evidence-based where possible
3. Simplicity and ease of application
4. Functionally-based
5. Conceptual and methodological congruity between and within organ systems.

Measures of permanent impairment are primarily based on diagnosis and then modified, based on several factors such as severity and functional limitation. Whether these new guides will supplant the 5th edition is not yet clear.

Use of the 5th or 6th version of "The Guides" will bring objectivity to the measurement of permanent impairment and protects the surgeon from influence of the patient or the employer and insurance carrier.

Summary

The care of the injured worker mirrors the care of all patients with upper extremity injury and illness. The additional superimposition of the legal framework of Workers' Compensation adds an extra dimension to the care of the injured worker. The upper extremity surgeon must be knowledgeable of the local regulations and must be perceptive to their influence on the patient, the workplace, and the surgeon, and maintain the ability to take the best care possible of the patient.

Access the complete reference list online at **http://www.expertconsult.com**

2. Szabo RM, King KJ. Repetitive stress injury: diagnosis or self-fulfilling prophecy? *J Bone Joint Am.* 2000;82:1314.

   This current concepts review is a sobering review of the lack of science surrounding the epidemic of repetitive motion injuries. Szabo logically in a step-by-step fashion updates the literature on the perspective of a hand surgeon regarding these diagnoses.

6. Tanaka S, Peterson M, Cameron L. Prevalence and risk factors of tendonitis and related disorders of the distal upper extremity among US workers: comparison to carpal tunnel syndrome. *Am J Ind Med.* 2001;39(3): 328–335.

   This study reviewed the results of a survey instrument in a large population and found that 0.46% of those people who had worked in the previous 12 months reported prolonged hand discomfort. 28% of these problems were thought by a medical person to be work related. The authors estimate there were 520 000 patients with work related musculoskeletal disorders of the distal upper extremity in 1988.

17. Lozano-Calderon S, Anthony S, Ring D. The quality and strength of evidence for etiology: The example of carpal tunnel syndrome. *J Hand Surg.* 2008;33A:525–538.

   The authors perform an exhaustive evaluation of the literature on the relationship between activity and carpal tunnel syndrome. Although it may not be prudent to use the guidelines of Hill as criteria, the authors have an extensive reference list and thoughtfully analyze the literature.

18. Harris I, Mulford J, Solomon M, et al. Association between compensation status and outcome after surgery: a mea-analysis. *JAMA.* 2005;293(13):1644–1652.

   An eye-opening article that documents what surgeons have known for years. Patients whose medical problems are attributed to the workplace have an inferior outcome. This manuscript looks at carpal tunnel syndrome as one example. It cries out to researchers, policy-makers, and society to try to understand and change this negative influence.

19. Manktelow RT, Binhammer P, Tomat LR, et al. Carpal tunnel syndrome: Cross-sectional and outcome study in Ontario workers. *J Hand Surg.* 2004;29A:307–317.

   This interesting study reports that ongoing symptoms after carpal tunnel release in the working population are common.

22. Rondinelli RD, ed. Guides to the Evaluation of Permanent Impairment. 6th ed. Chicago, IL: American Medical Association; 2008.

19

Rheumatologic conditions of the hand and wrist

Douglas M. Sammer and Kevin C. Chung

SYNOPSIS

- Rheumatoid arthritis is a systemic autoimmune inflammatory disease that affects the joints of the hand and wrist. Rheumatoid arthritis also affects the soft tissues, and can cause disease processes such as trigger finger and carpal tunnel syndrome.
- The diagnosis of rheumatoid arthritis is primarily clinical, and is supported by radiographic and laboratory studies. Although symptoms can usually be managed effectively with newer biologic medications, some patients require surgery to treat refractory pain or to improve hand function.
- Operations for rheumatoid arthritis can be broadly categorized into five groups: synovectomy, tendon surgery, soft tissue rebalancing, arthrodesis, and arthroplasty. Specific techniques described include: wrist synovectomy, tendon transfers for tendon rupture, soft tissue rebalancing, management of the distal ulna and DRUJ, wrist arthrodesis and arthroplasty, small joint arthrodesis and arthroplasty, and treatment of trigger fingers and carpal tunnel syndrome.

Introduction

Rheumatoid arthritis (RA) is a systemic autoimmune disease that affects 1% of adults (ranging from 0.33% to 6.8%, depending upon the population).[1] Although RA has many diverse clinical manifestations, the single underlying pathologic process is synovial inflammation, which progressively destroys joints and soft tissue leading to deformity and disability. Over the last 20 years, many advances in the medical management of RA have been made. New medications have improved the ability to control rheumatoid inflammation, and can dramatically slow or prevent disease progression.[2] In spite of these tremendous strides, the hand surgeon continues to play a crucial role in treating RA. Many patients continue to suffer from recalcitrant pain or disability despite maximal medical management, and may benefit from surgical intervention.

In addition to RA, there are a number of diverse rheumatologic disorders that commonly affect the hand and wrist. These include systemic lupus erythematosus (SLE), scleroderma, gout, and others. These disorders frequently require surgical intervention.

Basic science/disease process

Etiology

Though much is understood about the pathogenesis of RA, the cause remains idiopathic. That being said, RA is known to have a genetic component. This is demonstrated by the fact that RA has a much higher concurrence rate in monozygotic twins (15–20%) than in dizygotic twins (5%), with susceptibility transferred in an autosomal recessive mode.[3–5] In addition, there are certain ethnic groups such as the Pima Indians that exhibit a greater incidence of RA than the rest of the population, providing further evidence of a genetic component to RA.[6]

Many studies suggest that a multitude of genes play a role in contributing to susceptibility to RA. These include the class II major histocompatibility complex (MHC) genes and many others. The most well-understood genetic association is with the class II MHC genes, which may contribute up to 40% of the genetic component of RA.[7] One class II MHC gene in particular, human leukocyte antigen (HLA) DR4 is associated not only with increased risk of disease, but also with increased disease severity.[4]

In addition to genetics, gender influences the development of RA. RA is more common in women than in men, with a ratio of 2:1 to 3:1. Multiple laboratory and clinical studies suggest that hormones, and estrogens in particular, affect the development of RA. However, the exact role of estrogen in the development of RA is not known.[8]

Although the mechanisms are not well understood, the environment plays a role in the etiology of RA as well. Smoking is a risk factor for the development of RA,

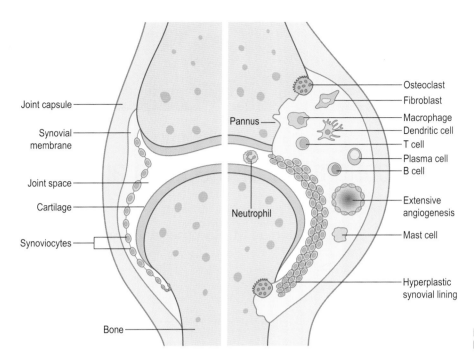

Fig. 19.1 The erosive synovial pannus consists of hypertrophic synovium and inflammatory cells.

particularly in susceptible men.[9] Coffee intake and exposure to silica have also been associated with RA.[4] In addition, infectious diseases likely act as a trigger in genetically susceptible individuals. Possible triggering agents include mycoplasma, enteric bacteria, Epstein–Barr virus, and others viral and bacterial triggers.[10–13] In summary, RA is an idiopathic disease, but which is known to have both genetic and environmental components. The genetic susceptibility and environmental triggers are complex and varied, and are not fully understood.

Pathogenesis

The target tissue of RA is the synovium. The disease process begins when an antigen, a trigger for RA, is presented to T-cells within the synovium. A complex interaction between macrophages, B-cells, T-cells, and synoviocytes ensues, orchestrated by systemic inflammatory modulators and local cytokines. The end result is the formation of proliferating inflamed synovium, or pannus *(Figs 19.1, 19.2)*. Once initiated, this process becomes systemic and self-sustaining, and does not require the prolonged presence of the trigger antigen. The synovial pannus produces proteolytic enzymes such as metalloproteinases, serine proteases, cathepsins, and aggrecanases that erode cartilage, bone, and supporting soft tissue structures. Cytokines secreted by the pannus activate osteoclasts in nearby bone, further contributing to bony erosions and joint destruction.[14–16]

Medical management

The medications used to treat RA include non-steroidal anti-inflammatory drugs (NSAiDs), corticosteroids, and disease-modifying antirheumatic drugs (DMARDs). In general, a combination of the above medications, with methotrexate as

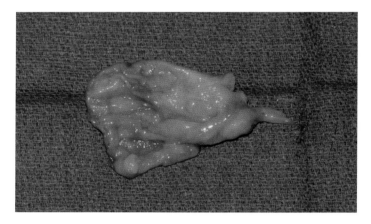

Fig. 19.2 Gross appearance of synovial pannus.

the basis, is used to control symptoms and the underlying disease. NSAIDs do little to affect the course of the disease, and are rarely used in isolation. They are effective, however, in treating symptoms such as joint pain, but must be used judiciously due to their gastrointestinal and renal side-effects. Corticosteroids on the other hand are very effective in treating both the symptoms of RA and the underlying disease process. They can be administered systemically or locally, in the form of a joint injection. However, long-term systemic use is associated with substantial morbidity. Because of this, a minimal clinically-effective dose is used. Often, corticosteroids are used briefly to control acute symptoms or flare-ups, and are then tapered as DMARDs begin to work. DMARDs include a diverse array of medications that can be divided into two groups: conventional DMARDs and biologic DMARDs.

The conventional DMARDs include methotrexate, leflunomide (Arava), azathioprine (Imuran), Plaquenil, and gold.[17] Methotrexate is the most commonly administered DMARD because of its effectiveness and favorable side-effect profile. It is generally taken orally once a week, in combination with folic acid in order to minimize side effects such as hepatotoxicity and bone-marrow suppression. Leflunomide (Arava) is a daily oral pyrimidine antagonist, with side-effects that include hepatotoxicity and marrow suppression. Plaquenil, an antimalarial drug that is effective in the treatment of RA, is taken daily and has few serious side-effects. Sulfasalazine is another common daily DMARD, and like many of the other conventional DMARDs it can cause leukopenia. Gold is rarely included in the antirheumatic regimen today due to significant side-effects and the need for intramuscular injections.

Biologic DMARDs are those that target tumor necrosis factor alpha (TNF-α) and interleukin 1 (IL-1), or the cellular components of the immune system. Etanercept (Enbrel) is an anti-TNF-α that requires once-weekly subcutaneous injections. Infliximab (Remicade) is a TNF-α blocker that is administered every 1–2 months, intravenously. Adalimumab (Humira) is a TNF-α blocker that is injected subcutaneously every two weeks. All three are very effective in treating RA, especially when combined with methotrexate.[18,19] However, the long-term toxicity of these new medications is unknown, and all three result in an increased susceptibility to infections.[20] Anakinra (Kineret) is a biologic DMARD that blocks IL-1 receptors, and requires daily subcutaneous injections. Like the anti-TNF-α biologics, it is associated with an increased susceptibility to infections. Rituximab (Rituxan) is an intravenously administered monoclonal antibody that targets certain B-cells, and lasts from many months up to a year. Abatacept (Orencia) is an antibody that targets T-cells, and requires a monthly intravenous injection.

The surgeon must be aware of the potential toxicities and side-effects associated with these medications. The preoperative evaluation of patients on DMARDs should include laboratory panels to screen for hepatotoxicity and bone-marrow suppression. In addition, the surgeon must weigh the risk of increased susceptibility to infection with the benefits of surgery.

The perioperative management of DMARDs and other rheumatoid medications is somewhat controversial and should be coordinated with the patient's rheumatologist. The perioperative cessation of DMARDs or corticosteroids can result in an acute deterioration (rheumatoid flare-up) that is poorly tolerated by the patient. In fact, the flare-up may be so severe that it affects the patient's ability to participate in postoperative rehabilitation.[21–23] In general, methotrexate should be continued throughout the perioperative period at its normal dose. Methotrexate does not appear to increase infection rates in patients with RA undergoing elective surgery.[21,22] Furthermore, corticosteroids, when used alone or in combination with methotrexate, do not affect wound infection rates and should not be stopped in the perioperative period.[23] Data on the other conventional DMARDs are more limited, and their perioperative dosing should be discussed with the patient's rheumatologist.

The appropriate perioperative management of biologic DMARDs, particularly the TNF-α inhibitors, is less clear. There are few data and no large studies to guide perioperative dosing of the biologic DMARDs.[22] Therefore, a conservative approach is recommended at this time. In general, the TNF-α inhibitors should be held 2–4 weeks before and after surgery.[22] Similarly, few data exist regarding the other biologics, and a similar approach is recommended.[24]

Diagnosis/presentation

The onset of RA is usually in the 3rd to 6th decade of life. The incidence of RA in young men is one-third that of women, but increases to be equal to that of women by the 6th or 7th decades of life. From the onset, RA tends to affect the hands and wrists. In fact, the metacarpophalangeal (MCP) joints, proximal interphalangeal (PIP) joints, and the wrist are often affected earlier and more frequently than other joints in the body.[2]

Diagnostic criteria have been described, and are useful in making the diagnosis of RA. They include: (1) morning stiffness = 1 h; (2) soft tissue swelling of three or more joints; (3) soft tissue swelling of hand joints (PIP, MCP, wrist); (4) symmetrical soft tissue swelling; (5) subcutaneous nodules (rheumatoid nodules); (6) seropositivity for rheumatoid factor (RF), and (7) erosions or periarticular osteopenia in hand or wrist joints. Four of the seven criteria should be present for diagnosis, and criteria (1) through (4) must be present for 6 weeks or longer. Morning stiffness, or stiffness after rest is common, and may be present for a number of hours, improving with hand use. The most sensitive findings are symmetric arthritis and arthritis of the hand joints. Classic radiographic changes, and the presence of rheumatoid nodules are less sensitive but very specific findings. RF is not only is a marker for RA, but also correlates with disease severity.[4] Although not one of the classification criteria, anticitrullinated protein antibodies (ACPAs) are very specific for RA, and are useful in confirming the diagnosis.[4,25] Like RF, ACPA seropositivity also correlates with disease severity.[26] In many cases, seropositivity to RF and ACPA develops prior to the onset of clinical disease. It should be noted however, that some patients with RA will convert to seropositivity after the onset of disease, and some patients with RA will never become seropositive.

RA usually develops in multiple joints slowly over a period of months, although atypical presentations are not unusual.[27] In some cases, symptoms can occur rapidly over a few days. When symptoms develop rapidly, the diagnosis of RA is often not considered, and septic arthritis or some other cause of acute-onset joint inflammation is initially suspected. In other cases, symptoms may involve one or two joints for some time before becoming polyarticular, confounding the diagnosis. Less commonly, some patients develop extra-articular disease (rheumatoid nodules, vasculitis, pericarditis, pleural effusion or interstitial disease, peripheral neuropathy, keratoconjunctivitis sicca, and many others), before synovitis and arthritis are evident.[4] Palindromic rheumatism is a rare variant of RA, in which symptoms begin in a single joint. Symptoms worsen and spread to other joints for a few days, then disappear in reverse order. Although the disease resolves in some patients, about half eventually develop classic RA.[28] Finally, it has been noted that some patients tolerate RA quite well; a presentation termed arthritis robustus. This tends to occur in athletes or heavy laborers who have little pain or disability in spite of severe radiographic changes.

Any joint in the body can be affected by RA, including the articulations of the ossicles of the middle ear.[29,4] However, joint involvement tends to follow a predictable pattern. Symptoms often begin in the MCP, PIP and wrist joints first, in part due to their high synovium to joint surface area ratio.[30] Larger joints like the knees, hips, shoulders and elbows are likely to be affected later in the disease process due to their lower synovium to joint surface area ratio.[31] Within the hand, the DIP joints are generally spared, possibly because of their relatively small absolute amount of synovium. The synovial lining of tendons is also affected by RA, and can result in a multitude of symptoms, including carpal tunnel syndrome, tendon rupture, tendonitis, and trigger digits.

It should be remembered that RA is a systemic disease with multiple extra-articular manifestations. Rheumatoid nodules, vasculitis, pericarditis, pleural effusion, interstitial pulmonary disease, peripheral neuropathy, and keratoconjunctivitis sicca are some of the more common extra-articular effects of RA. Although rheumatoid nodules are present in only a minority of patients with RA, they are a common reason for presentation to the hand surgeon. Rheumatoid nodules develop secondary to the same autoimmune process that occurs in the joints. They occur most often on extensor surfaces or areas of contact pressure such as the olecranon process. However, they can appear anywhere, including within internal organs such as the lungs, heart, or central nervous system.[32]

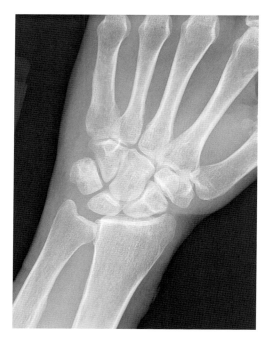

Fig. 19.3 PA radiograph of the left wrist, demonstrating early involvement of the DRUJ, as well as scattered carpal erosions from invasive synovitis.

Hints and tips: Diagnostic criteria for rheumatoid arthritis

Criterion	Details
1. Morning stiffness	1 h
2. Soft tissue swelling	3 or more joints
3. Soft tissue swelling	Symmetric
4. Soft tissue swelling of hand	MCP, PIP, wrist joints
5. Subcutaneous nodules	Rheumatoid nodules
6. Seropositivity	Rheumatoid factor (RF)
7. Typical radiographic findings	Periarticular erosions/ osteopenia, hand or wrist

Four of the seven criteria must be present, and criteria 1–4 must be present for at least 6 weeks.

Wrist involvement

Within the wrist and distal radioulnar joint (DRUJ), cartilage is degraded and bony erosions develop. Bony erosions occur first at sites of nutrient vessels and at the joint margins because there is no protective cartilage at these locations, thereby giving the invading pannus direct access to the bone.[33] Radiographic changes are first noted at the scaphoid waist, the ulnar styloid and the distal radioulnar joint (DRUJ) *(Fig. 19.3)*.[34,35] As the arthritis progresses, the radiocarpal joint becomes involved. Bony destruction tends to be more severe at the radiocarpal joint than the mid-carpal joint, although both joints are often involved.[36] In late stages, the volar lip of the distal radius becomes severely eroded, allowing proximal migration, volar translation and volar angulation of the lunate, with compensatory mid-carpal extension *(Figs 19.4, 19.5)*.[35,37]

The ligaments of the wrist and DRUJ are affected as well. As the pannus proliferates, it stretches and then directly invades the intrinsic and extrinsic wrist ligaments. Synovitis occurring at the scaphoid waist weakens the radioscaphocapitate ligament, leading to ulnar translocation of the carpus

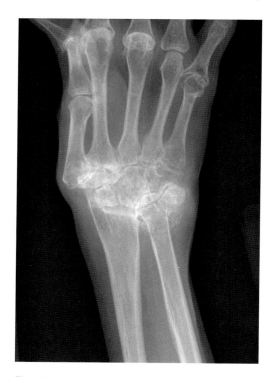

Fig. 19.4 PA radiograph of the right wrist, demonstrating severe involvement of the wrist.

(Fig. 19.6).[38] Destruction of the scapholunate ligament leads to carpal instability, and further contributes to ulnar translocation of the carpus. At the DRUJ, pannus invades the triangular fibrocartilage complex (TFCC), including the dorsal and palmar radioulnar ligaments, resulting in DRUJ instability and eventually dorsal dislocation of the ulnar head. Pannus also destroys the extensor carpi ulnaris (ECU) subsheath,

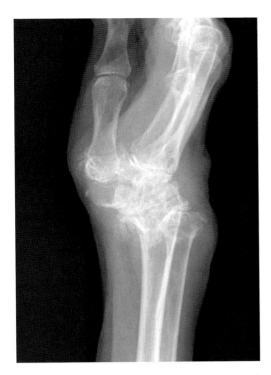

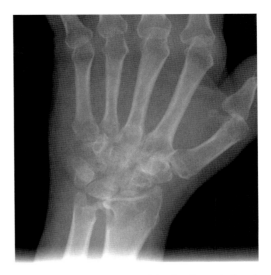

Fig. 19.6 PA radiograph of the left wrist, demonstrating ulnar translocation of the carpus. Note that the lunate no longer sits in the lunate fossa.

Fig. 19.5 Lateral radiograph of the right wrist, demonstrating destruction of the volar lip of the radius, with volar subluxation of the carpus.

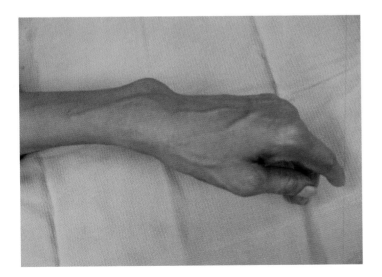

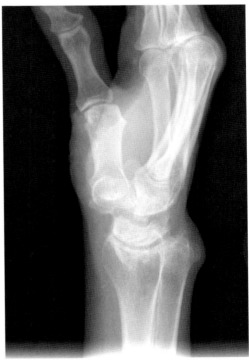

Fig. 19.7 Caput ulnae, with dorsal dislocation of the ulnar head and carpal supination.

Fig. 19.8 Lateral radiograph of the wrist, demonstrating a dorsally dislocated ulnar head.

resulting in volar subluxation of the ECU.[39,40] The ECU's function as a wrist extensor and ulnar deviator is lost, contributing to supination and radial deviation of the carpus. The combination of dorsal dislocation of the ulnar head, carpal supination and volar subluxation of the ECU is termed the "caput ulnae" *(Figs 19.7, 19.8)*.

End-stage wrist arthritis falls into three different clinical patterns, depending upon the degree of bony destruction and ligamentous instability.[41] These patterns are: (1) ankylosis; (2) arthritic stable, and (3) unstable (subdivided into ligamentous unstable and bony unstable). In the ankylosing wrist, the carpus undergoes autofusion. Frequently, ankylosis occurs with the wrist in acceptable alignment, although this is not always the case. In the arthritic stable wrist, the arthritis follows a pattern similar to that of osteoarthritis. Ligamentous destruction is limited, and the wrist remains stable over time.

In the unstable wrist, there is progressive malalignment. In the ligamentous unstable wrist, bony destruction is minimal, whereas in the bony unstable wrist, there is severe loss of bone resulting in instability and eventually dislocation.

On the dorsal aspect of the wrist, synovitis develops within the extensor tendon compartments *(Fig. 19.9)*. Depending upon the extent of the synovitis, there may be a bulge protruding beyond the distal and proximal margins of the extensor retinaculum, creating an hourglass appearance. Direct invasion of extensor tendons, combined with attritional wear over sharp bony edges at the ulna and DRUJ can lead to tendon ruptures. The extensor tendons to the small finger are usually affected first. Extensor tendon ruptures often progress radially, eventually affecting all digits. This ulnar to radial progression of extensor tendon ruptures is called the Vaughn–Jackson syndrome *(Fig. 19.10)*.[42] Tendon ruptures are sudden, and may not be painful. They can be difficult to identify in patients with severe deformity, and must be differentiated from volar subluxation of the MCP joint, radial nerve palsy, and extensor tendon subluxation at the MCP joint. On the volar aspect of the wrist, sharp erosions on the scaphoid can result in attritional rupture of the flexor pollicis longus (FPL) tendon, known as a Mannerfelt lesion *(Fig. 19.11)*.[43] Within the carpal tunnel, synovial pannus and tenosynovitis proliferate, creating a space-occupying lesion that results in carpal tunnel syndrome *(Fig. 19.12)*.

Finger and thumb involvement

In the fingers the MCP and PIP joints are primarily affected, with relative sparing of the DIP joints. As cartilage is degraded, joint space narrowing is seen. Pannus invades at the margins of the joints, resulting in marginal bony erosions. The joint capsule and collateral ligaments are initially stretched and then directly invaded by the synovial pannus, resulting in instability and deformity.

At the MCP joints, the typical pattern of instability is volar subluxation and ulnar deviation, and is the result of multiple forces.[44,45] Synovitis at the MCP joint erodes the dorsoradial portion of the joint capsule early in the disease process,

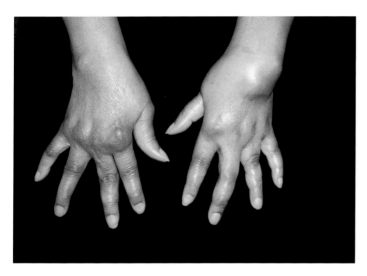

Fig. 19.9 Extensor tenosynovitis protruding from under the extensor retinaculum distally.

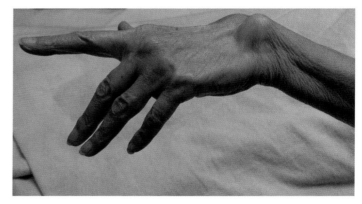

Fig. 19.10 Patient with Vaughn–Jackson syndrome, demonstrating extensor tendon ruptures associated with a caput ulnae.

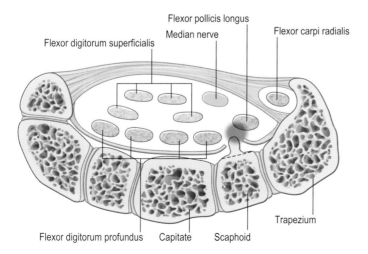

Fig. 19.11 Axial cross-section of the radial side of the wrist, demonstrating the Mannerfelt lesion. Note the proximity of the flexor pollicis longus tendon to the sharp erosion on the volar aspect of the scaphoid.

Flexor pollicis longus
Median nerve
Flexor carpi radialis
Flexor digitorum superficialis
Flexor digitorum profundus
Capitate
Scaphoid
Trapezium

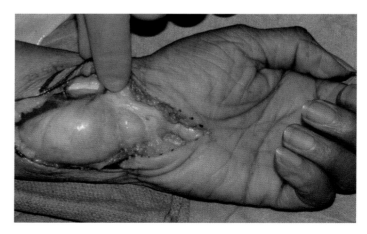

Fig. 19.12 Large proliferative flexor tendon tenosynovitis.

creating an early tendency towards ulnar deviation *(Fig. 19.13)* and volar subluxation *(Fig. 19.14)*.[46,47] Radial deviation at the wrist creates an ulnar approach of the extensor tendons to the MCP joints, which further contributes to ulnar deviation *(Fig. 19.15)*.[48] In addition, ulnar deviation forces during oppositional and key pinch stretch the dorsoradial portion of the capsule and the radial collateral ligament, particularly in the index and long fingers.[49] Finally, continued dorsoradial invasion of the pannus weakens the radial sagittal bands, causing ulnar subluxation of the extensor tendons between the metacarpal heads, which further increases ulnar deviation force on the MCP joints, and weakens extension power at the MCP joints *(Fig. 19.16)*.[35,50]

One of two patterns of finger deformity can occur, the swan-neck *(Fig. 19.17)* or boutonniere deformity *(Fig. 19.18)*. Although swan-neck deformity is more common, either deformity can occur and both can occur in the same hand. Swan-neck deformity can originate from pathology at the MCP joint, the PIP joint, or the DIP joint *(Fig. 19.19)*. At the DIP joint the terminal tendon insertion attenuates or erodes, resulting in a mallet finger. This causes an imbalance in the extensor mechanism, with increased extension force at the PIP joint. MCP flexion also contributes to increased pull of the central slip at the PIP joint. When these increased extension forces are combined with synovial disruption of the PIP volar plate, PIP hyperextension occurs, resulting in swan-neck deformity. Swan-neck deformity can originate at the PIP joint as well. Pannus stretches and erodes the volar plate and capsule, allowing hyperextension. Flexor tendon rupture may also contribute to a loss of flexion force at the PIP joint. The lateral bands slide dorsally, limiting PIP flexion. DIP joint flexion is a secondary phenomenon in this scenario, and is due to slack in the extensor mechanism combined with tightening

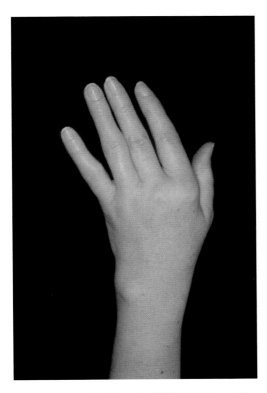

Fig. 19.13 Ulnar deviation at the MCP joints (ulnar drift).

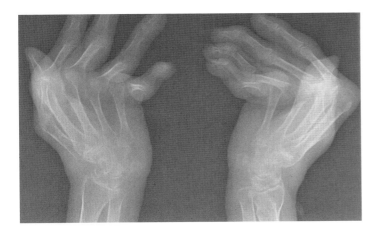

Fig. 19.14 Radiograph of bilateral hands, demonstrating flexion and volar subluxation of the MCP joints.

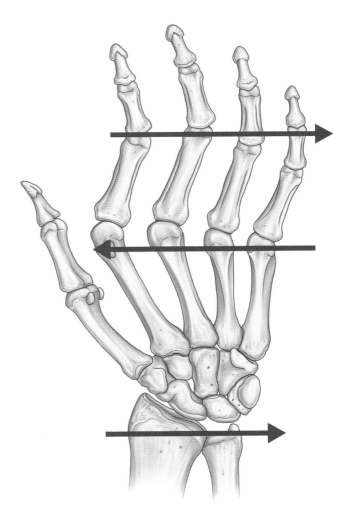

Fig. 19.15 Radial deviation and ulnar translocation at the wrist contribute to ulnar deviation at the MCP joints.

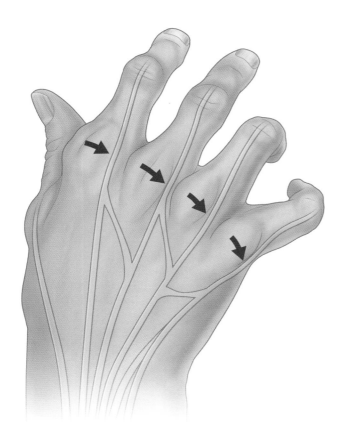

Fig. 19.16 The extensor tendons to displace ulnarly and volarly into the space between the metacarpal heads, making them ineffective as MCP extensors, and adding to ulnar deviation force.

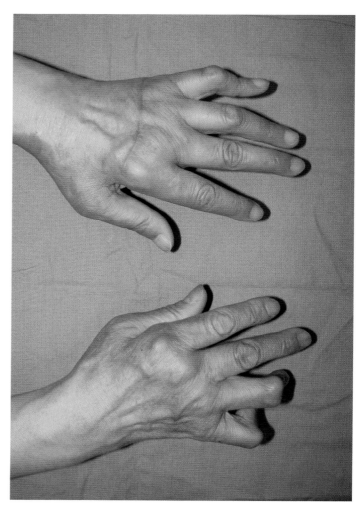

Fig. 19.18 Boutonniere deformity of the right ring and small fingers, and left small finger. Left ring finger demonstrates very early boutonniere deformity.

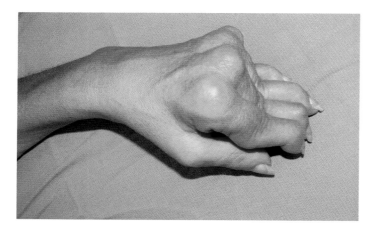

Fig. 19.17 Classic swan-neck deformities of all fingers, with MCP flexion, PIP hyperextension, and DIP flexion.

of the flexor digitorum profundus (FDP) from PIP hyperextension. MCP pathology can initiate the development of swan-neck deformity as well. Flexed MCP position results in excessive pull through the extensor mechanism. The intrinsics also tighten over time, thereby hyperextending the PIP joint when MCP extension is attempted. The lateral bands also migrate dorsally, contributing to the deformity. The most

debilitating result of swan-neck deformities is loss of flexion at the PIP joints, resulting in an inability to flex the fingers for pinching and grasping.

Boutonniere deformities are usually less debilitating than swan-neck deformities, because pinch and grasp are usually preserved. Unlike swan-neck deformities, boutonniere deformities always begin with pathology at the PIP joint **(Fig. 19.20)**. The initial insult is stretching, erosion, and rupture of the central slip insertion on the base of the middle phalanx. Attenuation of the dorsal capsule, transverse retinacular ligament and triangular ligament allows the lateral bands to sublux volar to the joint axis of rotation, becoming PIP flexors. The volar position of the lateral bands makes them even more effective extensors of the DIP joint, resulting in secondary DIP hyperextension.

Synovitis also develops within the flexor tendon sheath, and can lead to triggering or rupture of the flexor tendons. Trigger digits associated with RA are distinct in mechanism and pathology from nonrheumatoid trigger digits, and occur secondary to synovitis or small rheumatoid nodules in the flexor tendon.[51] The specific location of the synovitis or rheumatoid nodules determines the presentation of the rheumatoid trigger finger. A nodule located proximal to the A1 pulley

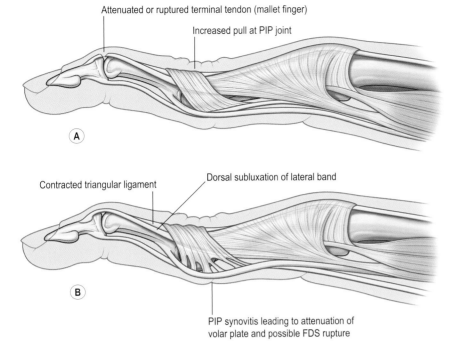

Attenuated or ruptured terminal tendon (mallet finger)

Increased pull at PIP joint

(A)

Contracted triangular ligament

Dorsal subluxation of lateral band

(B)

PIP synovitis leading to attenuation of volar plate and possible FDS rupture

Fig. 19.19 (A) Swan-neck deformity originating from a mallet finger, with subsequent increased extension force at the PIP joint. **(B)** Swan-neck deformity originating at the PIP joint, with volar plate attenuation and possible FDS rupture due to PIP synovitis, and subsequent dorsal subluxation of the lateral bands.

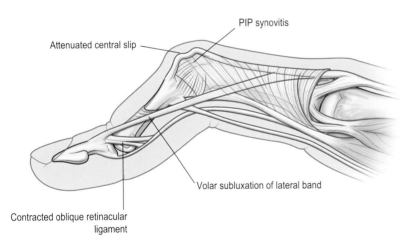

PIP synovitis

Attenuated central slip

Volar subluxation of lateral band

Contracted oblique retinacular ligament

Fig. 19.20 Boutonniere deformity secondary to synovitis at the PIP joint, with attenuation of the central slip, and subsequent volar subluxation of the lateral bands.

may present like a typical nonrheumatoid trigger finger with locking in flexion, or triggering during extension. A nodule just distal to the A2 pulley can result in the finger locking in extension, or triggering during flexion. Diffuse tenosynovitis or multiple nodules can result in swelling and loss of flexion and extension.[52,53]

Thumb deformity can be organized into five categories. Type I, the most common, is a boutonniere deformity with MCP flexion, IP hyperextension, and radial abduction of the metacarpal *(Fig. 19.21)*. Deformity begins when synovial pannus at the MCP joint erodes dorsally, attenuating and eventually rupturing the extensor pollicis brevis (EPB) tendon insertion, and displacing the extensor pollicis longus (EPL) ulnarly and volarly. Because of the loss of dorsal capsule and the loss of the EPB, the MCP joint flexes and subluxates volarly. Hyperextension at the IP joint occurs secondarily, and can be exacerbated in patients with an FPL rupture. Type III rheumatoid thumb deformity is a swan-neck deformity, and

is the second most common deformity, presenting with MCP hyperextension, IP flexion, and metacarpal adduction contracture. This deformity begins at the carpometacarpal (CMC) joint, with attenuation of the volar beak ligament. As the CMC joint subluxates or dislocates, metacarpal adduction occurs in a similar fashion to nonrheumatoid CMC arthritis. MCP joint hyperextension occurs secondarily as the thumb compensates for the adducted metacarpal, and is exacerbated by volar plate attenuation or erosion from pannus invasion.

Types II, IV, and V are less common, but do occur. Type II rheumatoid thumb includes MCP flexion and IP extension, but unlike a type I boutonniere deformity, there is dislocation or subluxation at the CMC joint. Type IV is a gamekeeper's deformity secondary to synovial pannus destruction of the ulnar collateral ligament. Type V is MCP hyperextension, and compensatory flexion at the IP joint, similar to a swan-neck deformity (type III) but without metacarpal adduction contracture.

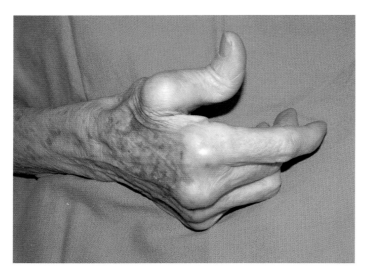

Fig. 19.21 Boutonniere deformity of the thumb.

Patient selection

Perioperative considerations

Care must be taken during the preoperative workup of RA patients, because many unique problems can impact the safety and timing of surgery. Airway management can be quite difficult. Temporomandibular joint arthritis can limit oral opening, making intubation difficult. Glottic narrowing can also occur due to inflammation or arthritis of the cricoarytenoid joints, creating further difficulty with airway management.[54] Atlantoaxial instability is another concern, and is quite common in patients with RA. Flexion of the neck during intubation in patients with significant instability can cause spinal cord injury or death. Therefore, preoperative cervical spine flexion-extension radiographs should be obtained in all rheumatoid patients preoperatively. Fiberoptic intubation with the patient in a cervical collar is recommended in patients with atlantoaxial instability.[55]

> **Hints and tips: Perioperative management of anti-rheumatic medications**
>
> | Medication | Recommendation |
> | --- | --- |
> | Corticosteroids | Continue at normal preoperative dosage |
> | | Provide stress-dose at time of surgery if taking >5–10 mg/day, or if recently stopped long-term corticosteroid use |
> | Methotrexate | Continue at normal preoperative dosage |
> | Other conventional DMARDs | Discuss with rheumatologist, but in general continue |
> | Biologic DMARDs | Discuss with rheumatologist, but in general hold for 2–4 weeks before and after surgery |

Cardiac function can be affected as well. Pericardial effusion, constrictive pericarditis, or conduction block can occur secondary to RA. In addition, RA patients are at increased risk for coronary artery disease. Pulmonary involvement may include rheumatoid nodules, pleural effusion, and interstitial disease. Patients with long-standing disease are at risk for Felty's syndrome, a combination of splenomegaly, neutropenia, and secondary thrombocytopenia. For the above reasons, RA patients undergoing surgery should have a thorough preoperative anaesthesia evaluation including an EKG, metabolic panel, complete blood count and differential, chest X-ray, and cervical spine radiographs.

> **Hints and tips: Preoperative workup for rheumatoid arthritis patients**
>
> - Preoperative anesthesia clinic visit for all, regardless of general medical condition
> - C-spine radiographs, including lateral flexion and extension views
> - 12-lead EKG
> - Chest X-rays
> - Complete blood count (CBC) with differential
> - Metabolic panel

Goals of surgery

The goals of surgery in RA patients are pain relief, improvement of function, prevention of progression, and improvement of appearance. In general, pain relief can be accomplished reliably by arthrodesis or arthroplasty. Because of this, pain is the primary indication for surgery in the rheumatoid patient. Improvement of function is less reliably accomplished, and although important, is a secondary indication for surgery. It is important to remember that deformity does not equal loss of function. Many patients have little pain and are able to function quite well in spite of severe deformity. These patients may not benefit from surgery. Slowing the progression of disease is a third priority, and is less often required in the era of effective DMARDs. However, in some situations, surgery is required to prevent progression of disease. For example, a Darrach procedure (resection of the distal ulna) and dorsal tenosynovectomy in the setting of an extensor tendon rupture can prevent or delay additional extensor tendon ruptures. Appearance is considered a last priority. However, aesthetic considerations should not be discounted as these issues are important to RA patients.

Sequence of surgery

In general, proximal problems within the upper extremity should be corrected first, particularly if they affect more distal problems. For example, wrist surgery should be performed prior to finger surgery, because the deformity at the wrist exacerbates the finger deformity. In practice however, the sequence of surgery may be dictated by patient preference. For example, a patient with severe swan-neck deformities, and a pain-free but ulnarly subluxated wrist may not accept the idea of wrist surgery before correcting the finger deformity. Another consideration is the mobility of the patient. Many RA patients use crutches or canes for ambulation, or may even be confined to a wheelchair, resulting in a loss of mobility during the recovery period after hand surgery. The surgeon should discuss these issues with the patient preoperatively so that preparations can be made.

Treatment/surgical technique

Operations at the wrist

Wrist synovectomy/dorsal tenosynovectomy

A minority of patients will have persistent wrist synovitis or dorsal tenosynovitis that is painful and unresponsive to at least 6 months of maximal medical treatment. Wrist synovectomy and/or dorsal tenosynovectomy may be effective in improving pain in these patients.[56,57] Whether this significantly slows the progression of disease is unknown.

A midline longitudinal incision is made over the dorsal wrist, and skin flaps are elevated at the level of the extensor retinaculum, preserving the radial and ulnar sensory nerves that lie within the subcutaneous tissue. If there is a large amount of synovitis, it can be seen deep to the attenuated extensor retinaculum *(Fig. 19.22)*. The extensor retinaculum is incised along the radial border of the first extensor compartment, leaving enough substance intact for later closure. The retinaculum is elevated in an ulnar direction to, but not into the sixth extensor compartment, exposing the extensor tendons. The extensor retinaculum is often very attenuated, and care should be taken to preserve its integrity during elevation. Extensor tenosynovectomy is then performed. Working systematically, each extensor tendon is retracted individually and synovium is excised with curved tenotomy scissors *(Fig. 19.23)*. In some cases, it becomes clear during tenosynovectomy that an extensor tendon rupture has previously occurred, and that the ruptured extensor tendon or tendons are held together by a mass of adhesions and synovial pannus. This

situation should be discussed preoperatively with the patient, as tendon transfers will be required. After completing the extensor tenosynovectomy, a posterior interosseous neurectomy may be performed to improve pain relief. The posterior interosseous nerve is identified on the floor of the fourth extensor compartment and a 2 cm segment is excised, with cauterization of the proximal stump.

If painful wrist synovitis is present, a ligament-sparing capsulotomy is made. Synovial pannus is identified at the radiocarpal and mid-carpal joints. With the wrist flexed and distracted, a synovial rongeur is used to remove all synovium within the radiocarpal and mid-carpal joints. Any sharp edges are smoothed with a curette or rongeur. If DRUJ synovitis is present, a longitudinal incision is made over the DRUJ, in the floor of the fifth extensor compartment. This incision can be extended 90° ulnarly just proximal to the TFCC if necessary for additional exposure. Pronation also improves exposure of the DRUJ. Synovial pannus is removed with a synovial rongeur. Sharp bony edges are smoothed with a rongeur to prevent tendon ruptures. The capsulotomy incisions are closed with 3-0 absorbable suture.

If any rough bony surfaces remain exposed after closure of the capsule, the retinaculum can be divided transversely, creating two ulnarly based retinacular flaps. One flap is sutured deep to the extensor tendons, covering the exposed bony surfaces. The other retinacular flap is closed dorsal to the extensor tendons, leaving the EPL transposed *(Fig. 19.24)*. Alternatively, if the ECU tendon is subluxated volarly, the retinaculum can be used to stabilize it. The ECU tendon is synovectomized and relocated to its normal position dorsal to the ulna. Half of the retinacular flap is placed deep to the ECU tendon, then wrapped back dorsally and radially and sutured to itself at the border of the fifth extensor compartment, securing the ECU dorsal to the wrist axis of rotation.

Postoperative care

The wrist is immobilized for 2–3 weeks, followed by initiation of motion. If the DRUJ was debrided a sugar-tong splint should be used to prevent forearm rotation. If the wrist or

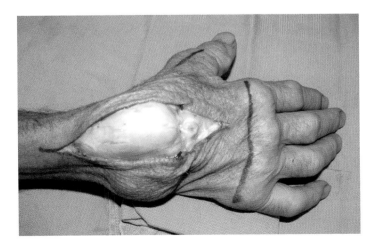

Fig. 19.22 Extensor tenosynovitis of the right wrist, with severely attenuated extensor retinaculum.

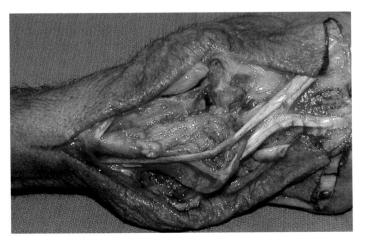

Fig. 19.23 The extensor tenosynovitis has been partially removed. Note the redundancy of the extensor tendons, which have been stretched by the long-standing tenosynovitis.

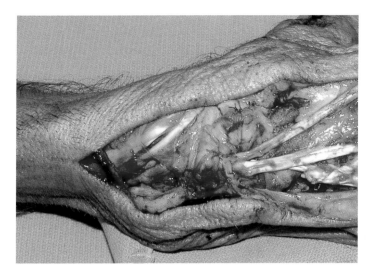

Fig. 19.24 One retinacular flap (the distal half of the retinaculum) has been placed deep to the extensor tendons to protect them from rough bony surfaces. The other flap (the proximal half of the retinaculum) has been sutured dorsal to the extensor tendons to prevent bow-stringing.

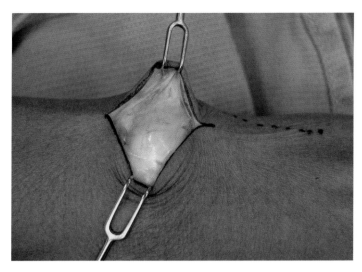

Fig. 19.25 Chevron incision made directly over the ulnar head, with skin flaps elevated and extensor retinaculum exposed.

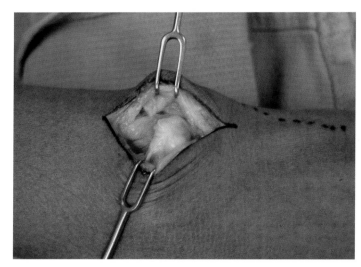

Fig. 19.26 The DRUJ and ulnar head have been exposed through an incision in the floor of the fifth extensor compartment.

DRUJ is unstable prior to surgery, a longer period of mobilization may be required.

Outcomes, prognosis, and complications

Synovectomy of the wrist or DRUJ usually relieves pain, but recurrence of synovitis is the rule rather than the exception, although the rate at which synovitis recurs is variable. Whether wrist synovectomy significantly alters the course of the disease is not known. Dorsal tenosynovectomy on the other hand likely prevents or delays the occurrence of extensor tendon ruptures.

Secondary procedures

If the patient develops recurrent painful synovitis after wrist joint synovectomy, a definitive wrist procedure such as arthrodesis may be indicated.

Hints and tips: Wrist synovectomy/dorsal tenosynovectomy
• Allow at least 6 months of maximized medical treatment prior to considering surgery • Concomitant PIN neurectomy may improve pain relief • Ensure that all rough bony surfaces are smoothed and covered with soft tissue

Distal ulna resection (Darrach procedure)

Distal ulna resection may be indicated for painful DRUJ instability, painful destruction of the DRUJ, or caput ulna syndrome with extensor tendon ruptures. It can be performed in isolation, but is often combined with extensor tenosynovectomy, extensor tendon repairs or tendon transfers, wrist arthrodesis, or wrist arthroplasty.

If performed in isolation, a 3 cm longitudinally oriented chevron incision is made over the dorsal aspect of the ulnar head *(Fig. 19.25)*. If combined with another wrist procedure, skin flaps and retinacular flaps are elevated, and extensor tenosynovectomies are performed as described above. A longitudinal incision is made in the floor of the fifth extensor compartment, with a 90° extension ulnarly just distal to the head of the ulna, and just proximal to the TFCC. Although it is often destroyed, when the TFCC is present, it should be preserved. The capsule is elevated off the ulnar head, and the ulnar head and neck are dissected subperiosteally with a 15-blade and Freer elevator *(Fig. 19.26)*. The ECU is usually subluxed volarly, and is elevated off the ulna during subperiosteal dissection. Hohmann retractors are used to provide exposure of the neck and head of the ulna. Once the ulnar head and neck have been exposed circumferentially, a sagittal saw is used to create a transverse osteotomy at the neck of the ulna, at the level of the proximal margin of the sigmoid notch of the radius. Any remaining soft tissue attachments are released, and the ulnar head is removed *(Fig. 19.27)*. The dorsal edge of the ulnar stump is then beveled with the sagittal saw, and rasped smooth to prevent tendon abrasion and rupture. Any remaining synovial pannus can now be easily accessed, and is debrided with a synovial rongeur.

Prior to closure, the ulnar stump should be stabilized and the normal relationship between the ulna and the carpus should be re-established or improved. The pronator quadratus is elevated subperiosteally from the volar ulnar aspect of the ulna, leaving its attachment to the radius intact. It is

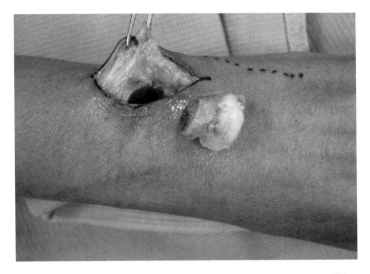

Fig. 19.27 The ulnar head has been removed. The distal end of the stump will be beveled dorsally.

important to keep the periosteum attached to the pronator quadratus. It is then delivered through the interosseous space and draped dorsally over the ulnar stump. The ulna is reduced volarly. While maintaining the ulnar stump in reduction, the pronator quadratus and its periosteum are sutured securely to the dorsal aspect of the ulnar stump, using bone anchors if necessary *(Fig. 19.28)*. In this position, the pronator quadratus serves as a buffer against impingement between the radius and ulna, and also helps prevent dorsal subluxation of the ulna.

Alternatively, a distally based slip of the ECU is elevated. The DRUJ capsule and periosteal flaps are closed with nonabsorbable sutures, and are imbricated tightly with the ulna reduced volarly. The slip of ECU is then woven through the capsule at the distal end of the ulna, and is then sutured to the dorsal ulnar aspect of the radius. This sling helps stabilize the ulnar stump, and also reduces carpal supination *(Fig. 19.29)*. Pre- and postoperative radiographs are shown in *Figure 19.30*.

Postoperative care

The patient is placed in a sugar-tong splint in supination for 2–3 weeks prior to allowing wrist motion and forearm rotation. If a tendon transfer is done, the patient should be splinted for 4 weeks.

Outcomes, prognosis, and complications

One potential complication after distal ulna resection is extensor tendon rupture due to attrition over the sharp dorsal edge of the osteotomy. This is prevented by beveling and rasping down the dorsal edge of the osteotomy, and by performing a soft tissue stabilizing procedure at the time of the Darrach procedure, in order to minimize dorsal subluxation of the ulnar stump. Another potential complication is painful radioulnar convergence and impingement, which tends to occur

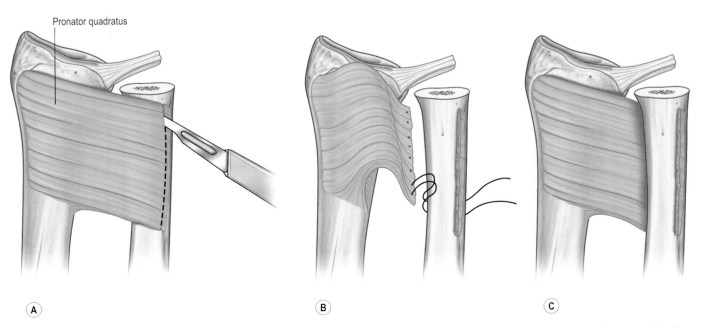

Pronator quadratus

(A) (B) (C)

Fig. 19.28 The pronator quadratus is released from the volar aspect of the ulna, passed through the interosseous space, and sutured to the dorsal aspect of the ulna.

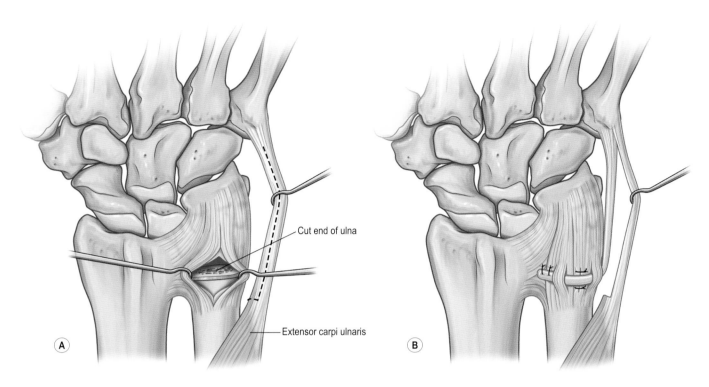

Fig. 19.29 Distally based slip of ECU is used to stabilize the ulnar stump.

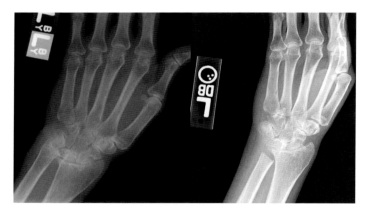

Fig. 19.30 Pre- and postoperative radiographs demonstrating resection of the ulnar head.

Hints and tips: Distal ulna resection

- Create a dorsal bevel after making the transverse osteotomy, and smooth with a rasp to prevent attrition ruptures
- Distal ulna resection should be performed at the time of extensor tendon transfers if the distal ulna was the source of extensor tendon rupture
- A stabilizing procedure should be performed to decrease recurrent dorsal subluxation, minimize radioulnar convergence, and reduce carpal subluxation.

during loading. Again, stabilization and/or padding of the distal ulna at the time of Darrach procedure as described above helps to minimize this.

Secondary procedures

Persistent painful instability or radio-ulnar impingement may be treated with a soft-tissue stabilization procedure using the ECU as described above. Alternatively, ulnar head implant arthroplasty may be considered to salvage the failed Darrach complicated by painful radio-ulnar impingement.

Partial wrist arthrodesis (radioscapholunate arthrodesis)

In some rheumatoid wrists, the radiocarpal joint becomes arthritic with relative preservation of the mid-carpal joint

(Fig. 19.31). In these patients, radioscapholunate arthrodesis may be indicated to treat refractory pain secondary to radiocarpal arthritis. Patients should understand that they will lose approximately 60% of wrist flexion-extension, depending upon the quality of the mid-carpal joint. In addition, patients should be consented for the possibility of complete wrist arthrodesis if the mid-carpal joint is found to be substantially arthritic at the time of surgery.

The skin and retinacular incisions are the same as described above. Extensor tenosynovectomies are performed if required, and a posterior interosseous neurectomy is performed. An H-shaped capsulotomy is made, exposing the radiocarpal and mid-carpal joints. Radiocarpal and mid-carpal synovectomies are performed. The quality of the mid-carpal joint is assessed, and the decision to proceed with radiocarpal fusion versus complete wrist fusion is made. The radiocarpal joint is

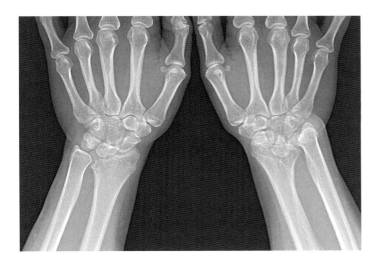

Fig. 19.31 Bilateral wrist radiographs demonstrating severe involvement of the radio-carpal joint, and relative sparing of the mid-carpal joint.

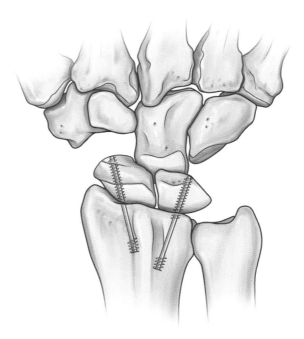

Fig. 19.32 Radiocarpal arthrodesis, with compression screws. The distal pole of the scaphoid is resected to preserve mid-carpal motion. Triquetrum excision is optional.

assessed as well. In some cases, the radioscaphoid articulation is preserved, allowing the surgeon to perform a radiolunate fusion, although in most instances the entire radiocarpal joint is arthritic. With the wrist flexed and distracted, a rongeur is used to remove the remaining articular cartilage and subchondral bone from the distal radius and the proximal articular surfaces of the lunate and scaphoid. The articular surfaces are prepared in this manner until bleeding cancellous bone is encountered. During joint surface preparation, the matching concave-convex surfaces of the radiocarpal joint should be preserved. The carpus is then reduced by maneuvering the lunate into neutral flexion-extension, correcting any scapholunate gap, and correcting ulnar translocation if present. The use of 0.062-inch K-wires as joysticks may be necessary for reduction. The scaphoid and lunate are temporarily held in reduction with 0.062-inch radiocarpal K-wires, and a mini c-arm is used to confirm carpal alignment. Next, the distal pole of the scaphoid is resected in order to improve mid-carpal motion. A transverse osteotomy is made at the proximal margin of the distal pole of the scaphoid using a reciprocating saw. The distal pole is then removed piece-meal with a rongeur.

Autologous cancellous bone graft is packed into the fusion site. This should be obtained from the iliac crest, or from the resected distal pole of the scaphoid and from the distal ulna if a Darrach procedure has been performed. Bone graft should not be harvested from the distal radius, as this reduces the stability of the radioscapholunate fixation. Fixation is achieved with headless compression screws that are inserted into the dorsal aspect of the distal radius, and driven distally and volarly into the scaphoid and lunate. Three or four compression screws are used, with two passing from the radius into the scaphoid, and one or two passing from the radius into the lunate *(Fig. 19.32)*. It is usually necessary to back out the temporary fixation K-wires in order to achieve compression. In addition, in order to achieve even compression when two screws are placed across one articulation, the screws should be simultaneously advanced. After screw placement, final c-arm views are used to confirm carpal alignment and screw position. The mid-carpal joint is directly examined to ensure

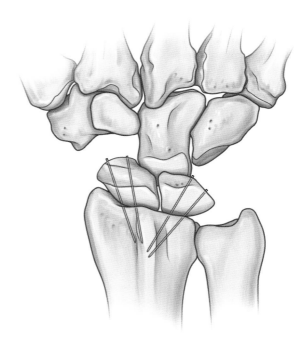

Fig. 19.33 Radiocarpal arthrodesis with K-wires.

that there is no screw penetration. If there is any concern about the stability of the fixation, supplemental K-wires can be placed. If the bone quality is too poor to support compression screws, as it often is in patients with rheumatoid arthritis, fixation can be performed with K-wires alone *(Fig. 19.33)*.

Other alternatives for fixation include staples or a T-shaped plate. The capsule is closed and the extensor retinaculum is closed with the EPL transposed.

Postoperative care

The wrist is immobilized until bony union occurs. Active and passive range of motion and strengthening exercises are initiated after bony union occurs.

Complete wrist arthrodesis

Complete wrist arthrodesis is an effective treatment for the painful and unstable wrist. However, the loss of wrist motion after complete arthrodesis can cause significant functional difficulty, particularly if the patient has a stiff contralateral wrist. Because of this, it should be reserved for patients with recalcitrant pain or debilitating instability or malalignment, in spite of maximum medical management, steroid injections, and wrist splinting.

In patients with high quality bone, a dorsal wrist fusion plate can be used *(Fig. 19.34)*. However, if bone quality is poor, Steinmann pin fixation may be performed.[58,59] The wrist is exposed as described above for radioscapholunate fusion. If indicated, a Darrach procedure is performed as described above. The radio carpal and mid-carpal joints are exposed. With the wrist flexed and distracted, a synovial rongeur is used to débride synovial pannus, allowing access to the articular surfaces. A rongeur is then used to remove articular cartilage and subchondral bone from the opposing articular surfaces, until bleeding cancellous bone is encountered *(Fig. 19.35)*. A small Steinmann pin is drilled retrograde into the radius in order to create a track for the final Steinmann pin. The starting point on the radius is chosen carefully, in order to allow the Steinmann pin to pass directly into the isthmus of the medullary canal without any angulation. The correct starting point is usually in the dorsal half of the radius articular surface, and near the interval between the scaphoid and lunate fossae. Fluoroscopy is used to confirm the position of the Steinmann pin. The small Steinmann pin is removed and exchanged for the largest diameter Steinmann pin that will fit into the medullary canal of the radius. The large Steinmann pin is removed from the radius and then it is drilled antegrade through the carpus, exiting the carpus at the 2nd or 3rd intermetacarpal space, and exiting the skin between the MCP joints. With the radius and carpus reduced, the Steinmann pin is tapped retrograde back into the radius, and through the isthmus of the medullary canal *(Fig. 19.36)*. It is cut distally at the skin, and then tapped 2–3 cm proximal to the level of the skin. If necessary, additional fixation with temporary k-wires can be used. Cancellous autograft is packed into the radiocarpal and mid-carpal joints. The capsule is closed with 3-0 absorbable sutures, and the retinaculum and skin are closed as described above. The wrist is immobilized until union occurs.

An alternative is to use two smaller Steinmann pins. The technique is similar to that described above, except that one pin passes through the second intermetacarpal space, and one passes through the third intermetacarpal space. An oblique K-wire can be added to augment the fixation. The pins are cut deep to the skin, and can be removed after bony union is achieved *(Figs 19.37, 19.38)*. If future MCP arthroplasty is planned, and there is no reason to preserve the articular

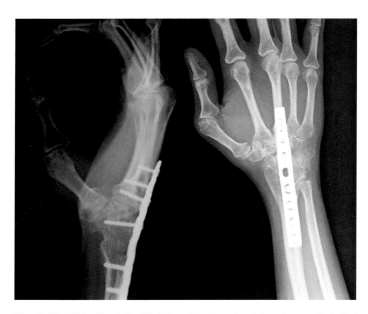

Fig. 19.34 Wrist arthrodesis with fusion plate. Use of a plate and screws is limited to patients with good bone quality.

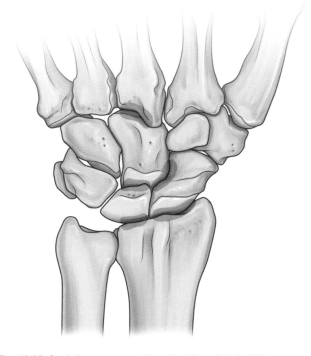

Fig. 19.35 Shaded areas represent the articulations that should be prepared for a complete wrist arthrodesis.

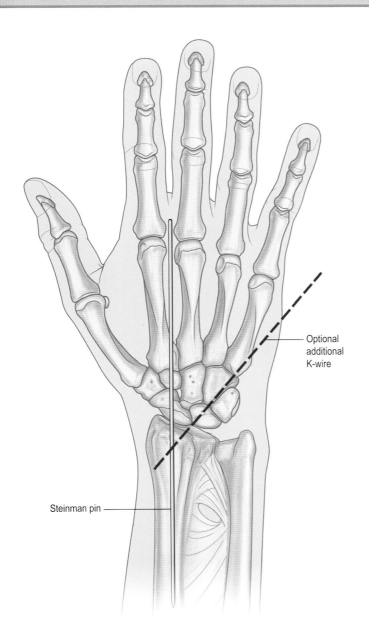

Optional
additional
K-wire

Steinman pin

Fig. 19.36 Wrist arthrodesis with a single Steinmann pin. The pin exits the carpus in the second intermetacarpal space, and is cut just below the skin for later removal. The oblique K-wire is optional.

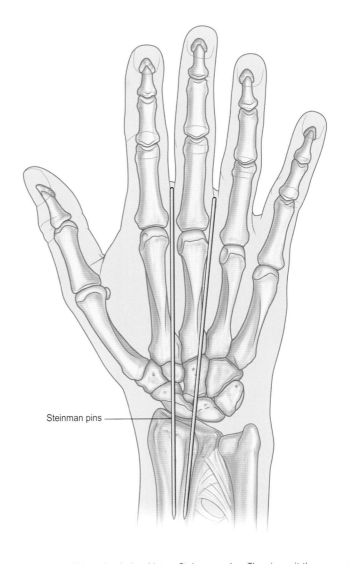

Steinman pins

Fig. 19.37 Wrist arthrodesis with two Steinmann pins. The pins exit the carpus in the second and third intermetacarpal spaces, and are cut just below the skin for later removal.

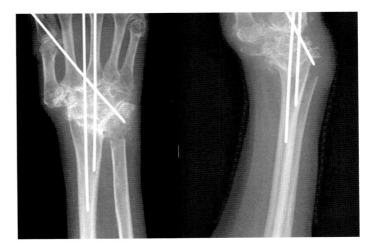

Fig. 19.38 Wrist arthrodesis with two longitudinal Steinmann pins, and a third oblique pin for added fixation.

surface of the metacarpal head, one pin can be advanced through the medullary canal of the long finger metacarpal, exiting the metacarpal head distally, and then tapped proximally into the radius after reduction. If a Steinmann pins is placed in the medullary canal of the long finger metacarpal, it should be tapped proximally to allow enough room for future MCP arthroplasty *(Figs 19.39, 19.40)*. As noted above, in patients with high quality bone a dorsal wrist fusion plate can be used. These plates allow compression across the wrist, and result in very stable fixation.

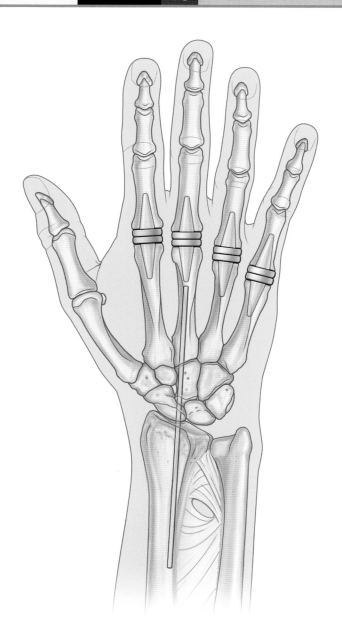

Fig. 19.39 Wrist arthrodesis with a single Steinmann pin placed in the medullary canal of the long finger metacarpal. Note that the length of the Steinmann pin should not prohibit future MCP arthroplasty.

Postoperative care

The wrist is immobilized until bony union occurs.

Outcomes, prognosis, and complications

Limited or complete wrist arthrodesis reliably treats pain in RA when used for appropriate indications. Although the complication rate is less than that for total wrist arthroplasty, minor complications such as delayed skin healing, prominent hardware, tendon irritation, neurapraxia, and pin-site issues are not uncommon. Potential major complications include infection, loss of fixation, and nonunion. A deep infection requires hardware removal, serial debridement, and intravenous antibiotics. Nonunion, if it occurs, may or may not be symptomatic.

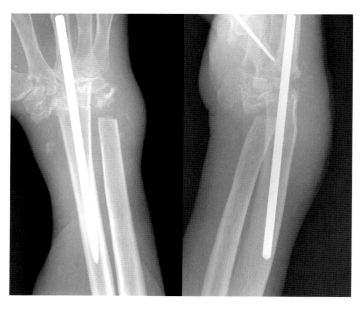

Fig. 19.40 PA and lateral radiographs demonstrating wrist arthrodesis performed with a single intramedullary pin. Note the large caliber of pin required to fill the medullary canal of the radius.

Secondary procedures

In some cases prominent hardware requires removal. Unless there is an indication for more urgent removal, this should be delayed for a year after union is achieved. After hardware removal, the wrist should be protected in a splint or cast for a minimum of 6 weeks.

Hints and tips: Partial or complete wrist arthrodesis

- Resection of all cartilage and subchondral bone, with exposure of bleeding cancellous bone, is critical in order to achieve union
- Compression screw or plate and screw fixation should be used only if bone quality is good, otherwise K-wires or Steinmann pins may be used for fixation
- Assessment of bony union may be difficult with plain radiographs. In this situation, computed tomography (CT scan) is ideal for confirming union.

Total wrist arthroplasty

Total wrist arthroplasty is effective at relieving pain in patients with rheumatoid wrist arthritis. However, in spite of recent advances, wrist arthroplasty is associated with a high complication rate. In order to minimize complications such as loosening, migration, and dislocation, wrist arthroplasty should only be performed in patients who place low demands on their wrists. In addition, arthroplasty is only indicated in wrists with good bone stock that will support an implant. Furthermore, the patient must have functioning wrist flexors and extensors to benefit maximally from wrist arthroplasty.

It is important to discuss complications such as infection, loosening, migration and dislocation with the patient, as well as the postoperative rehabilitation and long-term limitations that will be placed on wrist use. A number of implant designs are available worldwide. The most commonly used implants consist of cobalt chrome metal components, often with titanium plasma spray on the stems to improve osseointegration, and ultra-high molecular weight polyethylene on metal articulations. Because wrist implants are continually modified and refined, the details of the surgical technique change and the implant manufacturer's specific recommendations should be followed. The general steps of the operation are described below.

The dorsal wrist capsule is exposed as described above *(Fig. 19.41)*. A distally based U-shaped capsulotomy is created, leaving a cuff of capsule on the radius for closure *(Fig. 19.42)*. Radiocarpal and mid-carpal synovectomies are performed. A transverse carpal osteotomy is made, removing 2 mm of the head of the capitate, the proximal pole of the hamate, the proximal half of the scaphoid, and the entire triquetrum and lunate. With the wrist flexed, the surface of the radius is prepared using a guide and a burr or saw *(Fig. 19.43)*. Next, a

guide-wire is drilled into the radius. It should be in line with the medullary canal, with a starting point about 2–3 mm volar to the dorsal lip of the radius and near the interfossal ridge. The distal radius is then sequentially broached, keeping the broach aligned with the medullary canal. After broaching, the radial trial component is placed and impacted. If it is proud, further broaching or burring of the radius may be required. Next, the radial trial is removed, and the carpus is prepared. This step varies depending upon the implant used. After preparing the carpus, a trial reduction is performed with both the radial and carpal trial components. Articulation and range of motion are checked. Trials are removed, the wound is copiously irrigated, fresh towels are placed, and gloves are changed. The radial implant is placed first and impacted, and its position checked with fluoroscopy. Next, the carpal component(s) is placed and impacted, and the joint reduced *(Fig. 19.44)*. Hardware position and alignment are checked with fluoroscopy *(Fig. 19.45)*. Depending upon the implant design, carpal screws may be placed. Joint stability and ROM are checked, and final X-rays are taken. The tourniquet is let down, hemostasis is achieved, and the retinaculum is closed with the EPL transposed.

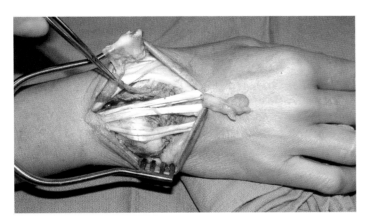

Fig. 19.41 A radially based retinacular flap has been elevated, exposing the extensor tendons. Synovectomy is being performed.

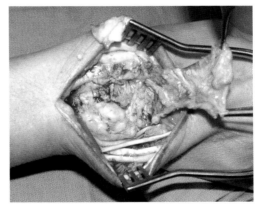

Fig. 19.42 A wrist capsulotomy has been made. The capsulotomy is U-shaped, and is distally based, providing full exposure of the wrist joint.

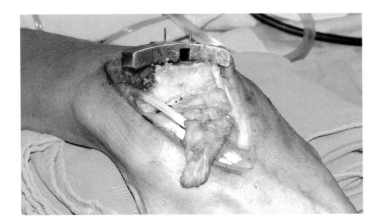

Fig. 19.43 An osteotomy has been made at the distal end of the radius. Note the saw-guide held in place with two K-wires.

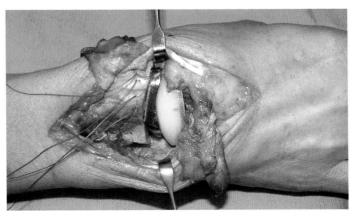

Fig. 19.44 The radial and carpal components have been seated, and the joint reduced. Final position of the implant.

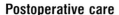

Fig. 19.45 PA and lateral radiographs demonstrating good position and alignment of the prosthesis.

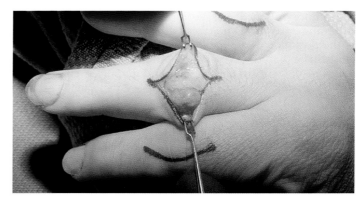

Fig. 19.46 A slightly curved incision has been made over the dorsal aspect of the PIP joint, and skin flaps have been elevated. The synovial pannus can be seen protruding ulnar to the central slip.

Postoperative care

The patient is splinted in 30° of extension for 2 weeks. ROM begins at 2 weeks under the guidance of a therapist, and protection of a removable splint for the next 6–8 weeks. Strengthening begins at 4–6 weeks. Patients are given a 20-lb lifting restriction, and sports and other heavy activities are prohibited. It is crucial for the patient to take preoperative antibiotics before dental, urologic, and gastrointestinal procedures, etc.

Outcomes, prognosis, and complications

Total wrist arthroplasty effectively relieves wrist pain. However, the surgeon and patient are accepting a higher complication rate in order to preserve wrist motion. Major complications include implant instability or dislocation, migration, infection, fracture, loss of alignment, and persistent pain.

Secondary procedures

Although revision arthroplasty may be attempted, failed total wrist arthroplasty is most reliably treated with complete wrist arthrodesis. Wrist arthrodesis after failed total wrist arthroplasty is not straightforward, due to scarring and loss of bone stock. Difficulty with fixation and delayed union are not uncommon.

Hints and tips: Total wrist arthroplasty

- Total wrist arthroplasty is a "high risk–high reward" operation. The patient is accepting a relatively high complication rate for the chance to preserve wrist motion
- The patient must be aware of life-time limitations on upper extremity use
- The patient must be instructed in taking antibiotics prior to dental, urologic, GI, and other invasive procedures or surgeries after total wrist arthroplasty.

Operations for the hand and fingers

MCP synovectomy and soft tissue reconstruction

Synovectomy and soft tissue reconstruction of the MCP joints is a temporizing operation, and synovitis and deformity usually recur. It is only indicated in patients with persistent synovitis that does not respond to at least 6 months of maximum nonoperative management who have radiographically intact joints, correctible deformities, and substantial dysfunction. Patients with adequate function should not undergo MCP synovectomy and soft tissue reconstruction, regardless of the presence of synovitis or deformity.

A transverse incision is made over the dorsal aspect of the MCP joints. Dissection is carried down to the extensor mechanism over each joint, using longitudinal spreading to protect the dorsal veins and sensory nerves. Often, the extensor tendon has subluxated ulnarly, and there may be attenuation or destruction of the radial sagittal band. The ulnar sagittal band is incised longitudinally, adjacent to the extensor tendon. A 15-blade is then used to separate the extensor mechanism from the underlying joint capsule. The capsule, which is usually very thin, is then incised transversely with a 15-blade, exposing the MCP joint. Synovial pannus is removed with a curette or small synovial rongeur. (It should be noted that PIP synovectomy can be performed as well for painful synovitis that is unresponsive to medical management, as demonstrated in *Figures 19.46 and 19.47*).

The finger is checked for intrinsic tightness. The PIP joint is passively flexed while the MCP joint is alternately held in flexion, and then hyperextension. Increased resistance to PIP flexion when the MCP is held in hyperextension indicates intrinsic tightness. In addition, ulnar sided intrinsic tightness is evaluated by testing the PIP joint with the MCP ulnarly versus radially deviated. If intrinsic tightness is present, an ulnar intrinsic release and cross-intrinsic transfer are performed.

On both sides of the finger, the soft tissue is elevated off the lateral bands using tenotomy scissors. The ulnar lateral band is divided distally and freed proximally to the musculotendinous junction. It is then transferred to the radial lateral band of the adjacent finger and secured with a modified Pulvertaft weave *(Fig. 19.48)*. The cross-intrinsic transfer should be tensioned with the finger in neutral alignment. In the small finger the abductor digiti minimi is released with a 15-blade at its musculotendinous junction. Finally, the extensor tendons are mobilized radially and relocated centrally over the MCP joints. The radial sagittal band of each joint is imbricated. The MCP joints are then passively ranged. If the extensor mechanism tends to re-subluxate, or if the radial sagittal band reconstruction is not secure, the extensor tendon should be sutured directly to the underlying joint capsule at the base of the proximal phalanx.

Postoperative care

A splint is applied with the MCP joints extended and in neutral radio-ulnar alignment. Active ROM in a dynamic MCP extension splint is begun once pain and edema have improved. A resting splint that holds the MCPs extended and in neutral alignment should be worn at night and at other times. Splinting can be weaned after 6–8 weeks, although night-time splinting may be continued indefinitely.

Outcomes, prognosis, and complications

Recurrence of synovitis and deformity should be expected over time. *Figure 19.49* demonstrates a patient before and 1.5 years after MCP synovectomy and cross-intrinsic transfer.

Secondary procedures

Recurrent synovitis and deformity that are painful or adversely affect hand use, are indications for arthroplasty.

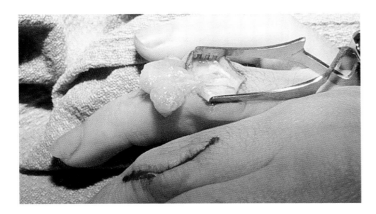

Fig. 19.47 Excision of the synovial pannus, working in a proximal to distal direction.

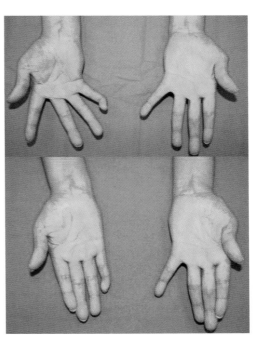

Fig. 19.49 Preoperative (above) and postoperative (below) views of both hands after cross-intrinsic transfers.

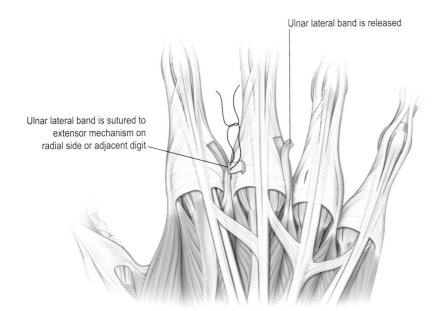

Ulnar lateral band is released

Ulnar lateral band is sutured to extensor mechanism on radial side or adjacent digit

Fig. 19.48 The ulnar lateral bands of the index, long and ring fingers are divided distally, and transferred to the radial lateral bands of the adjacent long, ring, and small fingers. The abductor digiti minimi of the small finger is divided.

MCP arthroplasty (silicone)

Video 1

MCP arthroplasty is indicated in patients who have pain or substantial loss of function due to MCP deformity and arthritis. If the patient has reasonable hand function without pain, arthroplasty is not indicated regardless of the degree of deformity. PyroCarbon implants or surface replacement arthroplasty (SRA) implants can be used in rheumatoid patients in certain situations *(Fig. 19.50)*. However, because of the soft tissue laxity and joint instability associated with RA, silicone arthroplasty is generally preferred. A silicone implant acts as a spacer and internal mold that becomes encapsulated, and thereby provides some degree of alignment stability. A number of silicone MCP implants are commercially available. Although there are some minor differences in design, the surgical techniques are similar.

A transverse incision is made across the dorsal aspect of the MCP joints. If only one joint is undergoing arthroplasty, a longitudinal incision can be used. The extensor mechanism is exposed as described above. Because of the alignment of the fingers, arthroplasty is performed at the index finger and progresses ulnarly. A longitudinal incision is made in the ulnar sagittal band adjacent to the extensor tendon. The extensor mechanism is elevated off the joint capsule, and the extensor tendon is retracted radially. If intrinsic tightness is contributing to ulnar deviation, an ulnar intrinsic release can be performed as described above. The capsule is incised longitudinally with a 15-blade and synovectomy is performed. The ulnar collateral ligament is released by separating its proximal insertion from the lateral aspect of the metacarpal head. If possible, the radial collateral ligament is preserved. The MCP joint is then maximally flexed, exposing the metacarpal head. A starter awl is used to open the medullary canals of the metacarpal and proximal phalanx, and fluoroscopy is used to confirm appropriate alignment *(Fig. 19.51)*. In order to center the awl in the medullary canal, the entrance point should be in the dorsal third of the articular surface *(Fig. 19.52)*. A transverse osteotomy is made in the metacarpal head just distal to the insertion of the collateral ligaments. The proximal phalanx is then brought into extension, and a transverse osteotomy is created at the proximal phalanx base, resecting only articular cartilage and subchondral bone *(Fig. 19.53)*. Conservative osteotomies should be made initially, as more bone can be resected later if necessary. The medullary canals of the metacarpal and proximal phalanx are broached sequentially until an appropriately sized implant can be

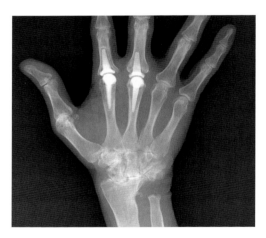

Fig. 19.50 Index and long MCP arthroplasties with PyroCarbon implants. The use of PyroCarbon implants should be limited to patients without soft tissue instability.

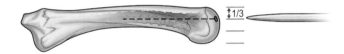

Fig. 19.52 In order to be in-line with axis of the medullary canal, the starting point should be created at the junction of the middle and dorsal third of the articular surface.

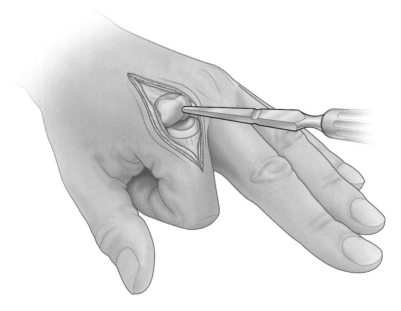

Fig. 19.51 A starter awl is used to open the subchondral bone at the head of the metacarpal and at the base of the proximal phalanx, in order to gain access to the medullary canal.

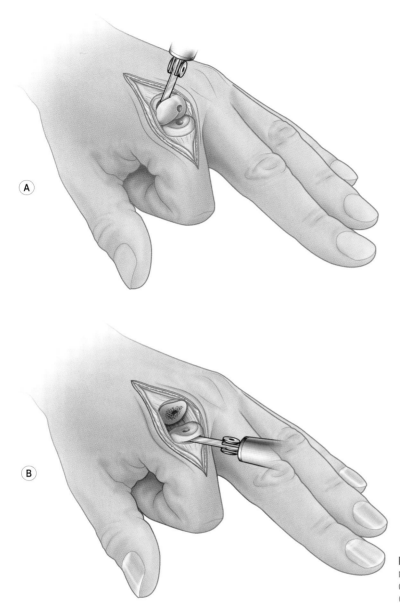

Fig. 19.53 A sagittal saw is used to create osteotomies of the metacarpal head and base of proximal phalanx. Conservative osteotomies should be made at first, and revised if needed. The collateral ligaments should be preserved if possible.

placed *(Fig. 19.54)*. Trials are used to select an implant that matches the diameter of the medullary canals and covers the entire exposed bony surface, but that does not overhang. When broaching the medullary canals, the broach should be oriented in such a way as to minimize the rheumatoid deformity. For example, in the index finger, the rectangular broach should be positioned high on the dorsal ulnar side of the base of the proximal phalanx, and low on the radial palmar side. This helps bring the finger into supination when the implant is place, and prevents pronation deformity. The small finger broaching should be done in the opposite manner to prevent supination deformity. After broaching is completed, a rasp is used to smooth all cortical surfaces that may come in contact with the implant. The trial is then placed and the joint is reduced *(Fig. 19.55)*. The transverse barrel should seat against both osteotomy sites, but should not be compressed. The joint is then passively ranged. If the implant is compressed during extension, further bone resection is required. There should be no bony impingement with flexion and extension. The trial is removed, and the wound is copiously irrigated. Using fresh powder-free gloves, the final silicone implant is placed. The radial collateral ligament is imbricated using 3-0 Ethibond sutures. If release of the radial collateral ligament was required, it must be sutured back to the periosteum or to bone holes created prior to implant placement. The capsule is closed, and the radial sagittal band is imbricated, centralizing the extensor tendon. A cross intrinsic transfer may be performed as described above.

Postoperative care

Postoperatively, the wrist is splinted in 20° of extension, and the MCPs are splinted in extension and slight radial deviation. The IP joints are left free. Once edema and pain have improved,

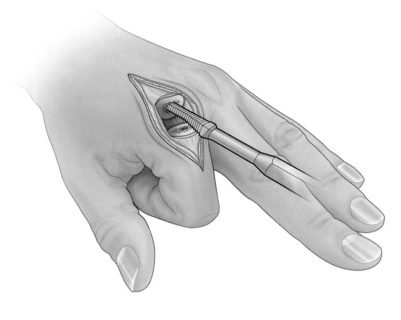

Fig. 19.54 The medullary canals are sequentially broached.

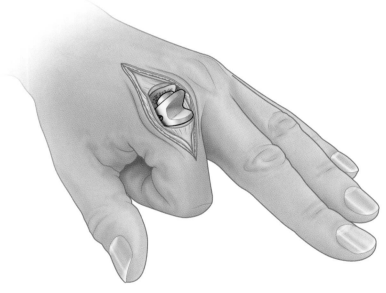

Fig. 19.55 Final position of the implant.

active motion with the guidance of a therapist is initiated. The patient wears an MCP extension splint in between exercises, and a dynamic MCP extension splint may be used for exercises if needed. Modifications of splinting position are frequently required, depending on the severity of the preoperative deformity, and on patient progress after surgery. Splinting is weaned at 6 weeks.

PIP arthroplasty

PIP arthroplasty can effectively relieve pain and improve alignment, while preserving joint mobility in patients with PIP arthritis. However, PIP arthroplasty is less reliable than MCP arthroplasty in terms of stability and correction of deformity. PIP arthroplasty should therefore be avoided in the index finger, which must resist strong ulnar deviation forces during pinch. It is most effective in patients with pain due to arthritis, who have relatively good soft tissue.

The procedure is similar to that for MCP arthroplasty described above. A dorsal longitudinal incision is made over the PIP joint, and skin flaps are elevated at the level of the extensor mechanism. The central slip is divided longitudinally from the mid-portion of the proximal phalanx to the central slip insertion, without disrupting the central slip insertion. The joint is flexed and a transverse capsulotomy is made. The collateral ligaments should be preserved if possible. If collateral ligament recession is required for adequate exposure of the joint, the collateral ligaments are repaired prior to skin closure. A transverse osteotomy is made in the head of the proximal phalanx just distal to the collateral ligament insertion. An osteotomy is not required at the base of the middle phalanx, but osteophytes should be removed and the articular surface smoothed. Bony resection should be conservative, and further resection can be performed later if required. A starter awl is used to open the medullary canals, and fluoroscopy is used to confirm correct alignment. Broaches are then used to sequentially broach up the medullary canals of the proximal and middle phalanges. Trials are used to select the appropriate implant size as described above. The appropriately sized trial is placed, the joint is reduced and ranged, and checked for instability or impingement. If required, further bony resection and re-broaching is performed. The trial is removed and bone edges are smoothed. The wound is copiously irrigated, gloves are changed, and the final implants are inserted. If required, the central slip and collateral ligaments are reattached to bone using sutures passed through bone holes drilled with a Kirschner wire. The bone holes should be created and the sutures passed prior to placing the final implant. The divided central slip is approximated with absorbable sutures, and the skin is closed.

Postoperative care

Patients begin motion postoperatively, as soon as edema and pain are improved. Splinting is continued for at least 6 weeks postoperatively. The position and type of splinting required vary substantially, depending upon the preoperative deformity and patient's postoperative progress.

Outcomes, prognosis, and complications

Although the outcomes reported in the literature are variable, silicone MCP arthroplasty has been demonstrated in multiple studies to effectively treat pain, correct ulnar drift, improve MCP joint arc of motion, and improve appearance. These effects are often maintained for years, although slow deterioration usually occurs. At the PIP joint, arthroplasty typically relieves pain, but is not as effective at correcting deformity or improving motion. Potential complications include recurrence of deformity, extension lag or loss of flexion, fracture of silicone implant, dislocation of implant, silicone synovitis, and infection. Recurrence may be due to soft tissue changes, implant fracture, or inappropriate positioning of implant.

Secondary procedures

Revision arthroplasty after implant failure is possible, but should be reserved for patients with loss of hand function that is directly correlated to the failure of the implant. Often, overall upper extremity function is decreased not because of implant failure, but because of ongoing changes at the wrist, elbow, or shoulder. Furthermore, a fractured implant often continues to function as a spacer, and the patient may not notice a change in joint function. When revision arthroplasty is performed, it is important to correct any issues that may have contributed to implant failure, such as soft tissue deforming forces, sharp bony edges, or inadequate bone resection.

Hints and tips: MCP and PIP arthroplasty

- Pyrolytic carbon or other surface replacement arthroplasties should be reserved for patients with stable joints and normal ligaments and soft tissue
- Most RA patients who require MCP or PIP arthroplasty should have silicone rather than surface replacement arthroplasty
- The surgeon should start with conservative osteotomies and broaching. More bone can always be resected if needed.

MCP and PIP arthrodesis

Arthrodesis of the MCP or PIP joint is a reliable method for treating refractory pain due to arthritis. Although motion is sacrificed, the complication rate of arthrodesis is less than that of arthroplasty, making it an attractive option in some clinical situations. Arthrodesis is most commonly indicated at the index or long finger PIP joint, where the ability to resist strong ulnar deviation forces during pinch is crucial.

The joint is exposed as described above for arthroplasty. The collateral ligaments can be divided in order to improve joint exposure. With the joint flexed, a rongeur is used to remove all articular cartilage and subchondral bone from the opposing articular surfaces, creating flat opposing cancellous surfaces. The flat cancellous surfaces must be created in such a way that when they are apposed, there is full contact between the two surfaces with the joint in the desired amount of flexion, without radial or ulnar deviation. Next, two parallel 0.035 or 0.045 inch K-wires are drilled across the joint, entering the cortical bone dorsally at least 1 cm proximal to the arthrodesis site, and angled volarly into the medullary canal of the distal bone. The K-wires should be advanced until they enter cortical or subchondral bone distal to the osteotomy site. Next, a 0.045 inch K-wire is used to create a transverse hole in the distal bone, 1 cm distal to the arthrodesis site. A 24-guage stainless steel wire is passed through the transverse hole in the distal bone. Both ends of the wire are then turned proximally, crossed over the dorsal aspect of the arthrodesis site and wrapped around the k-wires, creating a figure-of-eight *(Fig. 19.56)*. The free ends are twisted down with a needle driver until strong compression is achieved. The excess wire is then cut and bent down against the bone. The two K-wires are retracted 2 mm proximally, bent 90° and cut, and then tapped back in to prevent a sharp protruding K-wire. The extensor mechanism is repaired, and the skin is closed.

Postoperative care

Light active finger motion is allowed immediately and a splint is worn for comfort only. Heavy activity is allowed after union is achieved.

Outcomes, prognosis, and complications

MCP or PIP arthrodesis effectively relieves pain at the expense of motion. Often, the severely arthritic and painful joint has little motion prior to surgery, and in many cases hand function is improved rather than worsened after arthrodesis. Although the complication rate is lower than that of arthroplasty, complications are not unusual, and may include delayed union or nonunion, infection, skin flap compromise, and hardware related problems such as loss of fixation, palpability, and tendon irritation.

Correction of swan-neck deformity

Swan-neck deformity is more debilitating than Boutonniere's deformity because the fingers cannot be flexed into the palm for grasping objects. Swan-neck deformity can be divided into four types, based upon the degree joint mobility and arthritic changes. In a finger with type I deformity, full active PIP flexion is preserved, there is no intrinsic tightness, and patients have little if any functional problems. In a finger with type II deformity, intrinsic tightness is present. With the MCP in

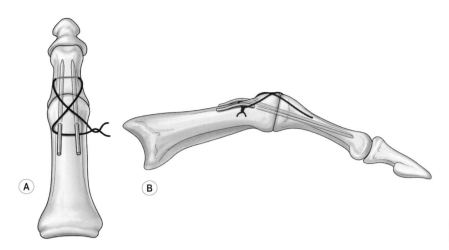

Fig. 19.56 K-wire and stainless steel wire configuration for tension band arthrodesis of the PIP joint.

ulnar deviation and flexion, PIP flexion is possible. However, if the MCP deformity is corrected by placing it in extension and correcting ulnar deviation, the ulnar intrinsics are tightened, and PIP flexion becomes more difficult. Fingers with type III deformity have more severe intrinsic tightness, and PIP flexion is difficult or impossible regardless of MCP position. In the type IV deformity substantial arthritic changes are present.

In type I deformities, a silver ring splint that prevents PIP hyperextension, while at the same time allowing PIP flexion, is adequate treatment. For type II deformities an intrinsic release and a PIP extension block are required. A Bruner incision is made over the PIP joint and the flexor tendon sheath is exposed. The ulnar intrinsics are exposed through the volar incision and are released as described above. A transverse incision is then made in the mid-portion of the A2 pulley. One slip of FDS is transected with tenotomy scissors as proximally as possible. The transected end which remains attached distally at the FDS insertion is passed through the slit in the A2 pulley, and turned distally. It is then sutured to itself near the FDS insertion through a small window in the flexor tendon sheath *(Fig. 19.57)*. This is tensioned so that the joint cannot be passively extended beyond 20–30° of flexion. If the MCP joint is subluxated and ulnarly deviated, MCP arthroplasty and soft tissue reconstruction should be performed as well. Persistent DIP flexion is treated with arthrodesis if necessary.

In type III deformity, the PIP joint is stiff regardless of MCP position. PIP flexion is limited not only by intrinsic tightness, but also because the lateral bands are fixed in a dorsal position. A dorsal skin contracture further complicates the deformity. The first goal is to regain passive mobility in the PIP joint. Serial casting or dynamic splinting should be used in an attempt to restore passive mobility. If passive mobility is restored, the type III swan-neck is converted to a type II swan-neck, and is treated accordingly. However, if nonoperative methods fail, passive motion must be restored surgically. A longitudinal incision is made over the PIP joint, with an oblique extension over the dorsal aspect of the middle phalanx. Skin flaps are elevated. A longitudinal incision is made on each side of the central slip, releasing the dorsally displaced lateral bands *(Fig. 19.58)*. The joint is passively flexed, and the lateral bands should slide volarly. If the joint cannot be flexed,

a dorsal capsulotomy and collateral ligament recession may be required. An intrinsic release is performed as described above. The PIP joint is then pinned in flexion. The skin is closed proximally, but the oblique distal portion of the incision is allowed to gap open and heal secondarily *(Fig. 19.59)*. This takes tension off the dorsal skin closure, and prevents skin necrosis.

In type IV swan-neck deformity with articular destruction, PIP arthrodesis is a reasonable option. In the ring and small fingers, PIP arthroplasty combined with an FDS sling is an alternative.

Postoperative care

The K-wire is removed and active and passive PIP motion within a dorsal blocking splint is initiated, as soon as finger edema is improved. After the finger has healed and passive mobility is restored, the swan-neck deformity can be treated with an FDS tenodesis. If present, MCP deformity should be corrected as well. Persistent DIP flexion is treated with arthrodesis.

Correction of boutonniere deformity

Boutonniere deformity is less functionally limiting than swan-neck deformity because the patient retains the ability to flex the finger for pinch and grasp. Furthermore, surgical treatment of boutonniere deformity creates the risk of converting a boutonniere deformity into a swan-neck deformity. Because of this, surgery should only be considered for moderate or severe boutonniere deformity that substantially affects hand function.

Stage I boutonniere deformity is mild, with only a slight extension lag at the PIP joint. The PIP joint is passively correctible, and the MCP joint is normal. There is little functional limitation. However, if DIP joint hyperextension is severe, it can be treated with an extensor tenotomy.[60] A longitudinal incision is made over the dorsal aspect of the middle phalanx. Skin flaps are elevated and the extensor mechanism is exposed. An oblique incision is made through the entire extensor mechanism at the level of the middle of the middle phalanx, allowing the DIP joint to flex. Care should be taken not to injure the oblique retinacular ligament. If a mallet deformity occurs, it is treated with a splint or with DIP arthrodesis. Finger motion

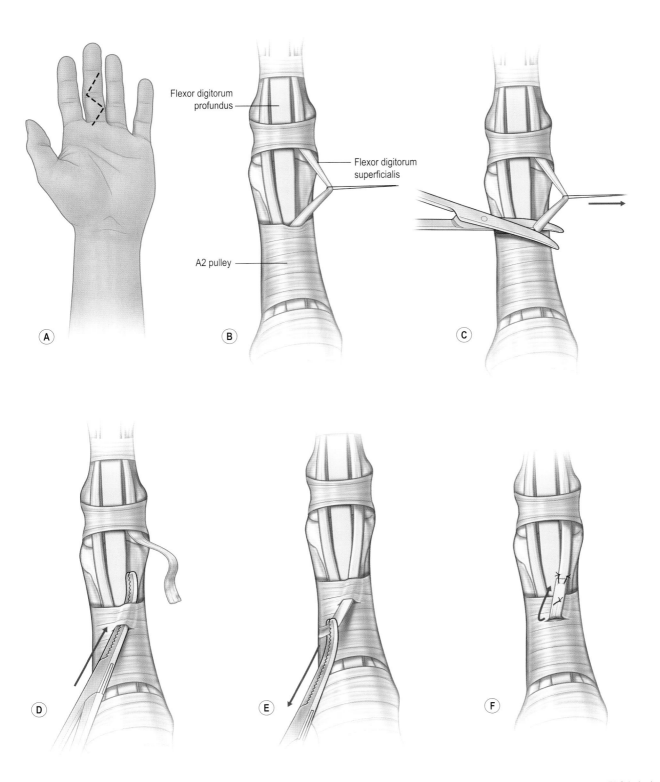

Fig. 19.57 Sublimis sling for correction of swan-neck deformity. A Bruner incision is made: **(A)** exposing the FDS and FDP **(B)**. One slip of FDS is isolated **(C)** and divided proximally **(D).** The FDS slip is then passed through an incision in the A2 pulley **(E,F)** and then sutured back on itself, creating a block to hyperextension of the PIP joint **(G,H).**

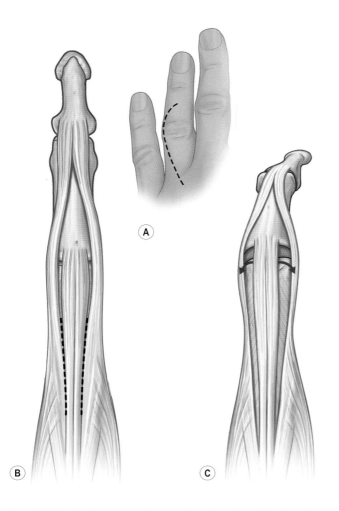

Fig. 19.58 An incision is made between the central slip and the lateral bands, allowing the lateral bands to relocate volarly with PIP joint flexion.

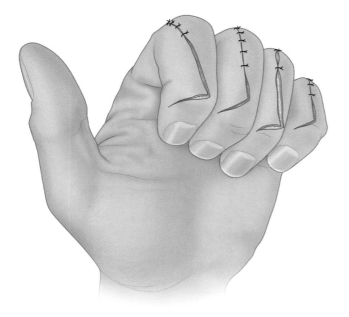

Fig. 19.59 When there is an insufficiency of dorsal skin in cases of long-standing swan-neck deformity, the distal portion of the incision is allowed to gap and heal secondarily.

is allowed immediately postoperatively. A dynamic PIP extension splint is worn for 6 weeks postoperatively.

Stage II boutonniere deformity involves a more severe PIP flexion contracture of 30–40°. MCP hyperextension is present, and DIP hyperextension is more severe. If the PIP joint is not passively correctible, serial casting should be attempted preoperatively. If serial casting fails to restore passive mobility, surgery is required to restore passive motion. Once the joint is supple, the boutonniere deformity can be corrected. A longitudinal incision is made over the PIP joint, and extended distally over the middle phalanx. An extensor tenotomy is performed as described above to allow DIP flexion. At the PIP joint, the goal is to shorten the central slip and correct the volar subluxation of the lateral bands. The central slip is transected 3 mm proximal to its insertion on the base of the middle phalanx, leaving enough for a later repair. A 15-blade is used to separate the central slip from the volarly subluxated lateral bands. A longitudinal incision is then made in the transverse retinacular ligament on each side of the finger, just volar to the lateral band. The lateral bands are then mobilized dorsally, and the PIP joint is brought into extension. The central slip is advanced distally towards the distal remnant at the central slip insertion. Excess central slip is excised, usually measuring about 5 mm in length, and the central slip is sutured to the remnant on the base of the middle phalanx using nonabsorbable sutures. Next, the lateral bands are sutured to the central slip using horizontal mattress sutures *(Fig. 19.60)*. It should be possible to passively flex the PIP joint after tendon reconstruction.

In severe boutonniere deformity, the PIP joint is severely flexed and cannot be passively extended. In many cases, the PIP joint is arthritic or the joint surfaces have remodeled. PIP arthroplasty combined with soft tissue reconstruction can be considered. However, in this situation PIP arthrodesis is probably the most reasonable option.

Postoperative care

The PIP joint is splinted in full extension for 4 weeks, and then finger motion is begun with a wire-foam dynamic extension splint during the day, and a volar PIP extension splint at night for 6 weeks.

Outcomes, prognosis, and complications

Outcomes after correction of swan-neck and boutonniere deformities are variable, and depend largely upon the severity of the original deformity. The most common complications are stiffness, recurrence, and pain. It should be emphasized that boutonniere deformity is in general a less debilitating deformity than swan-neck deformity, and the surgeon should be careful not to convert a boutonniere to a swan-neck by over correction.

Hints and tips: Swan-neck and Boutonniere deformities

- Swan-neck deformities can be more debilitating than boutonniere deformities
- The surgeon should be careful not to overcorrect a boutonniere deformity, thereby creating a swan-neck deformity

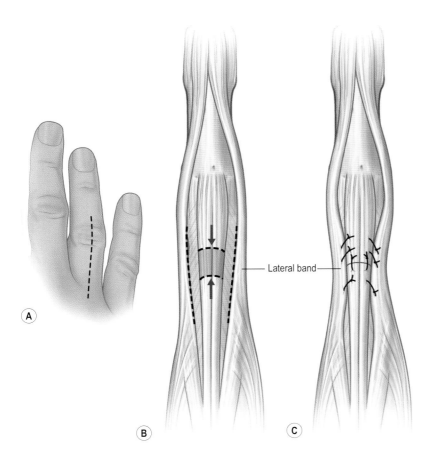

Lateral band

Fig. 19.60 Correction of boutonniere deformity. Excess central slip is excised and closed, and the volarly subluxated lateral bands are mobilized dorsally and sutured to the central slip. Care must be taken not to create a swan-neck deformity.

Correction of thumb deformities

The most common thumb deformity is a boutonniere's deformity (type I thumb deformity), with MCP flexion, IP hyperextension, and CMC abduction *(Fig. 19.61)*. Early in the disease process the joints are passively correctable, and splinting may be adequate treatment. If splinting fails to improve function, reconstruction of the extensor mechanism can be performed. A dorsal incision is made over the MCP joint, and the extensor mechanism is exposed. An incision is made between the EPB and EPL tendons, and tenosynovectomies of the attenuated or ruptured EPB tendon and of the volarly subluxated EPL are performed. A transverse capsulotomy is made, leaving most of the capsule attached distally to the base of the proximal phalanx. MCP joint synovectomy is performed. The EPL tendon is divided between the MCP and IP joints, and is mobilized proximally. This allows the IP joint to move into flexion. A small transverse incision is made in the distal aspect of the MCP joint capsule, just distal to the MCP joint. The MCP joint is then positioned in full extension, and the proximal EPL tendon is passed through the incision in the capsule. It is then turned proximally and sutured to itself under tension. The EPB is advanced and sutured to the base of the proximal phalanx and to the adjacent EPL tendon. The MCP joint is pinned in extension for 6 weeks. Motion at the IP joint is initiated immediately after surgery, but the IP joint is splinted in extension between exercises to prevent development of an extension lag. The MCP K-wire is removed

in 6 weeks, splinting is discontinued, and motion is initiated.

In more severe boutonniere deformities, the MCP and IP joints can become fixed or arthritic. Treatment depends upon the status of these two joints. If the IP joint is fixed in extension but the articular surfaces remain intact, joint release with EPL release is performed. If the IP joint is arthritic, arthrodesis is performed. The fixed or arthritic MCP joint is treated with arthrodesis if motion can be preserved at the IP joint. If IP joint arthrodesis is required, the MCP joint should be treated with silicone arthroplasty and extensor tendon reconstruction.

Swan-neck deformity (type III thumb deformity) is the second most common thumb deformity. Dorsoradial CMC subluxation occurs, and metacarpal adduction contracture develops, followed by MCP hyperextension and IP flexion *(Fig. 19.62)*. Early disease is treated with ligament reconstruction and tendon interposition (LRTI). More advanced disease is also treated with LRTI, but may also require a web-space release and adductor pollicis release. After trapezial resection, a 4-flap Z-plasty is designed in the first web-space. The skin is incised and skin flaps are elevated. If the skin release alone is not sufficient to allow contracture release, dissection is carried down to the adductor pollicis and first dorsal interosseous. The contracted fascial bands of the adductor pollicis and first dorsal interosseous are released. If necessary, the adductor pollicis is released from its origin on the third metacarpal. The LRTI is then completed. Significant MCP hyperextension is treated with MCP arthrodesis.

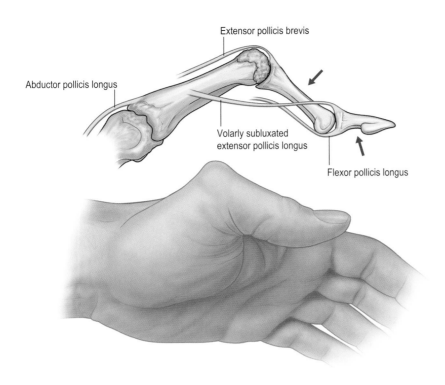

Abductor pollicis longus

Extensor pollicis brevis

Volarly subluxated extensor pollicis longus

Flexor pollicis longus

Fig. 19.61 Boutonniere deformity of the thumb. Synovitis at the MCP joint results in attenuation or rupture of the EPB near its insertion. The EPL is volarly subluxated.

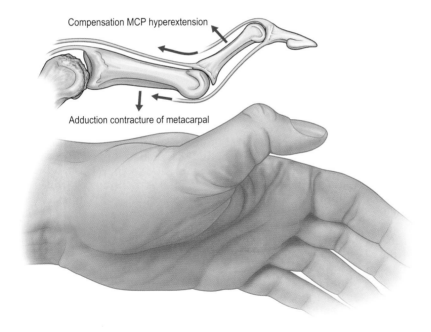

Compensation MCP hyperextension

Adduction contracture of metacarpal

Fig. 19.62 Swan-neck deformity of the thumb. Synovitis and subluxation at the CMC joint results in metacarpal adduction contracture and compensatory hyperextension at the MCP joint.

Treatment for type II and type V thumb deformities is individualized, and depends upon the specific deformity at each joint. Type IV deformity, or gamekeeper's thumb, is treated with MCP arthrodesis.

Postoperative care

A thumb spica splint is used to immobilize the thumb for 4–6 weeks postoperatively. After 4–6 weeks, splinting is weaned and active motion is initiated. Motion is advanced, light activity is allowed, and gentle strengthening is initiated gradually, as tolerated.

Outcomes, prognosis, and complications

As with finger deformities, outcomes are related largely to the severity of the deformity and the degree of arthritis present before surgery.

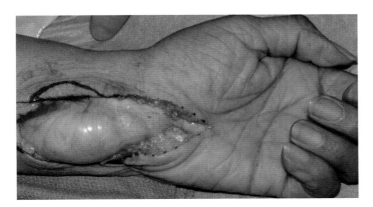

Fig. 19.63 Carpal tunnel release in patients with rheumatoid arthritis usually requires an extensive flexor tenosynovectomy using an extensile exposure.

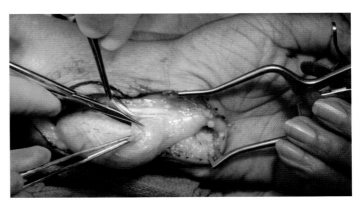

Fig. 19.64 Tenosynovectomy is performed one tendon at a time, while protecting the median nerve.

Tendon surgery and carpal tunnel syndrome

Carpal tunnel syndrome

Carpal tunnel syndrome is common in RA patients and is secondary to the mass-effect of proliferative flexor tenosynovitis within the carpal tunnel. Very mild and intermittent carpal tunnel syndrome can be treated with medical management of the RA, splinting, and steroid injections. However, significant, constant, or progressive symptoms should be treated surgically. Standard carpal tunnel release is generally inadequate. An extended carpal tunnel release with flexor tenosynovectomy is usually required.

A standard carpal tunnel release is performed, and the carpal canal is examined for the presence of synovitis. If synovitis is present, the incision is extended distally to the distal palmar crease in a zig-zag fashion, and proximally across the wrist crease in a zig-zag fashion, continuing at least 5 cm proximally in the forearm. Care is taken to keep the incision ulnar to the palmar cutaneous branch of the median nerve. Distal to the transverse carpal ligament, dissection is performed with tenotomy scissors, elevating skin flaps, while preserving the superficial palmar arch and the branches of the median nerve. Proximally, scissors are used to dissect down to the antebrachial fascia which is divided longitudinally, ulnar to the palmaris longus, exposing the full extent of the tenosynovitis *(Fig. 19.63)*. Next the median nerve is identified proximally, where there is less synovitis, and a vessel loop is passed around it. Next, flexor tenosynovectomies are performed, beginning with the FDS tendons and progressing to the FPL and FDP tendons *(Fig. 19.64)*. Each tendon should be addressed individually, working sequentially, and removing all hypertrophic synovium *(Fig. 19.65)*. The fingers should be flexed by retracting on the flexor tendons, one-by-one, to ensure that excursion is not limited. The median nerve is examined. Hypertrophic synovium is carefully removed from the nerve with tenotomy scissors, preserving the deep motor branch distally, and the palmar cutaneous branch proximally. Finally, the floor of the carpal tunnel is examined. Sharp bony erosions or osteophytes should be removed using a rongeur, and soft tissue or capsule sutured over the smoothed area. The skin is closed with horizontal mattress sutures.

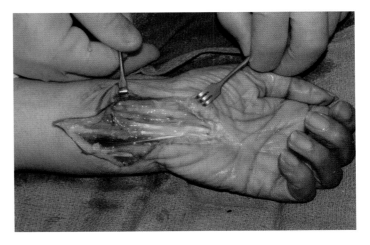

Fig. 19.65 The carpal tunnel is decompressed after tenosynovectomy.

Postoperative care

A volar forearm based wrist splint is applied for 2 weeks. Finger motion is initiated immediately. Full activity without restrictions may resume 5 weeks after surgery.

Outcomes, prognosis, and complications

Carpal tunnel release with flexor tenosynovectomy is effective at relieving carpal tunnel symptoms, particularly in patients who experience symptoms only intermittently, or who have had symptoms for a short period of time. Patients who have constant numbness, particularly if associated with 2-point discrimination changes or thenar atrophy, will have slow or even incomplete relief of symptoms. Complications will be more common with carpal tunnel release in this population, due to the presence of adhesions and synovitis within the carpal canal.

Secondary procedures

Recurrence of carpal tunnel symptoms is minimized by effective medical control of the RA. However, if tenosynovitis recurs and leads to recurrent carpal tunnel symptoms, repeat carpal tunnel release and tenosynovectomy is indicated in order to relieve pressure on the median nerve. Secondary surgery is tedious, and great care must be taken to avoid injury to the median nerve. The incision and initial dissection should begin a few centimeters proximal to the original incision, so that the median nerve can be identified in a tissue plane that has not been previously operated on. Dissection is then carried distally, protecting the median nerve while completing the flexor tenosynovectomy through the distal forearm and carpal tunnel.

Hints and tips: Carpal tunnel release

- Carpal tunnel syndrome may be the initial presenting complaint in RA
- RA patients typically require an extensile incision, with flexor tenosynovectomy
- A standard or limited-incision carpal tunnel release is generally not indicated, and will not treat the underlying pathology.

Flexor tendon ruptures

Flexor tendon ruptures present with an acute loss of finger flexion. However, in a rheumatoid patient with limited motion due to flexor tenosynovitis or joint destruction, a flexor tendon rupture may go unnoticed. A difference between the active and passive finger ROM is suggestive of rupture, but can also be due to flexor tenosynovitis or a rheumatoid trigger finger.

FPL rupture is common, and is due to a sharp bony edge on the volar aspect of the scaphoid (Mannerfelt lesion). The incision for flexor tenolysis is made as described above. Flexor tenolysis is performed. The osteophyte is removed with a rongeur, and the capsule closed over the area to provide a smooth gliding surface *(Fig. 19.66)*. If both ends of the ruptured tendon can be identified within the wrist and palm incision, a small bridge graft of palmaris longus or a strip of the FCR is used. It is weaved proximally and distally into the FPL using a Pulvertaft weave and 3-0 Ethibond horizontal mattress sutures to secure the weave. It is important to resect frayed and damaged tendon edges, and graft into healthy tendon. If grafting within the palm is not possible, tendon transfer is required. A Bruner incision is made on the long finger over the proximal phalanx. The FDS is divided 1.5 cm proximal to its insertion and retracted into the palmar wound. Another Bruner incision is made over the thumb IP joint. Dissection is carried down to the flexor tendon sheath, and the FPL insertion. The sheath is opened near the FPL insertion, and the FPL is retracted and delivered into the distal thumb incision. The FPL is divided transversely with scissors, leaving a 1 cm stump attached to the insertion. The FPL stump is then divided longitudinally in its mid-line along its entire remaining 1 cm length, along its insertion. A small amount of elevation of the central portion of the insertion is performed, but care is taken to keep most of the insertion intact. The volar aspect of the base of the distal phalanx is roughened with a small rongeur to provide a surface for tendon healing. The FDS is delivered through the fibro-osseous canal of the thumb using a pediatric feeding tube. Two suture anchors with 3-0

Ethibond are placed in the base of the distal phalanx, between the split halves of the FPL stump. The FDS is then laid down between the split halves of the FPL and secured to the bone by tying it down to the suture anchors. Next, the two halves of the FPL stump are brought around and volar to the FDS tendon, and sutured to the FDS tendon with horizontal mattress sutures, reinforcing the insertion. Tension should be set so that IP extension occurs with wrist flexion, and full flexion into the palm occurs with wrist extension.

An isolated FDS rupture does not necessarily result in significant functional loss. An end-to-side suture to an adjacent FDS is performed if the rupture occurs within the palm or carpal tunnel, using a Pulvertaft weave. Flexor tenosynovectomy and treatment of any sharp bone edges should be performed. If the FDS rupture occurs within the finger, a tenosynovectomy with resection of the FDS should be performed.

FDP rupture may also not result in severe functional loss, if isolated. Flexor tenolysis, and treatment of any sharp bony edges should be performed. If the rupture occurs within the palm or wrist, an end-to-side suture to an adjacent FDP is performed. If FDP rupture occurs within the finger and the FDS is functional, the FDP is resected. If the DIP joint hyperextends during pinch or grip, DIP arthrodesis is performed.

Rupture of both the FDS and FDP results in significant functional loss. If the ruptures are within the palm or carpal tunnel, end-to-side suturing of the FDP to an adjacent tendon is performed. Alternatively, a bridge graft can be used as described above for the FPL, with the FDS serving as a donor graft. If both tendons have ruptured within the flexor tendon sheath, a staged reconstruction can be considered. However, the outcome of staged flexor tendon reconstruction in patients with RA is often disappointing, and patients should be counseled that recovery of motion will be limited. In patients with arthritis of the IP joints, the best option is arthrodesis of the PIP and DIP joints in a functional position, with preservation of some finger motion at the MCP via the intrinsics.

Postoperative care

If tendon transfers are performed, the hand and fingers are immobilized in such a way as to take tension off of the transfer. The transfer is immobilized for 3–4 weeks, after which motion and retraining are begun under the guidance of a therapist. It should be noted that there is an increasing interest in early movement protocols following tendon transfer surgery, and this may result in improved outcomes or earlier recovery.

Outcomes, prognosis, and complications

Patients have the potential to maintain good finger function after isolated rupture of the FDS or FDP, if their pre-rupture finger function was good and if they receive appropriate treatment in a timely fashion. However, if pre-rupture finger function was limited, outcomes will be poor even if the rupture is treated appropriately. Outcomes after rupture of both the FDS and FDP are poor, regardless of pre-rupture finger function or the method of treatment.

Trigger fingers

Triggering can occur due to the presence of rheumatoid nodules or because of hypertrophic synovium. A very small

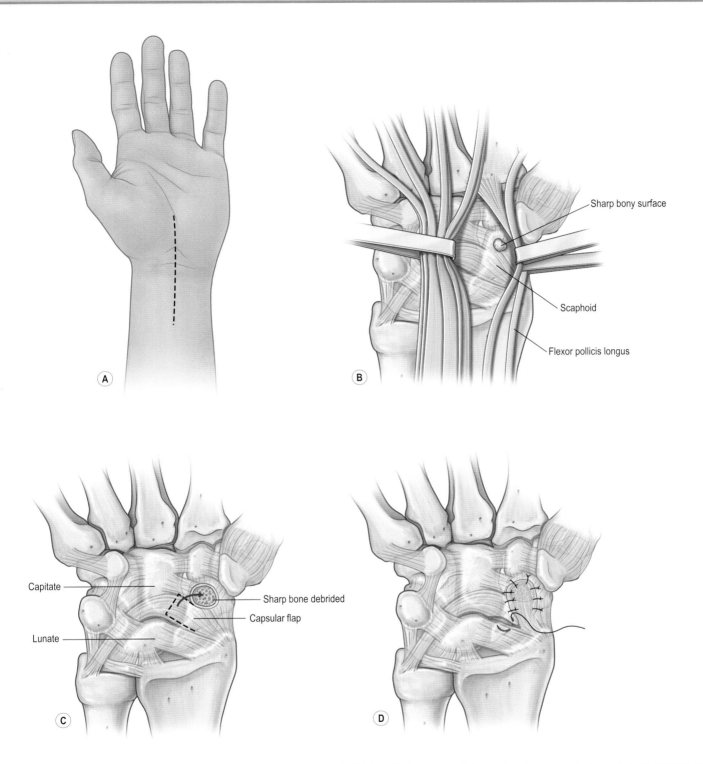

Fig. 19.66 Mannerfelt lesion. The osteophyte on the volar aspect of the scaphoid is identified and removed. Next, a flap of volar capsule is elevated and rotated to cover the rough bony surface.

nodule or synovitis can significantly affect tendon excursion and finger function. Furthermore, the location of the pathology is variable. Although the source of triggering can often be located preoperatively, the surgeon should plan for the possibility of an extensile incision.

The operation is performed under sedation and with local anesthetic, so that the patient can actively flex the finger after tenosynovectomy. A Bruner incision is made over the finger. Initially, the incision is limited to the suspected area of pathology, and can be extended later if necessary. Skin flaps are elevated and the flexor tendon sheath is exposed, preserving the neurovascular bundles. A window is made within the flexor tendon sheath at the level of the cruciate pulley, or at the A1 or A3 pulley nearest the pathology. The flexor tendons

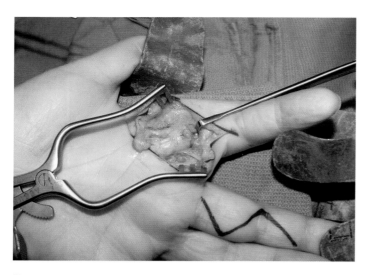

Fig. 19.67 Proliferative synovitis can be seen protruding through rents in the flexor tendon sheath.

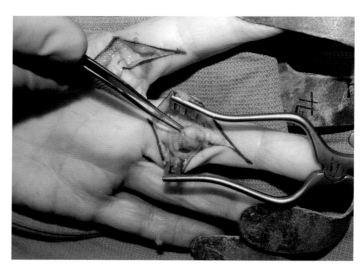

Fig. 19.68 A large piece of synovitis is being removed through a small opening in the flexor tendon sheath just distal to the A2 pulley.

are retracted out of the flexor tendon sheath individually through the window using a Ragnell retractor. Synovium is removed from the flexor tendons using tenotomy scissors or a synovial rongeur, taking care to preserve the vinculae *(Figs 19.67, 19.68)*. If a rheumatoid nodule is encountered, it is excised. If pathology is more extensive, more windows are created within the sheath at the cruciate, A1 or A3 pulleys, allowing full access to the tendons. Rarely, it is necessary to excise the FDS tendon in order to allow FDP excursion. Complete release of the A1 pulley is avoided to lessen the chance of abnormal pull of the flexor tendon that would contribute to ulnar deviation. The patient is awakened and asked to actively flex the finger. If active motion is less than passive motion, or if triggering has not resolved, the surgeon must search for further pathology.

Postoperative care

A light dressing is placed and active and passive motion is begun immediately postoperatively, including tendon gliding exercises.

Outcomes, prognosis, and complications

A good outcome is dependent upon identification and treatment of the cause of the triggering. In order to prevent the complication of persistent postoperative triggering, the surgeon must make sure that he or she has located and addressed all potential sources of triggering by having the patient actively range the finger prior to incision closure.

Extensor tendon ruptures

Extensor tendon ruptures most commonly occur at the wrist. They are due to a combination of erosive tenosynovitis and attritional wear over a sharp spicule of bone at the ulnar side of the wrist, often arising from the ulnar head or DRUJ. Rupture of the EPL is common as well. In addition to treating the rupture, it is critical to address the underlying cause in order to prevent subsequent ruptures.

A dorsal wrist incision is made, skin flaps are elevated, and the retinaculum is incised as described above. A dorsal tenosynovectomy is performed as described above. The ruptured tendon is identified, and soft friable ends are resected with tenotomy scissors until the proximal and distal stumps consist of healthy tendon. The cause of the rupture should be sought, and is usually related to a sharp edge of bone. Care should be taken to smooth down all bony surfaces. In many cases a Darrach procedure is indicated, and can be performed at this time as described above. Next, a retinacular strip is transferred volar to the extensor tendons to cover any remaining exposed areas of bone. Next, the tendon reconstruction is performed. Rarely, the tendon ends can be repaired primarily. In most cases, there is a substantial zone of injury that precludes direct repair.

The reconstruction depends upon the number of tendons ruptured. If the tendon(s) to a single finger is (are) ruptured, the distal stump(s) should be sutured to an adjacent tendon using an end-to-side Pulvertaft weave *(Figs 19.69, 19.70)*. Alternatively, the extensor indicis proprius (EIP) can be transferred in an end-to-end fashion to the ruptured tendon *(Fig. 19.71)*. For the EIP transfer, a longitudinal incision is made over the index MCP joint, extending distally to the middle of the proximal phalanx. Skin flaps are elevated, exposing the extensor mechanism. The interval between the ulnarly located EIP and the radially located EDC is identified and incised longitudinally, separating the two tendons. The sagittal band is carefully elevated off the EIP with a 15-blade, for later repair. The EIP is divided as far distally as possible, and retracted into the dorsal wrist incision. The distal stump of the EIP is sutured to the adjacent EDC, the sagittal band is repaired and the skin is closed. The EIP is then Pulvertaft weaved into the EDC and EDQ of the small finger. It is important to tension the transfer correctly, creating a natural cascade of the fingers. The wrist is passively flexed and extended, checking the tenodesis effect. With the wrist flexed, the MCP joint should easily come into full extension or slight hyperextension. With the wrist extended, it should be possible to passively flex the MCP joint. It is preferable to slightly

Video 2

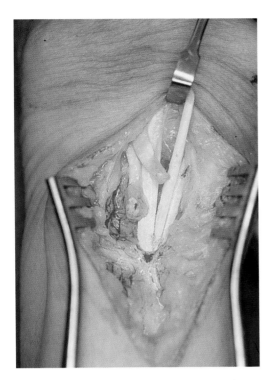

Fig. 19.69 The small finger extensors (EDC and EDQ) have ruptured at the level of the wrist, and their distal ends can be seen just distal to the extensor retinaculum.

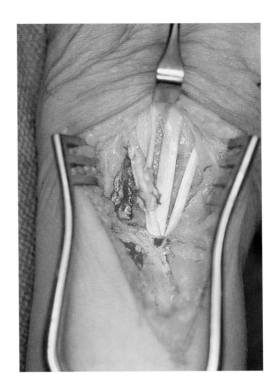

Fig. 19.70 The small finger extensors (EDC and EDQ) have been transferred end-to-side to the ring finger EDC.

over-tighten the transfer, as there will be some loosening with time.

If both the small and ring finger extensor tendons are ruptured, the ring finger EDC is transferred to the long finger EDC in an end-to-side fashion. The small finger extensors, however, will not reach the long finger EDC, and end-to-side transfer usually cannot be performed. Therefore, the EIP tendon is transferred end-to-end to the small finger extensors *(Fig. 19.72)*. The EIP is transferred to both the EDC and EDQ of the small finger, using a Pulvertaft weave. Again, setting tension properly is critical. The natural cascade of the fingers and the tenodesis effect are used as a guide to set the tension.

If three or four of the extensor tendons are ruptured, an FDS transfer is often performed. With three ruptures, the long finger EDC is sutured to the adjacent intact index EDC, and the ring FDS or EIP is used to restore extension of the small and ring fingers *(Fig. 19.73)*. With four ruptures, two FDS transfers are required. The long FDS is used to restore index and long finger extension, and the ring FDS is used to restore ring and small finger extension *(Fig. 19.74)*. For FDS harvest, a Bruner incision is made over the proximal phalanx of the appropriate finger. Skin flaps are elevated, and the flexor tendon sheath exposed. A small opening is made in the flexor tendon sheath, and the FDS is divided 1.5 cm proximal to its insertion. A longitudinal volar incision is made in the distal forearm proximal to the wrist flexion crease, and ulnar to the palmaris longus. Dissection is carried down to the FDS tendons, and the divided FDS is retracted into the wrist incision. The FDS is passed around the radial subcutaneous border of the wrist and delivered into the dorsal wrist incision. The transfer is completed and tensioned as described above.

EPL rupture is not always symptomatic, and may not require treatment. IP extension is usually preserved through the intrinsics, and MCP extension may or may not be lost. If MCP extension is lost and thumb function is affected, the EPL rupture is treated with an EIP to EPL transfer. The EIP is harvested as described above, and is retracted into the wrist incision. It is then passed distally to the dorsal aspect of the thumb, and transferred to the EPL with a Pulvertaft weave at the level of the metacarpal. It should be tensioned so that the MCP joint fully extends with the wrist flexed. With the wrist extended, it should be possible to passively flex the MCP joint.

Postoperative care

For finger extensor tendon transfers, the wrist and MCP joints are splinted in extension for 4 weeks. Active motion and retraining is begun under the supervision of a hand therapist after 4 weeks. Gentle passive flexion can be started at 6 weeks, and strengthening at 8 weeks. Full activity and discontinuation of extension splinting occurs at 12 weeks. The thumb is protected in a thumb spica splint with the MCP and IP joints extended for 4 weeks, after which motion is initiated.

Outcomes, prognosis, and complications

Restoration of MCP extension can be reliably achieved with tendon transfers in patients who have preserved MCP joints. In patients with volarly subluxed and arthritic MCP joints, it is preferable to restore joint alignment and passive mobility by arthroplasty and soft tissue reconstruction prior to performing tendon transfers. Any attempt to restore extension without first addressing MCP deformity or arthritis will result

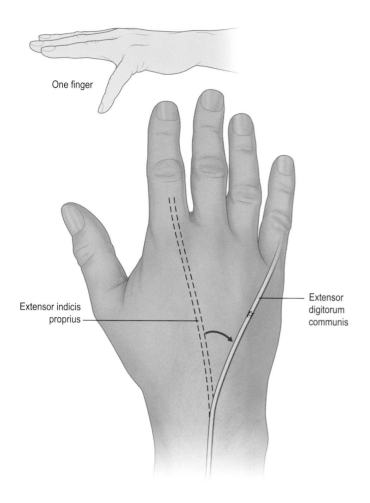

Fig. 19.71 Rupture of the EDC and EDQ to the small finger. The EIP is transferred to the small finger extensors.

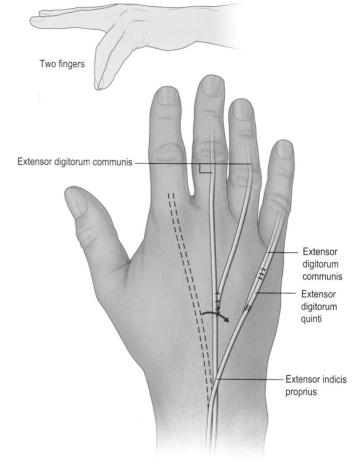

Fig. 19.72 Rupture of the small and ring finger extensors. The ring finger EDC is transferred end-to-side to the long finger EDC. The EIP is transferred end-to-end to the small finger extensors.

in sub-optimal outcomes. Recurrent rupture can occur, and is minimized by correcting the underlying causes, including extensor tenosynovitis, rough bony surfaces, and the caput ulna.

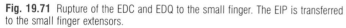

Hints and tips: Extensor tendon ruptures

- Once an extensor tendon rupture occurs, subsequent ruptures can occur in rapid sequence
- Although not an emergency, there is some urgency to treating the underlying cause
- The surgeon should be careful to treat the underlying cause of the rupture when performing tendon transfers for extensor tendon rupture
- The surgeon should have a low threshold for performing a distal ulna resection if there is concern that distal ulna or DRUJ pathology caused the ruptures.

Other rheumatologic disorders of the hand and wrist

Seronegative spondyloarthropathies

Seronegative spondyloarthropathies include Reiter's syndrome, psoriatic arthritis, ankylosing spondylitis, and inflammatory bowel disease associated arthritis. The most common seronegative spondyloarthropathy to affect the hands is psoriatic arthritis. Patients are usually RF negative, have an inflammatory arthritis, and have psoriasis (*Table 19.1*). Psoriasis affects 2% of the population and onset usually occurs in the 2nd decade of life.[61] Among patients with psoriasis, the prevalence of psoriatic arthritis is unknown, but ranges from approximately 5% to 40%.

Radiographic findings are diverse, and may include erosions and resorption, osteolysis, periostitis, ankylosis (often at the PIP joint), or juxta-articular bone formation. Radiographs may reveal a "pencil-in-cup" deformity at the DIP joint, which is the result of new marginal bone formation at the base of the

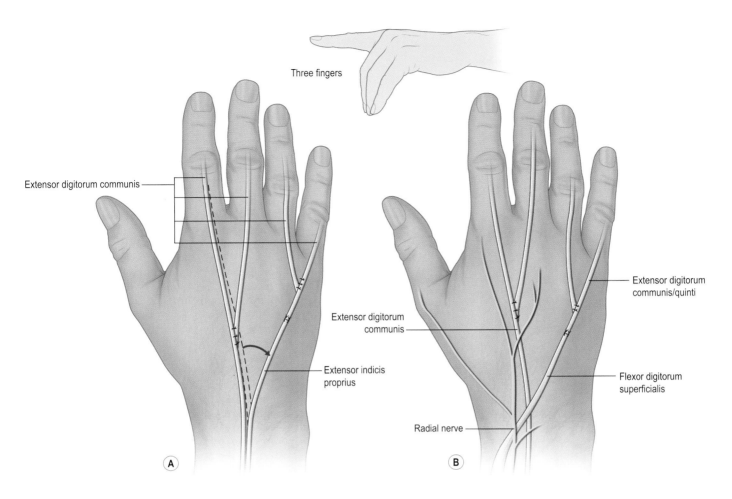

Fig. 19.73 Rupture of the long, ring, and small finger extensors. The EDC of the long finger is transferred end-to-side to the EDC of the index finger. The EIP **(A)** or the FDS **(B)** can be transferred to the small and ring finger extensors.

Table 19.1 **Characteristics of other rheumatologic conditions of the hand**

	Serology	Radiographs	Examination
Psoriatic arthritis	Negative	Erosions Resorption Osteolysis Periostitis Ankylosis (PIP) Juxta-articular bone formation Pencil-in-cup (DIP)	Psoriasis Nail abnormalities Dactylitis PIP flexion contracture Opera glass hand swan-neck deformity
SLE	ANA Anti-DNA, Antiphospholipid antibody Leucopenia Hemolytic anemia Thrombocytopenia	Preservation of joints Secondary OA	Deformity similar to that seen in RA Malar rash Discoid rash Serositis Other
Scleroderma	ANA Anti-centromere Anti-topoisomerase I Anti-RNA polymerase	Tuft resorption, Secondary OA	Cutaneous telangiectasia Raynaud's Cutaneous sclerosis Ischemic ulceration Joint contracture due to skin contracture
Gout	Hyperuricemia Negatively birefringent crystals (synovial analysis)	Sclerotic joint margins Overhanging edges Erosion from tophi (late) Joint destruction (late)	Red, hot, swollen joint MTP of great toe involvement Tophi

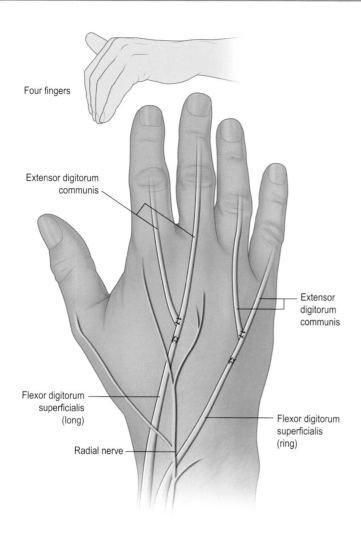

Four fingers

Extensor digitorum communis

Extensor digitorum communis

Flexor digitorum superficialis (long)

Radial nerve

Flexor digitorum superficialis (ring)

Fig. 19.74 Rupture of the extensor tendons to all four fingers. The long finger FDS is transferred to the index and long finger extensors, and the ring finger FDS is transferred to the ring and small finger extensors.

distal phalanx, combined with osteolysis of the head of the middle phalanx.

Joint involvement can be symmetric or asymmetric, and may be oligoarticular or polyarticular. The small joints of the hands and feet are most commonly affected, and DIP involvement is often a prominent feature of psoriatic arthritis. Although tenosynovitis and tendon ruptures are rare, inflammation at tendon insertions may occur. Another occasional finding is dactylitis, which involves swelling and inflammation of an entire digit. The nails also develop abnormalities. Pitting is the classic finding, although onycholysis, nail dystrophy, leukonychia, and hyperkeratosis can occur as well. The most common finger deformity is a PIP flexion contracture, with compensatory MCP hyperextension. This is not a true boutonniere deformity. Swan-neck deformities can occur secondary to a mallet finger. In the thumb, a boutonniere deformity can occur, and the CMC joint can become arthritic as well. Wrist arthritis and DRUJ arthritis can occur as well. Rarely, severe osteolysis, or arthritis mutilans, results in collapse of the fingers known as the "opera glass hand."

Swan-neck deformity is treated in a similar fashion to swan-neck deformity associated with RA. Severe fixed PIP flexion contractures are treated with arthrodesis. MCP extension contractures with associated joint destruction are treated with silicone arthroplasty. Arthritis mutilans is treated with arthrodesis, often requiring bone graft. Wrist involvement is treated with limited intercarpal fusions or complete wrist arthrodesis, depending upon the pattern of joint involvement. A Darrach procedure may be indicated for DRUJ arthritis.

Systemic lupus erythematosus

Systemic lupus erythematosus (SLE) is a systemic autoimmune disease, in which tissue damage is caused by autoantibodies and immune complexes. It affects five in 10 000 people in the United States, and women are affected much more frequently than men (9:1). African Americans and Latinos are affected more often than Caucasians, and tend to have a more severe disease process. Susceptibility is related to multiple genes. Many potential environmental triggers have been implicated, including Epstein–Barr virus (EBV) infection, multiple medications, dietary factors and bacteria.

The diagnosis of SLE is primarily clinical, and is supported by positive laboratory findings. Extra-articular manifestations are diverse and may include malar rash, discoid rash, photosensitivity, cardiovascular disease, oral ulcers, arthritis, serositis, proteinuria, seizures, psychosis, leukopenia, hemolytic anemia, thrombocytopenia, and many others. Seropositivity for antinuclear antibody (ANA) is very sensitive (95%), although there are cases of ANA-negative lupus. However, specificity is low and ANA may be positive in multiple rheumatologic diseases. Other supportive laboratory findings include anti-DNA, anti-Sm nuclear antigen, and antiphospholipid antibodies.

The IP joints, MCP joints, and wrist are commonly involved, and may be the initial presenting symptoms of the disease. Patients experience swelling, pain, effusion and morning stiffness. The arthritis associated with SLE is not erosive, and may not be deforming. If finger deformities do occur, they are very similar to those seen in rheumatoid arthritis. Volar subluxation and ulnar deviation occurs at the MCP joints, and swan-neck or boutonniere deformities may occur, but with an absence of destructive joint changes. In addition, tenosynovitis may occur, and may result in tendon ruptures. Synovitis within the carpal tunnel may lead to carpal tunnel syndrome. In addition, patients may develop subcutaneous nodules along the flexor tendons, histologically similar to those that develop in rheumatoid arthritis.

In many cases, the finger and wrist deformities that occur with SLE are passively correctable. In these cases splinting can be quite helpful. Intrinsic stretching can also be helpful to decrease MCP flexion and ulnar deviation. Because of poor soft tissue quality, soft tissue procedures alone are rarely successful, and the mainstays of surgery in the fingers are arthrodesis and arthroplasty, which can be combined with soft tissue procedures. Partial wrist arthrodesis or total wrist arthrodesis may be beneficial, depending upon the deformity and instability pattern. The Darrach procedure is often indicated for dorsal subluxation of the ulna, which can often cause attrition ruptures. Because of the many organ systems involved, patients must have a thorough medical workup and preoperative clearance.

Scleroderma

Scleroderma, or systemic sclerosis, is a disease of the connective tissue and small blood vessels that affects multiple tissues. It is rarer than either rheumatoid arthritis or SLE, with a prevalence of <300 per 1 million in the United States. Like most rheumatologic disorders it is more common in women than men, and onset typically occurs in the 3rd or 4th decade of life. The disease is idiopathic, but there is a genetic component and an environmental trigger is likely required to initiate the disease. Systemic sclerosis can present as limited cutaneous disease (often involving the fingers or hands), diffuse cutaneous disease, or CREST syndrome (calcinosis, Raynaud's phenomenon, esophageal involvement, sclerodactyly, and telangiectasias). Systemic sclerosis can affect the lungs, resulting in interstitial disease and pulmonary fibrosis. Cardiac, vascular, renal, gastrointestinal and other organ systems are also commonly involved. The diagnosis is clinical, and is supported by antibody testing. Nail fold capillary microscopy is also helpful. ANA, anti-centromere, anti-topoisomerase I, anti-RNA polymerase antibodies are all associated with systemic sclerosis.

Raynaud's phenomenon affects almost all patients, and is present in limited cutaneous, diffuse cutaneous, and CREST forms of the disease. Critical ischemia, however, occurs due to vascular disease related to the systemic sclerosis, and is not due to Raynaud's phenomenon. Occlusive vascular changes affect the medium sized vessels, and the ulnar artery in particular. Ischemic ulceration may occur in the fingertips, on the extensor surface over flexed joints, and in areas of calcinosis. Ischemia related resorption of the tufts can occur, and is termed acro-osteolysis. Cutaneous telangiectasia may be seen on the palm. Treatment of the vascular manifestations of the disease are outside the scope of this chapter.

Finger deformities are related to skin contracture, and to fibrosis and contracture of joint ligaments and capsule. Arthritis and joint destruction do not occur directly. If joint changes or arthritis are seen, they are usually osteoarthritic changes that occur secondary to prolonged deformity and abnormal motion. The most common deformity in the hand is PIP flexion contracture. These contractures can be severe, and dorsal skin ulceration can occur with tendon or joint exposure. MCP hyperextension occurs secondarily, and can become fixed as well. In addition, the first web space contracture is common. Soft tissue loss over joints should be treated conservatively, with Silvadene dressing changes and minimal debridement. Ultimately, bony debridement or amputation may be required. At times, skin breakdown occurs over an area of calcinosis. Removal with a curette and irrigation with saline is performed. For severe PIP contractures with intact overlying skin, arthrodesis may be indicated. Care should be taken when managing the skin, and minimal skin flap elevation should be performed. In addition, significant bony resection should be performed, in order to take tension off the overlying skin. A compression screw or removable K-wires should be used in order to avoid subcutaneous hardware. Dressings should be light, and noncompressive. Patients should be cautioned about the possibility of wound healing problems, potentially resulting in the need for amputation. At the MCP joint resection arthroplasty is indicated for severe fixed extension contracture. A volar longitudinal incision is made directly over the metacarpal head. Dissection is carried down to the flexor tendon sheath, retracting the neurovascular bundles radially and ulnarly. The A1 pulley is incised, and the flexor tendons retracted. A 15-blade is used to create a volar arthrotomy through the volar plate and joint capsule. Subperiosteal dissection is then performed, exposing the head and neck of the metacarpal. A sagittal saw is then used to resect the metacarpal head. Bony resection is performed until MCP flexion is possible. The skin is closed and the patient is splinted with the MCPs flexed. Motion is allowed as soon as skin healing has occurred. First web-space contracture is difficult to treat. Because of the stiff nature of the skin, Z-plasties are rarely successful, and the contracture must be treated more like a severe burn contracture. A long transverse incision is made in the first web space. Dissection is carried down to the adductor pollicis and first dorsal interosseous. Tight fascial bands are released with tenotomy scissors until the thumb can be abducted. If thumb CMC arthritis or CMC subluxation contributes to the adduction deformity, trapeziectomy can be performed through a separate incision. A full thickness skin graft is used to close the defect, and should be harvested from an area with minimal skin involvement.

Postoperative care

The thumb should be pinned in abduction for 6 weeks, followed by motion and intermittent splinting.

Crystalline arthropathy

Gout is characterized by recurrent bouts of acute arthritis, eventually progressing to chronic arthritis. It affects approximately 1% of the population, and is more common in men.[62,63] Risk factors include obesity, alcohol use, hypertension, renal disease, and certain medications like hydrochlorothiazide and cyclosporine. Triggers for an acute gout attack include physiologic stress, fever, surgery, dehydration, and alcohol use. In addition, foods that are high in purine increase the risk of a gout attack, including oatmeal, mushrooms, lentils and spinach.[64]

Gout begins with asymptomatic hyperuricemia, and then progresses to intermittent episodes of acute gout attacks. Initially gout attacks are monoarticular, and involvement of the MTP joint of the great toe is classic. The involved joint becomes swollen, red, and exquisitely painful. Initially radiographs may be negative. The acute attack may last from hours to many days. As gout progresses, it can become polyarticular, and systemic symptoms such as fever, chills, or sweats may be present. Hand and wrist involvement is common. Eventually chronic arthritis and tophi develop, with continued episodic acute attacks. In chronic gout radiographic findings include erosions with sclerotic margins, and overhanging edges of bone. Definitive diagnosis is made by arthrocentesis and identification of crystals with negative birefringence under polarized light microscopy.

Treatment is primarily medical and is guided by the rheumatologist. For an acute attack colchicine, indomethacin, or corticosteroids are often used. An intra-articular steroid injection is quite effective, and can rapidly relieve symptoms. It is particularly useful in elderly patients in whom colchicine should be avoided. Prophylaxis is provided by daily low-dose colchicine or indomethacin. In addition, xanthine oxidase inhibitors such as allopurinol, or uricosuric agents such as probenecid can be used to reduce serum uric acid levels. Chronic gouty arthritis is treated with selective arthrodesis of joints that are painful, or that have deformity that is affecting function. Large painful tophi, or tophi that are interfering with function can be excised.

Summary

Multiple diverse rheumatologic disorders exist, many of which commonly affect the hand and wrist. Although the medical management of rheumatologic diseases has dramatically improved, there are still many patients with recalcitrant pain and loss of function who may benefit from hand surgery. In most cases, arthritic pain can be effectively treated with arthrodesis or arthroplasty. Restoration of function is less reliably achieved, but is an important secondary goal. It is important for the patient to undergo a thorough medical and anesthesia workup prior to any surgery because of the many systemic manifestations associated with rheumatologic disorders.

Access the complete references list online at **http://www.expertconsult.com**

20. Bongartz T, Sutton AJ, Sweeting MJ, et al. Anti-TNF antibody therapy in rheumatoid arthritis and the risk of serious infections and malignancies: systematic review and meta-analysis of rare harmful effects in randomized controlled trials. *JAMA.* 2006;295(19):2275–2285.

24. Bongartz T. Elective orthopedic surgery and perioperative DMARD management: many questions, fewer answers, and some opinions. *J Rheumatol.* 2007;34(4):653–655.

    An excellent review of the current state of the evidence regarding perioperative DMARD management. An evidence-based, practical and conservative approach is recommended by the authors.

39. Linscheid RL, Dobyns JH. Rheumatoid arthritis of the wrist. *Orthop Clin North Am.* 1971;2(3):649–665.

41. Flury MP, Herren DB, Simmen BR. Rheumatoid arthritis of the wrist. Classification related to the natural course. *Clin Orthop Relat Res.* 1999; (366):72–77.

    The authors present a classification system for the rheumatoid wrist that is now commonly used and frequently referenced. This classification system uses radiologic indicators to divide wrists into those that are stable (types I and II) and those that are unstable (type III).

43. Mannerfelt L, Norman O. Attrition ruptures of flexor tendons in rheumatoid arthritis caused by bony spurs in the carpal tunnel. A clinical and radiological study. *J Bone Joint Surg Br.* 1969;51(2):270–277.

44. Flatt AE. Some pathomechanics of ulnar drift. *Plast Reconstr Surg.* 1966;37(4):295–303.

49. Flatt AE. *The care of the rheumatoid hand.* St. Louis: Mosby; 1974.

    An excellent historical overview of surgical treatments for the rheumatoid hand, as well as descriptions of the mechanics of the disease process.

50. Shapiro JS, Heijna W, Nasatir S, et al. The relationship of wrist motion to ulnar phalangeal drift in the rheumatoid patient. *Hand.* 1971;3(1):68–75.

51. Nalebuff EA. Surgical treatment of tendon rupture in the rheumatoid hand. *Surg Clin North Am.* 1969;49(4):811–822.

    A detailed description of the surgical management of tendon ruptures by a hand surgeon with extensive experience in treating patients with rheumatoid arthritis.

55. Urban MK. Anaesthesia for orthopedic surgery. In: Miller RD, Eriksson LI, Fleisher LA, et al, eds. *Miller's anesthesia.* Philadelphia: Churchill Livingstone; 2009.

20

Osteoarthritis in the hand and wrist

Brian T. Carlsen, Karim Bakri, Faisal M. Al-Mufarrej, and Steven L. Moran

 Access the Historical Perspective section online at
http://www.expertconsult.com

SYNOPSIS

- Osteoarthritis is characterized by a loss of articular cartilage.
- The development of osteoarthritis is a dynamic process that represents an imbalance between destruction and repair of the articular cartilage. It can resulft from trauma, such as an intra-articular fracture or a ligamentous injury that results in abnormal load-bearing characteristics or it can be idiopathic without an identifiable cause.
- Osteoarthritis can affect the entire joint, including the articular cartilage, subchondral bone, ligaments, joint capsule, synovial membrane, and periarticular muscles and tendons.
- Patients with osteoarthritis seek treatment because of pain, loss of function, or both. However, there is often a poor correlation between the patient's symptoms and radiographic findings.
- Osteoarthritis is more common in women. In the hand, the DIP joints of the fingers and the CMC joint of the thumb are most commonly affected followed in order by the finger PIP and MP joints.
- Radiocarpal arthritis is most commonly a result of traumatic injury and follows a regular progression over time as seen in SLAC and SNAC wrist arthritis patterns.
- Treatment of arthritis is directed toward alleviating pain and improving function.
- Treatment strategies include operative and nonoperative treatments. Nonoperative treatments include lifestyle modification, hot and cold therapy, splinting, oral or topical anti-inflammatory agents (NSAIDs), and alternative therapies (diet modification, ultrasound, TENS, and acupuncture)
- Surgical management of osteoarthritis includes load altering procedures, joint debridement and/or synovectomy, arthrodesis, and arthroplasty procedures.
- The appropriate type of operation varies depending on multiple factors including patient age, demands placed on the joint, the requirement for motion to perform one's activities of daily living or job requirements, patient desires, and the likelihood of success of restoring function and alleviating pain.

Introduction/epidemiology

- Osteoarthritis (OA) is a heterogeneous disease that includes conditions with different etiology, distribution, heredity, clinical presentation, and progression.
- It is characterized by mechanical and biological events that alter the homeostatic relationship of degradation and repair of the surrounding articular tissues.
- Although all joint tissues are involved, including the subchondral bone, it is damage to the articular cartilage that is the hallmark of the disease.
- Osteoarthritis is the most common rheumatologic disorder in the world. It affects all races, sexes and age groups.
- It is a major cause of adult morbidity. It is the cause of disability in 10% of the population over age 60.[1]
- In a study from Rotterdam, OA was found in 87% of persons age 55–65.[2]
- It is estimated that 21% of the population or 46.4 million Americans in 2005 were affected by osteoarthritis.[3]
- Symptoms of OA may include joint pain, swelling, tenderness, stiffness, and crepitus. OA is typically considered a noninflammatory condition to differentiate it from the inflammatory arthropathies such as rheumatoid and psoriatic arthritis.
- There is no cure for osteoarthritis and no effective method of altering the progression of the disease process.

This chapter will review the presentation, evaluation, and treatments of osteoarthritis as it presents in the various joints of the hand and wrist. Both nonoperative and operative approaches will be discussed, with particular attention to the indications and contraindications of specific treatments.

Basic science/disease process

Osteoarthritis (OA) is characterized by a loss of articular cartilage. It can be either primary or secondary in nature. *Primary OA* (idiopathic OA) occurs in the absence of antecedent trauma. The pathogenesis is likely heterogeneous; genetics, joint shape and underlying endocrine abnormalities can contribute. *Secondary OA* is the result of direct trauma to the joint and can occur as a result of fracture, dislocation or infection.

In order to understand the pathophysiology of osteoarthritis, one must first consider the normal anatomy and biochemistry of the synovial joint. Normal articular cartilage consists of an extensive extracellular matrix composed primarily of proteoglycans, collagens (predominantly type II), and water. While chondrocytes compose only 1% of the volume of the cartilage ECM, they are responsible for maintaining its architecture and composition. The matrix composed primarily of collagen, proteoglycans, proteins and glycoproteins. Cartilage proteoglycans belong to two major classes: large aggregating molecules (aggrecans), and smaller nonaggregating molecules. The aggrecan molecule consists of a central protein core with about 100 glycosaminoglycan (GAG) side branches composed of repeating, negatively-charged disaccharides. Aggrecan molecules form proteoglycan aggregates by linking with a long central hyaluronan molecule. The result is a very large molecule with 10^5 negatively-charged groups. These groups fill voids in the cartilage framework and create a high osmotic pressure in the framework, providing a stiff construct resistant to compression. Nonaggregating proteoglycans and other matrix proteins serve a variety of functions in the matrix including framework stabilization, regulation of fibrillogenesis, and matrix metabolism through chondrocyte interactions.[6] Such molecules include biglycan, decorin, fibromodulin, chondroadherin, cartilage oligomatrix protein, and fibronectin. The interstitial fluid provides an important function in terms of altering the cartilage friction coefficient with changes in pressure (load).[7]

Microscopically, articular cartilage can be divided into four zones based on the cartilage matrix composition and architecture.[8] Zone 1 is the most superficial zone and is called the superficial or tangential zone. Here, the chondrocytes are flat and oriented parallel to the articular surface. The collagen is condensed and proteoglycans are sparse. The thin collagen fibers are arranged parallel to the articular surface. This construct resists shear force and has been compared to a "tough skin" that protects the underlying intermediate and deep zones.[9] In zone 2, the intermediate zone, the chondrocytes are isolated or in isogenous groups and are surrounded by oblique collagen fibers. This zone is the thickest and is rich in proteoglycans. Proteoglycans are complex macromolecules composed of a protein core with attached glycosaminoglycan chains (chondroitin sulfate and keratan sulfate). The negative charge of the glycosaminoglycans accounts for the hydration and large swelling pressure of cartilage.[10] Zone 3 is the radiate layer and includes large, round chondrocytes oriented vertically with intervening radial collagen fibers. Zone 4 is the deepest layer or calcified layer. It lies adjacent to the subchondral bone and resists shear stress between cartilage and bone.[9] Between zone 3 and zone 4 is the *tidemark (**Fig. 20.1**)*. With age, articular cartilage becomes thin and there is relative

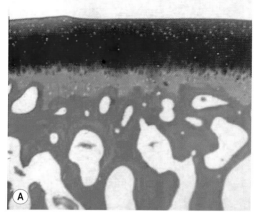

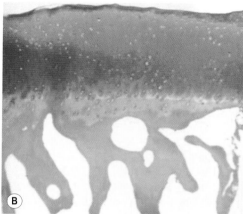

Fig. 20.1 Histological section of **(A)** normal and **(B)** abnormal cartilage. In the **(A)** normal joint articular cartilage is connected to the bone through a layer of calcified cartilage. The basophile line, or blue line, histologically separates the articular cartilage from calcified cartilage. The calcified cartilage receives nutrients through the epiphyseal vessel; the articular cartilage receives nutrients primarily through diffusion from the overlying joint fluid. **(B)** In joints affected by OA there is fraying in the superficial cartilage and decrease in articular cartilage thickness.

advancement of the tidemark zone that occurs together with replacement of calcified cartilage with bone.[11] The result of this anatomic design is a shiny and slippery surface with a friction coefficient lower than any prosthetic replacement. This remarkable construct is able to withstand millions of loading cycles each year with forces that may reach up to 18 MPa.[12]

In the healthy, homeostatic state, the chondrocyte responds to the mechanical and biochemical environment by altering the synthesis and degradation its macromolecules. Two groups of enzymes function to degrade the extracellular matrix: matrix metalloproteinases (MMPs) and *a d*isintegrin *a*nd *m*etalloproteinase with *t*hrombospondin-like motifs (ADAMTS). MMPs break down collagen and[13] ADAMTS functions to break down aggrecan. The main MMP in cartilage is MMP-13 that breaks down type II collagen and the main ADAMTS in cartilage are ADAMTS-4 and ADAMTS-5.[14,15] The regulation of matrix degradation and synthesis is poorly understood, but cytokines play an important role in both anabolic and catabolic pathways.[8,16,17] The interplay between these cytokines is complex. Anabolic activity seems to be a response of the structural needs of the matrix, as may occur in response to mechanical loading. Cytokines involved in the anabolic pathway include transforming growth factor-beta (TGF-β) and insulin-dependent growth factor I.[8] Catabolism within the matrix involves a complex cascade that includes interleukin-1, stromelysin, aggrecanase, and plasmin, in response to stimulation or inhibition by TGF-β, tumor necrosis factor, tissue inhibitors of metalloproteinases, tissue plasminogen activator, plasminogen activator inhibitor, and other molecules.[8]

Pathophysiology

Osteoarthritis involves all of the tissues around the synovial joint, including the articular cartilage, joint capsule, ligaments, subchondral bone, metaphyseal bone, and the muscles acting across the joint. However, the principle pathological change is that of loss of articular cartilage. Other changes are noted such as subchondral sclerosis, subchondral cyst formation and marginal osteophytes.[8,18,19]

The earliest microscopic findings of OA are that of fibrillation and fraying of the superficial zone cartilage along with decreased staining for proteoglycans in the superficial and transitional zones and in-growth of blood vessels into the tidemark from subchondral bone *(Fig. 20.1B)*.[8] Progression of the disease leads to clefts in the articular surface, fracture of the superficial cartilage and decrease in cartilage thickness. Enzyme activation leads to further destruction of the cartilage leading to complete loss of articular cartilage exposing dense, and eburnated bone.[8]

Associated with these changes of the cartilage, are alterations in the subchondral bone, specifically an increased density. This increased density can be seen as a sclerotic line on radiograph. These changes may be more pronounced at the joint periphery where the new bone formation may be so exuberant as to produce osteophytes. The exact pathophysiology of osteophyte formation is not known, however it may be related to the release of anabolic cytokines from the matrix that stimulate the abnormal bone and cartilage growth.[20,21]

The changes involving the joint also affect the periarticular tissues. The synovial membrane becomes inflamed as fragments of cartilage become embedded within them.[22] As the joint loses motion due to mechanical factors and pain, the capsule and surrounding ligaments become stiff due to myotendinous contraction and ongoing edema. The lack of motion and use can lead to muscle atrophy.[8]

Diagnosis

The most common symptoms of OA are pain, swelling and stiffness of the affected joint. Pain is the primary feature of the condition and is the focus of treatment. Examination confirms swelling, tenderness, and limited range of motion. In the case of post-traumatic arthritis, there may be joint instability associated with previous ligamentous injury.

Symptoms can dissipate with time and are not always correlated with the radiographic severity of disease. Osteoarthritis may also be present in the absence of pain. In a classic study

looking at arthritis among miners in their 40s, Kellgren and Lawrence found that only 24% of miners with radiographic OA had pain and 8% of radiographically normal knees had pain.

Radiographs are the most helpful test in making the diagnosis. In primary and secondary OA, joint spaces are narrowed radiographically due to a loss of radiolucent articular cartilage. Subchondral bone remodeling can manifest as increased density within the subchondral bone or sclerosis. Osteophytes and loose bodies may also be present *(Fig. 20.2)*.

In 1957, Kellgren and Lawrence described a grading system for the radiographic appearance of OA.[23] Findings considered included: (1) the presence of peripheral osteophytes; (2) periarticular ossicles (commonly found in association with DIP and PIP joints); (3) narrowing of joint cartilage and subchondral sclerosis; (4) small pseudocystic areas with sclerotic walls, typically in the subchondral bone, and (5) altered shape of the bone ends. The authors then classified the arthritis into five grades:[23]

1. Normal joint
2. Doubtful
3. Minimal (but definitely present)
4. Moderate
5. Severe.

This system has been broadly applied for grading osteoarthritis in various joints; unfortunately the grading system can be ambiguous as there are no specific cut-off criteria between

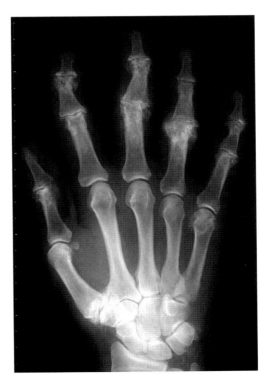

Fig. 20.2 PA radiograph of the hand of a 69-year-old male showing typical bony changes seen in advanced OA. Osteophyte formation is seen at the DIP and PIP joints and TMC joint of the thumb. Joint narrowing is seen within the fingers as well as evidence of subchondral sclerosis.

the grades. In a recent analysis by Schiphof and colleagues, the authors note inconsistency in the application of the grading system within multiple cohort studies and have recommended the development of a single validated classification system.[24]

Management of OA of the fingers

Hand and finger arthritis is one of the most common presentations of primary OA. Its onset is insidious with progressive aesthetic deformity followed by pain and functional limitation. Epidemiological studies of the joint-specific prevalence of hand arthritis consistently show the distal interphalangeal joint to be the site most frequently affected by OA, followed by the thumb CMC joint, and the PIP joint.[25] These studies typically defined OA based on the radiographic features described by Kellgren and Lawrence, which include the presence of osteophytes, joint space narrowing, subchondral sclerosis and subchondral cysts.[23]

Distal interphalangeal joint (DIP) arthritis

Diagnosis

Osteoarthritis of the distal phalangeal (DIP) joint is common and affects females more frequently than males. Clinically, patients present with enlarged joints and hard, knobby protuberances overlying the DIP joints of multiple fingers. These, so called, *Heberden's nodes* are pathognomonic for the condition and are attributed to osteophyte formation with overlying soft tissue thickening. These should be differentiated from a *mucous cyst*. A mucous cyst is a dorsal synovial cyst, often limited to a single digit. They are often associated with lateral deviation of the distal phalanx, and a limited range of motion *(Fig. 20.3)*.

Radiographically, joint space narrowing and osteophyte formation are common findings. However, the radiographic appearance of the DIP is not consistently associated with the patient's symptoms. Frequently, the only significant concern for the patient is the aesthetic appearance. Even patients with severe DIP deformity may have little pain or functional impairment and the presence of Heberden's nodes alone is not generally considered an indication for surgery.

Indications for surgery

The treatment of DIP OA is dictated by the severity of pain and functional limitation. Splinting allows the joint to be rested and protected from minor trauma. Splinting used in conjunction with oral or topical anti-inflammatory medication and lifestyle modification, are the mainstays of nonoperative treatment. This approach is usually sufficient to treat acute exacerbations of pain and swelling. Steroid injections can be attempted for temporary pain relief but are difficult to administer in such a small joint and multiple repeated injections are not a convenient as a long-term treatment plan. When intractable pain, deformity and misalignment are severe enough to interfere with precision pinch, oppositional pinch and global hand function, surgery is indicated.

The surgical options for treatment of severe DIP arthritis are essentially limited to arthrodesis, which is well tolerated in the DIP position. Although implant arthroplasty is technically feasible, it is not commonly performed because of concerns of long-term joint instability[26–30]

Biomechanical effects of DIP fusion

The normal range of motion at the DIP joint is 0–60°; however only 15% of digital flexion occurs at the DIP and the joint only contributes 3% of the overall flexion arc of the whole finger.[31] Thus of all finger joint fusions, DIP arthrodesis confers the least detrimental impact to hand motion, and is the well tolerated. One study of splint-simulated DIP fusion found a 20% reduction in grip strength which was attributed to the *quadriga effect*, as a result of the limited excursion of the FDP tendon in the fused digit.[32] Significant loss of grip strength has not been shown in clinical studies.

DIP arthrodesis

Indications

The single most common indication for arthrodesis is intractable pain at the DIP joint that has failed all conservative treatments. Other less common indications include chronic mallet deformity, missed flexor tendon avulsions or distal phalanx nonunions.

Techniques

A multitude of fixation techniques have been described,[33] including interosseous wiring,[34] percutaneous pinning, tension band wiring,[35,36] bio-resorbable pinning,[37] plating,[38] oblique lag screw fixation,[39] and axial compression screw fixation.[33,40] Regardless of the technique chosen, the joint is prepared in a similar manner and the requirements for a successful outcome are: (1) full apposition of the cancellous bone surfaces; (2) preservation of distal phalanx bone stock to allow for hardware purchase; (3) fusion in approximately 5–10° of flexion if possible, and (4) stable fixation.

Most techniques utilize a transverse skin incision overlying the joint. Oblique or axial extensions are made proximally and distally and skin flaps are raised to complete an H-shaped exposure centered over the joint. Alternatively, a mid-lateral or a Y-shaped dorsal incision can be used. Specific care should be taken to avoid injury to the germinal nail matrix located just distal to the extensor insertion. The extensor tendon and joint capsule are sharply divided in a transverse orientation, the collateral ligaments are divided, and the joint is maximally flexed to allow access to the articular surfaces.

With the base of the distal phalanx and the condyles of the middle phalanx exposed, a rongeur is used to remove dorsal

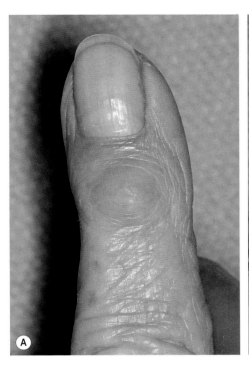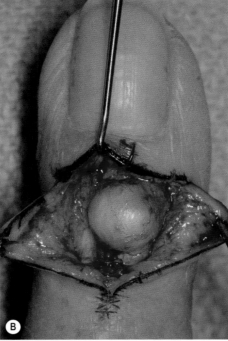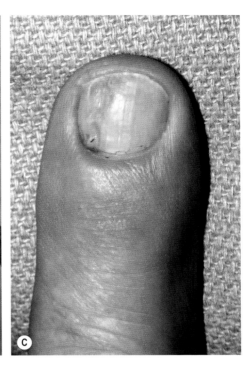

Fig. 20.3 Typical appearance of a mucous cyst in this 67-year-old female with DIP OA. **(A)** A mass is palpable over the joint. **(B)** The cyst is clearly seen at the time of surgical exploration. **(C)** Mucous cysts may also present with nail grooving, which results from pressure on the germinal and sterile matrix of the nail.

and lateral osteophytes. The articular surfaces are decorticated until cancellous bone is visualized. Alternatively, osteotomies can be created with a small oscillating saw to achieve precise apposition of the cancellous bone. If power saws or burrs are to be utilized, copious irrigation should be maintained throughout the cutting process to avoid the risk of thermally induced osteonecrosis which can elevate the risk of nonunion postoperatively.[41]

Interosseous wiring

Interosseous wiring involves securing the distal and middle phalanx together by means of one or two dental wires passed through bone tunnels. Interosseous wiring can be used to achieve some compression of the joint and is usually used in conjunction with K-wires for greater stability. Zavitsanos et al. described a technique which allows the K-wires to be completely buried, minimizing the risk of infection.[34]

K-wire fixation

After the joint is prepared, two crossed 0.045 inch Kirschner wires are passed across the joint. Alternatively, an axial K-wire and a single oblique wire can be used. A minimum of two wires needs to be used to prevent rotation. The wires are typically cut beneath the skin at the fingertip. This enables the patient to continue to use the finger in activities of daily living. The DIP joint is immobilized in a splint to protect the fusion. Once union is documented radiographically, the wires can be removed. Wire removal can be done in the office under digital block anesthesia.

Tension band wiring

With the joint surfaces prepared, two 0.045 inch K-wires are placed parallel across the joint. Distally, the pins are buried in the distal volar cortex of the distal phalanx while proximally the pins exit on the dorsal cortex of the middle phalanx. A transverse canal is made dorsal to the wires in the proximal distal phalanx. A 28-gauge dental wire is passed through this canal and secured proximally around the K-wires exiting on the dorsal proximal phalanx in a figure of eight fashion. The dental wire is twisted and secured and the K-wires are bent to assure the construct is as low profile as possible. The tension band construct is remarkably stable and early motion may be permitted in selected patients. If the hardware is bothersome it can be removed after bony union.

Axial compression screw

A single axial compression screw *(Fig. 20.4)* can be used to reliably achieve DIP joint fusion. A traditional lag screw technique can be used but will result in prominent hardware at the fingertip and is discouraged. Buried headless compression screws are preferred. The technique for the use of a threaded headless compression screw initially involves preparation of the joint surfaces followed by the placement of an antegrade axial K-wire through the distal phalanx exiting at the hyponychium. The bone surfaces are then coapted in the position of fusion and the same wire is drilled retrograde back into the middle phalanx. The position of the wire and arthrodesis are checked fluoroscopically, and a cannulated drill is used prepare the channel for screw placement. The appropriate screw size is determined through fluoroscopic measurement, and a cannulated, fully threaded; self-tapping screw is inserted in a retrograde fashion to complete the fusion *(Fig. 20.4)*.

The screw should be long enough to engage the cortical isthmus of the middle phalanx. Occasionally, the intramedullary canal of the middle phalanx is too wide for the thread to engage the endosteal cortex even at the isthmus (e.g., thumb),

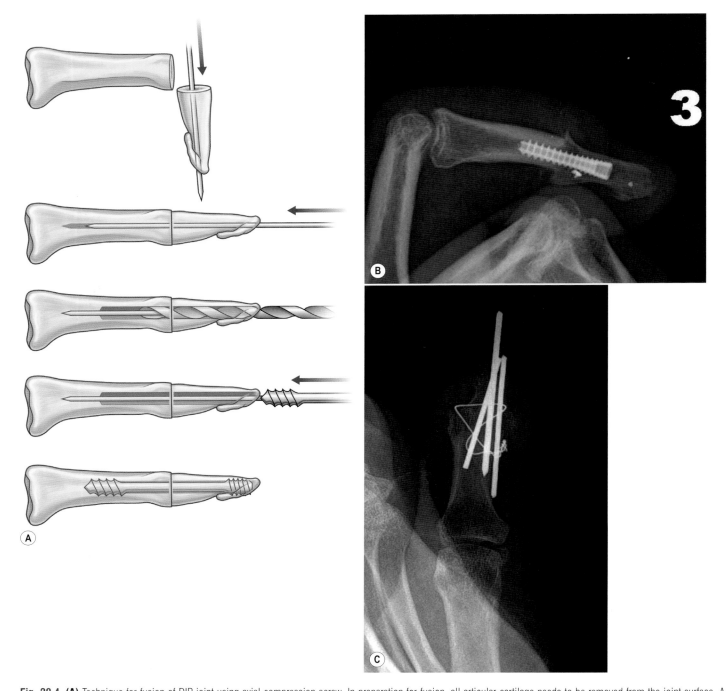

Fig. 20.4 (A) Technique for fusion of DIP joint using axial compression screw. In preparation for fusion, all articular cartilage needs to be removed from the joint surface. A K-wire is then driven retrograde out of the distal phalanx. The joint is then reduced in preparation for fusion and the wire is then driven across the DIP joint. A cannulated drill is used to prepare the bones for screw placement. The screw may then be placed over the wire to complete the fusion. **(B)** Final position of screw within joint. **(C)** DIP fusion may also be accomplished with the use of K-wires alone or tension band technique.

and the chances of a stable construct are reduced. Additionally, specific attention should be paid to the anteroposterior (narrowest) diameter of the distal phalanx to ensure that the screw thread diameter is not greater than this measurement, otherwise dorsal fracturing and nail bed deformity can occur.[42]

The major advantages of this technique over other methods of DIP fusion are buried hardware and stable fixation. Immobilization time with the use of compression screws has been shown to be significantly shorter when compared to other techniques for DIP fusion. Patients may often be splinted for only one to 3 weeks, allowing patients to return to work earlier.[43] One disadvantage of this technique is the difficulty in achieving the optimal prehensile position at the DIP as the joint is typically fused straight due to the conical shape of the screw. Other reported complications have included a single case of skin necrosis of the finger tip requiring secondary amputation;[44] this was likely due to unrecognized prominent hardware.

Complications of DIP fusion

Infection

Traditional fixation techniques for small joint arthrodesis include interosseous wiring, crossed K-wires or a combination of these techniques. The rate of deep infection and osteomyelitis with these techniques remains up to 20% in some studies.[45] Surgeons who prefer this technique should consider burying the K-wires during the consolidation phase, as infection and nonunion rates are much lower with buried techniques are utilized.[46]

Nonunion

Reported nonunion rates for DIP arthrodesis range from 0–20%. Several studies have reported low rates of nonunion with screw techniques[44,45,47–49] as well as traditional techniques,[46] however a clear relationship between fixation technique and the rate of nonunion has not been shown for DIP arthrodesis.[45]

Kirschner wire and interosseous wire techniques produce significantly less compression across the fusion site than compression screw techniques and compression itself has been shown to achieve more rapid fusion. In a biomechanical cadaver study comparing fixation techniques, the use of a single buried axial compression screw (Herbert screw) was shown to be superior in terms of fixation strength when compared to a combined K-wire/tension band technique.[42] Despite this biomechanical study, retrospective clinical studies have noted similar nonunion rates when comparing compression screws, interosseous wiring, and crossed K-wires techniques; it is thought that nonunion rates most closely correlate with the amount cortical bone and condition of the bone stock at the time of operative procedure.[45]

DIP arthroplasty

Distal interphalangeal joint arthroplasty is an uncommon procedure with few indications. The obvious advantage is maintained range of motion of the DIP, which may be beneficial in selected cases, e.g., in professional musicians.[30] There are few published series and these all report on the use of silicone interposition implants.[27–29] The largest series reported 38 DIP arthroplasties of which 10% were removed by 10 years. The average range of DIP motion was 33° with an average extension lag of 12°.[28]

Mucous cyst

Dorsal synovial cysts are commonly associated with DIP arthritis and develop in response to irritation of the joint by marginal osteophytes *(Fig. 20.3)*. Cysts slowly expand damaging the germinal matrix resulting in nail deformity and nail grooving. Progressive thinning of the overlying skin and recurrent inflammation are also common. Infection can be troublesome, as communication with the joint risks the development of septic arthritis and recurrently symptomatic cysts should be removed surgically.

Needle aspiration of the mucous cyst with subsequent corticosteroid injection of the DIP joint is appealing because it can be performed in the office setting with minimal morbidity.[50–52] Typically, the cyst is too small for effective needle aspiration and instead, multiple punctures are made with a 25-gauge needle and manual expression of the cyst fluid is performed. The joint may then be injected with a lidocaine and corticosteroid solution and wrapped snuggly for several days. This technique has been associated with a 60% resolution of the cyst.[50] However, one must observe careful sterile technique to minimize chance of infection into the joint space.

If the cyst recurs surgical excision can be performed. Our preferred surgical technique consists of marking the margins of the cyst under loupe magnification followed by excision of the cyst and overlying attenuated skin. The underlying inflamed synovium should be debrided and associated dorsal and marginal osteophytes are removed. Specific attention should be paid to preservation of the extensor insertion, which can be challenging as it may be significantly attenuated. Skin closure may require the use of local skin flaps in rare circumstances.[50,53–55]

Fritz et al. reported the results of surgical excision of 86 mucous cysts. Nail deformities were present in 29% of patients preoperatively.[56] Postoperative loss of extension of 5–20° at the IP or DIP joints was seen in 17% of patients. One patient developed a superficial infection and two developed a DIP pyarthrosis, eventually requiring DIP arthrodesis. A total of 7% of patients without preoperative nail deformity developed one postoperatively; however 60% of preoperative nail deformities were improved by the procedure. Recurrence was seen in 3% of cases and other complications included persistent swelling, pain, numbness, stiffness, and radial or ulnar deviation at the DIP joint.

Proximal interphalangeal (PIP) joint arthritis

Within the hand, the PIP joint is the third most frequently affected by OA. The joint is more commonly affected in females.[25] The PIP joint has been described as the "functional locus of the finger" as it produces 85% of intrinsic digital flexion and contributes 20% to the overall arc of finger motion.[57] Despite this, a full range of motion is not absolutely necessary for good hand function, and a 45–90° flexion arc allows for most activities.

As in DIP arthritis, PIP joints affected by OA are often enlarged and painful. Patients will complain of their inability to wear or remove rings from the affected fingers. *Bouchard's nodes* are pathognomonic for PIP OA and are bony protuberances at the joint, analogous to Heberden's nodes at the DIP joint. Range of motion at the PIP joint tends to be preserved until late in the disease process. Radiographic findings include joint space narrowing, subchondral sclerosis and osteophytes *(Fig. 20.2)*.

Management

Patients with occasional or minor symptoms are medicated with oral or topical non-steroidal anti-inflammatory drugs. Resting the joint by splinting in *extension* can be used to decrease pain in acute exacerbations. Intra-articular steroid injections can also be used to decrease pain but repeated injections are impractical for the long-term management of severely symptomatic patients. When nonoperative management strategies are insufficient to control the patient's symptoms, PIP joint OA is usually treated surgically, with either arthrodesis or implant arthroplasty. Vascularized joint transfer is technically feasible but uncommonly practiced due to significant donor site morbidity and inferior outcomes when compared with implant arthroplasty.[58-61]

The decision for PIP arthrodesis or arthroplasty is dictated by the patient's functional needs, desires to preserve PIP motion, and the requirements for lateral stability at the joint. The ulnar three digits are important for generating grip strength. Maximal grip strength requires almost full PIP flexion to avoid the quadriga effect. The index finger's relatively independent FDP function does not impose a significant quadriga effect on the remaining digits during grasp. In comparison, the index finger is used to generate oppositional and adduction pinch strength, which requires PIP lateral stability but little PIP motion if metacarpophalangeal joint motion is preserved. Therefore, the decision for arthrodesis versus arthroplasty may be different for each digit involved. For example, arthrodesis of the index finger PIP joint provides finger stability for pinch and is well tolerated; however for the ring and small finger PIP joints, implant arthroplasty may be preferred as PIP joint motion in these digits is important for grip function and strength. If fusion is to be performed on the PIP joints of the ulnar three digits care must be taken in placing the joints in enough flexion to preserve grip strength. A significant decrease in grip strength occurs when the PIP joint of the small finger is fused in less than 45° of flexion, and when the PIP joint of the middle and ring fingers are fused in less than 60° of flexion.[62]

PIP arthrodesis

PIP arthrodesis can be accomplished using the same techniques as described for DIP arthrodesis. The optimal position of PIP fusion varies according to the digit, with some authors recommending 40° of flexion for index, 45° for the long, 50 for the ring and 55° for the small finger *(Fig. 20.5)*;[63] however, this can be tailored according to the patient's occupation and recreational activities. Preoperative splints simulating fusion at various angles can be used to allow the patient to make a more informed decision.

Techniques

The PIP is approached dorsally through a longitudinal incision centered over the joint. The extensor tendon and joint capsule are split longitudinally and dissected radially and ulnarly. The central slip should be elevated subperiosteally off the base of the middle phalanx. The proximal origins of the collateral ligaments are divided and the joint is flexed to expose the joint surfaces. The bone ends are prepared using angled saw cuts on both phalanges. Alternatively, rongeurs or a burr can be used to create a concave-convex (cup and cone) configuration on the opposing bone surfaces. The digit is necessarily shortened by preparation of the bone surfaces. Prolapse of the volar plate in between the bone ends may

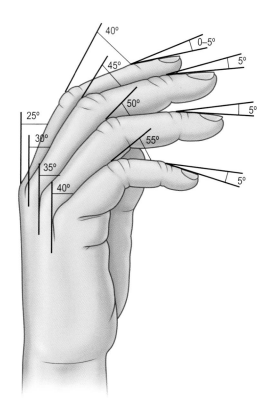

Fig. 20.5 Illustration of recommended fusion angles for DIP, PIP and MCP joints. DIP fusion angles are often performed with 0–15° of flexion. PIP fusion angles increase as one moves from the index to the small finger, to correspond with the natural cascade of the hand. Recommended fusion angles for the PIP joint have been 40° of flexion for the index, 45° for the long, 50° of flexion for the ring and 55° of flexion for the small. MCP fusion angles have been recommended to progress from 25° of flexion at the index to 40° of flexion at the small finger.

result in non union; the volar plate should be resected if this occurs. Fixation can be achieved by one of the following techniques:

Crossed K-wire technique

After preparation of the joint, two crossed 0.045 inch or larger Kirschner wires are passed obliquely across the joint in a coronal plane. Alternatively, an axial K-wire and a single oblique wire can be used. Similar to DIP fusion, the wires can be buried beneath the skin and removed once there is radiographic union. During this time, the joint is protected in an immobilizing splint.

Tension band wire technique

Tension band wiring uses a combination of K-wires and interosseous wire to achieve moderate stability and compression. After preparation of the joint, a transverse hole is drilled through the middle phalanx approximately 5 mm distal to the osteotomy and a 0.6 mm stainless steel wire is passed through the hole. Two parallel 1 mm K-wires are inserted across the joint, and left protruding through the dorsal cortex of the proximal phalanx. The steel wire is passed around the K-wires in a figure-of-eight fashion and tightened to produce compression of the construct. The wire ends and K-wires should be cut short and manipulated to lay flat on the dorsal cortex and prevent extensor tendon attrition.

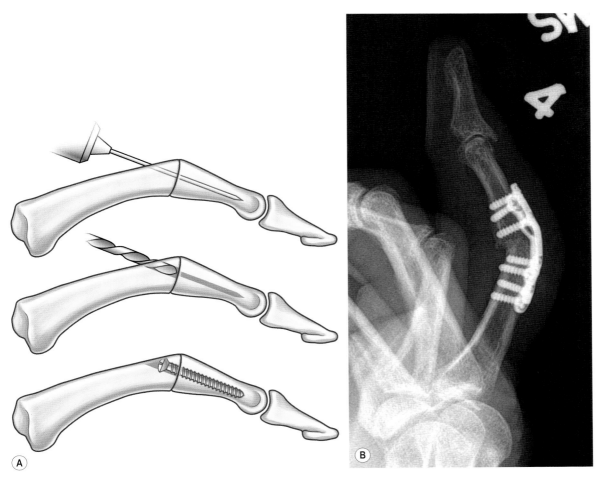

Fig. 20.6 Example of a PIP fusion with **(A)** headless compression screw and **(B)** dorsal plating technique.

The dorsal soft tissues are closed and a splint is applied. A splint is worn for protection until radiographic union.

Compression screw

Arthrodesis of the PIP joint can be accomplished by antegrade insertion of a headless compression screw across the prepared joint *(Fig. 20.6A)*. A K-wire is used to start a hole in the dorsal cortex of the proximal phalanx and oriented obliquely in a sagittal plane. The angle of insertion should correspond to the desired angle of fusion and the wire is inserted antegrade across the joint, into the middle phalanx. The position of the entry hole in the proximal phalanx should be at least 6 or 7 mm proximal to the joint to prevent fragmentation of the dorsal cortex, which can be a complication of this technique. The K-wire is used as a guide wire for the cannulated drill sequence required for the particular screw being used (as described above for DIP arthrodesis). Fluoroscopy is used to check alignment, and to choose an appropriately sized screw that is then inserted in an antegrade fashion, with the assistant holding manual compression of the bone surfaces. The thread should reach the cortical isthmus of the middle phalanx to achieve endosteal purchase. The dorsal soft tissues are closed and a bulky splint is applied. A thermoplastic splint can replace this after 7 days, which should be worn for approximately 3 weeks. The major advantage of this method of fixation is the substantial stability of the construct, which allows early mobilization, and less likelihood of hand stiffness *(Fig. 20.7A)*.

Plating

For severely osteoporotic bone, or for salvage of failed fusion attempts using other methods, PIP arthrodesis may be obtained using mini-plates (1.7 mm up to 2.7 mm). Newer plate designs allow for compression or locking screw placement which can significantly improve fixation in severely osteoporotic bone. Plates are applied using standard AO technique. Pre-contouring of the plates is required to achieve the appropriate angle *(Fig. 20.6B)*.

PIP arthroplasty

Arthroplasty will allow for some preservation of joint motion. Arthroplasty techniques consist of soft tissue interposition, silicone spacers and a variety of constrained and unconstrained implants. Soft tissue arthroplasties are mentioned for historical purposes but have been largely replaced by implants, silicone or other. Techniques for soft tissue arthroplasty have included resection of the head of the proximal phalanx,[64] volar plate interposition,[65] and perichondrial transplant arthroplasty.[66–68]

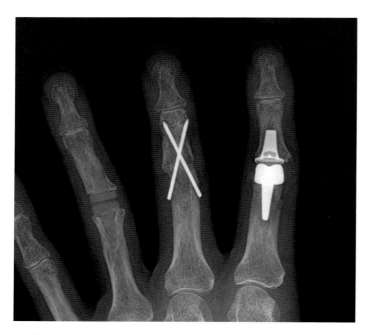

Fig. 20.7 AP radiograph showing an example of silicone arthroplasty of ring finger PIP joint in a 51-year-old woman. Note that distal stem of the implant is improperly positioned and not within the intramedullary canal. In this patient, improper placement of silicone joints in the long and index finger necessitated revision of these joints to a fusion of the long finger PIP joint with cross K-wires, and surface replacement arthroplasty of index finger PIP joint. (Courtesy of Marco Rizzo, MD).

Currently, there are two popular approaches to implant arthroplasty – interposition silicone spacers including the Swanson implant (Wright Medical Technologies, Arlington, TN) and NeuFlex implant (DePuy, Warsaw, IN); and surface replacement or total joint replacement implants such as the SR-PIP implant (Small Bone Innovations, New York, NY) and the PyroCarbon PIP (Ascension Orthopedics, Austin, TX). The success of PIP implant arthroplasty is largely dependent on the condition of the surrounding soft tissues including the collateral ligaments, tendons and volar plate. When these structures are preserved, implant arthroplasty has a higher success rate.

Silicone interposition arthroplasty

Silicone interposition implants consist of one-piece flexible, stemmed, hinged elastomer spacers that can be used in all digits after resection arthroplasty of the PIP joint. Swanson and Niebauer first devised these implants in the 1960s *(Fig. 20.7)*. The implant consists of a single silicone unit with a tapered proximal and distal stem with a central interposed flexion region, which is dorsally offset *(Fig. 20.8A)*. The implant does not function as a true joint but rather a spacer that is stabilized by the fibrous capsule, which develops around the implant. The implant glides or "pistons" within the medullary canals during movement and this was originally believed to disperse forces over a broader surface area potentiating the life of the implant. Newer implant designs have maintained the same general concept but have incorporated a 30° pre-flexed hinge between the proximal and distal stems to facilitate finger flexion.

Technique

The PIP joint can be exposed by one of three surgical approaches – dorsally, laterally or from the volar surface. We prefer a longitudinal dorsal approach in most cases, as it affords superior exposure to the joint and allows easier insertion of the implants. A 2–3 cm straight or curved dorsal incision is made over the PIP joint and continued through the center of the extensor tendon from mid-proximal phalanx until just distal to the insertion of the central slip on the middle phalanx. The two parallel halves of the central slip are then mobilized off the underlying middle phalanx. This produces radial and ulnar tendinous bands, each containing half of the central slip and a lateral band, which are allowed to sublux laterally when the middle phalanx is flexed, exposing the PIP joint. The joint is flexed to 90°, and osteophytes are removed as necessary. An alternative exposure of the PIP joint involves the use of Chamay technique, where a distally based flap of the extensor mechanism is elevated from proximal to distal *(Fig. 20.8)*. The flap is then repaired at the completion of the surgical procedure.[69]

A micro-oscillating saw is used to make a transverse osteotomy at the distal-most portion of the flare of the proximal phalanx, just proximal to the condylar insertion of the collateral ligaments. In general, no resection of the base of the middle phalanx is necessary. Specially designed awls and broaches (specific to implant system used) are used both proximally and distally to open the intramedullary canal to allow the largest size implant. After a trial implant is inserted, the joint is taken through a range of motion to assess stability and fit and the definitive implant is placed. The soft tissues are closed and the hand and wrist are immobilized in the intrinsic plus position. Within a week, the patient is provided a dynamic splint and motion is initiated in a supervised rehabilitation program.

Surface replacement arthroplasty with nonconstrained implants

The first PIP joint replacement prosthesis was described in 1959 by Brannon and Klein.[70] Numerous implant designs have since been produced and many have been abandoned due to implant failure, instability or high complication rates.[71–74] At present, the two designs available in the United States are made of metal or PyroCarbon.

Linscheid and Dobyns introduced the first nonconstrained PIP prosthesis in 1979 and this design is still available as the SR-PIP implant (Small Bone Innovations, New York – previously Avanta, San Diego).[75] The proximal component is made of a chromium-cobalt alloy with a polished articular surface, and the distal component has an ultra-high molecular weight polyethylene (UHMWPe) articular surface fixed to a titanium base and stem. The articulating surfaces is a tongue in groove configuration, similar to the PIP joints anatomic design. For this reason, the system is described by the manufacturer as "semiconstrained." This congruency adds to the lateral stability of the joint. The titanium stems are textured and are designed to "press-fit." However, noncemented implants have been shown to have a higher incidence of subsidence and loosening.[76]

Pyrolytic carbon implants have been developed for use in PIP joint. Pyrolytic carbon is a substance similar to graphite,

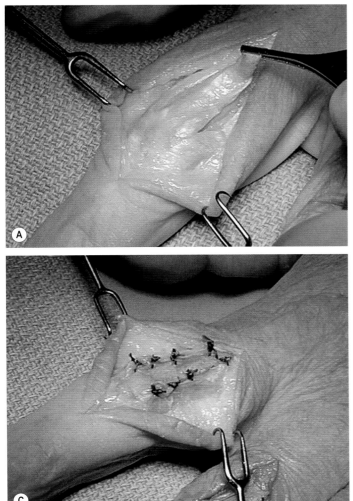

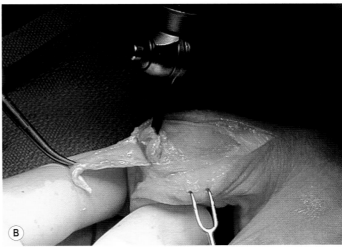

Fig. 20.8 The dorsal approach to the PIP joint involves either a longitudinal split of the extensor mechanism or the use of the Chamay approach. **(A)** The Chamay approach involves the creation of a distally based rectangular flap of extensor tendon. **(B)** The flap is mobilized distally and preserves the attachment of the central slip at the level of the middle phalanx. **(C)** This flap may then be repaired to the surrounding extensor mechanism at the end of the procedure.

which is formed by the high-temperature pyrolysis (thermal decomposition) of hydrocarbons, and their subsequent recrystallization as a surface coating. Pyrolytic carbon is used in joint arthroplasty as a 0.5–1.0 mm coating on a graphite substrate and 1% tungsten is added to produce radio-opacity. The elastic modulus of PyroCarbon (23 GPa) is a much closer match to that of cortical bone (29 GPa), than other implant systems (titanium 105 GPa, CoCr 230 GPa), thus it is presumed that there should be less subsidence. The pyrolytic carbon proximal interphalangeal – PyroCarbon PIP (Ascension Orthopedics, Austin, TX) is a noncemented, minimally constrained, 2-component, nonlinked total joint replacement implant. Joint stability is achieved as a function of the complementary shape of the component surfaces, but ultimately depends on surgical preservation of the collateral ligaments and soft tissues. Like the SR™ PIP arthroplasty, the device can be cemented at the surgeon's discretion.

Both the PIP pyrolytic carbon implant system (Ascension) and SR™ PIP arthroplasty (Small Bones Innovation) are approved for use by the FDA as Humanitarian Use Devices (HUD). Such devices are authorized for use in PIP joint arthroplasty when the patient:

"... has soft tissue and bone that can provide adequate stabilization and fixation under high-demand loading conditions after reconstruction; and needs a revision of a failed PIP prosthesis, or has pain, limited motion, or joint subluxation/dislocation secondary to damage or destruction of the articular cartilage."

Because these devices are used for HUD purposes, they use requires Institutional Review Board (IRB) approval. However, once approved, the IRB does not have to review and approve each individual case.

Patient selection

A trial of nonoperative management is recommended in all patients with PIP OA prior to discussing operative intervention. Unconstrained surface replacement implants rely on the preservation of the collateral ligaments for stability. Patients with gross ligamentous instability or who have damaged their collateral ligaments may not be appropriate candidates for arthroplasty and would be better served with fusion. Evidence of insufficient bone stock, inadequate intramedullary space, marked soft tissue compromise, or ongoing active or chronic infection, are all contraindications to implant arthroplasty, and an alternative surgical option should be pursued. Patients should be informed that average joint motion following arthroplasty is only 40–60°, and joint motion may deteriorate over time. Preoperatively, true AP and lateral radiographs are obtained of each PIP joint so that joints may be templated for implant sizes. Strong consideration must be given to PIP arthroplasty within the index finger PIP joint as this finger is subject to significant lateral force during pinch maneuvers.

Technique for nonconstrained or semiconstrained PIP arthroplasty

Surface replacement arthroplasty of the PIP joint can be performed through either a dorsal, lateral, or volar approach *(Fig. 20.9)*. Our preference is for the dorsal approach as it provides excellent exposure of the joint and facilitates implant placement. A 2–3 cm straight or curved dorsal incision is made over the PIP joint and continued through the center of the extensor tendon from mid-proximal phalanx until just distal to the insertion of the central slip on the middle phalanx. The 2 parallel halves of the central slip are then mobilized off the underlying middle phalanx. This produces radial and ulnar tendinous bands, each containing half of the central slip and a lateral band, which are allowed to sublux laterally when the middle phalanx is flexed, exposing the PIP joint. The joint is flexed to 90°, and osteophytes are removed as necessary.

A 0.035-inch K-wire is inserted into the dorsal ⅓ of the proximal phalanx head, and fluoroscopy is used to confirm a central position in the medullary canal. A starter awl is then used to enlarge the intramedullary canal. A cutting guide is then used to create a vertical osteotomy approximately 0.5–1 mm distal to the insertion of the collateral ligaments on the head of the proximal phalanx removing the articular cartilage. Next, the proximal phalanx is broached, until the medullary canal is filled with the largest broach possible. The lateral fluoroscopic view will be the first to show the size limitations of the intramedullary canal. Once the canal has been enlarged, a matched oblique cutting guide is used to create a back cut in the proximal phalanx, congruent with the sized implant shape. A proximal trial implant can then be inserted and checked radiographically for size and alignment.

Hyper-flexion of the joint then exposes the middle phalanx joint surface. Preparation of the middle phalanx proceeds similarly to the proximal phalanx with the goal of inserting the largest implant possible. Due to the increased amount of cortical bone in the middle phalanx a side-cutting burr is used to facilitate implant placement. Ideally the distal implant should be the same size as the proximal implant, but implants can be mismatched one size smaller or larger if necessary. The distal trial implant is then inserted and a good press fit is checked. Apposition of both the dorsal and volar collar of the prosthesis against the osteotomy is required for a good outcome.

Prior to final implant insertion, holes are drilled with a fine K-wire into the dorsal bony ridge on the middle phalanx and nonabsorbable sutures are placed to attach the central slip back to the bone. The distal implant is inserted and impacted, followed by the proximal implant, and the central slip is reconstructed using the previously placed sutures. If the collateral ligaments have been compromised during the implant placement, collateral ligament stabilizing sutures should be placed to prevent ulnar or radial laxity or hyperextension. The remainder of the tenotomy is closed longitudinally and the skin is closed with nonabsorbable sutures. A padded dorsal, blocking splint is applied in a neutral position.

Postoperative therapy for PIP arthroplasty

Patients must adhere to strict hand therapy follow-up for approximately 10 weeks following surgery and this should be discussed preoperatively, as poor therapy compliance will lead to poor outcome *(Fig. 20.10)*.[77] Hyperextension of the PIP joint must be avoided at all costs, and we therefore do not pursue complete joint extension, preferring to accept a 5–10° flexion deformity, as hyperextension will lead to joint dislocation.

During the first 2 postoperative weeks the patient is splinted or casted in full extension and minimal motion is

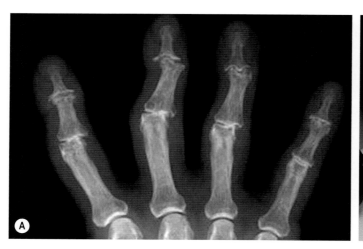
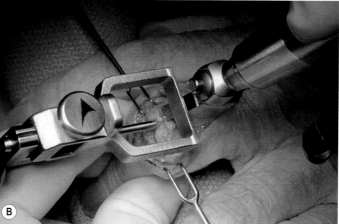

Fig. 20.9 (A) The PA radiograph of a 73-year-old woman with advanced OA of the PIP joints of the index through ring fingers, who has elected to under PyroCarbon arthroplasty of the index and long finger PIP joints. The arthroplasties were performed through a dorsal approach. **(B)** The proximal phalanx is prepared initially with the aid of a cutting guide to remove the articular surface.

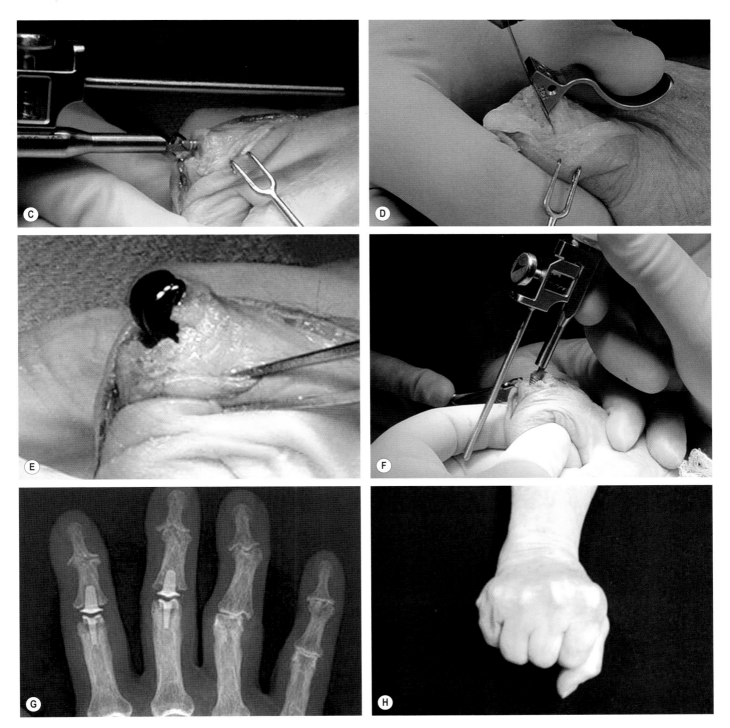

Fig. 20.9, cont'd (C) A broach is used to prepare the canal of the proximal phalanx so that it will accept the implant. **(D)** A back cut is then created in the proximal phalanx so the implant can be properly seated. **(E)** The proximal component is then trialed to access the fit and position. **(F)** A similar procedure is then performed on the middle phalanx. **(G)** PA radiographs showing results at 1 year and functional result. The ring finger PIP was not treated because it was not producing pain and still had reasonable motion **(H)**.

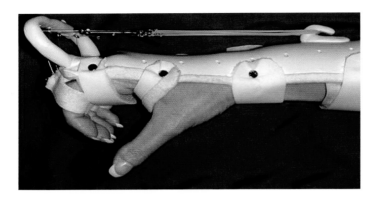

Fig. 20.10 The typical splints used when rehabilitating the PIP joints following surface replacement arthroplasty. The PIP joints are allowed protected flexion with passive extension for the first several weeks following surgery.

allowed at the PIP joint. Strict elevation is encouraged to manage swelling. The plaster splint is removed after 10–14 days and sutures are removed and the patient is allowed to start a short arc motion protocol allowing for 30° of flexion at the PIP joints. Flexion is gradually increased each week to achieve a goal of 70–90° of flexion by 6 weeks. Resting splints are discontinued after 6 weeks if there is no extension lag and active flexion is encouraged with no limits. Isolated pinching, deviation and rotation should be avoided during the rehabilitation phase. Buddy tapping may be used to increase motion of stiff joints.

Outcomes and complications of PIP arthroplasty

Successful implant arthroplasty of the PIP joint affords obvious benefits over arthrodesis; however, despite multiple advancements in implant design, uniformly predictable results have been difficult to achieve.[78] The major complications from PIP arthroplasty continue to be implant failure, instability and loss of motion. Pellegrini and Burton compared arthrodesis and silicone and metal arthroplasty in 43 patients and noted better pinch strength in the arthrodesis group especially in the index finger. Few revisions were necessary in the silicone arthroplasty group, however seven patients underwent revision of the metal prosthesis in order to improve lateral stability. All of these failed and required revision, and the authors concluded that arthrodesis remains the treatment of choice for the index finger, and silicone arthroplasty for the ulnar digits.[79]

Silicone implants have been used for PIP replacement for over 40 years with several large series' reported in the literature. Pain relief tends to be good and the degree of functional improvement and patient satisfaction is high; however, very few series' report improvement in range of motion. The reported incidence of implant fracture with silicone arthroplasty is variable, ranging from 5–44%, and rotational malalignment and lateral deviation may occur with longer follow-up.[80–82] The first large series of silicone interposition arthroplasty was reported by Swanson in 1972.[83] He reviewed 148 implants and there were no major complications. The series was later expanded to report 424 PIP joint arthroplasties. In this series, complete pain relief was achieved in 98% of patients, with an average increase in the arc of PIP motion of

10°.[84] Complications included bone resorption in 1.2% of cases and implant fracture in 5%. More recently, Takigawa et al. reviewed 70 implants with an average follow-up of 6.5 years and reported pain relief in 70%, improvement in extension from 32° to 18°, but no change in total active motion of the PIP joint.[85] Complications included fractures in 15% of the implants, and nine joints required revision. Patients rated their outcome as good in 25 joints, fair in 27, and poor in 18.

Lin et al. reviewed their experience of 69 PIP silicone arthroplasties done through a volar approach.[81] There was an improvement in the extension deficit from 17° to 8° but no improvement in overall arc of motion. Complete resolution of preoperative pain was noted in 67 of 69 joints and complications were observed in 12 joints, including five implant fractures and three cases of implant malrotation. More recent studies by Namdari and Weiss reported 4-year outcomes of 16 joint replacements using the pre-flexed NeuFlex silicone implant.[86] After an average 4-year follow-up, the mean range of motion was 61°, with 0° of extension lag. Pain relief was excellent or good in 84% and overall patient satisfaction was rated at 90%. Pettersson et al. compared this new implant with a traditional silicone implant design, and found better patient satisfaction but otherwise similar results.[87] Silicone interposition PIP arthroplasty remains popular and is often used as a benchmark comparison for newer surface replacement implants such as metal or PyroCarbon systems.

The outcomes of metal surface replacement arthroplasty was reported by Linscheid et al., where they described the outcomes of 66 cemented CoCr-UHMWPE surface replacement prostheses with an average 4.5-year follow-up.[71] In this study, the average arc of motion improved from 35 to 47°, and total pain relief was achieved in 85%. There were a significant number of complications, including five swan-neck deformities; five unstable joints; coronal deviation in four joints, and 12 joints required reoperation.

Jennings and Livingstone reviewed 43 metal surface replacement PIP arthroplasties with an average follow-up of 37 months, and found no change in arc of motion and a 25% revision rate.[88] Revision arthroplasties were generally performed for loosening of the components. They found a significantly higher loosening rate for uncemented components (39%) when compared with cemented components (4%). Johnstone et al. reported similar findings in their study.[76] Johnstone and colleagues noted a higher incidence of subsidence and component loosening in newer generation implants which were not cemented.[76] Luther et al. recently reported an average 27-month follow-up on 24 SR™ PIP arthroplasty.[89] They found that 14 joints required reoperation (58%), including four that required removal. Despite this, 70% were satisfied with their final functional results.[89]

The results of pyrolytic carbon arthroplasty for proximal interphalangeal joint replacement have been the subject of several recent studies.[90–94] Bravo et al. published the largest and most comprehensive study to date.[91] A total of 50 PIP PyroCarbon joint replacements were performed in 35 patients. The minimum follow-up was 27 months. The average age at the time of surgery was 53 years. Joints replaced included the index,[15] middle,[18] ring,[10] and small.[7] The mean preoperative range of motion was 40°, mean pinch and grip measurements were 3 and 19 kg, respectively, and the mean preoperative pain score was 6 by visual analog scale (0–10). Postoperatively, mean range of motion improved to 47°, mean pinch and grip measurements were 4 and 24 kg, respectively. Despite these modest improvements, the mean postoperative pain score was 1 and overall patient satisfaction was high (80%). Fourteen joints required additional procedures and the revision arthroplasty rate was 8%. There were no cases of implant infection. Notably, radiographic evidence of subsidence was noted in 20 joints although there was no apparent loosening.

Tuttle et al. also reported a retrospective series of 18 joint replacements in eight patients.[93] The average active range of motion was unchanged, however there were no cases of lateral instability. Complete resolution of preoperative pain was apparent in only eight cases. Complications included two dislocations evident at the first office visit; five contractures (with a motion arc of <35°), and eight squeaky joints. Wijk et al. reported 2-year follow-up on 53 PIP PyroCarbon arthroplasty procedures.[94] Range of motion and grip strength were unchanged postoperatively, however pain relief and occupational performance were improved and patient satisfaction was high. Revision surgery was required in seven patients, including two who required subsequent arthrodesis.

Chung et al. evaluated 14 patients (21 joints) prospectively. The mean arc of motion at 12 months was 38°, grip and pinch strength both improved postoperatively. Patient-rated outcomes were studied by questionnaire, showing a significant improvement in pain, satisfaction and esthetics outcome.[58]

Herren et al. performed 17 PyroCarbon PIP joint arthroplasty procedures for osteoarthritis, which were followed prospectively for a mean of 20.5 months.[95] All patients noted significant pain relief with a reduction in mean preoperative pain score of 7.6 on a 10-point VAS, to 1.3 at final follow-up. One patient required a revision procedure because of implant migration. Nunley et al. performed five PyroCarbon PIP arthroplasties on younger patients with posttraumatic arthritis.[92] These were followed prospectively for 1 year and were found to have no statistically significant improvement in pain or motion arc, however grip strength increased significantly postoperatively.

Branam et al. have published the only study comparing the outcomes of pyrolytic carbon implants with silicone implants for PIP arthroplasty.[90] This retrospective study compared outcomes of 19 PyroCarbon implants with 23 silicone implants. Although differences in final motion arc and pain relief were statistically insignificant, coronal plane deformity was more prevalent and more pronounced in patients who had silicone arthroplasty. Overall it is apparent that both joints provide benefits with regard to pain relief and preservation of some motion. The superiority of one type of implant over another has yet to be determined.

OA of the metacarpophalangeal (MCP) joint

Anatomy and biomechanics

The metacarpophalangeal (MCP) joint is a multiaxial condyloid joint that allows for flexion, extension, abduction, adduction, and a limited degree of circumduction. Circumduction or rotation is not a motion under active control, but is allowed for passively by the intrinsic joint mechanics. The joint contributes to 77% of the total arc of finger flexion.[96] The metacarpal head has been described as having a unique "cam" shape. However, this description is not true to its mechanical reality. A cam is mechanical link that translates rotational motion into linear motion or vice versa, typically with a rotating *eccentric* wheel. However, the head of the metacarpal is *round* and therefore, the analogy is not valid. The circular metacarpal head is offset volar to the access of the metacarpal shaft, which does result in differential tension of the collateral ligaments in flexion and extension. The unique three-dimensional shape of the head, being wider on its volar aspect, adds to the collateral ligament tension in joint flexion and limited lateral motion in this position. On the other hand, when the MCP joint is extended the collateral ligaments are lax and there is maximal abduction and rotation of the joint in this position.

The MCP joint capsule is composed of areolar tissue dorsally that is loosely reinforced by the extensor tendon and the sagittal band.[97,98] Laterally, the collateral ligaments support the joint, while the volar plate provides volar support. The intrinsic muscles provide only modest, secondary capsular support. The ulnar and radial proper collateral ligaments are fan-shaped, thick and wide, arising from the dorsal aspect of the metacarpal head and inserting into the volar aspect of the proximal phalanx. The accessory collateral ligaments are located volar to the origin of the proper collateral ligaments on the metacarpal head and interdigitate with the proper collateral ligaments distally. The collateral ligaments play a major role in stabilizing the MCP joint in all directions of joint displacement. The accessory collateral ligaments contribute primarily to abduction-adduction and rotational stability, while the volar plate prevents dorsal dislocation of the joint when fully extended. The dorsal capsule provides a very modest contribution to stability when the joint is in distraction and at the extremes of supination and pronation.[97,98]

Osteoarthritis (OA) affects the MCP joint less commonly than other hand joints and is usually secondary to injury or trauma, e.g., intra-articular fracture, septic arthritis, chronic repetitive trauma in setting of heavy labor occupations, and occasionally in metabolic disorders such as hematochromatosisi.[99–101] MCP OA usually affects the index and middle fingers.[99,100] Conservative treatment with splinting, hand therapy, non-steroidal anti-inflammatory drugs, and steroid injections is the first-line treatment of MCP OA. Surgery is indicated for stiffness and/or pain that are refractory to nonoperative treatments.

Resection and resurfacing arthroplasty

Resurfacing arthroplasty involves the resection of diseased metacarpal cartilage and bone, followed by the placement of soft tissue into the joint space to prevent direct bone contact. This procedure was used historically to treat MCP OA but now is reserved as a salvage procedure for cases of failed implant arthroplasty. Tupper[102] described the use of the volar plate for interposition arthroplasty. The volar plate is detached proximally from the metacarpal head before the diseased cartilage and bone of the metacarpal head is resected. This distally based volar plate is then attached to the dorsal edge of the osteotomy by means of sutures preplaced through drill holes in the metacarpal. Before the joint capsule is closed, the collateral ligaments are reattached using horizontal mattress sutures preplaced through drill holes on the sides of the distal metacarpal.[103,104] Other resection/interposition arthroplasty techniques using tendon and interosseous muscles have been described by Vainio[105] and Riordan and Fowler,[106] though not specifically for OA.

Costal perichondrium may also be used for joint resurfacing. After harvesting the perichondrium and cutting it to the size and shape of the joint surface, the perichondrial graft is secured by means of a horizontal mattress suture. There are limited and variable reports on the outcomes of using rib perichondrium for resurfacing arthroplasty.[67,107] A study by Seradge[67] noted poor outcomes in patients over 40 years of age and uniform failure in cases of reconstruction after septic arthritis. He concluded that such patients constitute a contraindication for the procedure. If perichondrium is to be used it should be oriented with the deep surface facing the joint as this is the chondrogenic surface. Similarly if the retinaculum or volar plate are used for resurfacing, the synovial (deep) surface should be oriented facing the joint.[107]

Implant arthroplasty

MCP implant arthroplasty is most commonly used in patients with rheumatoid arthritis. These patients tend to have a lower demand on the hands and therefore make implant arthroplasty more appealing. In distinction to patients with rheumatoid arthritis, patients with OA of the MCP joint tend to have preservation of the collateral ligaments and fewer issues with soft tissue imbalance and thus can be excellent candidates for implant arthroplasty of the MCP joint. Contraindications for MCP arthroplasty are similar to PIP arthroplasty. The index finger MCP joint can be considered for arthroplasty even in a manual laborer. MCP joint prostheses can be grouped into one of four basic groups: hinged designs, flexible (silicone) prostheses, surface replacement prostheses, and PyroCarbon implants.

Hinged prostheses

Metal-hinged prostheses are rarely used today. The 1953, Brannon and Klein prosthesis was the first prosthesis to be used for MCP arthroplasty.[70] This simple, uniaxial metal prosthesis resulted in bone resorption with subsequent finger shortening and loss of range of motion. In the 1970s and 1980s, the hinge implants evolved into multi-axial designs made of metal, polymers, or ceramics. The two-component ball-and-socket Griffith-Nicolle prosthesis[108] and ceramic prostheses[109,110] were strong enough to prevent fracture, but postoperative range of motion was too limited for adequate joint function.[108]

Silicone constrained prostheses

The Swanson prosthesis was the first silicone MCP joint prosthesis and has been in use since the 1960s.[111] This prosthesis has been widely used and studied, although primarily for rheumatoid arthritis (RA). The silicone elastomer is crosslinked which creates a rubber-like form to the implant. The implant acts as a dynamic spacer and not a true joint. The prosthesis is held in position by a process of fibrous

encapsulation, instead of osteointegration.[111] The prosthesis does not flex at the central hinge section until the joint has been flexed beyond 45°. Instead, in early flexion, the implant bends at the interface between the stem and the hinge.[112] This results in a high incidence of stem fracture. Beckenbaugh reported a fracture rate of 26% at 2.5 years when using the original Swanson MCP prosthesis. After this study, the silicone elastomer used in the prosthesis was modified to increase its tear propagation strength and its fatigue-crack growth resistance, and a newer, "High Performance implant" was released.[113] Kirschenbaum et al.[114] reported a 10% fracture rate within 8.5 years of insertion of the modified Swanson implant. Fracture rates of around 5–7% have been reported at 2–5-year follow-up.[115,116] Interestingly, many of these fractures do not require treatment as they go unnoticed by the patients.[114] Other complications with the implant have included implant deformation and silicone synovitis.[114,117,118]

The clinical experience with the Swanson implant in patients with RA constitutes the main body of the literature on this implant. However, Rettig et al.[119] reported their experience with silicone MCP arthroplasty in the setting of OA. While the experience in RA can shed some light on the management of patients with OA, the outcome of silicone arthroplasty in this population is likely to be different than patients with OA. They reported 100% patient-reported overall improvement with a mean MCP flexion of 59°. This small study consisted of 12 patients and 14 MCP joints. In contrast to the literature on Swanson implant failures in the setting of MCP RA, this study, albeit small, demonstrated no Swanson implant fractures in patients with OA.

The limitations of the Swanson implant in patients with RA have motivated the development of new silicone implant designs like Sutter (Avanta) and the NeuFlex (DePuy, Warsaw, IN) implants. Unfortunately, computer modeling has shown higher stresses in the Avanta design when compared to the Swanson implant,[120] and this has been confirmed clinically with observations of at least double the fracture rate in patients with RA.[121] Studies are more promising for the NeuFlex implant, an anatomically neutral silicone implant with a block-hinge design and a preformed 30° resting angle that approximates the relaxed MCP position. The logic for this design is that with the finger in repose, there is no stress on the implant, contrary to the Swanson design. In vitro studies also suggest that the NeuFlex implant has greater longevity than the Swanson implant before fracture.[122] Weiss et al.[123] compared MCP joint mechanism after NeuFlex, Swanson and Sutter arthroplasty and found that the mechanics of the NeuFlex implant most closely matched that of an intact MCP joint. Only one study[86] specifically examines the in vivo use of NeuFlex implants in OA of the MCP joint. At 4-year follow-up, NeuFlex implants were associated with a mean flexion arc of 65°, a mean extension lag of 3°, no implant fractures, and high patient satisfaction.[86] Despite the limitations of the Swanson MCP prosthesis, it remains the current "gold standard" to which other implants are compared. Not only is it effective in relieving pain and improving motion arc, but it is also relatively cheap and easy to place and remove (*Fig. 20.11*).[124–126]

Surface replacement prostheses

Silicone implants are inadequate in patients who place a higher demand on the MCP joint due to employment

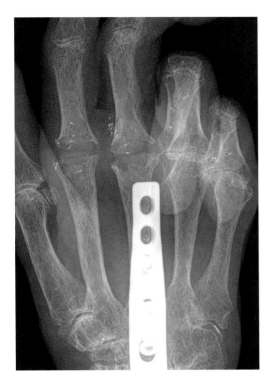

Fig. 20.11 Example of silicone MCP arthroplasties of the index and long finger in a 63-year-old woman who was suffering from post-traumatic arthritis.

or lifestyle. Surface-replacement prostheses are more appropriate in such patients unless the soft tissue around the MCP joint is inadequate to offer implant stability.[127–130] Surface-replacement prosthetics attempt to recreate normal joint anatomy. They vary in their design: a single-component silicone implant with a Dacron-coated stem;[127] a nonjoined, two-component pyrolite carbon implant;[128] a four-component polyethylene-titanium implant;[129] or a three-component titanium plate-silastic hinge implant.[130] Studies on surface replacement prostheses are small, consisting mainly of RA patients, with short postoperative follow-up. With the exception of a 20% fracture rate with the Hagert prosthesis, the surface replacement prostheses are associated with a high patient satisfaction, resolution of pain, improved cosmetic appearance, average range of motion of 47–60°, and a low fracture rate.[127–130] The main problem with these implants is instability and dislocation.[128]

Kung et al. developed a stable surface replacement arthroplasty implant based on cadaveric evaluation of normal MCP joint articular geometry.[131] The implant is a non-constrained, two-component implant with a hemi-spherical cobalt chrome alloy metacarpal component with and an ultra high molecular weight polyethylene phalangeal component. The head has lateral volar contours that increase lateral stability during flexion. Also, its arc of rotation is greater than that of an anatomical joint to decrease the risk of palmar subluxation. The stem of each component may be "press-fit" or secured into the intermedullary canal with bone cement. When mechanically tested at different angles, axial loads, and directions of motion, this semiconstrained MCP joint implant demonstrates more intrinsic stability than cadaveric MCP joints.[131]

PyroCarbon arthroplasty

Pyrolytic carbon, formed by the pyrolysis of a hydrocarbon gas, has an elastic modulus similar to cortical bone.[132] This makes the material ideal for implant-bone stress transfer, potentially reducing implant wear and subsidence.[132] The implant is stabilized by appositional bone growth and does not require cement fixation.[133] PyroCarbon implants require minimal bone resection and preserve the collateral ligaments allowing for greater distribution of compressive forces. However, such noncontraint prostheses are more likely to sublux or dislocate especially in the setting of sub-optimal soft-tissue support. It is for this reason that these implants are less stable in patients with RA. Cook et al. reported a 70% 16-year implant survival for the early PyroCarbon implant design. The patients in that study, the majority of whom had RA, had good outcomes.[134] A short-term study by Nunez and Citron[135] specifically focuses on the use of the implant in patients with OA; after a mean follow-up of 2.2 years, 10° of motion was gained, pain significantly improved, and there were no cases of implant failure. A 2007, a study by Parker and colleagues reported similar range of motion as previous reports.[134,136] A systemic review of the literature, however, suggests that PyroCarbon prostheses may provide no significant advantage over the Swanson implant with regards to postoperative motion and that complication rates of both implant designs may be similar.[58] Overall, PyroCarbon arthroplasty has been shown to decrease pain, improving extension lag and improve grip and pinch strength.[134,136]

Technique for MCP joint arthroplasty with PyroCarbon implant

Prior to surgery AP and lateral radiographs used to template the size of the implants needed for the surgical procedure, keeping in mind that most routine radiographs are magnified by 3%.[137] The MCP joint is exposed through a longitudinal incision, alternatively if several joints are to be replaced a transverse incision can be made as in the case of RA. The extensor mechanism is split centrally; alternatively it can be mobilized from the radial or ulnar aspect of the sagittal bands *(Fig. 20.12)*. If the extensor mechanism is divided from the sagittal bands for joint exposure, these structures will need to be reconstructed and the extensor mechanism must be centralized at the completion of the case.

Once the joint is exposed, a starter awl is used to identify the intramedullary canal of the metacarpal. An alignment guide is placed within the intramedullary canal and the cutting guide is attached to the alignment guide. Using the cutting guide a 27.5° back cut is created into the metacarpal head. The guide is then removed and the remaining osteotomy is completed by hand. The cutting plane of the guide is positioned 1.0–2.0 mm distal to the dorsal attachments of the collateral ligaments. Upon completing the metacarpal osteotomy, the proximal phalangeal base is prepared in a similar manner, however, the cutting plane is positioned 0.5–1.0 mm distal to the dorsal edge of the proximal phalanx and is tilted 5° distally from vertical. It is strongly recommended that a conservative osteotomy (limited to the joint's articular surfaces), be performed initially to avoid damage to the collateral ligaments. Additional metacarpal and proximal phalanx can

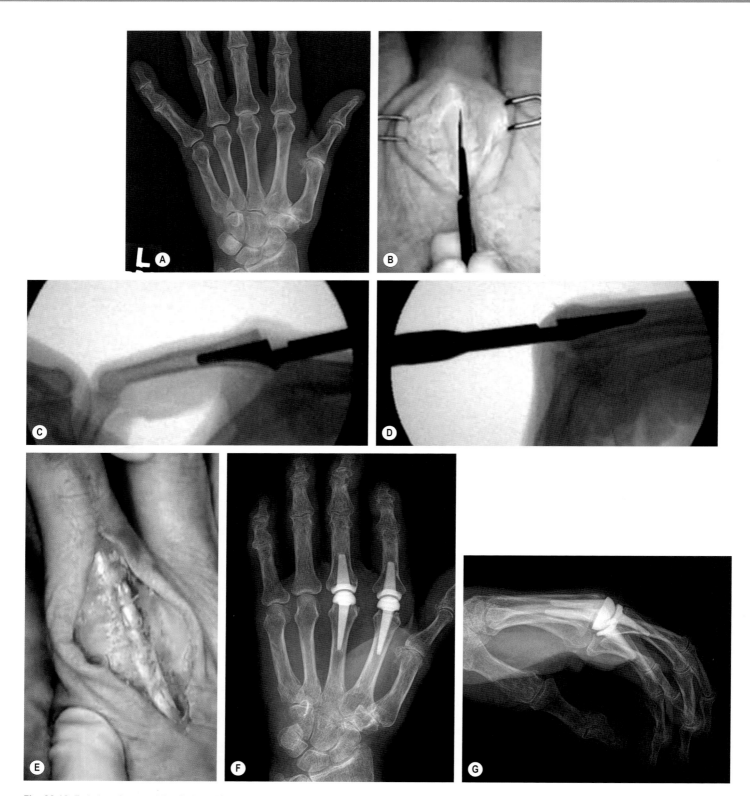

Fig. 20.12 Technique for use of PyroCarbon MCP joint arthroplasty. **(A)** PA radiographs of a 63-year-old male with OA of the MCP joint, as demonstrated radiographically by joint narrowing. **(B)** The surgical exposure is obtained through a longitudinal incision over the MCP joint. **(C)** The joint surfaces are prepared with a cutting guide similar to PIP joint arthroplasty. After the articular cartilage has been removed, the proximal phalanx is broached in preparation for implant placement. Broach position is verified with intra-operative fluoroscopy. **(D)** A similar procedure is performed on the metacarpal. **(E)** The final implants are placed and the extensor mechanism is reconstructed with braided suture with the finger held in extension. **(F,G)** Final position of the implants on PA and lateral radiographs 6 months following the surgery.

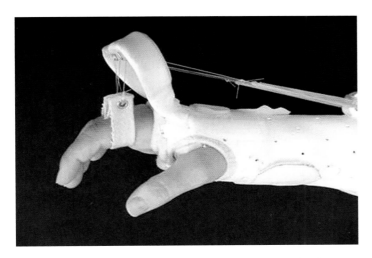

Fig. 20.13 Splint design for rehabilitation of surface replacement arthroplasty at the MCP joint.

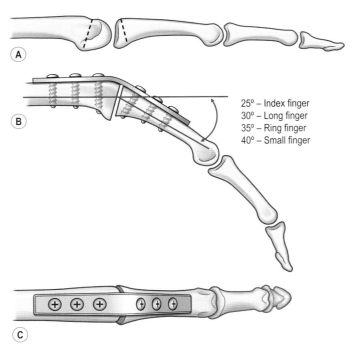

25° – Index finger
30° – Long finger
35° – Ring finger
40° – Small finger

Fig. 20.14 MCP joint fusion can be achieved with various techniques. Angled cuts in the proximal phalanx base and MCP head allow one to maximize surface contact and create appropriate fusion angles. MCP fusion angles increase as one moves from the index finger to the small finger. Recommended fusion angles for the MCP joints have been 25° of flexion for the index, 30° for the long, 35° of flexion for the ring and 40° of flexion for the small.

always be removed later if the joint space is too small to accommodate the implants.[137]

Following completion of the osteotomies the proximal phalanx is broached to accommodate the largest implant. The metacarpal is then broached to match the proximal phalanx. Trial components are then inserted and checked using fluoroscopy. Motion should allow for approximately 10–15° of hyperextension and full flexion. Impaction grafting with autograft or allograft can be used if there is any concern about implant seating against the intramedullary bone. When satisfied with the preliminary appearance of the trial implants and the MCP joint motion, the trials are removed, and permanent implants are press fit into the intramedullary canals. Unlike the PIP PyroCarbon joints, the MCP implants should not be mismatched for size, as this may produce edge wear on the implant. Care must be taken to assure the correct axial rotation of the component by verifying that the dorsal surface of the component is parallel to the dorsal surface of the proximal phalanx. To prevent volar subluxation or dislocation of the implant, a capsular repair is performed and the extensor tendon is centralized.

Postoperatively, the hand is placed in a volar splint with the wrist at 10–15° of dorsiflexion and slight ulnar deviation; the MCP joints are placed in full extension, and the PIPs may be left in slight flexion (5–10°).[137] Short arc (30°) MCP joint flexion is started on day 5–10. Flexion is increased weekly by 20° until full flexion is obtained. Nighttime and resting splints are worn for 6 weeks keeping the joint in full extension when not exercising to minimize and resultant extension lag *(Fig. 20.13)*.

MCP arthrodesis

Current implant arthroplasty techniques have made MCP arthrodesis a final resort in the treatment of MCP OA. MCP arthrodesis can be very debilitating, particularly if the other joints of the fingers have limited motion due to OA. Arthrodesis can be considered whenever arthroplasty is not possible due to inadequate soft tissue support or significant damage to the metacarpal or proximal phalanx bone stock. In general, the

MCP joints should be fused in increasing flexion starting with 25° of flexion for the index finger and adding an additional 5° of flexion for each finger as one advances in an ulnar direction *(Fig. 20.14)*. In preparation for arthrodesis, good cancellous to cancellous bone contact is essential and this may be achieved in a "ball-in-socket" or a flat surface configuration. There are many techniques for arthrodesis of the MCP joints. Intramedullary olecranon bone[138] and prosthetic pegs[139] have been described. Some 97–99% fusion rates have been reported with crossed Kirschner pin stabilization.[140,141] In contrast, intraosseous wiring is associated with a 9% nonunion rate[142] and an 8% nonunion was reported with AO screw arthrodesis.[143] Arthrodesis with miniplates has been reported to achieve 96% fusion rates *(Fig. 20.15)*.[144] Alternatively, tension band arthrodesis allows for another means of fixation with acceptable fusion rates.[145,146] Tension bands can transform distracting flexor tendon forces across an arthrodesis site to compressive forces dorsally, that stabilize the arthrodesis.

Vascularized joint transfer/costochondral replacement

Although not commonly performed, the MCP joint can be replaced with a free vascularized or pedicled transfer of another joint. When compared to implant arthroplasty, vascularized toe transfer is less effective in improving postoperative arc of motion.[58] Thus, in cases of OA of the MCP joint, vascularized joint transfers are only indicated in patients where implant arthroplasty is contraindicated or has already failed, in young manual workers where implants have a high failure

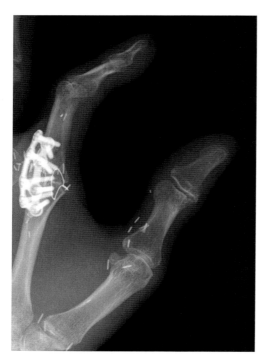

Fig. 20.15 Oblique radiograph of the index finger demonstrating an MCP joint fusion obtained with a dorsally applied mini-plate.

rate, and/or in cases where there is inadequate bone stock for implant arthroplasty.[147] Vascularized joint transfers are also recommended in children, as it is the only procedure that preserves the epiphyseal growth plate and allows for some longitudinal growth.[58] Better functional results in MCP joint reconstruction can be seen with the use of the second metatarsophalangeal joint.[148] After harvesting the flap, the whole second ray should be amputated for rapid recovery of normal gait. A small dorsalis pedis flap can be raised for any associated hand skin defects.

OA of the thumb

The thumb accounts for 50% of overall hand function and as such it is the most important digit in the hand.[31] Arthritis of the thumb can occur at the interphalangeal (IP), MP, or trapeziometacarpal (TM) joints. Arthritis of the interphalangeal joint is managed in a manner similar to that of the finger DIP joints as described above. One needs to decide the degree of flexion in which to fuse the joint and the method of fixation (K wires, 90–90 interosseous wiring, or headless compression screw fixation). The technique of joint debridement and fixation is essentially the same as with the finger DIP joints. Similarly, mucous cyst formation can be a complication of IP joint arthritis of the thumb. This is managed similar to a manner identical to that described for DIP arthritis above.

MCP joint arthritis of the thumb

Osteoarthritis of the thumb MCP joint is relatively uncommon and frequently the result of injury, particularly chronic radial or ulnar collateral ligament injury.[149] While arthroplasty may be an appropriate option for the thumb MCP joint in rheumatoid arthritis, MCP arthrodesis has been the standard of care for OA of the thumb MCP joint for more than 50 years.[150] MCP thumb joint fusion is well tolerated due to the large degree of motion at the thumb CMC joint. As with the IP joint of the thumb, MCP joint fusion can be accomplished by a variety of techniques that have been outlined above, such as tension band wiring, crossed K-wires, or plate fixation. The primary decision is what position the joint should be fused. The position must be functional, that is it should facilitate opposition to the fingers and not hinder the ability to oppose to the tip of the ring finger or small finger. This typically means fusing the joint in slight (15°) of flexion.[150] However, fusing the joint in slightly more flexion (20–40°) takes some work out of opposition for the CMC joint and may decrease the load across this joint and therefore be protective against the development of OA at this location or at least slow its progression.[150]

Trapeziometacarpal arthritis

Etiology and epidemiology

Osteoarthritis of the trapeziometacarpal (TM) joint of the thumb is very common, with a reported age adjusted prevalence of 7% in men and 15% in women.[151] In a retrospective study of patients presenting with distal radius fracture, the prevalence of TM arthritis rose steadily after age 40, with 91% of patients over 80 demonstrating arthritic changes (85% of men and 94% of women over age 80) While many patients remain relatively asymptomatic, a subset of patients will develop debilitating pain, thumb weakness and instability, severely limiting hand function. Many treatment options exist, including non-steroidal anti-inflammatory drugs (NSAIDS), splinting, and corticosteroid injections.[152–155] When conservative options fail, surgical treatment should be considered.

The effect of basal thumb OA on disability and mortality is modest, and as such, it is likely under-diagnosed in clinical practice.[151] Basal thumb arthritis usually involves the carpometacarpal joint, but the scaphotrapeziotrapezoid (STT) joint can also become involved. Combined CMC/STT disease is twice as likely to be symptomatic than isolated CMC arthritis.[156] Males with thumb arthritis are more likely to be symptomatic than females.[157]

Epidemiological studies suggest that basal thumb arthritis is most common in post-menopausal women. While the prevalence of radiographic thumb carpometacarpal OA among men is 7%, it is more than double that (15%) in women[151] and quadruple that in the postmenopausal population.[156] The discrepancy is not as wide when considering only symptomatic disease; 5% of men and 7% of women over the age of 70 years suffer from symptomatic basal thumb OA.[157] Among postmenopausal women with radiographic evidence of basal thumb arthritis, the majority have isolated CMC disease; 6% have isolated STT disease, and 23 % have combined CMC/STT.[156] The gender differential seen in this disease may be explained by anatomic differences in the joint. Female CMC joints have greater reciprocal articular surface curvatures and lower degree of surface congruity resulting in smaller contact areas with greater stresses.[158] Hormonal factors may also contribute to the development of basal thumb OA in females. Spector et al.[159] found an increased risk for the disease in women who had a hysterectomy. Interestingly, the relationship is not demonstrable with other hand joints, putting the validity of this relationship into question.[160]

Other risk factors for thumb CMC OA have been extensively studied. Obesity is a strong determinant of thumb CMC OA in both sexes.[151,161,162] Obesity causes OA by increasing the load on weight-bearing joints, however the first CMC is not a weight-bearing joint. Obesity may predispose to CMC osteoarthritis via a nonmechanical, biological mechanisms related to elevated serum lipids.[163] Unlike weight-bearing joints,[164,165] there is no independent association between thumb CMC OA and diabetes or hypertension.[160] Furthermore, while an association between thumb CMC OA and OA in weight-bearing joints has been reported by some investigators,[166-168] others have dismissed this relationship.[151] While thumb CMC OA is not specifically associated with heavy physical activity,[160] it is clearly associated with occupations requiring repetitive thumb use (especially in the absence enough rest breaks) and occupations that expose the thumb to greater than normal forces.

Family history is another strong predictor in the development of thumb CMC OA. In a classic twin study, Spector[169] provided clear evidence of a genetic link for the development of TM OA in females. Jonsson and colleagues[170] went on to suggest that the genetic influence increased with the severity of the disease.

Anatomy and biomechanics

The TM joint comprises the articulation between the trapezium and the base of the thumb metacarpal. The trapezium and first metacarpal base have reciprocal concavoconvex surface which resembles a biconcave saddle joint).[171] The trapezial surface is concave in an ulnar-radial direction and convex in a dorsopalmar direction. Reciprocally, the base of the first metacarpal is convex in an ulnar-radial direction and concave in a dorsopalmar direction. The radius of curvature of the metacarpal base is 34% greater than that of the trapezium and is thought to predispose to joint incongruity and instability.[172] The trapezial surface flattens and transforms from a saddle type to a semicylindrical type joint with advancing arthritis.[173] The scaphotrapezial (ST), trapeziotrapezoid and trapezium-index metacarpal joints are also considered as part of the basal joint of the thumb and can become involved in late stage OA.

Due to the bony incongruity and large cantilever forces, the CMC joint relies heavily on static ligamentous restraints for stability. Up to 16 ligaments have been identified;[172,174] however, the there are five major internal ligamentous stabilizers of the TMC joint; these ligaments are the dorsal radial ligament, posterior oblique ligament, first intermetacarpal ligament, ulnar collateral ligament and the anterior oblique ligament. The dorsal radial ligament prevents lateral subluxation. The posterior oblique ligament provides stability in flexion, opposition, and pronation. The first intermetacarpal ligament (IML) is taut in abduction, opposition and supination; it holds the first metacarpal tightly against the second metacarpal. The IML is joined by the ulnar collateral ligament,

which prevents lateral subluxation of the first metacarpal on the trapezium and controls for rotational stress. The fifth and most important ligament is the volar anterior oblique ligament with its deep (dAOL) and superficial (sAOL) components. The ligament arises form the volar tubercle of the trapezium and inserts on the volar aspect of the thumb. The AOL is taut in extension, abduction, and pronation; it controls pronation stress and prevents radial translation. The dAOL serves as a pivot point for the TMC joint and guides the metacarpal into pronation while the thenar muscles work in concert to produce abduction and flexion. These fibers limit ulnar translocation of the metacarpal during palmer abduction while working with the sAOL to constrain volar subluxation of the metacarpal (*Fig. 20.16*).[171,172,174]

The TM joint surface allows for biaxial movements – flexion/extension of the CMC and palmar abduction/adduction.[171] Capsular laxity allows for rotation of the metacarpal on the trapezium. Combined flexion, palmar abduction and rotation allow for opposition.[171] Cooney et al. radiologically demonstrated that the average total motions of the TM joint (defined as motions of the first metacarpal with reference to the third metacarpal) is 53° of flexion-extension, 42° of abduction-adduction, and 17° of axial rotation (pronation-supination).[175]

Diagnosis and classification

The diagnosis of TM OA is usually made from the history and physical examination. Radiographs are used to stage the

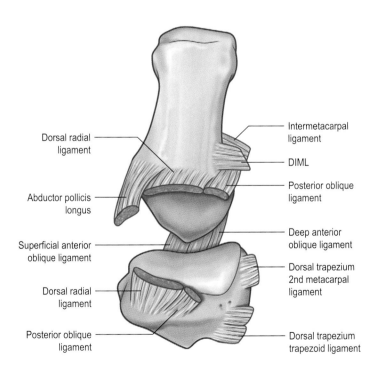

Fig. 20.16 Diagram of the trapezio-metacarpal joint looking from dorsal to palmar. A portion of the dorsal radial ligament (DRL) and posterior oblique ligament (POL) have been removed to show the palmar ligaments. The most important ligaments for thumb stability are the dorsal radial ligament (DRL), posterior oblique ligament (POL), ulnar collateral ligament (not depicted), first intermetacarpal ligament (IML), and the anterior oblique ligament, deep and superficial heads (DAOL, SAOL).

Intermetacarpal ligament

DIML

Posterior oblique ligament

Deep anterior oblique ligament

Dorsal trapezium 2nd metacarpal ligament

Dorsal trapezium trapezoid ligament

Dorsal radial ligament

Abductor pollicis longus

Superficial anterior oblique ligament

Dorsal radial ligament

Posterior oblique ligament

disease. When evaluating a patient with thumb base pain, the differential diagnosis is broad and includes: flexor carpi radialis (FCR) tendonitis, de Quervain's tenosynovitis, inflammatory arthritides, rheumatoid arthritis, gout, pseudogout, gamekeeper's thumb, radial sensory neuritis and radiocarpal or STT arthritis.

Basal joint arthritis typically presents in females 50–70 years old who complain of worsening thumb pain interfering with activities of daily living. Patients often complain that activities requiring opposition or pinch grip, such as opening jars or carrying heavy objects between the thumb and fingers, produce pain at the base of the thumb. Complaints of stiffness or pain at rest are usually indicators of late-stage disease. On physical examination, patients may show the following signs:[176,177]

a. *Shoulder sign*: classically reveals squaring or prominence at the base of the thumb (dorsoradial subluxation secondary to ligamentous laxity and the pull of APL on the base of the metacarpal)

b. *Point tenderness* at the CMC joint

c. *Grind test*: pain on axial compression with rotation of the metacarpal on the trapezium is pathognomonic of CMC arthritis

d. *Distraction test*: pain on thumb metacarpal base rotation and axial traction may be present in early stage disease due to joint capsule inflammation

e. *Adduction deformity*: in later stages of the disease, the metacarpal adopts an adducted posture and the patient may develop a subsequent contracture of the first web space

f. *Hyperextension deformity*: as a result of the adduction deformity or severe joint stiffness, there may be a compensatory hyperextension deformity of the thumb MCP joint

g. *Thumb weakness*: pinch strength is almost always diminished and functional hand width is often narrowed

h. *Carpal tunnel syndrome*: up to 43% of patients with TM OA may have evidence of median nerve compression on nerve-conduction studies.[178] The prevalence is even higher in women, worker's compensation patients, and those with diabetes mellitus. Given this high association, one should take great care to diagnose coexistent carpal tunnel syndrome in patients scheduled for basal joint surgery. If present carpal tunnel syndrome can be treated at the same time of TM OA surgery.[178]

AP, lateral, and oblique radiographs of the TM joint can be used to confirm the diagnosis and stage the disease. TM stress views (30° PA view with the patient forcefully pushing the radial aspects of their thumb tips against each other) can help assess the degree of joint subluxation and joint space loss.[179] Stess views also demonstrate the ST joint and the index finger TM joint very well. The Robert's view (AP view with the hand hyperpronated) also provides a clear image of all four trapezial articulations.[176] Only 28% of women who have radiographic signs of isolated TM arthritis and 55% of women with pantrapezial arthritis admit to symptoms of thumb arthritis, thus radiographic changes must always be correlated with physical signs prior to developing any treatment plan.[156]

There are two frequently used classification systems for CMC arthritis. The Eaton classification *(Table 20.1)*,[179] is most commonly used and is based on radiographic features alone. Individual symptoms may not correlate with the Eaton stage. In comparison, Burton classification *(Table 20.2)* is based on clinical and radiographic findings.[180,181]

The Eaton classification of TM OA follows the progressive changes that occur with progression of disease. In stage I the joint appears normal or slightly widened, associated with effusion or ligamentous laxity. In stage II there is slight narrowing of the joint associated with cartilage loss. Joint debris such as loose bodies and osteophytes may be seen, but measure less than 2 mm in size and sclerotic changes are minimal. In stage III, the joint space is markedly narrowed or obliterated, subchondral sclerosis and cystic changes are apparent, dorsal subluxation is variably seen, and osteophytes and debris exceed 2 mm in size. The STT joint is spared

Table 20.1 **Eaton classification**	
Stage	Radiographic characteristics
Stage I	Normal or slightly widened trapeziometacarpal joint Trapeziometacarpal subluxation up to $\frac{1}{3}$ of articular surface Normal articular contours
Stage II	Decreased trapeziometacarpal joint space Trapeziometacarpal subluxation up to $\frac{1}{3}$ of articular surface Osteophytes or loose bodies <2 mm
Stage III	Decreased trapeziometacarpal joint space Trapeziometacarpal subluxation >$\frac{1}{3}$ of articular surface Osteophytes or loose bodies ≥2 mm Subchondral cysts or sclerosis
Stage IV	Involvement of the scaphotrapezial joint or less commonly the trapeziotrapezoid or trapeziometacarpal joint of the index

(Data from Eaton RG, Littler JW. Ligament reconstruction for the painful thumb carpometacarpal joint. J Bone Joint Surg Am 1973;55(8):1655–1666.)

Table 20.2 **Burton classification**	
Stage	Findings
Stage I	Pain Positive grind test Ligamentous laxity Dorsoradial subluxation of CMC joint
Stage II	Instability Chronic subluxation Radiographic degenerative changes
Stage III	Involvement of the scaphotrapezial joint or less commonly the trapeziotrapezoid or trapeziometacarpal joint of the index
Stage IV	Stage II or III with degenerative changes of the MCP

(Reproduced from: Braun RM, Feldman CW. Total joint replacement at the base of the thumb. Semin Arthroplasty 1991; 2(2):120–129;[180] and Brunelli G, Monini L, Brunelli F. Stabilisation of the trapezio-metacarpal joint. J Hand Surg Br 1989;14(2):209–212.)

(normal) in stage III. However, in stage IV, there is pantrapezial arthritis with STT joint involvement in addition to those changes seen in stage III *(Fig. 20.17)*.[179]

Nonoperative treatment

Splinting alone may be effective in early stage disease. Reconstructive procedures aimed at providing pain relief, as well as restoring thumb motion and strength are usually necessary in the later stages. Regardless of stage at presentation, all patients should undergo a trial of conservative management prior to operative intervention. This includes activity modification, splinting, non-steroidal anti-inflammatory drugs (NSAIDs), and steroid injections.

Teaching patients to avoid aggravating activities of the thumb improves their pain control and overall function.[182] Patients should be advised to avoid twisting, lifting, gripping and pinching movements. Joint protection by dividing stress among multiple hand joint and using assistive devices preserves the integrity of the joint structure and improves joint function both in the short and the long terms.[183,184] Patients may be taught home hand exercises that aim to strengthen the thenar muscles, the abductor pollicis longus and the extensor pollicis longus (EPL). These exercises counter the flexion-adduction force of the adductor pollicis muscle, prevent adduction contracture of the first web space, and improve grip strength and global hand function.[183,185,186] The use of a joint protection arthritis education program with educational-behavioral teaching methods has proven beneficial in adherence, pain, disease status and functional ability in arthritis patients.[184] Such strengthening exercises, however, should only be recommended to patients with early stage OA without significant pain.

Splinting rests the joint and holds it in a position of maximum surface contact, thus increasing joint stability and diminishing mechanical stress.[187,188] This often decreases the associated acute inflammation and pain enough that an adequate level of function returns. A long opponens splint holds

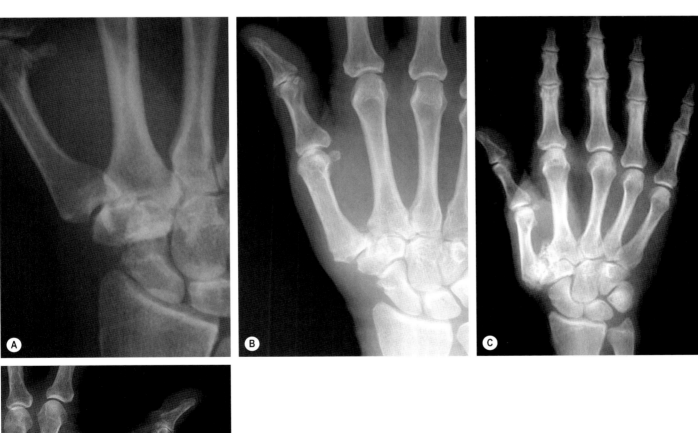

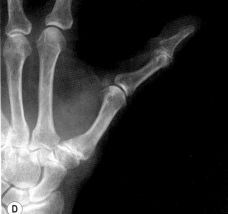

Fig. 20.17 Radiographs of Eaton stage I-IV TMC OA. **(A)** An example of stage I arthritis and displays a slightly widened TMC joint space due to ongoing synovitis. **(B)** An example of stage II arthritis with joint space narrowing and small osteophyte formation. **(C)** An example of stage III showing significant joint destruction and osteophyte formation but preservation of the STT joint. **(D)** An example of stage IV arthritis with narrowing and arthrosis at both the TMC and STT joints.

the thumb in palmar abduction with the MP joint in 30° of flexion and pronation and the wrist in 15° of extension. This shifts the center of pressure dorsally and away from the palmar side of the CMC joint that is susceptible to OA.[188] A short opponens splint by definition does not immobilize the wrist. A modified short splint that only immobilizes the CMC is also commercially available.[187] Although the long and short splints are equally effective, patients tend to prefer the less bulky design of the short splints.[189] Splints may be prefabricated neoprene or custom-fitted thermoplast.[190,191] While some authorities prefer the individualization and rigidity offered by the custom-fitted thermoplast splints,[191] neoprene splints offer greater pain relief and are generally preferred by patients over the more rigid splints.[190] Patients are instructed to wear the splints whenever they feel basal thumb pain whether it is day or night.[190] After 3–4 weeks, patients may notice a decreasing need for splinting. Recently, however, a randomized European trial suggested that patients with thumb CMC OA may need to be splinted longer (several months) before one can actually see significant improvement in their overall pain and disability.[192]

Medical therapy for basal thumb OA includes NSAIDs and intra-articular steroids. Systemic and topical NSAIDs help reduce synovitis, but they do not halt or reverse disease progression. There is no difference in the effectiveness of currently available NSAIDs.[193] Intra-articular steroid injections can be used to resolve synovitis refractory to activity modification, splinting, and NSAID therapy. When followed by three weeks of splinting, a 40% success rate for subjective symptom improvement has been reported.[194] While steroid injections seem to offer short term pain relief in early basal thumb OA,[195] their long-term effectiveness is uncertain.[196] Steroid injections should not be more often two to three times a year and should be used cautiously in very early stage disease as they can potentially accelerate arthritic degeneration. As demonstrated in a small 2004 randomized controlled trial, patients with stage IV disease are unlikely to benefit from steroid injections.[153] With increasing evidence that hyaluronic acid contributes to joint hemostasis[197] and reduces pain in patients with knee OA,[198] investigators have studies injections of hyaluronic acid into the thumb CMC joint. While studies suggest that hyaluronic acid may result in some basal thumb pain relief, there is no evidence that its effectiveness is superior to that of steroids.[199] Interestingly, a recent prospective, randomized, double-blinded trial[200] studying hyaluronic acid and steroid injections found no improvement in pain, strength, range of motion, or disability with either when compared with placebo. However, this study did not exclude patients with advanced stage disease, and follow-up was limited to 26 weeks.

The technique for CMC injection is straight-forward, however advanced disease associated with large osteophytes and distorted anatomy may present a challenge. The landmark for thumb CMC joint injections is the dorsoradial aspect of the proximal end of the first metacarpal.[191] The thumb is opposed against the little finger so that the proximal end of the first metacarpal is palpable. Traction is applied to the thumb in order to widen the CMC joint space. The CMC joint is then injected using a 25-gauge needle. The needle is inserted at a point proximal to the prominence at the base of the first metacarpal on the palmar side of the extensor pollicis brevis and the abductor pollicis longus tendons. The needle is

advanced distally until it penetrates the joint capsule.[191] Fluoroscopy can be used if the joint anatomy is distorted. The anatomical snuffbox should be avoided because it contains the radial artery and superficial radial nerve. Several corticosteroid preparations are commercially available. Betamethasone is water soluble and does not leave intra-articular precipitates behind.[191] About 1.5 milliliters of a 50/50 mix of betamethasone and 1% lidocaine without epinephrine may be used.[191]

Surgical procedures for stage I disease

Surgery for TM arthritis is indicated in patients with persistent pain, instability, and decreased function refractory to conservative therapy. The type of procedure used is dictated by disease severity, depending primarily on whether the cartilage of the CMC joint is unaffected (stage I) or shows signs of degeneration (stages II–IV). Attritional changes in the beak ligament cause hypermobility and synovitis that precede any cartilaginous degeneration.[201] The palmar articular cartilage neighboring the beak ligament is subject to compressive forces in early disease.[202] Attrition of the beak ligament results in dorsal translation of the contact area with subsequent cartilage degeneration.[202] The goal of surgery in early stage of disease is to stabilize the joint, preventing further subluxation, and to offload the palmar cartilage, preventing further degeneration.[203] Surgical procedures that are appropriate for such early stage CMC arthritis include arthroscopy, metacarpal abduction-extension osteotomy, and volar ligament reconstruction.

Thumb CMC arthroscopy

Not only is arthroscopy diagnostic in cases of basal thumb arthritis, but also it can serve as primary therapy in early disease or as adjunctive therapy in advanced stages.[204,205] Thumb CMC arthroscopy is viewed as a less invasive therapeutic intervention. Synovectomy, debridement, and thermal shrinkage capsulorraphy of the beak ligament may all be performed arthroscopically. Synovectomy and debridement are appropriate for early stage disease that failed conservative therapy.[204,205] Arthroscopic intervention is not recommended for more advanced disease with significant cartilage loss. Menon[206] described arthroscopic interposition arthroplasty (using tendon, fascia lata, or Gore-Tex® patch) with excellent results. Badia, however, cautions against arthroscopic interposition arthroplasty for stage 3 disease in young, active patients (who may benefit more from arthrodesis) and in low-demand patients (who may benefit more from trapeziectomy with or without ligament reconstruction).[204,205]

Thumb CMC arthroscopy is usually performed under regional anesthesia with tourniquet control.[204,205] A total of 5–8 pounds of longitudinal traction is applied on the thumb using a single finger trap. Joint distension is achieved by injecting 5 mL of normal saline into the joint under direct palpation. A radial portal (1-R) and an ulnar portal (1-U) are usually needed. The radial portal is placed just radial to the APL tendon, and the ulnar one is placed ulnar to EPL tendon. The DRL, posterior oblique ligament, and the ulnar collateral ligament are best evaluated using the radial portal. The ulnar portal allows for better assessment of the beak ligament.[204,205]

A short barrel, 1.9 mm 30° arthroscope and a full-radius shaver with suction are utilized.[204,205] A radiofrequency probe may be used to perform the synovectomy, the chondroplasty (in cases with focal cartilage wear), or the thermal capsulorraphy (in patients with ligamentous laxity). Performing an arthroscopic trapeziectomy in stage 3 disease requires burring away the articular cartilage and removing subchondral bone down to a bleeding surface. This increases joint space and allows for hematoma formation, optimizing tendon graft placement and adherence. A volar slip of APL or palmaris longus may be used as a tendon graft and is inserted into the joint space via a portal. The joint is protected in a thumb spica splint for 1–5 weeks depending on the pathology and the intervention.[204,205]

Dorsal wedge extension osteotomy

The volar compartment of the CMC joint is where compressive forces localize when the thumb is in its functional position of flexion and adduction.[202] One way to unload this compartment in early disease is to perform a dorsal, closing wedge osteotomy of the thumb metacarpal that extends and abducts the metacarpal away from the trapezial joint surface. Pellegrini and his colleagues[207] were the first to evaluate the biomechanical efficacy of a 30° dorsal wedge osteotomy. Their data suggested that the procedure is successful at offsetting the subluxing forces acting on the base of the metacarpal. This procedure was found to not only shift the joint load dorsally[207] but also tighten the dorsoradial ligament and reduce overall joint laxity.[208] In a cadaveric model of extension osteotomy, Shrivastava et al. demonstrated that the procedure reduced laxity in all directions (40% reduction in the dorsal-volar direction, 23% reduction in the radial-ulnar direction, 15% reduction when distracted, and 15% reduction in pronation-supination).[208] Because of the changes it creates in the articular forces, the procedure is contraindicated in cases of global joint instability and cases of nonreducible subluxation.

The technique for a dorsal wedge extension osteotomy is described by Tomaino.[209,210] After establishing regional anesthesia and Esmarch bandage exsanguination, tourniquet control is applied, and a 3 cm dorsal incision is made from the base of the thumb metacarpal distally. The dorsal sensory branch of the radial nerve and lateral antebrachial cutaneous nerve as well as the extensor pollicis longus tendon are identified and protected. The CMC joint is identified using a 25-gauge needle. A transverse arthrotomy may be performed to document normal joint surfaces if the radiographs are questionable or if there is crepitance on examination.[209,210] One centimeter distal to the joint, subperiosteal, circumferential dissection of the metacarpal is obtained. Using a microsagittal saw, a partial transverse osteotomy is performed in this location down to the volar cortex. A new saw blade is used to make a 30° osteotomy 5 mm distal to the first one. The two osteotomies are connected at the volar cortex completing a dorsally-based 30° wedge of bone that is removed. The distal metacarpal is extended and compressed against the base. The reduction is secured in place with K-wires[210] or two 11 × 8 staples.[209] Plates or tension band technique can be used for fixation as well. The periosteum and skin is then closed, and a thumb spica splint is placed for 10 days. A thumb spica cast (with the interphalangeal joint left free) is then placed for an additional four weeks. At around 6 weeks postoperatively, the cast is replaced with a forearm-based thumb spica Orthoplast splint, and the patient is instructed to start gentle TM motion.[209] Osteotomies heal at an average of 7 weeks.[210] Unless union is delayed, grip and pinch exercises are started 8 weeks postoperatively.[209]

Pain relief and improved hand function following extension osteotomy is likely related to both load transfer and increased joint stability. Some 80% of patients have good–excellent long-term pain relief.[203] At 2.1-year follow-up, grip and pinch strengths increase by an average of 8.5 and 3.0 kg, respectively.[210] At 6.8-year follow-up, 82% of patients have normal grip and pinch strengths.[203] This procedure also has the added benefit of correcting any adduction contracture that may be present. Overall long-term patient satisfaction with this procedure is reported at 91–93%.[203,210]

Volar ligament reconstruction

Since volar ligamentous laxity contributes to CMC joint instability and degenerative disease progression, early basal thumb OA can be addressed surgically by reconstructing the volar ligaments. Eaton and Littler described a technique for reconstructing the volar ligaments by passing the radial half of the FCR tendon through the base of the thumb metacarpal and then suturing it to the APL tendon. The procedure was initially described for the treatment of late disease;[179] however subsequent reports have confirmed the efficacy of the procedure in early disease.[211,212] This procedure is viewed by many as the first of choice for early disease when there is only early chondromalacia.[212] The presence of STT OA precludes use of this procedure.[211,212] This technique has been reported to slow the radiographic progression of the disease in up to 94% of female patients at 15-year follow-up.[212] This compares favorably with the 17% reported radiographic prevalence of stage III-IV disease in post-menopausal women in the general population.[156] While it eliminates long-term pain in only 29% of patients, patients with persistent pain tend to have only mild pain and are generally satisfied with the procedure.[212] The technique appears to be less effective in men and patients involved in worker compensation claims.[212]

Technique for Eaton–Littler procedure

Adequate thumb CMC joint exposure for volar ligament reconstruction usually necessitates a modified Wagner incision, which is a longitudinal incision that is located parallel to the long axis of the thumb metacarpal at the interval between the glabrous palmar and nonglabrous dorsal skin (Fig. 20.18).[213] The dorsal sensory branch of the radial nerve and branches of the lateral antebrachial cutaneous nerve crossing the operative field must be identified and protected. The radial edge of thenar muscles is elevated extraperiosteally off the metacarpal, exposing the trapezium, the metacarpal base and the CMC joint. The interval between EPL and extensor pollicis brevis is developed to expose the dorsal cortex of the metacarpal base. Using handheld awls or a cannulated drill over a K-wire, a tunnel is made in the metacarpal base in a dorsal to volar direction (perpendicular to the axis of the thumbnail, one centimeter distal to the dorsal surface of the joint aiming volarly just distal to the insertion of the beak ligament, and parallel to the articular surface). A 28-gauge stainless steel wire, or Huston tendon passer, is passed through the

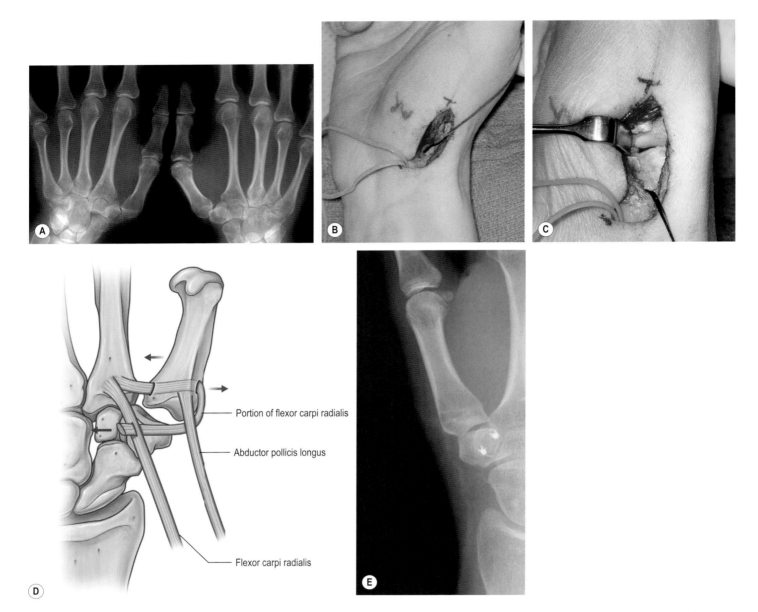

Fig. 20.18 Stress views of a 28-year-old female with right thumb pain and grade I radiographic changes **(A)**, showing evidence of joint instability of the right TMC joint. **(B)** The patient elected to undergo an Eaton–Little procedure for stabilization of the TMC joint. The procedure is performed through a modified Wagner incision, which is a longitudinal incision parallel to the long axis of the thumb, in the interval between the glabrous and nonglabrous skin. **(C)** Vessel loop is around the radial artery. The TMC joint is easily exposed through the incision. **(D)** A strip of the FCR is then passed through a bone tunnel parallel to the base of the thumb metacarpal. **(E)** An AP radiograph of the thumb showing restoration of TMC joint congruity.

tunnel from volar to dorsal and is used to pass the tendon through the bone.[213]

After incising the FCR tendon sheath longitudinally, the ulnar half of the FCR tendon is split longitudinally with a heavy suture.[213] The tendon slip is harvested using multiple transverse incisions on the volar forearm from the level of the wrist to the level of the musculotendinous junction. The tendon is divided proximally and delivered through the subfascial plane into the distal incision. The split is completed distally to the level of the trapezium. The FCR tendon slip is then delivered through the metacarpal base in a volar to dorsal direction using the previously placed wire or tendon

passer. After the tension is set, the tendon is secured to the periosteum of the dorsal cortex using 3-0 braided synthetic suture. The tendon is then secured beneath the APL tendon. The remaining tendon is directed volarly, looped around the FCR tendon, sutured to the FCR tendon, and finally redirected dorsally where it is sutured beneath the APL tendon. Although not absolutely necessary, the CMC joint may be further secured with K-wires. Finally, the thenar muscles are reapproximated, and the skin is closed.[213]

Postoperatively, the thumb is immobilized in a short arm thumb-spica cast for 4 weeks.[213] After that, the thumb is protected in a thermoplast long opponens splint which is removed for hand therapy. Active and active-assisted range of motion of wrist, thumb CMC, MP, and interphalangeal joints are performed in hand therapy.[213] Palmar abduction is started before radial abduction. During the first 2 weeks out of cast, opposition and flexion to the index and long fingers are encouraged. Strengthening is begun after four weeks of cast removal. This is started with minimal resistance putty and then gradually increased to unrestricted activity by 3 months postoperatively.[213]

Procedures for stage II–IV disease

In stage II–IV disease, there is loss of articular cartilage. In such cases joint salvage will not provide adequate pain relief. Surgical procedures to manage more advance disease can be grouped into four major categories, which include: (1) trapeziectomy; (2) trapeziectomy with soft tissue arthroplasty; (3) arthrodesis, and (4) Replacement of the TM joint (prosthetic arthroplasty). The goal of surgery is to reduce pain while maintaining thumb strength and motion.

Trapeziectomy alone

Complete excision of the trapezium is the earliest described surgical procedure for CMC arthritis. It was first described by Gervis in 1947 at the Royal Society of Medicine.[214] His work was published the next year in the *Postgraduate Medical Journal*.[215] The procedure has been shown to be effective at resolving joint pain.[216–218] The improvement in thumb pain allows for improvement in hand function despite some loss in grip and pinch strengths. Historical concerns with this procedure include the possibility of proximal migration of the thumb metacarpal producing painful metacarpo-scaphoid impingement[219–222] and thumb instability.[217,223,224] This has led to the development of stabilization and suspensionplasty procedures in an attempt to return more thumb stability and prevent trapezial supsidence.[222] Loss of trapezial space height has not been directly correlated with loss of grip or pinch strength.[219,220] In addition prospective studies have failed to show any difference in function or metacarpal subsidence when comparing simple trapeziectomy to soft tissue procedures[225,226] while partial trapeziectomy can be done, excising the whole bone is important in cases of STT disease.

Surgical technique for simple trapeziectomy

A dorsal approach to the thumb is usually employed.[221,227] Blunt dissection is undertaken down to the first dorsal compartment and then continued dorso-ulnarly to the radial artery. The artery and radial sensory nerves are dissected off the underlying CMC joint. The joint space can be identified by palpation and opened with a longitudinal capsulotomy that is ulnar to the first dorsal compartment, starting 5 mm on the metacarpal base and extending proximally until the scapho-trapezial joint is encountered. Longitudinal traction on the thumb may help visualization in cases of severe subluxation. The trapezium is identified by visualization of the saddle joint and the metacarpal base. Confirmation may be obtained with fluoroscopy. The trapezium is removed piecemeal from within the surrounding capsule using a rongeur, a knife, an elevator or an osteotome. Attention to the FCR tendon at the base of the wound is paramount to avoid inadvertent injury. The wound is irrigated, and all small bone fragments are removed before closing the capsule and skin.[221,227]

Postoperatively, the thumb is immobilized for 6 weeks, after which the patients are instructed to start range of motion exercises as they wean from using an elastic bandage splint over the course of 4 days.[227] The activity is advanced as tolerated over another ten days. Patients who, at that point, cannot touch the small finger metacarpal head with the tip of their thumb are referred to hand therapy.[227]

A variation of the simple trapeziectomy approach is trapeziectomy and distraction arthroplasty, also referred to as *hematoma arthroplasty*, as blood is thought to fill the space left by the removed trapezium, eventually forming scar.[221,227] A standard trapeziectomy is performed followed by temporary K-wire fixation of the thumb in a position of distraction, palmar abduction, and opposition for about 4 weeks. A single 1.6 mm (0.062 inch) K-wire is inserted percutaneously through the thumb and index metacarpal bases. The fixation is intended to promote dense hematoma formation and scarring in the area of the excised trapezium, hence reducing thumb subsidence. Transverse wire placement is preferred over a longitudinal as the latter may allow the thumb metacarpal to slide proximally along the wire into the trapeziectomy space.[221,227]

Unfortunately, as reported by Gray and Meals in 2007,[218] such fixation does not seem to prevent thumb subsidence. However, the procedure is associated with an 82% rate of pain resolution with an average of 11% and 21% increase in pinch and grip strengths, respectively. These results are equivalent to that of the more complex tendon interposition techniques. Despite its effectiveness, unless the patient is a low-demand elderly patient who does not have metacarpal subluxation,[228] some authorities do not recommend hematoma arthroplasty as a primary treatment and suggest that it be avoided in young patients who require strong grasp and pinch strengths for work.[217,229] However, recent comparative studies and a Cochrane review recommend trapeziectomy alone for the treatment of CMC arthritis since outcomes are similar among the different techniques but complications and cost are lower with trapeziectomy alone.[225,226,230]

Trapeziectomy with ligament reconstruction and/or tendon interposition

Several procedures for tendon interposition arthroplasty are available. These procedures consist of a complete or partial trapeziectomy and interposition of tendinous tissue in the trapeziectomy void. The different operations described for biological arthroplasty are distinguished by: (1) the choice of tendon used to fill the trapeziectomy void and prevent thumb subsidence, and (2) the choice of method used to stabilize the thumb following trapeziectomy. An attempt to reconstruct the intermetacarpal ligament anchoring the thumb metacarpal to the index metacarpal is known as *suspension arthroplasty*.

Video 1

Froimson's fascial arthroplasty is one of the first described interposition arthroplasties that did not include any element of ligament reconstruction. After a standard trapeziectomy, half of the FCR tendon is harvested, rolled up in an "anchovy" fashion, and used to fill the trapeziectomy space. Froimson[231] reported a 90% rate of pain relief at 88-month mean follow-up, but pinch power was reduced by 30%. Radiographically, the procedure resulted in a 50% decrease in the interval between the first metacarpal base and the scaphoid, but clinically the thumb shortening was minimal.[231]

Burton and Pelligrini[229] described a thumb ligament reconstruction performed with the radial half of the FCR tendon routed through the base of the thumb metacarpal, and the remaining length of the tendon was placed in the trapeziectomy void. This procedure has become known as the *ligament reconstruction and tendon interposition procedure* or LRTI and is one of the most common trapeziectomy soft tissue reconstructive procedures performed *(Fig. 20.19)*. At a mean 2-year follow-up, grip and pinch strengths increased19% compared with preoperative values.[229] At 9-year follow-up, thumb function improved further (grip strength 93%, tip-pinch strength 65%, and key-pinch 34%), suggesting that the procedure is not only durable but also improves thumb function for several years postoperatively.[232] Loss of trapezial space averaged 11% at 2 years[229] and 13% at 9 years postoperatively,[232] despite the interposition of a portion of the FCR tendon.

Another variation on LRTI is the Brunelli procedure.[181] Described in 1989, Brunelli utilized one of the slips of the APL tendons for the ligament reconstruction. The tendon is divided proximally, leaving its insertion intact. It is then passed through a tunnel created in the base of the thumb and index metacarpals and sutured to the second and third carpometacarpal ligaments. Tendon interposition may be achieved using a palmaris longus graft. Like ligament reconstruction with FCR, this form of ligament reconstruction has also been advocated for use in early (stage I) disease without performing a trapeziectomy.[181]

Other modifications to the trapeziectomy procedure have included the use of tendon slings or *suspensionplasties*. Suspensionplasties are thought to resist the sagittal plane collapse that occurs when the weakened arthritic thumb is loaded during pinch.[222] Weilby described a suspensionplasty that avoids the use of bony tunnels by simply weaving a slip of FCR around the APL and remaining FCR in a figure of eight fashion (see *Fig. 20.23*).[233] The procedure has been reported to relieve pain in 92% patients.[234] It affects thumb mobility in 12% patients, and while it improves grip and pinch strengths, recovery usually takes three to six months.[234]

Exposure for the Weilby suspensionplasty is accomplished using the modified Wagner incision previously described. The radial artery and sensory nerve are identified and protected. A radial slip of FCR is released at the level of its myotendinous junction and freed all the way distally to base of the metacarpal. A capsulotomy of the CMC joint is performed and followed by a trapeziectomy. If the scapho-trapezoidal joint appears arthritic on traction of the index and long fingers, a proximal trapeziectomy is performed.[222] The thumb is then held in distraction and radial abduction making sure the base of the first metacarpal is in line with the base of the second metacarpal. The slip of the FCR is then passed through a slit

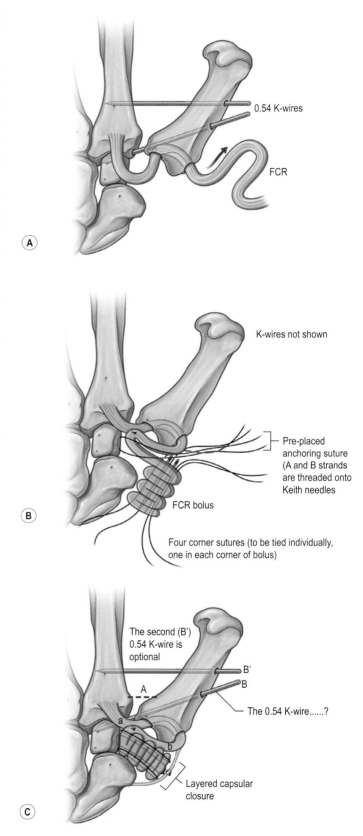

Fig. 20.19 The Burton and Pelligrini procedure begins with the removal of the trapezium, followed by the harvest of a portion of the FCR tendon. The tendon is passed through a drill hole created in the base of the metacarpal. The tendon is passed through the drill hole in a volar to dorsal direction. The remaining tendon end is then sewn to itself to stabilize the metacarpal base of the thumb. The remaining tendon is then placed into the space left by the resected trapezium to function as an interpositional spacer.

in the APL tendon. The tendon is then secured at its insertion through the APL. The remaining tendon is then passed in a figure of eight fashion around the APL and remaining FCR to form a firm sling at the base of the metacarpal. The tendon construct is secured with sutures and then the capsule and skin are closed.[233] This procedure may be performed alternatively with a slip of the APL passed through a slit in the FCR *(Fig. 20.20).*[235]

At around 10 days postoperatively, the thumb spica splint is replaced by a cast for another 3 weeks.[222] The patient is placed in a custom-made thumb spica splint when range of motion exercises are started at around 4 weeks postoperatively. Strengthening and opposition across the palm are delayed until around 8 weeks postoperatively. The splint is then weaned by 10 weeks.[222]

Despite variation in surgical technique, there seems to be minimal outcome differences between simple trapeziectomy, trapeziectomy with ligament reconstruction, and LRTI. When compared in a 2004 prospective randomized trial,[236] no difference in grip strength, pinch strength or thumb subsidence was noted at 8.2-month follow-up between patients who underwent trapeziectomy and ligament reconstruction alone and patients who underwent ligament interposition as well. A more recent Cochrane review[230] included nine studies involving 477 patients undergoing various procedures for basal thumb OA. The review concluded that, "while no procedure appears to be superior over another in terms of pain, physical function, patient satisfaction, or range of motion, there is insufficient evidence at this time to be certain." The review, however, did demonstrate that LRTI, when compared to simple trapeziectomy, is associated with 12% more adverse effects (including scar tenderness, tendon adhesion or rupture, sensory change, or Complex Regional Pain Syndrome Type 1). The small number of studies included in this review and the studies' unclear risk of bias have raised some doubts with regards to these results.[230]

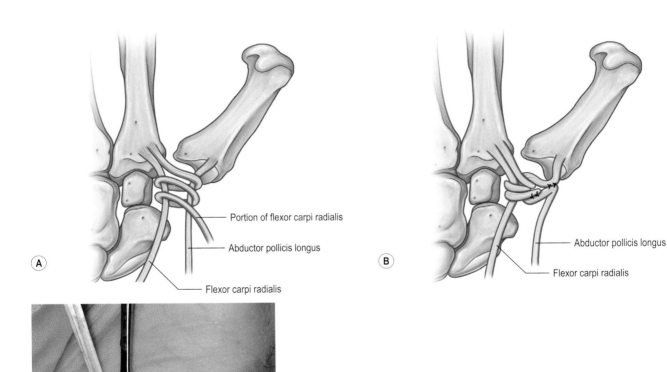

Portion of flexor carpi radialis

Abductor pollicis longus

(A)

Flexor carpi radialis

Abductor pollicis longus

(B)

Flexor carpi radialis

(C)

Fig. 20.20 The Weilby suspensionplasty uses a portion of the FCR to create a sling below the metacarpal base to prevent proximal migration of the thumb. The slip of the FCR is wrapped between the APL and the remaining slip of the FCR **(A,B). (C)** An intraoperative photograph of the weave being started by wrapping the slip of the FCR around the APL tendon.

Prosthetic arthroplasty

Silicone arthroplasty for the TM AO was introduced independently in the late 1960s by Swanson[237] and Niebauer.[238] The procedure had the theoretical advantage of minimizing proximal migration of the thumb metacarpal after trapeziectomy. Early reports showed good results in the short term;[237,239] however longer follow-up noted a high incidence of dorsoradial subluxation.[240] Subluxation continued to be a problem even after modifications in technique and implant design.[237,239,240] Reports of implant wear, silicone synovitis, and bone erosion also started emerging in the late 1980s.[241] With implant wear, investigators noted a 50% loss of implant height (especially on the ulnar border of the implant) at 4-year follow-up.[242] A 16% revision rate for silicone synovitis was also noted.[242] Because of these complications, silicone implant CMC arthroplasty fell out of favor with most surgeons. Recently, however, Bezwada and colleagues[243] showed that osteolysis, implant wear and subluxation did not directly correlate with clinical or subjective outcomes. In their study, they reported an 84% rate of patient satisfaction with and no radiographic evidence of synovitis.

Comparative studies are few, but in 2005, Taylor et al.[216] performed a retrospective comparison between patients undergoing silicone arthroplasty, resection arthroplasty (with and without ligament reconstruction), and arthrodesis for the treatment of TM OA. Taylor found no significant differences in the clinical outcomes between silicone arthroplasty and resection arthroplasty over 5-year period. In this study, the arthrodesis group was found to have a higher reoperation rate.[216] While the follow-up may not be long enough to document clinical deterioration of silicone implants,[244] this study suggests that silicone arthroplasty may be a reliable option for disabling, refractory basal thumb OA, especially in the low demand patient. A newly developed one-piece silicone implant that has been shown to be biomechanically superior to LRTI may expand the current indications for silicone arthroplasty in CMC OA.[245]

Other types of TM arthroplasty have included metallic prostheses mainly of a ball-and-socket design.[246] Constrained TM joint prostheses are more prone to loosening, while nonconstrained prostheses dislocate more easily.[246] The de la Caffiniere implant (ball-and-socket, cemented, semi-constrained prosthesis) is probably the most widely used and most studied.[247] The implant has a cobalt-chromium ball inserted into the shaft of the metacarpal and a polyethylene cup placed in the trapezium. Outcome studies have shown that patients with preoperative complaints of pain or instability do better than those with preoperative stiffness as their major complaint.[247] The implants have a 72–89% 16-year implant survival rate, with higher prevalence of loosening of the trapezial component and a greater need for revisional surgery in working-age men.[248,249] In lieu of a silicone prosthesis, this implant may be considered in women over the age of 60 years for whom joint stiffness is not a main complaint.[246,250]

Other TM joint prostheses have produced high failure rates over time and have fallen from favor due to loosening, heterotopic bone formation and subsidence.[251–253] More recent implant designs have focused on metacarpal resurfacing in hopes of producing a *hemiarthroplasty*. The PyroCarbon metacarpal replacement hemiarthroplasty (Ascension, Austin, TX)

has shown promise in grade II and III disease. Subluxation of the implant, however, is a likely complication if the trapezial cup is made too shallow *(Fig. 20.21)*.[254]

Trapeziometacarpal arthrodesis

With the success of the above reconstructive techniques, arthrodesis is now usually reserved for young (<50 years) high-demand patients who wish to maintain grip strength or as a salvage procedure for failed reconstructions. Although a previous report has suggested that mild pantrapezial arthritis is not an absolute contraindication for TM arthrodesis,[255] most authorities feel that the procedure should not be preformed in the setting of STT arthritis.[256–258] The optimal position to fuse the joint is 35° of radial and palmar abduction with 15° pronation and 10° of extension.[259] This position replicates the position of the thumb in a fully clenched fist with the distal phalanx of the thumb resting on the middle phalanx of the index finger. Methods for CMC arthrodesis include slotted bone grafts, cerclage wiring, tension band wiring, staples, K-wire fixation, and screw fixation.[259] Screw and plate fixation

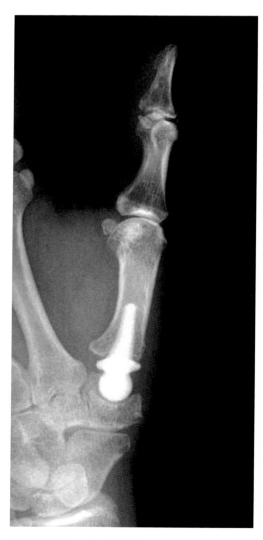

Fig. 20.21 Example of a PyroCarbon arthroplasty of the thumb TMC joint.

has a higher rate of complications requiring hardware removal.[260]

Technique for arthrodesis

The surgical exposure for CMC arthrodesis *(Fig. 20.22)* is similar to that of a trapeziectomy. The base of the thumb metacarpal is delivered into the incision by flexing and adducting the shaft.[259] The eburnated articular cartilage and bone of the trapezium and metacarpal base are removed, exposing the cancellous bone. Surfaces are molded to allow for maximum bone contact between the two ends. If K-wires are being used, three 0.045 wires are usually needed with one wire placed parallel to the long axis of the bones and the other two crossing at 15° to the axis. The K-wires should not extend proximal to the trapezium unless the trapezium is too osteopenic to hold stable fixation. K-wires are usually removed 6–8 weeks postoperatively. Postoperatively, patients are immobilized in a thumb spica until fusion is confirmed radiographically.[259]

Successful fusion will result in diminished thumb opposition and an inability to lay the hand flat.[259] Normal MP and ST joints, however, can compensate well for this limitation to allow for a functional thumb range of motion post-fusion. Post-fusion, MP joint and ST joint motions can increase by 75% and 25%, respectively.[256]

Common complications of CMC arthrodesis include nonunion, progression to peritrapezial arthritis, and symptomatic hardware requiring removal.[259] Radial sensory neuritis may also occur. Many nonunions are asymptomatic. Symptomatic nonunions may be treated with repeat arthrodesis, simple trapeziectomy, or LRTI.[259] In the literature, radiographic nonunion rates range from 6–12.5%[255,258,261–264] with one study reporting a nonunion rate as high as 50%.[265] There appears to be no correlation between nonunion rates and the use of bone grafts.[266] Rizzo and colleagues recently reported on the outcomes of 126 patients following TM arthrodesis. Over the average follow-up period of 11.2 years, the incidence of radiographic STT arthritis was noted to be 31% and MP arthritis was identified in 12.7% of patients.[266] Despite these high values, none of the patients with radiographic MP arthritis were symptomatic and only 6% of patients with STT arthritis were symptomatic.[266]

Despite its disadvantages and complications, patient satisfaction with TM arthrodesis is usually high with adequate recovery of pinch and grip strength postoperatively. While some have reported satisfaction rates as low as 60–78%,[261,264] most studies report a satisfaction rate >90%.[257,265,267] Although arthrodesis is generally recommended for younger patients, the procedure actually has favorable outcomes in patients over 50 years as well.[268]

OA of the wrist

Etiology

Osteoarthritis of the wrist may be primary (idiopathic) or secondary. Causes of primary OA include avascular necrosis of the lunate or scaphoid (Kienbock's or Preiser's disease, respectively), which can lead to degenerative changes throughout the wrist in later stages.[269,270] Congenital deformities, such as Madelung's deformity, can alter articular load patterns at the ulnocarpal, radiocarpal, and distal radial ulnar joints leading to the development of wrist OA. Perhaps the most common idiopathic OA of the wrist is that involving the scaphotrapezo-trapezoid (STT) joint. Epidemiologic studies note a very high incidence of STT arthritis in the general population. A radiographic and anatomic study by North and Eaton, demonstrated an incidence of STT arthritis in 34% of wrists.[271] Another cadaver study reported the incidence of STT arthritis in 83% of cadaver wrists.[272]

Secondary causes of osteoarthritis of the wrist usually are related to trauma, with scapholunate ligamentous injury, distal radius fractures, and united scaphoid fractures contributing most frequently to the development of secondary radio-carpal OA. Scapholunate interosseus ligament injury can lead to a progressive form of carpal instability which may lead to the development of *scapholunate advanced collapse* (SLAC) arthrtis.[273,274] In 1984, Watson and Ballet published a review of a 121 wrist radiographs with degenerative arthritis due to scapholunate advanced collapse, termed SLAC wrist.[273] This pattern accounted for 55% of all wrists with degenerative changes and was the most common pattern of wrist arthritis.

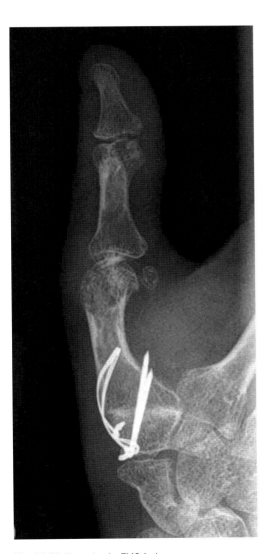

Fig. 20.22 Example of a TMC fusion.

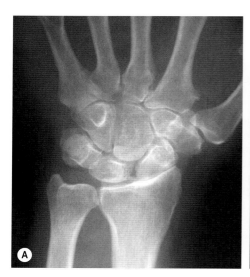
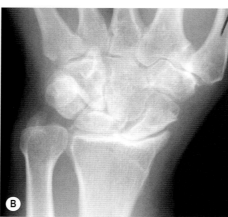
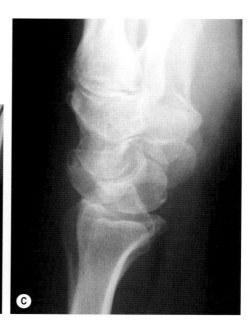

Fig. 20.23 Examples of SLAC arthritis. **(A)** An example of stage II SLAC changes. There is evidence of advanced arthritis at the radial styloid and radioscaphoid fossa, but the midcarpal joint is still relatively free of arthritic changes. **(B)** A PA radiograph of a wrist with stage III SLAC changes. In addition to arthritis at the scaphoid fossa, there is narrowing of the capitolunate articulation, and midcarpal arthritis. **(C)** A lateral wrist radiograph in the same patient showing significant midcarpal instability with a DISI pattern.

They found that arthritis initially involved the radial styloid (stage 1) and scaphoid waist then progressed to involve the proximal scaphoid and scaphoid fossa of the radius (stage 2) with arthritis finally being identified in the midcarpal joint at the lunocapitate articulation (stage 3).[273] Other authors have added a fourth stage which describes pan-carpal arthritis with diffuse involvement of the radiocarpal and midcarpal joints, with or without involvement of the distal radioulnar joint *(Fig. 20.23)*.[275–277]

The important point to note about SLAC arthritis is that the radiolunate joint is typically spared.[274–279] However, a recent publication by Lane et al. suggests that in a minority of cases (5–6% of SLAC wrists), the lunate fossa may be arthritic as well.[280] For this reason, it is important to assess the lunate fossa before committing to a particular reconstruction.

Wrist or forearm fracture can also lead to osteoarthritis of the wrist. The cause can be related directly to damage to the articular surface of the joint with an intra-articular fracture, with or without malunion. Alternatively, extra-articular distal radius fractures can result in malunion leading to abnormal joint wear.[281,282] Extra-articular distal radius fracture malunion can result in radial shortening, loss of radial inclination, loss of volar tilt, supination of the distal fragment, or radial or ulnar translation of the distal fragment. Each of these malunion patterns can result in abnormal load patterns across the wrist or adaptive malalignment deformities that can resemble instability patterns.[281,283] The end result of the abnormal load and wear may be osteoarthritis. In a classic report of intra-articular distal radius fractures, Knirk and Jupiter report 91% incidence of arthritis on late follow-up if there was any degree of articular step-off after fracture reduction and 100% incidence of arthritis (8/8) if there was >2 mm stepoff of the articular surface.[284] Only 11% of those wrists with a congruent articular reduction developed arthritis at late followup. The presence of wrist arthritis within this study adversely affected the clinical outcome.

The final major cause of wrist OA is the sequelae of untreated or mal-united scaphoid fractures. It is estimated that between 5% and 10% of all scaphoid fractures will fail to heal.[285] Scaphoid nonunion can lead to a pattern of carpal instability similar to that seen with scapholunate ligament injury.[286] Like the SLAC wrist, scaphoid nonunion can lead to wrist arthritis in a predictable pattern and is termed *scaphoid nonunion advanced collapse* (SNAC) arthritis.[279,285,287] There are three stages of SNAC arthritis that have been adapted from the description by Ruby et al.: Stage I involves arthritis at the radial styloid- and scaphoid articulation;[279,287,288] stage II involves progressive degeneration of the radioscaphoid articulation and scaphocapitate joint; stage III includes the pathology found in stages I and II but with progression to include the lunocapitate articulation *(Fig. 20.24)*.[279,288]

Patient evaluation

Evaluation of the patient with suspected wrist arthritis begins with a careful history and physical examination. Important aspects of the history include the mechanism of original injury, quality and location of the pain, and exacerbating and alleviating factors. It is important to note what measures the patient has already tried to treat the pain, such as splinting, steroid injection or NSAIDs. It is important to determine the degree to which the pain is affecting the patient's lifestyle and work, as this will dictate the decision to treat with nonoperative methods or proceed to wrist salvage. This is an important consideration as surgery may require a significant investment by the patient in terms of time off work due to immobilization and a potential loss of wrist motion. For these reasons, it is often advisable to see the patient

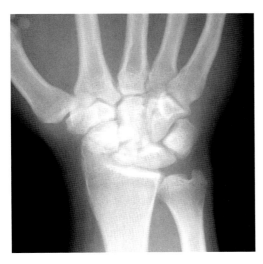

Fig. 20.24 A PA wrist radiograph of a patient with stage II SNAC arthritis.

on more than one occasion and sometimes follow them for years before embarking on a reconstruction. In the meantime, pain is managed with nonoperative means such as splinting, NSAIDs (oral and/or topical), and periodic steroid injections.

A critical evaluation of PA and lateral wrist radiographs is essential. In doing so, one should get a sense of the etiology of the OA, whether secondary or primary. One must note which articulations are involved and which are spared as this will dictate what surgical options are available, i.e., involvement of the lunocapitate articulation in the SLAC wrist. Involvement of the lunocapitate articulation should give one pause before proceeding with a proximal row carpectomy reconstruction as this will leave an arthritic capitate head behind to articulate with the lunate fossa. In this situation, a mid-carpal fusion, such as a scaphoidectomy and 4-corner fusion may be more appropriate. Further imaging such as a CT scan, MRI, or bone scan is not part of the routine evaluation, but may be indicated in select situations to evaluate for early signs of midcarpal arthritis. Another helpful diagnostic adjunct is a selective injection of lidocaine with or without steroid into the joint in question. This test can be potentially useful for diagnosis as well as treatment. A study by Bell et al. looked at the diagnostic utility of midcarpal lidocaine (with or without corticosteroid) injection in patients with chronic wrist pain.[289] They noted that patients with chronic wrist pain had an improvement in grip strength with the injection, whereas normal volunteers had a reduction in grip strength. In addition, those patients with an improvement of >6 kg or >28% improvement over baseline had a 73% sensitivity and 70% specificity of having intracarpal pathology at arthroscopy.

Surgical treatment

Surgery is directed at elimination of pain at the arthritic joint through debridement (radial styloidectomy), denervation (neurectomy), arthroplasty, or partial or total wrist arthrodesis. The specific treatment is carefully selected based on the patient's symptoms, expectations, pattern of arthritis, and functional demands. Biomechanical data is available to help predict the range of motion that may be predicted with proximal row carpectomy, mid-carpal joint fusion and radiocarpal joint fusion.[290,291] Based on these studies, mid-carpal fusion can result in a wrist with 50–67% of the motion of the normal side, radiocarpal fusion will provide only 33–40% of contralateral motion. If the distal pole of the scaphoid is removed following a radioscapholunate fusion an additional 15–20% of motion is possible.[276] Proximal row carpectomy can preserve 50–75% of contralateral wrist motion.[276]

Technique for dorsal approach to the wrist

The surgical approach to the wrist should account for the future likelihood of additional procedures should the selected initial treatment option fail. A total wrist fusion represents the ultimate salvage for wrist arthritis. Since this is typically performed through a longitudinal dorsal wrist incision in line with the third metacarpal, this approach is recommended for limited salvage procedures, such as partial wrist arthrodesis. Following the skin incision, full thickness flaps are raised in an ulnar and radial direction. The extensor retinaculum is opened over the third extensor compartment and the extensor pollicis longus tendon is transposed. The retinaculum is raised in a radial and ulnar direction. The second and fourth compartment tendons are retracted and the dorsal wrist capsule is exposed. A ligament sparing incision is made in the capsule (*Fig. 20.25*).[292,293] This incision creates a radially based flap in line with the dorsal radiotriquetral ligament and dorsal intercarpal ligament. This approach gives excellent exposure of the midcarpal joint as well as the scaphoid.

Radial styloidectomy

For patients with early SLAC arthritis where arthritis is confined to the radial styloid, radial styloidectomy may be performed as a conservative palliative procedure, either in isolation or in combination with other another procedure. Radial styloidectomy is usually performed subperiosteally through the anatomic snuffbox. It is important to preserve the volar attachment of the radioscaphocapitate ligament during the procedure which insert to the radial styloid. If more than a 6–10 mm of styloid is removed, the radioscaphocapitate ligament origin will be significantly compromised possible resulting in ulnar translation of the carpus.[294–296] The radial styloid fragment may be used as a bone graft for concomitant fusion procedures.

Neurectomy

Total denervation of the wrist is associated with improved pain without loss of motion and with minimal morbidity and convalescence.[297–299] Partial denervation of the anterior interosseous nerve (AIN) and posterior interosseous nerve (PIN) is possible through a single dorsal incision.[300] This procedure has been shown to provide partial relief of wrist pain in cases of radiocarpal arthritis with at an average of 31 months after surgery.[301] In a study of 20 patients, performed by Weinstein and Berger, only three patients required additional procedures for pain relief following AIN/ PIN neurectomy. Most patients in this study continued to have some wrist pain, but the majority (90%) were significantly improved. Prior to proceeding with neurectomy, patients should undergo

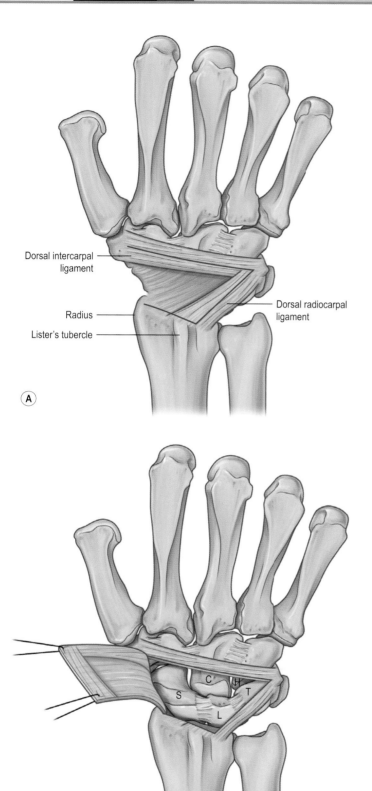

Fig. 20.25 Dorsal exposure to the wrist bones is accomplished through the use of a ligament sparing capsulotomy. **(A)** A triangular shaped flap is designed over the dorsum of the wrist capsule extending from the Lister's tubercle to the triquetrum and back to the upper third of the scaphoid. **(B)** The capsulotomy runs in line with the fibers of the dorsal radioscaphocapitate ligament and the dorsal intercarpal ligament.

a selective AIN/PIN block with long-acting anesthetic to verify that pain relief will be adequate. This allows the patient to assess the level of relief that may be expected from the denervation procedure.[301]

Proximal row carpectomy

Proximal row carpectomy (PRC) is an option when the proximal capitate articular surface and the lunate fossa of the radius are preserved *(Fig. 20.26)*. In other words, there is no arthritis at the mid-carpal joint or radiolunate joint. PRC entails removal of the entire proximal carpal row (scaphoid, lunate, and triquetrum) and results in the wrist functioning as a simple hinge joint. The capitate articulates with the lunate facet of the radius. The radius of curvature of the lunate fossa is larger than that of the capitate head and there is resultant incongruity at the new articulation. This incongruity may lead to articular wear between the capitate head and radius.

Proximal row carpectomy has some advantages over intercarpal fusions. It does not require a lengthy period of immobilization for an arthrodesis to heal. Krakauer et al. have compared proximal row carpectomy with intercarpal fusion.[302] They found that carpectomy preserved better motion, an average arc of 71° versus 54° for limited arthrodesis. Both types of procedure preserved reasonable strength and reduced pain.

There is limited data on long-term outcomes after PRC. Jebson and colleagues reported on 20 patients, 11 of who underwent PRC for osteoarthritis. Two patients in this series required wrist arthrodesis for persistent pain. The remaining 18 patients were evaluated at an average of 13 years following surgery. The average wrist range of motion and the average

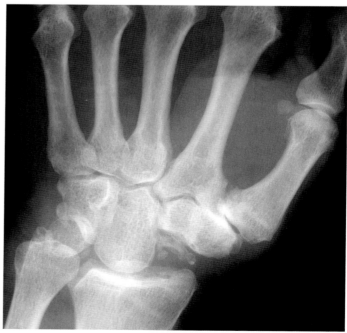

Fig. 20.26 A PA wrist radiograph of a proximal row carpectomy. A PRC involves the removal of the scaphoid, lunate and triquetrum. The lunate fossa of the radius and the articular surface of the capitate should be free of arthritic changes to maximize the outcome of this procedure.

maximal grip strength was 63% and 83%, respectively of the opposite extremity. Sixteen of the 18 patients had returned to their previous employment. Flattening of the capitate was present in 33% of patients and 22% of patients had some evidence of moderate to severe radiocapitate arthrosis. However, this finding did not correlate with patient satisfaction, wrist pain, or function.[303] DiDonna and colleagues have also published similar findings in a long-term outcome study of PRC with a minimum of 10-year follow-up. There were four failures (18%) requiring fusion at an average of 7 years following initial surgery. The average flexion extension arc was 72° with and average grip strength of 91% of the contralateral side. Of the 18 wrists that did not fail, all patients were either satisfied or very satisfied with the procedure with an overall DASH score of 9. Degenerative changes were seen in 14 of 17 wrists at the radiocapitate articulation at follow-up. However, like the findings by Jebson, this did not correlate with symptoms.[304]

Four-corner fusion

Scaphoidectomy and 4-corner fusion represents another method for treating midcarpal and radial sided wrist arthritis (*Fig. 20.27*). This procedure entails excision of the scaphoid and fusion of the mid-carpal joint (lunate, capitate, triquetrum, and hamate). This procedure does not require preservation of the lunocapitate articulation and therefore may be appropriate in more advanced stages of the SLAC/SNAC wrist; however, it does require preservation of the radiolunate articulation.[280] In 1984, Watson presented outcomes of his "SLAC procedure" for the SLAC wrist.[273] Although this SLAC wrist procedure was initially proposed to be used with a silicone

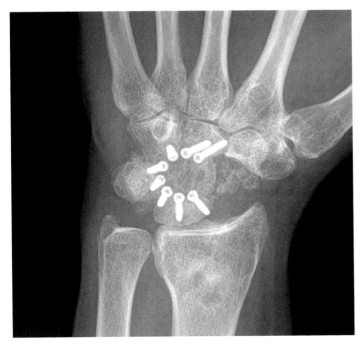

Fig. 20.27 A PA radiograph showing and example of a scaphoidectomy and 4-corner fusion. This wrist salvage option is indicated if there is evidence of arthritis at the midcarpal joint and the scaphoid fossa.

scaphoid implant, scaphoid excision without an implant works equally well and avoids the long-term risk of silicone synovitis. Potential advantages of 4-corner fusion over PRC include the retention of the native radiolunate interface. Preservation of the lunate and capitate preserves carpal height, which arguably maintains the resting muscle tension across the wrist preserving grip strength.[273,274]

Several studies have examined the functional outcome following 4-corner fusion.[302,305–308] Ashmead et al. have provided one of the largest series, reporting on 100 cases. In this series, final wrist flexion –extension arc averaged 53% of the contralateral side and final grip strength averaged 80% of the contralateral side. Nonunion occurred in only 3% of patients. And 51% of patients had total resolution of wrist pain, while 15% continued to have pain with daily activities or at rest.[305]

Techniques ensuring successful outcome have focused on adequate decortication of the four bony surfaces and correction of the dorsiflexed lunate to re-establish a collinear relationship between the lunate and capitate. Failure to correct lunate position can lead to limited wrist extension, hardware abutment and pain.[305,306] The use of bone graft has not been shown to clearly correlate with fusion rates nor has hardware choice; however hardware complications have been noted with pins, staples and circular plates.[302,307,309] In Vance et al.'s study, nonunion and impingement occurred in 48% of cases treated with circular plate fixation in comparison to a 6% rate with traditional fixation (K-wires, staples, or compression screws). Plate fixation was also associated with a higher rate of patient dissatisfaction.[309]

A variation of 4-corner fusion can involve capitolunate arthrodesis alone. Early attempts using this limited arthrodesis were associated with high rates of nonunion, most likely due to a smaller bony contact areas for successful bony fusion.[310–312] These results were significantly improved by Calandruccio and colleagues who combined capitolunate fusion with scaphoid and triquetral excision.[313] This procedure may provide for more wrist motion than four corner fusion but long-term data is still pending.

Total wrist arthrodesis and total wrist arthroplasty

In advanced arthritis where longstanding changes have resulted in injury to the midcarpal joint and the lunate fossa, wrist arthrodesis and wrist arthroplasty may be the only options for wrist salvage. Arthroplasty may be an enticing option because of the potential for motion preservation; however, the normal wrist functions through complicated interactions at multiple articulations across the wrist joints. It is impossible for a prosthesis to duplicate this complexity of motion and strength.[314] Therefore, there is a compromise that occurs for motion at the expense of strength. For these reasons, wrist arthroplasty is carefully selected only for those patients with low demand wrists or who have a fusion of the contralateral wrist.[315] Patients with rheumatoid arthritis as opposed to osteoarthritis of the wrist tend to match the patient profile more appropriately for total wrist arthroplasty. The choice of wrist arthroplasty is dependent on the patient's age, activity level, and status of the contralateral wrist.

Total wrist arthrodesis represents the ultimate salvage procedure for all types of wrist arthritis. It involves fusion of the radiocarpal, midcarpal and third carpometacarpal joint. Total wrist arthrodesis is an established method of achieving pain

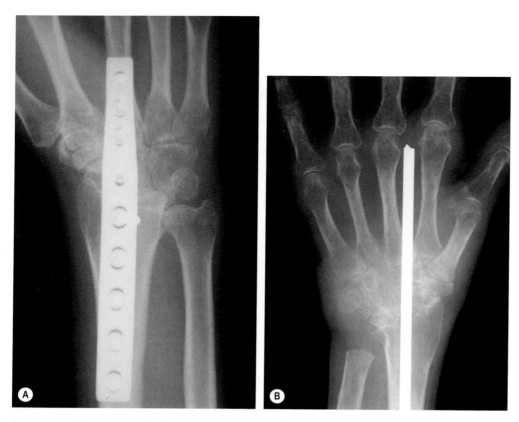

Fig. 20.28 (A) A complete wrist fusion may be accomplished with either the use of a dorsal plate or **(B)** the use of large intramedullary pins.

relief and maintaining strength in patients without alternative options such as those with pan-carpal arthritis. This procedure is typically performed with the use of a dorsal wrist fusion plate, but alternative methods have also been described using pins alone. Because the DRUJ is not involved in a standard wrist fusion forearm rotation is still possible. The ideal position for wrist fusion is in mild extension with mild ulnar deviation.[31] This position maximizes grip strength *(Fig. 20.28)*.

Wrist fusion is usually performed through a dorsal incision centered over the 4th extensor compartment. Decortication of the radiocarpal joint, midcarpal, and third finger CMC joint, have been recommended to obtain solid fusion throughout the carpus. Alternatively a proximal row carpectomy can be performed and the capitate can be fused to the lunate fossa of the radius. This technique can be beneficial for cases of profound wrist contractures, where decreasing the carpal height

may allow for improvement in wrist position; however it dramatically decreases the area of bony contact through which the fusion may occur. Bone graft is not necessary if good opposition between the bone ends is achieved but in difficult cases bone graft may be acquired from the iliac crest, radial styloid or any bones which are removed from the carpus at the time of fusion. During plate fixation, screws are ideally placed within the shaft of the third metacarpal and shaft of the radius. It is often possible to place additional screws into the capitate for additional fixation. Pin fixation, which lacks the rigidity of plate fixation, is usually achieved by placing long Steinmann or Rush pins through the intermetacarpal space of the index/long and long/ring fingers. Following fusion the wrist is placed into plaster immobilization for 6–8 weeks, or until bony consolidation is seen on plain radiographs.

Access the complete reference list online at **http://www.expertconsult.com**

174. Bettinger PC, Linscheid RL, Berger RA, et al. An anatomic study of the stabilizing ligaments of the trapezium and trapeziometacarpal joint. *J Hand Surg Am.* 1999;24(4):786–798.

This article provides a comprehensive and well-illustrated description of the ligaments stabilizing the trapezium and TMC joint. An anatomic study of 37 cadaver hands was performed identifying 16 ligaments with attachments at this important joint. Insertions, fiber orientations and positions

producing ligament tension are described for each ligament. A discussion of the biomechanical role and clinical relevance of the most important ligaments is presented.

212. Freedman DM, Eaton RG, Glickel SZ. Long-term results of volar ligament reconstruction for symptomatic basal joint laxity. *J Hand Surg Am.* 2000;25(2):297–304.

This is a 15 year follow-up study of 24 prearthritic hypermobile trapeziometacarpal (TMC) joints that underwent volar ligament reconstruction for symptomatic ligament laxity, after failed conservative therapy. At final followup, 17 patients (71%) complained of intermittent or daily pain, seven patients (29%) had no pain, and only two joints (8%) progressed to stage III radiographic arthritis. The authors present a thorough review of clinical, radiographic and intraoperative characteristics in relation to long-term clinical and radiographic outcomes of the procedure. They conclude that volar ligament reconstruction is indicated for the painful hypermobile TMC joint and limits the progression of degenerative arthritis.

224. Burton R. Basal joint arthritis. Fusion, implant, or soft tissue reconstruction? *Orthop Clin North Am.* 1986;17(3):493–503.

    This is a review article summarizing the relevant anatomy and clinical features of basal thumb arthritis. The author highlights some of the advantages and disadvantages of several surgical options, and discusses fundamental considerations for successful operative management.

226. Davis TR, Pace A. Trapeziectomy for trapeziometacarpal joint osteoarthritis: is ligament reconstruction and temporary stabilisation of the pseudarthrosis with a Kirschner wire important? *J Hand Surg Eur.* 2009;34(3):312–321.

    This is a randomized prospective study comparing two surgical treatment options for basal thumb arthritis. A total of 61 thumbs underwent trapeziectomy, LRTI, K-wire immobilization and 6 weeks of splinting and 67 thumbs underwent trapeziectomy alone and 3 weeks of immobilization with a soft bandage. Outcome measures included pain, DASH scores, and thumb and grip strengths, which were all assessed at 3 and 12 months. Detailed results are presented and no significant difference between the procedures was detected in any of the outcomes measures.

228. Barron OA, Glickel SZ, Eaton RG. Basal joint arthritis of the thumb. *J Am Acad Orthop Surg.* 2000;8(5): 314–323.

    This review article is presented by leaders in the study of basal thumb arthritis. The basic science, diagnosis and classification of the condition are reviewed in detail. A treatment algorithm is presented and their techniques for volar ligament reconstruction, and ligament reconstruction tendon interposition (LRTI) are reviewed and illustrated.

266. Rizzo M, Moran SL, Shin AY. Long-term outcomes of trapeziometacarpal arthrodesis in the management of trapeziometacarpal arthritis. *J Hand Surg Am.* 2009; 34(1):20–26.

    The authors performed a 33-year retrospective study of trapeziometacarpal (TMC) arthrodeses performed at Mayo Clinic. Amongst 241 procedures reviewed, they included 126 thumbs with adequate pre- and postoperative clinical and radiographic data at an average 11-year follow-up. They report improvement of preoperative pain scores, oppositional and appositional pinch strength, and grip strength (p < 0.01). There was no significant change of any thumb motion arc. Nonunion rate was 13% and was unrelated to the use of bone grafting. Radiographic progression of STT arthritis was seen in 39 thumbs, only eight of which were symptomatic. This study presents detailed long-term

    outcomes of TMC arthrodesis, providing level IV evidence for the management of TMC arthritis.

283. Linscheid RL, Dobyns JH, Beabout JW, et al. Traumatic instability of the wrist. Diagnosis, classification, and pathomechanics. *J Bone Joint Surg Am.* 1972;54(8): 1612–1632.

    This is a seminal article from 1972 that presents the foundation for study of carpal instability. The authors' describe wrist instability that develops as a result of scapholunate and other carpal ligament injuries in addition to instability from fracture dislocations, scaphoid fractures, and fractures of the distal radius and ulna. They provide the earliest comprehensive dialogue of the diagnosis of carpal instability. The article includes clinical and radiographic data, a detailed discussion of the biomechanics of carpal instability, and proposal of the now accepted classification of dorsal and palmar intercalated segment instability. The radiographic parameters and nomenclature presented in this article remain in use today. The article has been recognized as a "classic orthopaedic reference" and a summary was republished in the Journal of Bone and Joint Surgery in 2002.

304. DiDonna ML, Kiefhaber TR, Stern PJ. Proximal row carpectomy: study with a minimum of ten years of follow-up. *J Bone Joint Surg Am.* 2004;86A:2359–2365.

    The authors retrospectivey evaluate the long-term results of 22 proximal row carpectomy procedures performed for the treatment of scapholunate advanced collapse, scaphoid nonunion with advanced collapse or Kienbock's disease. Outcomes were assessed by means of followup radiographs, objective measurement of motion and grip strength, and the DASH questionnaire. Their surgical technique is reviewed and results at a minimum 10 year followup (average 14 years) are presented. There were four failures (18%) at an average of 7 years, all of which occurred in patients younger than 35 years. The authors report a wrist motion arc of 72° and grip strength of 91% of that of the contralateral side in the 18 (82%) successes. They conclude that proximal row carpectomy is a viable motion-preserving procedure for advanced carpal arthritis that provides satisfactory long term results in most patients, and advise against it in patients younger than 35 years.

305. Ashmead 4th D, Watson HK, Damon C, et al. Scapholunate advanced collapse wrist salvage. *J Hand Surg Am.* 1994;19(5):741–750.

    The authors present a substantial series of 100 scaphoid excisions and 4-corner fusions with an average 4-year follow-up. Long-term subjective, clinical and radiographic data is presented. At the time of follow-up, 91% of cases had significant improvement in pain levels, and no patient described their pain as worse. Flexion/extension averaged 72(, and grip strength was 80% that of the contralateral side. Nonunion occurred in only three cases and only two instances of radiolunate destruction were noted, both in conjunction with ulnar translation of the carpus. Outcomes with and without the use of silicone scaphoid spacers were found to be similar.

308. Wyrick JD, Stern PJ, Kiefhaber TR. Motion-preserving procedures in the treatment of scapholunate advanced collapse wrist: proximal row carpectomy versus

four-corner arthrodesis. *J Hand Surg Am*. 1995;20(6): 965–970.

This is a retrospective cohort study comparing proximal row carpectomy (PRC) with 4-corner fusion for scapholunate advanced collapse. Two cohorts of 19 patients each (from separate institutions performing exclusively either PRC or 4-corner arthrodesis), were compared. The cohorts were well matched and the authors found significant improvement in function and pain with both procedures. Postoperative motion and functional outcomes were similar in both procedures. The authors discuss the surgical techniques, outcomes and controversies related to the two procedures.

21

The stiff hand and the spastic hand

David T. Netscher

SYNOPSIS

- Flexion and extension contractures may result from contractures of structures volar or dorsal to the joint, capsular/pericapsular structures, and bony deformity.
- Non-operative treatment is more effective in the early phase following injury and includes splinting, extremity elevation, compression gloves, moist heat, and ultrasound.
- Surgery is indicated for residual flexion contractures refractory to nonoperative measures.
- Checkrein ligament release is key in PIP joint flexion contracture surgery.
- Postoperative splint application maintains surgical correction.
- Salvage procedures for PIP joint flexion include disarticulation at the PIP joint or bone shortening with PIP joint fusion.
- In the spastic hand, nonsurgical treatment for cerebral palsy includes splinting, occupational therapy, intramuscular botulinum toxin A and intrathecal baclofen.

Introduction

Hand stiffness arises as a result of flexion and extension contractures of the small joints of the hand. Limitation of extension or flexion may be both active and passive or active alone. The appropriate treatment should be decided following clinical evaluation of what tissue needs to be addressed. This chapter will first outline the general principles of evaluation and treatment of contractures, followed by specific treatment of spasticity and Volkmann's ischemic contracture. Some less common causes of stiffness and contractures will also be reviewed. A separate entity, the spastic hand, will also be reviewed.

The stiff hand

Diagnosis/patient presentation

Flexion contracture *(Fig. 21.1)*

This may result from tightness in one or more of the structures on the palmar aspect of the joint[1,2]:

- Skin: Contracture from scarring results from lacerations or palmar burns
- Palmar fascia: Dupuytren's contracture is the classic example
- Flexor tendon sheath: Shortening and contracture may occur
- Flexor tendon: This is due to tendon shortening or tendon adhesions. Temporary joint fixation in a particular position with locking and release by painful manipulation may result from a trigger finger within the tendon sheath but also may occur within the joint especially at the metacarpophalangeal (MP) joint (intracapsular tumors, loose bodies, osteophytes, articular surface distortions).

Capsular and pericapsular structures

Collateral ligament

The collateral ligament at the proximal interphalangeal (PIP) joint is taut in all positions of the joint and collateral ligaments are taut in flexion only at the MP joints.[3] Thus, collateral ligament shortening never produces a flexion contracture at either joint. However, collateral ligament adherence to the lateral aspect of the proximal phalanx when the finger is flexed, does play a role in PIP joint flexion contracture.

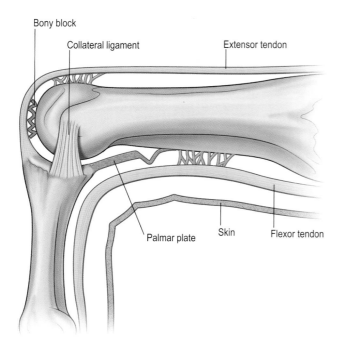

Fig. 21.1 Flexion contracture may result from tightness of structures volar to the joint, including skin, flexor tendon sheath, tendons, volar palmar plate, and accessory collateral ligaments. In addition, a bone block may impede joint motion, whereas dorsal tendon adhesions may limit the ability to extend the joint.

Volar plate

When other structures are the primary cause of the flexion contracture, the volar plate becomes contracted at an early stage, especially at interphalangeal joints.

Accessory collateral ligaments, transverse retinacular ligaments, and intrinsic tendons

Contracture of accessory ligaments, adherence of fibers of the transverse retinacular ligament to the collateral ligaments, and adhesions of intrinsic tendons in the lumbrical canals may cause flexion of MP joints.

Dorsal adhesions

Generally with flexion contracture, tightness of structures on the flexor aspect of the joint exists. However, joint extension may sometimes be prevented by incongruity of articular surfaces or adhesion of dorsal capsule or of an extensor tendon to the articular surface of the head of the proximal bone. In such a case, there is not only a flexion contracture but also limitation of flexion.

Bone

Bone block or exostosis can also cause flexion contracture.

Extension contracture

Limitation of flexion (extension contracture) *(Fig. 21.2)* can be caused by one or more structures on the dorsal aspect of the joint.[1,2] However, they too can result from a "jamming" effect of volar structures that block flexion, such as a bone block or palmar plate adhesions.

Skin

This usually results from scar contracture.

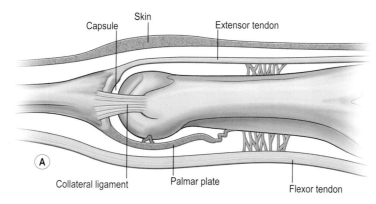

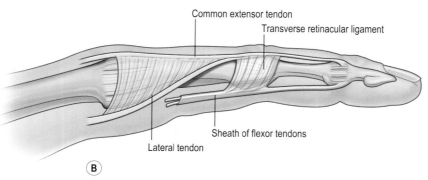

Fig. 21.2 (A) Extension contracture may result from tightness of dorsal structures, including skin, extensor tendons, collateral ligaments and joint capsule, and well as from a bone block. Volar structures may also impede the ability to flex the joint. **(B)** In addition, adhesions in the lumbrical canal and of the transverse retinacular ligament fibers may impede both flexion and joint extension.

Long extensors
Tendon shortening or adhesions limit joint flexion. With extensor tendon adhesions, active extension of the joint is limited or absent, and active extension falls short of passive extension.

Intrinsic muscles
Intrinsic contracture may follow ischemia, or muscle fibrosis may occur for nonischemic reasons (rheumatoid arthritis, cerebral palsy). The "intrinsic plus" position of the hand results in which the fingers are flexed at the MP joints and extended at the interphalangeal joints.[3] A "saddle deformity"[4] results from adhesions between lumbrical and interosseous muscles. With active intrinsic contraction, painful impingement on the deep transverse metacarpal ligament occurs with limitation of flexion (the transverse metacarpal ligament is the "saddle" and the two muscles are the "legs of the rider.")

Capsular and pericapsular structures

Dorsal capsule
The dorsal capsule may become scarred and contribute to extension contracture.

Collateral ligaments
Adhesions to the head of the proximal bone may limit flexion. In contrast to flexion contracture, which is more common in interphalangeal joints (especially proximal), stiffness in extension from collateral ligament shortening is more likely at MP joints. Collateral ligaments at the MP joints are relaxed in extension and taut in flexion.[5] Loss of MP joint flexion can come about simply from immobilization in the incorrect, extended position. Collateral ligaments are at their tightest (the cam arc effect of the metacarpal head) at a range between 70° and 90° flexion.

Volar plate
Flexion is prevented by volar plate adhesions to the palmar surface of the proximal bony head. Palmar plate adhesions and collateral ligament tightness may both be causes of MP joint extension contracture.[1] They may be distinguished from each other. If the collateral ligaments are contracted, finger abduction–adduction in extension (normally about 45°) is greatly reduced. When palmar plate is the sole cause, attempted passive flexion produces an opening of the dorsal aspect of the joint. The volar lip at the base of the proximal phalanx jams against the adherent volar plate, and the unaffected (loose) collateral ligaments allow the flexion force to rock the dorsal lip away from the metacarpal head, felt as a subtle dorsal recess between head and base. This sign should always be sought intraoperatively as a residual impediment to passive flexion after tight collateral ligaments have been released.

Painful resistance to passive PIP joint flexion may indicate volar plate injury (volar plate test).[6] Pain results from synovial involvement, and the most common cause is volar plate avulsion with or without a small bone fragment torn from the base of the middle phalanx. Positive volar plate test at 6–9 months following injury indicates that volar plate repair of the middle phalanx may be necessary.

Transverse retinacular ligaments
Transverse retinacular ligaments may be adherent to the lateral capsular ligament at the PIP joint.

Flexor tendon adherence
Flexor tendon adherence within the sheath may be sufficiently bulky to block full flexion of the interphalangeal joint.

Bone

This may be a true block or result from intraarticular incongruity. Chondral fractures may not be radiographically apparent and so may present a diagnostic problem (*Fig. 21.3*). Persistent waxing and waning joint swelling with limited

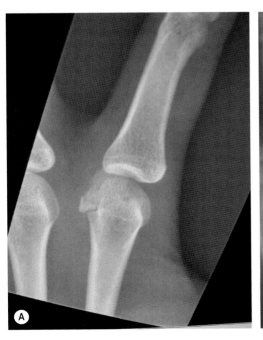
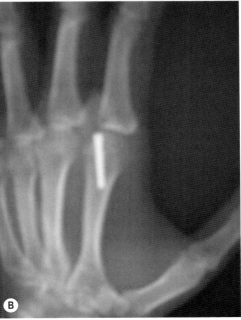

Fig. 21.3 (A) This patient had an osteochondral fracture involving the metacarpal head after a finger "jam" and presented with inability to flex at the MP joint and joint swelling. The fracture involved about one-third of the articular surface but was still attached by a single collateral ligament. **(B)** Bone fixation restored perfect joint function.

flexion may result from a chondral fracture, which is more likely at the MP joint. Questioning of the patient may lead to recollection of an injury that could have caused the proximal phalangeal base to impinge on the metacarpal head. Surgical exploration may reveal the chondral fracture and consequently loose body in the joint. Computed tomography scanning may help in arriving at the correct diagnosis.

Seesaw effect

This results when a contractural element spans two joints. Presence of this sign helps in the diagnosis of structures that potentially contribute to a stiff joint.[7] If one joint in a contracted system is flexed, the other joint can then be extended, and vice versa. This is seen, for example, when a longitudinal volar skin scar crosses both proximal and distal interphalangeal joints. The DIP joint can be extended only if the PIP joint is flexed. A similar effect is seen with adherent extrinsic flexor or extensor tendons *(Fig. 21.4)*. For example, flexion of MP joints in the presence of a flexor tendon adhesion over the proximal phalanx has no effect on the flexion contracture of the PIP joint. If the adhesion lies proximal to the MP joint, flexion of that joint results in correction of the contracture apparently present in the PIP joint. Furthermore, with flexor tendon adhesions, passive flexion of the affected joint exceeds active flexion, provided the extensor tendon is healthy. Similarly, in the presence of a Volkmann contracture of the flexors in the forearm, passive extension of the finger joints is reduced with the wrist extended and not if the wrist is flexed.

If the extrinsic extensor tendon is adherent to the metacarpal, the limitation of extensor tendon excursion distal to that joint prevents simultaneous flexion of MP and PIP joints. This is the test for extrinsic tightness *(Fig. 21.5A)*.[8,9] The test of

Bunnell for intrinsic tightness results from the seesaw phenomenon in which the band acts across two joints but is an extensor of one joint and a flexor of the adjacent joint.[10] If the intrinsic musculotendinous system is foreshortened, extension of the MP joint either actively or passively increases the tone in the system and restrains flexion of the PIP joint. This is tested by passively extending the MP joint and passively flexing the PIP joint *(Fig. 21.5B)*. If flexion of the PIP joint is greater when the MP joint is flexed than when it is extended, intrinsic tightness is present. In the swan-neck deformity, not only is there an extension contracture of the PIP joint, but that joint hyperextends because of volar plate laxity. There is dorsal displacement of the lateral bands at the PIP joint. This slackens the distal tension on the extensor mechanism because of the fixed attachment of the central tendon at the PIP joint. Thus there is unopposed force of the flexor digitorum profundus at the distal joint, which then drops into flexion *(Fig. 21.6A)*.[9]

A similar volar to dorsal seesaw effect occurs at the DIP joint secondary to action of the oblique retinacular ligament and lateral bands, resulting in extension contracture at that joint. This occurs with the boutonniere deformity. When the central tendon insertion into the dorsal base of the middle phalanx ruptures or attenuates, the PIP joint drops into flexion and the lateral bands move volar to the axis of motion of that joint.[11] They will foreshorten and adhere in that position. Excess extensor pull that secondarily bypasses the PIP joint is imposed dorsally at the DIP joint with consequent recurvature at that joint *(Fig. 21.6B)*. The oblique retinacular ligament is an extensor of the DIP joint and a flexor of the PIP joint.[11] It also foreshortens and this permits the DIP joint to be flexed as long as the PIP joint is maintained in flexion. Passively extending the PIP joint brings the DIP joint into extension,

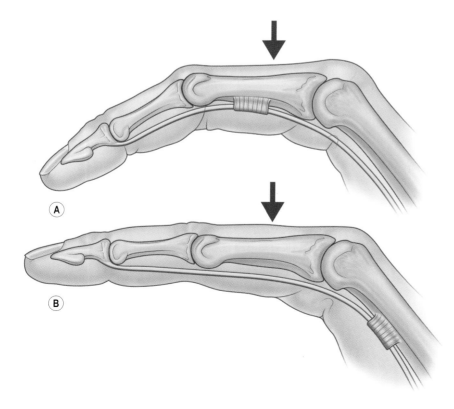

(A)

(B)

Fig. 21.4 By adjusting the joints proximal to the joint that appears to be the cause of the contracture, the primary problem may be revealed. **(A)** If a patient had a PIP flexion contracture, flexion of the MP joint in the presence of flexor tendon adhesion at the proximal phalanx has no effect on the PIP flexion contracture. **(B)** If the flexor tendon adhesion is proximal to the MP joint, flexion of that joint will result in correction of the PIP joint contracture.

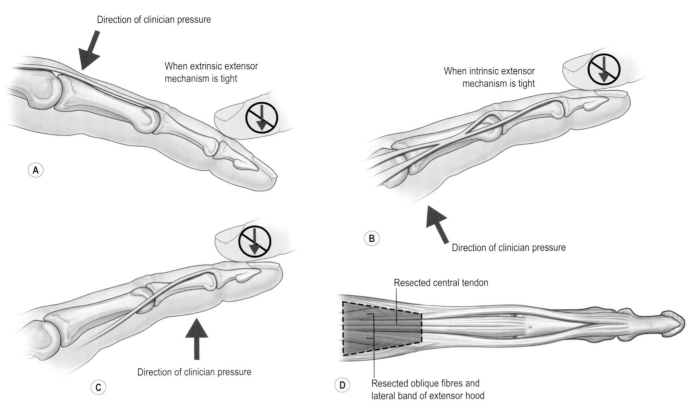

Fig. 21.5 (A) Test for extrinsic tightness. When the MP joint is flexed (arrow), passive PIP joint flexion is increasingly difficult. **(B)** Test for intrinsic tightness. When the MP joint is extended (arrow), passive PIP joint flexion is more difficult. **(C)** Boutonniere test. The oblique retinacular ligament is foreshortened so that when the PIP joint is extended (arrow), passive DIP joint flexion is difficult. **(D)** Central slip tendon excision is performed for extrinsic extensor tightness and wing tendon excision (oblique fibers and lateral bands) for intrinsic tightness — either of which might cause PIP hyperextension.

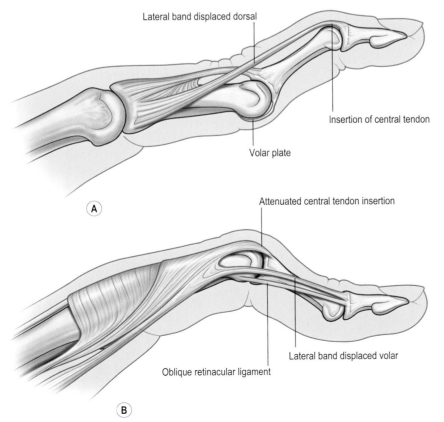

Fig. 21.6 (A) Swan neck deformity with hyperextension at the PIP joint. Dorsal displacement of the lateral bands slackens distal extensor tension, and so the unopposed flexor digitorum profundus draws the DIP joint into flexion. **(B)** Boutonniere deformity. The PIP joint drops into flexion because of central slip attenuation, and the lateral bands move volar. Excess extensor pull bypasses the PIP joint and hyperextends the DIP joint. The oblique retinacular ligament foreshortens.

making passive flexion increasingly more difficult. This maneuver is the Boutonniere test *(Fig. 21.5C)*.

Volar plate and collateral ligament changes

Changes in the volar plate and collateral ligaments occur with flexion contractures. Flexion and extension contractures can occur at the PIP joint. In contrast, at the MP joints, extension contractures occur, but flexion contracture is rare due to volar plate and collateral ligament anatomy. The volar plate at MP joints is different anatomically from that of interphalangeal joints.

The protected position of MP joints is in flexion. The cam and volar flare shape of the metacarpal head places collateral ligaments in greatest tension during flexion *(Fig. 21.7)*. The MP joint volar plate has criss-crossing bands of fibers that expand with joint extension and are collapsible with flexion.[6] Thus, the volar plate at the MP joint is considerably longer in extension than in flexion *(Fig. 21.8A)*.

In contrast, the interphalangeal joint collateral ligaments do not change in tightness with joint flexion and extension. The volar plate is relatively uncollapsible. Rather, the volar plate slides proximally and distally with flexion and extension of the joint *(Fig. 21.8B)*. The volar plate is not attached to the proximal phalanx as this would prevent full extension. The assembly lines are the two ridges on the volar lateral surfaces of the phalanx to which are attached the flexor sheath, Cleland ligaments, Grayson ligaments, oblique retinacular ligaments, and transverse retinacular ligaments, and the transverse metacarpal ligament and MP joint volar plate more proximally. Normally, there is no ligament structure between the volar plate of the PIP joint and the assembly line or extension of that joint would not be possible. Two bands (checkreins)[6,12,13] form between the lateral proximal volar plate and the assembly lines after injury. These are pathologic structures

(Fig. 21.9). They are thicker at the base attached to the volar plate and have a thinner longer proximal apex attached to the assembly line. The communicating artery of the vincula system passes deep to the checkreins. With interphalangeal joint contracture it is the checkreins that mainly prevent extension. Division of these checkreins and accessory collateral ligaments enables extension at the interphalangeal joint to be achieved when surgery is required. It is virtually never necessary to divide collateral ligaments.

Basic science/disease process

Injury, infection, excessive immobilization, and inappropriate splinting of the hand all predispose to joint stiffness. The initial response to any insult of the hand is edema formation. Unless edema accumulation is prevented, joints assume the posture in which their ligaments are most relaxed.[1,14,15] Ligament contracture and fibrosis then cause joints to become immobile in this position *(Fig. 21.10)*, which is:

- Wrist: flexion
- Thumb: adduction
- MP joint: extension
- PIP joint: flexion

This is the negative or injured hand position; wrist position and MP joint posture are the keys to its development. When the wrist is allowed to flex, increased tone in the extrinsic extensor tendons causes MP joints to extend. When nearly fully extended, the MP joint has maximum capsule and collateral ligament laxity as well as intracapsular fluid capacity. When the MP joint is fully flexed, intracapsular fluid capacity is minimal and the ligaments are taut. After injury, edema fluid drives the MP joints hydraulically into extension. In this position, tension is increased in the flexors and decreased in

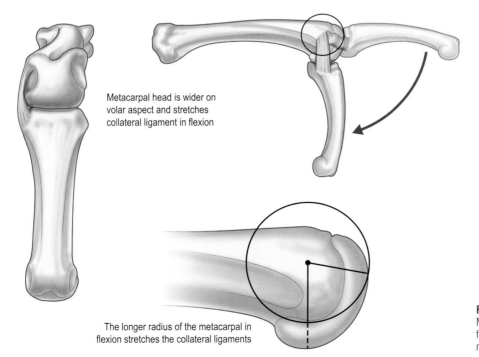

Metacarpal head is wider on volar aspect and stretches collateral ligament in flexion

The longer radius of the metacarpal in flexion stretches the collateral ligaments

Fig. 21.7 Cam-like action of the collateral ligaments at the MP joint. Collateral ligaments are in greatest tension during flexion because of the cam and volar flare shape of the metacarpal head.

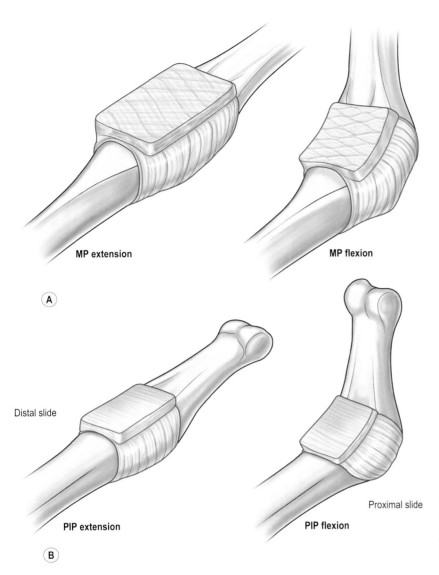

MP extension

MP flexion

(A)

Distal slide

PIP extension

PIP flexion

(B)

Proximal slide

Fig. 21.8 (A) Criss-crossing bands of fibers make up the MP joint volar plate, and these allow expansion with joint extension. **(B)** The volar plate at the PIP joint is relatively uncollapsible. In contrast to the MP joint, the PIP volar plate slides proximally and distally with joint flexion and extension.

the extensors. Thus, fingers flex at PIP and DIP joints. There is no hydraulic drive at PIP or DIP joints because there is only minimal change in collateral ligament tightness and fluid capacity of flexed versus extended interphalangeal joints. Positional changes in interphalangeal joints are thus secondary to changes in MP joints. Slight wrist flexion occurs in the neglected edematous hand because total power of flexors exceeds the extensors.[16] Post-burn claw contractures from dorsal hand burns similarly drive the MP joints into fixed extension and the PIP joints into flexion. Thus, the traumatized hand, susceptible to joint stiffness, must be appropriately immobilized by placing it in the intrinsic plus position with MP joints in flexion and interphalangeal joints in extension.

Patient selection

These measures may be more effective early on after the injury during the edema phase and subsequent collagen phase of wound healing when fluid can be displaced and collagen remodeled. Once a scar and fibrosis have reached maturity, it is less likely to respond to nonoperative measures. These measures include splinting. Other hand therapy endeavors such as edema reduction (by extremity elevation and compression gloves), moist heat, and ultrasound may enhance the beneficial response achieved by splinting.[17] Splinting involves the application of a nonelastic force in the direction of the desired correction. Initial splinting displaces tissue fluid during 5–12 min. This is the rapid gain phase of splinting. Only once this tissue edema has been displaced can the external forces of the splint result in collagen remodeling. Rapid deformity recurrence after a period of splinting should not discourage the patient because this is due to redistribution of tissue fluid originally displaced by exercise. Only if prolonged, will splinting eventually have the desired effect on collagen.[18] As weeks pass, patients notice that less time and force are necessary to achieve the desired result and that the finger returns to its contracted position more slowly and less severely after splint removal. Finally, active muscle contraction may be able to achieve complete joint range of motion, and the patient may then experience only morning stiffness that finally progressively resolves.

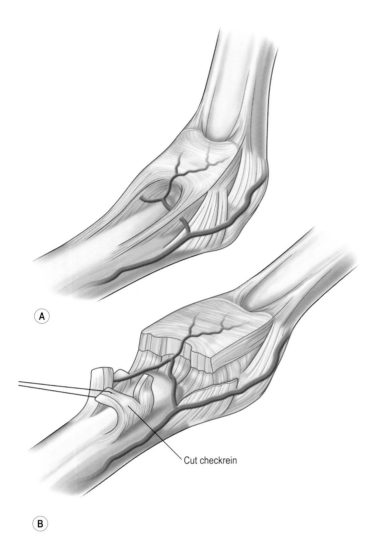

(A)

(B)

Cut checkrein

Fig. 21.9 (A) Checkreins are attached by a broad base to the volar plate, and a tapering apex is attached to the assembly line. **(B)** Release of the PIP flexion contracture requires excision of the checkreins, with care taken not to injure the transverse communicating vessel between the two digital arteries.

For PIP joint flexion contractures, the patient may wear a nighttime progressive static splint *(Fig. 21.11)*. With a Joint-Jack (Joint-Jack Company, East Hartford, CT 06118), the patient tightens the screw every 2 or 3 min as tolerated, starting 1 h before bedtime. The screw can then be loosened half a turn at bedtime for comfort. A Joint-Jack may be difficult to keep in position on the little finger because its proximal base tends to rock off the ulnar border of the palm. In that case, a custom palm-based thermoplastic splint with Velcro straps that can be tightened over the PIP joint may be appropriate. High compression foam built into the brace supports the distal phalanx. For PIP joint flexion contractures of more than 60°, these splints may be inappropriate because they will place undue extension stress on the DIP joint. These splints must be fitted with care to avoid hyperextension stress at the DIP joint. The volar distal pressure should be on the volar plate of the DIP joint and not at the fingertip. Splints such as WireFoam finger extension splints (DeRoyal LMB Hand

Rehab Products, San Louis Obispo, CA 93406) are less bulky and may be more acceptable for daytime use by the active patient. Serial finger casting, with a new cast replaced every three days, may be helpful in a difficult, seemingly unresponsive case or when PIP joint flexion is >60°.

PIP joint extension contractures rarely occur as pure joint contractures. They nearly always involve structures other than joint capsule, such as extensor mechanism adhesions. A joint strap may be placed around the middle phalanx and the finger positioned in maximum passive flexion *(Fig. 21.12)*. With time, the strap is tightened to increase flexion. Snug Coban wrapping about the palm and finger can accomplish the same objective.

A variety of flexion splints are available that place a static flexion force across MP joints when there are extension contractures at those joints. One such chronic progressive flexion splint is the Knuckle-Jack splint (Joint-Jack Company, East Hartford, CT 06118).[7]

Treatment/surgical technique

PIP joint flexion contracture of more than 70° is unlikely to respond effectively to nonoperative therapy alone. Furthermore, once a plateau in improvement has been reached with nonoperative measures and there is still a functionally impairing residual deformity, surgery is indicated. Radiographic changes within a joint or an obstructing bone block may also persuade one to undertake surgery. Once swelling has resolved, and if the joint range of motion reaches an abrupt stop rather than having a gradual increase in resistance to passive motion, clinical judgment would make one believe that maximum benefit has been reached from splinting.

PIP joint flexion contracture

It is important to first evaluate whether there is shortage of skin. Prolonged joint contracture, even without soft tissue scar, may result in longitudinal shortening of soft tissues. One may decide to make a mid-volar longitudinal incision that is broken up into multiple Z-plasties as the access incision. For severe accompanying soft tissue contracture, a transposition flap from the dorsolateral surface of the homolateral digit (Joshi flap)[19] or crossfinger flap from an adjacent finger, or homodigital island flap may be planned.[20] If there is no soft tissue deficit, any conventional volar zig-zag type surgical approach may be used.[21]

Shortened checkrein ligaments are the primary abnormality.[12,13] If a flexor tendon injury was the initiating event, a flexor tenolysis or secondary repair may be required. The flexor sheath just distal to the A2 pulley and the checkreins are cut free from their attachments to the proximal edge of the volar plate *(Fig. 21.9)*. Gentle passive extension may be required to break up other adhesions after checkrein resection to achieve full joint extension.

A "jumping" sensation is occasionally noted as the PIP joint is fully extended once checkrein release has been done. This is secondary to a cam effect of the collateral ligament and is relieved by cutting only the most dorsal fibers of both collateral ligaments.[6]

Tightness of the oblique retinacular ligaments may also contribute to the PIP joint flexion contracture, especially in association with DIP joint hyperextension in the boutonniere

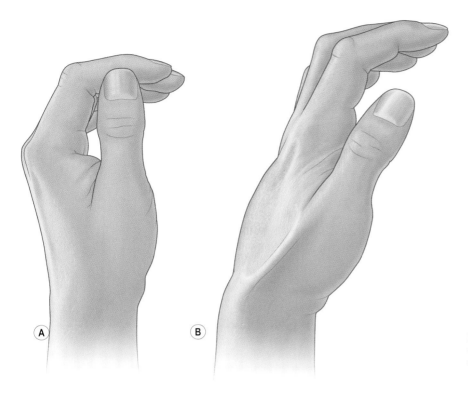

Fig. 21.10 (A) Posture of the relaxed uninjured hand.
(B) Edema accumulates in the available space on the dorsum of the injured hand, drawing the wrist into flexion, the MP joints into hyperextension, the PIP joints into flexion, and the thumb into adduction.

deformity. Transection of the oblique retinacular ligament is then indicated.

PIP joint extension contracture

A mid-dorsal longitudinal curvilinear surgical incision affords the luxury of not needing to close the entire incision proximally or distally, provided an adequate soft tissue flap covers the extensor mechanism. In this way, soft tissue closure will not limit the flexion achieved as a result of the joint release. A dorsolateral skin incision may also adequately expose the extensor hood.

The transverse retinacular ligament fibers are divided and the lateral band is elevated while the central slip insertion is preserved.[2,6] The dorsal joint capsule is incised and the joint passively flexed. Extensor tendon adhesions to the dorsum of the proximal phalanx are released. If the jump phenomenon occurs after dorsal capsulotomy, the most dorsal fibers of both collateral ligaments are cut until there is no residual jumping. In the presence of severe intraarticular fibrosis, both collateral ligaments may need to be divided and a small dissector used to free volar plate adhesions (without detaching the volar plate from its distal insertion).

Partial resection of the appropriate portion of the extensor mechanism in carefully selected cases is helpful in those patients who have intrinsic tightness or extrinsic extensor tendon tightness (see *Fig. 21.5*). In patients with extrinsic extensor tightness, the central tendon portion is resected. In those with intrinsic tightness, only the lateral bands and oblique fibers of the extensor hood are resected.[22] Sagittal band fibers are left intact because they are the prime method

through which extension is transmitted to the MP joint from the extensor mechanism

Once the finger has been stiff in extension, the flexor tendons frequently become adherent in their bed. The operator should return and check function of these tendons by making a counterincision in the palm or forearm.[2,6] By placement of traction on the flexors, the fingers should fully flex. Failure for this to occur necessitates performance of a flexor tenolysis as well. An excellent method of anesthesia administration when performing a tenolysis, is to use the tumescent technique of local anesthesia infiltration using a mixture of lidocaine with epinephrine added. This enables the so-called "wide-awake" method of local anesthetic infiltration, avoiding the paralytic effects of prolonged tourniquet ischemia or of a regional block, and ensuring full cooperation of the patient. The end point of the tenolysis or joint release is achieved only when the patient can actively reproduce normal function on the operating table.[23]

MP joint extension contracture

A longitudinal dorsal skin incision is used. Sagittal band hood fibers are retracted distally and the dorsal capsule is transected.[2,6,24] As the joint is flexed passively, one may note that the tight collateral ligament cannot pass over the condyles on the volar aspect of the metacarpal head. In such circumstances, it is necessary to transect the collateral ligaments proximally at their attachments to the metacarpal head. It may be necessary, as with extension contractures of the PIP joint, to free volar plate adhesions by inserting a blunt dissector into the volar plate pocket dorsal to that structure. If the

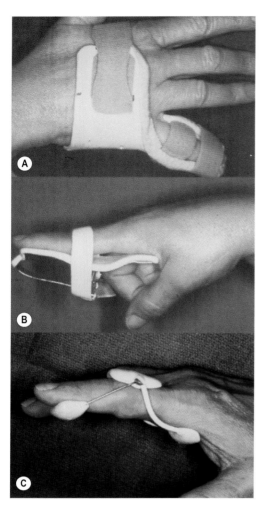

Fig. 21.11 (A) Custom palm-based night PIP extension splint. **(B)** Joint-Jack splint. **(C)** WireFoam PIP extension splint.

jump phenomenon is encountered, it is managed in a fashion similar to that of the PIP joints.

Postoperative care

Extremity elevation reduces postoperative edema. A postoperative splint applied during the first week maintains the restored joint position. Thereafter, active mobilization is begun. Daily application of splints as well as a continuous night splinting is sometimes necessary for several weeks to months postoperatively to help minimize the risk of contracture recurrence. Continuous passive motion (CPM) may be a useful modality to maintain joint motion but it is not a substitute for maintaining active motion and tendon gliding and excursion.

Outcomes, prognosis and complications

Full extension of PIP joint flexion contractures after operative release occurs in 96% of cases.[12,13] There is frequently relapse, though not complete recurrence, of the deformity despite adequate release and good postoperative management. After

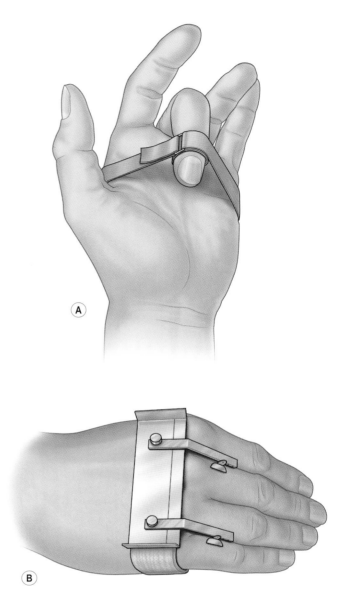

Fig. 21.12 A flexion strap can be progressively tightened around the hand and finger for treatment of a PIP joint extension contracture.

PIP joint flexion contracture release in patients with Dupuytren contractures, there is reported relapse in those with severe contractures from a preoperative mean of 78° to a postoperative mean of 36°.[25] With severe PIP flexion contractures, one can seldom expect to regain normal extension, although the deformity can be improved.

Neurovascular injury may occur during surgical release. However, even if there has not been a sharp injury to the digital neurovascular structures, ischemia to the finger may result from neurovascular overstretch when the finger has been previously flexed for a long time. Skin flaps may be thin and ischemic and develop postoperative necrosis. Necrotic skin flaps may leave tendons and their sheaths exposed and in danger of desiccation, necessitating secondary soft tissue reconstruction. Skin flap marginal necrosis may also lead to secondary wound healing and adverse scarring with relapse of contractures.

Excessive and unwarranted attempts at release of the volar plates, accessory collateral ligaments, and collateral ligaments, and use of excessive passive extending force in treatment of PIP joint flexion contracture may result in the joint subluxing into hyperextension. This results in a significant postoperative problem and the finger must then be held in a flexed position until adequate scarring heals the torn ligaments.

Cartilage necrosis may result at the distal end of the proximal phalanx when it is brought into full extension from a flexed position because of excessive pressure now applied on the fully extended joint surface.[26] Risk of overstretched neurovascular ischemia and cartilage necrosis may be heightened if a Kirschner wire has been used to temporarily fix the PIP joint in extension to maintain the contracture release.

A hyperextending force of the DIP joint by an improperly placed Joint-Jack splint that applies excessive pressure on the fingertip may cause iatrogenic functional problems at the DIP joint. Dysesthesias to the fingertip, stiffness in both flexion and extension, and reflex sympathetic dystrophy are potential complications of contracture release.

Secondary procedures

A relapse of a functionally impairing PIP joint flexion contracture may necessitate disarticulation amputation at the PIP joint or bone shortening at the PIP joint arthrodesis site with fusion in a more favorable position. Either of these two options may be considered in the primary treatment of the patient who is too frail to undergo any other surgical management or the patient who lacks the motivation needed for successful postoperative management. The patient who is a heavy smoker and has a longstanding severe flexion contracture (more than 70°) of the PIP joint may also potentially be best served by PIP joint disarticulation amputation or perhaps fusion.

The spastic hand in cerebral palsy

Diagnosis/patient presentation

Treatment of cerebral palsy necessitates accurate assessment of the clinical problem, nonsurgical modalities, as well as surgical treatment. Overall upper extremity function is classified by the 9-level House activity scale *(Table 21.1)*.[27] Surgical intervention has been shown to improve limb function by 2.6 functional levels.

Patient selection

The age of the patient is important and the child should be at least 6 or 7 years old to cooperate with the preoperative assessment and postoperative therapy. The type of palsy is important and may be spastic, ataxic or choreoathetotic. The last is a contraindication to tendon transfers. Surgery for athetoid patients usually will involve only joint stabilization through fusions such as at the MP joint of the thumb. The patients who derive the most benefit from surgery usually have spastic hemiparesis.[28] A hand with poor sensibility is less likely to be used after reconstructive surgery. Some

Table 21.1 House functional classification for cerebral palsy

Grade	Designation	Activity level
0	Does not use	Does not use
1	Poor passive assist	Uses as stabilizing weight only
2	Fair passive assist	Can hold onto object placed in hand
3	Good passive assist	Can hold onto object and stabilize it for use by other hand
4	Poor active assist	Can actively grasp object and hold it weakly
5	Fair active assist	Can actively grasp object and stabilize it well
6	Good active assist	Can actively grasp an object and then manipulate it against other hand
7	Spontaneous use, partial	Can perform bimanual activities easily and occasionally uses the hand spontaneously
8	Spontaneous use, complete	Uses hand completely independently without reference to the other hand

Reproduced with permission from House JH, Gwathmey FW, Fidler MO. A dynamic approach to the thumb-in-palm deformity in cerebral palsy. J Bone Joint Surg 1981; 63A:216–225.

believe that an intelligence quotient of >70 is desirable if surgery is contemplated, but others feel that intellect is less important.[29,30]

Nonsurgical treatment

Nonsurgical modalities include splinting, occupational therapy and pharmacologic intervention. Splinting may help prevent joint contractures. This requires a high level of compliance from patients and caregivers. It may also be a necessary component of postoperative management. Many medications have been used, some of which have significant adverse drug reactions. The most commonly used are intramuscular injection of botulinum toxin A and intrathecal baclofen. Botulinum toxin injection relaxes muscles that may then be responsive to splinting and stretching in therapy.

Surgical technique

The typical spastic posture of the upper limb includes shoulder internal rotation, elbow flexion, forearm pronation, wrist flexion and ulnar deviation, thumb-in-palm, and clenched fist *(Fig. 21.13)*. A thorough preoperative analysis of the pattern of spasticity is required and assessment of joint contractures which may need to be released. Assessment of passive range of motion must be done slowly to overcome muscle spasticity. Joint contractures are assessed by evaluating biarticular muscles. Thus, positioning the wrist joint in flexion will allow passive finger extension if there is no joint contracture.

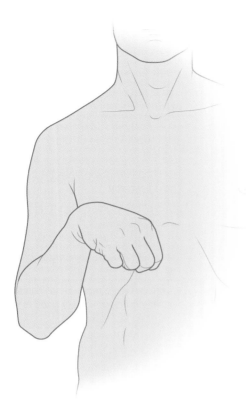

Fig. 21.13 Typical spastic hemiplegic posture of the upper extremity shows shoulder internal rotation, elbow flexion, forearm pronation, wrist flexion and ulnar deviation, thumb-in-palm, and clenched fist deformities.

Spastic muscles need to be either released or weakened by lengthening to correct muscle imbalance around joints. At the wrist, there is usually poor volitional control of ECRL, ECRB and ECU and there is spastic overpull of FCR and FCU. One next assesses which muscles are weak or have poor motor control. These flaccid muscles need to be augmented by tendon transfer. Finally, assess which muscles are available for transfer. Those under good voluntary control are the best for tendon transfer though transfer of a spastic muscle may weaken the overpowered side and utilize it to strengthen the weaker side of the unbalanced joint. Severe joint contractures or joint instability may necessitate joint fusion.

Surgical treatment options by type of deformity

Shoulder

Shoulder surgery is rarely indicated. Occasionally, Z-lengthening of pectoralis major through a delto-pectoral incision is done together with Z-lengthening of the subscapularis (or simple division by myotomy or recession from the scapula which maintains subscapularis integrity) may be necessary. With a tight adduction contracture, there may be a soft tissue deficit requiring flap reconstruction (although this is more frequently necessary with tight shoulder adduction contractures that may occur with spastic posttraumatic or stroke brain injury). Latissimus dorsi and teres major transfer to the

posterolateral humerus at the greater tuberosity is seldom required as is an external rotational humeral osteotomy.

Elbow

Mild flexion contractures may be improved simply by the necessary surgical procedures directed towards forearm pronation and wrist flexion (flexor-pronator muscle slide; or flexor aponeurotic release-FAR) as these muscles cross the elbow. More significant flexion contractures (usually >40° or 50°) demand attention to biceps, brachialis, and possibly brachioradialis. Antecubital soft tissue paucity may become apparent after the release, necessitating Z-plasty or even a flap *(Fig. 21.14)*. If brachioradialis needs to be released, this can be done distally and the muscle turned up into the antecubital fossa for wound coverage and a skin graft placed over it.

Lacertus fibrosus is released and Z-lengthening of the biceps tendon done. If residual unacceptable contracture remains, then stepwise release of brachialis (which is weakened by intramuscular incision into the fibrous septae) and of the brachioradialis (either proximally or distally) is performed.[28,31] Postoperative elbow extension splinting is done for 4 weeks, followed by progressive range of motion and intermittent extension splinting.

Forearm pronation

This deformity has been classified into four groups:[28,32]

- Group I: Active supination beyond neutral
- Group II: Active supination less than neutral
- Group III: No active supination; free passive supination, but with active pronator teres
- Group IV: No active supination; tight passive supination.

When treating the forearm pronation deformity in isolation, recommendations are: no surgery for group I; pronator quadratus release with or without FAR for group II; pronator teres release for group III, and pronator quadratus release and FAR for group IV. FAR consists of excision of a 2 cm transverse strip of fascia from the flexor-pronator mass as well as division of all fascial septae. This allows muscle fibers to be stretched, so releasing myostatic contracture without cutting tendons. Pronator teres rerouting involves taking down the distal insertion with a distal cuff of periosteum and then rerouting it through an interosseous membrane window and reattaching to the dorsoradial side of the radius with a suture anchor. Alternatively, a Z-tenotomy of pronator teres distal insertion is done, rerouting the distal segment around the radial side of the radius and reattaching the two ends.

However, often the forearm pronation deformity cannot be taken out of context with the wrist and finger flexion deformities. A flexor-pronator muscle slide used for the latter problems will often significantly improve forearm pronation as will the Green FCU transfer for active wrist extension.[33]

Wrist flexion

It is important to note the amount of digital flexor tightness that is also present. Digital flexor tightness can be quantitated by measurement of the Volkmann angle *(Fig. 21.15)*. The wrist is flexed with the digits held extended. Wrist is then passively extended as much as possible while keeping digits extended. Full wrist extension can be accomplished in the absence of

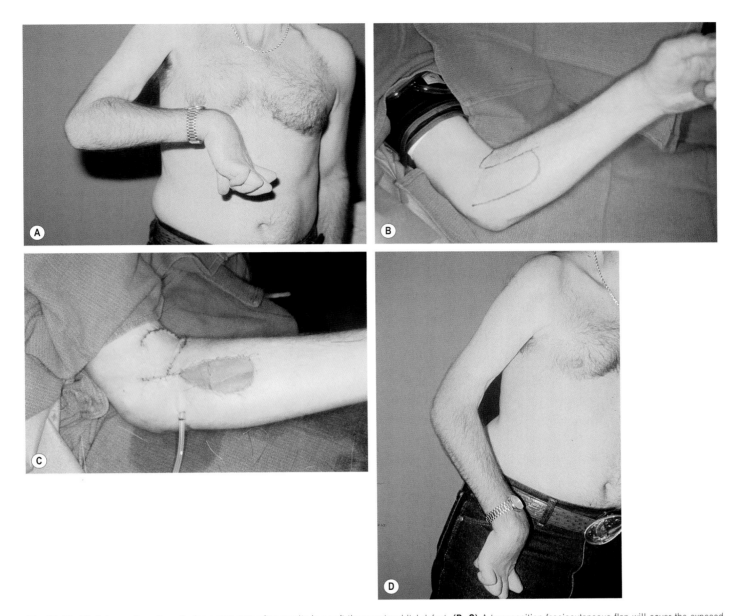

Fig. 21.14 (A) Release of an elbow flexion contracture often results in a soft tissue antecubital defect. **(B, C)** A transposition fasciocutaneous flap will cover the exposed vital structures in the antecubital fossa and then the donor defect over the proximal forearm muscles can be replaced with a split thickness skin graft. **(D)** Final elbow extension accomplished.

flexor tendon tightness. With digital flexor contracture, the wrist cannot be extended to neutral. As digits are extended, with wrist extended, one can assess selective digital spasticity. When PIP joint extension is limited, FDS spasticity is suspected (FDP spasticity may also be present). If full PIP joint extension is possible, but DIP joints do not extend, FDP spasticity is present.

The Zancolli classification of active finger and wrist extension is helpful *(Table 21.2)*.[34] In the patient with active wrist extension, spastic wrist flexion, and no significant digital flexor tightness, a FAR procedure along with fractional lengthening of the FCU, Z-lengthening of the FCR, and release of palmaris longus may be required. In contrast, the patient with flexed fingers, but relatively little spasticity of wrist flexors, may benefit from fractional lengthening of the involved finger flexors. If the fingers can be extended only with the wrist in moderate flexion, then one can perform wrist flexor releases and additional finger flexor fractional lengthening. However, a flexor-pronator muscle slide will address simultaneous wrist and finger flexion and the forearm pronation deformity *(Fig. 21.16)*.

Only once the acute flexor spasm has been released, may one then be able to accurately assess if there is active wrist extension. This may be addressed by ECU transfer to ECRB. Alternatively, the author has found that FCU can be transferred (and will have sufficient strength) several months after a flexor-pronator muscle slide has been performed. This may greatly improve grasp by removing the habitual grasp pattern of simultaneous wrist flexion. The fingers and wrist and elbow are splinted for four weeks postoperatively with

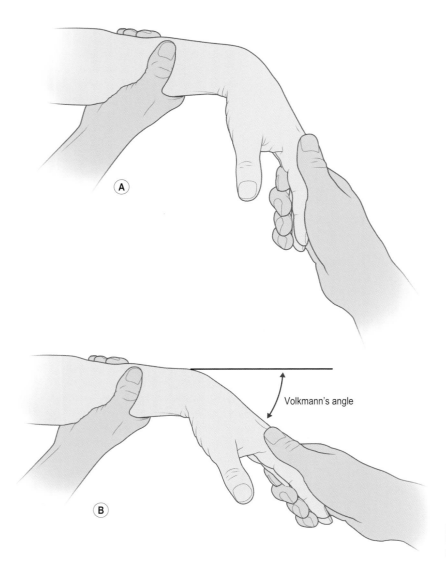

Fig. 21.15 Volkmann test for digital flexor tendon tightness. When wrist extension is less than neutral (Volkmann's angle), surgical intervention is indicated.

Volkmann's angle

Table 21.2 Zancolli classification of active finger and wrist extension

Level	Designation	Description
1	Minimal flexion spasticity	Can completely extend the fingers with a neutral position of the wrist or with <20° of flexion
2	Moderate flexion spasticity	Fingers can be actively extended but only with >20° of flexion
2A		Can actively extend, partially or totally the wrist with the fingers flexed
2B		Cannot actively extend the wrist with the fingers flexed because of flaccid paralysis of the wrist extensor muscles
3	Severe flexion spasticity	Cannot extend the fingers even with maximal flexion of the wrist

Reproduced with permission from Zancolli EA, Zancolli ER Jr. Surgical management of the hemiplegia spastic hand in cerebral palsy. Surg Clin North Am 1981; 61:395–406.

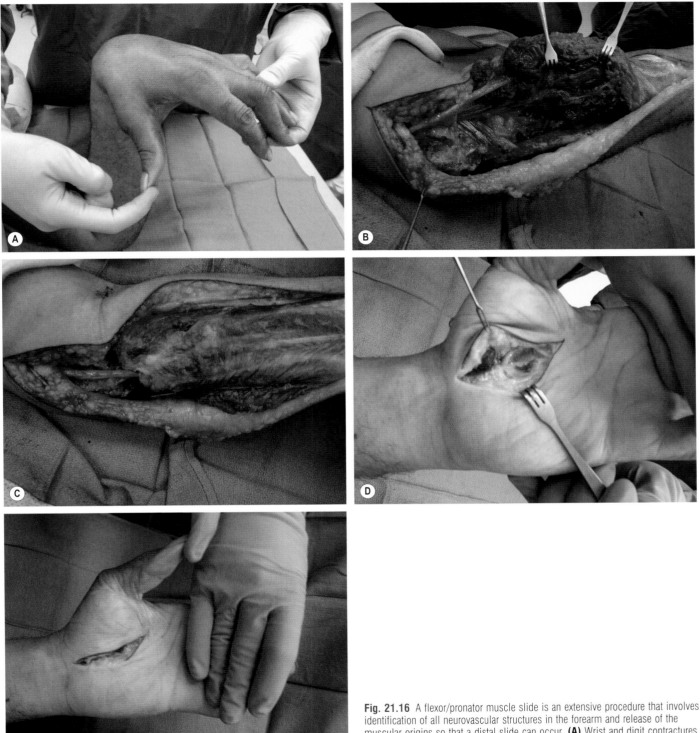

Fig. 21.16 A flexor/pronator muscle slide is an extensive procedure that involves identification of all neurovascular structures in the forearm and release of the muscular origins so that a distal slide can occur. **(A)** Wrist and digit contractures. **(B)** Muscle origin releases. **(C)** Muscle advancement. **(D)** Thenar intrinsic release. **(E)** Passive correction accomplished.

continued wrist splinting for another six weeks and night positional splinting of the fingers.

Wrist fusion by proximal row carpectomy (PRC) and using those removed carpal bones for graft is reserved for very severe wrist flexion contractures (often with a nonfunctional hand). Shortening accomplished by PRC may reduce the need to shorten finger flexors.

Correction of wrist and finger flexion deformities may unmask intrinsic hand tightness. A simultaneous thenar release can be done through a curvilinear thenar incision (avoiding the median motor nerve branch), but the author prefers to address finger swan neck deformities at a later date.

Thumb

Deformity as described by House and modified by Tonkin et al.[35] is a useful classification *(Table 21.3)*. If the deformity is adduction without MP or IP joint deformity, then release of adductor pollicis is performed in conjunction with first webspace Z-plasty. Release of the dorsal fascia or even first dorsal interosseous release may also be required. If there is tight thumb adduction with MP joint flexion (without significant IP joint deformity) then also release the flexor pollicis brevis though the same incision.[36] If both MP and IP joints are flexed together with thumb adduction, then add FPL lengthening through a separate incision, performing either fractional lengthening or Z-lengthening (for more severe IP joint flexion).

In a patient who does not have sufficient antagonistic strength, tendon transfers will be needed to augment these previously described releases. One must assess extrinsic thumb extensor function. If there is a functioning EPL and weak abduction, rerouting EPL is helpful. EPL is transected proximal to the IP joint, the extensor mechanism is repaired, and the proximal end is rerouted through the first dorsal compartment and reattached to the radial side of the extensor mechanism, so changing its vector direction.[30] If there is no EPL function, brachioradialis to APL transfer can be performed.

With MP joint hyperextension instability then either a volar tenodesis or capsulodesis of the joint must be done or MP joint fusion performed.

Finger swan-neck deformity

If there is mild deformity, secondary to intrinsic spasticity, extrinsic silver ring splints may be used, or intrinsic muscle slide performed *(Fig. 21.17)*. With a concomitant thumb adductor spasticity, and if a temporary ulnar nerve block favorably affects both the thumb-in-palm deformity and intrinsic finger spasticity, then one may on occasion consider ulnar motor neurectomy in Guyon's canal. With more severe PIP joint instability, an FDS distal slip tenodesis secured to the proximal phalanx works well *(Fig. 21.18)*.[37]

The spastic hand following stroke and traumatic brain injury

Patient selection

The principles of assessment and treatment are very similar to cerebral palsy. Procedures for flexed fingers are divided into functional procedures or those that are hygiene procedures.[38] The results of surgery are better when deformities are corrected early before fixed joint contractures have developed. Surgery should not be considered as a treatment of last resort. "Nonfunctional" surgical procedures may actually help overall bodily function. For example, in spite of not having active function in the upper extremity after spastic releases, dressing may be facilitated or positioning the hand on a walker may improve ambulation.

Finger nails may dig into the palm and palm skin may be macerated. Clenched fist is often accompanied by a flexed wrist. Assess for active finger flexion. If the PIP joints flex while DIP joints remain extended, there is spasticity in the FDS rather than FDP.

Surgical technique

If there is skin maceration and no volitional flexion, then significant lengthening of flexor tendons is required and superficialis-to-profundus (STP) transfer is performed. At best, a mass action grasp pattern is achieved with the STP transfer and at worst, passive restraint to extension is accomplished rather than a "floppy hand" with joint instability if simple tenotomies were to be performed. Associated procedures may be required such as thenar release and Z-lengthening of wrist flexors.

If there is volitional control of extrinsic finger flexors, and if the degree of flexion contracture is less severe, then fractional lengthening of FDS, FDP and even FPL is done by sharply incising the intramuscular tendon fibers. A short volar splint may be used for postoperative comfort, but active exercises are begun immediately. A flexor-pronator muscle slide may sometimes be used for a more global correction of flexed elbow, forearm pronation, wrist and finger flexion.

Table 21.3 Modified House classification of thumb deformity

Type	Deforming forces	Thumb position
1. Intrinsic	Adductor pollicis 1st dorsal interosseous Flexor pollicis brevis	Metacarpal adduction MCP joint flexion IP joint extension
2. Extrinsic	Flexor pollicis longus	MCP joint flexion IP joint flexion Metacarpal adduction less marked
3. Combined	Adductor pollicis 1st dorsal interosseous Flexor pollicis brevis Flexor pollicis longus	Metacarpal adduction MCP joint flexion IP joint flexion (True "thumb-in-palm" deformity)

Reproduced with permission from Tonkin MA, Hagrick NC, Eckersley JR, et al. Surgery for cerebral palsy part III: Classification and operative procedures for thumb deformity. J Hand Surg 2001; 26B:465–470.

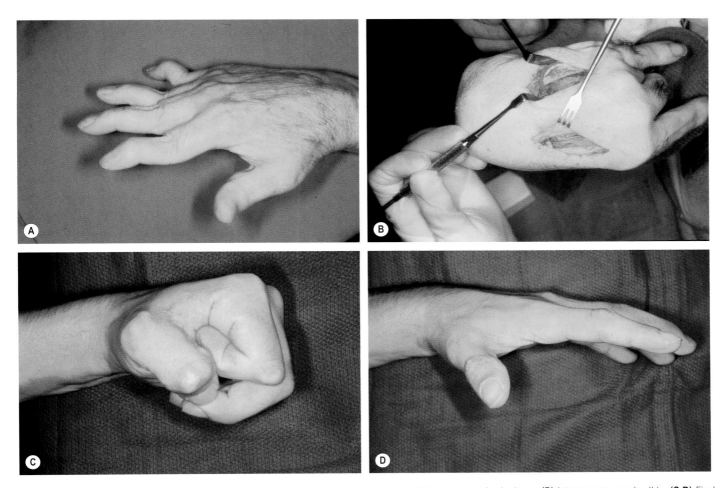

Fig. 21.17 (A) Patient with residual swan neck deformities and intrinsic muscle contractures following more proximal release. **(B)** Interosseous muscle slide. **(C,D)** Final ability to flex and extend the fingers.

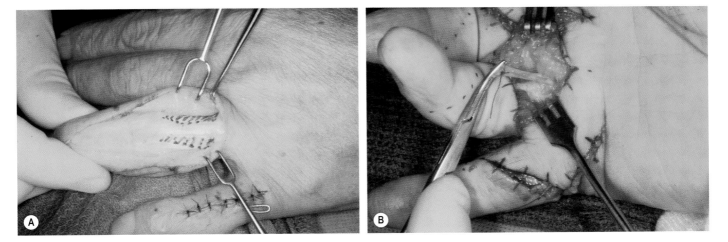

Fig. 21.18 A residual hyperextension swan neck deformity at the PIP joint may be treated by **(A)** a proximal intrinsic release and **(B)** tenodesis using a distally based slip of FDS that is rerouted back around the origin of the flexor tendon sheath or anchored into bone of the proximal phalanx.

Conclusions

Contractures in the upper extremity result not only from joint pathology but also from disorders of periarticular disorders as well as tendon adhesions and muscle imbalance. The correct treatment is predicated on making the appropriate diagnosis. A variety of specific disorders are known to lead to contractures, but the most common conditions that the hand surgeon will have to treat are the consequences of trauma. Meticulous postoperative therapy and splinting are essential to optimize best functional outcome.

Access the complete references list online at **http://www.expertconsult.com**

1. Lister G. *The hand: diagnosis and indications*, 3rd edn. New York: Churchill Livingstone; 1993:191–198.

2. Curtis RM. Stiff finger joints. In: Grabb WC, Smith JW, eds. *Plastic surgery*, 3rd edn. Boston: Little Brown; 1979:598–603.

3. Smith RJ. Nonischemic contractures of the intrinsic muscles of the hand. *J Bone J Surg*. 1971;53A: 1313–1331.

   This is a classic article that very lucidly describes the pathologic anatomy and treatment of the disorders of the intrinsic hand muscles.

10. Eaton RG. The extensor mechanism of the fingers. *Bull Hosp Joint Dis*. 1969;30:39–47.

    Another classic article that has stood the test of time and is recognized for its practical approach to the extensor mechanism and contributions to finger contractures.

12. Watson HK, Light TR, Johnson TR. Check-rein resection for flexion contracture of the middle joint. *J Hand Surg*. 1979;4:67–71.

    This article describes in detail the role of the volar plate in PIP flexion contractures and the importance of identifying the pathologically disordered checkrein ligaments.

19. Joshi BB. Dorsolateral flap from same finger to relieve flexion contracture. *Plast Reconstr Surg*. 1972;49:186–189.

28. Lomita C, Ezaki M, Oishi S. Upper extremity surgery in children with cerebral palsy: review article. *J Am Acad Orthop Surg*. 2010;18:160–168.

    This is a very concise article that is packed with practical information. It is a systematic review that includes spasticity of the elbow, forearm, wrist, thumb, and fingers in sequence.

30. Manske PR. Redirection of extensor pollicis longus in the treatment of spastic thumb-in-palm deformity. *J Hand Surg*. 1985;10A:553–560.

32. Gschwind CR. Surgical management of forearm pronation. *Hand Clin*. 2003;19:639–655.

35. Tonkin MA, Hagrick NC, Eckersley JR, et al. Surgery for cerebral palsy part III: Classification and operative procedures for thumb deformity. *J Hand Surg*. 2001;26B:465–470.

    Another practical guide that classifies thumb deformity into "intrinsic" and "extrinsic" contractures or a combination of the two. This analysis of the deformity then translates into a useful surgical treatment algorithm.

22

Ischemia of the hand

Hee Chang Ahn and Neil F. Jones

SYNOPSIS

- Upper extremity ischemia is caused by many etiologies and may be classified into acute and chronic cases.
- A precise understanding of arterial anatomy is pertinent to preoperative diagnosis, patient selection, and operative procedure.
- A history of cold intolerance, Raynaud's phenomenon and frequency of ischemic pain is important. Color changes, ulcerations and infections are evaluated.
- Noninvasive vascular examination includes measurement of fingertip temperatures, Doppler ultrasound, segmental arterial pressures and capillaroscopy.
- Various pharmacologic agents can be used to counteract the sympathetic effect on the muscular layers of the arterial wall in a conservative medical approach.
- Surgical intervention is directed at interrupting the sympathetic innervation of the muscle layer, by physical dilatation of the obstructed lumen, or by microsurgical reconstruction of the occluded lumen.

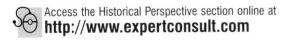

Access the Historical Perspective section online at
http://www.expertconsult.com

Introduction

Hand ischemia occurs when the vascular system is no longer able to transport blood efficiently because of trauma, constriction, obstruction, or vasospasm. It is the critical vascular event that results in eventual tissue necrosis and even amputation without proper management. Compared with the lower extremity, the symptomatology and presentation is varied in

the upper limb and it is frequently underdiagnosed. Upper extremity ischemia is caused by many etiologies[1] and may be classified into acute and chronic cases *(Box 22.1)*. Any microvascular injury that diminishes the vascular flow induces the acute ischemic conditions of the hand. Systemic, congenital and genetic problems also cause chronic ischemic conditions. Raynaud's phenomenon is a well-known vasospastic condition that affects 5–10% of the general population.[2,3] Primary Raynaud's disease occurs in the absence of any underlying condition whereas secondary Raynaud's syndrome is associated with other vasospastic conditions.

Fuchs classified arterial disease according to the three arterial layers: the intima, media, and adventitia. Several of the most frequent pathologic processes (atherosclerosis, intimal hyperplasia) originate in the intimal layer. Endothelial disruption produces thrombotic occlusion and embolization.[4] The media consists of smooth muscle cells, fibroblasts and elastic tissue. Atherosclerosis also influences the loss of tissue integrity. The media can become chronically dilated in a diffuse (ectasia) or localized (aneurysm) pattern. The adventitia is involved in diffuse pathologic entities (arteritis, Buerger's disease). Jones categorized hand ischemia into subgroups of acute and chronic disease. There are multiple causes of upper extremity ischemia *(Box 22.1)*[1] but a classification system based on the underlying pathophysiologic mechanism responsible for producing the ischemia would seem to be most appropriate as a rationale for suitable treatment. Jones described five main pathophysiological mechanisms of hand ischemia: emboli, thrombosis, occlusive disease, vasospasm, and low flow states.[5]

Regardless of its causes, ischemia of the hand is manifested by color and temperature changes, pale fingers, cold intolerance, numbness, digital ulcerations and gangrenous changes. Despite appropriate treatments, such as smoking cessation, cold avoidance, biofeedback techniques, and pharmacological therapy, ischemia commonly progresses to the eventual consequence of amputation.[6–11] This chapter provides an insight to accurate diagnosis and appropriate treatment to avoid devastating tissue losses.

Raynaud's phenomenon

Raynaud's disease is a rare disorder but it is an important cause of upper limb ischemia. This entity is often confused with Raynaud syndrome. Raynaud's phenomenon in patients with upper extremity ischemia is common and classically consists of an orderly progression of color changes (white, blue, and then red) and symptoms in the affected hand secondary to vasospasm. Pallor is followed by a cyanotic appearance, and culminates with reactive hyperemia and burning pain or dysesthesias. This classic pattern occurs in about two-thirds of affected patients. In 1932, Allen and Brown proposed that Raynaud syndrome/phenomenon be differentiated from Raynaud's disease in that no underlying organic cause can be found in Raynaud's disease.[14] They listed the following criteria as necessary for the diagnosis of Raynaud's disease:

1. Bilateral symptoms
2. Absence of gangrene
3. No evidence of underlying organic disease
4. Symptoms present for at least 2 years.

Merritt,[15] and Blunt and Porter[16] argued that these criteria are confusing and perhaps obsolete, considering that Raynaud's phenomenon can be present for an average of 11.5 years prior to diagnosis of an underlying connective tissue disease.[17] Furthermore, in one study using sensitive laboratory testing of patients with Raynaud's disease, more than one-half of patients were found to have some evidence of an underlying systemic disease.[18]

The relationship between vasospasm in Raynaud's phenomenon and occlusive disease continues to be controversial. Some researchers have suggested that occlusive disease may initiate vasospasm via humoral and/or sympathetic mediators. This concept is supported by the fact that excision of the occluded arterial segment in patients with traumatic ulnar artery thrombosis (hypothenar hammer syndrome) will improve the digital vasospasm often seen in this disorder.[19] Vasospastic symptoms in patients with connective tissue disorders may also be related to an underlying abnormality of the vessel wall. Intimal hyperplasia, thrombosis, fibrosis, embolism, adventitial thickening, aneurysm formation, and calcification have all been found in patients with Raynaud's phenomenon.[20,21] The question remains whether these changes are responsible for the vasospastic symptoms or merely potentiate vasospasm initiated at another site. Therefore, bypass of distal arterial occlusions may not only provide oxygen delivery via increased blood flow to the hand but also may remove a potential source of vasospasm.

Basic science

Anatomy

Embryology

The limb buds appear at 4 weeks of embryonic life as lateral swellings and the forearm vasculature evolves through several stages between 4 and 8 weeks (see Ch. 25). A median artery, ulnar artery and radial artery arise in order from the brachial artery at the elbow, but the median artery involutes as the radial and ulnar arteries provide the majority of blood flow to the hand.

Arterial system in the forearm, hand, and digits

Variations in the vascular pattern of the deep and superficial palmar arches and the common digital arteries are frequent. Therefore, a precise understanding of arterial anatomy is pertinent to preoperative diagnosis, patient selection and operative procedure.

Superficial palmar arch

The superficial palmar arch may be classified as either "complete" or "incomplete." This classification provides the simplest understanding of the anatomy of the arches.[22] Gellman et al. defined an arch to be complete if there was an anastomosis between the vessels constituting it and an incomplete arch as having an absence of communication or anastomosis between the vessels constituting the arch.[23] Coleman and Anson also described an incomplete superficial arch as one "in which the contributing arteries do not anastomose, or when the ulnar artery fails to reach the thumb and index finger."[22] Koman et al.[24] also reported a complete arch in 78.5% of extremities. Gellman et al. reported a complete arch in 38 of 45 specimens studied (84.4%). In contrast to these studies, Fazan[25] reported that only 43% of right hands and 52% of left hands had complete arches.

Multiple variations of the superficial palmar arch have been classified into subgroups. According to Gellman's study, complete arches have been divided into five subgroups.

- Type A: The radioulnar arch is formed by anastomosis between the superficial volar branch of the radial artery and the continuation of the ulnar artery.
- Type B: The superficial arch is formed by a continuation of the ulnar artery and even provides common digital vessels to the thumb and index web space.
- Type C: The median and ulnar arteries combine to form the superficial arch without a contribution from the radial artery.
- Type D: This is characterized by all three vessels (radial, median, ulnar) contributing to the arches.
- Type E: A branch from the deep palmar arch communicates with an ulnar artery initiated superficial arch.

The main branches from the superficial palmar arch are the three common digital arteries to the index-middle, middle-ring, and ring-small finger web spaces[22,26] and the proper digital artery to the ulnar border of the small finger.[23,27,28] When the princeps pollicis artery and a vessel to the radial side of the index finger (index radial digital artery), originates from the superficial palmar arch, this should be named as the first common digital artery.[27,29]

Deep palmar arch

The deep palmar arch is less variable than the superficial arch. The radial artery forms the deep arch when it passes from dorsal to palmar by piercing the two heads of the first dorsal interosseous muscle. The arch then curves along the bases of the metacarpal bones. The deep arch may anastomose with one or both volar branches of the ulnar artery.[23,30] At least one of the deep volar branches was present in all individuals in a recent study. The deep palmar arterial arch travels across the palm, deep to the flexor tendons, at the level of the carpometacarpal joints to connect with a deep arterial branch from the ulnar artery.[22,31] The deep palmar arch gives rise to as many as five palmar metacarpal arteries that pass distally to the level of the metacarpal heads, where they branch dorsally to join the dorsal metacarpal arteries and also connect to the common digital artery through a small palmar arterial branch. Nystrom et al. described three palmar and three dorsal arches which connect the four forearm arteries (ulnar, median, radial, and interosseous arteries). Dorsal metacarpal arteries which originate from the dorsal carpal arches pass to their respective web spaces distally, where they join perforating vessels from the palmar circulation.[32]

The most consistent of the dorsal vessels supplying the dorsal carpal rete, which consists of numerous small, thin vessels (0.3–0.5 mm), is the radial dorsal carpal branch. It branches off the radial artery 10–15 mm distally to the radial styloid.[23]

When the superficial arch is well developed, the deep palmar arch is correspondingly less developed and vice versa. A reciprocal inverse relationship was also found between the common palmar digital arteries and the palmar metacarpal arteries.[22,30,33,34]

Digital arteries

The ulnar digital arteries of the thumb and index finger are larger than the radial digital arteries. The radial digital artery is larger in the ring and small fingers. The difference between the radial and ulnar digital arteries is statistically significant only in the border digits. The anatomy of the thumb digital arteries is unique. The blood supply of the thumb comes mainly from the princeps pollicis artery, the terminal branch of the superficial palmar arch, and the first dorsal metacarpal artery. There are numerous sources of blood supply from the radial and ulnar arteries, including the palmar ulnar, palmar radial, dorsal ulnar and dorsal radial arteries. The first palmar metacarpal artery is absent in about 2% of patients.[22,31] This accounts for the tolerance to ischemia by the thumb due to numerous collateral blood vessels.

According to the Hagan–Poiseuille's law, the blood viscosity, diameter, length and the pressure gradient influence flow through the digital arteries, and larger digital arteries can carry more blood. Strauch and de Moura described the numerous interconnections between the digital arteries beyond the metacarpophalangeal joints. These connections play an important role in hand ischemia if segmental arterial obstruction develops.[34]

Micro-arterial system

Microvascular vessels are defined as having a diameter of <100 μm. Their role is to deliver oxygen and nutrients at a cellular level. They consist of nutritional capillary and thermoregulatory vessels.[33] In the digits, 80–90% of the total flow passes through thermoregulatory beds and 10–20% are involved in capillary nutrition.[35] In pathologic states, cellular hypoperfusion leads to ischemic symptoms and imbalance in the distribution of thermoregulatory and nutritional flow resulting in cell death or damage.

Physiology of blood flow

Hemodynamics

Koman et al.[24] described macrovascular structures that are defined as vessels >100 μm. Their function is to deliver nutrients to the microvascular beds, provide adequate capacity for arteriovenous thermoregulatory flow and drain nutritional and thermoregulatory beds.

Cellular control mechanisms

Blood flow does not only follow principles of fluid dynamics. There is compensation between arterial dilatation, collateral vessels, and resistance in the peripheral circulation. In a normal extremity, blood flow in the hand depends on sympathetic tone, metabolic demands, environmental events, local factors, and circulating humoral mediators. Alpha-adrenergic control is the dominant control arm of vasoconstriction, however vasodilatation is initiated by endothelium-derived relaxing factor. Active vasoconstriction and vasodilatation may be initiated by a central control process mediated through peripheral neural structures or circulatory factors or by local autoregulation, which is metabolic or myogenic. Metabolic autoregulation occurs in response to local metabolic needs and is mediated by decreased oxygen and build-up of adenosine and potassium.[36] Myogenic autoregulation is mediated via transmural pressure and stretch-operated calcium channels.[37] The microcirculation is also affected by endothelial factors within blood vessels. The endothelium plays a major role in control of vasomotor tone and blood fluidity, lipid metabolism and finally angiogenesis. The endothelium has been recognized as an active tissue responsible for elaborating both vasodilatory and vasoconstrictor substances. Endothelial cells respond to differences in intravascular pressure due to variations in the size of the lumen by releasing endothelium-derived relaxing factor.[38] Endothelium-derived relaxing factor produces active vasodilatation, and endothelin is a potent vasoconstrictor. Both compounds are released from the endothelial cells to regulate vascular flow. Endothelial cells can also release thromboxane A2, prostacyclin, and the molecule of thrombomodulin and heparin sulfate.

Pathophysiology

As described previously, Fuchs classified arterial disease according to the three arterial layers: intima, media, and adventitia. Several pathologic processes (atherosclerosis, intimal hyperplasia) originate from this intimal layer. Endothelial disruption produces thrombotic occlusion and embolization.[4] The media consists of smooth muscle cells, fibroblasts and elastic tissue. Atherosclerosis leads to loss of tissue integrity, and the media becomes chronic dilated in a diffuse (ectasia) or localized (aneurysm) pattern. The adventitia is involved in diffuse pathologic conditions (arteritis, Buerger's disease).

A classification system based on the underlying pathophysiological mechanism responsible for producing the ischemia would seem to be most appropriate as a rationale for determining treatment. The pathological processes that produce ischemia in any end organ (and the hand can be considered such an end organ) are emboli, "sludging" of blood in low flow states, thrombosis, external compression, intimal proliferation progressing to occlusion (arteriosclerosis), and vasospasm.[5]

Emboli

Large emboli from the heart due to atrial fibrillation or myocardial infarction lodging at the bifurcation of the brachial artery are best managed by embolectomy by a vascular surgeon. However, smaller emboli or "micro-emboli" dislodged from an ulcerated atherosclerotic plaque in a large artery may lodge in the distal radial and ulnar arteries and digital arteries, and result in digital ulcerations or gangrene.

Trauma

Traumatic causes of ischemia can be occupational, iatrogenic, or secondary to an injury. Hypothenar hammer syndrome (HHS) first described by Van Rosen in 1934 is an uncommon cause of secondary Raynaud's phenomenon, and occurs mainly in patients who use the hypothenar part of their hand as a hammer.[39]

Because of its anatomic configuration within Guyon's canal, the ulnar artery is particularly vulnerable to mechanical injury. The hook of the hamate bone presses against the superficial palmar branch of the ulnar artery in Guyon's canal, leading to the development of progressive periadventitial scarring, damage to the media, disruption of the internal elastic lamina, intimal damage, and subintimal hematoma of the ulnar artery. These events are postulated to be the pathophysiological mechanism whereby repetitive trauma causes thrombosis in competitive athletes (volleyball, karate, handball, and baseball).[40–42]

'Vibration white finger' or vibration-induced Raynaud's phenomenon is also related to repetitive trauma in workers who frequently use drills, jackhammers and chain saws. High frequency vibration is assumed to affect the response of the sympathetic vasoconstrictor nerves and receptors, not only to mechanical but also to thermal induced pain.[43,44]

Radial artery catheterization frequently results in radial artery thrombosis, although it is frequently asymptomatic because of communication between the radial and ulnar arterial systems. However, if the patient has an incomplete superficial palmar arch, distal ischemia may occur.[23] Cardiac catheterization via the brachial artery may result in thrombosis and distal emboli, with an incidence of approximately 0.6%.[45]

Arteriovenous shunt operations in renal failure patients may also result in hand ischemia. The arteriovenous shunt may redirect a critical volume of blood flow away from the hand, resulting in a "steal" phenomenon producing severe motor and sensory deficits.[46,47]

Systemic disease

Systemic disease may produce distal hand ischemia and/or Raynaud's symptoms, including connective tissue disease, vasculitis, malignancy, septicemia, arteriosclerosis, Buerger's disease, polycythemia, cryoglobulinemia, and chemical toxicity.[15]

Diagnosis/patient presentation

Evaluation

Evaluation of vascular competency should define the patient's vascular anatomy and function under stressed and unstressed conditions. Therefore, a combination of studies is needed. Most importantly, a complete history and physical examination is essential in establishing a diagnosis. Investigations including noninvasive or invasive vascular studies may be required for exact evaluation of the patient's status.

The patient's symptoms, and studies such as Thermoscan, color Doppler and angiogram are carefully reviewed to identify those patients who require surgical intervention.

History and physical examination

A history of cold intolerance, Raynaud's phenomenon (Fig. 22.1), and frequency of ischemic pain is important, as is smoking history; occupation involving repetitive injury or vibration trauma, and systemic disease including diabetes,

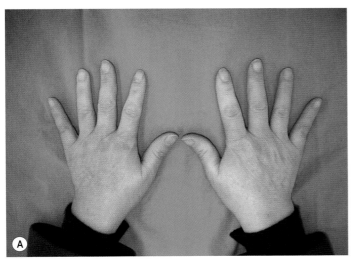 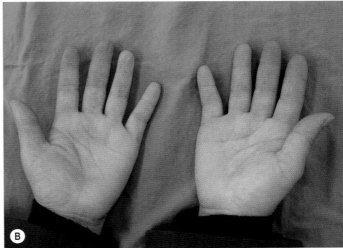

Fig. 22.1 Triphasic color changes. **(A)** Fingers turn white. **(B)** Fingers turn purple.

cardiac disease, arrhythmias, drug use, blood dyscrasias and peripheral neurological abnormalities. Unilateral Raynaud's symptoms are especially suspicious and are usually indicative of occlusive disease on the affected side.

McCabe *et al.* and Troum *et al.* developed a questionnaire that can be used to assess the severity of cold sensitivity and quantify the magnitude, duration, and frequency of vasospastic symptoms and their effect on function.[48,49]

A thorough examination of the upper extremity for previous trauma, old scars or operative incisions, skin color, temperature, presence of digital ulcers, and motor and sensory evaluation of the three peripheral nerves should be routine. Observation of blood flow in the fingernails may help to diagnose ischemia due to connective tissue disease.[25,50]

Palpation may detect an abnormal mass or thrill. The brachial, radial and ulnar arterial pulses are also palpated. The Allen test allows rapid evaluation of the patency of radial and ulnar arterial inflow into the hand. A digital Allen test can occasionally be performed either by forcing blood out of the finger or by sequential compression of the digital arteries.[51,52]

Color changes, ulcerations and infections are evaluated. Nonhealing ulcerations and/or impending gangrene associated with unilateral Raynaud's symptoms are presumptive evidence of thrombosis or embolism.[25,53]

Diagnostic investigations

Noninvasive vascular examination includes measurement of fingertip temperatures, Doppler ultrasound, segmental arterial pressures and capillaroscopy.

Capillaroscopy

The capillaries of the nail fold can be examined directly by specialized dynamic videophotometric capillaroscopy, which provides measurements of capillary diameter, red blood cell velocity and total flow. It can be difficult to perform in 10–12% of individuals due to anomalous vessel orientation, varying length of capillary loops, hyperkeratotic skin or dense pigmentation. Dynamic capillary videomicroscopy allows direct assessment of nutritional perfusion and arteriovenous

shunting, and provides objective evidence of the effects of systemic disease on the microcirculation and objective confirmation of any improvement with medical intervention.[25]

Ultrasound

The pencil Doppler probe can also be used to assess the patency of the distal radial and ulnar arteries at the wrist and the dorsal branch of the radial artery as it passes through the web space, the superficial palmar arch, the common digital arteries and each proper digital artery on the radial and ulnar aspects of each digit. Jones found the pencil Doppler probe to be the simplest, most informative technique providing precise determination of the patency of the arterial structures. Doppler evidence of occlusion of either the distal radial or ulnar arteries is one of the primary criteria for proceeding to invasive arteriography.[1,5]

Segmental arterial pressures of the brachial artery at the elbow and the distal radial and ulnar arteries at the wrist may be measured with a pencil Doppler probe. A Radial-Brachial Index (RBI) and a Digital-Brachial Index (DBI) can be calculated with a value of ≤0.7 indicating that arterial outflow to the hand is decreased.[54]

Duplex ultrasonography

A Duplex ultrasonogram is noninvasive, repeatable, and can be used for follow-up investigation. Its most important advantage is presenting real time blood flow information *(Fig. 22.2)*.[55,56]

Isolated cold stress testing

Cold stress testing was developed to provide an evaluation of the digital response to physiologic stress. Digital temperatures or digital plethysmography (pulse volume recordings) are measured before, during, and after application of a cold stress-immersion in cold water or a cold chamber at 4°C.[57] If the fall in digital temperature or drop in pulse volume recording can be partially ameliorated by a prior injection of local anesthetic, this implies that vasospasm is a likely mechanism for the ischemia.

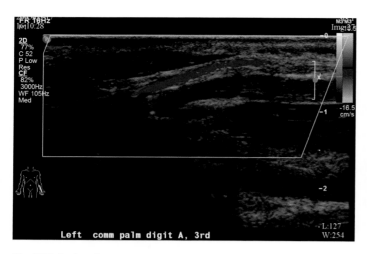

Fig. 22.2 Duplex ultrasonogram.

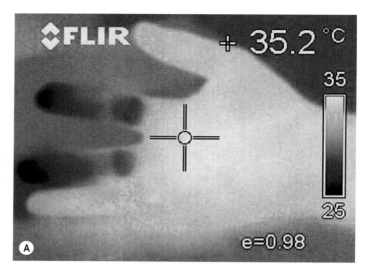

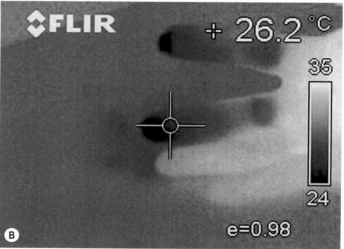

Fig. 22.3 Infrared thermography. (A) Normal temperature in the palm. (B) Ischemic fingers.

Infrared thermography

Infrared thermography (IRT) provides a measure of the decreased skin temperature of patients with hand ischemia due to decreased superficial skin blood flow.[44] The advantage of IRT is that it is noninvasive, easy to use and inexpensive *(Fig. 22.3)*. However, it is influenced by the ambient temperature, and skin temperature itself does not reveal the condition of a blood vessel and cannot visualize the site of stenosis.

Angiography

Potential disadvantages of conventional angiography include bleeding, allergic response to the contrast media, and X-ray exposure. A major problem with invasive angiography is the vessel spasm induced by the contrast media *(Fig. 22.4)*.[23,56,58] This can be circumvented by performing angiography under a brachial plexus block or by preventing vasoconstriction by intra-arterial injection of 4 mg phentolamine.[59]

Angiography defines the site and extent of thrombosis or occlusion of the distal radial and ulnar arteries and even the common digital and proper digital arteries.[23,58] Jones[5] has suggested some criteria for angiographic investigation of upper extremity ischemia as follows: (1) Unilateral Raynaud's phenomenon; (2) progressive digital ulceration or gangrene despite good medical management; (3) recurrent digital ulceration; (4) Doppler evidence of occlusion of a major inflow artery, and (5) acute onset of ischemic symptoms.

MR and CT angiography

More recently, high-resolution contrast enhanced MR angiography and CT angiography continue to be refined to compete with conventional angiography.[60] Even though enhanced MR angiography and CT angiography are noninvasive, the resolution still does not allow the same visualization of the digital arteries compared with conventional angiography. Currently, if the surgeon requires accurate visualization of the digital arteries, conventional angiography is still preferred *(Fig. 22.5)*.

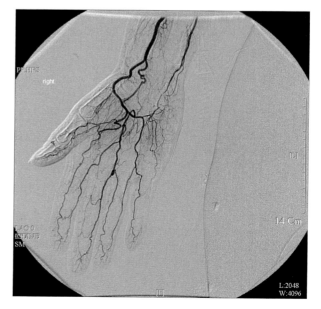

Fig. 22.4 Brachial angiography showing localized occlusion of the ulnar artery.

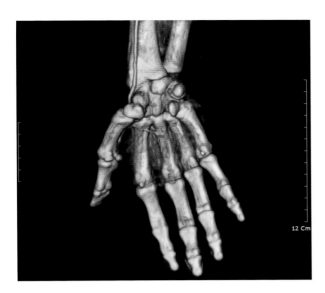

Fig. 22.5 CT angiography.

Patient selection

Acute ischemia

Acute arterial injury

Acute ischemia of the hand may occur following laceration of the brachial, radial, and ulnar arteries. Closed vascular injuries are often caused by high energy trauma with accompanying fractures.[61] High energy trauma may cause hemorrhage, thrombosis, incomplete vessel injury with development of an aneurysm, compartment syndrome, or progressive thrombosis and distal embolization.[62] Specific injuries of the upper extremity that may result in ischemia of the hand include shoulder dislocation, posterior dislocation of the elbow and supracondylar fracture of the humerus. Diagnosis is usually not difficult in patients with significant hemorrhage and distal ischemia. Undetected injury to noncritical vessels may result in a false aneurysm or formation of an arteriovenous fistula.[63] Thal described the indications for operative exploration.[64]

Physical findings of a pulsatile hematoma, a thrill, an audible bruit, decreased peripheral pulses, or associated neurologic deficits are very important, but the presence of a distal pulse is not reliable in the evaluation of vascular integrity *(Box 22.2)*. Immediate diagnosis is crucial in patients with acute ischemia of the hand, and this has been accomplished most expeditiously with Doppler examination and angiography.

Arterial emboli

The heart is the most common origin for arterial emboli. Acute onset of pallor, pain, coolness, paresthesias and pulselessness should lead to strong suspicion for embolism. Ischemia will produce muscle paralysis after an embolus proximal to the forearm muscles, but paralysis is not present in distal emboli. Segmental arterial pressures are helpful, and arteriography of the entire upper extremity will determine if there is a more proximal arterial source of emboli and also will help differentiate embolism from acute arterial thrombosis.[70]

Iatrogenic injuries

- Cannulation of the radial artery
- Catheterization through the brachial artery
- Harvest of radial artery for coronary artery bypass
- Harvest of the radial forearm flap
- Drug injection injury
- Acquired arteriovenous fistula – for dialysis in renal failure.

Cannulation injury

Radial artery cannulation injuries have increased because of the increased frequency of arterial blood pressure monitoring. Repeated injury to the radial artery can cause acute thrombosis with distal embolization, pseudoaneurysm, and arteriovenous fistula. Because of concomitant endothelial injury in cannulation injuries of the radial artery, immediate resection of the involved segment and reconstruction with an arterial or vein graft is more effective than thrombectomy with small Fogarty catheters.

Arterial injection injuries

Self-inflicted or inadvertent drug injection arterial injuries result in severe acute ischemia due to chemical endarteritis, arterial blockage by acid crystals, activation of the clotting cascade, and secondary vasospasm which causes severe vasoconstriction and widespread thrombosis. Diagnostic modalities are the same as in other vascular injuries.[65]

Acquired arteriovenous fistula

Arteriovenous fistulas may occur following trauma or infection but are usually created surgically to provide vascular access for patients undergoing hemodialysis.[66] End-to-end radial artery to cephalic vein anastomosis may result in both ischemic and neurological complications related to a "steal" phenomenon.[67] Side-to-side anastomosis (radiocephalic arteriovenous fistula) also may reduce digital blood flow to the thumb because of proximal shunting.[68] Dialysis access-associated "steal" syndrome occurs in 2–4% of surgically created arteriovenous fistulas.[69] Diagnosis is usually obvious. For traumatic or post-injection fistulas, Duplex sonogram imaging, technetium scanning or MR angiography are diagnostic. Arteriography is usually not necessary unless embolization is selected as a treatment option.

Chronic ischemia

Arterial thrombosis

The ulnar artery is the most common site for thrombosis in the upper extremity. The anatomy of Guyon's canal leaves the ulnar artery vulnerable at the hook of the hamate.[54]

Repetitive trauma may damage the intima and cause hypothenar hammer syndrome. Ischemic pain or paresthesias in the ulnar two digits, color changes and tenderness are the usual signs at presentation. Allen's test will show poor inflow through the ulnar artery. Digital plethysmography (pulse volume recordings) quantifies the degree of compromised perfusion. Duplex sonogram or MR angiography will reveal occlusion of the ulnar artery. Arteriography may show the diagnostic "corkscrew" sign of hypothenar hammer syndrome due to alternating segmental stenoses.[71]

Radial artery thrombosis occurs much less frequently compared to ulnar artery thrombosis. Ischemic pain and cold intolerance are confined to the thumb and index finger. Diagnostic modalities are similar to those described for ulnar artery thrombosis.

Vibration-induced "white finger syndrome" represents thrombosis of the digital arteries, and occurs most frequently in the index finger. A digital Allen test is helpful but an ultrasonogram and angiography is diagnostic.[44]

Aneurysm

Upper extremity aneurysms may be divided into two types. True aneurysms contain three layers of the arterial wall whereas a false aneurysm or pseudoaneurysm lacks endothelial cells. A true aneurysm occurs most frequently in areas of repetitive trauma or is related to atherosclerosis. A pseudoaneurysm is usually the result of a penetrating injury.

A painless, palpable mass is highly suspicious of an aneurysm but signs and symptoms of ischemia are very uncommon. Rarely nerve compression may cause pain or sensory abnormalities. An aneurysm is readily identified by a Doppler duplex ultrasonogram. Arteriography defines the extent of involvement and allows for evaluation of collateral flow for preoperative planning.[72]

Arteritis

Buerger's disease

Buerger's disease or thromboangiitis obliterans is an inflammatory disease of the small and medium sized vessels of the upper and lower extremities.[73] Diagnosis is dependent on five

criteria: (1) smoking history; (2) onset before 50 years age; (3) arterial lesions below the knee; (4) upper limb involvement or migratory phlebitis, and (5) absence of atherosclerotic risk factors other than smoking. Surgical treatment by interposition or bypass vein grafting has been ineffective because the process occurs in the very distal vessels.

Connective tissue disorders

- Systemic sclerosis (scleroderma)
- Mixed connective tissue disease
- Systemic lupus erythematosus
- Wegner's granulomatosis.

Ischemic symptoms in connective tissue disorders should be investigated with noninvasive modalities first, such as segmental arterial pressure measurements, pulse volume recordings, and cold stress testing. Angiography is necessary if surgery is contemplated.

Vasospastic disease

1. Primary Raynaud's disease
2. Secondary Raynaud's syndrome.

As described previously, the medical literature relevant to vasospastic disease or Raynaud's syndrome is confusing and at times misleading. Koman[24] described the criteria of Raynaud's disease and Raynaud's phenomenon (*Box 22.3, Table 22.1*).

Vasospastic conditions are either defined as primary with absence of an identifiable etiology or secondary associated with an underlying cause. Based on this terminology, Raynaud's disease is primary and all other conditions are secondary.[25] The vessels in primary Raynaud's disease are not diseased, hence the prognosis is benign. Because the structure of the artery is normal, arterial reconstruction is not necessary, but occasionally patients who are refractory to medical treatment may be candidates for cervical sympathectomy or digital sympathectomy.

In comparison to primary Raynaud's disease, secondary Raynaud's syndrome has a more severe prognosis, which is primarily related to the severity of the underlying disease.[15] Surgical treatment of the ischemia in secondary Raynaud's syndrome includes digital sympathectomy and arterial reconstruction.

BOX 22.3 Criteria defining Raynaud's disease

- Characteristic triphasic digital color changes
- Bilateral hand movement
- Absence of occlusive disease
- Absence of gangrene or trophic changes (fingertip trophic findings permissible)
- Absence of identifiable systemic disease (e.g., collagen vascular disorder)
- Symptoms at least 2 year's duration
- Female predominance

Data from Dabich L, Bookstein JJ, Zweifler A, *et al*. Digital arteries in patients with scleroderma. Arteriographic and plethysmographic study. Arch Intern Med. 1972;130(5):708–714.

Table 22.1 Raynaud's disease versus Raynaud syndrome

Characteristics	Disease	Syndrome
History		
Triphasic color change	Yes	Yes
Age >40	No	Yes
Progression rapid	No	Yes
Underlying disease	No	Yes
Female predominance	Frequent	Occasional
Physical examination		
Trophic findings	Infrequent	Frequent
(ulcer, gangrene)		
Abnormal Allen test	No	Common
Asymmetric findings	Infrequent	Frequent
Laboratory testing		
Blood chemistry	Normal	Frequently abnormal
Microangiography	Normal	Frequently abnormal
Angiography	Normal	Frequently abnormal

Reproduced with permission from Koman LA, Ruch DS, Smith BP, et al. Vascular disorders. In: Green DP, Hotchkiss RN, Pederson WC, eds. Green's operative hand surgery. New York: Churchill Livingstone; 1999:2254–2302.

Treatment

A detailed history, physical examination and differential diagnosis are the first steps in the management of ischemia of the hand. An arteriogram is essential to evaluate the arterial system of the entire upper extremity from the aortic arch to the digital arteries. The aims of treatment are to restore blood flow to an ischemic limb, prevent thromboembolic complications and preserve hand function by avoiding secondary muscle ischemia and necrosis through compartment syndrome.

Treatments are selected according to the cause of ischemia,[25] with options ranging from environmental modification to surgical intervention. Various pharmacologic agents can be used to counteract the effect of humoral factors on the muscular layers of the arterial wall in a conservative medical approach, whereas surgical intervention is directed at interrupting the sympathetic innervation of the muscle layer or by physical dilatation of the obstructed lumen or by microsurgical reconstruction of the occluded lumen.

Nonsurgical treatment

Environmental modification

Cessation of smoking, avoidance of cold exposure and limitation of activities which precipitate symptoms are fundamental. Cigarette smoking increases vasoconstrictor tone and alters blood coagulability; both are detrimental to a patient with ischemic disease. Nicotine patches may be used because they do not impair nutritional blood flow.[25] It is important that patients are aware of the relationship between cold and emotional stress and the reflex vasospasm in their hands.[57] Most patients intuitively avoid these circumstances but should also be instructed in protective techniques.

Medical management

Pharmacological agents

Drug therapy is aimed at mitigating the sympathetic hyperactivity in vasospastic and occluded arteries. Topical nitroglycerine is a simple first-line treatment in an attempt to relieve the pain associated with digital ulcerations. Currently, calcium channel blockers are the optimal choice for vasospastic symptoms,[74] by preventing calcium influx in vascular smooth muscle cells, which, in turn, ameliorates sympathetically driven vasoconstriction. Nifedipine, 10–30 mg orally three times a day, or in a long-acting form (30–60 mg/day) sustained-release capsules once or twice a day is most commonly used.[11]

Both tricyclic antidepressants and selective serotonin reuptake inhibitors have also proved efficacious in the treatment of chronic pain due to ischemia. However, some drugs that directly affect sympathetic tone (α-adrenergic antagonists) are often difficult for patients to tolerate due to their side-effects.[75,76] Local anesthetic blockade and intra-arterial vasodilators such as reserpine and guanethidine have been used systemically and by local injection, but long-term benefit has not been achieved.[77]

For treatment of obstructive Raynaud's syndrome, vasodilator drugs that alter prostaglandin metabolism (prostaglandin E1, prostacyclin and its analogues), and rheologic agents (aspirin[Rx], pentoxifylline[Rx], piracetam) have been advocated.[15] Some success has been reported with intra-arterial administration of prostaglandin E1, a potent vasodilator and inhibitor of platelet aggregation.[73]

Recently, Van Beek et al. described a novel use for Botox (Botulinum toxin A) in the management of vasospastic disorders.[74] Injection of botulinum toxin A into the hand appears to have a beneficial effect on intractable digital ulcerations and rest pain in patients with severe vasospastic disorders.

Thrombolytic therapy

Thrombolytic agents may be helpful for an embolic occlusion of a small vessel, especially if the agent is administered shortly after the acute embolic event. They can also be used preoperatively as an adjunct to vessel repair by lysing clot that is obscuring an underlying vascular abnormality (e.g., aneurysm), permitting the surgeon to plan reconstruction of the vessel abnormality.[78] Successful salvage of hand ischemia events has also been described with a combination of PGE1 and local fibrinolytic therapy with tissue plasminogen activator (rt-PA).[79] Although some authors[80] have doubted the benefit of fibrinolytic agents for treatment of a preformed thrombus in a small (0.82–1.5 mm) vessel, low-dose streptokinase has been shown to be clinically effective for a thrombus in the hand if the drug is administered locally as a continuous infusion within 36 hours after the onset of symptoms.[81] Anticoagulation using intravenous heparin to prevent the propagation of thromboemboli and permit early lysis of thrombotic arterial occlusions should be instituted intraoperatively.[82–84] The role of low-molecular weight heparin in contrast to intravenous heparin has not been addressed thus far. McClinton made the following suggestions to increase the likelihood of success; initiate the infusion as soon as possible, be alert to the effect of systemic anticoagulation, and proceed with surgical exploration if no lysis occurs after the initial 2-h high-dose treatment. Steroids and iloprost (a prostacyclin analogue with potent vasodilating and antiaggregant properties) have anecdotal results.[82,84] The role of phosphodiesterase inhibitors such as sildenafil has yet to be determined.

Biofeedback

Biofeedback training to develop central nervous system control over peripheral autonomic functions involves instruction in techniques that allow the conscious regulation of autonomic body processes. This entails consciously increasing digital blood flow or temperature.[85]

Biofeedback improves symptoms most effectively in patients with Raynaud's disease, vasospasm from nonneural or nonvascular etiology, and Raynaud's phenomenon with adequate collateral circulation. However, it tends not to be helpful in secondary vasospastic disease.

Thermal biofeedback is effective in primary vasospastic disease increasing digital flow, raising digital temperatures, and reducing cold-induced symptoms 2–3 years after treatment.[15,25,86]

Surgical treatment

Surgical intervention should be considered in patients who are refractory to medical treatment. Surgical options include reconstruction or bypass of occluded vessels by microvascular reconstruction with or without vein grafts and/or modification of sympathetic tone.[49,87–89] Sympathetic tone may be reduced by (1) proximal cervicothoracic sympathectomy, (2) Leriche sympathectomy (resection and ligation of a thrombosed or occluded arterial segment), (3) peripheral periarterial sympathectomy, and (4) new techniques in balloon angioplasty with periarterial sympathectomy.

Embolectomy

Emboli can be removed through a brachial arteriotomy and passage of catheters both proximally and distally. Number 2 or 3 Fr Fogarty catheters can usually be threaded all the way into the hand. If distal pulses do not return following restoration of flow, completion angiography is mandatory.

In high-flow arteriovenous malformations when emboli diminished the blood flow, initial attempts to preserve the fistula and relieve the vascular steal were aimed at reducing flow across the fistula by narrowing the fistula with bands. Even with precise intraoperative monitoring, this technique failed because of a high rate of fistula thrombosis.[90] Berman et al.[91,92] reported successful distal revascularization-interval ligation in more than 90% of patients.

Sympathectomy

When medical management has failed to control rest pain, or there is impending infarction of digits, or nonhealing of ischemic ulcerations, digital artery sympathectomy is indicated.

Most of the sympathetic nerves in the upper extremity emerge from the spinal cord with the ventral roots of the second and third thoracic nerves[93] and are widely dispersed in the brachial plexus to the forearm and hand.[88,94] Cervical sympathectomy has a long history in the treatment of secondary vasospasm, but has currently lost favor because it has a high relapse rate and is essentially of no benefit in connective tissue disease.[15,93] Pick[94] first noted in his dissections of the sympathetic nervous system that some of the sympathetic nerves bypass the sympathetic trunk and pass first with proximal somatic nerves and then in the periarterial adventitia to the digits. Failure of cervical sympathectomy for upper extremity vasospastic disease may be due to branches that bypass the cervicothoracic sympathetic trunk and are not interrupted during the operative procedure of cervical sympathectomy.[88,89]

Sympathetic nerve branches pass from the peripheral nerves to adjacent arteries at intervals along the extremity and travel in the perivascular tissue including the large and easily identifiable nerve of Henle. This nerve accompanies the ulnar artery along its course from forearm to the hand, supplying several large segments to the ulnar artery.[95] Pick[94] identified individual sympathetic nerve branches to the arterial structures from the wrist to the digits, providing a basis for the current approach to surgical sympathectomy of the hand and digits.[96] This anatomic concept has provided the basis for two types of peripheral sympathectomy.

Leriche sympathectomy (arteriectomy)

Leriche advocated excision and ligation of the thrombosed or diseased arterial segment to improve collateral circulation and interrupt the vasomotor disturbance. If there is adequate collateral flow, excision of a thrombosed arterial segment without reconstruction, interrupts sympathetic control over the distal vessels and reduces vasospasm. Several surgeons determine intraoperatively whether adequate collateral flow exists (e.g., after excision of a segment of ulnar artery) by measuring digital arterial pressures.[54,86,97] Zook et al.[98] have applied the Leriche sympathectomy concept to the digits by excising segments of occluded digital arteries when digital artery bypass was not possible.

Periarterial sympathectomy

Flatt[88] first introduced the concept of a sympathectomy at the digital level to apply its effect more distally in the extremity. Surgical stripping of the adventitia from arteries to interrupt the sympathetic innervation to the smooth muscle in the vessel media has been tried in situations of acute vasospasm following trauma or during microsurgery. However, this technique may be ineffective because of the vasoconstrictive effect on the smooth muscle by humoral factors, including catecholamines encountered in ischemic conditions.

By directly removing the sympathetic nerve input from the arteries, it is possible to block alternative sympathetic pathways or receptor upregulation. Flatt divided connections carrying sympathetic nerve fibers between the digital nerve and digital artery by stripping a 3–4 mm long segment of adventitia from the common digital artery; Eight patients had variable relief of their symptoms. Wilgis[10,89] extended this surgical dissection to include a 2 cm segment of the common and proper digital arteries and used preoperative anesthetic blockade to predict which patients would benefit from the procedure. Both

Flatt and Wilgis noted symptomatic relief in patients with primary vasospastic disease but did not achieve consistently good results in patients with connective tissue diseases.

Jones[99] introduced a more radical digital sympathectomy, with an extended digital sympathectomy for patients with connective tissue disease both to interrupt the sympathetic fibers and to remove fibrous tissue that encircles and compresses the arteries. Both the radial and ulnar arteries at the wrist are exposed and stripped over a 3 cm distance. The incision for the ulnar artery is extended into the palm in an inverted J-shaped fashion so that the entire ulnar artery and superficial palmar arch can be stripped of adventitia and sympathetic nerve fibers. The common and proper digital arteries are stripped from their origin to the base of the fingers, but not as far as the proximal interphalangeal joint, under the operating microscope. If the thumb and index finger are involved, the dorsal branch of the radial artery[100] is stripped from the anatomic snuffbox to the origin of the deep palmar arch. The high incidence of ulnar artery occlusion has been previously mentioned in connective tissue disorders. In such patients, if there is sufficient distal arterial runoff, microsurgical bypass grafting from the proximal ulnar artery to the superficial palmar arch or common digital arteries can be performed.[15,99,101] Koman *et al.*[102] demonstrated that sympathectomy can increase the percentage of nutritional blood flow with resultant healing of ulcers and gangrene.

The authors suggest that two different sympathectomy procedures should be considered depending on the severity of the disease: In a limited digital sympathectomy, adventitia is stripped from the radial and ulnar digital arteries and common digital arteries. In an extended, radical digital sympathectomy, adventitia is stripped from the radial and ulnar arteries, the common digital arteries and the proper digital arteries (*Figs 22.6, 22.7*).[104]

Because of the myogenic nature of the spasm, treatment may not just be directed towards the autonomic nervous system. The principle of mechanical dilatation is based on the observation of Bard,[103] who noticed that a vessel in a state of tonic contraction may respond by reflex dilatation when mechanical dilatation is applied. Vessel constriction should not be treated by physical dilatation until the nature of the lesion has been determined, intimal damage with or without thrombosis has been excluded, and if pharmacologic treatment has been ineffective. A closed technique may be tried initially in which heparinized saline solution is injected under pressure between occluding vascular clamps. An arteriotomy may be required and the vessel dilated with a small Fogarty catheter.

Arterial reconstruction

For small partial arterial injuries, closure in a transverse direction prevents narrowing of the lumen. Even with significant (up to 60%) arterial narrowing after transverse closure, flow is not affected.[110] A vein patch can be used to close a more extensive partial injury.[64,86] Sharp arterial transections can often be repaired end-to-end if the vessel ends are mobilized sufficiently. More extensive untidy arterial injuries commonly require a reversed vein graft interposed between the proximal and distal arterial ends. The cephalic, basilic, distal greater saphenous, and distal lesser saphenous veins are used most frequently. Some 10–30% more length of vein than is

estimated, is harvested and then the vein graft is reversed or the valves incised. For axillary and brachial arterial injuries, the greater saphenous vein is preferred.[63,64] A local forearm vein can be used for distal brachial, radial, and ulnar artery repairs when the extremity has not sustained significant additional soft tissue trauma. If forearm trauma precludes use of a local vein graft, leg or dorsal foot veins are used.[63]

Arterial reconstruction for symptomatic thrombosis or occlusion can be managed by ligation alone, excision with end-to-end repair, or excision and interposition grafting. Surgical indications include (1) absence of an alternative arterial inflow, (2) two or more levels of occlusion that compromise potential collateral flow, (3) thrombosis extending beyond the origins of the common digital vessels, and (4) incomplete deep and superficial arches. The major indication for arterial reconstruction is inadequate perfusion with a DBI (digital brachial index) of <0.7; If an appropriate risk-benefit ratio exists, arterial reconstruction should be performed.[25]

Surgical techniques include:

1. *In situ* and nonreversed vein grafts
2. Interposition reversed vein grafts
3. Interposition arterial grafts
4. Arterialization of venous flow
5. Free omental transfer.

The goal of arterial reconstruction is to increase digital blood flow and restore nutritional flow. Successful arterial reconstruction in patients with underlying collagen vascular disease increases total digital blood flow and nutritional flow, diminishes symptoms, and promotes healing of ulcers. Regardless of the etiology, the level and extent of occlusion, the adequacy of collateral flow, and any component of sympathetic overactivity obviously influence the results of reconstruction for arterial thrombosis and occlusion.

Jones advocated that if by stringent clinical and angiographic criteria, segmental thrombosis or occlusions are identified in the distal radial and/or ulnar arteries and the superficial palmar arch, and if adequate distal "run off" can be demonstrated in the common digital arteries, microsurgical revascularization should be considered in patients with symptomatic hand ischemia unresponsive to medical management.[5] Jones described four basic vein graft configurations that have evolved for revascularization of the hand, and this classification may be helpful in planning surgery.[1]

For short segmental occlusions or thrombosis of the ulnar artery in Guyon's canal, end-to-end anastomosis of a vein graft or arterial graft from the ulnar artery in the distal forearm to the distal ulnar artery just proximal to the superficial palmar arch is classified as a type I configuration.

Occlusion of the distal radial artery is much rarer in comparison to ulnar artery occlusion. End-to-end anastomosis of a vein graft or arterial graft from the distal radial artery in the forearm to the deep palmar arch or princeps pollicis artery in the thumb–index web space is classified as a type II configuration.

If the superficial palmar arch is involved but the common digital arteries are spared, reconstruction of the superficial palmar arch may become necessary with end-to-end anastomosis of the vein or arterial graft to the ulnar artery in the distal forearm and end-to-side anastomoses of the common digital arteries to the interposition vein graft. This type III

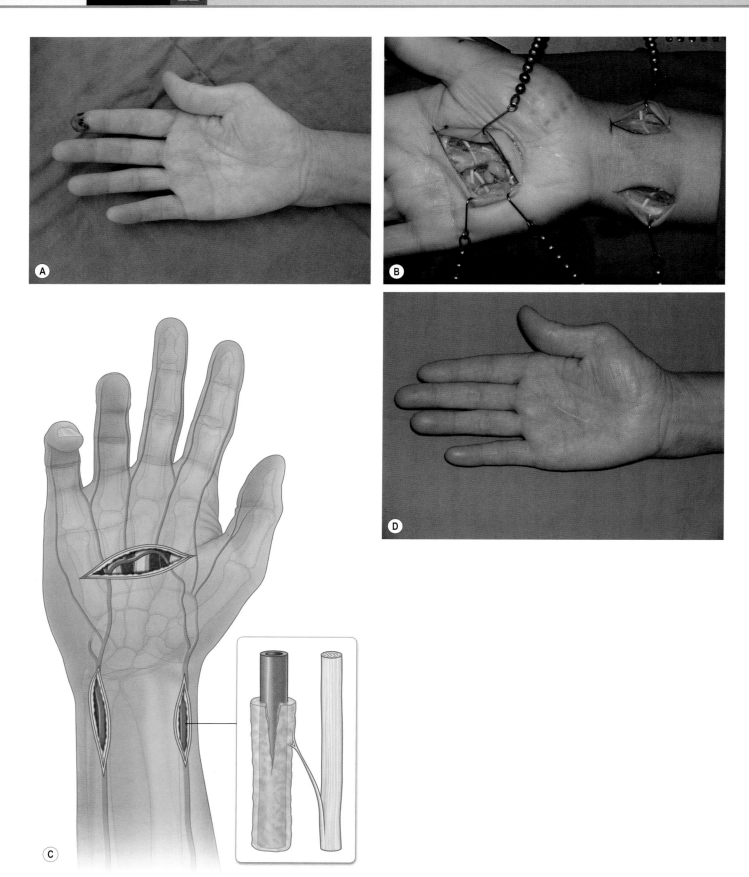

Fig. 22.6 Limited digital sympathectomy. (A) Preoperative. (B) Operative view.
(C) Schematic drawing. (D) Postoperative view.

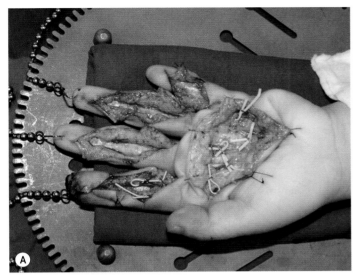

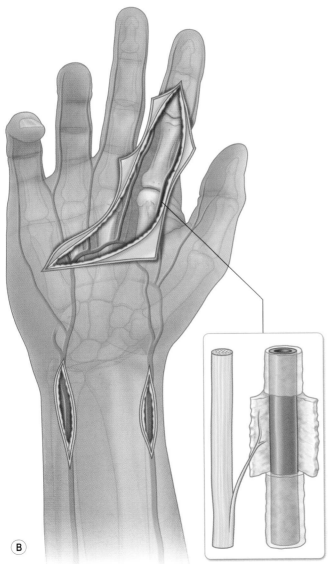

Fig. 22.7 Radical digital sympathectomy. (A) Radical sympathectomy of common and proper digital arteries in the palm and digits. (B) Schematic drawing of radical digital sympathectomy.

Table 22.2 Wake Forest classification of occlusive/vasospastic/vaso-occlusive disease

Group	Etiology	
I	Raynaud's disease	Idiopathic
II	Raynaud's syndrome	Collagen vascular disease
A	Adequate circulation	
B	Inadequate circulation	
III	Secondary vasospasm/ occlusive disease	Vascular injury
A	Adequate circulation	Occlusion/embolus
B	Inadequate circulation	
IV	Secondary vasospasm	Nonvascular injury
		Nerve/bone/soft tissue damage

Reproduced with permission from Koman LA, Ruch DS, Smith BP, et al. Vascular disorders. In: Green DP, Hotchkiss RN, Pederson WC, eds. Green's operative hand surgery. New York: Churchill Livingstone; 1999:2254–2302.

configuration is commonly required in systemic disease manifest by secondary Raynaud's disease. In this situation, a deep inferior epigastric arterial graft may be more useful than a vein graft. The deep inferior epigastric artery has numerous branches which can be used to reconstruct a new palmar arch with end-to-end anastomoses to the common digital arteries. End-to-end anastomoses are easier to perform compared with end-to-side anastomoses if an interposition vein graft is used which may also cause turbulent flow.

There are other technical advantages to using an autologous deep inferior epigastric artery graft. The size match between the inflow ulnar artery and the proximal epigastric artery is excellent.[111] The deep inferior epigastric artery tapers as it gives off branches and the size of these distal branches is a close match for anastomoses to the common digital arteries (Fig. 22.8).

In a type IV configuration, two interposition vein grafts or two deep inferior epigastric artery grafts are used to revascularize the superficial palmar arch or common digital arteries from the distal ulnar artery and the deep palmar arch or princeps pollicis artery from the distal radial artery.

In the Wake Forest classification of occlusive/vasospastic/vaso-occlusive disease (Table 22.2), Koman et al. recommended that arterial reconstruction is indicated in patients with refractory symptoms and inadequate collateral circulation (groups IIB and IIIB), and should be individualized in groups IIA and IIIA.[24]

Aneurysms

Treatment options include: (1) resection and ligation;[108] (2) excision of the damaged wall and "patch" grafting; (3) resection with end-to-end repair, and (4) resection with an interposition graft, depending on collateral flow and vasomotor tone.[109]

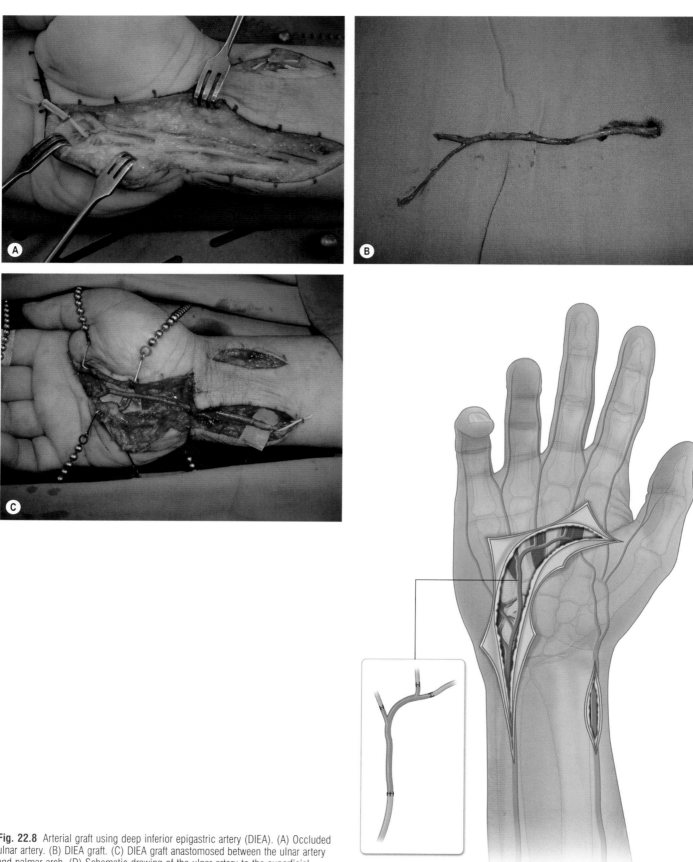

Fig. 22.8 Arterial graft using deep inferior epigastric artery (DIEA). (A) Occluded ulnar artery. (B) DIEA graft. (C) DIEA graft anastomosed between the ulnar artery and palmar arch. (D) Schematic drawing of the ulnar artery to the superficial palmar arch reconstruction.

Early excision of true or false aneurysms of the radial or ulnar arteries is strongly advocated to prevent distal embolization. An intraoperative digital/brachial artery index <0.7 after aneurysm excision indicates the need for arterial reconstruction.[54] Postoperative care and surgical outcomes are similar to those after reconstruction of ulnar artery thrombosis (*Fig. 22.9*).

Mycotic aneurysms are secondary to hematogenous or local bacterial infection that weakens the vessel wall and virtually all are now due to intravenous drug abuse.[72] Infection producing a soft tissue swelling overlying an artery should be evaluated for the possibility of a false aneurysm to avoid an ill-advised incision and drainage procedure. If clinical examination is not conclusive, duplex scanning should be diagnostic. Excision and ligation of the artery are preferred if the feeding vessel is not critical to limb survival, otherwise excision and vein bypass around the infected area will restore arterial inflow.

Balloon angioplasty for stenotic lesions

Ahn applied the technique of balloon angioplasty for treating patients with secondary Raynaud's syndrome who had an arterial stenosis of their radial and ulnar arteries diagnosed by arteriography.[112] After adventitial stripping of the affected radial and ulnar arteries, palmar arch, and common digital arteries, vessel dilatation was performed using a PTCA balloon catheter. The balloon was inserted through a branch of the ulnar artery and advanced from the main artery through Guyon's canal, into the palmar arch, and common digital arteries. Sequential dilatation of any stenotic segment was performed by inflation of the balloon to six atmospheres for 40 seconds.

Balloon catheter dilatation is a useful adjunct procedure and may potentiate the effects of digital sympathectomy. The technique can also be used for incomplete arterial occlusions up to 15 cm in length and may eliminate the need for interposition vein grafts (*Fig. 22.10*).

Other surgical options

Surgeons have investigated alternative options to salvage severely ischemic limbs when standard arterial bypass procedures are not possible. Two salvage procedures for impending digital loss are reversal of blood flow through the upper

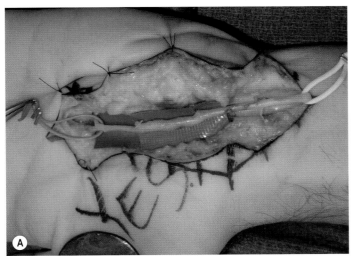

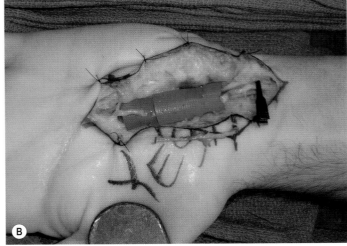

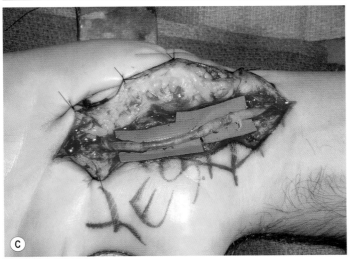

Fig. 22.9 Ulnar artery aneurysm treated by resection and interpositional vein graft. (A) Aneurysm. (B) Resection. (C) Interpositional vein graft.

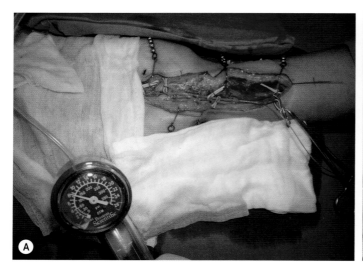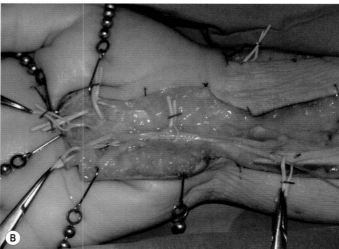

Fig. 22.10 Balloon angioplasty. (A) Ballooning of stenotic ulnar artery. (B) Ballooning of the palmar arch.

extremity veins and vascularized omental transfer to the dorsum of the hand.

King *et al.*[105] reported arterialization of the venous system of the upper limb based on in situ vein bypass. In situ vein bypass is a standard vascular surgery technique that involves complete exposure of the chosen vein and ligation of all its branches. A small valvulotome is used to divide each half of the bicuspid valves in the vein all the way to the metacarpal heads distally. The vein is then anastomosed to a proximal artery (usually end-to-end to the brachial artery), shunting arterial blood through the vein into the hand. Patients are heparinized after this procedure. Pederson has used the concept of reverse venous flow to improve vascularity in severe hand ischemia. He anastomosed the distal portion of either the radial or ulnar artery to suitable hand veins thereby creating a reverse flow situation in an attempt to improve capillary perfusion. He reported his personal experience in over 20 cases, and showed significant improvement in pain and ulceration after the procedure.[106,107]

The recipient vein is prepared by removing the valves at the level of the metacarpal necks. The cephalic vein is well suited for this procedure because it has great interconnections with the dorsal venous system of the hand, which potentially allows for a single proximal anastomosis. Arterial branches are then ligated and the proximal end-to-side anastomosis is performed. Postoperative thrombosis and swelling of the limb may result.

A new blood supply can be supplied indirectly to the hand, by a second technique. A free omental flap is harvested and placed beneath the dorsal skin of the forearm and hand, and the superior gastro-epiploic artery and vein anastomosed to the brachial artery and cephalic vein at the elbow.[106,107]

Treatment algorithm

All patients with chronic ischemia of the hand should obviously be treated pharmacologically with topical nitroglycerin, calcium channel blockers, vasodilators, and possibly botulinum toxin.[74] Patients with ischemic pain often follow an intractable course and surgical intervention is frequently inevitable. Established gangrene, osteomyelitis and septic arthritis usually require a digital amputation. Amputations are effective in relieving patients' pain, for which they are very grateful.

Arteriography, MR angiography or Duplex ultrasound will allow delineation of the exact site and extent of any stenosis or complete occlusion, and assist in surgical planning. Indications for arteriography with the intent of surgical revascularization include the following:

- unilateral Raynaud's phenomenon;
- progressive digital ulceration or gangrene despite good medical management;
- recurrent digital ulceration; and
- Doppler evidence of occlusion of a major artery.[5]

Specific indications for surgical intervention in patients with chronic ischemia of the hand have been suggested.[5,99] Options for surgical intervention include digital sympathectomy, balloon angioplasty and microsurgical revascularization using interposition vein grafts or arterial grafts. In some patients these procedures can be combined.

In a patient with Raynaud's phenomenon unresponsive to pharmacological treatment, if angiography reveals no evidence of occlusion of the main inflow radial and ulnar arteries and satisfactory visualization of the three common digital arteries, digital sympathectomy should be considered.[99,104]

If angiography reveals stenosis or occlusion of the radial or ulnar arteries over a distance of <3 cm, balloon angioplasty may be considered so that expansion of the vessel lumen may increase digital blood flow. Balloon angioplasty can also be combined with radical sympathectomy.

If angiography demonstrates segmental occlusions of the main inflow radial and/or ulnar arteries but there is satisfactory "run-off" in the common digital arteries, microsurgical revascularization of the superficial palmar arch from the ulnar artery and much less frequently microsurgical revascularization of the deep palmar arch from the radial artery can be considered.

Despite more complicated harvesting, a deep inferior epigastric artery graft may allow end-to-end anastomoses of the branches of the arterial graft to the common digital arteries, whereas an interposition vein graft requires end-to-side anastomoses. However, the more extensive the involvement of the ulnar or radial arteries, the more likely that an interposition vein graft rather than an interposition arterial graft is required.[112]

If the symptoms of chronic ischemia are localized to a single finger and angiography reveals a discrete segment of occlusion of a proper digital artery, resection of the segment of proper digital artery and reconstruction with an interposition vein graft or arterial graft may occasionally be considered *(Fig. 22.11)*.[113] Balloon angioplasty of a stenotic common digital artery or proper digital artery is very difficult and may result in vessel rupture.[112]

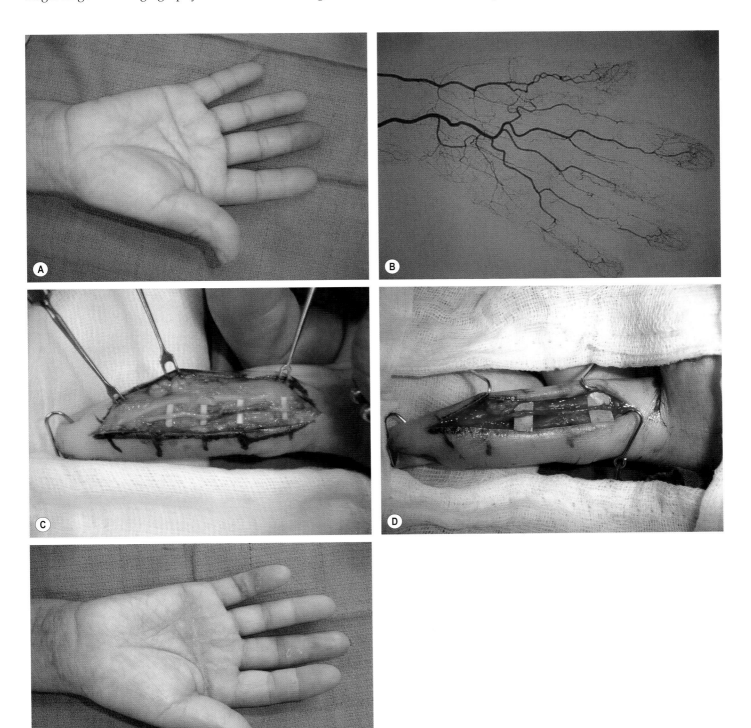

Fig. 22.11 Proper digital artery reconstruction with reverse vein graft. (A) Preoperative. (B) Angiogram showing occlusion of the proper digital arteries to the middle finger. (C) Occlusion of the ulnar digital artery. (D) Resection and interposition vein graft. (E) Postoperative.

Postoperative care

After microsurgical revascularization procedures, a single bolus of heparin (1000–2400 IU, IV push) is administered immediately before the microsurgical clamps are removed and either heparin is maintained for 7 days, or dextran 40 is administered intravenously at 25 cc/hour for 5 days. If there is extensive intimal damage or vascular compromise, full heparinization and conversion to Coumadin is advisable. A bulky hand and forearm dressing with a dorsal plaster of Paris splint is applied with the hand in a functional position. A drain is left in place for 12–36 hours. Circulation to the finger tips is assessed every hour for 6 hours and then every 4 hours for 24 hours. Critical arterial reconstructions are monitored in the same way as replantations. Changes in color and capillary refill; temperature monitoring (loss of >2°C in 1 hour); pencil Doppler monitoring or pulse oximetry can be used. If sedation is required, chlorpromazine (25 mg orally three times daily) is prescribed. The patient obviously discontinues smoking, and avoids caffeine consumption. The patient is discharged home on aspirin 81 mg daily and continued for up to 3 months.

Sutures are removed at 10–14 days postoperatively. The hand is protected for 2–6 weeks in a lightweight splint and the patient is instructed to avoid any trauma to the surgical site. Some residual cold sensitivity, soreness, pillar-type palm pain, and ulnar nerve irritability are expected. Return to work is based on job type after 6–12 weeks, no athletic or work restrictions are necessary if the patient is asymptomatic.

Outcomes, prognosis and complications

Complications after surgical intervention for ischemia of the hand include impaired healing of the incision, dehiscence, infection, stiffness of the fingers, and specifically after microsurgical revascularization, thrombosis of the anastomoses.

After digital sympathectomy, patients usually report improvement in their symptoms of pain and cold tolerance, reduction in the frequency and severity of Raynaud's episodes and healing of digital ulcers.[99,119]

Microsurgical revascularization increases distal arterial perfusion, reduces symptoms of ischemic pain, promotes healing of ulcers and prevents progression to gangrene in hands without adequate collateral circulation.[99] Koman et al. have demonstrated that this is due to an increase in the ratio of nutritional to total flow without increasing total microvascular perfusion within digits.[102] Patency rates of 80–90% can be expected of interposition vein grafts for hypothenar hammer syndrome, but thrombosis of the grafts can occur and symptoms return in longer follow-up. Of 106 interposition vein graft reconstructions of the ulnar artery, 87 (82%) remained patent.[40,97,114–117]

The prognosis for patients with chronic ischemia of their hands depends on the etiology, the severity, the response to treatment and progression of the underlying condition.[99,118] Prognosis seems to be worse in patients with diabetes and renal vascular disease. Hartzell et al. reported that long-term follow-up of 27 patients, revealed that while digital sympathectomy healed digital ulcers and decreased the number of ulcers in vasospastic disease in autoimmune patients, the efficacy was much lower in patients with vasospasm secondary to atherosclerosis. This might explain why the prognosis is worse in patients with underlying diabetes.[119] Patients with chronic ischemia of their hands due to scleroderma show improvement after digital sympathectomy and microsurgical revascularization, but because of progression of the underlying disease, there is a significant recurrence of digital ulcers 2 years after surgery.[21] Therefore, these procedures should be considered palliative rather than curative. Since digital sympathectomy and microsurgical revascularization cannot usually be repeated, recurrence of digital ulcerations may ultimately require amputations. Jones[99] has suggested that the hand be considered an "end organ" just like the heart, brain and kidneys and therefore hand ischemia may reflect similar pathology in these other organs.

Secondary procedures

Secondary procedures after digital sympathectomy or microsurgical revascularization are rare because of the postoperative scarring from the original operation. Revision surgeries at the same location are usually not advised. Digital amputation or even ray amputation would be a last option should the ischemia progress.

Access the complete references list online at **http://www.expertconsult.com**

1. Jones NF, Emerson ET. Interposition vein graft configurations for microsurgical revascularization of the ischemic hand. *Tech Hand Up Extrem Surg.* 1999;3(2):121–130.

    Despite the various causes of upper extremity ischemia, the presenting symptoms are usually predictable. These symptoms constitute acute ischemia, digital ulcers and gangrene, Raynaud's phenomena, or claudication with

exercise. For segmental arterial occlusive diseases in selected patients, microsurgical revascularization with bypass vein grafts may be effective. This study reviews such cases that are bypassable with vein grafts, and proposes a classification system for distal upper extremity bypass vein grafts.

5. Jones NF. Acute and chronic ischemia of the hand: pathophysiology, treatment, and prognosis. *J Hand Surg Am.* 1991;16(6):1074–1083.

Fifty patients with acute and chronic ischemia of the hand were investigated using various methods over 4 years. For many causes of the ischemia, medical management with emergent intra-arterial streptokinase, heparin, or dextran was used, along with nifedipine and pentoxifylline in chronic cases. Surgical treatment such as stellate ganglion blocks, microsurgical revascularization, and digital sympathectomy was used. Eighteen patients underwent amputation due to end-stage gangrene, and long-term follow-up revealed 20% incidence of recurrent digital ulcerations.

10. Wilgis EF. Evaluation and treatment of chronic digital ischemia. *Ann Surg.* 1981;193(6):693–698.

    Forty-two patients were evaluated and treated for chronic digital ischemia. Manifestations of pain, severe cold intolerance and occasional tip ulceration were seen despite conservative treatment of vasodilators, tobacco abstinence, and beta-blockers. Direct microvascular reconstruction, thermal biofeedback and digital sympathectomy were performed with improvement in 70% of patients.

21. Jones NF, Imbriglia JE, Steen VD, et al. Surgery for scleroderma of the hand. *J Hand Surg Am.* 1987;12(3):391–400.

    Out of 813 consecutive patients with scleroderma, 31 underwent one or more surgical procedures. Raynaud's phenomenon and digital tip ulcerations were controlled with vasodilators and meticulous local wound care. Frank gangrene was usually managed conservatively until autoamputation, but 23 digital amputations had to be performed. Digital sympathectomy and micro-revascularization were performed in selected patients. Arthrodesis was performed in patients with severe digital contractures.

24. Koman LA, Ruch DS, Smith BP, et al. Vascular disorders. In: Green DP, Hotchkiss RN, Pederson WC, eds. *Green's operative hand surgery.* New York: Churchill Livingstone; 1999:2254–2302.

    Symptomatic vascular disorders of the upper extremity interfere with health-related quality of life, diminish function, and have a negative impact on patients and society. Although less prevalent than ischemic lesions of the lower extremity, heart, or brain, upper extremity vascular morbidity is a significant social burden. Aberrant microvascular flow secondary to acute or chronic trauma, congenital deformity, systemic processes, or genetic influences affect over 10% of the general population and 20–30% of premenopausal women. Pain, cold intolerance, numbness, ulceration, or gangrene can result from these vascular insufficiencies or incompetencies. Abnormal perfusion may occur secondary to congenital or acquired events that affect vascular structures, vascular function, or both. Vascular insufficiency occurs due to blood flow compromise with decreased cellular perfusion and resultant cell damage, cellular injury, and pain. Various approaches to diagnosis and management of vascular disorders based on physiologic factors are covered.

88. Flatt AE. Digital artery sympathectomy. *J Hand Surg Am.* 1980;5(6):550–556.

89. Wilgis EF. Digital sympathectomy for vascular insufficiency. *Hand Clin.* 1985;1(2):361–367.

99. Jones NF. Ischemia of the hand in systemic disease. The potential role of microsurgical revascularization and digital sympathectomy. *Clin Plast Surg.* 1989;16(3):547–556.

101. Jones NF, Raynor SC, Medsger TA. Microsurgical revascularisation of the hand in scleroderma. *Br J Plast Surg.* 1987;40(3):264–269.

102. Koman LA, Smith BP, Pollock FE Jr, et al. The microcirculatory effects of peripheral sympathectomy. *J Hand Surg Am.* 1995;20(5):709–717.

118. Hartzell TL, Makhni EC, Sampson C. Long-term results of periarterial sympathectomy. *J Hand Surg Am.* 2009;34(8):1454–1460.

23

Complex regional pain syndrome in the upper extremity

Ivica Ducic and John M. Felder III

SYNOPSIS

- Complex regional pain syndrome (CRPS) is a regional pain syndrome occurring mostly in extremities after trauma that displays chronic regional pain, neurosensory changes, and features of dysautonomia, inflammation, and dystonia.
- The pain of CRPS may include an element of sympathetically maintained pain (SMP), sympathetically independent pain (SIP), or both.
- The emerging model for the pathogenesis of CRPS suggests a triad of nerve injury, peripheral sensitization, and central sensitization.
- Contemporary thinking suggests that CRPS I (reflex sympathetic dystrophy: RSD) is frequently related to small-caliber nerve pathology, even when a specific, discrete peripheral nerve injury is not identifiable by traditional means.
- Diagnosis of the syndrome rests on specific history and physical exam findings, and the lack of other plausible explanations. Various adjunctive testing measures serve mainly to characterize further an individual's disease and create an individualized approach to therapy.
- Diagnosis of CRPS should always prompt a thorough search for underlying nerve injury, such as nerve compression syndromes or neuromas which can be surgically treated.
- Early recognition and multidisciplinary management, including physical rehabilitation, pharmacologic and procedural pain management, psychological consideration, and peripheral nerve surgery evaluation, are crucial for effective treatment.
- When CRPS is due to identifiable nerve injury, treatment of nerve injury should be a primary treatment for the syndrome.
- A variety of peripheral nerve surgery techniques are indicated for treatment of CRPS, including neurolysis, nerve reconstruction, neuroma resection, and denervation. With proper patient selection, these techniques can provide effective and enduring therapy.
- Much of the burden of CRPS is due to changes mediated by the central nervous system (CNS). The peripheral nerve surgeon is most effective by preventing peripheral pathology from progressing to central changes.
- Understanding the scientific rationale for the new theories behind the development of CRPS provides a logically based directive for peripheral nerve surgeons to become more involved in managing this disorder.

Introduction

Few chronic medical problems are more frustrating for the physician and patient than severe and unremitting pain. Frustration develops not only when there is an inability to control symptoms, but also due to a poor understanding of their cause

"Complex regional pain syndrome" or CRPS is the moniker given to a disorder that is clinically challenging because it typifies these frustrations. Although the disorder is predominantly one of chronic pain, the full spectrum of its symptomatology and the mystifying sequence of pathophysiology that leads to its development have proven so confusing that even its name and diagnosis are a subject of debate. CRPS type I, formerly known as reflex sympathetic dystrophy (RSD), may develop after any noxious insult, but most commonly after an orthopedic extremity injury, such as a sprain or fracture, and/ or related treatments. CRPS type II, formerly known as causalgia, develops specifically after a nerve injury. Both are characterized by persistent pain, but unlike typical postinjury pain or typical neuralgia resulting from a nerve injury, the pain of CRPS may spread to a region beyond the zone of the original insult, may be maintained by adrenergic activity, and may encompass more than the territory of a single nerve. The pain of CRPS is constantly present but is often exacerbated by the presence of tactile allodynia or hyperpathia, to the point where patients may shield or hide the affected body part for fear of it being touched. In addition, the patient develops an array of symptoms, such as edema, osteopenia, vasodysregulation, temperature dysregulation, hyper- or hypohidrosis, or muscle dystonia, that are alarming to patients and physicians because they are more typically associated with autonomic or neurologic dysfunction than with physical injury (see

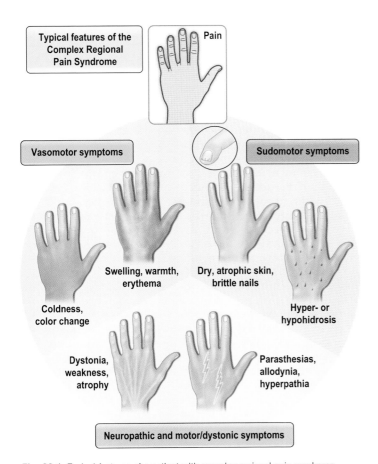

Fig. 23.1 Typical features of a patient with complex regional pain syndrome.

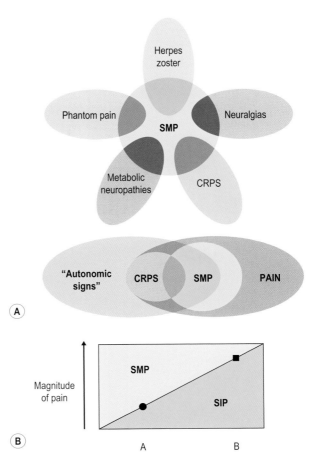

Fig. 23.2 International Association for the Study of Pain diagram of complex regional pain syndrome (CRPS). SMP, sympathetically maintained pain; SIP, sympathetically independent pain. (Adapted, with permission, from Stanton-Hicks M, Jänig W, Hassenbusch S, et al. Reflex sympathetic dystrophy: Changing concepts and taxonomy. *Pain.* 1995;63:127–133.)

Figure 23.1 for a summary of the complex of symptoms of CRPS). These changes, and possibly the disease process itself, lead many patients to develop comorbid anxiety, depression, and personality changes. Taken together, the pain and associated symptoms have the potential to be debilitating and isolating, and may either spontaneously resolve or progress to a chronic, unremitting form.

Theories for the underlying cause of the syndrome and their attendant epitaphs have ranged from those of peripheral nervous dysfunction (e.g., "causalgia"), of autonomic hyperactivity ("RSD"), of exaggerated inflammatory response ("Sudeck's osteodystrophy"), and even psychologic hysteria, among others. Each has found its supporters, but has failed to account for the entire clinical picture. The most contemporary terminology, CRPS, attempts to unify previously separate diagnoses under a less specific but more sensitive umbrella by removing from its name etiologic references (such as "reflex," "sympathetic," or "dystrophy") that are suggestive of underlying models of pathogenesis whose validity have never been borne out. It makes provisions to include disparate features such as sympathetically maintained pain (SMP) *(Fig. 23.2)* and nerve injury, without requiring their presence for diagnosis. Although the name "CRPS" and its diagnostic criteria were developed at a consensus conference of pain specialists in 1994 *(Table 23.1)*,[1] even these are not universally agreed upon,[2,3] with many authors preferring the older terms "RSD" and "causalgia."

Although multiple theories still coexist, progress is being made in rejecting convenient yet unfounded theories on the etiology of CRPS and developing research-based models that will do a better job both defining the disorder and its risk factors, and yielding more appropriate therapies.[4] The most compelling possibility is that all cases of CRPS are caused by some form of peripheral (somatic and/or autonomic) nerve damage. The empiric observation that both forms of CRPS may have identical clinical manifestations but that type II is brought on by a recognizable nerve injury (whereas the symptoms of type I are not as closely linked to a specific cause) is suggestive of a role for nerve injury in both types. As well, there is mounting research evidence to suggest that peripheral nerve damage, whether of large recognizable nerves or of smaller distal fibers, may be the inciting incident in a cascade of events that ultimately leads to the clinical syndrome of CRPS.[5–7] This chapter will explain how CRPS is linked to nerve injury, and why this provides a logical directive for the involvement of peripheral nerve surgeons in its treatment.

Pathophysiology

There is no consensus regarding the pathophysiologic mechanisms underlying the development of CRPS. However, most pertinent to peripheral nerve surgeons is the emerging model

Table 23.1 International Association for the Study of Pain criteria for diagnosis of chronic regional pain syndrome (CRPS)

CRPS type I (reflex sympathetic dystrophy)

1. Type I is a syndrome that develops after an initiating noxious event
2. Spontaneous pain or allodynia/hyperalgesia occurs, is not limited to the territory of a single peripheral nerve, and is disproportionate to the inciting event
3. There is or has been evidence of edema, skin blood flow abnormality, or abnormal sudomotor activity in the region of the pain since the inciting event
4. This diagnosis is excluded by the existence of conditions that would otherwise account for the degree of pain and dysfunction

CRPS type II (causalgia)

1. Type II is a syndrome that develops after a nerve injury. Spontaneous pain or allodynia/hyperalgesia occurs and is not necessarily limited to the territory of the injured nerve
2. There is or has been evidence of edema, skin blood flow abnormality, or abnormal sudomotor activity in the region of the pain since the inciting event
3. This diagnosis is excluded by the existence of conditions that would otherwise account for the degree of pain and dysfunction

(Reproduced from Stanton-Hicks M, Janig W, Hassenbusch S, et al. Reflex sympathetic dystrophy: changing concepts and taxonomy. Pain 1995;63:127–133.)

of CRPS as the ultimate result of untreated nerve injury. We propose the three components of this model: (1) peripheral nerve injury; (2) peripheral sensitization; and (3) central sensitization *(Fig. 23.3)*.

The two most common mechanisms of nerve injury are either from an acute trauma (including surgery), such as by crush, stretch, or transection, or from chronic compression *(Fig. 23.4)*, as is often seen in upper and lower extremity compression syndromes like carpal, cubital, radial, or tarsal tunnel. Nerve injuries may spontaneously recover, or they may result in neuroma, or compression neuropathy – two permanent disruptions in nerve architecture that generate chronic pain. In the case of trauma, the result of nerve injury is often a painful neuroma, where the cut or crushed end of a nerve grows aberrant sprouts in an attempt to regenerate *(Fig. 23.5)*. These sprouts become tangled in surrounding connective tissue, failing to regenerate along their normal course, and causing chronic pain. A variant of this pattern is the neuroma in continuity, where the nerve is not transected, but a crush injury disrupts the internal fascicular organization of the nerve; scar tissue then forms within the nerve, blocking the regeneration of axonal sprouts and creating a neuroma.[8,9] The other end point of nerve injury that causes chronic neuropathic pain is compression neuropathy *(Fig. 23.4)*. Compression neuropathy causes nerve ischemia and degeneration by physical pressure on the nerve, which occludes blood flow as well as axonal transport. Compression neuropathy may occur in the setting of a naturally tight anatomic tunnel exacerbated by tissue edema/hypertrophy (such as

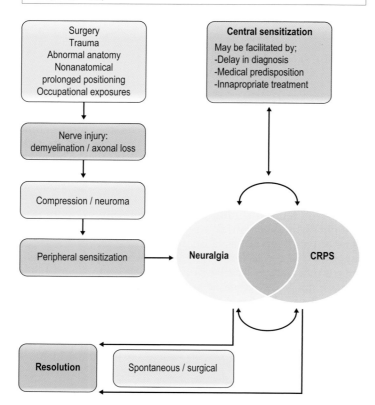

Fig. 23.3 Model for the development of complex regional pain syndrome (CRPS) from nerve injury. Nerve injury is followed by peripheral sensitization, which progresses to neuralgia. Via central sensitization, there is a regional spread of pain and activation of other inappropriate responses, leading to CRPS. The condition may resolve spontaneously, or with surgical treatment of the underlying nerve injury.

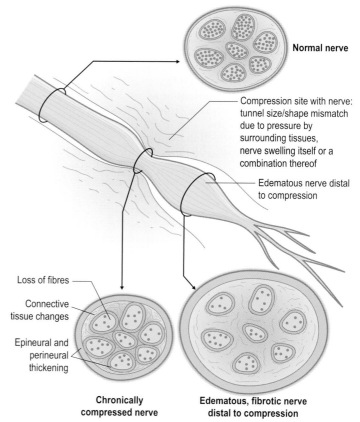

Fig. 23.4 Model of nerve compression.

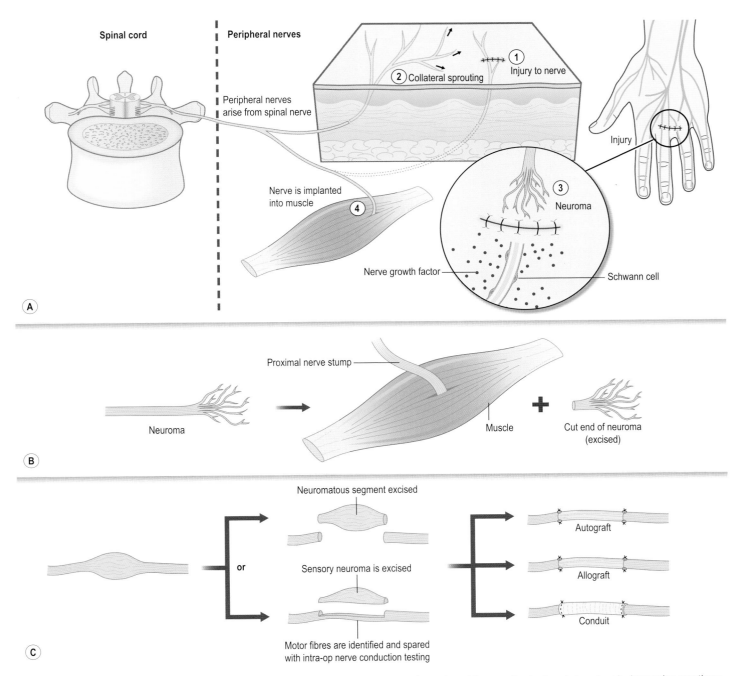

Fig. 23.5 Model of neuroma and neuroma in continuity. **(A)** Painful neuromas arise when normal neural repair/regeneration is disrupted, such as by intervening scar tissue. **(B)** The treatment for painful neuroma is resection of the neuroma with implantation of the proximal nerve stump into a muscle. **(C)** Neuroma in continuity is characterized by internal architectural derangement of an intact nerve. The segment containing neuroma can be selectively or totally resected, and then repaired using grafting or conduit.

occurs with overuse syndromes and trauma), or may be the result of nerve entrapment in scar tissue following trauma. Clinically recognizable neuromas or large-nerve compression neuropathies can be the basis for CRPS type II (causalgia), whereas damage to clinically undetectable small distal fibers is likely the basis of CRPS type I (RSD),[4,5,10,11] which does not classically include a nerve injury.

Not all nerve injuries progress to CRPS. Some may never be painful, or may be only briefly painful. Some may cause chronic neuropathic pain in the distribution of the injured nerve, but never lead to the regional spread, dysesthesias,

trophic changes, and associated dysautonomic symptoms that characterize CRPS. The first step towards the development of CRPS after nerve injury comes with the onset of peripheral sensitization, defined as a progressive increase in the response of peripheral nociceptors to repeated stimuli.[12] This increasing sensitivity of nociceptive afferents is brought about both by autosensitization, wherein activation of the receptor itself reduces its own activation threshold, and by heterosensitization, where mediators such as inflammatory cytokines (e.g., prostaglandin E_2, bradykinin) and neurotrophic factors increase excitability of the neuronal membrane without activating transducers. In both cases, transduction threshold is reduced, making it easier for an action potential to occur. Noteworthy in the case of CRPS, whose clinical features include regional spread of pain and pain in response to sympathetic stimuli, is the concept that peripheral sensitization does not only affect the injured nerve, which is often distally malfunctioning and/or incapable of producing positive signals. Instead, neighboring nerve endings are sensitized, and there is experimental evidence showing that damage to a nerve causes early and spontaneous ectopic firing of adjacent, uninjured C-fibers. These fibers also develop reduced threshold for ectopic firing; particularly, they become sensitive to alpha-adrenergic activity.[13,14]

The end result of peripheral sensitization is both an increase in the pain experienced by the patient, as well as an amplification of nociceptive input entering the CNS. Left untreated, and in a chronic form, prolonged and increased nociceptive input to the CNS triggers modulation in central pain pathways, resulting in central sensitization. Central sensitization results in enhanced responsiveness of central pain transmission neurons, which either outlasts the initiating input or requires only a low-level peripheral drive to maintain it.[12] Thus, pain which began from a physical insult in the periphery can become centrally generated by the CNS even in the absence of any continued peripheral stimulus. Because the mechanisms underlying this modulation involve changes in receptor (e.g., N-methyl-D-aspartate (NMDA) receptors) expression akin to the long-term potentiation associated with memory in the hippocampus, they are long-lasting and make the disorder difficult to reverse at this point.

Taken together, this combination of nerve injury, peripheral sensitization, and central sensitization can explain many of the perplexing disease features of CRPS. Features of the syndrome that were previously assumed to be the result of abnormal sympathetic outflow can be explained by distal small-fiber loss due to nerve injury. Distal small nerve fibers are mixed in function, consisting of not only sensory (A-delta and C fibers) components, but sympathetic axons, and neuroeffector peptides (e.g., substance P, and calcitonin gene-related peptide) that regulate tissue function. Small fiber loss may cause denervation of distal limb arteriovenous shunts, with loss of resting tone and opening of the shunts.[5] This could lead to the asymmetric limb warmth and hyperperemia associated with RSD, while causing paradoxical hypoperfusion of deeper tissues,[15] contributing to deep pain. That some CRPS-affected limbs appear blue and cold rather than warm and hyperemic may be explained by eventual supersensitivity of denervated vessels to circulating catecholamines. The sudomotor instability (hypo- or hyperhidrosis) often seen in RSD/CRPS I is also explicable by nerve injury leading to denervation of sweat glands, which are normally innervated by cholinergic sympathetic small fibers. Sweat glands of CRPS I patients have been shown on pathologic examination to be denervated of these cholinergic sympathetic small fibers, but have aberrant ectopic sprouting of adrenergic innervation from nearby nervi vasorum; thus, they may both sweat insufficiently from direct neural stimulation and yet sweat excessively in response to circulating catecholamines.[5,16]

Remaining disease features are accounted for by peripheral and central sensitization. As previously mentioned, the process of peripheral sensitization can reduce activation threshold as well as induce expression of adrenergic receptors on nociceptive fibers adjacent to an injured nerve[13,14]; this phenomenon helps to account for both SMP and regional spreading of pain. Spreading of pain and hypersensitivity to regions beyond the injured tissue is also accounted for by the mechanisms of central sensitization, wherein a centrally sensitized neuron can generate pain outside the distribution of the stimulating peripheral input by increasing the excitability of its synapses with multiple other central neurons.[12,17] Finally, innappropriate sensitization of both peripheral and central afferents leads to the hyperpathia and allodynia that are characteristic of the pain in CRPS.[12,18]

Patient presentation

Epidemiology

CRPS occurs with an estimated incidence of 26.2 per 100 000 person-years,[19] with a published range of 5.46–26.2 per 100 000 person years.[19,20] Published estimates indicate that CRPS I makes up 97% of cases in the general population, with CRPS II being more common in certain subpopulations such as the military as a result of gunshot wounds and shrapnel injuries.[19] However, experience in the surgical literature suggests that CRPS II may be underdiagnosed or frequently misdiagnosed as CRPS I.[6,7] The syndrome may occur in any age group, although the peak prevalence seems to be in middle age, suggesting that many cases actually resolve and do not progress to a chronic form with disability.[19,20] Females are affected at least three times as often as men,[19,20] for unclear reasons.

Precipitating events

The most common precipitating events for CRPS I are extremity fractures (e.g., distal radius fractures) and sprains, although surgery, tendon injuries, and crush injuries are also common causes. Seemingly minor or innocuous events, such as phlebotomy, can also be causes, as can nontraumatic insults such as tumors, infarctions, and vasculitis with mononeuropathy multiplex. For known cases of CRPS II, nerve compression syndromes and penetrating injuries (including surgery) are common causes. For both types of CRPS, the upper extremity is more often involved than the lower extremity (60% versus 40%), although as a group, CRPS of the extremities make up the vast majority of cases, with head, trunk, and visceral involvement being possible but rare.[21,22] This distribution is in keeping with an underlying etiology of nerve injury, since the axial pattern and proximity to hard tissues of extremity nerves make them more vulnerable to injury than trunk nerves. Upper extremity involvement may be more frequent than lower extremity involvement due to the smaller receptive fields and greater density of innervation in the arm than the leg.

Patient characteristics

The only high-powered study to examine medical history prior to the onset of CRPS found an association between a history of migraines, asthma, neuropathies, osteoporosis, and menstrual cycle-related problems and the later development of CRPS.[23] Although the cryptogenic nature of the disease as well as the emotional changes it may produce in patients have caused suspicion for a hysterical or psychological underpinning in CRPS, multiple studies have studied the association of psychological factors with CRPS onset and found no evidence in support of CRPS as a psychologically mediated disease, or of the idea that certain psychological profiles are predisposed to its development.[23–25] With this being said, it is important to keep in mind that emotional and psychological changes such as anxiety and depression do develop in chronic CRPS as a consequence of central sensitization, and therefore may be a presenting feature of the disease.

Diagnosis

CRPS is a clinical diagnosis that should be made based on history and physical examination findings. There are several proposed diagnostic criteria, with the 1994 International Association for the Study of Pain (IASP) criteria *(Table 23.1)* being most frequently cited. Several modifications of these criteria have been proposed in an attempt to improve specificity.[26]

For the peripheral nerve surgeon, the question of whether or not a patient meets certain CRPS criteria is far less important than the question of whether the patient's pain will respond to surgical intervention. Evaluation by the peripheral nerve surgeon should consist of a thorough search for the presence of an underlying nerve injury (compression or neuroma) that may have initiated the syndrome, and then an assessment of whether surgical treatment of the nerve injury is likely to improve that patient's symptoms.

Nerve injuries are identified by the combination of history, physical exam, and electrodiagnostic testing. History should be focused on whether or not the patient recalls a traumatic or surgical event in the area that may have caused a nerve injury. If the pain began after a previous surgery, the operative note should be requested and reviewed for mention of nerve injuries. The history should also clarify exactly the type of pain, and the distribution of pain; every attempt should be made to clarify whether the pain rests in the distribution of one or more peripheral nerves, or whether regional spread outside of specific nerve distributions has occurred. Associated symptoms such as the presence of edema, vasodysregulation, sudomotor instability, and weakness or dystonia may also be inventoried, although their significance to the peripheral nerve surgeon is somewhat less. Finally, it is crucial to elicit an account of the time passed since the initial insult, and the length of time that the full syndrome of CRPS, if present, has been active. Patients with newer-onset CRPS (less than 3–6 months) who are still in the process of nerve injury and peripheral sensitization are much more likely to benefit from surgical repair of peripheral pain generators than those with chronic CRPS whose pain has become centrally generated. Other factors in the history that favor a good response to surgery are a discrete traumatic event responsible for the initiation of pain, and a well-localized source of pain.

Physical examination should be performed concurrently with the history to augment the identification of nerve injuries. Physical exam begins with a search for outward scars or signs of trauma to the painful region. The presence of any of the typical inflammatory, dysautonomic, or atrophic features of CRPS should be noted *(Figs 23.6 and 23.7)*. The location of the patient's pain as described in the history should then be mapped on to the surface of the body, and this region should

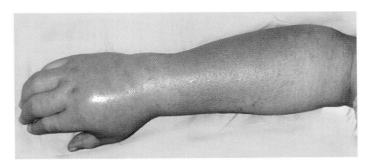

Fig. 23.6 "Acute, inflammatory" complex regional pain syndrome.

be scrutinized by the examiner for a correlation to specific peripheral nerve distributions. When the distribution of the pain does not match a known peripheral nerve distribution, either multiple overlapping nerve territories may be implicated, or the regional spread of pain via sensitization may have occurred. Once the region of pain has been clarified on physical exam, the presence of a Tinel's sign in nerves within the region should be tested for by tapping over any known anatomical compression points, obvious scars, or suspected sites of painful neuromas. The presence of a positive Tinel's sign (a tingling sensation radiating distally from the site of percussion) helps to localize cutaneous neuromas, and signals a greater likelihood of response to surgery for nerve compression injuries, presumably by indicating the presence of surviving neurons distal to the point of injury.

If a cutaneous neuroma is suspected based on history and physical exam, the likelihood that the symptoms of CRPS will resolve with resection and implantation of the neuroma should be assessed using nerve block with local anesthetic. This is performed by infiltrating the region proximal to the suspected neuroma with local anesthetic (the nerve itself is not injected). The response is considered positive when there is a postblock to preblock reduction in pain by greater than or equal to 5 points on a visual analog scale (score of 0–10, with 10 being the worst pain). If a single block fails to produce pain relief, the possibility that a nearby nerve with an overlapping sensory territory is also involved should be investigated by a new block of the suspected adjacent nerve. If the pain remains after sequential block of all possible sensory nerve territories, then there is presumed to be a fixed central mechanism (e.g., dorsal column, thalamus) for the pain and peripheral nerve surgery is unlikely to be of benefit.[6]

A special note should be made for CRPS that localizes to a particular joint, such as often occurs after joint injury (e.g., wrist fracture) or surgery (commonly knee surgery). After orthopedic evaluation has ruled out biomechanical joint problems, these cases should be treated by the peripheral nerve surgeon as suspected injuries to joint afferent fibers, and the office workup for these patients should be analogous to that for cutaneous neuromas, with response to surgery being predicted by nerve blocks of the joint afferents and surgical therapy, if warranted, being partial joint denervation.[6,7,27,28]

The final tool in the diagnostic workup used by peripheral nerve surgeons to identify nerve injury and predict response to treatment is electrodiagnostic neurosensory testing (NST). NST in the context of CRPS is indicated mainly for the detection and evaluation of nerve compression syndromes. Although accepted and widespread in their use, traditional

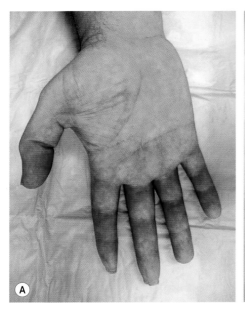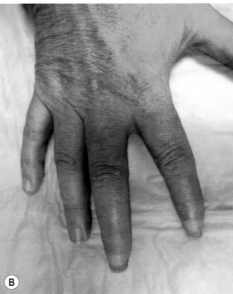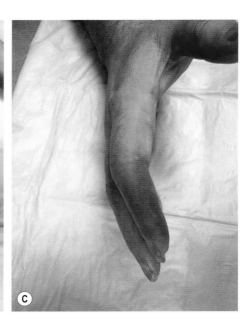

Fig. 23.7 Subtle visual findings of chronic complex regional pain syndrome I. This patient was examined 18 months following crush injury to the index and middle fingers with distal phalanx fractures, treated nonoperatively. Despite bony union, the patient went on to develop severe hyperesthesia, allodynia, pain, and cold intolerance of the index and middle fingers. **(A)** Prominent mottling of the skin which is exacerbated with dependent positioning. Edema and distal tapering of the index and middle fingers are also noted, with brittle fingernails that are overgrown on the affected fingers due to hypersensitivity with trimming. **(B)** Dorsal view again showing edema and tapering as well as trophic changes of the skin, with a thin, shiny appearance as well as loss of the distal interphalangeal joint flexion creases on the index and middle finger. Brittle, overgrown nails are again noted. **(C)** Lateral view showing prominent discoloration. Notice that the exam findings and distribution of pain fit a regional pattern not in any one nerve territory. The patient is under consideration for a spinal cord stimulator. (Courtesy of Dr. Kenneth Means, Curtis National Hand Center, Baltimore, MD.)

electrodiagnostic testing modalities such as electromyography and nerve conduction studies are too painful for CRPS patients, who often suffer from severe hyperpathia and allodynia. Additionally, these tests can have a high false-negative rate for detecting small-fiber disease, which may represent the bulk of CRPS I cases along with CRPS II cases due to neuromas of smaller cutaneous afferents. A less painful and more sensitive test is the quantitation of cutaneous pressure thresholds for one- and two-point discrimination throughout the nerve distributions in question. This can be performed using the Pressure-Specified Sensory Device (PSSD), which has been shown to have improved sensitivity compared to nerve conduction studies[29] for the detection of compression neuropathies while being as painless as possible (the device exerts gentle dull pressure without penetrating the skin or giving an electrical stimulus). NST can be used to document the presence of a suspected nerve lesion, to quantify its severity, and to monitor recovery through a period of observation or postoperatively.

Adjunctive diagnostic measures

There is no objective laboratory study specific for CRPS. However, a variety of adjunctive diagnostic tests have traditionally been used in an attempt to support or clarify the diagnosis of CRPS. These tests are useful for the primary care provider or the interdisciplinary team, where they can be used to define a particular patient's unique constellation of disease manifestations and therefore develop a rationally tailored medical treatment plan that addresses not only pain, but also associated symptoms that also impact quality of life such as inflammation, edema, dystonia, and SMP.

Tests commonly used to search for evidence of the inflammatory process in CRPS are X-ray and bone scanning. X-ray may reveal the cortical and cancellous osteopenia (Sudeck's), and subchondral cysts that are commonly associated with the generalized inflammation in early CRPS; if found on X-ray, osteopenia can be treated appropriately (e.g., with bisphosphonates) to reduce morbidity. Of course, occult arthritis or biomechanical joint problems may also contribute to CRPS and should be treated appropriately if detected on X-ray. Radionuclide bone scan with technetium-labeled diphosphonate will also show abnormalities in many CRPS patients. The test is divided into three phases, with diffuse uptake of tracer in the delayed image (phase 3) reportedly correlating well with the diagnosis of CRPS.[30–33] Although this costly test has been advocated as being quite specific for CRPS, it is by no means sensitive in all cases, and a negative bone scan does not rule out the diagnosis; thus, the test is of little use to the peripheral nerve surgeon and serves mostly to help establish the diagnosis of CRPS in cases where clinical criteria may not be clear and there is no other clear cause for the patient's symptoms. Other imaging modalities, such as magnetic resonance imaging, are helpful to exclude other causes (e.g., biomechanical) of regional pain and to assess deep-tissue edema, but do not produce CRPS-specific findings.

Vasomotor function can be assessed with either comparative temperature measurements between contralateral limbs or with laser Doppler flowmetry, a noninvasive technology where Doppler shifts in laser light reflected off the skin surface can be used to quantify the velocity of small-vessel bloodflow.[34] This technique is a research more than a clinical tool and adds little to the treatment algorithm. Sudomotor dysfunction can likewise be quantitated with the resting sweat output or quantitative sudomotor axon reflex test.[35–38] Tests for vasomotor and sudomotor dysfunction may help to define the extent of a patient's autonomic features and justify a role for adjunctive therapies such as pharmacologic sympatholysis, but they do not diagnose CRPS, are not required for initiating treatment, and have no part in the peripheral nerve surgeon's approach to the disease.

The final group of adjunctive diagnostic procedures that may be employed in CRPS patients are sympatholytic procedures for the diagnosis of SMP. An important concept clarified by the IASP consensus conference that created the name "CRPS" is that the diagnosis of CRPS does not require the presence of SMP. In other words, of all patients with CRPS, some will have a very pronounced painful response to sympathetic stimuli, while others will have pain that is completely independent of sympathetic stimulation; still others will have some combination of SMP and SIP. This stands in contradistinction to earlier conceptualizations of the disease, such as "RSD," where heightened pain in response to sympathetic stimuli was thought to be the defining feature of the disorder. Therefore, sympatholytic procedures in CRPS are said to be diagnostic of SMP itself, which is a component or feature of the larger disorder, and not diagnostic of CRPS. There are a variety of procedures available, all aimed at interrupting sympathetic outflow to the affected region. The simplest is a systemic infusion of phentolamine (a potent, short-acting alpha-adrenergic antagonist) which temporarily reverses the pain of many patients with SMP. Another frequently employed procedure is the sympathetic nerve block (SNB), achieved by injecting local anesthetic at the level of the stellate ganglion (SGB), or lumbar sympathetic chain (LSB) for pain in the upper versus lower extremity, respectively.

Overview of treatment options

The principles of effective treatment for CRPS are early diagnosis and intervention, multidisciplinary management, individualized pain management, and the use of less invasive treatment before invasive or morbid treatment. Each CRPS patient, having complex needs, should be managed from the outset by a team of practitioners, who can each provide support and address these needs individually, with the overall aim of controlling pain and symptoms enough to allow participation in a desensitization and rehabilitation program.

Relatively underemphasized in the literature has been the role of the peripheral nerve surgeon, and part of the aim of this chapter is to clarify exactly how, when, and why peripheral nerve surgeons should be involved in the management of CRPS. The peripheral nerve surgeon should not serve as the primary care provider or coordinator for patients with CRPS; however, as demonstrated in *Figure 23.8*, referral to and evaluation by a peripheral nerve surgeon should occur early after diagnosis as part of the team management of CRPS. This is because the value of a surgical consultation lies in the potential to diagnose and treat nerve injuries definitively (compression neuropathies or neuromas) that may be the cause of CRPS before the syndrome has had sufficient time

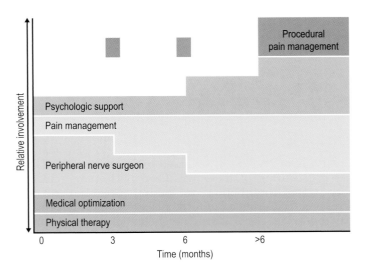

Fig. 23.8 Changing the paradigm for multidisciplinary management of complex regional pain syndrome.

to progress from peripheral to central sensitization (as was discussed under pathophysiology, above). The window for this intervention is generally within the first 3–6 months; once sensitization of the CNS has occurred and the pain becomes centrally generated, surgery to correct peripheral nerve insults is likely to be ineffective. Therefore, although multidisciplinary management and rehabilitation should commence from the outset of symptoms, the first 3–6 months should be dominated by an effort to diagnose and treat underlying nerve injuries before they lead to a potentially irreversible progression of disease.

Physical therapy and rehabilitation

The concept of "functional restoration" through physical therapy and rehabilitation has become regarded as the most pragmatic and broadly applicable treatment for CRPS available. An exaggerated but telling view of the overall interdisciplinary approach to CRPS is that the primary utility of other types of nonsurgical treatment (e.g., pharmacotherapy and procedural pain management) is to reduce pain sufficiently to allow participation in functional restoration programs. A full description of the scope of and recommended approach to rehabilitation in CRPS is beyond the scope of this chapter and has been well described elsewhere,[27] but generally is led by physical and occupational therapists, with the goals of therapy being to normalize sensation, promote normal positioning, decrease muscle guarding, minimize edema, and increase functional use of the extremity. Also involved are recreational and vocational therapists, who play an important role in returning the debilitated CRPS patient to normal social and vocational activities, which is important to minimize the distress and isolation brought on by the potentially extreme symptoms of CRPS.

Psychological support

Although several cross-sectional and retrospective studies have evaluated the underlying psychological traits of CRPS patients and found no definite evidence for psychologic dysfunction as being causative of CRPS,[23–25] lingering doubts remain as to the full association between psychological comorbidities and the onset and maintenance of CRPS. In addition, there is a reasonable theoretical mechanism to explain how emotional distress can exacerbate the pain of CRPS: emotional distress and pain by themselves are enough to provoke catecholamine release into the systemic circulation; since peripheral afferents become sensitized and up-regulate adrenergic receptors after adjacent nerve injury, it is possible that the circulating catecholamines released in response to emotional cues cause firing of these sensitized nociceptors, creating more pain, contributing to central sensitization, and increasing the likelihood of further catecholamine release in a self-amplifying cycle. Thus, the potential for appropriate psychological therapy to impact the level of suffering in CRPS is great and may operate at multiple levels in the disease process.

Pharmacologic therapy

Many upper extremity surgeons, when initially confronted with CRPS, will empirically prescribe a steroid taper in the hopes of countering the inflammatory process. However, the full range of pharmacotherapy for CRPS draws upon a diverse array of drugs to address cooperatively the many different comorbid manifestations of this disease. Management of these drugs often reaches a level of complexity requiring supervision by a pain management specialist and hence, a full review of the subject is beyond the scope of this surgical text.[39] The approach to management can be summarized, however, by recommending that specific agents are chosen to target specific troublesome aspects of patient presentation, such as using nonsteroidal anti-inflammatory drugs and steroids to treat inflammation, opioids for intractable pain, antidepressants or anxiolytics for depression and anxiety, anticonvulsants for allodynia/hyperalgesia, and bisphosphonates for osteopenia. The intensity of pharmacotherapy is generally initiated at the lowest level required, and then increased as required to reach the goal of successful participation in rehabilitation. For a detailed review of this subject, readers are referred to the Complex Regional Pain Syndrome Treatment Guidelines published by the Reflex Sympathetic Dystrophy Syndrome Association (available at www.rsdsa.org).[26]

Procedural and interventional therapies

A wide variety of interventional therapies, including nerve blocks, drug infusions, and implantable pain treatment devices, are available for the treatment of CRPS. These therapies are generally initiated on an individual basis as needed to relieve pain and allow successful mobilization of the extremity and participation in rehabilitation. Interventional therapies also have an important role perioperatively, where they may reduce the risk of postoperative pain exacerbations by putting the somatosensory and autonomic nervous systems to rest before and during the trauma of surgery *(Fig. 23.8)*.

The most prevalent of the interventional therapies are pharmacologic blockades. Although simple peripheral nerve blocks with local anesthetic may be used to control pain (especially in the context of diagnosis, as described above), the pharmacologic blocks more traditionally associated with CRPS are performed with sympatholytic agents to control dysautonomic symptoms and pain in those patients with a significant component of SMP. Sympatholysis can be accomplished either regionally or systemically; typically, a systemic infusion of phentolamine (a potent, short-acting alpha-adrenergic antagonist) is used to confirm the diagnosis of SMP. Thereafter, sympatholysis can be accomplished intermittently in the affected extremity with either SNB or intravenous regional anesthesia (IVRA).

SNB is achieved by injecting local anesthetic at the level of the stellate ganglion (SGB), or lumbar sympathetic chain (LSB) for pain in the upper versus lower extremity, respectively. The pain relief following SNB generally outlasts the effect of the local anesthetic, and may be long-lasting in some cases.[26] Although frequently employed, the effectiveness of SNBs has not been definitively proven in the literature.[40,41] Therefore, despite various published report opinions, the role for SNB has been and continues to be determined on an individual basis: if the block provides good analgesia in a patient, then a short series of blocks in conjunction with active reactivation physiotherapy should be regarded as appropriate therapy.[26,42]

IVRA is accomplished by injecting an anesthetic or sympatholytic agent into a tourniquetted extremity, to allow regional distribution. Commonly used agents include adrenergic modifiers (guanethidine, reserpine, bretylium, and clonidine), local anesthetics (lidocaine), and anti-inflammatory medications (hydrocortisone and ketorolac). These can be used alone or in combination, and success has been reported with various modifications of the basic technique,[43] however most large studies to examine the topic have found a lack of evidence for the effectiveness of IVRA.[44–49]

For patients failing intermittent blocks and requiring longer-term anesthesia or sympatholysis of the affected extremity, indwelling anesthetic infusion catheters provide another alternative for pain control. For upper extremity involvement, the catheter is placed in the axilla, with the tip positioned to block the brachial plexus; for lower extremity involvement, an epidural infusion catheter is used. Commonly used medications include bupivacaine, clonidine, and opioids, with published evidence for epidural clonidine being the strongest for sympatholysis.[50] Indwelling catheters can be titrated to the level of pain, using local anesthetics to provide complete sensorimotor block, and then titrating down the level of local anesthesia to allow motor function, while adding sympatholytics and opioids to maintain analgesia. Though potentially very effective, the use of indwelling catheters is limited by the risk of infection, which restricts their prolonged use.[26]

Emerging therapies

Intravenous ketamine infusion therapy

Although currently restricted to case reports and small trials, the use of ketamine is both promising and interesting because it is a rational therapy directed at the mechanism of long-term pain in CRPS, as understood in the current model of pathogenesis of the disease (outlined above). Namely, ketamine antagonizes NMDA receptors, a subtype of neuronal receptor believed to underlie the central sensitization of CRPS. Preliminary studies have shown that extended infusions of ketamine are capable of reducing pain, although further study is needed to determine the place of this therapy in the treatment algorithm for CRPS.[51,52]

Botulinum toxin

Botulinum toxin (BTX) is a recent addition to the armamentarium for procedural treatment of neuropathic pain and has generated a lot of excitement owing to encouraging results in several early randomized controlled trials (RCTs) and animal experiments. With its well-known effect of relaxing skeletal muscle by preventing presynaptic release of acetylcholine from motor neurons, BTX has been successfully used for decades in the management of chronic pain of musculoskeletal origin. BTX is increasingly recognized as having pleiotropic properties and may help to alleviate pain by several mechanisms.[53–56]

Botox for CRPS can be given either locally/subdermally, or as part of an SNB.[54,57–59]

Invasive pain management therapies

Invasive therapies for CRPS include implantable stimulators and sympathetic ablation. All of these therapies carry a greater risk to the patient than the noninvasive therapies described above since they are surgical in nature and involve alteration or destruction of native tissues. Therefore, these therapies should be reserved for cases where less invasive therapies have failed, or where surgical indications for peripheral nerve surgery were not met.

Of the implantable stimulators, spinal cord stimulators (SCS) are the most well studied. These devices consist of a small array of electrodes surgically implanted in the epidural space and connected to an adjustable generator device. By stimulating the dorsal columns and dorsal horns, they are able to produce a sensory change that is perceived as diminished pain by the patient. A high-profile RCT has been published showing the effectiveness of SCS in reducing pain as compared to physical therapy alone.[60] However, a follow-up study of the same cohort showed that the efficacy of the these devices falls off after 3 years of use, making them impractical as a permanent solution.[61] Therefore, these costly devices should not be the first line of invasive therapy, but rather should be viewed as an option for relief of intractable chronic pain when the patient is not a candidate for peripheral nerve surgery, or if surgery fails.[62–64]

The other type of invasive therapy that has been historically employed for treatment of CRPS is sympathetic ablation, either via surgical sympathectomy, by injection of neurolytic chemicals such as phenol, or by radiofrequency ablation[65–68] of the stellate or lumbar ganglia. However, although there have been case series advocating each of these techniques and many isolated reports of successful long-term pain control for patients with SMP, these techniques should be approached with hesitancy both because they carry with them the risk of continued pain via "postsympathectomy neuralgia" and because there is a paucity of evidence-based data to support lasting positive outcomes after these procedures.[69]

Of the invasive therapies, peripheral nerve surgery is the only means currently available to address the cause of the problem in CRPS (by deactivating peripheral pain generators), and therefore should be viewed as a first-line therapy in applicable cases. In contrast, implantable stimulators and sympathectomy should be approached with the recognition that they will not reverse the disease state; instead, they serve as a last resort for obtaining relief of symptoms in chronic cases of CRPS where all other measures have failed and progressive central sensitization has ruled out peripheral nerve surgery as a viable option.

Peripheral nerve surgery for CRPS

Patient selection for surgery

As summarized in *Figure 23.9* and described in the section on physical examination above, patient selection for surgery is focused on ruling out all other potential causes for the patient's symptoms, and then identifying patients with nerve injuries that are likely to respond to surgical therapy.

Patients referred to a peripheral nerve surgeon should have already undergone a thorough evaluation by a PCP, relevant surgical specialist, neurologist, and or anesthesia pain specialist including the appropriate diagnostic studies as described above, to establish CRPS as the cause of symptoms and to rule out mimickers like radiculopathy or polyneuropathy. Among patients with true CRPS, the type (e.g., I or II) is not a reliable criteria to determine surgical candidacy. Rather, candidates will be identified by the results of physical examination, response to blocks, and NST (when indicated) as defined above and illustrated in *Figure 23.9*. Because many cases of CRPS spontaneously resolve, patients should initially undergo a period of observation and conservative therapy for 3 months (6 weeks to 6 months range, individually tailored) after the onset of symptoms; if there is a lack of improvement, then surgery should be planned at 3 months. If improvement is seen clinically or on NST, then it is reasonable to continue nonsurgical therapy with interval reassessments, planning for surgery at 6 months if there is no improvement *(Fig. 23.9)*.

Perioperative management

Traditionally, surgeons have been cautioned against operating on any patient with active CRPS, or even with a history of CRPS, for fear of causing a recurrence or exacerbation of symptoms. Diverse recommendations have been made as to the appropriate time to wait before operating on a CRPS patient: some authors have suggested waiting a prescribed length of time from the onset of symptoms (e.g., 1 year), others recommend obtaining complete control of symptoms, regardless of chronology, while still others have emphasized the need to reverse specific disease features, such as edema or vasodysregulation, before surgery.[70] Unfortunately, such recommendations have not been based on prospective randomized trials, and have not been studied in patients who are undergoing surgery specifically for the treatment of nerve injuries suspected to be underlying their CRPS. Therefore, as in many aspects of CRPS treatment, there is no uniform consensus guideline as to when it is safest to operate on CRPS patients and what specific preventive measures should be taken in the perioperative setting.

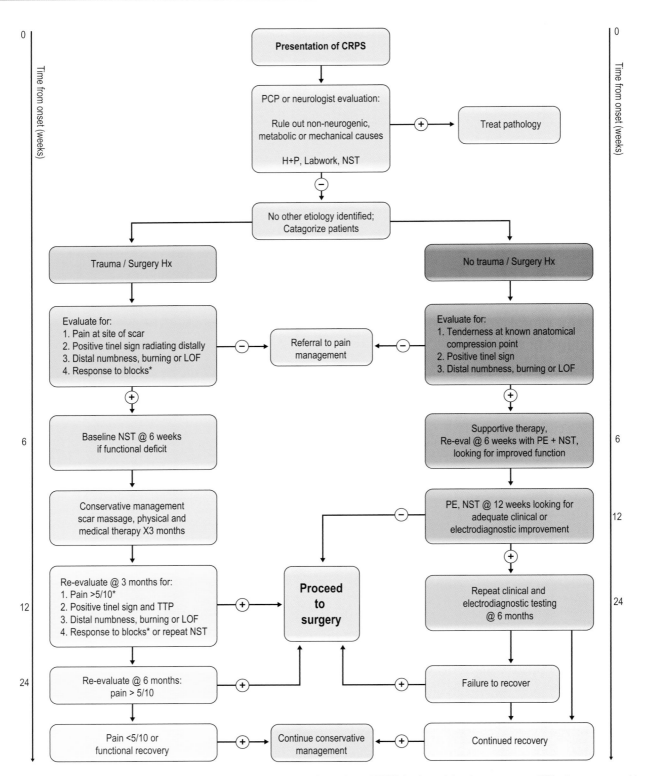

Fig. 23.9 Workup and treatment of the patient with complex regional pain syndrome (CRPS) by the peripheral nerve surgeon. PCP, primary care provider; H+P, history and physical; NST, neurosensory testing; Hx, history of; LOF, loss of function; PE, physical examination.

The risk that symptoms may recur or be exacerbated by the pain of surgery in CRPS patients is, however, a real one,[43,71] and merits some form of intervention to minimize it. Perioperative management of CRPS should always involve consultation with anesthesia or pain management, both for pharmacologic management and for the administration of

procedural pain control in the perioperative setting. The general idea is to prevent sensitization and sympathetic activation with a durable regional anesthesia and, when applicable, sympatholysis, that begins before the incision and extends through the period of postoperative acute pain. Various authors have advocated SNB,[72] IVRA,[48] local anesthetic nerve block, and brachial plexus[73] or epidural catheterization[6,7,74] for perioperative control of pain. The decision of which technique to use will depend on what has worked for the patient in the past (e.g., SNB will only be effective for patients with SMP), and the familiarity of the involved anesthetist with the applicable techniques. However, indwelling catheters (of the brachial plexus for upper extremity CRPS and epidural catheters for lower extremity CRPS) are the most versatile option for regional anesthesia, with the ability to titrate not only the degree of anesthesia, but the length of anesthesia (from hours to days), and the degree of sympatholysis by the inclusion of agents such as clonidine along with a local anesthetic or opioid. The largest published case series specifically to study peripheral nerve surgery for treatment of compression syndromes and neuromas in CRPS patients have all used indwelling catheters in conjunction with general anesthesia and have reported successful perioperative pain control as well as low rates of complication and recurrence, making this technique a good starting point for future prospective studies of the effectiveness of perioperative pain control in CRPS.[6,7,73,74]

Surgical technique

The usual gamut of peripheral nerve surgery techniques are applicable in CRPS and will be employed as the individual scenario demands. This is summarized in *Figure 23.5*. Pain after nerve injury can be the result of a compression neuropathy (nerve entrapment), neuroma, or neuroma in continuity.

Compression neuropathies are of recognizable, named nerves and occur in known anatomic tunnels, as summarized in *Table 23.2*. The treatment for compression neuropathies is neurolysis, a surgical release of the surrounding scar or connective tissue that is causing the entrapment *(Fig. 23.10)*.

Neuromas may be of larger, named nerves, as is the case in CRPS II (causalgia), or may be of smaller cutaneous afferent fibers, as is often the case in CRPS I. CRPS that localizes to a joint may be the result of neuromas forming in damaged joint afferents. In any case, the treatment of a neuroma always involves excision of the neuroma at the distal stump of the injured nerve, with implantation of the cut end into muscle *(Fig. 23.11)*. In the case of joints, this may involve partial denervation of the joint by neurectomy and implantation of multiple joint afferents, as summarized in *Table 23.3*.

Crush injuries that do not transect the nerve can create a neuroma in continuity, as described in the pathophysiology section above *(Fig. 23.12)*. These are best treated by surgery with intraoperative nerve conduction studies to identify and selectively resect the sensory fibers of the neuroma, while leaving motor fibers intact *(Fig. 23.5)*. If selective resection of sensory fibers is not possible, then the entire neuroma in continuity may be resected, and the resultant gap repaired with a nerve allograft, nerve autograft, or artificial nerve conduit tube to allow regrowth of the nerve fascicles along their severed tracts *(Fig. 23.5)*.

Postoperative care

The interdisciplinary team should be closely involved in the care of the postoperative CRPS patient. An anesthesiologist or pain specialist should continue to provide somatosensory and sympatholytic blockade through procedural pharmacologic intervention during the acute postoperative period. CRPS patients undergoing peripheral nerve surgery should be encouraged to make an early return to physical therapy programs and mobility of the affected area, usually following suture removal.

Outcomes

Among the large volume of literature produced on the topic of CRPS, peripheral nerve surgery has been relatively understudied. While certain surgical procedures such as SCS and sympathectomy, for control of pain and sympatholysis, respectively, have generated extensive discussion in the literature, surgery for repair of nerve insults generating peripheral pain in CRPS has been examined in only a few scattered retrospective case reports and case series. Published guidelines and reviews generally fail even to mention peripheral nerve surgery as an option.[26,75,76] Therefore, the only evidence available to perform an outcomes analysis of peripheral nerve surgery for the treatment of CRPS is either completely anecdotal, or relatively "low-level," on the ladder of evidence-based medicine. As such, whether or not peripheral nerve surgery should be routinely employed for the treatment of CRPS is a question that will remain controversial until high-quality RCTs are performed to answer it. Despite the current lack of RCTs, there is reason to emphasize the important role

Table 23.2 Nerve compression syndromes involved in complex regional pain syndrome in the upper extremity

Nerve	Site of compression
Brachial plexus	Thoracic outlet
Median nerve	Carpal tunnel
Anterior interosseous nerve	Pronator teres
Ulnar nerve	Cubital tunnel, Guyon's canal
Radial sensory nerve	Anterolateral forearm
Posterior interosseous nerve	Radial tunnel
Radial nerve	Humeral shaft

Table 23.3 Joint denervation surgery in the upper extremity

Joint	Denervated nerves
Wrist	Anterior and posterior interosseous nerves
Lateral elbow	Joined branches of the posterior cutaneous nerve of the forearm
Medial elbow	Radial nerve branch to the medial epicondyle along intermuscular septum
Shoulder	Lateral pectoral nerve

We would refer readers to the following sources for more detailed descriptions of joint denervation technique:
Dellon AL. Partial joint denervation I: wrist, shoulder, and elbow. Plast Reconstr Surg 2009;123:197–207.
Dellon AL. Partial joint denervation II: knee and ankle. Plast Reconstr Surg 2009;123:208–217.

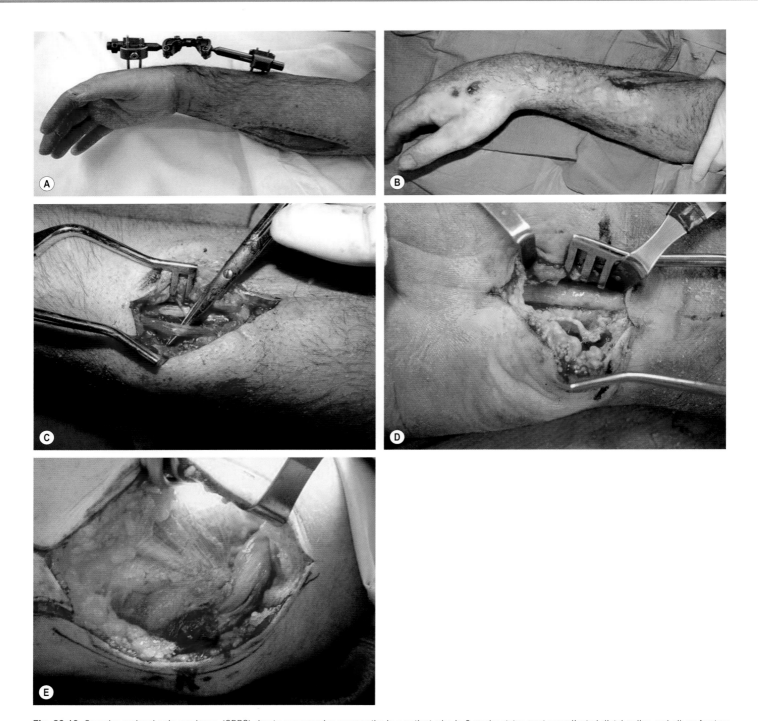

Fig. 23.10 Complex regional pain syndrome (CRPS) due to compression neuropathy in a patient who is 6 weeks status post complicated distal radius and elbow fracture with compartment syndrome requiring forearm fasciotomies. **(A)** Preoperative view: clinical presentation included persistent pain, edema, hyperesthesia, and skin color and trophic changes. **(B)** Dorsal view after removal of external fixator, showing fasciotomy scar. **(C)** Neurolysis of the radial sensory nerve in the dorsoradial forearm, where it was found to be compressed in scar tissue at the old fasciotomy site. **(D)** Neurolysis of the median nerve at the carpal tunnel. **(E)** Neurolysis of the ulnar nerve at the cubital tunnel (performed at a later date for continued symptoms of ulnar neuropathy); the ulnar nerve was both compressed in scar tissue and entrapped in aberrant musculature between the olecranon process and medial epicondyle. Preoperatively, the patient had been diagnosed with "reflex sympathetic dystrophy," but following all three neurolyses, the symptomatology of "reflex sympathetic dystrophy" was completely reversed, suggesting that the patient actually had CRPS II due to nerve compression.

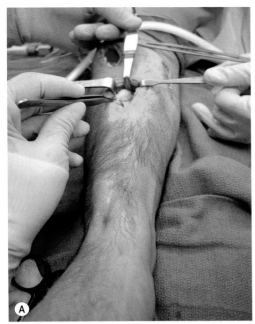

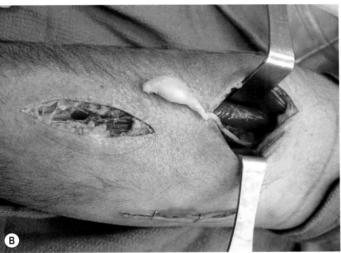

Fig. 23.11 The case of a patient who, for 20 years following open reduction internal fixation (ORIF) of a right distal radius fracture, had chronic regional pain, stiffness, and paresthesia diagnosed as "reflex sympathetic dystrophy." On physical exam, he had tenderness over the median nerve at the proximal forearm, the posterior interosseous nerve (PIN) at the proximal forearm, and tenderness with a positive Tinel's sign over the radial sensory nerve (RSN) and lateral antebrachial cutaneous nerve (LABC) at the site of his old scar. Prior to presentation, the patient had had a previous resection of a radial sensory nerve neuroma but continued to have regional forearm pain. **(A)** Intraoperative view following median nerve and PIN decompression showing a large neuroma of the RSN, probably due to inadequate implantation to muscle following previous resection. **(B)** Detail of RSN neuroma. The neuroma was excised and the proximal nerve stump buried in muscle. The patient was also found to have a neuroma of the LABC entangled in the scar of his old ORIF site. This example illustrates the need to treat cases of regional pain as presumed complex regional pain syndrome II and search for a correctable nerve injury before labeling patients as having complex regional pain syndrome I/"reflex sympathetic dystrophy."

that peripheral nerve surgery should assume in the treatment algorithm for CRPS. An increasingly accepted pathophysiologic model emphasizing peripheral nerve injury[4,5] makes peripheral nerve treatment a logical directive. Moreover, the individual experiences of high-volume peripheral nerve surgeons and the published case series (about 10 in total) that have focused specifically on neurolysis and neuroma resection for treatment of CRPS both show promising results.

Traditionally, surgery for CRPS was mostly limited to cases of causalgia (CRPS II), and earlier published case series reflect this. In 1985, Zhu and colleagues, based on intraoperative observations in patients with causalgia, developed a hypothesis of intraneural "hypertension" as the cause of the causalgia syndrome in patients with gunshot wounds. After building experimental support for their hypothesis in animal experiments, they proceeded to perform nerve decompression in 14 patients who had suffered explosion or gunshot injuries. They operated at an average of 66 days after injury, performing either epineural or intrafascicular neurolysis, and reported "symptomatic relief" in 13 of 14 patients, with relief occurring anywhere between immediately and 4 months following surgery.[77]

Grundberg et al.,[78] Jupiter et al.,[79] and Ducic et al.[74] report series of patients with symptoms of CRPS and demonstrable injuries of named (e.g., median, ulnar, tibial) peripheral nerves that responded to surgery (see annotated references).

Smaller case reports and case series have reported similar conclusions for both CRPS I and II. Inada and colleagues have reported multiple cases wherein CRPS has been relieved by excision of a neuroma or neuroma in continuity followed by gap reconstruction with a resorbable conduit.[80,81]

Citing clinical experience and a review of relevant literature,[11,82] Placzek and colleagues also suggest that many cases of CRPS II may be misdiagnosed as CRPS I, thus contributing to delay in identification and treatment of recognizable nerve injuries.[83] The largest and most recent case series yet published examining peripheral nerve surgery for CRPS echo and extend this theme. Dellon and colleagues have proposed the same and report two case series demonstrating that many so-called cases of CRPS I can be treated with peripheral nerve surgery.[6,7]

Overall, the summary suggestion of publications studying peripheral nerve surgery for the treatment of CRPS is that, when employed in the setting of an identifiable peripheral nerve lesion, it is likely an effective treatment for reducing or eliminating both the pain and dysautonomic/inflammatory syndrome of CRPS as well as helping to restore functionality to the affected extremity. It also appears that some cases of CRPS I, a disease widely presumed to have no role for surgical treatment, may in fact be due to peripheral nerve lesions that can be identified and treated, reversing symptoms.

Secondary procedures

For patients with CRPS who have undergone peripheral nerve surgery for treatment of a nerve compression or neuroma and fail to have resolution of symptoms, there are few secondary surgical options. Patients with strong clinical and electrodiagnostic evidence of nerve injury that have

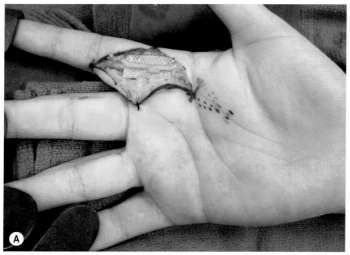

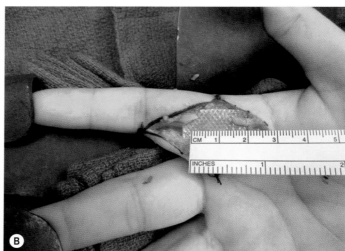

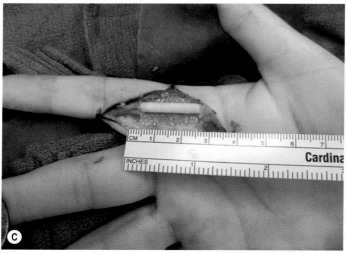

Fig. 23.12 Excision and reconstruction of a neuroma in continuity. Patient diagnosed with "reflex sympathetic dystrophy" after a crush injury to the palm suffered from chronic regional pain, stiffness, and limited use of the hand. Local anesthetic block alleviated symptoms and confirmed diagnosis of neuroma. **(A)** Operative exposure of index-finger ulnar digital nerve neuroma-in-continuity. **(B)** The nerve gap resulting from excision of the neuromatous segment is measured and an appropriately sized conduit is selected. **(C)** Reconstruction with nerve conduit. (Courtesy of Dr. Matthew L. Iorio, Department of Plastic Surgery, Georgetown University Hospital, Washington, DC.)

undergone neurolysis without clinical response may be candidates for a neurectomy of the involved nerve with implantation of the proximal stump to muscle; however the role for this procedure has not been well defined. This certainly can be considered only if the nerve is not a functionally critical nerve, in which case the resulting morbidity would outweigh the benefit.

Patients failing peripheral nerve surgery more than likely have either a "true" CRPS I (not at all related to an identifiable nerve injury) or have an entirely centrally generated syndrome. This may particularly be the case for patients with long-standing (greater than 6 months) CRPS, where the process of central sensitization has created long-term changes in activation threshold and synaptic strengthening among neurons in the CNS. In this scenario, it is intrinsically sensible that removal of a peripheral pain source, such as a nerve injury, will have little effect on the production of symptoms. Such patients, however, may be appropriate candidates for interventions such as the SCS (discussed separately above), which are aimed at masking centrally transmitted pain signals.[60,61] SCS should be implemented after at least 6 months of symptoms, with the recognition that its effectiveness in controlling pain has been shown to decrease over time, losing statistical significance at 3 years.[61]

Surgical and ablative (e.g., radiofrequency or phenol) sympathectomy is advocated by some practitioners for long-term relief of pain in patients with a significant and refractory component of SMP that has proven responsive to temporary sympathetic block. In general, ablative sympathetic techniques are not currently recommended to treat chronic CRPS due to questionable outcomes, and the potential risk for developing deafferentiation syndromes or "postsympathectomy neuralgia." This stance has been supported by a Cochrane database systematic review of the available studies.[83] Nonetheless, the decision to move ahead with these techniques may be reached as a consensus between patient and experienced practitioner if it appears to be the only means of relief for otherwise intractable SMP. When indicated, ablation by radiofrequency appears to be the most promising option because it is less invasive than surgical techniques and more controllable than neurolytic solution injections.[26]

The prospect of amputation for intractable CRPS is, of course, viewed as a last resort. Most available evidence indicates that the results of amputation are unpredictable, especially for the relief of pain. Amputation is unlikely to allow a trouble-free use of prosthesis in the affected limb and may lead to recurrent RSD after surgery. Therefore, prudence and published evidence suggest that amputation be reserved for the most extreme of circumstances and performed only for implications beyond pain alone, such as infection control or to improve residual function; when performed, amputation should be at the most proximal feasible level that preserves limb function while excluding all symptomatic tissues.[84]

Conclusion

In summary, the disease features of CRPS are diverse, but the syndrome is dominated by unremitting severe pain that may be sympathetically mediated, sympathetically independent, or both. The most current models of pathogenesis for the syndrome highlight the roles of nerve injury, followed by peripheral and central sensitization of the nervous system. CRPS is diagnosed clinically and patients should always be cared for by a multidisciplinary team. Because nerve injury is a potentially reversible cause of the symptoms of CRPS, the involvement of a peripheral nerve surgeon and a thorough search for treatable nerve injuries should occur early in the course of disease. Treatment for CRPS should progress along a stepladder of noninvasive to invasive therapies, with careful monitoring, active pain control, and physical rehabilitation playing a large role in the early disease course, since many cases will resolve with such measures alone. Peripheral nerve surgery is indicated in patients who have a clinically identifiable nerve compression or neuroma and whose CRPS fails to respond to conservative therapy; surgery consists of neurolysis for compression neuropathies or excision and implantation/reconstruction for neuromas. The timing of surgery can vary; it has to be individually tailored towards the patient's condition. It can be indicated only a few days after documented or highly suspicious nerve injury following surgery or trauma, or it can take place any time between 6 weeks and 6 months, depending on the pain severity and level of functional deficit. Although surgery will not be indicated or helpful for every case of CRPS, future efforts should be focused on performing high-quality, randomized controlled trials to establish the validity of peripheral nerve surgery in this disease, hopefully providing a rational and effective treatment for many patients who may otherwise be burdened with the distress and isolation of chronic pain.

1. Stanton-Hicks M, Janig W, Hassenbusch S, et al. Reflex sympathetic dystrophy: changing concepts and taxonomy. *Pain*. 1995;63:127–133.

4. Oaklander AL. RSD/CRPS: the end of the beginning. *Pain*. 2008;139:239–240.
   This paper is an important review of basic and clinical science evidence that supports the theory of CRPS I as arising from small-fiber nerve injuries.

5. Oaklander AL, Fields HL. Is reflex sympathetic dystrophy/complex regional pain syndrome type I a small-fiber neuropathy? *Ann Neurol*. 2009;65:629–638.

6. Dellon AL, Andonian E, Rosson GD. CRPS of the upper or lower extremity: surgical treatment outcomes. *J Brachial Plex Peripher Nerve Inj*. 2009;4:1.

7. Dellon L, Andonian E, Rosson GD. Lower Extremity Complex Regional Pain Syndrome: Long-term Outcome after Surgical Treatment of Peripheral Pain Generators. *J Foot Ankle Surg*. 2010;49:33–36.
   Dellon and colleagues, in two publications, propose that many cases of CRPS II (e.g., identifiable nerve injury) may be misdiagnosed as CRPS I, and that any case of CRPS, regardless of whether previously diagnosed as type I or II (reflex sympathetic dystrophy or causalgia) should be considered for treatment by peripheral nerve surgery, so long as the patient shows preoperative evidence of nerve injury. In their studies, nerve injury was evidenced by failure of 6 months of conventional therapy, response to nerve blocks with local anesthetic, and documentation of nerve compression by results of neurosensory testing and a positive Tinel sign at sites of anatomic narrowing. Using these methods in two separate case series, a group of surgical candidates was identified among patients diagnosed with CRPS of the upper or lower extremity, and patients underwent neurolysis,

resection of neuromas with implantation to muscle, partial joint denervation, or some combination of the above procedures. Both series (one of 70 patients and another of 13) report about 80% "good" or "excellent" response rate to surgery, as defined by pain reduction on a visual analog scale, reduced dependence on narcotics, and return to activity.

19. de Mos M, de Bruijn AG, Huygen FJ, et al. The incidence of complex regional pain syndrome: a population-based study. *Pain*. 2007;129:12–20.

26. Harden RN, Broatch J, Bruehl S, et al. Complex Regional Pain Syndrome: Treatment Guidelines. wwwrsdsaorg [serial on the Internet]. 2006: Available from: http://www.rsds.org/3/clinical_guidelines/index.html.

27. Dellon AL. Partial joint denervation II: knee and ankle. *Plast Reconstr Surg*. 2009;123:208–217.

28. Dellon AL. Partial joint denervation I: wrist, shoulder, and elbow. *Plast Reconstr Surg*. 2009;123:197–207.

74. Ducic I, Maloney Jr CJ, Barrett SL, et al. Perioperative epidural blockade in the management of post-traumatic complex pain syndrome of the lower extremity. *Orthopedics*. 2003;26:641–644.
    Ducic and colleagues, in a report advocating the use of perioperative epidural blockade for peripheral nerve surgery in patients with reflex sympathetic dystrophy of the lower extremity, describe a series of 4 patients who underwent either neurolysis of the common, superficial, and deep peroneal nerves, neurolysis of the tibial and plantar nerves, resection of leg afferent neuromas (saphenous or calcaneal nerve), denervation of the sinus tarsi, or a combination of these procedures. At postoperative follow-up, all 4 patients reported a reduction in preoperative pain and 2 of 4 patients achieved independence from narcotics.

78. Grundberg AB, Reagan DS. Compression syndromes in reflex sympathetic dystrophy. *J Hand Surg Am.* 1991;16:731–736.

    Grundberg and colleagues report a series of 29 patients with upper extremity "reflex sympathetic dystrophy" refractory to medical treatment who had clinical and electrophysiologic evidence of nerve compression. After peripheral nerve decompression (22 at carpal tunnel, 5 at cubital tunnel, 1 at Guyon's canal, and 1 herniated cervical disk), all patients showed improvement in pain, mobility, and grip strength.

79. Jupiter JB, Seiler 3rd JG, Zienowicz R. Sympathetic maintained pain (causalgia) associated with a demonstrable peripheral-nerve lesion. Operative treatment. *J Bone Joint Surg Am.* 1994;76:1376–1384.

    Jupiter et al. reported on 9 patients with causalgia and electromyogram evidence of nerve dysfunction who were treated with surgical decompression, nerve repair, continuous sympathetic block, or a combination of these procedures with rotation of a muscle flap over the nerve in an attempt to enhance blood supply in the area and reduce perineural scarring. In addition to surgical treatment, this group emphasized perioperative sympatholysis with an indwelling stellate ganglion or lumbar sympathetic block. The nerve lesions involved the median nerve at the wrist, ulnar nerve at the elbow, radial digital nerve of the index finger, and posterior tibial nerve at the ankle. Mean preoperative duration of symptoms was 17 weeks, and all 9 patients were reported to have a reduction in pain within the first 72 hours of surgery and no recurrence at 48-month follow-up.

24

Nerve entrapment syndromes

Michael Bezuhly, James P. O'Brien, and Donald Lalonde

SYNOPSIS

- Diagnosis of nerve compression syndromes should be based on a thorough clinical evaluation, including history of vocational and nonvocational activities.

- Electrodiagnostic testing should be used primarily to confirm the clinical diagnosis or rule out other pathology.

- Carpal tunnel syndrome (CTS) and cubital tunnel syndrome are among the most common clinical entities evaluated by the hand surgeon.

- Carpal tunnel release and cubital tunnel release under local anesthesia alone are safe and time- and cost-effective, as well as convenient for patients.

- Current evidence suggests that ulnar nerve transposition is no better than simple decompression alone in the treatment of cubital tunnel syndrome.

- Uncommon nerve entrapment syndromes such as quadrilateral space syndrome and suprascapular nerve compression should be considered in the differential diagnosis of chronic shoulder pain.

Introduction

- Chronic nerve entrapment syndromes in the upper extremity are common and their occurrence is only likely to increase as risk factors such as diabetes, obesity, and advanced age become more prevalent in the general population.

- In most cases, the diagnosis can be readily made on the basis of history and physical examination.

- For more atypical presentations, consideration should be given to other neurologic conditions that mimic nerve entrapment syndromes such as mononeuritis, Parsonage–Turner syndrome, and motor neuropathies; not only will these conditions not respond to surgical decompression, they may in fact be exacerbated by operative management.

- When the diagnosis is unclear, electrodiagnostic tests and imaging can be of benefit.

- The purpose of the current chapter is to provide the reader with a comprehensive review of the pathophysiology, diagnosis, and treatment of nerve entrapment syndromes of the upper extremity.

Pathophysiology of chronic nerve compression

Given the associated morbidity of nerve biopsy in patients, most of our current understanding of the histopathologic changes associated with nerve entrapment syndromes stems from animal model studies. A consistent finding in these studies is that the severity of pathologic changes is dependent on the magnitude and duration of compression. An initial breakdown in the blood–nerve barrier is observed, followed by endoneurial edema.[1] Along with perineural thickening, this edema may lead to the deposition of Renaut bodies within the substance of the nerve, further increasing endoneurial pressure. Increased endoneurial pressure disrupts the microneurial circulation, thereby inducing dynamic ischemia in the nerve.[2]

Clinically, these histopathologic changes correspond to paresthesias and an elevation in the static cutaneous sensory threshold as measured by Semmes–Weinstein monofilament testing. With increased compression, localized demyelination occurs followed by more diffuse demyelination.[3] Demyelination is followed by remyelination. Schwann cells, stimulated by mechanical forces, proliferate and deposit thinner myelin.[4] At this stage, patients will experience muscle weakness and will demonstrate increased pressure thresholds for quickly adapting fibers on vibrometry; two-point discrimination, measured in millimeters, remains unchanged. Superficial fascicles tend to undergo demyelination earlier and may explain varying patient symptoms within a single nerve distribution. In early CTS, for example, patients are more likely first to experience paresthesias in the long and ring fingers as the fascicles to these digits are most superficial within the median nerve. Unlike acute crush injuries, Wallerian degeneration is not seen until chronic nerve entrapment is particularly advanced.[5,6] Only at this stage are anesthesia and muscle atrophy observed.

The double-crush phenomenon is an important concept in chronic nerve entrapment. First proposed by Upton and McComas, the double-crush concept holds that compression of a peripheral nerve at one site increases susceptibility to compression at another site along the same nerve.[7] This phenomenon appears to be the result of the disruption of anterograde or, in the case of reverse double crush, retrograde axoplasmic flow of neurotrophic factors.[8] The double-crush phenomenon has been demonstrated experimentally in animal models of chronic compression.[9–12] Clinically, numerous examples of multiple sites of compression along the same nerve have been described and include reports of cervical disk disease and median nerve compression, CTS and pronator syndrome, and cubital tunnel syndrome and ulnar nerve compression in Guyon's canal.[13–16] The double crush concept suggests that two simultaneous points of compression, each of which might be insufficient to cause symptoms on its own, could together produce symptoms. In this way, decompression of one of the two sites might be sufficient to address a patient's symptoms. The most distal nerve compression is typically decompressed first as it is usually the site of the more severe compression and lower surgical risk. If decompression in the distal extremity fails to relieve symptoms, decompression of the more proximal site, such as the intervertebral space or brachial plexus, should be considered.

Electrodiagnostic studies

Depending on systemic factors as well as the location and degree of compression, patients with nerve entrapment syndromes can present with a constellation of symptoms. Given the wide variability in symptoms, numerous attempts have been made at creating standardized diagnostic approaches to these conditions. For example, consensus groups have tried to establish a definitive list of symptoms for the diagnosis of CTS.[17,18] Provocative tests such as Phalen's, Tinel's, and two-point discrimination tests might also be helpful in diagnosing CTS and other compression neuropathies; however, the positive predictive value of such tests alone is low.[19–21] When an atypical presentation or comorbidities cloud the clinical picture, symptom criteria and provocative tests can be combined with electrodiagnostic studies to make the diagnosis.

Two aspects of electrodiagnostic tests are most often used to diagnose nerve entrapment syndromes: nerve conduction studies (NCS) and electromyography (EMG). Of the two studies, the former are especially helpful. An NCS is performed by placing two electrodes on the skin, along the course of the nerve (**Fig. 24.1**). The first electrode is used to stimulate a peripheral nerve to fire, and the second electrode is used to record the characteristics of the generated action potential at some distance away from the stimulation point. The electrodes typically detect only larger, faster-conducting fibers. NCS provide a number of helpful measurements. Amplitude represents the size of the response and is roughly proportional to the number of depolarizing axons in the nerve. Latency is the delay in response following stimulation. Conduction velocity is determined by dividing inter-electrode distance by the latency.

For sensory nerves, recording electrodes are typically placed proximally along the nerve, toward the spinal cord, yielding a sensory nerve action potential (SNAP). For mixed motor-sensory and pure motor nerves, the recording electrodes are placed distally along the nerve toward or at the target muscle, providing a compound nerve action potential or compound motor action potential (CMAP), respectively.[22,23] Another useful parameter elicited by NCS is the F wave. F waves are produced by antidromic conduction of the artificially stimulated action potential back to the anterior horn cells, which then discharge and send impulses back down the nerve following the CMAP. Decreased F-wave latencies suggest more proximal lesions within the nerve, such as plexopathies and radiculopathies, which may contribute to a double crush.[24]

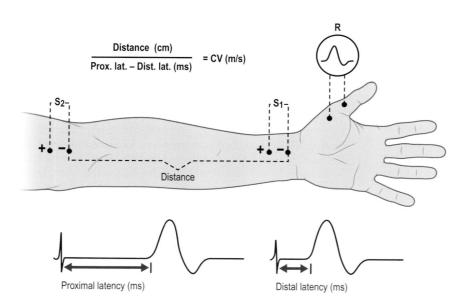

$$\frac{\text{Distance (cm)}}{\text{Prox. lat. – Dist. lat. (ms)}} = \text{CV (m/s)}$$

Proximal latency (ms)

Distal latency (ms)

Fig. 24.1 Method for determining the median nerve motor conduction velocity (CV) in the forearm, recording at the thenar eminence.

EMG studies assess the integrity of muscle function. Because muscle integrity is dependent on innervation, these studies help determine whether axonal damage has occurred. An electrode is inserted into a muscle, at which a slight activity is observed as the muscle membranes are induced to depolarize by the electrode. The needle is then moved from point to point within the muscle to test for fibrillation potentials, which signify abnormal twitching of denervated muscle fibers. Next, the needle is kept in a single position to check for fasciculations, which are random action potentials generated by the motor unit. Finally, the integrity of the neuromuscular junction and nerve is checked by recording motor unit potentials (MUPs) during a voluntary contraction. The amplitude of the MUPs is proportional to the number of activated muscle fibers in a given motor unit.

In the early stages of chronic nerve compression, an increase in latency and a decrease in nerve conduction velocity are observed as focal demyelination occurs.[22,23,25] CMAPs and SNAPs triggered distal to the compression site exhibit little to no decrease early in nerve entrapment syndromes. Over time, however, axonal damage occurs at the compression site, resulting in decreases first in SNAPs and later in CMAPs. As further axonal loss takes place, EMG studies demonstrate increased insertional activity, fibrillation potentials, positive sharp waves, or fasciculations. Axonal sprouting produces collateral reinnervation, the hallmark of which are short, high-amplitude "giant" MUPs on EMG. Following decompression, remyelination occurs and nerve conduction velocities typically return to normal with loss of "giant" MUPs.

Compression of the median nerve

Carpal tunnel syndrome

CTS is the most common nerve entrapment syndrome in the upper extremity, with an estimated incidence in the US of 1–3 cases per 1000 subjects per year and a prevalence of 50 cases per 1000 subjects per year.[26] The economic burden from lost wages and productivity and treatment costs is considerable.[27] Despite the prevalence of CTS, debate remains over the accurate diagnosis and optimal treatment of the condition.

Anatomy

The anatomic boundaries of the carpal tunnel are defined dorsally by the carpus, and volarly by the transverse carpal ligament (TCL), which spans from the hamate and triquetrum on the ulnar side to the scaphoid and trapezium on the radial side. The median nerve and flexor tendons (flexor pollicis longus (FPL), four flexor digitorum superficialis (FDS) and four flexor digitorum profundus (FDP) tendons) pass through the carpal tunnel. The median nerve is the most superficial structure within the canal. The median nerve may divide in the forearm or split within the carpal tunnel. Both presentations are associated with a persistent median artery. The recurrent motor branch to the thenar muscles usually arises off the median nerve in an extraligamentous position distal to the TCL (46–90%) *(Fig. 24.2)*. Less frequently, the motor branch originates from beneath the TCL (subligamentous, 31%) or perforates the TCL (transligamentous, 23%).[28] The palmar

cutaneous branch typically arises off the radial aspect of the median nerve 5–6 cm proximal to the distal wrist crease. Additional branching pattern variations of the recurrent motor branch and palmar cutaneous branch have been described.[29]

Etiology

In the vast majority of CTS cases an underlying etiology cannot be identified. Women are more often affected than men.[30] On histologic examination of idiopathic CTS, tenosynovial tissue demonstrates increased edema and fibrous thickening with minimal inflammation. Compression tends to be greatest at a point 1 cm distal to the distal wrist crease where the TCL is thickest.[31] In rare instances, structural causes such as a persistent median artery, ganglion cyst, hemangioma, or proximal lumbrical origin can increase pressure within the carpal tunnel.

Systemic conditions, such as renal failure, thyroid disease, rheumatoid arthritis, and diabetes mellitus, may also predispose patients to CTS. CTS can occur in up to 45% of pregnant women during the third trimester but usually resolves postpartum.[32] In the pediatric population, mucopolysaccharidoses are a frequent cause of CTS.[33] To date, the only strong evidence linking occupation to CTS has been among operators of handheld vibratory tools.[34] Scientific support for a causative role for other repetitive work activities (e.g., typing) in the development of CTS is otherwise lacking.[35]

Diagnosis/patient presentation

A thorough history and physical examination are central to the diagnosis of CTS. Patients with CTS report nocturnal pain, numbness and tingling in the thumb and radial fingers. Paresthesias are usually triggered by activities involving sustained wrist flexion or extension. Shaking and wringing of the hands tend to alleviate symptoms. Bilateral symptoms are common. Occasionally, paresthesias can radiate proximally along the median nerve to the forearm and may even involve the ulnar digits.

Threshold sensory tests such as Semmes–Weinstein monofilament measurements tend to be more sensitive for detecting early CTS than innervation density measurements.[36] Manual testing of abductor pollicis brevis muscle strength as well as grip and pinch strength can also be helpful. Thenar atrophy has a high predictive value in CTS, but is rarely observed.[37]

Several provocative tests should be considered to aid in the evaluation of CTS. Tinel's sign is elicited by gently percussing over the median nerve at the carpal tunnel. A positive sign is present if the patient describes an electrical shock sensation in the median nerve distribution. The low specificity and sensitivity of the sign may in part be due to the wide intra- and interexaminer variability with which it is elicited.[38] Phalen's test is performed by having the patient place the elbow on a table and flex the wrist for 60 seconds. The test is considered positive if the patient reports paresthesias in the median nerve distribution. Durkan's median nerve compression test involves direct compression of the median nerve at the carpal tunnel for 30 seconds. A positive test is obtained if the patient reports numbness or tingling in at least one of the radial digits.[39] Other less frequently used provocative tests include the reverse Phalen's and tourniquet tests.[40] For multiple

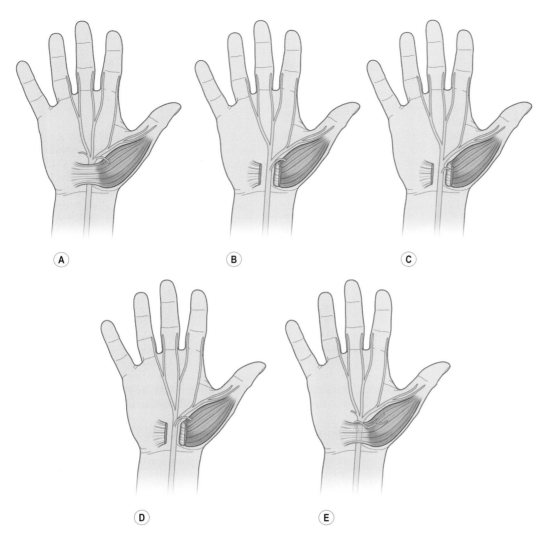

Fig. 24.2 Variations in median nerve anatomy in the carpal tunnel. **(A)** The most common branching pattern of the motor branch is extraligamentous. **(B)** Subligamentous branching pattern of the motor branch. **(C)** Transligamentous course of the recurrent motor branch. **(D)** The motor branch can rarely arise from the ulnar border of the median nerve. **(E)** The motor branch can also lie superficial to the transverse carpal ligament.

reasons, including poor study design, variability in outcome measures and small datasets, no single test has been identified to diagnose CTS consistently. Of the above maneuvers, Durkan's compression test performed with a calibrated pressure device demonstrates the highest sensitivity (89%) and specificity (96%).[39] The sensitivities and specificities of Tinel's sign and Phalen's test are lower.[19–21]

Given the utility of patient symptoms and physical findings, attempts have been made to develop formal clinical criteria for the diagnosis of CTS. Graham *et al.* generated a list of six clinical criteria (CTS-6) for the diagnosis of CTS, based on a validated statistical analysis of recommendations by an expert panel. The six criteria included: (1) nocturnal numbness; (2) numbness and tingling in the median nerve distribution; (3) weakness and/or atrophy of the thenar muscles; (4) Tinel sign; (5) Phalen's test; and (6) loss of two-point discrimination.[41] Similarly, an American Academy of Orthopaedic Surgeons (AAOS) panel reviewed the available literature and developed recommendations for diagnosing CTS;

high-level evidence was lacking to support the majority of recommendations.[42]

CTS remains a clinical diagnosis, and the role of electrodiagnostic and imaging studies remains complementary. Electrodiagnostic tests are routinely performed, yet their validity is largely unproven. These studies have been shown to be poor predictors of symptom severity or functional impairment.[43] Patients with clinical evidence of CTS and negative NCS studies have been shown to have identical clinical improvement after surgery as patients with positive NCS findings.[44] Electrodiagnostic tests are most useful in ruling out other pathology, monitoring treatment response in complicated cases, or making the diagnosis when the patient is a poor historian. Distal motor and sensory latencies greater than 4.5 and 3.5 ms, respectively, are generally considered positive.[45] Routine radiographs have a low yield for underlying abnormalities.[46] Ultrasound examination of the cross-sectional area of the median nerve shows some promise in predicting clinical symptoms while obviating the need for more invasive electrodiagnostic studies; however, for this diagnostic tool to be useful, validated normative data must first be established.[47,48]

Patient selection

Nonoperative treatment

As underscored by AAOS treatment recommendations, there is a role for both nonsurgical and surgical modalities in the management of CTS *(Table 24.1)*.[49] Splinting is the most widely used nonsurgical modality. On the basis of two well-designed studies, splinting has been shown to be more effective than no treatment at relieving symptoms for at least 3

Table 24.1 American Academy of Orthopaedic Surgeons clinical practice guidelines for the treatment of carpal tunnel syndrome (CTS): recommendations

1. Nonsurgical treatment is an option for early CTS. Surgery is an option when there is evidence of median nerve denervation
2. A second nonsurgical treatment or surgery is recommended when initial nonsurgical treatment fails after 2–7 weeks
3. There is no evidence to support specific treatment recommendations for CTS associated with diabetes, cervical radiculopathy, hypothyroidism, polyneuropathy, pregnancy, rheumatoid arthritis, or CTS in the workplace
4a. Local steroid injection or splinting is recommended prior to treatment with surgery
4b. Oral steroids and ultrasound are also options for treatment
4c. Carpal tunnel release is recommended for treatment of CTS based on level I evidence
4d. Heat therapy does not have evidence to support its use in CTS
4e. Other nonsurgical treatment modalities are not recommended for treatment of CTS
5. Surgical treatment with complete division of the flexor retinaculum is recommended, regardless of the technique used
6. Skin nerve preservation, epineurotomy, flexor retinacular lengthening, internal neurolysis, tenosynovectomy, and ulnar bursa preservation are not recommended in the performance of carpal tunnel surgery
7. Use of preoperative antibiotics is an option that may be decided upon by the surgeon
8. Wrist immobilization is not recommended postoperatively after routine carpal tunnel release. No recommendation is made regarding use of postoperative rehabilitation
9. It is suggested that physicians use one or more patient response tools to assess results after carpal tunnel treatment in performing research

months.[50,51] No difference has been demonstrated between continuous splinting and nocturnal splinting alone.[52]

Steroid injection is another commonly used nonsurgical treatment that has been extensively reviewed.[53] Steroid injection provides greater clinical improvement in symptoms 1 month after injection compared to placebo.[54,55] In addition, local injection provides superior symptom relief compared to systemic steroid administration for up to 3 months.[56] Two local corticosteroid injections do not provide significant added clinical benefit compared to one injection.[57] Steroid injection in combination with splinting has also been shown to be better than splinting only at 6-month follow-up.[58] Although systemic corticosteroids have been shown to provide clinical improvement, concerns remain over the risk of steroid-related complications.[59]

Ultrasound has also been shown to be an effective treatment.[60] High-level evidence is lacking to support other nonsurgical modalities including iontophoresis, laser therapy, heat therapy, diuretics, vitamin B, and nonsteroidal anti-inflammatories (NSAIDs).

Treatment/surgical technique

Surgery is the treatment of choice when nonsurgical treatments have failed or when abductor pollicis brevis and/or sensory denervation is advanced. Release of the TCL may be performed using an open or endoscopic technique. Open carpal tunnel release (OCTR) is the most common method of decompression and can be performed under general, intravenous regional (Bier block), or local infiltration anesthesia.

Video 1,2

The wide-awake approach (local infiltration without sedation or tourniquet) has been shown to be safe and cost-effective and is the preferred method of the authors.[61,62] Tumescent field infiltration of 20 mL of 1% lidocaine with 1:100 000 epinephrine is performed *(Fig. 24.3)*. A 3-cm incision is made in line with the flexed ring finger paralleling the thenar crease and ending just distal to the distal wrist flexion crease. The palmar fascia and TCL are incised longitudinally to expose the median nerve. In cases where a prominent palmaris brevis muscle is present, the senior author attempts to preserve it, dividing the TCL deep to it *(Fig. 24.4)*. The ligament and forearm fascia releases are extended distally to

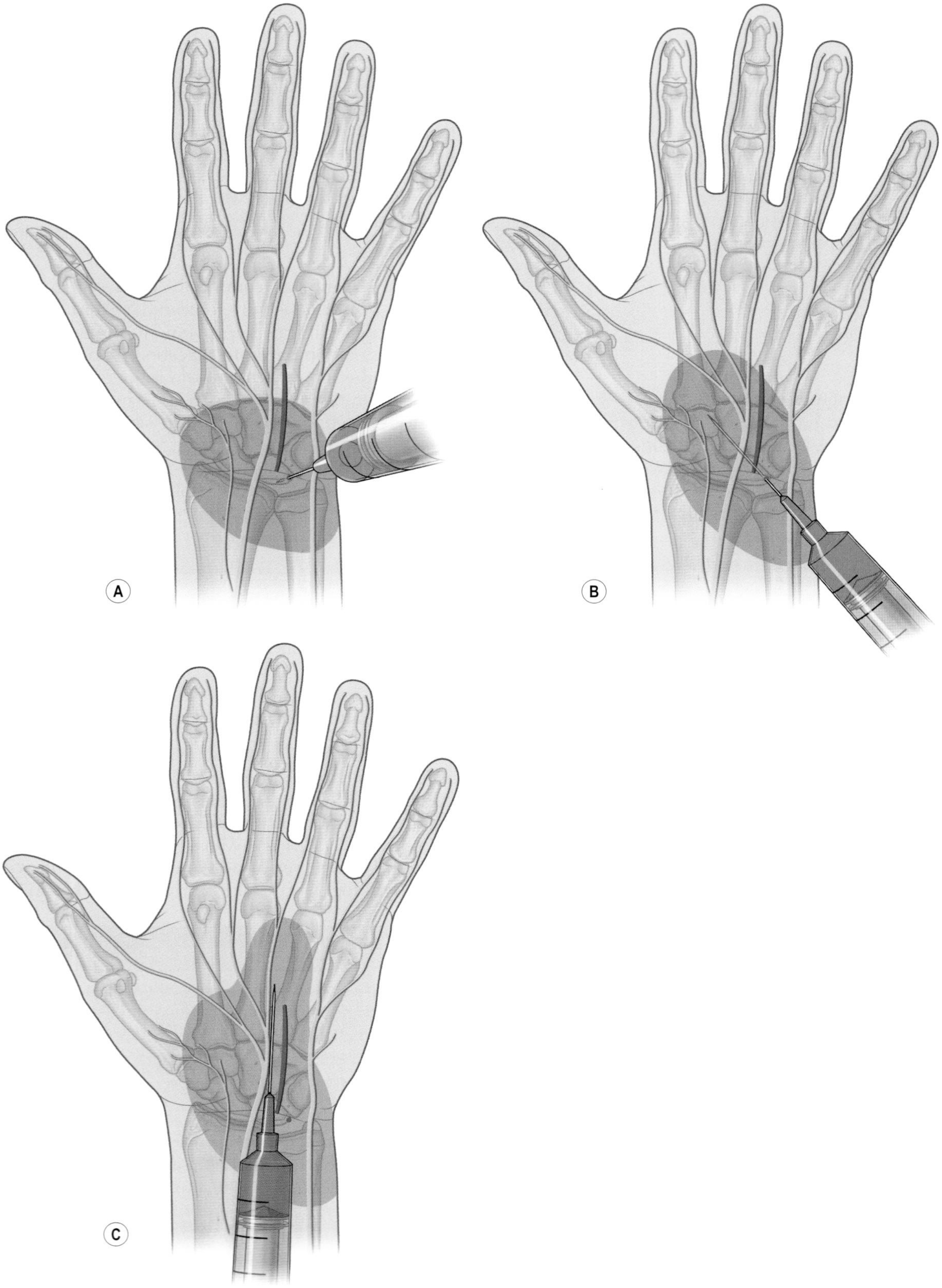

Fig. 24.3 Method of local anesthesia infiltration for the wide-awake approach to open carpal tunnel release. **(A)** Up to10 cc of 1% lidocaine with 1:100 000 epinephrine local anesthetic is infiltrated superficial and deep to the antebrachial fascia of the distal volar forearm, producing a clear wheal proximal to the planned incision. **(B,C)** Infiltration then continues distally deep superficial to the proximal transverse carpal ligament under the incision. Paresthesia induction is contraindicated as the needle can damage nerve fascicles.

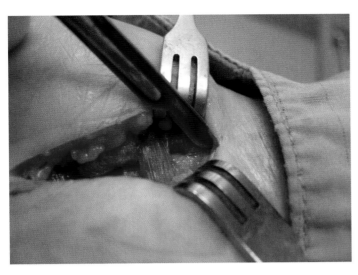

Fig. 24.4 Preservation of prominent palmaris brevis or thenar muscles during open carpal tunnel release. The senior author has found that postoperative pain and grip strength are improved with preservation of palmaris brevis or thenar muscles encountered during dissection with no compromise of decompression. The transverse carpal ligament is divided deep to the muscle under direct visualization.

divide all distal TCL fibers completely in the fat pad and proximally beneath the wrist flexion crease for about 1 cm into the forearm. Placement of the incision ulnar to the thenar skin crease avoids the palmar cutaneous branch, while direct visualization of the median nerve allows identification of an anomalous origin of the motor branch. The authors prefer to perform skin closure using buried intradermal 5-0 absorbable monofilament sutures, thereby obviating the need for suture removal (as shown in video 2, which also contains detailed advice provided to patients intraoperatively). A light dressing only is applied, as postoperative splinting has not been shown to improve pain relief or surgical outcome.[63] Patients are allowed to remove the dressing and shower the day after surgery. A new dressing may be applied for padding and protection for up to a week. Patients are advised to elevate and rest the hand for the first two postoperative days. In most cases, ibuprofen and acetaminophen provide sufficient analgesia over this time. After the second postoperative day, any residual pain is usually the result of overexertion; a gradual return to full activities is advised with pain serving as a guide. Most patients can return to full work activities by 8 weeks. Patients are advised that mild discomfort at the operative site and decreased grip strength can persist for several more months.

Endoscopic carpal tunnel release (ECTR) techniques were developed in an attempt to avoid problems occasionally experienced following OCTR, namely scar tenderness and pillar pain. Popular approaches include the dual-portal technique of Chow and the single-portal technique of Agee.[64,65]

Using the Chow technique, proximal and distal incisions are made deep to the TCL. The endoscope and blade assembly are passed from the proximal incision through the distal incision, deep to the TCL. The distal TCL is released using a probe knife. A second cut is made in the midsection of the TCL with a triangular knife and joined to the first cut using a retrograde knife. The endoscope is then repositioned and in a similar fashion the probe knife used to cut the proximal TCL. A retrograde knife is inserted into the midsection of the TCL and drawn proximally to complete the release.

In the Agee ECTR, a small transverse skin incision is made at the ulnar border of the palmaris longus tendon, midway between the flexors carpi ulnaris and radialis and proximal to the wrist flexion creases. A distally based forearm fascia flap is elevated to reveal the proximal edge of the TCL. With the wrist in extension, the endoscopic blade assembly is inserted into the canal in line with the ring finger. The TCL is visualized and divided distally to proximally.

Both OCTR and ECTR are practiced widely, with proponents of both techniques continuing to debate the merits of one over the other. A common argument in favor of ECTR over OCTR has been reduced postoperative pain and a shorter return to vocational activities. Although these findings have been borne out in some studies,[66,67] other studies show that any differences between techniques in patient symptoms, function, and satisfaction equalize by 1 year.[68,69] Supporters of OCTR have in turn cited a higher incidence of postoperative neurovascular complications as a reason to avoid ECTR.[70] More recent studies have failed to support this higher risk in ECTR.[66–69,71] Cost has been another factor in the debate between OCTR and ECTR. A 1998 cost-effectiveness analysis comparing the two techniques concluded that ECTR is cost-effective provided major complications occur 1% less often than in OCTR.[72] Previous prospective studies have not shown a substantial cost difference between the techniques if the cost of ECTR equipment is excluded.[66–68]

Outcomes and complications

Nonsurgical management has clearly been shown to provide short-term relief of CTS; however long-term studies of these modalities is lacking.[53,57,59] Long-term outcome studies have focused on surgical treatment. Several studies have examined factors to predict response to carpal tunnel release. Burke *et al.* used a validated self-assessment tool to demonstrate that severity and not duration of symptoms preoperatively was the greatest predictor of degree of improvement.[73] While advanced thenar wasting and complete anesthesia are not likely to resolve following surgery, pain associated with CTS typically does, regardless of its duration. Although response to carpal tunnel release is widely held to be worse among elderly and diabetic patients, this has not been borne out by a number of recent studies.[74–76] Overall, outcomes following carpal tunnel release are excellent, with patient satisfaction, symptom relief, and functional improvement observed in more than 94% of cases.[75,77]

Hints and tips

Patients can be advised that, although carpal tunnel release relieves most of the numbness most of the time in most patients, it does not relieve all of the numbness all of the time in all people. If constant numbness has been present for an extended period of time, return of normal sensation after carpal tunnel release is less likely. Surgery may be helpful in alleviating shoulder, arm, elbow, or forearm pain associated with the numbness.

Complications of carpal tunnel release include, but are not limited to, injuries to the motor and palmar cutaneous branches and main trunk of the median nerve; hypertrophic scarring; pillar pain; superficial palmar arterial arch injury; incomplete TCL release; tendon adhesions; infection; wound hematoma; stiffness and recurrence. The most common complication with OCTR is pillar pain (25%), followed by laceration of the palmar cutaneous branch of the median nerve.[78] Incomplete TCL release is the most frequent complication of ECTR.[66] Recurrent CTS symptoms are seen in up to 20% of cases.[79] Revision carpal tunnel surgery generally results in less favorable outcomes. Revision techniques described include complete division of the TCL, nerve grafting or neurolysis with fat transfer, muscle transfer or vein wrapping.[79,80]

Median nerve compression in the proximal arm and elbow

Diagnosis/patient presentation

Compression of the median nerve in the forearm is far less common than CTS. Once formed by the terminal divisions of the medial and lateral cords of the brachial plexus, the median nerve travels medial to the brachial artery, giving off no branches to muscles above the elbow. In the distal upper arm proximal and medial to the medial epicondyle, a supracondylar process, with its attached ligament of Struthers, can be found in over 1% of the population; as the median nerve travels deep to the ligament of Struthers it can be compressed *(Fig. 24.5)*.[81] As it enters the forearm, the median nerve can become compressed at several other sites proximal to the carpal tunnel, including the bicipital aponeurosis or lacertus fibrosis, anomalous muscles (such as Gantzer's muscle, an accessory FPL muscle), and anomalous arteries. Most common of the median nerve entrapment syndromes in the forearm are

pronator syndrome and anterior interosseous nerve (AIN) syndrome.

Pronator syndrome

Pronator syndrome is very uncommon when compared with CTS. It results from the compression of the median nerve as it passes between the two heads of the pronator teres or under the fibrous edge of the FDS arch. Patients typically present with aching pain in the proximal volar forearm with paresthesias extending into the median nerve distribution distally. These sensory symptoms can make discriminating between pronator syndrome and CTS challenging. In the latter condition, however, sensation in the palmar cutaneous nerve distribution is preserved as this nerve branch arises proximal to the carpal tunnel. Another helpful clinical maneuver is to have the patient attempt to pronate the neutral forearm against resistance; if symptoms are elicited during this maneuver as the elbow is extended, compression at the level of pronator teres should be suspected.[82] If pain or paresthesias are triggered by resisted flexion of the fully supinated forearm, the lacertus fibrosus may represent the site of compression. Finally, if resisted contraction of the FDS to the long finger reproduces symptoms, the FDS fibrous arch is a more likely compression point. The examiner must take care during resisted tests not to elicit signs from unrelated pathology such as wrist osteoarthritis. Electrodiagnostic tests should be considered to exclude other sites of compression, but are not very helpful in the diagnosis of pronator syndrome itself.

Anterior interosseous nerve syndrome

Also known as Kiloh–Nevin syndrome, after the individuals who first fully described the condition, AIN syndrome results from the isolated compression of the AIN under the fibrous arch of the FDS or the pronator teres.[83] Patients with AIN

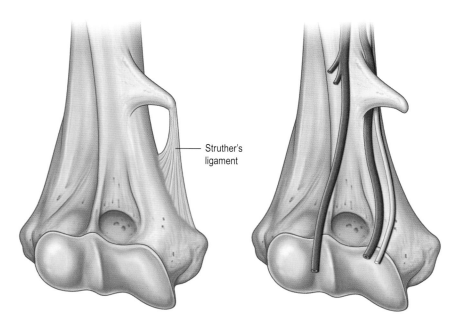

Struther's ligament

Fig. 24.5 Ligament of Struthers. This proximal site of compression of the median nerve is formed by a supracondylar bony process and a ligament that extends to the medial humeral epicondyle.

syndrome will describe weakness of pinch, which affects activities such as picking up small objects and writing, without sensory loss. There may be a history of forearm pain preceding the motor weakness. If instead there is a history of transient shoulder pain following a viral infection that precedes the motor weakness, the surgeon should consider the possibility of Parsonage–Turner syndrome (brachial neuritis). These two entities need to be distinguished as the management of AIN syndrome is directed toward the elbow and forearm. In a patient with rheumatoid arthritis, rupture of the FPL needs to be ruled out by ultrasound, magnetic resonance imaging (MRI), or exploration of a small portion of FPL under local anesthesia.

Because the AIN innervates the FPL, FDP to the index and middle fingers, and pronator quadratus, patients with a complete AIN palsy should exhibit no motor function in these three muscles unless a Martin–Gruber connection or ulnar contribution to the middle finger FDP is present.[84] In incomplete AIN palsy, isolated FPL involvement is most typically observed. Severe weakness of FPL and the index finger FDP results in a characteristic inability to make an "OK" sign. More subtle weakness of these muscles can be demonstrated by having the patient hold a piece of paper between the thumb and index finger against resistance; with an AIN palsy, the patient will compensate by keeping the thumb interphalangeal and index distal interphalangeal joints extended. Electrodiagnostic studies may be helpful in ruling out more proximal lesions such as a brachial neuritis. MRI has been described but is not widely used in the diagnosis of AIN syndrome.[85]

Patient selection

Nonoperative treatment

Conservative management such as avoidance of aggravating activities, rest, and use of NSAIDs has been shown to be effective in both pronator and AIN syndromes. Up to 70% of patients diagnosed with pronator syndrome respond to nonsurgical treatment.[86] When nonsurgical approaches fail, or when a clear anatomic cause such as a tumor is identified, surgical decompression of the median nerve in the forearm should be considered. Controversy remains over the appropriate period to continue conservative treatment before considering surgical intervention. Although most authors recommend surgical exploration after 12 weeks of persistent symptoms despite nonsurgical treatment, spontaneous recovery has been shown to occur as long as 1 year following symptom onset.[87–89]

Treatment/surgical technique

For both pronator and AIN syndromes, access to the median nerve in the forearm is obtained through a zigzag or lazy-S incision over the antecubital fossa. Decompression is begun proximal to the antecubital crease in order to identify the median nerve easily and explore for a ligament of Struthers. Decompression in the forearm includes release of the bicipital aponeurosis and the proximal edge of the FDS arch *(Fig. 24.6)*. The superficial or humeral head of the pronator teres is then released fully or lengthened using a step cut. The arm can be immobilized for 1 week in a well-padded posterior splint with the elbow at 90° and the forearm in neutral.

Compression of the ulnar nerve

Ulnar nerve compression in Guyon's canal

Anatomy

Ulnar nerve entrapment in Guyon's canal, also known as ulnar tunnel syndrome, is very uncommon. Guyon's canal is defined radially by the hamate, volarly by the volar carpal ligament, dorsally by the TCL, and ulnarly by the pisiform and flexor carpi ulnaris (FCU); more distally, nerve branches course deep to the hypothenar muscles *(Fig. 24.7)*. Depending on the location of the compression with Guyon's canal, symptoms may be a combination of motor and sensory (zone I), purely motor (zone II), or purely sensory (zone III).

Zone I contains both volar sensory and dorsal motor fibers and extends from the proximal edge of the volar carpal ligament distally to the bifurcation of the ulnar nerve. Zone II transmits the deep motor branch of the ulnar nerve. It extends from the level of the bifurcation to the fibrous arch formed by the flexor and abductor digiti minimi muscles radially and distally. Soon after passing under the fibrous hypothenar arch, the deep motor branch wraps radially around the hook of the hamate and passes beneath the pisohamate ligament where it can become compressed. Zone III is located ulnar to zone II and is bordered volarly by palmaris brevis and dorsally by the hypothenar muscles. The superficial branch contained in zone III is predominantly sensory with only a few motor fibers to palmaris brevis. Loss of palmaris brevis function is rarely, if ever, noticed by patients, and so for practical reasons the superficial branch is considered to be purely sensory.

Etiology

The most common cause of ulnar nerve compression at the wrist is external compression by a space-occupying lesion, most commonly a ganglion.[90] The zone within which the ganglion arises can typically be determined on the basis of patient symptoms and clinical examination alone.[91] Tumors such as giant cell tumor, neurilemmoma, and lipoma may also give rise to ulnar tunnel syndrome.[92] Numerous cases of anomalous hypothenar muscles impinging on the ulnar nerve have been reported.[93–95] Hypothenar hammer syndrome can be associated with compression of the ulnar nerve in Guyon's, most commonly within zone III.[96] Other less common causes of ulnar nerve compression at Guyon's canal include rheumatoid arthritis and carpal fractures.[97–100]

Diagnosis/patient presentation

Patients with ulnar nerve compression in Guyon's canal typically present with a history of paresthesias in the small and ring fingers, ulnar-sided pain, or decreased grip strength. A history of wrist trauma or vocational exposure to repetitive hand vibration is not uncommon. Patients with ulnar nerve entrapment at the wrist also frequently suffer from CTS; carpal tunnel release can often eliminate ulnar symptoms as it has been shown to decompress Guyon's canal indirectly.[101]

Physical examination should include a thorough sensory assessment. The absence of dorsoulnar hand sensation suggests a site of compression proximal to the branching of the

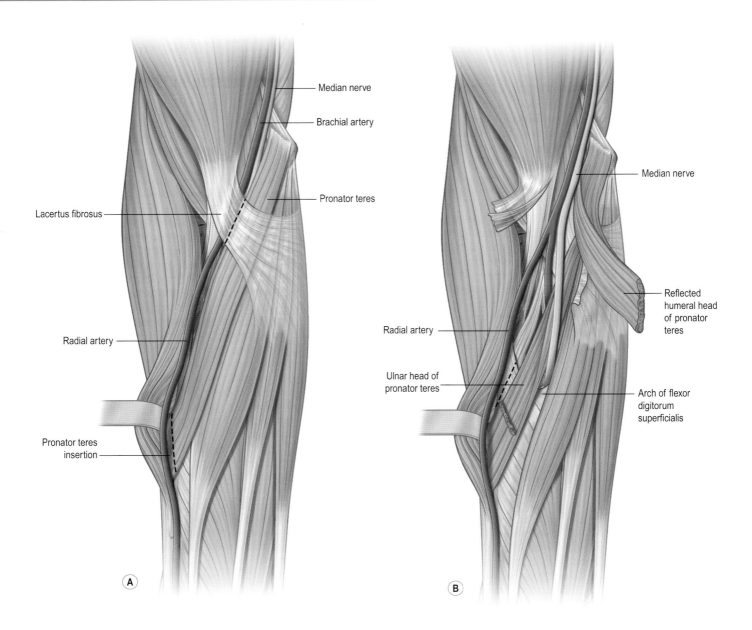

Fig. 24.6 Decompression of the proximal median nerve. **(A)** The lacertus fibrosis is divided. **(B)** The exposed deep head of the pronator teres and fibrous arch of the flexor digitorum superficialis (FDS) are also divided to decompress the median nerve fully.

dorsal sensory branch of the ulnar nerve. The motor exam should include both intrinsic and extrinsic muscle function. The first palmar and dorsal interossei, the lumbricals to the ring and small fingers, and the adductor pollicis are the most commonly affected muscles in ulnar tunnel syndrome. A vascular examination should include an Allen test to assess for potential ulnar artery thrombosis (hypothenar hammer syndrome). Palpation of the ulnar wrist may reveal a ganglion, tumor, aneurysm, or carpal fracture. On the basis of sensory and motor symptoms, the zone of nerve compression can be clinically determined.

Computed tomography and MRI can help delineate bony and soft-tissue pathology, respectively. Electrodiagnostic tests

can help to confirm the diagnosis and localize the compression site.[102]

Treatment/surgical technique

Although conservative methods such as NSAIDs and splinting are often an option, if an anatomic cause of nerve compression is present, surgical intervention is warranted. A 6–7-cm incision is marked between the hook of the hamate and pisiform extending into the ulnar forearm. Proximally, the FCU is retracted ulnarly to expose the ulnar artery and nerve that are then traced distally. The volar carpal ligament and palmaris brevis are incised. A careful examination is made for any

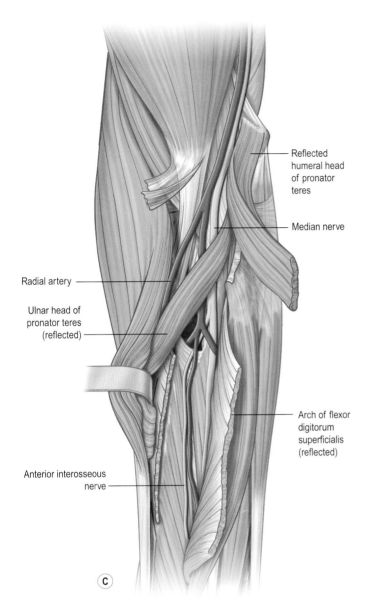

Reflected humeral head of pronator teres

Median nerve

Radial artery

Ulnar head of pronator teres (reflected)

Anterior interosseous nerve

Arch of flexor digitorum superficialis (reflected)

(C)

Fig. 24.6, cont'd (C) The radial origin of the FDS is elevated to expose the anterior interosseous nerve through its entire course.

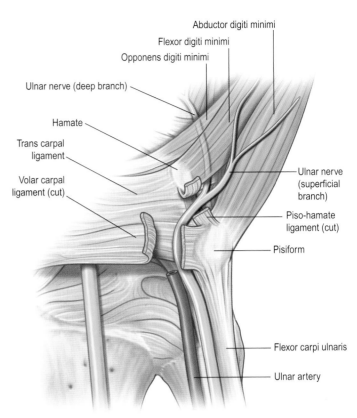

Abductor digiti minimi
Flexor digiti minimi
Opponens digiti minimi

Ulnar nerve (deep branch)

Hamate

Trans carpal ligament

Volar carpal ligament (cut)

Ulnar nerve (superficial branch)

Piso-hamate ligament (cut)

Pisiform

Flexor carpi ulnaris

Ulnar artery

Fig. 24.7 Guyon's canal. The relationship of the ulnar nerve and artery to the hook of hamate, pisiform, opponens digiti quinti, abductor digiti quinti, flexor digiti quinti, and flexor carpi ulnaris is clearly depicted.

ganglion or tumor. The deep motor branch is subsequently decompressed by dividing the fibrous edge of the hypothenar muscles and any fascial bands arising from the hook of hamate. The sensory branch is then traced superficial to the fibrous hypothenar arch where it is most commonly impinged upon by an aneurysm or thrombosis of the ulnar artery.

Postoperatively, patients are allowed to remove the dressing and shower the day after surgery. A dressing may be reapplied for padding and protection for a week. Patients can return to work when they no longer experience pain while performing their duties, usually by 8 weeks.[103]

Cubital tunnel syndrome

Compression of the ulnar nerve at the cubital tunnel is very common and second only to CTS in incidence. The diagnosis of cubital tunnel syndrome is primarily clinical, as electrodiagnostic tests can often be negative despite significant symptoms and exam findings. A thorough understanding of the anatomy of the ulnar nerve about the elbow is key to the treatment of this condition. Various surgical techniques for the decompression of the ulnar nerve are currently in use, with no definitive gold-standard procedure.

Hints and tips

Patients can be advised that the results following cubital tunnel surgery are not as good as those following carpal tunnel surgery and that numbness (or muscle power) may not improve significantly after surgery. By performing cubital tunnel surgery, we may at least prevent further nerve damage and disease progression.

Anatomy

The ulnar nerve is a terminal branch of the medial cord formed by the C8 and T1 nerve roots. In the upper arm, the ulnar nerve travels posterior to the medial intermuscular septum anterior to the medial head of the triceps. The arcade of Struthers is a deep brachial fascial band that joins the intermuscular septum and invests the ulnar nerve approximately

8 cm proximal to the medial epicondyle. This is the first potential site of ulnar nerve compression about the elbow. The medial antebrachial cutaneous nerve passes posterior to the ulnar nerve immediately proximal to or at the epicondyle; injury to this nerve can result in significant postoperative pain. The ulnar nerve travels posterior to the medial epicondyle and medial to the olecranon to enter the cubital tunnel. The tunnel roof comprises a tight fascial layer that extends from the FCU to the arcuate ligament of Osborne, while the floor is defined by the ulnar collateral ligament. Upon exiting the cubital tunnel, the ulnar nerve travels into the forearm between the ulnar and humeral FCU heads, then deep to the deep flexor pronator aponeurosis.

Diagnosis/patient presentation

A thorough history should include the onset of symptoms, presence of grip or pinch weakness, numbness, aggravating and alleviating activities, comorbidities (i.e., diabetes, peripheral neuropathies), and previous elbow trauma. Perhaps the single most important feature on history, however, is the chronicity of the symptoms. Intermittent symptoms elicited by elbow flexion are likely due to transient ischemia of the nerve and will respond well to treatment. Constant numbness or weakness responds less predictably to surgery. Numbness and paresthesias are the most common presenting features in early cubital tunnel syndrome, with pain developing later in the condition. Patient complaints of loss of dexterity suggest intrinsic muscle weakness.

The extent of muscle dysfunction can be classified using the scale developed by McGowan[104] and later modified by Dellon.[105] According to this classification, grade I dysfunction is characterized by transient paresthesias and subjective weakness. Grade II dysfunction presents with intermittent paresthesias and objective weakness. Grade III is defined by constant paresthesias and measurable weakness. In advanced cubital tunnel syndrome, intrinsic muscle paralysis develops, leading to a number of telltale clinical signs *(Table 24.2)*.

Table 24.2 **Clinical signs of ulnar nerve palsy**	
Duchenne's sign (claw or intrinsic-minus deformity)	Hyperextension of proximal phalanx with flexion of middle and distal phalanges caused by paralysis of lumbricals and interossei muscles
Masse's sign	Flattening of the dorsal transverse metacarpal arch caused by hypothenar paralysis and loss of fifth metacarpal supination
Wartenberg's sign	Ulnar deviation and weak adduction of the small finger caused by unopposed pull of extensor digiti minimi
Froment's sign	Hyperflexion of thumb distal phalanx and supination of index during attempted key pinch caused by atrophy of adductor pollicis and first dorsal interosseous muscles
Jeanne's sign	Hyperextension deformity of thumb metacarpophalangeal joint caused by compensatory instability

The two most commonly performed provocative tests for cubital tunnel are Tinel's sign and the elbow flexion pressure test. The sensitivity of Tinel's sign is 70%, while that of the elbow flexion pressure test is 98%.[106] The latter test is considered positive if symptoms are elicited after 60 seconds of digital pressure applied over the cubital tunnel with the elbow in flexion. More recently, Cheng *et al.* described the scratch collapse test.[107] The test is performed by having the patient resist bilateral shoulder internal rotation. The examiner then "scratches" over the site of suspected ulnar nerve compression and then immediately repeats resisted internal rotation. If nerve compression exists, the patient's affected extremity will briefly lose resistance and "collapse."

Radiographs should be obtained to assess for elbow arthritis, instability, or posttraumatic deformity. Electrodiagnostic testing is helpful in confirming the diagnosis or ruling out a peripheral neuropathy or other sites of compression. An ulnar nerve motor conduction velocity across the elbow of less than 50 m/s is generally considered positive. Eversmann held a relative motor conduction velocity decrease of 33% to be indicative of cubital tunnel syndrome.[108] Electrodiagnostic results must be interpreted carefully, however, as they have been shown to have a false-negative rate of more than 10% in the setting of cubital tunnel syndrome.[109] In recent years, ultrasound has emerged as a potentially promising diagnostic tool in cubital tunnel syndrome.[110]

Patient selection

Patients with mild or intermittent symptoms can often be successfully treated with activity modification, splinting, and physiotherapy (nerve mobilization techniques).[111] Nocturnal splinting to prevent elbow flexion of more than 45° can be particularly helpful. Surgical intervention should be considered if nonoperative modalities fail to improve symptoms after more than 2–4 months.[103]

Treatment/surgical techniques

Controversy persists as to the optimal surgical management of cubital tunnel syndrome, a fact underscored by the numerous techniques currently used by experienced surgeons to treat the condition. These techniques include *in situ* and endoscopic decompression, submuscular transposition, intramuscular transposition, subcutaneous transposition, and medial epicondylectomy.

Simple decompression

Our preferred approach at this time is open *in situ* decompression. A 6–10-cm incision is made along the course of the ulnar nerve between the olecranon and medial epicondyle. We prefer to perform this procedure using the wide-awake approach (local infiltration without sedation or tourniquet). Field infiltration of 40–60 mL of 0.5% lidocaine with 1:200 000 epinephrine is performed beginning 8–10 cm proximal to the medial epicondyle to ensure anesthesia in the medial antebrachial cutaneous nerve distribution. Care should be taken to avoid branches of this nerve during subsequent dissection. Beginning proximally, the arcade of Struthers is released, followed by Osborne's ligament and the FCU fascia. The ulnar nerve is left undisturbed in its bed. The elbow is placed through a range of motion to check for any

Video 3,4

residual compression sites or subluxation of the nerve. If the latter is present, in the senior author's experience, transposition of the nerve is indicated.

Endoscopic decompression

Endoscopic decompression techniques make use of a small 15–35-mm incision over the ulnar nerve at the level of the condylar groove.[112–114] Tunneling forceps are used to create a space superficial to the fascia covering the nerve and deep to the subcutaneous tissue. An endoscope is placed in this space and blunt scissors used to release any points of constriction over the nerve under direct visualization.

Submuscular transposition

With elbow flexion, the ulnar nerve is placed under tension and compression as the cubital tunnel volume decreases. The goal of transposition is to move the nerve anterior to the axis of elbow flexion, thereby decreasing tension on the nerve. Critics of this technique feel that dissection of the nerve from its bed compromises the segmental blood supply of the nerve.[115] Transposition may also lead to more local numbness and discomfort than simple decompression due to the sacrifice of a greater number of local cutaneous and articular sensory branches; it is certainly the authors' impression that patients experience faster resolution of local numbness and pain following simple decompression compared to transposition.

As in simple *in situ* decompression, the proximal nerve is identified and traced distally following release of the arcade of Struthers. To prevent the formation of a new compression site proximally, a segment of the intramuscular septum is excised; care must be taken to avoid injury to the venous plexus associated with the septum. The nerve is then unroofed to the level of the deep flexor pronator aponeurosis. A vessel loop is placed around the nerve to provide gentle traction while the nerve is dissected free from its bed and transposed anterior to the medial epicondyle. The motor branches to the FCU and the FDP are preserved. The flexor pronator muscle mass is divided 1–2 cm distal to the medial epicondyle. The median nerve must be identified and preserved. The flexor pronator mass is repaired over the transposed nerve with a stepwise lengthening technique to avoid causing a new compression site.

Intramuscular transposition

Intramuscular transposition is another technique used in combination with anterior transposition. Instead of elevating the entirety of the flexor pronator muscle mass to maintain the ulnar nerve anterior to the medial epicondyle, the intramuscular technique involves making a groove in the flexor pronator mass. Opponents of the technique feel that the absence of a natural tissue plane results in a scarred bed around the nerve that can itself lead to nerve compression.[103,116]

Subcutaneous transposition

After anterior transposition, many surgeons prefer to leave the nerve in a subcutaneous position. Instead of elevating the flexor pronator mass, the ulnar nerve is instead maintained in its transposed position by suturing the loose epineurium to the forearm fascia. Alternatively, a small sling can be created by suturing the subcutaneous tissue from the anterolateral skin flap to the fascia overlying the medial epicondyle, or by suturing a strip of elevated muscle fascia to the overlying dermis; care must be taken to avoid forming an iatrogenic point of compression with this maneuver. To prevent subluxation of the nerve back into its native bed, the roof of the cubital tunnel may be reapproximated *(Fig. 24.8)*.

Medial epicondylectomy

In the medial epicondylectomy technique, the nerve is dissected as in a simple *in situ* decompression. The medial epicondyle is exposed in a subperiosteal plane, maintaining the origin of the flexor pronator mass with the periosteum. The anteromedial edge of the epicondyle is scored with an osteotome. The epicondylectomy is performed along a plane midway between the sagittal and coronal planes of the humerus, all the while preserving the attachments of the ulnar collateral ligament. The flexor pronator origin is then reattached over the epicondylectomy site[103] *(Fig. 24.9)*.

Outcomes and complications

Controversy over the optimal operative management of cubital tunnel syndrome is ongoing, with numerous comparative studies demonstrating no statistical difference in outcomes with any given technique. Simple decompression has been shown to be effective in treating cubital tunnel syndrome, with results equivalent to those of anterior transposition.[117–120] Goldfarb *et al.* recently demonstrated a 93% success rate with *in situ* decompression; the patients who failed to respond to simple decompression were subsequently successfully treated with anterior submuscular transposition.[121] Similarly, a retrospective study comparing medial epicondylectomy alone with medial epicondylectomy and

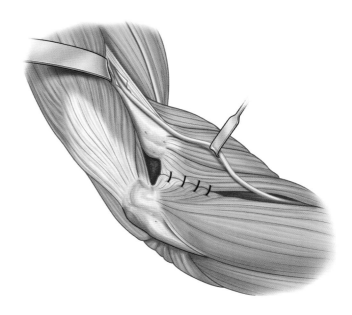

Fig. 24.8 Subcutaneous transposition technique. The arcade of Struthers and flexor carpi ulnaris has been released to prevent compression of the ulnar nerve. Subluxation of the nerve back into its original bed can be prevented by closure of the cubital tunnel roof following transposition.

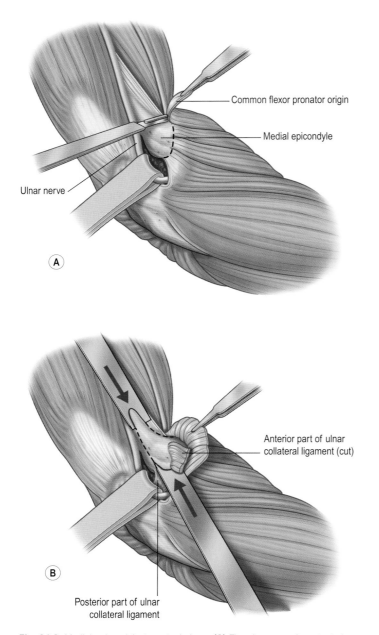

Fig. 24.9 Medial epicondylectomy technique. **(A)** The ulnar nerve is protected while the common flexor pronator origin is elevated from the medial epicondyle. **(B)** The proper plane of the osteotomy is between the sagittal and coronal planes.

anterior subcutaneous transposition showed no statistical differences.[122]

Two recent meta-analyses compared the outcomes of simple decompression and anterior transposition techniques.[123,124] Both failed to find a significant difference between surgical techniques, although the latter study did observe a trend toward improved outcomes with anterior transposition.[124] The major limitation of meta-analyses in cubital tunnel syndrome remains a lack of reliable, reproducible, and valid outcome measures.[125]

The posterior branch of the medial antebrachial cutaneous nerve is at potential risk of injury during both simple decompression and anterior transposition. Injury to the nerve can result in a painful neuroma and hyperesthesia.[126] Ulnar nerve subluxation following simple decompression can lead to persistent pain and is addressed by anterior transposition. Hematoma is more frequently observed following the endoscopic technique than open approaches.[113,114] Medial epicondylectomy is complicated by persistent elbow pain in up to 45% of patients.[127]

Recurrent or unrelieved symptoms are much more frequent than with CTS. Incomplete decompression is effectively addressed through a thorough reassessment for points of persistent compression followed by an anterior transposition.[128] If there is a significant amount of perineural scarring associated with symptoms, the addition of soft-tissue coverage in the form of a muscle flap, fat flap, or vein wrapping may be considered.[129,130]

Compression of the radial nerve

Entrapment neuropathies involving the radial nerve are relatively uncommon, with an annual incidence of 0.003%[131] Compression syndromes involving the superficial radial nerve (Wartenberg's syndrome), and the posterior interosseous nerve (PIN and radial tunnel syndromes) are well described.

Superficial radial nerve compression (Wartenberg's syndrome)

Anatomy

The superficial sensory branch of the radial nerve arises from the bifurcation of the radial nerve in the proximal forearm. It travels down the forearm immediately deep to the brachioradialis. It emerges into the subcutaneous plane approximately 9 cm proximal to the radial styloid by passing between brachioradialis and extensor carpi radialis longus (ECRL) *(Fig. 24.10)*. It is at this point that the nerve is at greatest risk of compression. It provides sensation to the dorsum of the three radial digits proximal to the proximal interphalangeal joints. In 1932, Wartenberg described a series of 5 patients with isolated compression of the superficial sensory radial nerve and termed this condition "cheiralgia paresthetica."[132] Today the condition is more commonly referred to as Wartenberg's syndrome.

Diagnosis/patient presentation

Patients with Wartenberg's syndrome report isolated pain or dysesthesias over the dorsoradial aspect of the hand. The presence of motor weakness suggests a more proximal site of compression. There may be a preceding history of trauma to the area (i.e., handcuffs, forearm fracture). It is important to differentiate Wartenberg's syndrome from de Quervain's tenosynovitis; in the former condition, pain is present at rest and exacerbated by pronation, while in the latter pain is elicited with changes in thumb and wrist position. A Tinel's sign over the superficial sensory radial nerve is the most common exam finding, but may also be positive in patients with neuritis of the lateral antebrachial cutaneous nerve. Electrodiagnostic testing is of limited value in Wartenberg's syndrome.

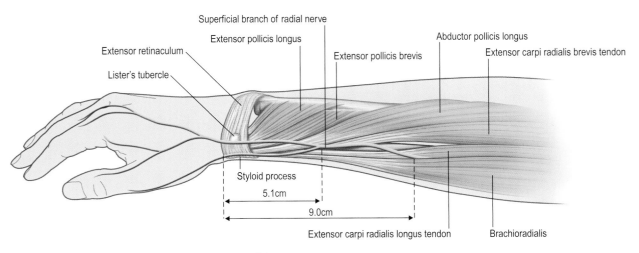

Fig. 24.10 Anatomy of the superficial sensory branch of the radial nerve.

Patient selection

Spontaneous resolution of symptoms is common in Wartenberg's syndrome. Indeed, many cases respond by simply eliminating the inciting factor, such as a tight watchband or bracelet. Rest, splinting, and NSAIDs are also effective. Evidence to support the use of corticosteroids is limited.[133,134]

Treatment/surgical technique

In patients who fail to respond to up to 6 months of nonoperative treatment, surgical decompression may be considered. A longitudinal incision is made slightly volar to the Tinel's sign, thereby avoiding injury to the lateral antebrachial nerve and preventing tethering of the incision scar over the superficial radial nerve. The fascia between the brachioradialis and ECRL is divided and the superficial radial nerve freed from its bed. Postoperative care may involve a desensitization program. An overall success rate of 74% has been reported following surgical decompression.[134]

Posterior interosseous nerve compression in the proximal forearm

Anatomy

The PIN arises from the bifurcation of the radial nerve in the proximal forearm. The PIN is a motor-only nerve that innervates the extensor muscles and abductor pollicis longus distal to the elbow. The PIN does not innervate the ECRL, brachioradialis, or anconeus muscles; these muscles instead receive their innervation from the radial nerve proximally. Immediately distal to the bifurcation, the PIN travels through the radial tunnel, a 5-cm space defined by the capsule of the radiocapitellar joint dorsally, the ECRL and extensor carpi radialis brevis

(ECRB) muscles laterally, the biceps tendon and brachialis muscles medially, and the brachioradialis volarly.

Within the area of the radial tunnel there are five potential sites of compression: (1) fibrous bands to the radiocapitellar joint between the brachialis and brachioradialis; (2) the recurrent radial vessels, or so-called leash of Henry; (3) the proximal edge of the ECRB; (4) the proximal edge of the supinator, or so-called arcade of Fröhse; and (5) the distal edge of the supinator. The arcade of Fröhse is felt to be the most common site of PIN compression. Compression of the PIN gives rise to two different compression syndromes, PIN and radial tunnel syndromes. The management of these two syndromes is identical.

Posterior interosseous nerve syndrome

Diagnosis/patient presentation

Patients with PIN syndrome present with loss of finger and thumb extension, most often due to compression of the PIN at the arcade of Fröhse.[135] Wrist extension is preserved, albeit with radial deviation, as innervation to the ECRL is unaffected. Partial PIN lesions can also be observed, with isolated weakness of the ulnar extensors observed with compression of the medial PIN branch, and weakness of the radial extensors and abductor pollicis longus seen with compression of the lateral branch.[136] Extensor tendon rupture or subluxation may mimic PIN syndrome, but can be readily ruled out by evaluating for an intact passive tenodesis effect. Lipomata are the most common tumor causing PIN syndrome.[137] Other sources include ganglia, rheumatoid synovitis, septic arthritis, and vasculitis.[136,138,139] Although the diagnosis of PIN syndrome is a clinical one, EMG testing is helpful both to confirm the diagnosis and monitor motor recovery following treatment.

Radial tunnel syndrome

Like PIN syndrome, radial tunnel syndrome results from compression of the PIN. In contrast to patients with PIN syndrome, radial tunnel syndrome patients complain of lateral proximal forearm pain with no discernible motor weakness. The syndrome must be distinguished from lateral epicondylitis. In lateral epicondylitis tenderness is localized to the ECRB insertion, while in radial tunnel syndrome the point of tenderness is 3–4 cm distal over the mobile wad.[140]

Compression of the PIN can be increased through combined elbow extension, forearm pronation, and wrist flexion. Pain relief after the administration of a combination of local anesthetic and corticosteroid near the point of tenderness helps to confirm the diagnosis.[141] Many still debate whether the pain experienced in radial tunnel syndrome is in fact due to nerve compression. Skeptics point to the fact that radial tunnel syndrome is unlike other common entrapment neuropathies in that focal tenderness does not follow the distribution of the affected nerve, and is not associated with a neurologic deficit. Furthermore, there are no objective imaging or electrodiagnostic findings to define the pain syndrome.[142] Those claiming that radial tunnel syndrome is a compression syndrome conjecture that the pain may be the result of compression that is sufficient to affect unmyelinated and small myelinated afferent fibers but not larger myelinated efferent motor fibers.[143]

Patient selection

Nonoperative treatment

Conservative management such as avoidance of aggravating activities, rest, splinting, stretching, and use of NSAIDs has been shown to be helpful in both PIN and radial tunnel syndromes.[144] No optimal duration of conservative management has been determined due to a paucity of randomized controlled trials. If activity modification is unsuccessful, an injection of local anesthetic and corticosteroid as described above may be therapeutic. Indeed, one study showed a 72% response rate to local injection in patients with radial tunnel syndrome at 6 weeks of follow-up; in the majority of these responders, pain relief persisted for more than 2 years.[145]

Treatment/surgical technique

Surgery is recommended for PIN syndrome if there is no appreciable improvement in motor function by approximately 3 months. If surgery is delayed for approximately 18 months, fibrosis of muscles innervated by PIN will occur, making tendon transfers the only viable option. Delays of even a few months may also compromise motor recovery in PIN syndrome. Both anterior and posterior approaches have been described for decompression of the PIN. Regardless of the approach adopted by the surgeon, all five potential compression sites mentioned above should be addressed.[103] The anterior approach involves a curvilinear or zigzag incision beginning proximal to the lateral epicondyle and continuing in the interval between the biceps and brachioradialis muscles and then curving 2 cm above the elbow flexion crease, over the mobile wad, and then medial to the border of the brachioradialis (*Fig. 24.11*). The fascia along the brachioradialis muscle is divided and retracted while retracting the biceps and pronator teres medially. The radial nerve is identified in the interval between the brachialis and brachioradialis then traced distally. Fibrous bands overlying the PIN and the edge of the ECRB are released. The leash of Henry and the arcade of Fröhse are divided. The mobile wad muscles are retracted to expose the superficial head of the supinator, which is then divided.

A posterior brachioradialis-splitting approach has also been described.[146] Beginning 1 cm distal to the elbow flexion crease, a longitudinal or curvilinear 6-cm incision is made over the mobile wad. The brachioradialis–ECRL interval is identified by a fascial stripe as well as by the darker color of the brachioradialis. Blunt dissection is carried down to the radial nerve. The superficial sensory radial nerve is found on the undersurface of the brachioradialis and protected. The arcade of Fröhse is readily identified and divided. Other points of compression are identified and released as described above.

Outcomes and complications

Hashizume *et al.* demonstrated full recovery in 16 of 17 patients who underwent surgical decompression of the PIN after symptom onset.[147] In contrast, Vrieling *et al.* noted a good to excellent response in 75% in patients in a smaller study.[148] The differences in outcomes may be due to the fact that in the former study patients underwent surgery at a mean of 2.5 months sooner following symptom onset than in the latter study.

The role of surgical decompression in radial tunnel syndrome remains unclear. In their systematic review of observational studies, Huissstede *et al.* noted the success of surgical decompression ranged from 67% to 92%.[149] This variability in success rates may be due in part to the presence of concomitant lateral epicondylitis in some patients; other studies have shown poorer outcomes among patients with coexistent lateral epicondylitis.[150,151] Similarly, poorer outcomes following surgical decompression for radial tunnel syndrome have been observed among patients receiving workers' compensation.[152]

Thoracic outlet syndrome

The term "thoracic outlet syndrome" (TOS) was first coined by Peet *et al.* in 1956 and referred to the compression of neurovascular structures in the interscalene triangle.[153] Since this original description, TOS has come to represent a number of different clinical entities resulting from the compression of the brachial plexus or subclavian vessels as they pass from the cervical area into the axilla and upper arm.

Because of the heterogeneity of clinical presentations and etiologies, the true incidence of TOS is uncertain, but is thought to range from 3 to 80 cases per 1000.[154] The diagnosis and treatment of TOS involves a multidisciplinary approach and may require that the plastic surgeon work closely with members of other disciplines such as physiotherapy, occupational therapy, neurosurgery, neurology, vascular surgery, orthopedic surgery, and psychiatry.

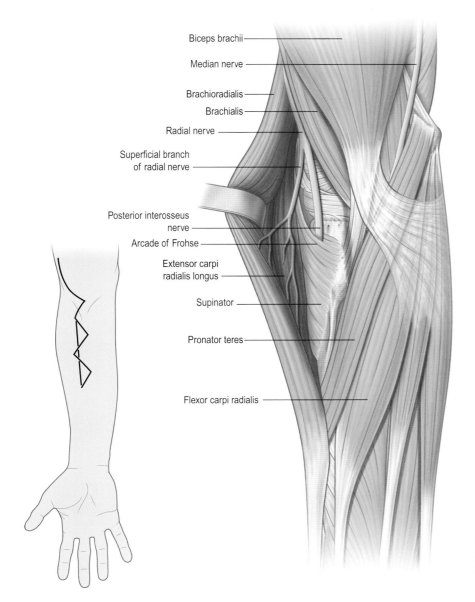

Biceps brachii
Median nerve
Brachioradialis
Brachialis
Radial nerve
Superficial branch of radial nerve
Posterior interosseus nerve
Arcade of Frohse
Extensor carpi radialis longus
Supinator
Pronator teres
Flexor carpi radialis

Fig. 24.11 Anterior approach to the posterior interosseous nerve. This provides good exposure of the radial tunnel when the point of compression cannot be localized to the arcade of Frohse. The zigzag incision provides a wider exposure, but may be less cosmetically acceptable to the patient.

Anatomy

As they course from the base of the neck to the axilla, the brachial plexus and subclavian vessels may become compressed at a number of sites *(Fig. 24.12)*. The first and most common site of potential compression is the interscalene triangle, defined by the anterior scalene muscle anteriorly, middle scalene posteriorly, and first rib inferiorly. The costoclavicular triangle is the second site of potential compression. Its borders are defined by the middle third of clavicle anteriorly, first rib posteriomedially, and upper scapular border posterolaterally. Finally, the subpectoralis minor space is located inferior to the coracoid.

Etiology

Anatomic abnormalities of the thoracic outlet are relatively common, but rarely result in a TOS.[155,156] Anatomic causes of neurovascular impingement in TOS include anomalous muscles, cervical ribs, and fibrous bands. As described by Roos, fibrous bands can arise from a cervical or rudimentary first thoracic rib, cervical transverse process, suprapleural membrane, or scalene muscle.[157] Motor vehicle accidents or cervical trauma, as seen in some sports, likely contribute to the pathogenesis of TOS by causing fibrosis of the muscles of the interscalene triangles.[158]

Etiopathology can be used to classify TOS. The two basic types of TOS are vascular and neurogenic. The vascular type can be further divided into venous and arterial, while the neurogenic type can be subclassified into "true" and "disputed" subtypes.[159] The "disputed" neurogenic subtype is the major source of controversy regarding TOS, and accounts for greater than 97% of patients diagnosed and treated for TOS.[156] As there are no set diagnostic or objective criteria, nor any obvious mechanical impediment to vascular flow or nerve conduction in this subtype, treatment of "disputed"

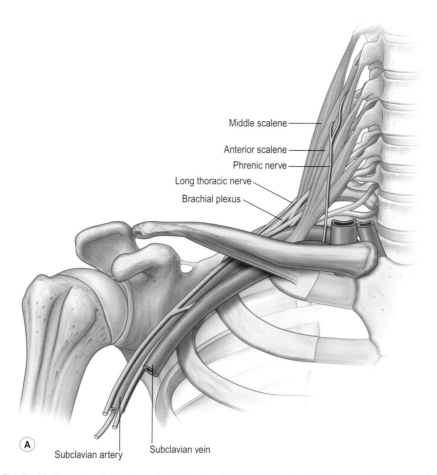

Middle scalene
Anterior scalene
Phrenic nerve
Long thoracic nerve
Brachial plexus

Subclavian artery   Subclavian vein

(A)

Fig. 24.12 Thoracic outlet anatomy. **(A)** Anatomic relationship of the brachial plexus, subclavian vessels, bony structures, and scalene muscles.

neurogenic TOS has focused primarily on nonoperative modalities.

Diagnosis/patient presentation

The diagnosis of TOS can be made on the basis of history, physical examination, provocative tests, diagnostic imaging, and electrodiagnostic testing. In general, the diagnosis of TOS is made through the exclusion of other conditions, including cervical disc disease, Pancoast tumor, peripheral compression neuropathies (i.e., CTS and cubital tunnel syndrome), Parsonage–Turner syndrome, rotator cuff injuries, and vasospastic disorders.[160]

On history, patients will typically complain of pain in the shoulder, upper back, and neck with radiation into the upper arm. Paresthesias and numbness are commonly described, particularly of the ulnar border of the forearm and hand. Physical appearance can provide helpful clues to the diagnosis of TOS. The typical patient will sit with the neck flexed, shoulders forward and internally rotated. Female patients may be particularly large-breasted. Distended superficial veins, edema, and cyanosis of the shoulder and arm may suggest the presence of Paget–von Schrotter syndrome (exertional thrombosis of the subclavian vein). Pallor and coolness with diminished pulses may suggest an arterial TOS. Muscles should be assessed for tone and bulk to rule out a "true" neurogenic TOS.

A number of provocative tests have been described to aid in the diagnosis of TOS, and are each relatively nonspecific and evaluate vascular integrity.[161,162] Wright's hyperabduction test assesses for compression at the level of the subpectoralis minor space *(Fig. 24.13)*. With the patient seated, the radial pulse is palpated. The arm is then hyperabducted; a decrease or loss of the radial pulse indicates compression of the axillary artery. The Halstead maneuver tests for compression at the costoclavicular triangle. The patient places the arms at the sides and protrudes the chest, thereby narrowing the thoracic outlet. The radial pulse is assessed for diminution. The costoclavicular compression test can be performed following the Halstead maneuver by applying downward compression on the clavicle and traction on the arm *(Fig. 24.14)*. Adson's test assesses for compression in the interscalene triangle. The radial pulse is palpated while asking the patient to rotate the head and elevate the chin to the tested side. If there is a decrease in the pulse, it suggests compression of the neurovascular bundle by the anterior scalene muscle or cervical rib. Roos' or the elevated arm stress test test also assesses

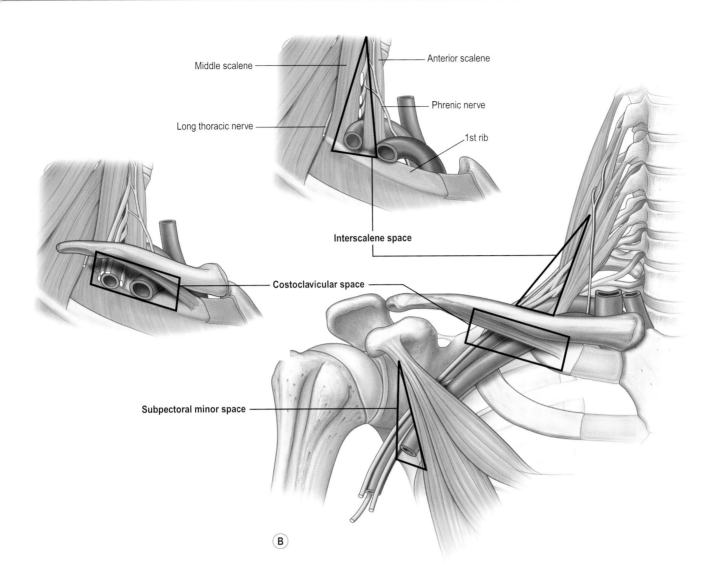

Middle scalene
Anterior scalene
Phrenic nerve
Long thoracic nerve
1st rib
Interscalene space
Costoclavicular space
Subpectoral minor space

(B)

Fig. 24.12, cont'd (B) The three anatomic triangles or spaces of the thoracic outlet, which serve as points of potential neurovascular compression.

the interscalene triangle and is performed by having the patient abduct and externally rotate the arm at 90° while repeatedly opening and closing the fist for 3 minutes; the test is considered positive if the maneuver rapidly reproduces symptoms.

Electrodiagnostic tests can be helpful in confirming "true" neurogenic TOS or ruling out other pathologies.[154] Recently, Machanic and Sanders demonstrated that medial antebrachial cutaneous nerve measurements might serve as an objective measure of neurogenic TOS.[163] Vascular TOS can be identified with venography or arteriography or by noninvasive techniques such as duplex ultrasonography and magnetic resonance arteriography or venography.[159] Cervical spine and chest radiographs are important to identify bony abnormalities, namely cervical ribs and prominent cervical transverse processes.

Patient selection

Nonoperative treatment

Conservative modalities are the primary treatment of patients with "disputed" neurogenic TOS, and may also be of benefit in mild cases of "true" neurogenic and vascular TOS. Symptom relief is reported in 90% of patients with nonoperative interventions only, with poorer outcomes being related to obesity and workers' compensation.[164] Nonoperative treatment may be conceptualized as being composed of four stages.[165,166]

In stage I, pain control is the major focus, with the judicious use of muscle relaxants, mild narcotics, and antiepileptic medications. Nutritional counseling, diet, and exercise programs are initiated during stage I and continue through subsequent stages. In stage II, stretching and relaxation exercises are

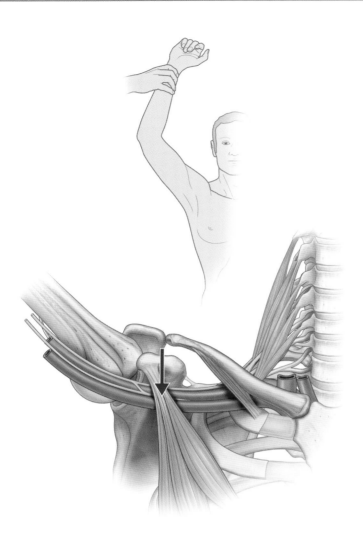

Fig. 24.13 Wright's hyperabduction test. Clinical symptoms or dampening of the radial pulse are elicited with hyperabduction and external rotation of the upper extremity.

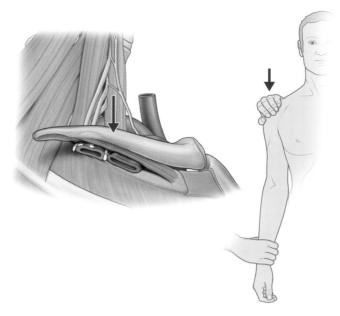

Fig. 24.14 Costoclavicular compression test (Halstead maneuver with clavicular compression).

introduced for correction of the abnormal forward-head posture seen in TOS. Weight loss programs and cardiovascular conditioning continue. In stage III, muscle strengthening and endurance training are undertaken with a goal of returning the patient to the premorbid level of function. In stage IV, a home program is introduced and a plan for returning to work instituted.

Treatment/surgical technique

When conservative management fails or when there is an obvious anatomic cause for a patient's symptoms, surgical decompression is advised. A wide variety of procedures have been described for TOS, including first-rib resection, anterior scalenectomy, and combinations of the two through transaxillary, supraclavicular, infraclavicular, and transthoracic approaches.[167]

The supraclavicular approach is preferred by the authors. Dissection is undertaken under loupe magnification with the patient supine and the neck in slight extension. Paralytic agents are avoided. An incision is made 2 cm cephalad and parallel to the clavicle. The supraclavicular nerves are identified deep to the platysma and preserved. The omohyoid is then divided and the fat pad of Brown retracted. The lateral portion of the sternocleidomastoid muscle is divided. The scalene muscles and brachial plexus are identified. The phrenic nerve and long thoracic nerves are identified and preserved on the anterior scalene and middle scalene muscles, respectively. The scalenes and any associated fibrous bands of Roos are released. The trunks of the brachial plexus are mobilized. The first rib and any cervical ribs are identified and divided in their midportion, then carefully rongeured back. A small drain is kept in place for 24 hours and the arm placed in a sling. Complications of the procedure include injury to the brachial plexus, phrenic nerve, or supraclavicular nerves; pneumothorax; and vascular injury.

Outcomes, prognosis, and complications

Wide variability in outcomes has been reported following the surgical management of TOS, likely due to the heterogeneity of clinical entities represented by TOS. Sanders and Hammond demonstrated that using a supraclavicular approach, the success of scalenectomy and brachial plexus neurolysis is not significantly improved by rib resection.[168] The 5-year success rate for scalenectomy with or without rib resection is approximately 70%. In contrast, a review by Landry *et al.* demonstrated no significant difference between neurogenic TOS patients treated with first-rib resection and those who did not have surgery in terms of symptoms or return to work.[169]

Other nerve compressions of the upper extremity

Quadrilateral space syndrome

Anatomy and etiology

Compression of the axillary nerve in the quadrilateral space is rare, but well described. The quadrilateral space is defined by the teres minor superiorly, the surgical neck of the humerus laterally, the long head of triceps medially, and the upper border of the teres major inferiorly *(Fig. 24.15)*. The axillary nerve and the posterior circumflex humeral artery travel through this space. After traveling along the subscapularis muscle, the axillary nerve winds around the neck of the humerus and into the quadrilateral space. In this region, it branches into an anterior division that innervates the middle and anterior deltoid, and a posterior division. The posterior division supplies motor innervation to the posterior deltoid and teres minor and sensory innervation to the lateral aspect of the upper arm.

Any condition that reduces the cross-sectional area of the quadrilateral space can lead to compression of the axillary nerve. Reported anatomic causes include a ganglion, muscle hypertrophy, scapular fracture, and glenoid labral cysts; however, fibrous bands are the most common cause of compression.[22,170–173]

Diagnosis/patient presentation

Patients with quadrilateral space syndrome present with a gradual increase in poorly localized pain over the anterolateral shoulder, paresthesias over the deltoid, and weak shoulder abduction.[174] Tenderness is almost always noted over the quadrilateral space posteriorly and pain can be elicited by having the patient abduct and externally rotate the shoulder. In severe cases, wasting of the deltoid may be present.

Electrodiagnostic studies have been shown to be insensitive but specific for quadrilateral space syndrome.[175] Based on their original report, Cahill and Palmer held that angiography was the investigation of choice; occlusion of the posterior circumflex humeral artery that accompanies the axillary nerve through the quadrilateral space was considered pathognomonic of the condition.[174] More recently, MRI findings of teres minor denervation atrophy muscle have been considered confirmatory of the diagnosis.[176,177]

Patient selection

In cases of quadrilateral space syndrome where a clear anatomic cause is not identified, 3–6 months of activity modification, NSAIDs, and strengthening exercise are often effective in relieving pain and restoring function. In patients with significant deltoid atrophy or with a clear structural compression, however, a nonsurgical approach is unlikely to be of benefit.

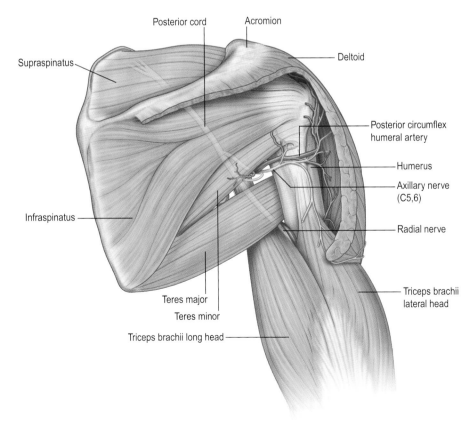

Fig. 24.15 Anatomic boundaries and contents of the quadrilateral space.

Treatment/surgical technique

The patient is placed in the lateral decubitus position and the quadrilateral space approached through a posterior vertical incision centered over the point of maximal tenderness. Alternatively, the quadrilateral space can be found at the intersection between the line from the acromion to the medial epicondyle and a second line at the groove between the posterior deltoid and triceps muscles.[178] Once skin flaps are elevated, the inferior border of the deltoid is identified and partially detached from the scapular spine to expose the quadrilateral space. The axillary nerve is identified and fibrous bands around it sharply divided; partial resection of the teres minor or major muscles or triceps may be required to widen the quadrilateral space adequately. The deltoid is repaired and a drain placed.

Suprascapular nerve compression

Anatomy and etiology

Compression of the suprascapular nerve is an uncommon entity. The suprascapular nerve innervates the supraspinatus and infraspinatus muscles and provides sensation to the coracoacromial ligament, acromioclavicular and glenohumeral joints, and, rarely, the skin of the lateral arm.[179]

From its origins from the upper trunk of the brachial plexus, the nerve courses through the posterior cervical triangle to reach the suprascapular notch *(Fig. 24.16)*. The suprascapular notch is a bony concavity medial to the coracoid process whose superior border is defined by the transverse scapular ligament. As the nerve passes deep to the ligament it is particularly susceptible to compression. Upon exiting the suprascapular notch, the nerve travels along the supraspinatus fossa, providing motor branches to the overlying supraspinatus muscle, before reaching the spinoglenoid notch. This depression at the lateral base of the scapular spine serves as a second common site of suprascapular nerve compression. A spinoglenoid ligament has been identified with variable frequency that may further impinge on the nerve.[180] Just beyond the spinoglenoid notch, the suprascapular nerve makes a medial turn around the base of the scapular spine to innervate the infraspinatus muscle.

Diagnosis/patient presentation

Suprascapular compression neuropathy should be suspected in younger athletes or laborers who perform repetitive overhead activities. Patients commonly present with dull posterolateral shoulder pain and dysfunction. The diagnosis can be delayed by months as treatment is erroneously directed towards the cervical spine, rotator cuff, or glenohumeral joint. Pain may be exacerbated by arm adduction and internal rotation that tighten the spinoglenoid ligament.[181] In advanced cases, supraspinatus and infraspinatus muscle wasting with weakness of shoulder external rotation and abduction may be observed. With suprascapular notch entrapment, the acromioclavicular joint and supraspinatus fossa may be tender to palpation.

When clinical examination and routine imaging are equivocal, pain relief following an injection of local anesthetic into

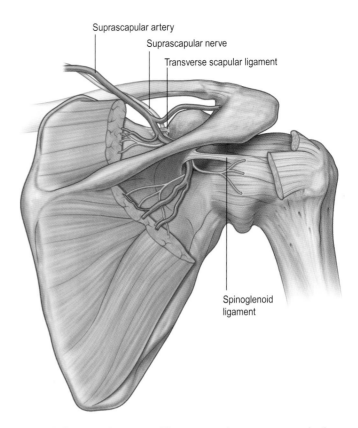

Fig. 24.16 Suprascapular anatomy. The suprascapular nerve passes under the transverse scapular ligament and through the suprascapular notch. Similarly, the spinoglenoid notch is covered by the spinoglenoid ligament. Both ligaments can compress the suprascapular nerve.

the suprascapular notch may help to localize the point of entrapment.[182] Nerve conduction and EMG studies may also be obtained but carry an increased rate of false-negative and positive findings.[183]

Routine radiographs should be obtained to rule out potential bony causes of entrapment. MRI studies are useful in delineating the extent of muscle atrophy as well as identifying potential soft-tissue etiologies or associated rotator cuff tears.

Patient selection

Most patients with suprascapular neuropathy have an underlying etiology of overuse. In these patients, most authors agree that 6–12 months of activity modification, NSAIDs, and strengthening exercise is adequate to relieve pain and restore function in up to 80% of patients.[184] In patients with significant muscle atrophy or with a clear structural compression, however, a nonsurgical approach is unlikely to be of benefit and may in fact lead to further dysfunction.[185]

Treatment/surgical technique

Traditionally, the suprascapular notch has been decompressed via a trapezius-splitting incision along the scapular spine.[186] The supraspinatus muscle is retracted posteriorly to expose the suprascapular vessels and suprascapular nerve superior and inferior to the transverse scapular ligament, respectively. If the nerve continues to be compressed following division of the ligament, the notch may be further widened using a burr. Open decompression of the spinoglenoid notch is carried out through a deltoid-splitting incision starting 4 cm medial to the posterolateral corner of the acromion. The infraspinatus muscle is retracted inferiorly to expose the spinoglenoid ligament and notch.[187]

More recently, less invasive techniques have been developed. Iannotti and Ramsey have described the arthroscopic decompression of the suprascapular nerve at the spinoglenoid notch.[188] Bhatia and colleagues demonstrated an arthroscopic approach to the suprascapular notch.[189] Subsequently, Lafosse et al. showed low morbidity and clinical and EMG improvements with this approach in a series of 10 patients at a mean 15-month follow-up.[190]

Access the complete references list online at **http://www.expertconsult.com**

2. Mackinnon SE. Pathophysiology of nerve compression. Hand Clin. 2002;18:231–241.

4. Tapadia M, Mozaffar T, Gupta R. Compressive neuropathies of the upper extremity: Update on pathophysiology, classification, and electrodiagnostic findings. J Hand Surg Am. 2010;35:668–677.
   This article summarizes the current developments in the basic science of chronic nerve compression and provides a review of the double-crush phenomenon as well as electrodiagnostic tests.

7. Upton AR, McComas AJ. The double crush in nerve entrapment syndromes. Lancet. 1973;2:359–362.

26. Bickel KD. Carpal tunnel syndrome. J Hand Surg Am. 2010;35:147–152.
   This review examines the ongoing challenges in developing clinical criteria for the diagnosis of carpal tunnel syndrome as well as reviewing current treatment approaches.

41. Graham B, Regehr G, Naglie G, et al. Development and validation of diagnostic criteria for carpal tunnel syndrome. J Hand Surg Am. 2006;31:919–924.

61. Lalonde D, Bell M, Benoit P, et al. A multicenter prospective study of 3110 consecutive cases of elective epinephrine use in the fingers and hand: The Dalhousie project clinical phase. J Hand Surg Am. 2005;30:1061–1067.

62. Leblanc MR, Lalonde J, Lalonde DH. A detailed cost and efficiency analysis of performing carpal tunnel surgery in the main operating room versus the ambulatory setting in Canada. Hand (N Y). 2007;2:173–178.

The authors examine the benefits of the wide-awake approach to carpal tunnel release compared to carpal tunnel surgery performed in the main operating suite under general anesthesia in terms of cost and overall efficiency. The wide-awake approach to carpal tunnel release allows the hand surgeon to improve productivity without compromising patient safety or outcomes.

69. Macdermid JC, Richards RS, Roth JH, et al. Endoscopic versus open carpal tunnel release: A randomized trial. J Hand Surg Am. 2003;28:475–480.

124. Macadam SA, Gandhi R, Bezuhly M, et al. Simple decompression versus anterior subcutaneous and submuscular transposition of the ulnar nerve for cubital tunnel syndrome: A meta-analysis. J Hand Surg Am. 2008;33:1314.e1–12.
   In their meta-analysis of all available comparative or randomized controlled studies examining the surgical management of cubital tunnel syndrome, the authors found no statistically significant differences, but rather a trend toward an improved clinical outcome with transposition of the ulnar nerve as opposed to simple decompression.

148. Vrieling C, Robinson P, Geertzen J. Posterior interosseous nerve syndrome: Literature review and report of 14 cases. Eur J Plast Surg. 1998;21:196–202.

165. Novak CB. Thoracic outlet syndrome. Clin Plast Surg. 2003;30:175–188.
   This publication provides a thorough review of the pathophysiology, diagnosis and management of thoracic outlet syndrome with a particular focus on the nonoperative modalities involved in the treatment of "disputed" neurogenic thoracic outlet syndrome.

25

Congenital hand I: Embryology, classification, and principles

Michael Tonkin and Kerby Oberg

SYNOPSIS

- Consistency of terminology is necessary for optimal communication.
- Limb outgrowth and patterning are controlled by specific signaling centers within the developing limb bud via the activation and interaction of molecular messengers.
- Anomalies of limb development result from:
  - spontaneous mutation of genetic material
  - inheritance of abnormal genes
  - subtle or gross insult to the limb bud.
- The anomaly may be isolated or syndromic.
- The Swanson/International Society for Surgery of the Hand (IFSSH) classification is unable to incorporate satisfactorily alterations consequent on the increasing knowledge of the molecular basis of limb development, but continues to be the classification relied upon by most surgeons. An alternative approach incorporates an understanding of the mechanism of insult and the site within the developing limb which is primarily affected.
- Assessment and treatment are specific for each child and family but are based on a detailed understanding of the processes of limb development, the psychological and physical effects of limb anomalies, and simple surgical principles.

Introduction

Limb development

The upper limb bud appears during the fourth week of development as an outgrowth on the sides of the embryo. Cells of the somatic lateral plate mesoderm form the skeletal framework of the limb, while mesoderm from the somite migrates in to form the muscular component and contributes to the limb's vascular network. Over the next 4 weeks, growth and differentiation transform the limb bud into an elegant asymmetric organ that is one of the defining features of the human species. The limb bud growth and differentiation are under the control of signaling centers, specialized areas within the limb which dictate, in concert, the appropriate sequential events of development.

The establishment of signaling centers and their subsequent behavior are under genetic control. The genes and the morphogens (proteins) they encode control the process of limb growth and differentiation and act as messengers between signaling centers and developing cells.

As knowledge of the process of limb development becomes more sophisticated, an understanding of the causation of limb anomalies becomes clearer.

Genetic mutations can disrupt the molecular function of a number of proteins orchestrating limb development, including secreted proteins (ligands), ligand receptors, and transcription factors. The mutation may be inherited or may arise spontaneously. Environmental factors, including mechanisms such as thalidomide, which resulted in an epidemic of limb malformations during the 1960s, radiation, nutritional defects, and infections may affect the molecular pathways of development or be responsible for a more gross insult resulting in tissue hemorrhage and/or necrosis. For example, if such direct damage occurs obliterating the apical ectodermal ridge (AER), an important signaling center that directs limb outgrowth, transverse truncation will result.

Classification

Congenital anomalies in the hand demand a reproducible and consistent terminology, a universal language which allows discussion of complex clinical entities, indications for treatment, and comparisons of results.

Swanson's classification was adapted as the standard system by which congenital hand anomalies are described by the IFSSH in 1976.[1] It is derived from ideas existing in the 1970s regarding limb embryology and is largely based on morphological appearance. Knight and Kay[2] have presented an extended version, attempting to incorporate a list of all congenital anomalies. Regrettably, this classification, based as it is on appearance and relying on knowledge available in the 1960s and 1970s, is intrinsically unsuited to alterations based on causation and etiology at a molecular level. It is perhaps time to consider alternatives.

Ideally, an overall classification of congenital hand anomalies would be based on etiology, with such a classification indicating the site in the molecular pathway and/or the anatomical site in the limb bud and the time at which the aberration occurs.

It would reflect whether the fault is a problem of longitudinal outgrowth, lies within one of the axes of differentiation, and affects primarily the hand plate alone or the whole upper limb. It is probable that the causation of some anomalies will confound our attempts to assign an etiology.

Assessment and principles of treatment

It is clear that the terminology applied to our efforts should reflect a language common to, and understood by, the geneticist, the anatomist, the pathologist, and the surgeon. For this reason, these authors have chosen to link the terminology of embryology of the limb bud at the molecular level, the terminology of dysmorphology, and the terminology of classification. This consistency would appear to provide less controversy in a rapidly changing field of knowledge. Furthermore, such an approach is of benefit when attempting to explain to parents how the limb normally forms and how any particular anomaly may occur. This process plays a vital role in the assessment of any specific anomaly and leads to a sensible plan of management.

Limb development (embryology)

Overview of upper limb morphogenesis

Around day 26 (4 weeks) after fertilization (Carnegie stage 12), the upper limb bud appears as an oblong ventrolateral bulge on the body wall between somites 9–12 (C5–8) **(Fig. 25.1)**.[3] The emerging limb bud is composed of somatic lateral plate mesoderm covered by ectoderm. Subsequent limb bud growth and differentiation are described in terms of three coordinate axes: proximodistal, dorsoventral (dorsovolar), and anteroposterior (or radioulnar) **(Fig. 25.2)**, each controlled by distinctive regions – signaling centers.

The ectoderm overlying the distal edge of the limb bud at the dorsovolar boundary thickens and forms a distinct ridge of stratified ectoderm, the AER.[4] The thickened AER is critical for proximodistal outgrowth and also adds mechanical rigidity to the distal rim of the limb bud, flattening it along the dorsovolar axis. Excision of the AER in chicken embryo limb buds prevents further proximodistal outgrowth and results in limb truncation.[5] Underlying the AER, the distal mesoderm exhibits robust proliferation and has been termed the progress zone (PZ). Cells in the PZ ultimately differentiate into specific cell types and are directed to specific positions within the limb.

The dorsal ectoderm is a critical signaling center for directing formation of dorsal and volar characteristics of the limb. Excision and rotation of dorsal ectoderm cause the formation of dorsal structures on the limb ventral surface.[6] Another

Table 25.1 Timing of hand formation

Time after fertilization	Hand development
27 days	Development of arm bud
28–30 days	Further development of arm bud
34–36 days	Elongation of arm bud
34–38 days	Formation of hand paddle
38–40 days	Early separation of digits
44–46 days	Digits separated
Week 9–10	Formation of fingernails begins

(Reproduced from: Gupta A, Kay SPJ, Scheker LR, editors. The growing hand: diagnosis and management of the upper extremity in children. London: CV Mosby; 2000, p. 25.)

collection of mesodermal cells at the distal ulnar (posterior) margin is called the zone of polarizing activity (ZPA). Although not morphologically distinct, these cells direct radioulnar patterning and coordinate asymmetric limb patterning with the other signaling centers during development. Removal of the ZPA in animal models leads to loss of the ulna and the ulnar digits.[7] Conversely, transplantation of these cells to the anterior (radial) aspect of limb buds of chicken embryos will result in formation of a mirrored complement of ulnar digits radially.[8]

Over the next week, the limb bud expands and elongates, particularly along the proximodistal axis **(Table 25.1)**. By day 33 of development (Carnegie stage 14), differential growth and programmed cell death transform the distal portion into a paddle-shaped hand plate. There is also progressive mesodermal condensation along the proximodistal axis, forming a tripartite skeleton composed of a proximal section, the stylopod (shoulder girdle and humerus), a middle section, the zeugopod (radius and ulna), and a distal section, the autopod (hand). The joints become fully evident about day 51 (Carnegie stage 20) when the elbow and wrist joints flex and by day 56 (end of eighth week, Carnegie stage 23), the major morphologic features of the limb are complete **(Fig. 25.1)**.

The molecular control of limb outgrowth and patterning

During early embryonic development, Hox transcription factors set up a segmental body plan along the cranial–caudal axis.[9] By the fourth week of development the presumptive upper limb fields are established, triggering the expression of Tbx5, Wnt3, and Fgf10 which initiate limb formation.[10] Tbx5 determines forelimb identity, while Wnt3 and Fgf10 induce mesodermal proliferation and limb outgrowth. Mesodermal Fgf10, in conjunction with ectodermal radical fringe (R-fng) at the apical dorsovolar boundary, induces ectodermal thickening to form the AER.[11–13] Formation of the AER initiates the expression of AER-related Wnt and Fgf proteins (including Fgf2/4/8/9/17)[14,15] which, in turn, act on the mesoderm just underneath the AER to sustain Wnt3 and Fgf10 expression in the PZ. This reciprocal loop of ectodermal and mesodermal Fgf/Wnt proteins promotes progressive proximodistal

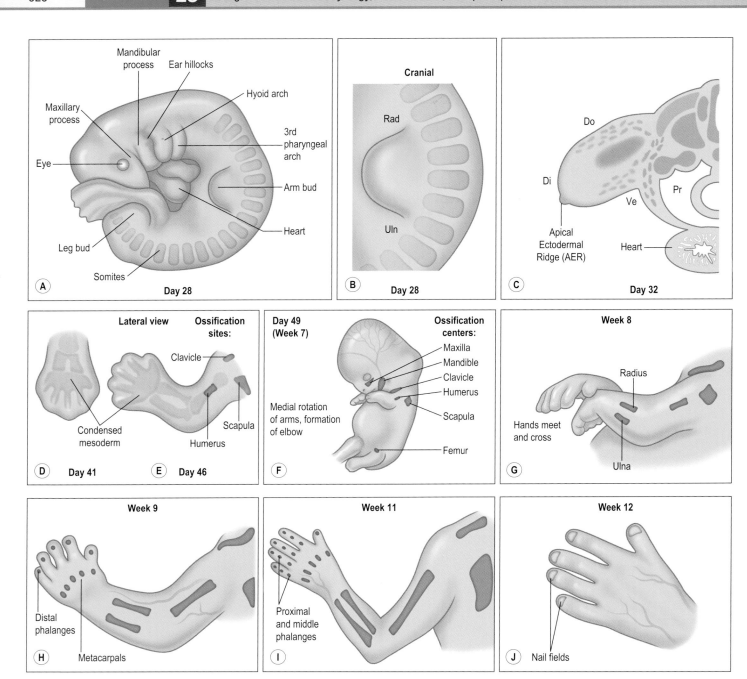

Fig. 25.1 Upper limb and hand development. **(A)** Human embryo at Carnegie stage 13 (about 28 days of development), showing early limb buds. **(B, C)** Cross section through an upper limb bud at 32 days of development (Carnegie stage 14), showing dorsal (Do)-ventral (Ve) limb bud flattening and the thickened apical ectodermal ridge at the distal tip of the limb bud (that runs along the dorsal-ventral border from anterior to posterior). **(D)** The handplate at 41 days of development (Carnegie stage 17). The scalloped edge conforms to the condensing digital mesenchyme. **(E)** Limb at 46 days of development (Carnegie stage 19). Separate fingers are evident. The proximal limb skeleton is well developed and ossification has begun in the humerus and shoulder girdle. **(F)** The embryo at 49 days of development (Carnegie stage 20), showing ossification centers in the upper limb, lower limb, and face. Note that upper limb development is more advanced than lower limb development. **(G)** Upper limbs at week 8 (Carnegie stage 22). The fingers are completely separate and ossification centers have developed in the forearm, i.e., radius and ulna. **(H)** The upper limb at week 9 (Carnegie stage 23). Metacarpal and distal phalangeal ossification has begun. **(I)** The upper limb at week 11. Ossification in proximal and middle phalanges is now evident in addition to distal phalanges and metacarpals. **(J)** The hand at week 12, showing developing nail fields (nails become visible during week 16). (Portions redrawn from England MA. A colour atlas of life before birth. London: Year Book Medical Publications, 1983.)

outgrowth[16,17] *(Fig. 25.3)*. In the absence of Wnt3 or Fgf10 limbs fail to develop and tetramelia results.[18,19] Application of Fgfs to the distal chick limb bud after AER removal will return proximodistal limb outgrowth.[15] Within the PZ, mesodermal cells persist in an undifferentiated or receptive state, allowing the signaling centers to direct their fates.

The ZPA in the posterior (ulnar) limb mesoderm secretes a potent morphogen, sonic hedgehog (Shh), that regulates radi-oulnar patterning[20] *(Fig. 25.3)*. Shh induces posterior (ulnar) proliferation of the limb bud expanding its width.[21,22] Moreover, Shh posteriorizes (ulnarizes) the developing forearm and defines the identity of the ulnar four digits. In a

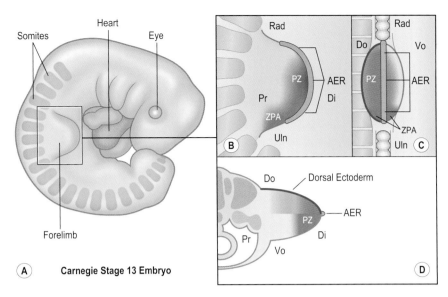

Fig. 25.2 Limb bud coordinate axes and signaling centers: **(A)** The forelimb (boxed region) of a Carnegie stage 13 embryo depicting the three coordinate axes – each with its own signaling center: the apical ectodermal ridge (AER) coordinating proximodistal (Pr-Di) outgrowth and differentiation; dorsovolar (Do-Vo) asymmetry is regulated by dorsal ectoderm; radioulnar asymmetry is controlled by the zone of polarizing activity (ZPA). Within the progress zone (PZ) the fate of mesodermal cells is determined by these signaling centers. The axes and signaling centers are shown in three different orientations: **(B)** dorsal view, **(C)** lateral, end-on view, and **(D)** axial cross-section. (Modified from Oberg KC, Greer LF, Naruse T. 2004. Embryology of the upper limb: the molecular orchestration of morphogenesis. Handchir Mikrochir Plast Chir 36:98–107.)

Proximodistal asymmetry

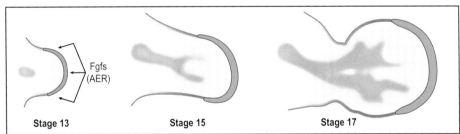

Radioulnar asymmetry

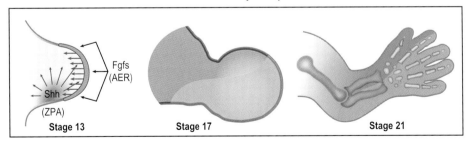

Dorsovolar asymmetry

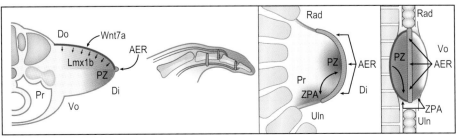

Fig. 25.3 Morphologic impact of signaling centers. Upper panel: role of apical ectodermal ridge (AER)-related Fgfs (orange) on skeletal outgrowth (humerus, blue; radius and ulna, green; hand, magenta). Middle panel: role of Shh secretion from the zone of polarizing activity (ZPA): influence on the forearm and digits (depicted in purple). Lower left panel: role of Wnt7a (medium green) and Lmx1b (light green), from the dorsal ectoderm and mesoderm respectively, in tendon and ligament formation in a digit. Do, dorsal; Vo, volar; Pr, proximal; Di, distal; PZ, progress zone. Lower right panel: illustration depicting communication between signaling centers – reciprocal Shh-Fgf loop (white bidirectional arrow). Wnt7a influence on Shh expression (white unidirectional arrow). Rad, radial; Uln, ulnar.

naturally occurring chicken mutant, limb-specific Shh expression is lacking and the upper limbs develop without ulnas and without digits.[23] Application of exogenous Shh to the posterior (ulnar) aspect of the limb bud can fully recover normal limb morphology. Furthermore, application of Shh to the anterior margin produces mirrored duplication of ulnar digits radially.[20]

The AER and the ZPA are also closely linked by a reciprocal feedback loop that maintains Shh expression at the distal posterior (ulnar) border of the limb bud adjacent to the AER during progressive outgrowth.[24–26] Removal of the AER causes regression of Shh expression and ablation of the ZPA induces a loss of Fgf signaling.[25] Secretion of Wnt7a from the dorsal ectoderm induces the homeodomain transcription factor Lmx1b in the underlying mesoderm and asymmetrically dorsalizes the developing limb[13,27,28] *(Fig. 25.3)*. Wnt7a also contributes to the maintenance of Shh secretion from the ZPA[29] linking the dorsovolar and radioulnar axes. Removal of dorsal ectoderm reduces Shh expression and disrupts posterior (ulnar) patterning.[30] Thus, Shh plays a pivotal role during limb development linking dorsovolar, proximodistal, and radioulnar axes during outgrowth.[30]

Around the end of the fifth week of development the hand plate becomes visible. Interplay between Hox transcription factors (particularly Hoxd9-13 and Hoxa9-13) and Shh establishes digit number and identity[31–34] *(Fig. 25.4)*. Shh also induces an ulnar to radial (posterior to anterior) gradient that appears to involve Bmps in at least two roles in the formation and differentiation of digits. First, Bmps induce programmed cell death or apoptosis via discrete interdigital signaling centers, in part by repressing Fgf expression in the overlying AER.[35–37] In addition, Bmps play a role in completing digital identity via the phalanx-forming region, a region overlying the distal digital anlagen that regulates Sox9 expression and chondrogenesis.[38] Applying a Bmp-laden bead or transplanting Bmp expressing interdigital tissue from the third interdigital space to the second transforms the second digit into a third digit.[35] The phalanx-forming region also maintains digit-associated Fgf expression in the overlying AER for continued digital outgrowth.[38] However, it is still unclear how the various members of the Bmp family (Bmp2/4/5/6/7 and Gdf5/6) and their receptors (BmpR1a, BmpR1b) that are expressed in the digital and interdigital mesenchyme establish periodic thresholds that alternate between chondrogenesis and apoptosis. With regression of the phalanx-forming region and loss of overlying Fgf, the terminal phalanges form at the distal tip of each digit, invoking a unique poorly characterized mechanism that includes membranous ossification in addition to anlagen formation.[39,40]

The development/differentiation of specific tissues

Limb bud formation and the progressive morphologic changes evident externally are accompanied by differentiation of various tissues internally that are regulated by the coordinate signaling centers described above. Differentiation of these tissues is coincident, but will be discussed separately to add clarity and to relate timing of formation to tissue-specific malformations.

Limb vasculature

As the limb bud grows, nutrients and oxygen are needed to maintain rapid cell proliferation and the secretory activity of the signaling centers. Induction of a primitive vascular system in the limb begins with transformation of mesoderm into angioblasts, cells that express the basic helix-loop-helix transcription factor Tal-1 and the vascular endothelial growth factor (VEGF) receptor Flk1.[41] A dense meshwork of primitive vascular channels forms *de novo* from angioblasts in the limb mesoderm.[42,43] Angioblasts formed in nearby somites also migrate into the limb bud and contribute to the formation of new limb vessels through continued vasculogenesis.[44] As angioblasts aggregate, differentiate into endothelium, and form primitive vascular tubes, new vascular markers emerge. Flk1 persists to allow further remodeling by VEGF, Tal-1 diminishes and VE-cadherin, a cell–cell adhesion molecule, is up-regulated.

The primitive vascular network undergoes significant remodeling as the limb develops. By stage 13, the vascular channels coalesce proximally to form a central artery (subclavian) that connects to the dorsal aorta via the seventh intersegmental artery[45] and two peripheral veins form that drain into the posterior cardinal system.[43] In addition to vasculogenesis, angiogenesis, i.e., vessel sprouting from a preformed vessel, also contributes to the definitive architecture of the limb vasculature.

Construction of the vascular pattern is under the direction of the coordinate signaling centers and involves the regulation of specific VEGF family members and VEGFR3 receptors.[45–47] The final vascular pattern progresses from proximal to distal

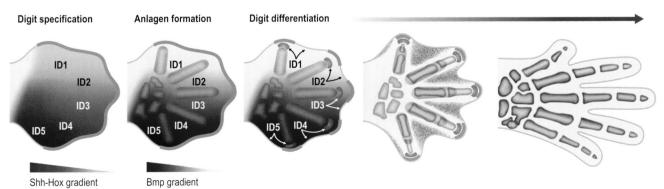

Fig. 25.4 Hand plate development. Progressive stages of hand development. ID, interdigital region. The phalanx-forming region is shown in pink capping the digital anlagen. Apical ectodermal ridge, orange; black speckling of interdigital regions, apoptosis.

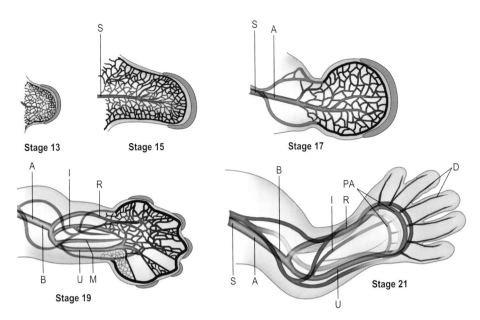

Stage 13 **Stage 15** **Stage 17**

Stage 19 **Stage 21**

Fig. 25.5 Vasculogenesis of the developing upper limb. Progressive vascular remodeling from Carnegie stage 13 through 21, showing: subclavian artery (S), axillary (A), brachial (B), median (M), radial (R), ulnar (U), interosseous (i), palmar arches (PA) and digital (D) arteries (red). Note the primitive vascular plexuses persist distally on the radial aspect at stage 19. The veins have also remodeled during this period, from a distal sinus and anterior (radial) and posterior (ulnar) marginal veins, into the distinctive veins of the limb (illustrated in blue).

(Fig. 25.5) – with formation of the axillary artery by stage 17 and the brachial and major forelimb branches by stage 19. The median artery is prominent in the forearm.[48] Distally the capillary plexus persists. Ulnar differentiation precedes radial differentiation and is evident distally by the radial artery merging with an extensive primitive capillary plexus radially, while the ulnar side of the axis is already forming the palmar arch which communicates with the ulnar associated capillary plexus.[49] The median and interosseous arteries decrease in size. The median artery degenerates, providing blood supply to the median nerve only.[48]

The vascular network must include arteries, capillaries, and veins. The diameter of each is dictated by blood flow, blood pressure, shear stress, and the accumulation of vascular smooth muscle around the vessel.[42] Formation of vascular smooth muscle around limb arteries lags behind vessel formation by about 2 days. It is unclear whether these muscle cells are derived from the endothelial cells or are condensations of the surrounding mesoderm. Furthermore, the mechanism underlying differential smooth-muscle accumulation in arteries and veins is unknown. Arteries are also differentiated from veins by the expression of Ephrin B2, a membrane-bound ligand, while the Eph-B4 receptor highlights veins. Presumptive capillaries will be negative to both Ephrin B2 and the Eph-B4 receptor.

By stage 21 the major vessel architecture is complete. The majority of vascular anomalies arise between stage 17 and 21, i.e., between days 41 and 52 or largely within the seventh and early eighth week of development. Lymphatics follow a similar course, albeit less well delineated, and are also composed of angioblasts that migrate into the limb from somitic mesoderm.[44] A defining molecular difference in lymphatic vessels is the coexpression of PROX-1 and LYVF-1.[50]

Skeletogenesis

Under the influence of the limb signaling centers, Sox9, a high-mobility group transcription factor, is up-regulated in a targeted population of limb mesoderm.[51] Sox9 transforms these cells into chondrogenic precursors and induces condensation, the first step in limb skeletogenesis.[52,53] Chondrogenesis occurs in a proximal to distal progression *(Fig. 25.6)*. The expression of Sox5 and Sox6 is required for further differentiation of chondrogenic precursors into chondrocytes to form cartilage anlagen.[54]

At precise locations within the forming skeletal anlagen, synovial joints form. Hoxa transcription factors (Hoxa9-13) exhibit expression patterns along the proximodistal axis that correlate with skeletal segmentation.[54] In addition, several molecules are known to participate in the process of joint formation, including Wnt14 and Gdf5. The first morphologic evidence of joint formation is the compact cellular condensation called the interzone that expresses Wnt14.[55] In addition, Gdf5 is induced in the proximal portion of the interzone, covering the distal end of the proximal anlagen.[56,57] The central region of the interzone begins to expand, accumulates hyaluronan, and becomes hypocellular in a process termed cavitation.[58,59] The two cellular regions of the interzone begin to differentiate into the opposing articular cartilage surfaces. Patterning signals and movement work in concert to shape the joint into its definitive morphology[57] *(Fig. 25.7)*. Mesoderm surrounding the developing joint condenses to form the joint capsule.[60]

Endochondral ossification converts the cartilage anlagen into the skeletal framework of the growing limb. This process is under precise regulation and involves Runx2, Twist1, Fgfs, Indian hedgehog (Ihh), and vascular endothelial growth factors (Vegfs).[53] Chondrocytes are induced to proliferate, undergo hypertrophy, and then die, leaving an extracellular cartilage matrix. This matrix is subsequently invaded by blood vessels, osteoclasts, and differentiating osteoblasts. Osteoblast differentiation is also under the control of Runx2 and Osterix (Osx), a bone-specific transcription factor.[61] Ossification begins within the diaphysis of anlagen at the primary ossification center during early fetal development. Subsequently, vascular invasion of the proximal epiphysis occurs, followed by the distal epiphysis forming secondary ossification centers later in development. Each metacarpal

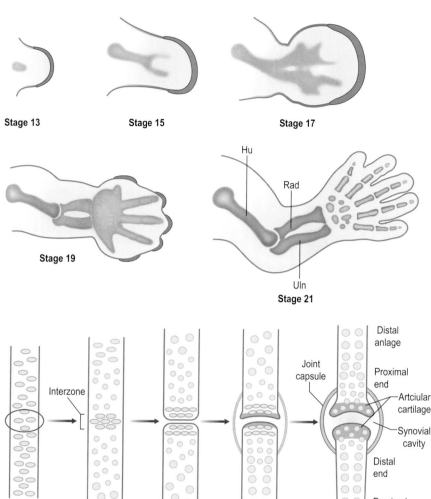

Stage 13

Stage 15

Stage 17

Stage 19

Hu

Rad

Uln

Stage 21

Fig. 25.6 Skeletogenesis of the developing upper limb. By Carnegie stage 17, there is partial rotation of the humerus (Hu, blue) at the shoulder and the elbow joint is starting to form. Radius (Rad, green); Ulna (Uln, green); Hand, magenta.

Distal anlage

Joint capsule

Proximal end

Artciular cartilage

Synovial cavity

Distal end

Proximal anlage

Interzone

Joint site determination

Interzone formation + Chondrocyte differentiation

Cavitation

Morphogenesis

Joint formation

◯ Chondrogenic precursors
○ Chondrocytes

Fig. 25.7 Joint formation. (Modified from Pacifici M, Koyama E, Iwamoto M. Mechanisms of synovial joint and articular cartilage formation: recent advances, but many lingering mysteries. Birth Defects Res C Embryo Today 2005;75:237–248.)

and digital phalanx has two ossification centers, a primary center within the diaphysis and a single secondary center that develops postnatally.

Bony malformations are most likely to involve the disruption of Sox9 and the progressive proximal to distal anlagen formation, i.e., radiohumeral synostosis would occur earlier in development than polydactyly or syndactyly.

Myogenesis

Muscular development of the upper limb is a coordinated effort between segment-specific tendon primordium, migrating myocytes, and migrating motor neurons.[62,63] There are three phases to myogenesis.[64] Embryonic myogenesis establishes the primary myotubes and the basic muscle layout. Later, a second wave of myogenesis occurs with secondary myofibers surrounding primary myofibers and contributing to the bulk of the muscle mass present at birth. Finally, satellite cells which take up residence in the basal lamina

surrounding myofibers will contribute to postnatal growth and muscle regeneration.[65]

During early limb bud formation, limb mesoderm condenses to form the proximal tendon primordium (PTP), establishing a target and an initial scaffold for migration of myocytes.[62] Myocyte precursors of the limb arise from the dorsolateral aspect of associated somites (the dermomyotome subdivision) and express the Pax3 transcription factor. Muscle precursors for the limb and body wall express c-Met, a surface receptor that is modulated by scatter factor initially emanating from the lateral plate mesoderm and then later from other sites, including the PZ. Scatter factor acts as a chemoattractant to promote myocyte precursor migration. A population of the myocyte precursors further differentiates into limb-specific precursors, demarcated by Lbx1 expression[66] *(Fig. 25.8)*.

During embryonic myogenesis, limb-specific myocytes migrate into the proximal limb bud, initially as dorsal and ventral masses *(Fig. 25.8)*. Continued migration, however, is not haphazard; rather myocyte precursors are directed into muscle anlagen by the tendon primordium, e.g., the ventral

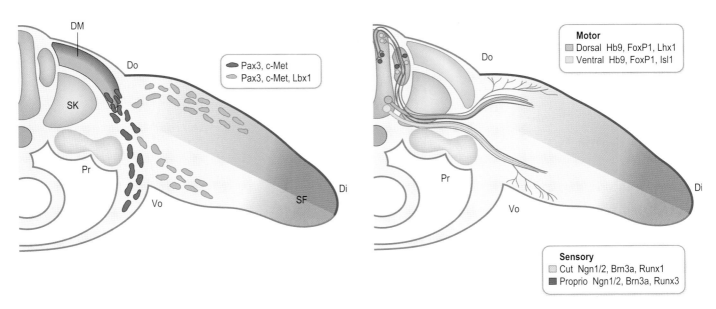

Fig. 25.8 Early neuromuscular development in the upper limb. **(A)** Dorsovolar view of presumptive myocyte migration into the limb from the lateral aspect of the dermomyotome (DM) – molecular markers listed in gray box. **(B)** Motor and sensory projection of processes into the developing limb. SK, sclerotome; SF, scatter factor; Do, dorsal; Vo, volar; Pr, proximal; Di, distal; Cut, cutaneous; Proprio, proprioception.

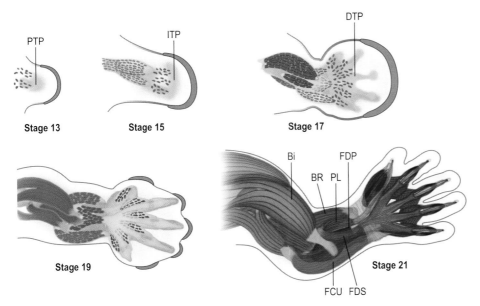

Fig. 25.9 Muscular development in the upper limb. Progressive myocyte migration and muscle formation between Carnegie stages 13 through 21 showing the ventral or volar surface. Note the resting flexed position of the upper limb in the stage 21 embryo rotates the upper arm so that the elbows shift from dorsal to caudal and the forearm rotates medially at the elbow. The palmaris longus and flexor carpi radialis are not shown. PTP, proximal tendon primordium; ITP, intermediate tendon primordium; DTP, distal tendon primordium; Bi, biceps; Tri, triceps; B, brachialis; BR, brachioradialis; PL, flexor pollicus longus; FDP, flexor digitorum profundus; FCU, flexor carpi ulnaris; FDS, flexor digitorum superficialis.

mass migrates into the biceps and brachialis under the direction of the PTP *(Fig. 25.9, Carnegie stage 15)*. With continued proliferation and differentiation, the myocytes up-regulate MyoD and Myogenin, declaring their commitment as myocytes. These myocytes will then coalesce to form fibers and begin to produce myosin filaments. Satellite cells, important for later growth and muscle regeneration, take up residence just under the basal lamina of the developing myofibers.[65] Concurrently, the tendon primordia further define the shape of specific muscles with discrete tendinous attachments. For example, expression of Lmx1b within the dorsal tendons directs the unique pattern of extensor attachments[67] and it is likely that each upper limb muscle is shaped by a unique combination of patterning factors.[68]

As in other aspects of upper limb development, there is progressive differentiation from proximal to distal. Thus, as the muscles of the upper arm take shape, migrating myocytes invade the forearm to associate with the PTP and a new mesodermal condensation forming at the presumptive wrist, the intermediate tendon primordium. In the forearm, the superficial muscles differentiate before the deep muscles. By Carnegie stage 17, the distal tendon primordia form and associate with migrating myocytes destined to be muscles of the hand *(Fig. 25.9)*. The intrinsic muscles arise from five embryonic muscle layers, which differentiate and fuse in a complex but logical manner.[69,70] Following embryonic myogenesis, a second wave of myocyte precursors migrate into the limb and coalesce around primary myofibers, forming secondary

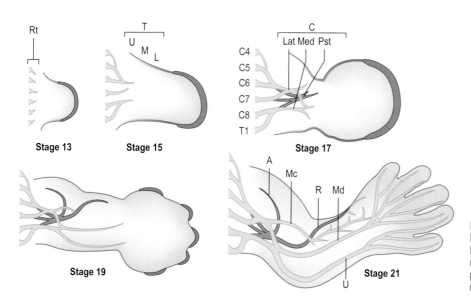

Fig. 25.10 Nervous development in the upper limb. Progressive innervation of the upper limb and formation of the brachial plexus. Rt, nerve roots; T, trunks; U, upper; M, middle; L, lower; C, cords; Lat, lateral; Med, medial; Pst, posterior; A, axillary; Mc, musculocutaneous; R, radial; Md, median; U, ulnar.

myofibers and adding bulk to the muscle masses as the fetus grows. It is during this secondary or fetal myogenesis that formation of motor endplates occurs and neuromuscular communication begins, further differentiating the forming muscle with slow and fast fiber types.[71,72]

Innervation

Outgrowth of nerves into the limb bud lags behind muscle migration *(Fig. 25.10)* and involves both motor and sensory neurons.[73] Motor neurons are specified early during spinal cord development by exposure to Shh, initially from the notochord and later from the floor plate of the developing neural tube.[74,75] Motor neurons begin to express a combination of transcription factors (e.g., Hb9/Mnx1, Lhx3/4) that promote motor neuron migration into discrete columns within the spinal cord and direct their axons to specific muscle groups.[63] Within the limb fields (specified by Hox6 in the forelimb and Hox10 in the hindlimb), a Hox accessory factor, FoxP1, is expressed that assists in deciphering the subsequent Hox-specific code within the limb for appropriate axon targeting.[76] As the axons of the motor neurons enter the limb, those expressing Lim1 (Lhx1) will project into the dorsal Lmx1b-expressing compartment of the limb to target dorsal extensor muscle groups. The remaining axons express Isl1 and will enter the ventral compartment to target flexor muscles of the limb.

Sensory processes accompany the axons of motor neurons into the limb. The cell bodies of sensory neurons reside within the dorsal root ganglion (DRG) which is derived from neural crest cells. Specification of sensory neurons within the DRG is characterized by up-regulation of neurogenin1 and 2 (Ngn1/2) and brain-specific homeobox/POU domain protein 3A (Brn3a). Furthermore, cuntaneous sensory neurons also express a runt homeodomain transcription factor 1 (Runx1), while neurons involved in proprioception express Runx2.

The nerve roots, containing motor and sensory processes from C4 to T1, coalesce to form a meshwork or plexus which eventually leads to the formation of three major trunks in the upper limb – upper, middle, and lower *(Fig. 25.10, Carnegie stage 15)*. The segregation of dorsal and ventral processes as the nerves project into the limb divides the plexus into dorsal (posterior) and ventral (anterior) divisions which form the posterior, lateral, and medial cords, whose names relate to their anatomic positions in the adult. The posterior cord gives rise to the axillary and radial nerves. The lateral cord gives rise to the musculocutaneous nerve and contributes to the median nerve. The medial cord forms the ulnar nerve and combines with processes from the lateral cord to form the median nerve.

The initial trajectory of processes is independent of neuromuscular communication and instead depends on a combinatorial expression of transcription factors that guide processes to targets expressing specific patterning factors within the limb.[73] However, during secondary or fetal myogenesis, patterning factors, motor endplate formation, and neuromuscular communication are required for fiber-type differentiation and survival of both muscles and nerves.[63,68,71]

Anomalies of limb development and their classification

Background

Congenital anomalies in the hand and upper limb demand a reproducible and consistent terminology, a universal language which allows discussion of complex clinical entities, indications for treatment, and comparisons of results. The terminology of dysmorphology offers a basis for understanding the etiology of congenital limb anomalies.[77] A malformation is an abnormal formation of tissue resulting from abnormal cell formation. Deformation differs from a malformation as the insult is to cells which have already formed normally. It is a deformation of normal tissue. Dysplasia is a lack of normal organization of cells into tissue. Dysmorphologists describe a fourth term, disruption. As this process involves alteration of tissue which is already formed, for the purposes of classification it is reasonable to include those conditions which are considered to be disruptions alongside those considered to be deformations. Although the pathogenesis of some specific anomalies remains obscure, the concept of separating malformations, deformations, and dysplasias provides a sound structure for categorizing congenital upper limb anomalies.

Ideally, a classification of congenital hand anomalies would be based on etiology, with such a classification indicating the site in the molecular pathway and/or the anatomical site in the limb bud at which the aberration occurs, and one which also is indicative of the timing of the causative disruption.

The first classification was probably that of Isidore St. Hilaire in 1832.[78] This introduced terms such as "phocomele" (seal limb), "hemimele" (part of the limb missing), and "ectromele" (limb absence). Frantz and O'Rahilly based their classification on skeletal appearance.[79] They introduced the concepts of terminal and intercalary defects, subsequently adding the subcategories of transverse and longitudinal deficiencies and including the involvement of pre- or postaxial position within the limb.[79] Kelikian has summarized the contributions of many authors in his classic text, *Congenital Deformities of the Hand and Forearm*, but acknowledged that "We have not as yet attained enough latitude of knowing about congenital hand anomalies to formulate a comprehensive classification."[80]

The currently accepted surgical classification of upper limb anomalies is that based on the proposals of Swanson *et al.* in 1968.[81] This was refined by Swanson and colleagues in 1976[1] and 1983,[82] was accepted by the IFSSH and expanded by Knight and Kay in 2000[2] and Upton in 2006[83] to encompass all anomalies. Recently an increasing number of surgeons, pathologists, and geneticists working in the field of congenital limb anomalies have questioned the adequacy of this classification and have suggested alternative approaches.[84–87]

Problems of the Swanson/IFSSH classification

The IFSSH classification is derived from an understanding of normal embryological development that was available in the 1960s and 1970s. The system is based upon clinical and radiological assessments which describe failures in certain anatomical structures. The two major groups of this classification do offer an indication of the timing of the causative insult by separating "failure of formation" from "failure of differentiation." However, formation and differentiation occur together, and it may be impossible to determine whether any specific anomaly is one or the other. Furthermore, the need to create separate groups for "duplication," "undergrowth," and "overgrowth" is illustrative of the inherent limitations of using these descriptive terms as components of a classification system, as these anomalies could also be considered as failures of formation and/or differentiation.

A system based on appearance is unable to incorporate changes based on our increasing understanding of etiology and causation at a molecular level. Attempts to do so create contradictions which are difficult to resolve. A consideration of central clefting and symbrachydactyly is illustrative. The IFSSH classification places central clefting of the hand within the "failure of formation" group as a "central longitudinal deficiency." However, many would not view this condition as a longitudinal deficiency in the manner of radial and ulnar longitudinal deficiencies for the following reasons: the limb anomalies are usually confined to hands and feet; the terminology erroneously suggests the presence of a central axis within the developing limb; the elegant experimental work and clinical observations of Miura,[88] Ogino,[89] and others have drawn attention to the association of clefting with syndactyly and polydactyly *(Fig. 25.11)*. Consequently, the Japanese

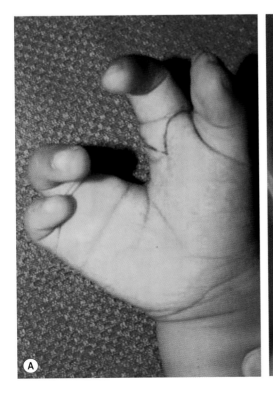
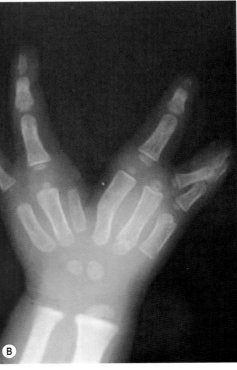

Fig. 25.11 (A, B) Clinical and radiological appearance of the association of clefting, syndactyly, and polydactyly.

Society for Surgery of the Hand (JSSH) has introduced an extra group within the IFSSH classification, this being an "abnormal induction of rays."[90] Although the introduction of this new group is attractive and well based, such modifications of the IFSSH classification introduce significant contradictions.

In this new subclassification of the JSSH, central polydactyly becomes an "abnormal induction of rays." However, radial and ulnar polydactyly remain under the group "duplication." Morphologically, the process of duplication, be it central, radial, or ulnar, appears to be similar *(Fig. 25.12)*. All could be considered as an "abnormal induction of rays."

Syndactyly, be it simple or complex with phalangeal synostosis, is moved from "failure of differentiation" to "abnormal induction" *(Fig. 25.13)*. Yet under the system proposed by the JSSH, symbrachydactyly, which has a component of syndactyly, becomes a "transverse failure of formation." Brachydactyly, which may include symbrachydactyly as a subcategory, remains within group 5, "undergrowth." Carpal synostoses and symphalangism remain within "failure of differentiation," although they both occur commonly in symbrachydactyly. All could be considered as an "abnormal induction of rays." Indeed, a longitudinal radial deficiency in the forearm could be considered as an abnormal induction of forearm radial structures. Whether any particular condition is a failure of formation, a failure of differentiation, or an abnormal induction may well be a dated and unhelpful concept, the differences being those of semantics.

In the search for evidence to support the suggestion that syndactyly, central polydactyly, and clefting should be classified within a single and new group, it is helpful to review those conditions with these characteristics which have a

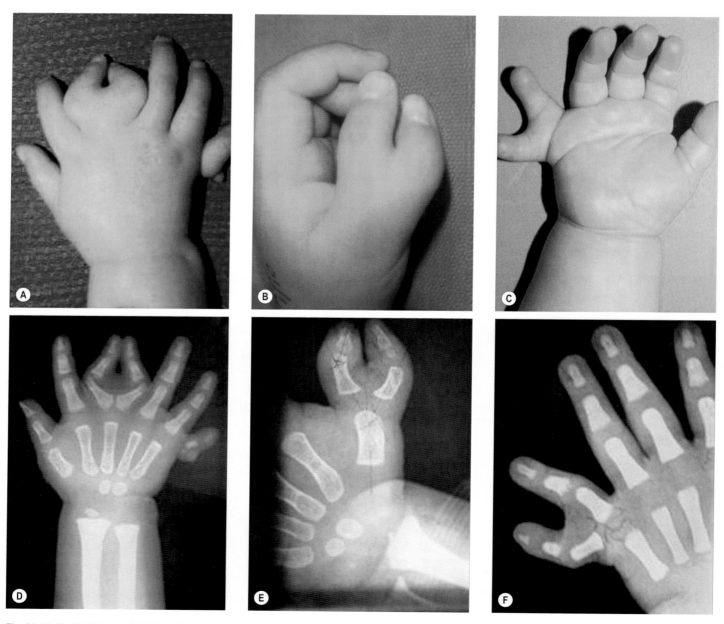

Fig. 25.12 (A–C) Clinical and **(D–F)** radiological appearance of central, radial, and ulnar polydactyly at the proximal phalangeal level.

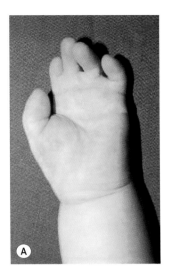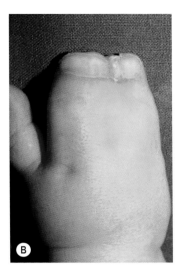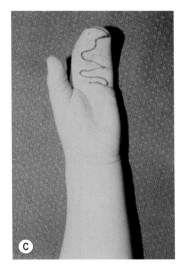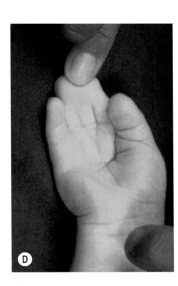

Fig. 25.13 Syndactyly in association with **(A)** symbrachydactyly short finger type; **(B)** mitten hand; **(C)** ulnar longitudinal deficiency; **(D)** Greig cephalopolysyndactyly syndrome.

known genetic basis. Synpolydactyly (syndactyly type II) is caused by an identified gene – HoxD13 – mapped to a known chromosomal locus – 2q31-32.[91] Clefting has not been described as an association of this genetic abnormality. Central longitudinal deficiency (clefting or split-hand/foot malformation) is also inherited in an autosomal-dominant manner. Its locus is known and differs from that of the synpolydactyly gene mutation. Type I syndactyly, in which there is nonseparation of digits 3 and 4 in the hands, often accompanied by nonseparation of digits 2 and 3 in the feet, also involves an abnormal gene, not yet identified, but which has been mapped to yet another locus.[92] From this, it becomes apparent that a particular phenotype may result from abnormalities in several genes at different chromosomal loci in one or many of the complex pathways involved in normal hand development, rather than from one constant gene abnormality. There may also be variations in phenotypic expression of single-gene mutations. It would appear that complex interactions involving formation of extra digits and joining of those digits are associated with cleft formation.[93] However, it is less certain that an inexorable teratogenic sequence obligatorily links isolated cases of polydactyly and syndactyly with clefting.[94]

The separation of symbrachydactyly from brachydactyly, noted above, also imposes apparent contradictions. The JSSH considers symbrachydactyly to be synonymous with "transverse failure of formation" and therefore suggests that symbrachydactyly be moved from group 5, "undergrowth," to group 1 of the IFSSH classification.[90,95] This necessitates combining transverse deficiencies, in which terminal ectodermal elements are absent, with symbrachydactyly, in which the initial deficiency is middle phalangeal and, even in severe cases, terminal elements – nail and terminal phalangeal remnants – remain *(Fig. 25.14)*. The Japanese allow for this by adding a "peripheral hypoplasia type" to the five types of the symbrachydactyly subclassification, so that all transverse deficiencies are included as a form of symbrachydactyly. Others consider this to be contradictory, believing symbrachydactyly to be a distinct entity, and to have a clear definition of intersegmental failure, which does not encompass terminal transverse deficiencies.[96] Regardless, the term "undergrowth"

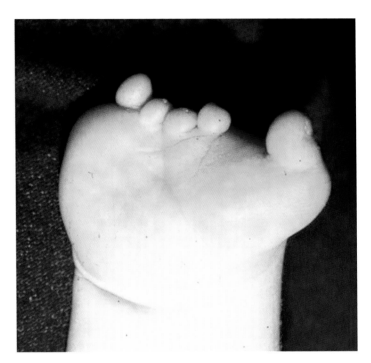

Fig. 25.14 Symbrachydactyly monodactylous type with terminal ectodermal elements.

represents an appearance only and is unable to embrace the above concepts.

The groups documented as "duplication," "overgrowth," and "constriction ring syndrome" suffer from similar limitations. It is becoming clear that increasing problems with the current classification demand an alternative approach.

A modified classification

All anomalies are placed within one of three groups defined at the beginning of this section: group 1, malformations; group 2, deformations; and group 3, dysplasias *(Table 25.2)*.

Table 25.2 Modified classification of congenital anomalies of the hand and upper limb

I. Malformations

A. Failure in axis formation and differentiation – entire upper limb
1. Proximal–distal outgrowth
   Symbrachydactyly
   Transverse deficiency
   Intersegmental deficiency
2. Radial–ulnar (anterior–posterior) axis
   Radial longitudinal deficiency
   Ulnar longitudinal deficiency
   Ulnar dimelia
   Radioulnar synostosis
   Humeroradial synostosis
3. Dorsal–ventral axis
   Nail–patella syndrome

B. Failure in axis formation and differentiation – hand plate
1. Radial–ulnar (anterior–posterior) axis
   Radial polydactyly
   Triphalangeal thumb
   Ulnar polydactyly
2. Dorsal–ventral axis
   Dorsal dimelia (palmar nail)
   Hypoplastic/aplastic nail

C. Failure in hand plate formation and differentiation – unspecified axis
1. Soft tissue
   Syndactyly
   Camptodactyly
   Trigger digits
2. Skeletal deficiency
   Brachydactyly
   Clinodactyly
   Kirner's deformity
   Metacarpal and carpal synostoses
3. Complex
   Cleft hand
   Synpolydactyly
   Apert hand

II. Deformations

1. Constriction ring syndrome

III. Dysplasias

1. Macrodactyly
2. Limb hypertrophy
3. Tumorous conditions

The anomalies which are documented under groups 1, 2, 3, and 5 in the IFSSH scheme become malformations (group 1). This classification scheme does not attempt to separate an abnormal formation from an abnormal differentiation. Malformations are subdivided according to whether the insult affects the upper limb as a whole or the hand plate alone, and whether it primarily involves one of the three axes of growth and patterning described in the preceding section of this chapter. This approach incorporates an understanding of the mechanism of insult and the site within the developing limb which is primarily affected, as suggested by Manske, Oberg,

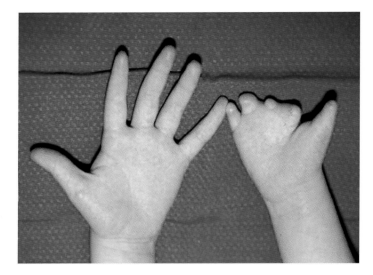

Fig. 25.15 Symbrachydactyly with short arm, hand, and fingers.

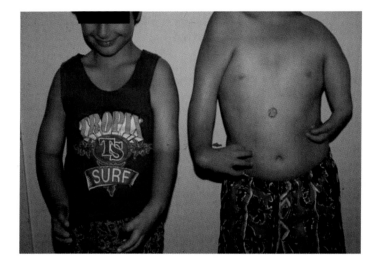

Fig. 25.16 Radial longitudinal deficiency affecting arm, forearm, hand, and digits of both limbs in brothers with Holt–Oram syndrome.

and others.[86,87] Symbrachydactyly, for instance, is an example of abnormal tissue formation and differentiation within the proximal–distal axis, as are the other transverse failures of formation *(Fig. 25.15)*. Radial longitudinal deficiency involves primarily the radial–ulnar axis *(Fig. 25.16)* and loss of dorsalization of hand and upper limb structures in nail–patella syndrome involves the dorsal–ventral axis. In all of these anomalies the whole of the upper limb may be involved, e.g., thumb hypoplasia with radial aplasia. Duplications which affect the whole of the upper limb, such as ulnar dimelia, are malformations with abnormal axial patterning within the radial–ulnar axis. All of these are classified within group 1A and according to the axis involved.

Alternatively, the primary defect may reside within the hand plate alone, and not involve proximal limb components but still affect one of the axes of development. This approach allows incorporation of IFSSH group 3 "duplications," radial and ulnar polydactyly, into a group which indicates intuitively the anatomical site and the axis in which the aberration occurs *(Fig. 25.17)*. The triphalangeal thumb may best be included in this group. Dorsal dimelia of the little finger is an example of hand plate involvement involving the dorsal–ventral axis *(Fig. 25.18)*. All of these conditions are classified within group 1B.

Other anomalies involve a primary defect within the developing hand plate, but one which does not primarily target one of the axes of patterning. These are classified within group 1C. The cleft-hand complex, isolated syndactyly, and central synpolydactyly are examples. This satisfies the concern that cleft-hand complex is not a longitudinal deficiency but rather a primary insult to the hand plate *(Figs 25.11 and 25.19)*.

Group 2 in *Table 25.2* allows the classification of amniotic band sequence (constriction ring syndrome) as a deformation, separating it from the malformations of group 1. The insult affects a part already formed *(Fig. 25.20)*.

Group 3, dysplasias, includes many otherwise difficult-to-classify conditions which have previously been listed according to their appearance. Limb hypertrophy and macrodactyly which is consequent upon tumour formation are examples *(Fig. 25.21)*, as are the other tumorous conditions. All of these were previously classified either as a "failure of differentiation" (tumorous conditions) or purely as a descriptive term – "overgrowth" for macrodactyly or limb hypertrophy. There may be dissent as to whether these conditions are in fact malformations or deformations. Indeed, increasing knowledge may demand their future transfer to either group 1 or group 2. This classification allows such adjustments.

This classification has the advantages of allowing inclusion of all groups within a logical framework; of utilizing a common terminology; and of indicating a site of anatomical insult in the developing or developed limb bud. The common descriptive terms, used in the IFSSH classification and which are familiar to all surgeons, are then placed within this framework. Each common descriptive diagnosis, such as radial longitudinal deficiency, retains its surgical subclassification, i.e., groups 0–4 for radial aplasia and Blauth groups 1–5 for thumb hypoplasia. These surgical subclassifications are discussed in subsequent chapters devoted to specific anomalies.

Although aberrations in some molecular pathways have been identified as causative of specific anomalies, it is not yet possible to develop a classification which relates cause and effect at the molecular level for all limb anomalies. Furthermore, the complex interaction between the various signaling centers and the cascades of molecular pathways which they control must be appreciated. Hence, any disruption of one signaling center or pathway will have consequences within other signaling centers and pathways, both upstream and downstream. However, many, but not all, of the current contradictions and flaws find solutions in this method of classification, which also allows adaptation based on evolving knowledge. Of importance is the necessity to utilize a system which allows recording of all anomalies present in any particular child. It is not a contradiction to document more than one diagnosis per child.

Assessment of the child and family

There are great rewards in treating children who are unfortunate enough to be born with hands we recognize as less than perfectly formed. Adaptive ability in the child is quite extraordinary, such that some question the wisdom of surgical interference for many presentations. Furthermore, initially, the hand is normal to the child. It is a growing awareness of the

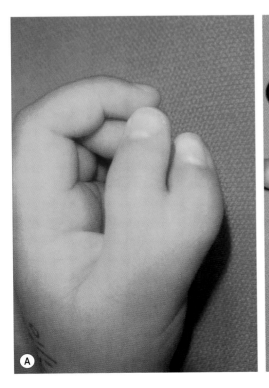
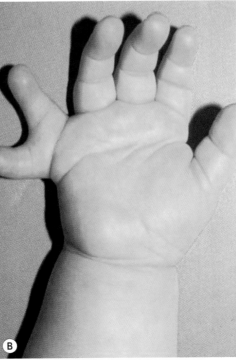

Fig. 25.17 (A, B) Radial and ulnar duplications demonstrate involvement of radial and ulnar axial abnormalities within the hand.

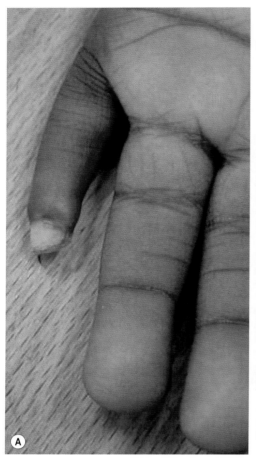

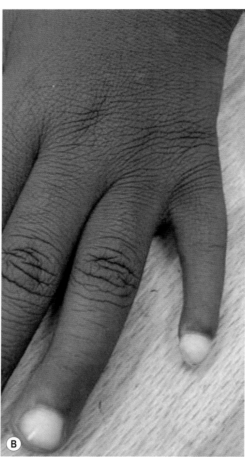

Fig. 25.18 Dorsal dimelia of the little finger.

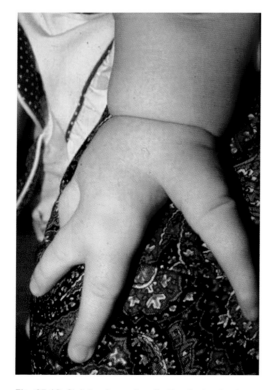

Fig. 25.19 Cleft-hand complex affecting the hand only.

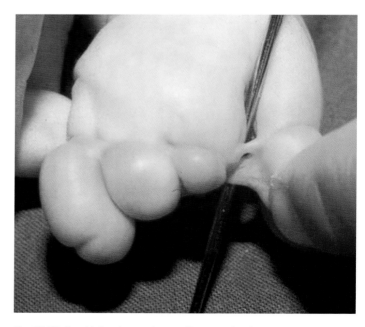

Fig. 25.20 Constriction ring syndrome with acrosyndactyly.

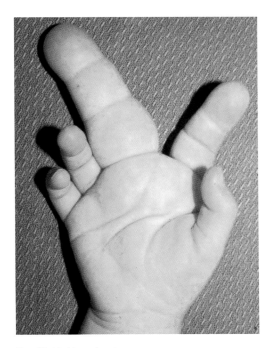

Fig. 25.21 Macrodactyly.

Table 25.3 Development of hand control

Hand control	When achieved (months)
Grasp small objects by ulnar–palm prehension	4
Grasp by partial thumb opposition	5
Transfer objects between hands	6
Grasp by full thumb opposition	7
Bang an object on a flat surface	7
Drink from cup held in hand with assistance	9–10
Pincer grasp	12
Scribble with crayon	13–15
Throw ball	18
Build a tower with 4–6 blocks	24

(Reproduced from: Gupta A, Kay SPJ, Scheker LR, editors. The growing hand: diagnosis and management of the upper extremity in children. London: CV Mosby; 2000, p. 51.)

"normal" environment which alters the child's perception. However, it is the observation of many that the child reflects the attitudes of others. If parents, relatives, friends, doctors, or therapists consider the problem to be overwhelming, the child will be more likely to have a problem.

For the surgeon, the opportunity to observe the development of the child and hand function during growth and learning provides a satisfaction which cannot be underestimated. Decision-making must be precise and involve parents and child such that all develop a confidence that the treatment is both appropriate and in capable hands. Few surgical fields allow greater application of surgical principles to the management of deformity and loss of function. The aim is to achieve optimal hand function – prehensile grasp and dexterity of fingers and thumb for fine activity – whilst also striving for optimal appearance.

The involvement of family doctor and pediatrician, therapist, and psychologist in the overall management of child and family is necessary. The geneticist can assist in identifying inheritance factors and advise regarding risk of recurrence for subsequent children. Specialist medical care is often required, as involvement of systems other than the musculoskeletal system is common. Specifically, cardiac, hematological, neurological, gastroenterological, and urological systems must be investigated for abnormalities. Many syndromic patterns have been described and alert the surgeon and treating physicians to probable associations. Finally, support groups can be of significant benefit. Often parents and children find great solace and encouragement from discussing their problems with others with similar afflictions.

The clinic

A calm, private, and warm environment is conducive to optimal assessment. Parents, often young, may be overwhelmed by the medical and paramedical attention that has been directed towards them and their child. At the initial introduction, the child and parents should not be confronted by too many foreign faces, perhaps the surgeon and one other only. Minimally, the surgical congenital hand clinic should also have immediate access to experienced occupational therapists and physiotherapists. In developed societies, an assessment of all other systems has been completed or is in progress before consultation with the hand surgeon. However, it is vital that the treating surgeon has sufficient understanding of the processes of normal and abnormal limb development and is sensitive to the association of other system anomalies with specific hand and upper limb anomalies. The parents expect and should receive information from the surgeon regarding the cause and mechanism of dysmorphogenesis; the likelihood of recurrence in subsequent children, and the likelihood of recurrence in future children of the presenting child; a description of the dysfunction the child is likely to confront in the future; and the possible methods and timing of procedures aimed at improving function and appearance. Photographs and models of pre- and postoperative example cases are beneficial in demonstrating expected outcomes. They also provide reassurance that surgery is not disfiguring.

History

Following introductions, a preliminary examination through observation alerts the surgeon to possible diagnoses and associations. A detailed history of the pregnancy, its duration and any untoward events, the lie of the child *in utero* and the method of delivery and birth weight provide valuable information. The presence of a positive family history of limb anomalies in siblings, parents, and the relatives of parents is suggestive of an inherited disorder. The surgeon should always question as to whether there are anomalies in other systems and whether a general pediatric review has been performed. The need for further specific system review may become apparent during the assessment.

Examination

Observation of the child at play provides much information, which may be withheld if the surgeon approaches a direct physical examination of the child either too early in the assessment process or too brusquely.

An understanding of developmental milestones is integral to recognition of delayed or abnormal functional development *(Table 25.3)*.[97] The child's upper limb movements are mainly reflexive at birth. There is a rudimentary grip via digit flexion. The thumb is clasped within the palm but exhibits reflex extension when startled.[98,99]

The development of prehension is well summarized by the work of Erhardt and Lindley.[100] These patterns are depicted in *Figure 25.22*. They demonstrate the development from

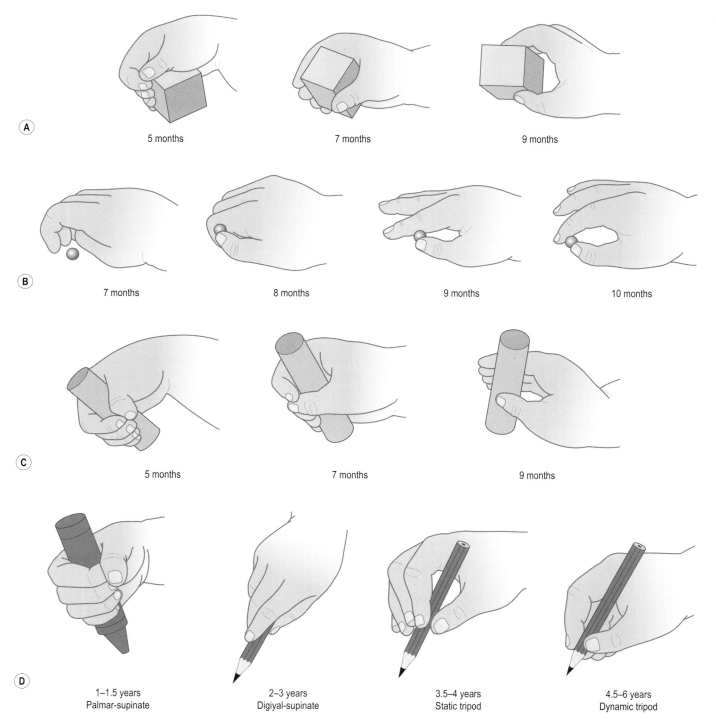

A 5 months   7 months   9 months

B 7 months   8 months   9 months   10 months

C 5 months   7 months   9 months

D 1–1.5 years
Palmar-supinate

2–3 years
Digiyal-supinate

3.5–4 years
Static tripod

4.5–6 years
Dynamic tripod

Fig. 25.22 (A–D) The development from rudimentary grasp, utilizing an ulnar power grip to precision function radially incorporating the thumb. (Redrawn after Erhardt RP. Developmental hand dysfunction: theory, assessment, and treatment, 2nd edn. San Antonio: Therapy Skill Builders, 1994.)

rudimentary grasp utilizing an ulnar power grip, to precision function radially incorporating the thumb. *Figure 25.23* demonstrates the change in weight-bearing through the upper limbs over the first 5 months of life.

Determination of hand dominance is usually not possible in the first year or so but becomes apparent by age 5.[101–103]

A general examination includes observation of the facial appearance with specific attention to eyes, ears, mouth, and jaw, examination of the spine and lower limbs, observation and palpation of the chest wall and abdomen where appropriate, and examination of all four limbs.

It often allays the child's distrust for the surgeon to take the mother's hand, gently examine this and return it to its owner, before attempting the same with the child. The experienced examiner will note any deformity and size discrepancy, diminished passive and active ranges of motion in any particular joint, often in association with poorly developed or absent skin creases, and joint instability. Some changes are subtle. A close examination of a child with second-web syndactyly in the feet may reveal subtle webbing of the third webs in the hands. This may also be present in the hands of the parent(s). Obvious thumb hypoplasia in one hand may be accompanied by subtle changes in the other.

All findings must be precisely recorded. Tracings, measurements of girth, and clinical photographs provide objective data for comparison at subsequent assessments.

Investigations

The mainstay of investigation is radiological. Plain X-rays should be requested for the specific anomaly with which the child presents but should be extended to a broader skeletal survey as indicated. Of course, the immature skeleton will not reveal the complete picture. For instance, the Wassell classification of thumb duplication relies on relative skeletal maturity to distinguish a type 1 from a type 2. The bony connection present in the former may not be apparent at the base of the terminal phalanges in initial X-rays until ossification of a cartilaginous connection has occurred. In most instances, X-rays should be repeated immediately prior to surgical intervention as the skeletal appearance may have changed. It is helpful to have available in the clinic sample hand X-rays and charts which detail the timing of appearance of ossification centers and closure of growth plates *(Fig. 25.24)*.[104,105] The method of Greulich and Pyle[106] and that of Tanner *et al.*[107] are

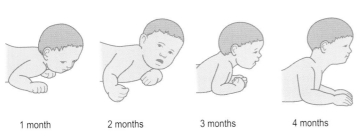
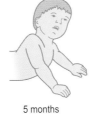

| 1 month | 2 months | 3 months | 4 months | 5 months |

Fig. 25.23 Change in weight-bearing through the upper limbs through the first 5 months of life. (Redrawn after Erhardt RP. Developmental hand dysfunction: theory, assessment, and treatment, 2nd edn. San Antonio: Therapy Skill Builders, 1994.)

Ossification centres

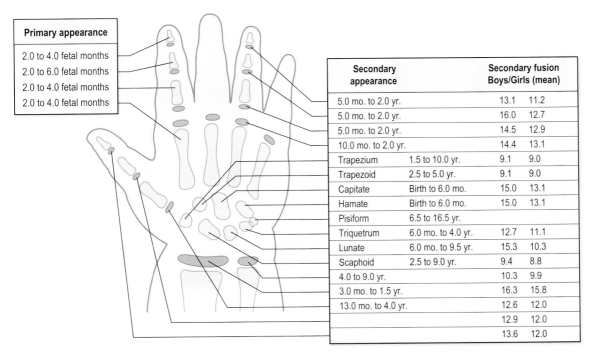

Primary appearance
2.0 to 4.0 fetal months
2.0 to 6.0 fetal months
2.0 to 4.0 fetal months
2.0 to 4.0 fetal months

Secondary appearance		Secondary fusion Boys/Girls (mean)	
5.0 mo. to 2.0 yr.		13.1	11.2
5.0 mo. to 2.0 yr.		16.0	12.7
5.0 mo. to 2.0 yr.		14.5	12.9
10.0 mo. to 2.0 yr.		14.4	13.1
Trapezium	1.5 to 10.0 yr.	9.1	9.0
Trapezoid	2.5 to 5.0 yr.	9.1	9.0
Capitate	Birth to 6.0 mo.	15.0	13.1
Hamate	Birth to 6.0 mo.	15.0	13.1
Pisiform	6.5 to 16.5 yr.		
Triquetrum	6.0 mo. to 4.0 yr.	12.7	11.1
Lunate	6.0 mo. to 9.5 yr.	15.3	10.3
Scaphoid	2.5 to 9.0 yr.	9.4	8.8
4.0 to 9.0 yr.		10.3	9.9
3.0 mo. to 1.5 yr.		16.3	15.8
13.0 mo. to 4.0 yr.		12.6	12.0
		12.9	12.0
		13.6	12.0

Fig. 25.24 Timing of appearance of ossification centers and closure of growth plates. (Reproduced from Upton J. Classification of upper limb congenital differences and general principles management. In: Mathes SJ (ed.) Plastic Surgery, 2nd edn, vol. 8. Philadelphia: Elsevier, 2006, p. 27.)

the most commonly used for measurement of skeletal maturation. In the former, the patient's radiograph is matched with an atlas image of the appropriate age.[106] One must be careful to differentiate actual age and maturity. The Tanner and Whitehouse method is more complex and is based on the rate of development of 19 individual bones.[107] Both methods suffer from the problem of variation between races. Progress is delayed in European children in comparison with those from Africa and North America.[108] Poor nutrition results in slower maturation. Maturation in girls is more rapid than in boys by 2 years.

Fluoroscopy, tomography, and arthrography may all have a limited place in the assessment of the pediatric hand, often more for injury than for congenital anomaly. Computed tomography and magnetic resonance imaging have replaced many of these modalities but do require sedation or general anesthesia for the child. Ultrasonography has many characteristics that make it an ideal imaging modality in that there is no ionizing radiation, and it is painless and inexpensive. However, it is operator-dependent and differentiation between tissues can be problematic. It is helpful in assessing cartilaginous contours prior to ossification.

Vascular studies, such as angiography, magnetic resonance angiography (MRA), or Doppler flow studies, may be considered prior to procedures involving vascularized tissue transfer, including toe transfers, particularly to parts with anomalous anatomical development. In particular, angiography and MRA, although uncommonly performed, may be indicated in some specific vascular reconstructions and for assessment of vascular tumors.

It is beyond the scope of this chapter to detail a complete investigation of all systems of the child with congenital limb anomalies. The incidence of associated anomalies is high. For instance, thrombocytopenic absent radius, Fanconi's anemia, Holt–Oram syndrome and the VACTERLS association may accompany a longitudinal radial deficiency. A cardiac echogram, renal ultrasound, and blood examinations are routine.

Diagnosis

Following the assessment and investigations, a classifiable diagnosis is usually evident. The surgeon, with assistance from medical colleagues, will have determined whether the anomaly is isolated or syndromic; whether a genetic abnormality is present through either a spontaneous mutation or an inheritance pattern; and whether there has been an abnormal formation of tissue, a breakdown of normal tissue, or a lack of organization of cells into normal tissue.

Principles of surgical management

Indications

When considering surgery the following question must always be asked: "Is reconstructive surgery likely to improve function and/or appearance with minimum risk?" That a part is incomplete or inadequate is not in itself an indication for surgical reconstruction.

Function

A stable shoulder, arm, elbow, and forearm enable appropriate positioning of the hand in space for function. The instability, deformity, and shortening of radial longitudinal deficiencies, for instance, severely compromise hand function. Hand function itself depends on the ability to use a mobile thumb ray against other parts of the hand, ulnar digits for grasp and radial digits for precision pinch. Adequate digit length, stability, and motion are necessary components of optimal hand use. Surgical decisions may be best guided by a simple assessment, asking whether the size and number of digits are appropriate, whether deformity requires correction, whether stability is a problem, and whether an improvement in mobility would benefit.

Some decisions regarding surgery are relatively easy. Most parents and children will request that an extra digit be removed, particularly if it gets in the way (*Fig. 25.25*). Occasionally social and/or religious mores will dictate otherwise. Removal of a type 3 hypoplastic thumb, with subsequent pollicization of the index finger, may prove to be less palatable for parents, as they fear a decision which results in four rather than five digits. As a principle, when confronted with the option of reconstruction or removal of a part, it is perhaps wiser to advise reconstruction if the part is incorporated into the child's activities, even if in an inefficient manner. The child and surgeon may benefit from the opinions of others who are experienced in this field of surgery. Advice from a knowledgeable colleague is particularly reassuring.

It is often not possible to restore normal function, even for what would appear to be a straightforward reconstruction of a Wassel type 1 thumb duplication, in which some joint instability and some compromise in interphalangeal joint motion may remain postoperatively. For complex duplications, full function and normal size are difficult to achieve, and pollicization never creates a normal thumb. Trigger thumb release should result in normal use and appearance. Clinodactyly of the little finger may represent no functional deficit preoperatively. Surgical interference should be carefully considered. Surgery for camptodactyly may improve extension at the expense of full flexion.

Appearance

The stigmata associated with an abnormal appearance are obvious. The hands are expressive and communicative. Deformity of a part is often more obvious than its absence and its correction may clearly result in an improved appearance for all eyes (*Fig. 25.26*). However, for many severe deformities it is simply not possible to create a normal-looking hand. Surgery to improve appearance in these cases must be undertaken realistically. Whether the appearance is improved, remains the same, or is poorer following surgery is simply in the eye of the beholder. Toe transfer for symbrachydactyly is one procedure which excites argument, with some adamant that appearance is improved and some adamant that it is not and that appearance should not play a role in decision-making. Probably the argument is irrelevant. The hand remains different regardless of the surgical reconstruction and

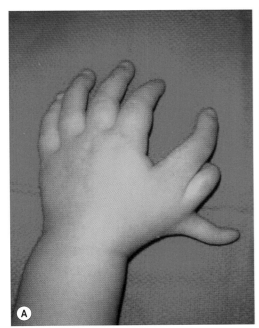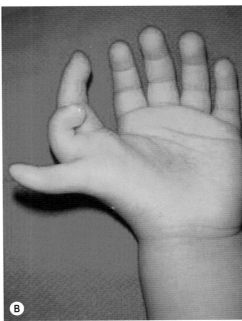

Fig. 25.25 The obvious deformity of thumb triplication.

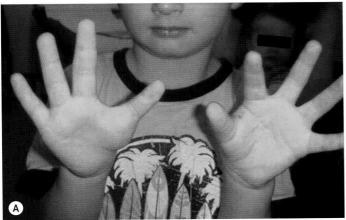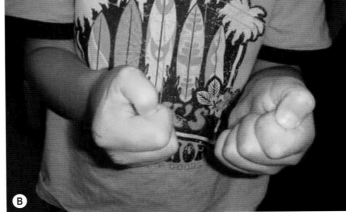

Fig. 25.26 (A, B) Pleasing appearance and function following pollicization.

the surgeon should not impose his or her views regarding appearance. Postoperative questionnaires in which patients and parents state their belief in an improved appearance are often flawed, as many psychological factors are involved, including that of guilt in having given birth to a "less than normal" child and the responsibility of having made a decision to subject that child to surgical intervention.

It is the responsibility of the surgeon to provide advice based on training, experience, and a knowledge of the literature. However, should that advice be rejected, the doctor–patient/parent relationship must not become adversarial. Repeated assessments over a period of time will usually lead to an agreeable solution.

Timing

The question of timing is vexatious. Surgical results may be compromised by the technical difficulties of procedures on small structures in early life. This must be balanced against the principle of providing the child with a final result as early as possible, such that learned patterns of use do not compromise optimal function following appropriate surgical reconstructions. It is a reasonable approach to allow the child to adapt to the new hand as early as possible. However, cortical plasticity allows significant adaptation at older ages and, if the surgeon is doubtful that the surgery is indicated or the parents demand delay, it is preferable to wait. If functional

Table 25.4 **Common practice relating to timing of specific surgical procedures**

Condition	Procedure	Timing
Syndactyly	Release	12 months
– Simple	Release	6 months
– Unequal digits with bony tether	Release	6 months
– Including thumb	Sequential simultaneous bilateral releases	Begin at 6 months
– Apert's acrosyndactyly		
Constriction ring syndrome	Release	Immediate
– Digit at risk	Release	6 months
– Acrosyndactyly		
Floating digit(s)	Excision	3 months
Thumb duplication	Reconstruction	12 months
Postaxial or central polydactyly	Reconstruction	12 months
Absent or inadequate thumb	Pollicization	12–18 months
Thumb hypoplasia	Reconstruction	12–18 months
Central longitudinal deficiency	Reconstruction	12–18 months
Symbrachydactyly	Toe phalangeal transfer	12–24 months
	Vascularized toe transfer	2–3 years
Radial longitudinal deficiency	Distraction	3–6 months
	Stabilization	6–12 months
Clinodactyly	Physeolysis	4–6 years
	Osteotomy	Late
Camptodactyly	Joint and soft-tissue release	12–18 months
– Fixed with joint changes	Release and transfers	After 2 years
– Soft tissue		
Trigger thumb	Release	After 12 months

(Reproduced from Tonkin MA. An introduction to congenital hand anomalies. Handchirurgie 2004;36:75–84.)

improvement is unlikely and if the indication for surgery is one of a questionable improvement in appearance, perhaps the child should make this decision for him- or herself at an older age.

Parents may wish to defer surgery in the hope that there is something new on the horizon which will, if not cure, at least improve the outcome. It is the surgeon's responsibility to encourage hope but to discourage unrealistic expectations. Having failed to make a decision at the optimal time, these decisions rarely become easier with further passage of time. Web pages are full of information, some beneficial, some not. Some is simply advertising.

Table 25.4 details common practice as it relates to timing of specific surgical procedures, although it is recognized that more urgent treatment of life-threatening conditions will delay hand surgery.[109] It will be seen that many anomalies are treated within the first 2 years of life. In principle, the development of progressive deformity is an indication to operate earlier. An example is a syndactyly of the fourth web with terminal phalanx fusion *(Fig. 25.27)*. Release of the first web, such as in an Apert hand, should be early. It is beneficial to complete most surgical procedures prior to school age, particularly in those instances in which appearance is significantly improved, such that teasing and ridicule by other schoolchildren are minimized. However, some procedures, such as minor revision surgery for the Apert hand or limb

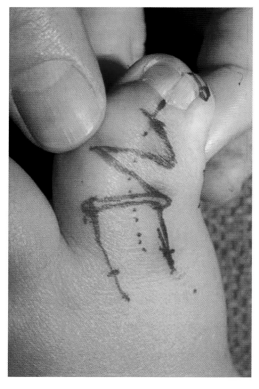

Fig. 25.27 Deformity of ring finger secondary to a four-five syndactyly.

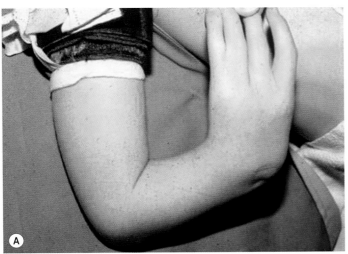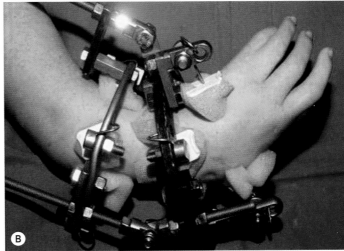

Fig. 25.28 (A, B) Correction of deformity and length for radial longitudinal deficiency at age 8.

lengthening for the short forearm of a radial longitudinal deficiency, may be indicated at an older age *(Fig. 25.28)*.

Finally, expectations of all involved must be realistic. Despite the rewards for surgeon, child, and family following surgery for congenital limb anomalies, an apparently successful and pleasing surgical result may be compromised by recurrent deformity, inadequate growth, uncontrolled growth, or the development of instability or immobility. At the time of operation the surgeon needs to be aware of the presence of factors which may, with time, subsequently alter the early result. In principle, these require correction at the initial surgery.

Access the complete references list online at **http://www.expertconsult.com**

1. Swanson AB. A classification for congenital limb malformations. *J Hand Surg*. 1976;1:8–22

   This is a widely cited classification scheme for congenital anomalies of the limb. The rationale for its design and use is presented.

9. Burke AC, Nelson CE, Morgan BA, et al. Hox genes and the evolution of vertebrate axial morphology. *Development*. 1995;121:333–346.

   Hox genes are known to play a role in anterior–posterior segmental identity. This study describes in situ hybridization and immunolocalization data in chick and mouse embryos demonstrating correlation between Hox expression and morphological boundaries.

15. Martin GR. The roles of FGFs in the early development of vertebrate limbs. *Genes Dev*. 1998;12: 1571–1586.

21. Towers M, Mahood R, Yin Y, et al. Integration of growth and specification in chick wing digit-patterning. *Nature*. 2008;452:882–886.

   This manuscript discusses a series of experiments investigating the role of Sonic hedgehog expression gradients in influencing digit development in a chick wing model. The molecular mechanisms explored provide perspective in understanding human congenital limb anomalies.

25. Laufer E, Nelson CE, Johnson RL, et al. Sonic hedgehog and Fgf-4 act through a signaling cascade and feedback loop to integrate growth and patterning of the developing limb bud. *Cell*. 1994;79:993–1003.

   Sonic hedgehog and Fgf-4 were experimentally regulated to clarify the role these molecules play in early limb development. A positive-feedback loop between the posterior mesoderm and the apical ectodermal ridge is described to mediate their expression.

62. Kardon G. Muscle and tendon morphogenesis in the avian hind limb. *Development*. 1998;125:4019–4032.

   A temporal series of chick embryos was stained and examined to establish morphogenetic developmental patterns. Experiments highlighting the role of interaction between different tissue types (e.g., muscle and bone) in development are presented.

77. Jones KL. Morphogenesis and dysmorphogenesis. In: Jones KL, ed. *Smith's Recognizable Patterns of Human Malformations*. 6th ed. Philadelphia PA: Elsevier Saunders; 2006:783–795.

87. Oberg KC, Feestra JM, Manske PR, et al. Developmental biology and classification of congenital anomalies of the hand and upper extremity. *J Hand Surg [Am]*. 2010;35:2066–2076.

98. Erhardt R. Developmental Hand Dysfunction: Theory, assessment, and treatment. 2nd ed. San Antonio: Therapy Skill Builders; 1994.

26

Congenital hand II: Disorders of formation (transverse and longitudinal arrest)

Gill Smith and Paul Smith

SYNOPSIS

- These are the most likely upper limb anomalies to be detected prenatally.
- The conditions encompassed are divided into transverse and longitudinal arrest, although this division has little to do with either etiology or treatment.
- Repeated observation of the child is the most useful evaluation of the functional capability of each upper limb, aided by the Great Ormond Street Ladder (see *Fig. 26.1*). This may demonstrate capabilities not noticed earlier due to development, achievement of milestones and progressive myelination of the peripheral nervous system.
- Most of these conditions are static with changes largely related to growth or surgical intervention. Early surgical intervention is indicated where deformity is progressive, for primary skeletal realignment or where growth will produce skeletal malalignment.

 Access the Historical Perspective sections online at **http://www.expertconsult.com**

Congenital transverse arrest

Key points 1

- Rare congenital abnormality
- Etiology may be sporadic or environmental
- Commonly occurs at level of upper arm or wrist
- Most transverse deformities will not require surgery. They may benefit from good quality prostheses for which they should be referred early.

Introduction

The birth of a disabled child is devastating for the parents. They will have many questions including those about the likely etiology of the condition. They may be looking for someone to blame. They frequently come with false hopes, encouraged by the media, about the possibilities of hand transplantation and stem cell technology. At this stage, the family may not be able to see beyond the child's structural absence, to accept them as an individual in their own right.

The plastic surgeon may be able to assist in answering questions but, most importantly, they may act as a useful link to a disablement services team. This team of physiotherapist, occupational therapist, psychologist, prosthetist, orthotist and rehabilitation physician will be essential for the ongoing care of this child. They will help the parents accept their child and then, can look at ways of providing aids for the future. They may be able to put them in touch with other parents with children with similar disabilities or suggest parent run organizations which are specifically for the child with limb anomalies.

Occasionally, after full assessment by the rehabilitation team *(Fig. 26.1)*, the plastic surgeon is asked to remove tissue/nubbins or make some surgical adjustment to the stump to make prosthesis fitting easier.

Sometimes, the parents themselves request to have the apparently useless tissue on the terminal part of the limb removed. When left alone they become favored by the child and there is a later reluctance to have them removed.

Basic science/disease process

The level of transverse arrest is defined by the level of skeletal absence but there may be residual soft tissue beyond that point such as small nubbins. There are probably two main groups; those where there is a defect in limb formation and those where there is intrauterine amputation after limb formation.

Longitudinal development of a limb is dependent on the apical ectodermal ridge (AER). For the limb to fail to form, there has been an interruption in signalling with fibroblast growth factors (FGF 2, 4, or 8) to the progress zone which

The Great Ormond Street ladder of functional ability

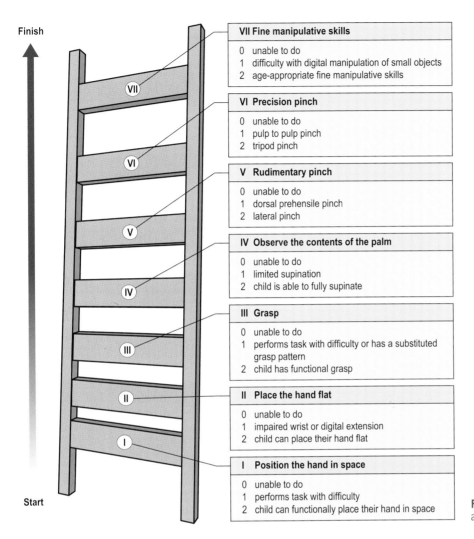

Finish

VII Fine manipulative skills

0 unable to do
1 difficulty with digital manipulation of small objects
2 age-appropriate fine manipulative skills

VI Precision pinch

0 unable to do
1 pulp to pulp pinch
2 tripod pinch

V Rudimentary pinch

0 unable to do
1 dorsal prehensile pinch
2 lateral pinch

IV Observe the contents of the palm

0 unable to do
1 limited supination
2 child is able to fully supinate

III Grasp

0 unable to do
1 performs task with difficulty or has a substituted grasp pattern
2 child has functional grasp

II Place the hand flat

0 unable to do
1 impaired wrist or digital extension
2 child can place their hand flat

I Position the hand in space

0 unable to do
1 performs task with difficulty
2 child can functionally place their hand in space

Start

Fig. 26.1 The Great Ormond Street Ladder allows rapid assessment of upper limb function in complex cases.

supports the AER, sometime in the period between week 5 and week 7 *in utero*, depending on the level of the transverse arrest.

With the exception of the teratogenic effect of thalidomide, etiological factors causing a failure of limb formation are largely unknown but may include genetic factors (there has been shown to be an autosomal recessive gene in Angora goats, which produces a deficiency of the distal limb segment[1]), chromosomal aberrations or environmental factors.

After limb formation, amniotic bands wrapped tightly around the limb, trauma producing a rupture of amnion or iatrogenic factors like laser ablation may produce an intrauterine loss.

Diagnosis/patient presentation

The patient presents with a congenital amputation *(Fig. 26.2)* which can occur at any level (humeral, proximal forearm,

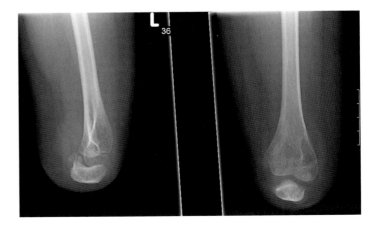

Fig. 26.2 Transverse arrest.

carpal or metacarpal). It may be bilateral – the left side is affected more at least twice as often as the right. Males are more commonly affected than females.

The diagnosis is usually straightforward at proximal levels but at the level of the carpus and metacarpals, there is frequently disagreement in terminology between transverse arrest and symbrachydactyly. Where there are distal nail elements or nail ghosts present on very short digital sacs, this represents symbrachydactyly but in the absence of these, the two conditions may be indistinguishable. If amniotic bands are present elsewhere, then the amputation is likely to be the result of a severely constricting band in utero. Rarely, a proximally situated amniotic band will have caused sufficient interruption to molecular signalling to create a distal hypoplasia which resembles a symbrachydactyly, with distal nail elements present. The management depends on the type of symbrachydactyly (*Fig. 26.3*).

From a treatment point of view, it makes no difference except where other limbs are affected, so the terminology is of academic interest only.

With the advent of fetoscopic laser ablation for twin to twin transfusion, an iatrogenic cause of intrauterine limb loss should be considered where there is a history of this procedure. The mechanism is probably via disruption of the amnion creating bands rather than by the laser itself.[2]

Patient selection, treatment/surgical technique and postoperative care

Transhumeral level

Options for treatment here are between different prostheses, starting with a passive prosthesis. As the child develops active function, the passive prosthesis is replaced with a body-powered cable-controlled or myoelectric prosthesis.

Forearm level

Any treatment is usually restricted to functional and cosmetic prosthetics. The Krukenberg procedure[3] has been used in this condition, particularly when bilateral, to provide a pincer grip between the two forearm bones. The interosseous membrane is extensively released and the defect skin grafted. This procedure has not been readily accepted by either surgeons or families because of the cosmetic deformity it creates in what is already an abnormal limb and is more appropriate in

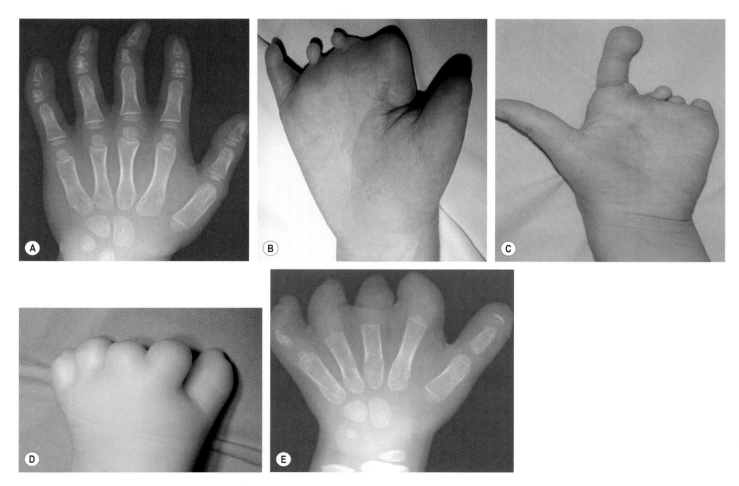

Fig. 26.3 (A) Short finger type symbrachydactyly; **(B)** cleft hand type symbrachydactyly; **(C)** monodactylous type symbrachydactyly with free toe transfer; **(D)** peromelic type symbrachydactyly; **(E)** radiograph of peromelic symbrachydactyly.

traumatic loss in adults where prostheses are unavailable and adaptation is more difficult.

Carpal level

Once again, prosthetics are the mainstay of management. From a surgical point of view, where there is sufficient carpus to be able to provide some intercarpal movement, a double free toe transfer may provide the ability to grip broader objects but is unlikely to be able provide a fine pincer movement due to the limited range of motion within the transfer. Inability to cup the palm, in the presence of a restricted motion distally in the toe transfers may limit the ability to provide a fine pinch.

Metacarpal level (symbrachydactyly)

Where all metacarpals are present, the simplest option is to deepen the first web to create some form of crude pinch (phalangization). However, although a simple procedure, the pinch is a crude lateral pinch, opposition is not possible and grasp is limited due to the poor span. There are two main alternative surgical options that may improve function further, each of which has a role and the decision to perform one rather than the other is frequently related to parental factors:

- Free phalangeal transfer (FPT) ± distraction augmentation manoplasty (DAM)
- Single or double free vascularized toe transfer.

Free phalangeal transfer may be done at any age but it is claimed, that to obtain near normal growth within the phalanx, this must be undertaken within the first 2 years of life. However, there is no substantial evidence to support this. In our experience, growth plates remain open even if transferred at up to 7 years of age. This procedure is only appropriate where there is a sufficiently large soft tissue envelope and does best where the metacarpals form a normal cascade rather than where the central metacarpals are more deficient, forming a V shape.

First, a pocket must be created by dividing the longitudinal fibrous bands that extend to the tip of the soft tissue nubbin from the flexor-extensor tendon confluence over the metacarpal head. It is only then that the true extent of the soft tissue envelope becomes apparent. The surgeon needs to be wary of those nubbins with a constricted base that will not provide sufficient width to accommodate a phalanx.

It is necessary to harvest a whole phalanx since a partial phalanx inserted into the pocket will be prone to resorption *(Fig. 26.4A)*. The phalanx needs to be taken together with an

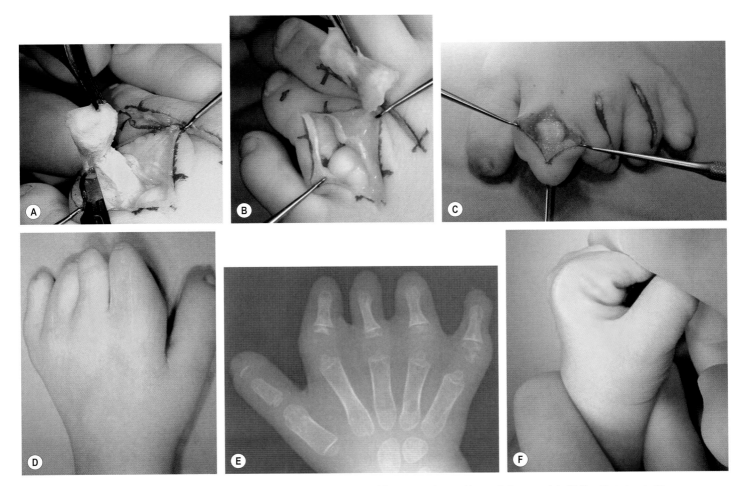

Fig. 26.4 (A,B) Free phalangeal transfer. Bone was harvested with periosteum intact; **(C)** bone was inserted into soft tissue pocket; **(D,E)** patients hand with symbrachydactyly post free phalangeal transfer; **(F)** range of passive motion post free phalangeal transfer.

intact periosteal envelope but the authors do not try to preserve the volar plate and collateral ligaments *(Fig. 26.4B)*. The phalanx is inserted into the soft tissue envelope *(Fig. 26.4C)*. The phalanx is sutured onto the flexor-extensor hood which covers the metacarpal head. The flexor/extensors are not divided. A single K-wire is passed through the phalanx and the centre of the metacarpal head. Four weeks later, this is removed and active and passive movement is encouraged in the new metacarpophalangeal (MCP) joints *(Fig. 26.4D–F)*.

The extensor and flexor tendons in the donor toe should not be sutured together but there is no consensus on how to deal with the toe donor site defect. It has been suggested that inserting an iliac crest bone graft to the toe at the time of harvest may limit the donor site defect in the longer term.

Distraction augmentation manoplasty is considered as a secondary procedure when the child is old enough to participate in the decision and comply with all that this involves. In our experience, 8 years old is the earliest age that this is likely. Not all patients undergo this stage and so results are in a highly selected group. For this to be successful, the length of

the bone being distracted must be a minimum of 10 mm long, it must be stable on the metacarpal and, for the fingers, the range of motion in the MCP joints must be >60°. In the thumb, the carpometacarpal joint must be stable. A distraction frame is applied to the bone with two Kirschner (K) wires or threaded pins fixing each bone proximally and distally *(Fig. 26.5A,B)*. A subperiosteal corticotomy is performed between the proximal and distal fixation points *(Fig. 26.5C)* and the bones are distracted by 4 mm. Postoperatively, distraction is begun after 1 week at 1 mm/day, with weekly radiographs to monitor progress *(Fig. 26.6)*.

Once the required soft tissue length is obtained, a further procedure is performed to bone graft the resultant defect with bone graft from the metatarsals, harvested subperiosteally *(Fig. 26.7)*. This rapid soft tissue distraction differs from distraction osteogenesis (callotasis) in the rapidity of distraction and need for bone grafting into the sheath of osteoid that forms. Its advantage is the shorter time needed with the distractor in place in bone on which it may have a tenuous hold. Other authors[4] have suggested that in children bone grafting is unnecessary but that has not been our experience where awaiting bone formation

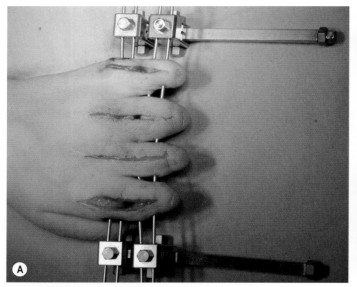

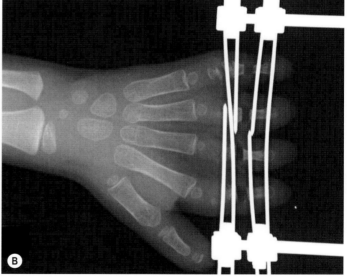

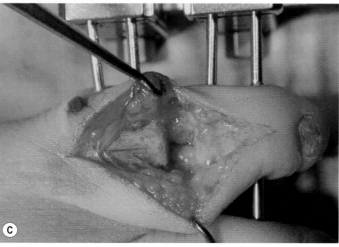

Fig. 26.5 (A,B) Application of fixator for distraction augmentation manoplasty. **(C)** Corticotomy prior to distraction.

first web, rather than trace the dorsal metatarsal artery on the dorsum of the foot. Here, it can be clearly seen if the toe has a dorsal or plantar dominant blood supply and the vessel can be dissected retrogradely, once identified, and its dominance established. Removal of the whole of the second metatarsal gives better access when dissecting the toe than leaving the base and also allows easy closure of the resultant cleft in the foot to leave an acceptable donor site. Ideally, there are two teams present so that one can close the foot, while the other proceeds with the transfer(s).

The toe is K-wired in place on the hand, tendon and nerve repairs are performed and microsurgical anastomosis of arteries and veins is carried out; the level of this and hence the size of the vessel is dependent on multiple factors but it is preferable to avoid the need for vein grafts but also to avoid too long a vessel that may kink and adversely affect flow.

After microsurgical anastomosis in the hand, the surgeon needs to take care to avoid tension in closure of the wounds and it is better to place a skin graft than accept tension that may compromise perfusion.

The free toe transfer needs to be monitored post-operatively and if there is sign of vascular compromise, may need urgent re-exploration.

Outcomes, prognosis, and complications

Prosthetics

If arrest is at the level of the upper arm, use of prostheses is frequent. If this is bilateral, the child may be disinclined to use prostheses and use the feet instead.

If the arrest is at the forearm level, prosthetic use is often limited to task-specific and cosmetic prostheses.

Free nonvascularized phalangeal transfer

Free nonvascularized phalangeal transfer for symbrachydactyly will have a poor outcome if:

1. There is inadequate space in the digital sac for the transferred proximal phalanx
2. If the transferred proximal phalanx is shortened to fit into the digital sac; it will be then be resorbed if the medullary cavity is exposed
3. If there is disruption to the periosteal covering on the proximal phalangeal transfer
4. If the transfer is sutured to divided flexor and extensor tendon, in other words, disruption of the dorsal hood, will lead to an imbalance between adjacent toes.

In terms of growth outcomes, it is often stated that the transfers should be undertaken below 18 months of age but in our series of over 100 free nonvascularized phalangeal transfers this did not prove to be the case and we found open epiphyses were maintained even in transfers up to the age of 7 years.[5] It is impossible to comment on whether or not the growth plates close prematurely because in all the published series the numbers are simply not enough to make a reasonable assumption. The viability of non-vascularized phalangeal transfers is assured provided they have a periosteal covering and there is no tension in the digital sac.

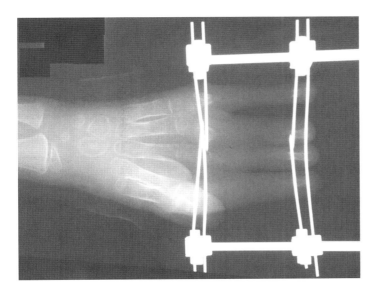

Fig. 26.6 After distraction and ready for bone grafting.

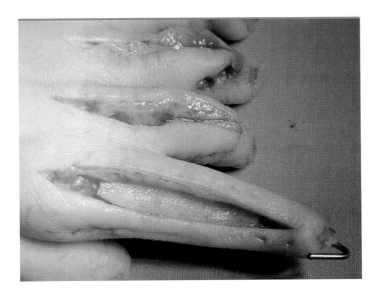

Fig. 26.7 Bone grafting, post-distraction.

has increased the number of complications with failure of fixation and resulted in some loss of the initial length obtained.

Free toe transfer is suitable in those cases where there are toes present that are suitable to harvest, the family will accept the loss of one or both second toes and there are no contraindications to microvascular tissue transfer. One or two toes may be transferred simultaneously in a single procedure or sequentially in two procedures. There is no known benefit in performing this surgery before the age of 2 years and most surgeons would prefer to do it later than this. The site at which the toes should be placed depends on the individual hand anomaly.

For the procedure, the hand must first be dissected out to find suitable tendons, nerves and vessels and decide on the length of these that is required from the donor. To approach the blood supply to the second toe it is easier to explore the

Where the metacarpals are of equal length with a good soft tissue envelope, free phalangeal transfers remain quite stable and can achieve up to 90° of motion at the new "MCP joint." However, with uneven lengths of metacarpals, the direct placement of free phalangeal transfers onto the metacarpal heads will often lead to angulatory deformity and subluxation.

Distraction augmentation manoplasty

The secondary phase of distraction augmentation manoplasty is difficult and is prone to complications with regard to pin tract infections. The rapid distraction is relatively straightforward provided that the proximal phalanges are large enough to accommodate two pins proximal to the osteotomy site and two pins distal to it. Trying to attempt to distract multiple digits simultaneously using the same pins and a single fixator tends to compromise one digit whereas multiple fixators may not be feasible because of their bulk.

With regard to the digits that are produced this are often thin and more prone to fracture, but the children concerned value the digits enormously *(Fig. 26.8)*. From a functional point of view, they improve the control of the flat hand, span and grasp of large objects. Psychological benefit to these children is from having four digits of equal length which move well at the MP joints. It is important to understand that the MCP joints that are created by the nonvascularized phalangeal transfers do achieve up to 80° of motion frequently.

Foot donor site (free phalangeal transfer)

Long-term follow-up is essential and it has become apparent to us recently that although the donor site in the toes initially shows surprisingly little deformity and looks satisfactory for up to 7 years, after 7 years very significant deformities can make themselves apparent. This is especially in terms of shortening, which only deteriorates in adolescence and

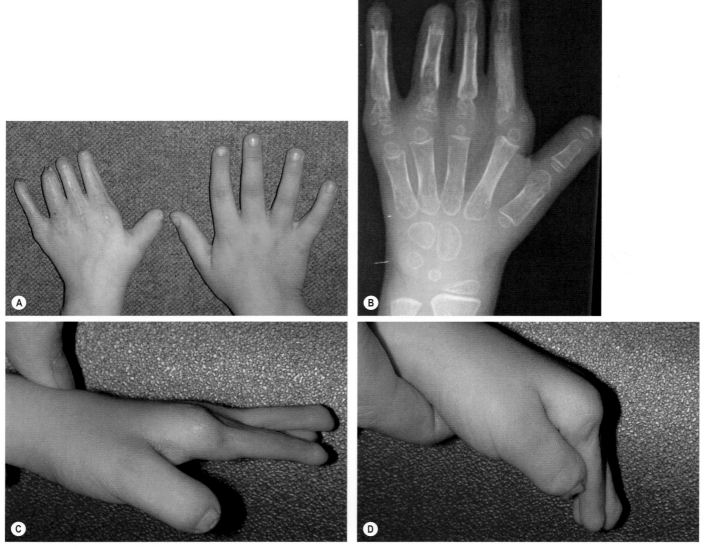

Fig. 26.8 (A–D) Results after distraction augmentation manoplasty.

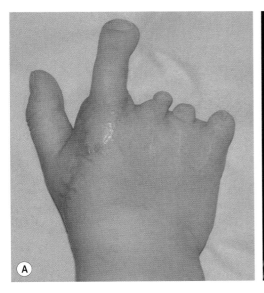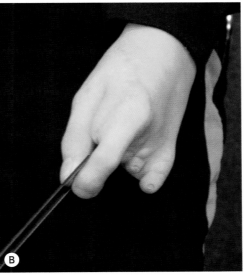

Fig. 26.9 (A,B) Free vascularized toe transfer.

functional issues related to shoe fitting may occur. These may result in toe amputation.

Bourke and Kay[6] utilize a dowel-shaped bone graft from the iliac crest, with its apophysis, to replace the proximal phalanx in the foot and this may well be a very sensible approach but requires long-term study to assess its efficacy.

Outcomes of free toe transfer

Survival of a free toe transfer is now >95% but there is a steep learning curve and initially up to 20% of cases need early re-exploration.

Three-quarters of the children will be expected to undergo secondary procedures including tenolysis and pulp debulking.[7] Despite tenolysis, the active range of motion remains significantly less than the passive range although it appears better when the transfer is done in the older child.[8] Recovery of protective sensation in the transferred digit is expected although, two-point discrimination and light touch sensation appear to recover better when the transfer is under the age of 8 years. The transfers are naturally incorporated into use, although their grip and pinch strength are less than on the normal side.[9]

The majority of children, when there has been appropriate counselling and discussion prior to surgery, have physical and psychological benefits from toe transfer *(Fig. 26.9)*. Problems in the child may be anticipated where the parents are poorly adjusted to the hand anomaly.[10]

The donor site morbidity from free toe transfer depends on which toe is chosen and the number of toes taken from each foot. The authors do not harvest more than one toe from each foot where the foot is to be preserved. Their preference is the second toe transfer because, after closure of the defect as a ray amputation, this provides an excellent aesthetic and functional foot, particularly if the harvest is bilateral. Gait does not appear to be affected in the long term.

Secondary procedures

Occasionally, the prosthetist or the child will request removal of nubbins to make prosthesis fitting easier or for cosmetic reasons – this is a remarkably infrequent occurrence as prosthetic fitting has improved hugely and the nubbins are sensate and often used by the patient. They may request removal due to cold intolerance.

DAM may be requested after previous free phalangeal transfer to increase the length of the digits to increase span and help with specific tasks. This may result in the web spaces being expanded distally and so further web release may be required once distraction is completed. If a child is likely to want DAM, it is best to defer web release until after this is complete.

Tenolysis and pulp-plasty may be required in the majority of free toe transfers to improve the range of motion of the digits allowing fine opposition and to make the appearance of the toes on the hand less toe-like. The overall range of motion remains limited (average 40°) and is usually less than can be achieved with FPT but it is within a useful functional range.

Congenital longitudinal arrest

Key points 2

- Longitudinal deficiencies are often associated with other anomalies which may be life-threatening, disabling or minor.
- The degree of disability is variable and is notably greater where the deformity is bilateral when even the basic functions of the hand can be impaired (see *Fig. 26.1*).
- Longitudinal deficiencies usually benefit from surgery both for functional and aesthetic reasons.
- Surgery is ideally completed by school age; this lies within period of most rapid growth. Early surgery may prevent progression of deformity and allow early skeletal realignment.
- Any surgery has the potential of impairing growth.
- Surgical tissue augmentation, tendon or muscle transfer, will not improve overall strength but will redistribute it to allow more normal function.

- Strength may be increased with free digital transfer where existing tendons can be brought into play to improve pinch and grip strength.
- Although there is research looking at untreated cases, there is little work showing the long term outcome of treated cases.

Phocomelia

Key points 3

- Represents an intercalary segmental failure of formation
- The mainstay of treatment is with therapist, orthotist and prosthetist.

Introduction

Phocomelia describes an intercalary failure of formation, where there are distal structures present but a long bone, such as the humerus or radius and ulna, is largely absent *(Fig. 26.9)*. Short finger type symbrachydactyly represents an intercalary deficiency but with smaller bones absent – these cases are not included usually within the term phocomelia.

Basic science/disease process

Although phocomelia is mainly sporadic, there are some problems with the same underlying genetic basis which produce four limb abnormalities which may be phocomelic. This includes Roberts syndrome, which is caused by mutation in the ESCO2 gene on chromosome 8, inherited in an autosomal recessive fashion.[12] The ESCO2 genes are important in producing the ESCO protein product required for attachment of sister chromatid cohesion during S phases to allow chromosomal separation during cell divisions. In Roberts syndrome, the protein is abnormal so the chromatids attach poorly and cell division is delayed.

Phocomelia has been mimicked in chick limb buds by exposure to X-irradiation. It was thought that this caused a patterning defect as the cell's identity was determined by its time spent in the progress zone. More recently, research has suggested that both thalidomide and X-irradiation cause defects due to a time-dependent loss of skeletal progenitors which do not survive or differentiate.[13] It is known that antiangiogenic analogues of thalidomide induce chick limb defects. It is likely that thalidomide prevents angiogenesis and this would be expected to cause upstream changes in limb morphogenesis.[14]

Diagnosis/patient presentation

There are three main types of phocomelia:
- Type I: hand attached directly to the trunk (complete phocomelia)
- Type II: short forearm attached to trunk (proximal phocomelia)
- Type III: short humerus attached to hand (distal phocomelia).

Both upper limbs are affected, although this may be to different degrees. When all four limbs are affected, the prognosis is more guarded. Phocomelia may be isolated or may be associated with other more serious congenital anomalies that may be the deciding factor in overall prognosis.

The clavicle and scapula may be abnormal in addition to the glenoid, which is hypoplastic. In type III, it may be difficult to distinguish between a severe radial or ulna longitudinal deficiency and phocomelia especially in cases with TAR syndrome who typically have extremely short forearms. Many have abnormalities proximal or distal to the segmental defects which suggest that those cases considered to be phocomelia may, in fact, fit better into a diagnosis of longitudinal dysplasia *(Fig. 26.10)*.[15]

In Roberts syndrome, there are severely shortened segments of all limbs especially the forearms and lower legs. The upper limbs are usually more affected than the lower limbs. There may be knee and elbow contractures. There is not always the full complement of digits, and those present may be abnormal. There are facial dysmorphisms, including microcephaly hypertelorism, downward slanting palpebral fissures, micrognathia, cleft lip and palate, a beaked nose, and small nostrils. There may be cerebral, heart, kidney and genital anomalies. Overall, growth is slow pre and post natally and there is some intellectual impairment. SC phocomelia used to be thought to be a separate entity but is now considered to be a milder variant of Roberts syndrome.

Patient selection

There is little place for surgical intervention here, except when excessive bone growth interferes with orthotic or prosthetic fitting. The occupational therapist and orthotist are key members of the team involved in finding ways to maximize the child's independence and functional abilities. There may however, be some activities where they need assistance. This is more likely to be the case where the lower limbs are also affected.

Treatment/surgical technique

The surgeon must work with the prosthetist and orthotist to enable the fitting of suitable artificial aims but his contribution is secondary to theirs in these patients management.

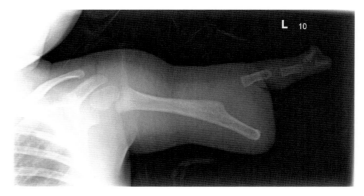

Fig. 26.10 Phocomelia.

Many children with normal lower limbs will use these to perform tasks for which the normal child would use their upper limbs. Many will use prosthetics or orthotics for certain specific tasks and discard them in favor of the remains of their sensate upper limbs and supplemented by their lower limbs for the rest of the time. Despite the restrictions of insensibility and weight that cause them to discard the functional prostheses, they may still desire non functional prosthetic arms for cosmetic reasons on occasion.

Postoperative care

Any surgery carried out should be with the aim of allowing orthotic and prosthetic fitting and use as soon as possible afterwards. Primary wound healing without the need for skin grafting or complex bony external fixation is required.

Outcomes, prognosis, complications

The prognosis is better where the condition is isolated and confined to the upper limbs. In Roberts syndrome, life expectancy depends on the severity of the associated systemic anomalies.

Secondary procedures

These are bony stump revisions that may be required throughout growth.

Radial hypoplasia or aplasia

Key points 4

- Radial ray dysplasia is a spectrum from minor size discrepancy in the thumb to complete absence of the thumb and radius. In any case of thumb hypoplasia, the proximal forearm and the contralateral thumb should be carefully evaluated.
- Cardiac and hematological associations need to ruled out.
- The prognosis is poorer when associated with syndromes.
- Treatment may range from simple tendon transfers to complex soft tissue and bony distractions.
- Soft tissue distraction makes wrist centralization or stabilization technically easier.
- Stabilization retains motion at the "wrist" but is inherently unstable.
- Centralization is stable but relatively immobile.
- Tendon transfers are always required in all but a small group of type I radial club hand.
- Wrist stabilization should precede thumb reconstruction.
- The role of forearm lengthening is yet to be defined but in the presence of a wrist stabilization or an unstable wrist is likely to produce recurrent deviation.

Introduction

Longitudinal radial deficiency or radial ray dysplasia, often referred to as "radial club hand" encompasses a spectrum of abnormalities of the preaxial border of the upper limb, where the hand lies deviated radially, flexed and pronated at the distal end of a shortened forearm. There is a combination of a lack of bony support on the radial side with carpal and musculotendinous abnormalities. Forearm rotation is reduced or absent, the elbow abnormal, the ulna may be bowed, the radiocarpal articulation unstable or absent, the carpus abnormal, the thumb absent or hypoplastic, and other radial digits may be stiff and abnormal. The only digit expected to be normal is the little finger which retains mobility in even the most severe cases. Any understanding of this condition to devise treatment strategies has to take into account the variety of tissues involved and not purely emphasize the bony abnormality.

The milder deformities rarely need surgical intervention but the management of the more severe deformities is both difficult and controversial. These patients do not have a functional radiocarpal articulation as their carpus is suspended on the radial and volar aspect of the ulna. The length of the ulna is reduced to 60% of normal.[16] Any attempt to use the fingers effectively is limited by the instability at the "wrist." Surgery is aimed primarily at creating a stable ulnocarpal connection by a combination of bony realignment and soft tissue release and rebalancing to allow the long digital flexors to function more effectively, whilst preserving forearm length and ulna growth. The aim is to improve the position of the limb on the Great Ormond Street Ladder of functional ability (Fig. 26.1).

When the condition is bilateral, functional disability is greater as it is in syndromic cases. Even in the absence of a syndrome, there is frequently association with other anomalies. Other systemic problems may delay the diagnosis as well as the treatment of these deformities.

The best estimate of prevalence is 1:100 000 live births[17] but this was in a Scandinavian population group and it may vary between populations.

Basic science/disease process

The etiology of radial club hand is still uncertain with both genetic and environmental factors likely to have an influence. Bilateral cases are more likely to have a syndromic association. Some of the many syndromes which include a radial ray deficiency may have a genetic basis. These may be transmitted as an autosomal dominant or recessive condition but are usually the result of a sporadic mutation.

Multiple environmental factors have been implicated. Thalidomide exposure between days 38 and 45 is a known etiological factor[19] and this also produces a higher incidence of other skeletal deficiencies. Valproic acid has been associated with radial defects, as part of the fetal valproic syndrome.[20] Phenobarbital[21] and ethanol[22] have also been implicated in radial defects.

In fetal white leghorn chickens, radial ray deficiencies may be produced by cauterization in the distal preaxial area, and ulnar ray deficiencies by cauterization in the distal postaxial area.[23] The critical periods for both radial and ulnar ray deficiencies are the same; from immediately after the formation of the wing bud to before the formation of the digital plate. Busulfan, an antimitotic agent, given to pregnant rats can induce defects similar to those seen in humans with radial club hand.[24]

Tickle *et al.*[25] have suggested that the polarizing region that determines anteroposterior patterning in the limb, produces a morphogen that diffuses across the limb bud. The quantity of morphogen that a single cell was exposed to would determine the identity of the ray into which it developed. A deficiency would prevent ray development. Experimentally, similar defects have been created in chick wings and both retinoic acid[26] and expression of the sonic hedgehog gene[27] have been shown to reproduce signalling of the polarizing region. However, it is unlikely that the situation is as simple as that. Sonic hedgehog gene is critical in regulating the function of the zone of polarizing activity but this is controlled by several factors including Hoxb-8 and Hand2 and is only induced due to signalling from the apical ectodermal ridge, probably by fibroblast growth factor. The maldevelopment of a limb may be related to several different interruptions to this pathway.

Diagnosis/patient presentation

The patient presents at birth with short pronated forearms, possibly stiff elbows, floppy "wrists" with radial deviation of the hand on the forearm, stiff radial digits and abnormal or absent thumbs *(Fig. 26.11)*. The severe deformities are usually picked up on initial neonatal check by the pediatrician and investigations to exclude associated problems should be instituted by them. It is slightly more common in males than females[28] and the right side is affected twice as much as the left.[29]

Some degree of bilateral involvement is common but this is often not symmetrical. The contralateral side must be closely inspected in the child with an apparent unilateral radial club hand as the radial ray dysplasia on the other side may comprise of a small amount of thenar muscle hypoplasia which would otherwise be easily overlooked in concentrating on the forearm deformity. This mildly hypoplastic thumb is likely to become the dominant one so any surgery to strengthen and improve this should be a priority.

Radial ray dysplasia was classified by Bayne and Klug *(Table 26.1, Fig. 26.12)* into four types although this takes no

account of the associated radial ray dysplasia in the carpus and hand.

The type I deformity may be missed *per se* but is usually referred to the hand surgeon due to associated absence or hypoplasia of the thumb. The deficiency of the radius is not obviously radiologically, but the child holds the hand radially deviated and flexed on the forearm. This is especially noticeable when they are putting any force through the hand, so may become more evident when picking up a toy. Although these patients often improve without surgery to the wrist, it should be noted that this tendency to collapse into flexion and radial deviation with load bearing is persistent to some degree. The thumb hypoplasia may vary in degree but, with the exception of TAR patients, a severe forearm deformity is associated with a marked thumb hypoplasia.

Another chapter concentrates on thumb hypoplasia but it should be noted that, since radial ray dysplasia is a spectrum of disorder, even in mild cases of thumb hypoplasia, there may be abnormalities present in the carpus and in the distal radius that may not be evident until the teenage years. The trapezium is likely to be small, the scaphoid absent or deficient, the trapezoid small and carpal coalitions are seen in the ulnar side of the wrist.

Similarly, the elbow is not normal in radial ray dysplasia, although it is affected less than the wrist. This is seen

Table 26.1 Bayne and Klug classification of radial longitudinal deficiency

Type	Radiological appearance
I	Late appearance of radial distal epiphysis
II	Small radius with proximal and distal epiphyses
III	Small proximal radius
IV	Complete radial aplasia

After Bayne LG, Klug MS. Long-term review of the surgical treatment of radial deficiencies. J Hand Surg Am. 1987;12(2):169–179.

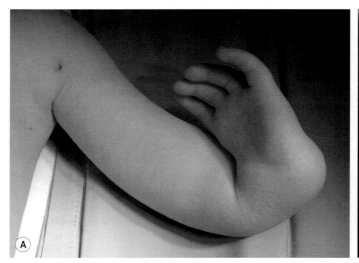
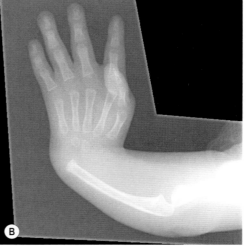

Fig. 26.11 (A,B) Radial ray dysplasia.

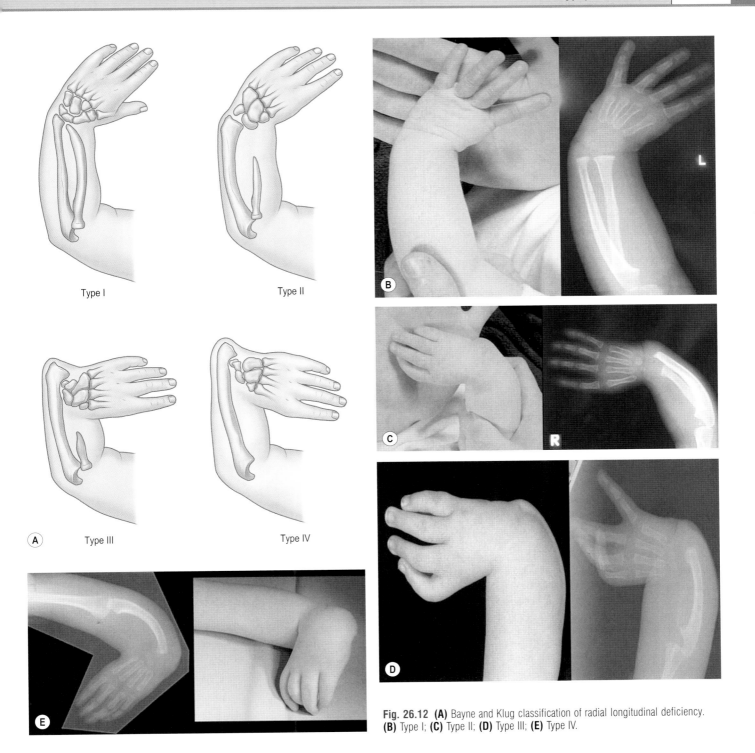

Fig. 26.12 (A) Bayne and Klug classification of radial longitudinal deficiency. **(B)** Type I; **(C)** Type II; **(D)** Type III; **(E)** Type IV.

increasingly with growth in the severely deficient cases who may demonstrate clinical evidence of subluxation of the humeroulnar articulation in extension. Radiological investigation shows a shallow acetabulum with a poor developed coronoid process and, to a lesser extent, olecranon. Humeral abnormalities parallel the severity of the radial defect. Forearm rotation is normally absent in types III and IV and reduced in types I and II. The patients compensate by the use of shoulder internal and external rotation,

There are a myriad of syndromic conditions associated with radial ray dysplasia, the diagnosis of many of which require a clinical geneticist's advice. However, there are certain groups of associated features that the surgeon should be aware of and seek to exclude. These include the hematological disorders of Fanconi's anemia and thrombocytopenia absent radius syndrome (TAR), Holt–Oram syndrome, and VATER syndrome. Patients with TAR syndrome may be distinguished as they have bilateral short forearms, bilateral radial club hand, usually type IV, and functional but abnormal thumbs. Other patients with this severity of radial dysplasia have absent or severely hypoplastic thumbs.

All these conditions may affect the timing and nature of surgical intervention on the upper limbs and hence the need for awareness of them when planning surgery.

Patient selection

There may be factors which determine whether or not a patient is selected for surgical treatment at all and these center around associated conditions. Such associated conditions as cardiac anomalies may prevent or severely delay the inception of treatment for radial club hand. Assuming that the child's general condition is suitable for surgery, then the surgical approach may be governed by mobility of the elbow. Many authors view the stiff elbow as a contraindication to any surgical centralization of the wrist because they feel that this may prevent the hand reaching the mouth. The authors' views reflect the comments of Lamb who noted that, when preoperative splintage was utilized on the wrist, elbow movement often increased. In the senior author's view, a stiff elbow is resolved by centralization of the wrist and this is not a contraindication. This view is based on experience of the treatment of 142 cases of types II-IV radial club hand.

The stiffness and degree of radial deviation and the grade of radial club hand will then determine the surgical approach.

- Grade 1: This requires simple tendon transfer, many of them do not even require this but will simply respond to splintage or may have so little radial deviation that intervention is judged not to be worthwhile.
- Grade 2: These are the most difficult of all. There is a residual radius, the temptation is to try and lengthen the radius by osteotomy and distraction and possible bone grafting to provide a proper radiocarpal joint. In the authors' experience, this is exceedingly difficult and may have to be repeated several times during growth. In several cases, the radial remnant has eventually had to be removed and the case treated as though it was a type 4.
- Type 3: Small proximal radius. This is best converted to a Type 4 by removing the radial anlage.
- Type 4: Complete radial aplasia. Our preference here is for centralization with a carpal slot after distraction lengthening and internal tendon transfers to rebalance, together with K-wire fixation on a temporary basis.

Treatment/surgical technique

The initial treatment in all grades of radial club hand involves teaching stretching exercises to the parents and these should be undertaken several times a day. As soon as it is possible to apply a splint this should be undertaken to produce retention of the daytime gain at night. Such splints require frequent adjustment and are difficult to apply to very young children. In the younger the child passive stretching is more important than splintage. This sort of standard advice may now be outdated by the advent of preoperative soft tissue distraction.

Once the child has reached a size where a soft tissue distraction device can be attached to the skeleton, a uniaxial fixator with a multiaxial joint or a multiaxial distractor may be applied. The authors consider that either will give similar results in primary cases but that the latter may be preferable in difficult revision cases. A distraction fixator is applied between the ulna and the second metacarpal on the radial side to begin the process of soft tissue distraction. A significant amount of distraction is undertaken at the time of the application of the fixator, this is then left for a week and distraction recommenced after that at 1 mm a day *(Fig. 26.13)*. The initial intraoperative distraction has been quite rapid and the subsequent distraction is significantly slower. This can be split into multiple episodes each day if it is easier for the family or more comfortable for the child. The parents are taught pin site care.

Once the hand has been distracted enough the carpus will translocate onto the distal end of the ulna but radiology is a trap for the unwary because the uncalcified carpal bones can be misleading and a straight forearm and hand may be obtained whilst the carpus remains subluxed on the volar aspect of the ulna and there is residual overlap.

Once a suitable position has been achieved, it is maintained there for one month following which wrist fixation is undertaken. This may either be a classical centralization with a carpal slot *(Fig. 26.14)* or a stabilization, which is often called

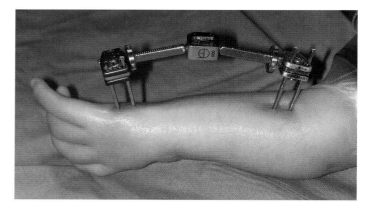

Fig. 26.13 Radial club hand with fixator applied completing soft tissue distraction.

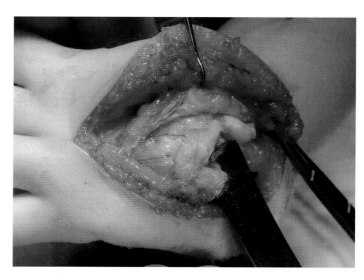

Fig. 26.14 Creation of a carpal slot for the ulna head.

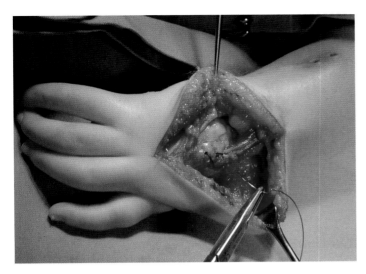

Fig. 26.15 Transfer of dorsoradial muscle mass in wrist stabilization for radial club hand.

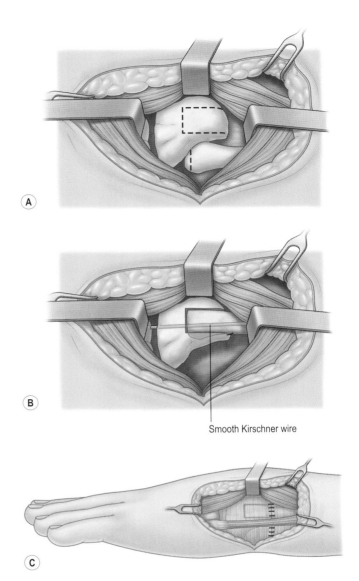

Smooth Kirschner wire

Fig. 26.16 After soft tissue release, a defect is created in the carpus, with radial and ulnar pillars, into which the ulna head is K-wired in place, by means of a long longitudinal and shorter oblique K-wire.

radialization. A radialization is essentially a balancing of the carpus on the ulna (a nonslotted centralization). In either process a tendon transfer is required, in fact the main part of the operation is the muscular rebalancing by transferring the dorso-radial muscle mass into extensor carpi ulnaris *(Fig. 26.15)*. The longer the fixator is left in place with a distraction force the more remodelling will be seen in the ulna and this in the majority of cases will correct an ulnar bowing but may not completely correct the orientation of the distal end of the ulna.

Centralization involves the alignment of the 3rd metacarpal with the ulna but with the deliberate creation of a notch in the carpus that is likely to result in a fusion between the proximal carpal row and the distal end of the ulna or a fibrous union *(Figs 26.16, 26.17)*.

Stabilization or radialization involves rebalancing the hand on the end of the ulna so that the second metacarpal is in alignment with the ulna and the tendon transfer of the dorsoradial muscle mass rebalancing the internal forces producing a more ulnar pull and a more ulnar vector *(Fig. 26.17)*. Radialization is thus poorly named as it is truly an ulnarization but the authors prefer to consider it as a nonslotted centralization. Unfortunately, it involves a balancing act and this is an unstable equilibrium *(Fig. 26.18)*, whereas a carpal slot centralization is stable *(Fig. 26.19)*. In reviewing our results for stabilization, there is a tendency for the rebalancing to fail and the wrist to be pulled back into radial deviation and to sublux volarly. This occurred in 50% of cases, and we are now much more likely to choose a stable centralization over an unstable stabilization (radialization).

All of these corrections are retained in position with a temporary K-wire *(Fig. 26.20)*. The definition of temporary varies, in our experience we leave these wires in for a minimum of 6 months but often for a year. Lamb used to leave his K-wires in for many years.

The whole aim of stabilization or radialization is to maintain adequate forearm length to reduce the possibility of impairment of growth at the distal end of the ulna and to

retain motion at the new pseudo wrist joint. These are admirable aims and other authors have attempted to achieve these by vascularized transfers to replace the radius. Both vascularized and non vascularized transfers of the head of the fibula have been attempted and Vilkki has utilized free vascularized metatarsophalangeal joint transfers, however the numbers involved in these cases has been very small.[30] In our experience in the 142 cases that we have cared for over a 25-year period, we have found the modern approach to centralization, following soft tissue distraction, to be satisfactory. Preoperative distraction lengthening enables the surgeon to largely ignore the skin problems and complicated incisions, such as the bi-lobed flap utilized to reduce ulnar soft tissue excess and increase radial deficiency in the skin, are rendered obsolete by

Centralization   Radialization

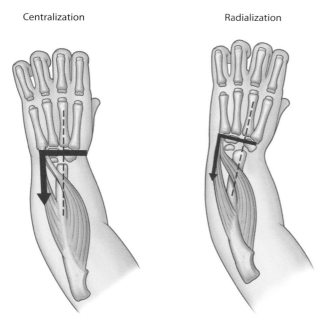

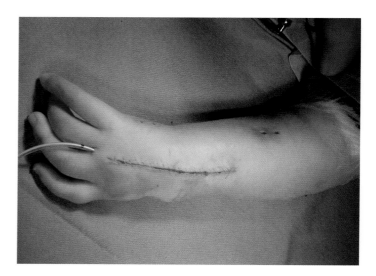

Fig. 26.20 Radial club hand post-wrist stabilization procedure.

Fig. 26.17 In centralization: a carpal slot is created to insert the ulna head aligned with the third metacarpal. In radialization: there is no carpal slot and alignment is with the second metacarpal. In both, balance is maintained with a tendon transfer of the dorsoradial muscle mass to extensor carpi ulnaris.

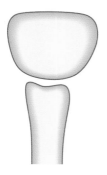

Fig. 26.18 Radialization is a balancing act and provides an unstable equilibrium.

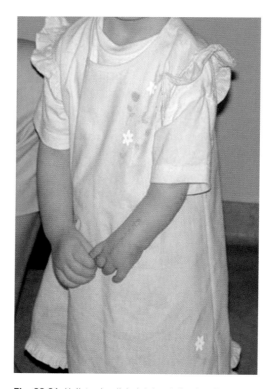

Fig. 26.21 Unilateral radial club hand showing discrepancy in forearm growth.

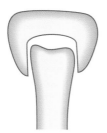

Fig. 26.19 Centralization involves the formation of a carpal slot and forms a stable equilibrium.

the soft tissue distraction. A straightforward linear incision is all that is required, which is simpler in the primary case but also should revision surgery be required later. The soft tissue distraction of the dorsoradial muscle mass and the ability to place the carpus on the distal end of the ulna makes centralization technically much easier and less traumatic. By always

undertaking a significant muscle transfer internally the combination of the rebalancing of forces internally and the stable design of a carpal slot produce results which are considerably better than those that have been achieved in the past.

All patients with radial club hand will have short forearms on the affected sides *(Fig. 26.21)*, some will desire ulnar lengthening to correct some or all of the discrepancy, this is a time consuming procedure, which should only be undertaken once the wrist is completely stable and the thumb has been operated on if required. In highly selected patients it may bring functional and cosmetic gains which they consider worthwhile.

The later ability to undertake forearm lengthening allows one to achieve a final result which is very satisfactory considering the severity of the initial deformity and at the present time distraction lengthening, centralization, muscle transfer and later forearm lengthening remain the mainstay of treatment and other techniques have yet to prove that they are worthwhile.

Postoperative care

Bleeding from the bony osteotomy sites is inevitable so suction drainage is essential. A significant amount of swelling can occur at the wrist and the plaster applied at operation should be checked frequently within the first week. Once the swelling has completely settled, a splint can be manufactured to replace the plaster.

All of these patients require considerable hand therapy in the post operative period, they also require removal of the K-wire at 6 months to a year and mobilization of the ulnocarpal joint will often give about 20° of flexion. It is advisable to utilize splinting for at least a year after surgery mainly to prevent the child from falling and traumatizing the area.

Once the K-wire has been removed the splint may be utilized for any occasions where falls are liable to occur and nocturnally. Some form of splinting is nearly always required intermittently until skeletal maturity.

Outcomes, prognosis, complications

Growth disturbance in the forearm has been demonstrated in past series. It has been shown that the unoperated forearm in radial club hand is often only 60% of normal length but Heikel[16] showed that surgery reduced this length to 40%. In our series, we found that preoperative distraction actually increased ulnar growth but whether this is an effect that is maintained long term requires a follow-up of at least 16 years. If the disturbance of growth is minor this can be dealt with by lengthening at a later date, but if it is major then it is catastrophic, but is virtually never seen nowadays. Many of the centralizations performed in the past have been little short of carpectomy and insertion of the residual carpus onto the end of the ulna. This has probably been the case because of the difficulty of undertaking the centralization. Buck-Gramcko showed that radialization would only work in less severely affected cases of radial club hand.

Minor pin site infections, treated by antibiotics, are frequent during the distraction phases but deep infection is a rarity. The scars formed by the distraction process are likely to initially be thick and hypertrophic but usually settle spontaneously. The forces across the wrist prior to tendon transfer are considerable and breakage of the external fixator pins, cutting out of the pins through the bone or fracture of the metacarpal or ulna are not unknown. K-wires may often break but if they do it indicates that there may be imbalance of forces at the wrist, the same can occur with plates though these should not be used except in a final wrist fusion, in failed cases.

Secondary procedures

Recurrent radial deviation of the ulnocarpal junction is seen less often these days and in the past was most often due to failure to internally rebalance the musculotendinous forces but a failure to release the deep fascia from mid dorsal to mid palmar area on the radial side may also be grounds for recurrence. Slight angulation of the distal ulna head may be problematic, even though the rest of the ulna is straight. Curvature of the ulna if significant but with a good distal ulnocarpal relationship may require a wedge resection to correct it. In some recurrent deformities where the carpus is re-deviating radially and volarly the use of a spatial frame and distraction lengthening of the soft tissues prior to bony fixation is useful. Once the ulnocarpal relationship is stable and the thumb no longer requires any surgical intervention it is then possible to consider forearm lengthening with a spatial frame.

The authors would normally correct radial deviation of ≥30°. More frequently nowadays, the problem is principally of a flexion deformity which may be improved by a dorsal wedge resection of the ulna proximal to the epiphysis and extensor shortening or, if there is barely any motion, by epiphyseal sparing wrist arthrodesis.

Forearm lengthening is best performed with a spatial frame to allow multi-axial distraction and continued use of the hand during distraction to stimulate new bone formation. It is often performed with temporary stabilization of the wrist with a plate which may lead to arthrodesis of the wrist which may compromise the result of earlier wrist surgery. It is important that the wrist is stable prior to bony lengthening or deviation will reoccur but the use of a plate across the ulnocarpal joint is possibly the best way to achieve this. Re-deviation may require rebalancing at the end of distraction to maintain functional positioning. Throughout the process regular hand therapy is required to maintain digital motion and care should be taken to watch for elbow dislocation where a single bone is being distracted in the presence of both. The rate of complications, which is considerable, increases with progressive gain in length and it is likely that the gain in length will be less if distraction is repeated.

Central ray deficiency

Key points 5

- Most common of the longitudinal deficiencies
- Deficiencies are located chiefly distal to the long bones within the hand plate
- Recent changes in the classification are confusing and unsatisfactory
- Hands are functionally good but an aesthetic disaster
- When functionally poor, there are limited surgical options for improvement
- Duplication and syndactyly may be present in addition to central absence
- Often affects the feet, is bilateral and autosomal dominant

Introduction

Central deficiencies involve a spectrum of anomalies where there is a deficiency of bony and soft tissue structures centrally in the hand plate. Despite lying within the category

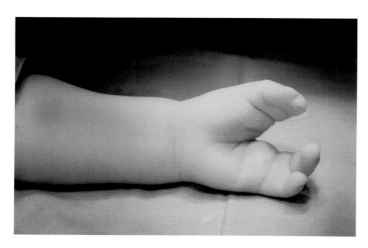

Fig. 26.22 Typical cleft hand with central deep V-shaped cleft and ectrodactyly.

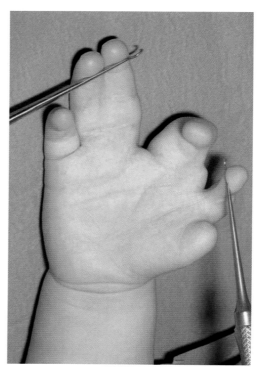

Fig. 26.23 Cleft hand with radial duplication and central syndactyly.

of longitudinal aplasia, the cleft hand deformities rarely affect structures proximally to the wrist, although carpal coalitions and radioulnar synostosis may be associated, and their position in the classification has stimulated much debate.

All authorities are, however, agreed with Flatt's[31] comment that the cleft hand is "a functional triumph and a social disaster", as these hands often have little functional limitation but the cosmetic deformity is eye-catching *(Fig. 26.22)*.

Basic science/disease process

Clefting is produced by a defect in the apical ectodermal ridge centrally or medially. Those known to be genetically related, such as in split hand/split foot, have defects in genes related to the formation of the apical ectodermal ridge. Split hand/split foot is caused by multiple loci including SHFM1, SHFM2, SHFM3, SHFM4, SHFM5 and mutations in TP63.[33]

Maisel's centripetal theory suggested a spectrum of increasing suppression with radial progression but this does not account for some of the clinical associations. Ogino's[34] work with teratogens in rats has shown an association of clefting with syndactyly and polydactyly, which is frequently seen clinically. This is related to teratogens producing local cell death and interrupting molecular signalling pathways that organize the limb and produce apoptosis, focally interrupting the apical ectodermal ridge. Blauth and Falliner[35] summarizes this as suggesting that an insult to the apical ectodermal ridge with or without underlying mesenchyme produces lack of differentiation (syndactyly), exaggerated differentiation (polydactyly) or defect formation (clefting) according to the nature and severity of the insult.

Diagnosis/patient presentation

Manifestations vary from a minor soft tissue cleft with a full complement of osseous components, and without the absence of a digit, to severe suppression where only a single ulnar digit remains. Any number of digits may be missing but the little finger always remains. Absence of the middle finger including its metacarpal produces a typical deep V-shaped cleft.

It has been suggested that the diagnosis of cleft hand can only be made where there is a complete osseous deficiency of the middle finger ray. The authors consider that this adds confusion and would prefer to view clefting as related to a spectrum of AER injury, as Ogino has demonstrated, which would include incomplete forms and associated radial polydactyly and syndactyly *(Fig. 26.23)*. This suggests that clefting should really sit in the classification within failure of differentiation rather than failure of formation of parts.

Syndactyly is likely to occur in the webs adjacent to the cleft, most commonly between the ring and little finger. Where there is complete syndactyly, this is more likely to be in the central digits and there may be synostosis with shared flexor tendons, pulleys and neurovascular bundles, which makes separation retaining function difficult. There may be deviation and rotation of the digits adjacent to the cleft with the presence of delta phalanges and broader proximal phalanges than would be expected. The ring finger, in particular, usually has a flexion contracture and so does the index finger where the first web is very narrow.

Transverse or obliquely lying bones which articulate distally with adjacent rays are frequently found and necessitate surgical intervention as the cleft will widen with growth, creating increasing deformity. There may also be cartilage remnants in the first or second web, which may be attached to and may further distort growth if not removed. These will not be visible on radiograph but will be easily palpable.

There is frequently a deficiency of the first web – in the most severe cases there is complex syndactyly of the thumb and index finger. This is frequently deficient and Manske's[36] classification of cleft hands is based on the severity of this deficiency *(Table 26.2)*.

Table 26.2 Manske's classification of cleft hands

Type	Description	Characteristics
I	Normal web	
IIA	Mildly narrowed web	
IIB	Severely narrowed web	
III	Syndactylized web	
IV	Merged web	Index ray suppressed
V	Absent web	Ulnar rays only present

After Manske PR, Halikis MN. Surgical classification of central deficiency according to the thumb web. Am J Hand Surg. 1995;20(4):687–697.

Table 26.3 Syndromes associated with central longitudinal deficiency

DeLange dwarfism
Oculodigital complex
Orodigital complex
Otodigital complex
Silver–Russell syndrome
EEC syndrome

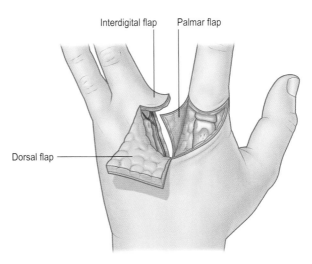

Fig. 26.24 Simple cleft closure technique where first web is adequate.

Cleft hands are most frequently bilateral and are associated with cleft feet in approximately one-third of cases. There are a number of syndromes associated with central deficiency of which EEC syndrome is the most frequent in our practice *(Table 26.3)*.

Patient selection

Discussion regarding treatment should reflect that there is a risk of losing some functional capability to improve aesthetics. Some families will not desire treatment as they have seen the functional capabilities of others affected in the family and also the effects of previous sometimes ill-advised surgery.

Surgery is strongly advised in the presence of transversely lying bones or cartilage remnants, as the cleft will widen with growth and this will affect function and worsen aesthetics. This is particularly the case in the feet where shoe-fitting will otherwise become an increasing problem or in the hand, where there is a palpable cartilage tether to the growth of a digit, usually the index finger.

The most functionally beneficial procedure for the hand is to ensure a good first web space but what is required to provide this varies with the complexity of the deformity.

Closure of the cleft can improve the appearance of the hand but risks creating scissoring of the digits. Release of simple syndactyly is worthwhile and skin graft can be harvested from the cleft to provide a good color match. Complex syndactyly release where there is proximal synostosis may risk losing motion due to the need to reconstruct pulleys and share flexor tendons.

Where the hand is very deficient, free toe transfer may be applicable to provide additional motors but the vascular supply to the toe and to the hand may be aberrant and the presence of proximal motors is uncertain, although something

is more reliably present than in symbrachydactyly. In clefting syndromes affecting the feet and the hands, orthopaedic surgeons may wish to remove the great toe to fit shoes and the opportunity should not be lost to reconstruct a missing thumb.

Treatment/surgical technique

The strongest indication for treatment in cleft hands is the presence of transverse lying bones. Care needs to be taken here to avoid destabilization of involved joints. Correction of camptodactyly of adjacent fingers is not usually helpful but it is worth examining tendon insertions at the time of excision of transverse bones or closure of the cleft to release aberrant ones which may help in preventing further deformity.

A simple soft tissue cleft should be closed with a small flap from the index finger *(Fig. 26.24)* to avoid a longitudinal scar in the web which would lead to a V-shaped deformity. The underlying transverse metacarpal ligament should be reconstructed using the adjacent A1 pulleys but there needs to be a soft tissue correction towards the centre of the bone or dorsally with either tendon graft or sutures through the periosteum to prevent scissoring of the digits with closure of the cleft. Where there is a hypoplastic third metacarpal, the cleft may sometimes be closed without need to transpose the second metacarpal.

The Snow–Littler[37] procedure *(Fig. 26.25)* involves the transposition of a palmar based flap from the cleft to supplement the first web, release of the first dorsal interosseous and adductor pollicis and simultaneous osteotomy and transfer of the index finger into the position of the first ray. This is technically demanding, may compromise the vascularity of the index finger and the long palmar flap moves poorly and may necrose distally. Modifications of this technique have been developed, with that by Miura and Komada[38] being the most popular *(Fig. 26.26)*. Their technique involves a dorsally based flap which therefore moves with greater ease and is technically easier.

Toe to hand transfer may be useful to provide a thumb but, where the feet are affected, the digit may be abnormal and have a restricted range of motion. It may be necessary to obtain vascular imaging of the hand and foot preoperatively to establish the pattern of vascularity.

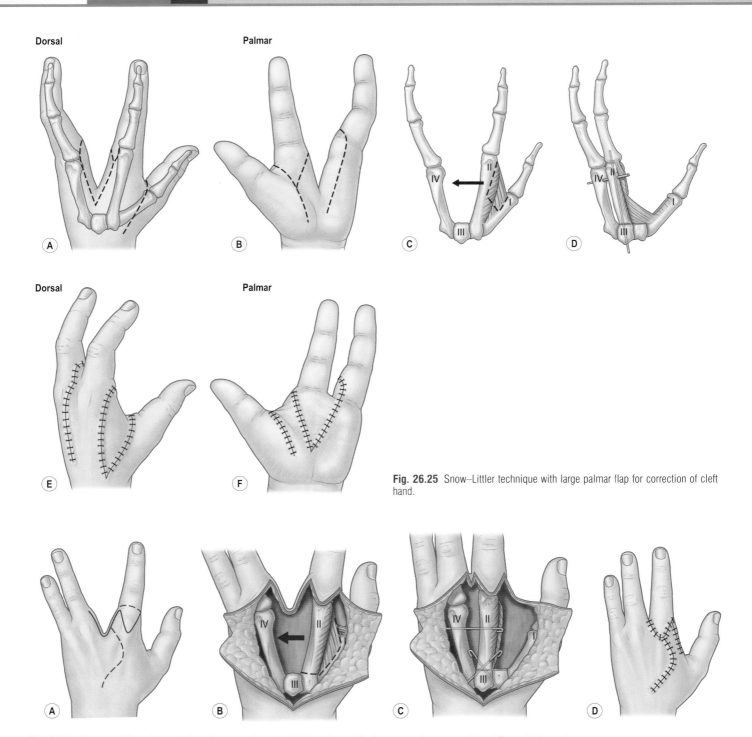

Dorsal   Palmar

A   B   C   D

Dorsal   Palmar

E   F

Fig. 26.25 Snow–Littler technique with large palmar flap for correction of cleft hand.

A   B   C   D

Fig. 26.26 Miura and Komada's technique for correction of a cleft hand is technically simpler than the traditional Snow–Littler technique.

Postoperative care

The authors treat almost all their congenital hand patients with a bulky boxing glove bandage attached to the skin by taping, rather than an above elbow cast. This is easy to change, difficult to escape from and not dangerous to others if used as a weapon. Once the wounds are healed, the child is given a C-shaped splint for night-time for three months to maintain the first web.

Outcomes, prognosis, and complications

Overall, the outcome of surgery for cleft hands is good, although, with growth, there is commonly slight widening of the gap where the cleft has been closed. There is a risk of digital loss, or ischaemia producing poor growth, from the Snow–Littler procedure and the authors have not seen good results from attempts at correcting camptodactyly of the index or ring fingers.

Release of complex syndactyly with synostoses may compromise range of motion of the digits with the sharing of available tendons and pulleys.

The results from free toe transfer are dependent on the deficiencies of the digit transferred so would not be expected to equal those for other indications, either aesthetically or functionally.

Secondary procedures

There may be the need to correct rotation or angulation of the digits by osteotomy, particularly in the presence of abnormal epiphyses.

Ulnar hypoplasia or aplasia

This is the rarest of longitudinal deficiencies. It affects the whole upper extremity, most severely at the elbow and hand. Functionally, most children adapt well except in some syndromic cases, but the aesthetics are poor for both static and dynamic appearance.

Introduction

This condition, often termed ulnar club hand, covers a spectrum of disorders where the ulna is deficient, the elbow is abnormal, and there are an associated variety of hand anomalies. Compared with other longitudinal defects, there are a greater variety of clinical appearances. The wrist is not normal but shows greater stability than in radial club hand whereas the elbow is always more severely affected.

Ulnar club hand is around 10 times less frequent in occurrence than radial club hand. The condition is bilateral in about half of cases but rarely symmetrical. The hand deformities may affect both post-axial and pre-axial borders but do not necessarily correlate with the severity of proximal limb deformity.[39]

Basic science/disease process

The exact cause is unknown but it is likely to be as a result of a problem earlier *in utero* than radial deficiency, probably during weeks 5–6 of development.

Similar deficiencies have been induced in rats experimentally using busulphan tetralogic agents[40] and acetazolamide[41] and in fetal white leghorn chickens by cauterization of the post-axial are of the limb bud immediately after formation of the limb bud but before that of the hand plate.[42] There is disruption to the zone of polarizing activity, probably due to a loss of sonic hedgehog function, which prevents the development of an ulna.

Commonly ulnar club hand is an isolated finding in an otherwise healthy child although cardiovascular anomalies have been reported and ulnar dysplasia is also seen as part of a number of syndromes that are inherited, usually in an autosomal dominant or recessive manner *(Table 26.4)*.

Diagnosis/patient presentation

Patients with ulnar deficiencies present with a wide variety of congenital upper limb appearances and complaints. These

Table 26.4 Syndromes associated with ulnar longitudinal deficiency

Syndrome	Associated abnormalities
Cornelia de Lange syndrome	Microcephaly, cleft palate, cardiac defects, severe developmental delay
Schinzel syndrome	VSD, pyloric stenosis, anal stenosis, reduced sweating
Weyer ulnar ray oligodactyly syndrome	Midline craniofacial anomalies, fibular defects, renal and splenic abnormalities
Ulnar mammary syndrome	Hypoplasia of breasts nipples and apocrine glands, abnormal teeth and genitalia
Femoral-fibular-ulnar deficiency syndrome	Short stature, fibula hypoplasia, talipes equinovarus
Ulnar fibula dysplasia	Short stature, fibula hypoplasia, mandibular hypoplasia
Klippel–Feil syndrome	Short webbed neck, cervical vertebral abnormalities

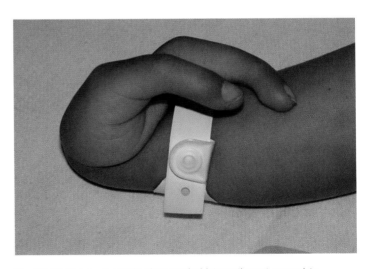

Fig. 26.27 Ulna ray dysplasia where surgical intervention not appropriate.

usually relate to the hand and elbow, although shoulder deficiency may also be present. The poor aesthetics of the upper limb may distract both parents and clinician from appreciating the limb function *(Fig. 26.27)*.

The most common classification system is the Bayne classification *(Table 26.5, Fig. 26.28)*. Although this concentrates on the degree of ulnar deficiency and is simple to apply, it does not account for any involvement of the rest of the upper limb nor does it determine treatment or likely functional outcome.

An alternative classification that relates better to possible treatment strategies for the forearm was suggested by Paley and Herzenberg *(Table 26.6)*.[43] Since there are similarities, it is important to be clear which classification is being used.

Table 26.5 Bayne classification of ulnar longitudinal deficiency

Bayne classification	Ulnar deficiency
I	Ulnar hypoplasia
II	Partial ulnar aplasia
III	Total ulnar aplasia
IV	Radiohumeral synostosis

After Bayne LG, Klug MS. Long-term review of the surgical treatment of radial deficiencies. J Hand Surg Am 1987; 12(2):169–179.

Table 26.6 Paley and Herzenberg classification of ulnar longitudinal deficiency

Paley and Herzenberg classification	Ulnar deficiency
I	Ulnar hypoplasia with distal epiphysis intact
II	Partial ulnar aplasia – absent distal ⅓
III	Partial ulnar aplasia – absent distal ⅔
IV	Total ulnar aplasia
V	Radiohumeral synostosis

(After Paley D, Herzenberg JE. Distraction treatment of the forearm. In: Buck-Gramcko D, ed. Congenital malformations of the hand and forearm. London: Churchill Livingstone; 1998:90–92.)

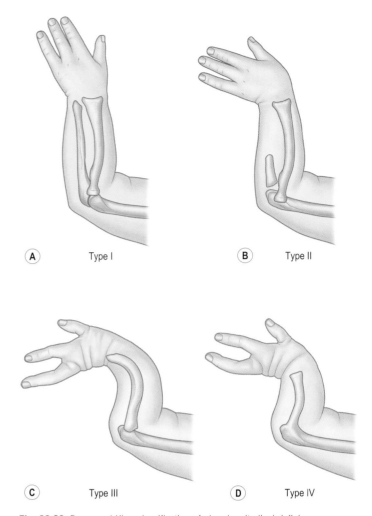

Fig. 26.28 Bayne and Klug classification of ulnar longitudinal deficiency.

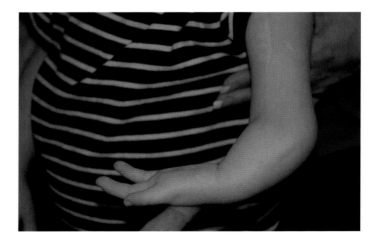

Fig. 26.29 Ulna ray dysplasia where humeral osteotomy has helped to position the hand better in space.

The limb may be positioned such that the hand faces backwards *(Fig. 26.29)*. The elbow may be fixed in either extension or flexion with synostosis affecting radiohumeral or ulnohumeral segments. Alternatively, the elbow may move but be unstable. The range of motion and its arc may vary with the degree of ulna deficiency although frequently there is a lack of full elbow extension.

In mild cases, the elbow may appear to function well until teenage years when the child may develop a lump on the posterolateral aspect which becomes painful and unsightly. This represents a dislocated radial head.

The forearm is short and the radius may be bowed with the radial head dislocated and the hand appearing ulnar deviated. Pronation and supination are restricted or absent depending on the severity of ulna deficiency and the presence or absence of associated radioulnar synostosis.

The wrist is relatively stable compared with the elbow, although the skeletally mature wrist will show carpal hypoplasia and coalitions. It may be ulnarly deviated although this is rarely progressive and is mild compared to the deviation seen in radial club hand. The pisiform is always absent and, as may be, the hamate, triquetral, capitate and trapezoid.

Hand abnormalities are expected. The absence of some digits (ectrodactyly) being the most frequent anomaly. Unlike in radial ray dysplasia, there may be both preaxial and postaxial abnormalities with thumb and first web deficiencies being common and often combined with post-axial hypoplasia and occasionally pre-axial duplication *(Fig. 26.30)*.

The post-axial border of the hand is always affected but commonly where several digits are missing both pre-axial and post-axial digits are missing. The thumb is often hypoplastic to some degree, lies in the same plane as the fingers and syndactyly with other digits is frequent. The digits that remain may be normal but they often have either camptodactyly or a deficiency of long flexor tendons. They may demonstrate

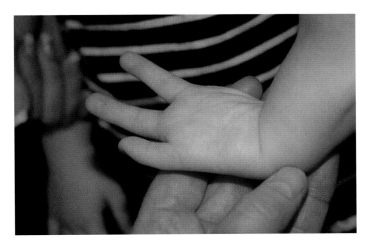

Fig. 26.30 Ulnar deficiency with concomitant radial deficiency in the hand.

Table 26.7 Paley and Herzenberg classification and treatment algorithm

Paley and Herzenberg type	Treatment
I without radial head dislocation	Repeated ulnar lengthening or radial shortening or both, with correction of radial bow
I with radial head dislocation	Repeated ulnar corrective osteotomy and radial shortening or ulnar corrective osteotomy and lengthening
II	Bone transport of ulna distally to support carpus
III	Creation of one bone forearm
IV	Corrective radial osteotomy
V	Osteotomy at elbow to improve elbow position and forearm osteotomy to improve rotation

After Paley D, Herzenberg JE. Distraction treatment of the forearm. In: Buck-Gramcko D, ed. Congenital malformations of the hand and forearm. London: Churchill Livingstone; 1998:90–92.

complete syndactyly and there may be a suppressed digit between them, although this pattern may fit better with a cleft hand. In a three digit hand, it is usually the thumb, middle and ring fingers which are the most likely to be present.

The arterial anatomy of the limb may be altered with an absent radial artery in half of cases and a persistent median artery in 16.7%. This is associated with abnormalities of the deep palmar arch and digital arteries. This only occurs where there is dysplasia of the ulna.

Function depends on the exact pattern of limb deformity, whether it is bilateral and on any associated developmental delay. Both power grip and key pinch are reduced compared with normal individuals, as are timed dexterity tests. However, adaptation produces good function in the majority of individuals.

Patient selection

This is dependent on the individual anatomy with the surgeon's aim to improve function between thumb and digits. It is the varied abnormalities of the hand that occupy most of the surgeon's time in this condition as this is where he can most reliably improve functional capability. Elbow and forearm procedures, although frequently requested are less reliable in improving function and are more controversial.

The outcome will also depend on the intellectual capability of the patient but it is rare that surgical procedures are determined by this.

Treatment/surgical technique

Surgery needs to first address the position that the limb can occupy in space. Humeral rotation osteotomies may reposition the hand so it lies within the child's sight. This is usually performed below the deltoid insertion. Attempts to release the elbow and gain range of motion have been tried at less than 6 months of age but results have been poor with a gradual loss of the motion obtained at operation. Elbow arthroplasty has not been found to be useful here. If the elbow is poorly positioned, humeral osteotomy may allow a change of position to allow certain tasks but the surgeon must be wary that this may deprive the child of other functions.

Radial head dislocation is being treated in some centers with distraction lengthening of the ulna but the ability to reposition the radial head in joint may not reflect its ability to stay there. Long-term follow-up is required to assess whether this is worthwhile since the relatively poor ulna growth will require this to be repeated several times during childhood. Radial head excision before skeletal maturity is associated with disruption of the forearm mechanics and the interosseous membrane with the development of wrist pain and deformity. The radial head is often excised, if dislocated, during adolescence but the long-term result of excision is likely to be similar, albeit not so severe, effects on the forearm and wrist. The production of a one-bone forearm is an option if elbow instability is severe.

Early excision of the fibrocartilaginous anlage at the distal end of the ulna has not been shown to be effective in preventing radial bowing but is still controversial and continues to be performed sporadically. Care has to be taken to protect the ulna nerve and artery and it is not necessary to excise the whole length of the anlage but a segment needs to be removed. Correction of the radial bow by osteotomy with or without ulna lengthening is worthwhile to improve the aesthetic appearance and may be done through the ulnar incision used for excision of the anlage.

A potential algorithm for treatment has been proposed in relation to the Paley and Herzenberg classification as shown in *Table 26.7* but the authors would caution that long-term results on these children are unknown and application of the same principles to radial longitudinal deficiencies, where the emphasis has been on skeletal realignment without discussion of the soft tissue anomalies and forces applied by them, has failed to correct the deficiency in the long term and has produced a group of children who have undergone multiple interventions without sustained long-term benefit.

Correction of the hand deformities is most likely to produce functional benefit *(Fig. 26.31)*. The hand deformities need to

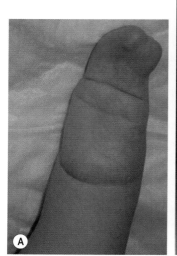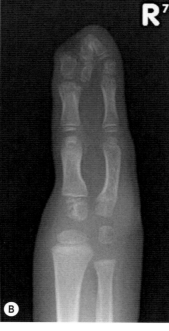

Fig. 26.31 (A,B) Ulna ray dysplasia where surgical intervention may assist function.

be addressed according to individual needs but are likely to include surgery to improve the first web, release of digital syndactyly and metacarpal osteotomies to provide pulp to pulp opposition of the existing fingers and thumb. Usually, this is possible using a standard syndactyly type release with full thickness skin grafting early on with later osteotomies. In the most severe cases, where the adductor pollicis is likely to need extensive release, microsurgical free flaps may be needed to provide a sufficiently large web space between the thumb and fingers.

Metacarpal or phalangeal osteotomies, to rotate the digits to provide opposition pinch, need to be performed at an age where there is sufficient bone stock to provide two point fixation and therefore control rotation. In the two digit hand, it is rarely possible to achieve pulp to pulp opposition with rotation osteotomy of the first metacarpal alone and the authors would expect to need to operate on both digits to turn them towards each other.

Occasionally in the absence of a thumb, pollicization may be required but this may be resisted by the parents as the

post-axial digits may also be deficient and they may be unwilling to risk surgery on one of the remaining better functioning digits or to lose the normal appearance of a three or four digit hand in order to make a thumb. Free toe transfer to create a thumb is dependent on having sufficient spare motors to make this useful.

Where there is thumb duplication, this may be addressed normally but there may be instances where the hand is so abnormal, that operating on the thumb duplication may adversely affect hand function without any significant overall aesthetic benefit. It this case, surgical intervention is contraindicated.

Postoperative care

The requirement for dressings, therapy and splintage is dependent on the procedure performed. Any attempt at ulna lengthening is likely to need repeating multiple times. All patients need follow-up until skeletal maturity.

Outcomes, prognosis, and complications

As most surgeons only have small series of these patients with widely differing patterns of involvement, the outcomes of surgery at skeletal maturity are largely unknown. However, functional adaptation appears good where the patient is nonsyndromic.

In teenage years, the appearance of the forearm, elbow and hand is inclined to attain greater significance for the patient than previously. This is an appropriate time to consider adjustment of the positioning of the elbow if required for certain tasks but it is worth first assessing where prosthetics may help. Scarring from previous surgery is most likely to become tight in the teenage growth spurt and may require revision.

This may be combined with revision of areas around the nail folds that may be problematic for functional or aesthetic reasons.

Any procedure that attempts to equalize the lengths of the radius and ulna is likely to need repeating multiple times during skeletal growth. It also harbors a risk of tightening long digital flexors, worsening wrist stability and dislocating an unstable elbow.

Secondary procedures

The mainstay of surgical procedures would be repeated distraction for radial head dislocation or to increase forearm length. Otherwise, further surgery is largely be related to minor revisions for web creep after syndactyly release.

Access the complete references list online at **http://www.expertconsult.com**

9. Schenker M, Wiberg M, Kay SP, et al. Precision grip function after free toe transfer in children with hypoplastic digits. *J Plast Reconstr Aesthet Surg.* 2007;60(1):13–23.

   The authors examined in detail the precision grips of the microvascular toe transfer in 13 patients: they concluded that sensory recovery was to normal if performed before the age of

8 years, that all adapted grip to object weight but malalignment of the digit could affect efficacy of the transfer in use. They postulated that the lack of intrinsic muscles was partly to blame.

15. Goldfarb CA, Manske PR, Busa R, et al. Upper-extremity phocomelia re-examined: a longitudinal dysplasia. *J Bone Joint Surg Am.* 2005;87(12):2639–2648.

The authors reviewed the notes and radiographs of 41 patients with 60 extremities diagnosed with phocomelia – all could be reclassified into severe forms of radial or ulnar longitudinal dysplasia – none had a true intercalary deficiency.

16. Heikel HVA. Aplasia and hypoplasia of the radius: studies on 64 cases and on epiphyseal transplantation in rabbits with the imitated defect. *Acta Orthop Scand.* 1959;39(Suppl):1–154.

    This is one of the first large series detailing the anatomy and the natural history of radial club hand.

18. Petit JL. Remarques sur un enfant nouveau-ne, dont les bras e-taient difformes. In: *Memoires de l'Academie Royale des Sciences.* Paris: Imprimere Royale; 1733:17.

19. Lamb DW. Radial club hand. A continuing study of sixty-eight patients with one hundred and seventeen club hands. *J Bone Joint Surg Am.* 1977; 59(1):1–13.

    This remains a seminal piece of work about the subject and its management and includes advice about the stiff elbow and problems with recurrence in a volar direction – subjects which are still discussed today.

38. Miura T, Komada T. Simple method for reconstruction of the cleft hand with an adducted thumb. *Plast Reconstr Surg.* 1979;64:65–67.

    The authors describe their skin incisions used to transpose an index finger in an ulnar direction in a simpler fashion than the Snow–Littler technique.

27

Congenital hand III: Disorders of formation – thumb hypoplasia

Joseph Upton III and Amir Taghinia

SYNOPSIS

- The thumb ray is the prime ray of the hand – its size, position, mobility, independence, and relations to the other digits are critical to function.

- The thumb is considered hypoplastic if any portion of the ray, skeletal or soft tissue, is deficient or absent.

- Growth and function of the thumb in the first year of life follows a predictable pattern.

- Although new procedures have expanded options for reconstruction, standard procedures such as first web space deepening, tendon transfers, and collateral ligament reconstruction remain predictable and reliable.

- Pollicization continues to be the treatment of choice for severe hypoplasia with a nonfunctional carpometacarpal joint, the floating thumb, and the absent thumb.

- Associated conditions of thumb hyperplasia include VACTERL, Fanconi anemia and other hematologic abnormalities, Holt–Oram syndrome, and thrombocytopenia absent radius (TAR) syndrome

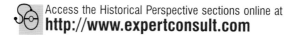

Access the Historical Perspective sections online at
http://www.expertconsult.com

Introduction

The hypoplastic thumb represents a wide spectrum of functional and aesthetic differences. Before classification and management of the deficient thumb, a careful surgeon must assess its: (1) size; (2) position; (3) relation to other fingers of the hand; (4) osseous components; (5) joint integrity and stability; (6) intrinsic and extrinsic musculotendinous units; (7) first web space depth and width; (8) associated malformations of the hand and elsewhere, and (9) functional consequences for the child. A thumb should be considered hypoplastic when there is a deficiency of any one or all structures that contribute

to the "normal" thumb. In the past, all definitions were restricted to the radiographic appearance alone; however, presently, we understand that soft tissue deficiencies also contribute to the overall diagnosis.

For the first 3 months of life, the thumb is adducted and flexed within the palm and serves primarily as a pacifier. By 9 months of age, though, this first ray gains its independence and mobility from the palm, and at a year of age, it has become a crucial portion of the hand.[1] In the normal hand, the strength and mobility needed for a wide variety of pinch and grasp functions rapidly develop, and by the time the baby is ambulatory, the thumb is used creatively and independently to manipulate the environment.

As relied upon in the past, a complete evaluation of the osteoarticular column will require plain radiographs. Normal primary ossification centers of the phalanges and metacarpal of the thumb appear in the second to fourth fetal months, but abnormalities of the skeleton of the thumb (e.g., triangular bones) may not be seen radiographically until well into the first or second year of life. Secondary ossification centers within the epiphyses of the thumb normally appear between 13 months to 4 years of age.[2] The delayed appearance of both primary and secondary ossification centers in the hypoplastic thumb is highly relevant to the diagnostic process because their appearance is often delayed in proportion to the degree of hypoplasia.

Basic science/disease process

Incidence

The true incidence of thumb hypoplasia is difficult to determine due to the large number of congenital malformations within which a hypoplastic thumb is a component part. All reported reviews are subject to study of the genetic composition of the patient population as well as any discrepancies of nomenclature and sampling. Entin[15,16] reported a 16%

incidence of thumb hypoplasia in his Canadian patients, while Flatt published an 11.2% incidence of thumb abnormalities and a 3.6% incidence of thumb hypoplasia or aplasia.[3] We have seen a 37% incidence within our entire registry, which includes many additional categories.[17] The majority of the children treated surgically are those with radial dysplasia – with and without a partial or complete absence of the radius. We have also seen a large incidence in syndromic patients, such as those with the Apert syndrome, who are commonly referred to large children's hospitals for treatment of their multiple malformations.

Etiology

Because radial or preaxial longitudinal deficiencies occur in many conditions with a wide variety of etiologies, the causes for these malformations span the entire spectrum of genetic, environmental, teratogenic and other factors (Table 27.1). Therefore, consultation with a genetic specialist is strongly recommended, and referral to standard genetic textbooks or the OMIM website[18] is a must for any responsible hand surgeon.

Associated conditions

The many potential associations with thumb and radial hypoplasias and aplasia may involve any organ system within the body. Most significant are those with the cardiovascular, gastrointestinal and genitourinary involvement. Associated hematologic problems, specifically Fanconi anemia, can be detected early but usually become clinically apparent later in childhood. The most common of these associated conditions is outlined herein.

Table 27.1 Thumb/radial hypoplasia/aplasia associations

	Frequent in	Occasional in
Thumb[a]/radial[b] hypoplasia/aplasia	Aase syndrome[a,b] Baller–Gerold syndrome[a,b] Facio-auriculo-vertebral spectrum[a] Fanconi syndrome[a,b] Holt–Oram syndrome[a,b] Levy–Hollister syndrome[a,b] Nager syndrome[a] Radial aplasia-thrombocytopenia (TAR) Syndrome[a,b] Roberts–SC phocomelia syndrome[a,b] Rothmund–Thomson syndrome[a] Townes syndrome[a] VACTERL association[a,b] 13q-syndrome[a] EEC syndrome	Cat-eye syndrome[b] de Lange syndrome[a,b] Fetal aminopterin effects[a] Feta; valporate effects[a] Fibrodysplasia ossificans Progressive[a] MURCS association[a] Najer syndrome[b] Seckel syndrome[b] Trisomy 13 syndrome[b] Trisomy 18 syndrome[b]
Metacarpal hypoplasia – first[c], all[d]	CHILD syndrome[d] Coffin–Siris syndrome[d] Cohen syndrome[d] Diastrophic dysplasia[c] Dyggve–Melchior–Clausen syndrome[c] Grebe syndrome[d] Oro-palato-digital syndrome, type II[d] Partial trisomy 10q syndrome[c] Poland anomaly[d] Ruvalcaba syndrome[d] Short rib-polydactyly, Majewski type[d] Short rib-polydactyly, non-Majewski type[d] Tricho-rhino-phalangeal syndrome[d] Trisomy 9p syndrome[d] 5p-syndrome[d] 18q-syndrome[d]	de Lange syndrome[c] Larsen syndrome[d] Robinow syndrome[d] Triploidy syndrome[c]
Broad thumb	Apert syndrome Carpenter syndrome Pfeiffer's syndrome Rubinstein–Tabyi syndrome Saethre–Chotzen syndrome	Robinow syndrome Trisomy 13 syndrome

Modified from Jones KL. Smith's recognizable patterns of human malformations, 5th edn. Philadelphia: WB Saunders; 1997.
The [a,b,c,d] refers to the hypoplasia/aplasia associations of the listed syndromes. For example, Aase syndrome has both thumb and radial hypoplasia but Nager syndrome has just thumb hypoplasia.

VACTERL

These children may have a wide spectrum of anomalies, including: *V*ertebral malformations; *A*nal atresia or hypoplasias; *C*ardiovascular anomalies; all degrees of *T*racheo-esophageal fistuli; *E*sophageal atresia; *R*enal malformations, and *L*imb abnormalities – which in the upper extremity involve all degrees of radial dysplasia. A patient does not need to fulfill every category on this list to be considered VACTERL.

Fanconi anemia and other hematologic abnormalities[19]

Fanconi (FA) children develop all degrees of a pancytopenia, which can be life-threatening.[20,21] Most are small with slow growth. Although many other organ systems may be abnormal, deficiencies of the thumb and, to a lesser extent, the entire radial ray are the most common and are present at birth in over half of these cases. Although in the past FA children were rarely diagnosed early in life, this condition can now be diagnosed at birth with a DEB test.[20,22] However, because this test involves an unstable gas, butane, it is not available in all medical centers. Other types of treatable childhood anemias, such as the Blackfan type, may occur in the later childhood years and are easily distinguished by routine hematologic tests including the DEB.[21] Treatment of FA children with oxymetholone and prednisone therapy has a 70% response rate, and nonresponders can be treated with bone marrow transplantation.[20]

Holt–Oram syndrome

Two pediatricians, Dr Holt in Philadelphia and Dr Oram in London, independently described the association of congenital heart disease and radial longitudinal defects of the upper limb, and their names have subsequently been associated with all degrees of congenital cardiovascular malformations and radial dysplasias. Interestingly, there is no correlation between the severities of the anatomic deficiency in one system relative to the other. Common to the upper limbs are a stiff hypoplastic thumb joined to a stiff index digit by a complete simple syndactyly, radial deficiencies, and proximal radioulnar synostoses. Often, hypoplasia of the glenohumeral joint is not diagnosed until adolescence when shoulder abduction is diminished.

Thrombocytopenia absent radius syndrome (TAR)

This unique group of children may be born with normal hematologic parameters, but they usually have a low platelet count, which may decrease rapidly during the first year of life. They are easily distinguished from other types of radial dysplasia due to the presence of a thumb despite all degrees of radial deficiencies. The thumb is hypoplastic, and extrinsic flexion and extension vary tremendously. Thenar intrinsic muscles are usually present and provide some palmar abduction by age 2 years of age. The low platelet count commonly reaches normal levels by ages 4–5 years, and the clinical results from centralization are among the best.

Diagnosis and patient presentation

Classification

The varying degrees of differences between hypoplastic thumbs have been classified in a number of ways that have few common characteristics.[23] Nevertheless, a well-accepted classification system has emerged that guides treatment. The five designated types of thumb hypoplasia-aplasia are shown in *Figure 27.1*. These anomalies are commonly associated with radial (preaxial) dysplasia, and the majority of congenital hand surgeons consider most types of thumb with a normal radius as part of this spectrum. It is well recognized that there are concomitant soft tissue anomalies that accompany the skeletal abnormalities. Since the correlation of soft tissue and skeletal deficiencies has been so well defined, this refined system works very well for clinical decision-making.

Hypoplasia of the thumb is associated with many other congenital differences, specifically central and transverse deficiencies. Because the anatomical make-up of the thumb does not always allow for easy categorization under the current system, we have included five additional categories,[17] which include the constriction ring syndrome, central deficiencies, radial duplication, the five-fingered hand, and short skeletal rays. In these conditions, the thumb ray usually has characteristic deficiencies that would fall into the German type II and III hypoplasia categories[24] and the anatomical abnormalities relevant to clinical decision-making will be presented here.

Clinical presentation (types of hypoplasia)

In the past, routine radiographs were the sole tool used for diagnosis of the hypoplastic thumb. However, this mode of assessment did not reveal any detail about the normal and abnormal soft tissue structures of individual hands. Therefore, surgeons today use a more complete analysis of intrinsic muscles, web space size, intrinsic muscles, extrinsic tendons, joint stability, and function – all of which impact directly upon treatment.

Type I: mild hypoplasia

In this most mild type of hypoplasia, the thumb is slender and slightly shorter than a normally configured first ray *(Fig. 27.2)*. The phalanges and metacarpal can be slightly thinner than

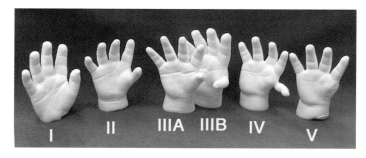

Fig. 27.1 Thumb hypoplasia. Molds of the right hand in six children with the five classic types of thumb hypoplasia are displayed. Type III has been subclassified into two categories: one with (IIIA) and intact CMC joint and one without (IIIB) an intact CMC joint. The type IV is often called the *pouce flottant* or floating thumb.

Type I

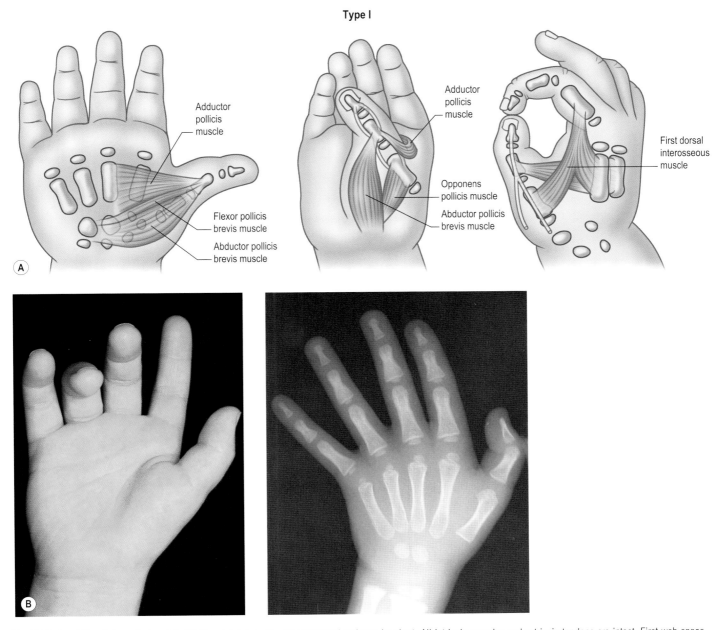

Fig. 27.2 Type I thumb hypoplasia-mild. **(A)** The skeletal ray is well segmented and may be short. All intrinsic muscles and extrinsic tendons are intact. First web space narrowing is minimal to moderate. **(B)** Clinical appearance and **(C)** radiograph of a child who did not require any surgical correction. Although his thenar muscles are weak, there were no significant functional problems.

usual, but the trapezium and scaphoid are present and the distal radius and styloid process are not affected. The interphalangeal (IP), metacarpophalangeal (MP), and carpometacarpal (CMC) joints are stable and exhibit normal passive and active motion. While there may be a slight hypoplasia and weakness of the abductor pollicis brevis (AbPB), opponens pollicis (OP) and lateral head of the flexor pollicis brevis (FPB) muscles, all intrinsic muscles are present.[24] The joints, ligament and capsules, tendons, nerves, and vascular structures are all normal, and there may be minimal narrowing of the first web space.

Type II: moderate hypoplasia

The metacarpal and phalanges are all present but small, and the trapezium, trapezoid, scaphoid, and – to a lesser extent – lunate may be hypoplastic. The first web space is short with the thumb adducted, the ulnar collateral ligament at the MP joint lax, and median innervated thenar muscles underdeveloped or occasionally absent *(Fig. 27.3)*.[25] Normally, the flexor pollicis brevis (FPB) and opponens pollicis (OP) are innervated by the median nerve, but the FPB varies, reported to be 40% median, 48% ulnar, and 12% both median and ulnar.[26]

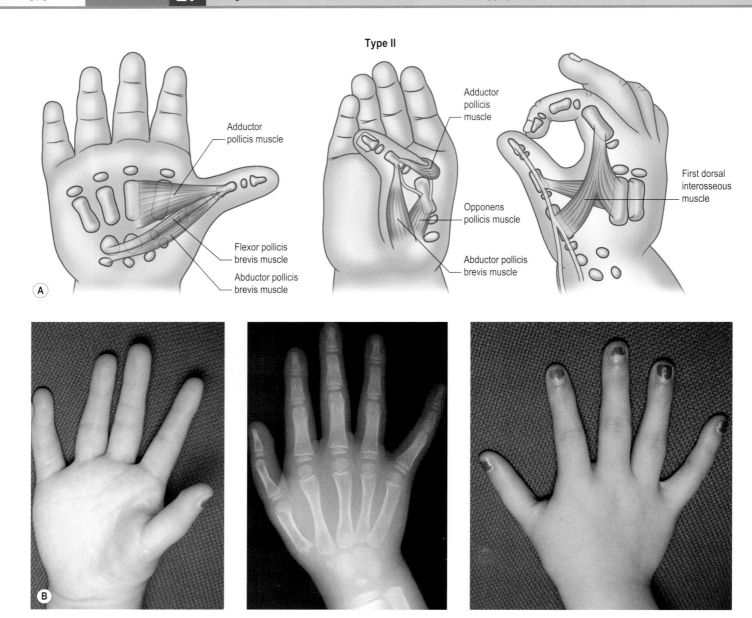

Fig. 27.3 Type II thumb hypoplasia-moderate. **(A)** There is minimal to moderate shortening of the skeletal ray. All bones are present and ligaments at the MP joint may be lax. The ulnar innervated intrinsic muscles, AddP and first DI (second metacarpal origin) are strong, and the median innervated intrinsics are very weak. Anomalous anatomy is common. Adduction contractures from fibrous structures and MP joint instability accompany a deficient first web space. **(B)** Clinical appearance and radiograph of a child with a type II hypoplasia of the right hand. The thenar intrinsic muscles are hypoplastic, the first web space tight, and the thumb much narrower than normal. Key pinch was weak, and the patient could not hold heavy objects between the thumb and digits. In addition, the ulnar collateral ligament was weak at the MP joint.

The ulnar innervated intrinsics, particularly the adductor pollicis (AddP), pull the metacarpal into adduction and narrow the first web space, which when explored surgically has tight fibrous bands between muscle groups. Type II thumbs contain two neurovascular bundles, and the recurrent motor branch of the median nerve is consistently found.

Many different muscle and tendon anomalies seen on the radial side of the hand have been identified in conjunction with the type II and IIIA thumbs. In fact, the clinical designation of a given thumb may vary greatly due to this large spectrum of soft tissue abnormalities. Obviously, the absence of interphalangeal (IP) or metacarpophalangeal (MP) flexion or extension creases in a slender thumb is the best clinical indicator of flexor and/or extensor abnormalities. Within this designation, many variations of the long flexor to the thumb (FPL) may be found. Both the tendon and the muscle belly of the FPL may be abnormal,[27] may have proximal duplications,[28–32] and may have a more radial distal insertion.[30] In some patients, one can observe this muscle originating from the index profundus tendon,[29] the transverse carpal ligament, or the fascia of the thenar intrinsics and inserting into the flexor sheath[28] and/or the extensor mechanism.[33] In other cases, this muscle may be absent entirely.[9,34–38] Some of these anomalies may represent abnormal radial wrist extensors or short thumb abductors instead of malformed or malpositioned terminal thumb flexors.[39] Occasionally, a small abnormal "musculus lumbricalis pollicis" muscle may extend from the thumb origin across the first web space and attach to the flexor system of the index finger.[40] We have seen this peculiar (atavistic) muscle extending across the first web space in children with the Freeman–Sheldon syndrome and in complex thumb duplications at the metacarpal level.

In addition, the extrinsic extensors may have abnormal insertions,[41,42] extend over the MP joint in a noncentralized position, and reveal abnormal connections with the extrinsic flexor.[31,33,40,43] These abnormal insertions of both flexor and extensors, combined with their deviated course, conspire to make both tendons act primarily as radial deviators and not primary flexors or extensors. In addition, the lax ulnar collateral ligament at the MP joint results in an abduction of the phalangeal portion of the thumb. Tupper has called this "pollex abductus" and noted that when these muscles contract, there is no IP flexion or extension, only abduction or radial deviation of the thumb. Many anatomical variations of this structure exist, but the functional result is the same (Fig. 27.4). A recent paper by Graham et al. has summarized the large list of muscle and tendon abnormalities, which often originate in the forearm.[31] Although type II thumbs may present with these intra-tendinous connections, the abducted posture and wide degree of muscle and tendon anomalies are primarily seen with type IIIA thumbs (Fig. 27.4). When followed proximally to the wrist and forearm level, many of these tendons have abnormal origins and long muscle bellies that extend well beyond the wrist into the metacarpal region.

Type III: severe hypoplasia

In these cases, the degree of skeletal shortening and narrowing is much more pronounced, particularly at the metacarpal level (Figs 27.5, 27.6). The hand and wrist may be radially deviated due to hypoplastic/aplastic carpal bones. The trapezium is usually very small, and frequently the scaphoid is absent. The distal radius is smaller in size and the styloid process absent, giving the radius a blunted appearance.[44] The extreme amount of anatomic variation within this group prompted Manske and colleagues to subdivide this group into type III-A with a full-length metacarpal and an intact CMC joint and type III-B with a tapered first metacarpal and no CMC joint.[45] Buck-Gramcko has included an additional variation which we shall call type III-C thumb which possesses only the metacarpal.[46] There are no tendons or muscles in this variant, and the skin bridge is much wider than that seen in type IV. In the B and C variants, a fibrous band may connect the hypoplastic metacarpal to a cartilaginous nubbin that represents either a trapezium or metacarpal base. Often, a small abductor pollicis tendon attaches to this remnant.

Median innervated intrinsic muscles are either severely hypoplastic or absent entirely; however, if they are present, they may actively flex the MP joint. The ulnar innervated adductor pollicis (AddP) pulls the metacarpal medially. The MP joint is lax on both radial and ulnar sides and anatomically either collateral ligament and the volar plate may be severely hypoplastic or missing. The small thumb with a short web space is abducted at the MP joint due to the frequent pollex abductus deformity. The radial origin of the first dorsal

interosseous from the thumb metacarpal is more severely affected than that from the index metacarpal. In the forearm, radial head is usually hypoplastic and commonly subluxed, occasionally dislocated.

Abnormal anatomy is the rule. The many intrinsic and extrinsic anatomical variations described within the type II group may exist with greater degrees of hypoplasia. Usually, the extrinsic flexor and extensor are present and weak, but in some cases they may be missing.[34,38,41] The flexor retinaculum is poorly developed with either attenuation or absence of the major pulleys. In some patients, the motor branch of the median nerve is absent, and there may only be one neurovascular bundle.[29] The radial origin of the first dorsal interosseous to the index finger is severely hypoplastic, and the first web space is severely restricted. Pollex abductus anomalies are common and must be recognized if IP flexion and/or extension is to be achieved.

Type IV: floating thumb

These thumbs (pouce flottant, French; pendeldaumen, German) arise distally from the palm and usually lie along the radial midaxial border (Fig. 27.7). They are attached only by a soft tissue pedicle, which has been described by Littler as "Nature's own neurovascular pedicle," due to the presence of a digital artery, two vena comitantes, and one or two nerves within the skin bridge.[47] There may be anomalous vascular or neural rings, involving neurovascular structures[1,5] that could affect the outcome of a pollicization. There is no metacarpal, and two small phalanges tend to be present within the soft tissue envelope, which contains a nail. It is important to note that a diminutive nail represents the presence of a distal phalanx. Intrinsic muscles do not insert onto these bones. A first dorsal interosseous muscle (abductor indicis) may be detected by abduction of the index finger. At the carpal level, the trapezium and less often the scaphoid are missing. The radial styloid may be absent, but the distal end of the radius is normal in most of these children.

Type V: aplasia

The thumb is completely absent in this category (Fig. 27.8). In half of our patients[48] and half those reported by Flatt,[49] there is an associated deficiency of the radius. When the radius is normal, the index digit is normal and has strong abduction at the MP joint due to the presence of a strong first dorsal interosseous muscle (e.g., abductor indicis). Many of these children with a normal radius will demonstrate "auto pollicization." The pulp of the index finger widens and the digit pronates and sits in a more abducted position resulting in a widening of the intermetacarpal space and attenuation of the intermetacarpal ligament. At best, this posture is a poor substitute for normal key pinch. In the case of a deficient radius, the index ray is stiffer, shorter, and often joined by a simple syndactyly to the long digit. There is a direct correlation between the degree of radial hypoplasia and the index finger deficiencies; the index ray is never normal when there are significant associated radial deficiencies. In these hands, the degree of stiffness decreases from the radial to the ulnar digits and the fifth finger is always the best on the hand.

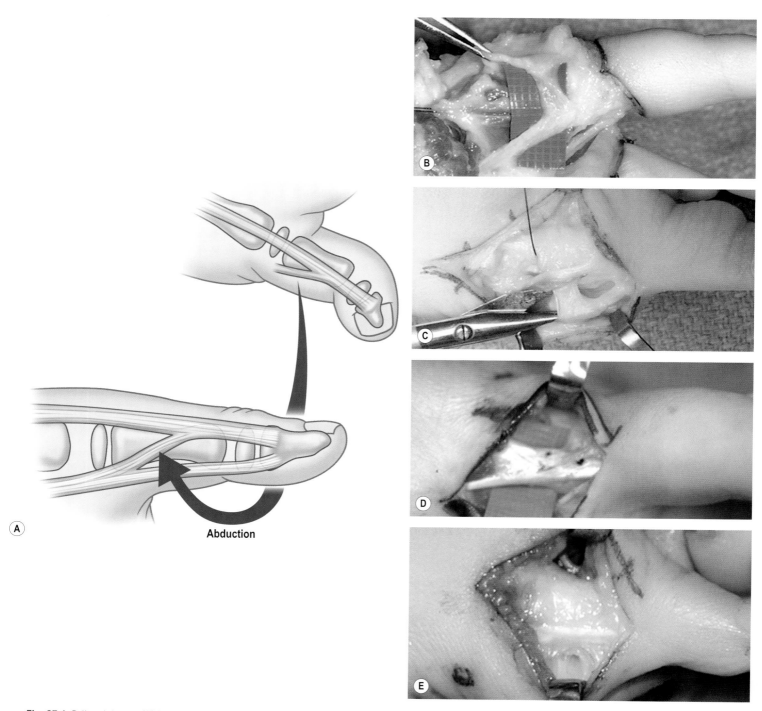

Fig. 27.4 Pollex abductus. **(A)** In severe type II and many type III thumbs, there may be very little, if any, IP joint flexion and there may be a radial deviation of the thumb at the MP joint. This is due to the abduction force created by the combined action of the extrinsic flexor and extensor tendons joined by intertendinous connections, the "pollex abductus." **(B-E)** Within types II and III thumb hypoplasias (and proximal thumb polydactylies), a very wide spectrum of intra-tendinous connections may vary between a wide, loose, almost areolar band (top) to a complete coalition the flexor and extensor into a single tendon. With excursion from either the flexor or extensor side, the resultant movement in all these thumbs is abduction of the MP joint.

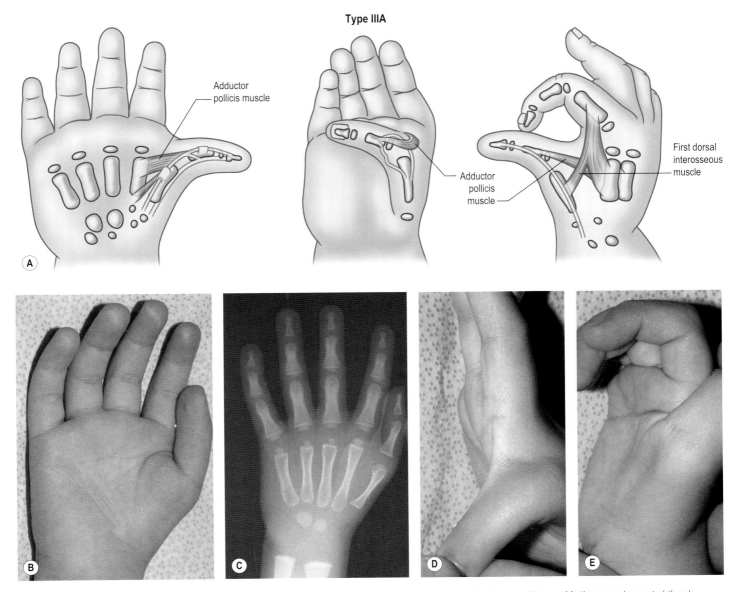

Type IIIA

Adductor pollicis muscle

Adductor pollicis muscle

First dorsal interosseous muscle

Fig. 27.5 Type IIIA thumb hypoplasia-severe. **(A)** These thumbs exhibit more severe skeletal hypoplasia, including the carpal bones. Median nerve innervated thumb intrinsic muscles are severely hypoplastic or absent, and the ulnar-innervated muscles are present but weak. Extrinsic tendons are abnormal, the "pollex abductus" deformity is frequent, the first web space is small, and the MP joint is unstable (more on the ulnar than the radial sides). The CMC joint and thumb metacarpal are intact in IIIA thumbs. **(B-E)** The clinical appearance and radiograph show a short slender metacarpal, an intact CMC joint, severe hypoplasia of the thenar eminence and a lax MP joint. The absent IP flexion crease is indicative of a deficient or absent FPL.

Type VI: central deficiencies: cleft hand and symbrachydactyly thumb

Cleft hand (typical)

Cleft hand is characterized by hypoplasia or aplasia of the central ray(s) of the hand thus forming a "V" or funnel-shaped cleft *(Fig. 27.9)*. All degrees of simple syndactyly of the first web are seen, resulting in moderate to severe deficiencies of the first web space. In addition, all degrees of hypoplasia, extending to aplasia of the central two rays, may exist.[9] The ulnar two digits in the ring and fifth positions are commonly webbed with simple syndactylies. The thumb in the cleft hand anomaly is usually slightly small with all components of the osteoarticular skeleton present. A Blauth type II thumb classification would be appropriate for the strict constructionist.[24] The wrist and forearm bones are normal, and the median innervated thenar intrinsics are present. The major deficiency of the thumb in this form of hypoplasia is that the ulnar innervated intrinsic muscles are severely hypoplastic or absent. In particular, the ulnar innervated adductor pollicis is usually severely hypoplastic or absent, and the first dorsal interosseous is moderately hypoplastic and contracted. The presence or absence of the third metacarpal is often an excellent

Type IIIB

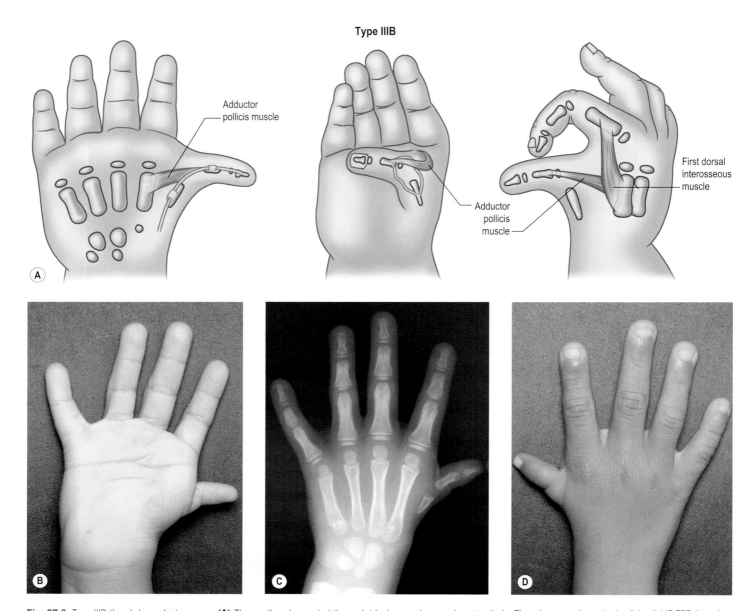

Fig. 27.6 Type IIIB thumb hypoplasia-severe. **(A)** The median- innervated thenar intrinsic muscles are absent entirely. There is severe hypoplasia of the AddP, FPB-lateral head, and the ulnar origin of the first DI. The CMC joint articulation of the proximal metacarpal is absent. The MP joint is very lax or absent on both radial and ulnar sides. Flexor and extensor extrinsic tendons are severely hypoplastic or absent. **(B, D)** Clinical appearance and **(C)** radiograph shows a 4-year-old patient with a well formed but functionless floppy thumb. There is no skeletal stability or extrinsic flexion or extension. Very small flexor or extensor tendons may be present and can result in some movement.

indicator of the status of the adductor pollicis muscle. Finally, the extrinsic flexor and extensor musculotendinous units to the thumb tend to be unaffected. ⊕ FIG **27.9** APPEARS ONLINE ONLY

In another variation of typical cleft hand, thumb polydactylies at all levels may be observed. The more distal type I and II polydactylies[50] are often associated with the absence of index phalanges that have an intact metacarpal. Super digits and transversely oriented tubular bones at the distal metacarpal level with complete absence of the index (and long) digits are often seen in this variation[51] With more proximal type III, IV and V polydactylies, the central (third) ray is often severely hypoplastic or absent.[52,53] Triphalangeal rays may also be

encountered with the proximal duplications at the metacarpal level.

Symbrachydactyly thumb

We refer to these atypical cleft hands as symbrachydactyly *(Fig. 27.10).* This form of deficiency is always unilateral, with varying degrees of hypoplasia of the central three rays of the hand. Nubbins with minute nail complexes may be present on the distal border of the palm, representing the index, long and ring fingers, but commonly these central three digits are completely absent with varying degrees of hypoplasia of the central three metacarpals. ⊕ FIG **27.10** APPEARS ONLINE ONLY

Type IV

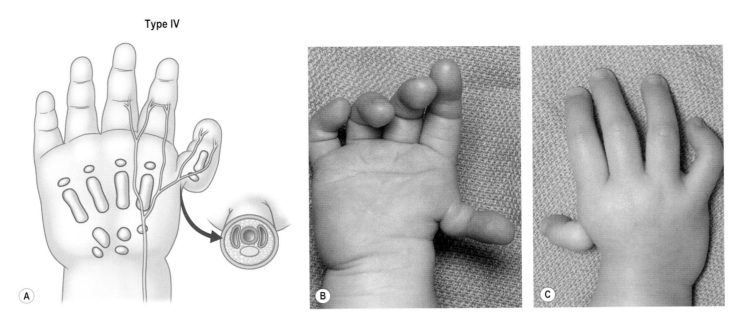

Fig. 27.7 Type IV thumb hypoplasia-floating thumb. **(A)** The hypoplastic thumb is attached to the hand only by a soft tissue bridge, which contains neurovascular structures and rarely hypoplastic tendons and fascia. There is no skeletal connection. **(B, C)** The attached thumb is small with diminutive phalanges and a nail. There is no active flexion or extension. The radial deviation of the wrist and hand is due to hypoplasia of the trapezium, scaphoid and lunate.

All degrees of variation exist, and no two hands are identical. The thumb in this condition is invariably smaller with severe hypoplasia or aplasia of the phalangeal components. Occasionally, a metacarpal and distal phalanx are present with a flail thumb at the MP joint level. With an intact third metacarpal, a functional adductor pollicis muscle is often present. Most of these thumbs have very weak adduction power. Usually, the median innervated thenar intrinsic muscles are intact and range from small to normal in size. The thumb CMC joint is well segmented and mobile, and the IP joint of the thumb may exhibit decreased passive and active motion due to weak extrinsic flexor and extensors. Upon exploration, the FPL tendon often courses to a hypoplastic or absent muscle belly in the distal forearm. In the severely hypoplastic thumb, there is marked limitation of MP and CMC motion, an absent IP flexion crease, and only a rudimentary FPL tendon. The anomalies seen with the extrinsic flexors and extensors are similar to those described for the types II and IIIA hypoplastic thumbs. The fifth ray is usually the best in the hand with intact intrinsic and extrinsic musculotendinous units. Frequently, this digit has a radial clinodactyly and a completely unstable MP joint, and the entire hand is hypoplastic. Radius and ulna are present and of equal length but may be small in comparison to the opposite limb.

Type VII: constriction ring syndrome

Amniotic band sequence (constriction ring syndrome, Streeter's dysplasia) is a condition that can affect one or all limbs and less commonly the face. As defined by Patterson,[54] limb involvement can result in any of the following deformities: (1) simple constriction rings, which may be partial or circumferential; (2) constriction rings with distal deformity, with or without concomitant lymphedema; (3) acrosyndactyly (distal fusion, fenestrated syndactyly); or (5) amputation(s) *(Fig. 27.11)*. ⊛ FIG **27.11** APPEARS ONLINE ONLY

Hypoplasia of the thumb is seen in this condition when there is a deficiency in the length of the thumb, which may have a transverse failure of formation at any level. Occasionally, the existing skeletal and soft tissue components of the first ray may be hypoplastic. The hallmark of the amniotic band sequence is that the anatomy proximal to the level of amputation or level of congenital amputation is normal. Either superficial or deep constriction rings around the thumb can be associated with hypoplasia or lymphedema of the distal segment of the digit with hypoplastic nail remnants and slender, truncated phalanges present. Acrosyndactyly is usually seen to involve the central three rays of the hand but can also involve the thumb and fifth finger. Amputation of the thumb in this condition is the major cause of partial aplasia of the thumb and can occur at any position along its length. The most practical way to analyze the amputation is to place it at one of three levels: (1) distal to IP joint; (2) proximal phalanx, and (3) metacarpal *(Fig. 27.11)*. Motion of the IP joint is usually severely affected – even with amputations or deep constriction rings distal to it.

Type VIII: five-fingered hand

In this type of hypoplasia, the thumb is smaller in width and longer in length and has the characteristics of a finger. As the radial border digit, it lies in the same plane as the ulnar four digits and is nonopposable. It is usually the same length as the adjacent index finger. The digit is slender and may be joined to the index finger in an incomplete simple syndactyly. A severe deficiency or nonexistent first web is often present, and some type of transverse metacarpal ligament is also present. The skeletal anatomy is similar to that of the index ray: a metacarpal with a distal growth center and three phalanges with proximal growth centers. The scaphoid is usually absent or hypoplastic. The thenar musculature (AbPB, FPB, OP muscles) are also absent as is the adductor pollicis

Type V

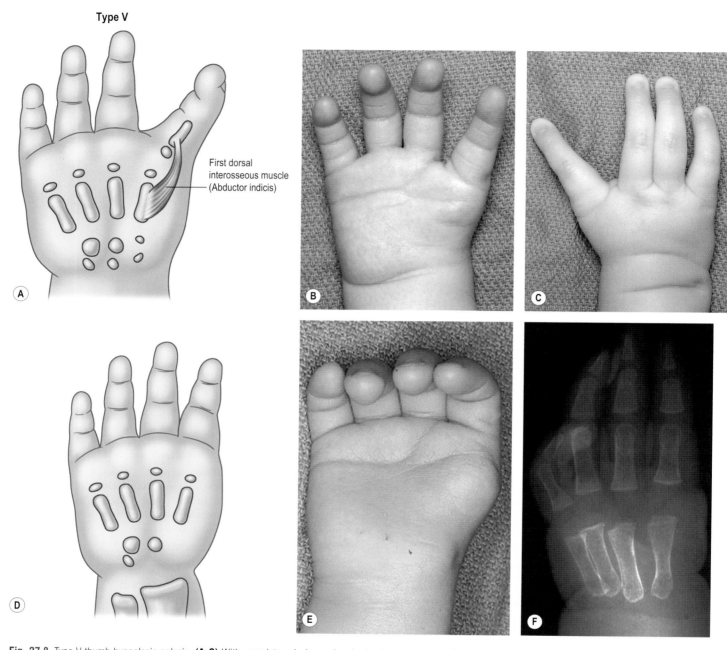

First dorsal
interosseous muscle
(Abductor indicis)

Fig. 27.8 Type V thumb hypoplasia-aplasia. **(A-C)** With complete aplasia, no thumb structures are present. In approximately half of these patients, the radius is normal. The trapezium, trapezoid, and scaphoid are often hypoplastic and a strong 1st DI (abductor indicis) pulls the index digit in abduction and in as much pronation as the intermetacarpal ligament will allow. **(D-F)** Index digits, which are not abducted, are often stiff at the interphalangeal joints and are commonly associated with some degree of radial hypoplasia or aplasia. The amount of stiffness decreases from radial to ulnar digits. Accordingly, the ring and small fingers are always the most functional components of these hands.

(AddP). Instead, the usual digital intrinsics are present – namely, a lumbrical, palmar, and dorsal interosseous *(Fig. 27.12)*. The extrinsic flexors and extensors mimic those of the normal fingers. Because the radial digit lies in the same plane as the other fingers in the hand, manipulation of objects is usually performed by utilizing lateral scissoring between the first two digits – or between the second and third if a first web syndactyly is present. Left untreated, those patients without a first web syndactyly tend to attenuate the transverse metacarpal ligament and "autopollicize" into an abducted and slightly pronated posture. ⊛ FIG **27.12** APPEARS ONLINE ONLY

Type IX: radial polydactyly

Despite the level of arborization, each partner thumb is hypoplastic to varying degrees, with the radial duplicate usually being the most severely affected. The complexity of the deformity and, therefore, the surgical correction increases as the level of the duplication progresses proximally. Associated triphalangia of the ulnar partner further complicates any surgical reconstruction. Specific abnormalities in each thumb are seen in the nail plate, the osteoarticular column, and both the intrinsic and extrinsic musculotendinous units. The nail plate of each duplicate is always more narrow than that of the unaffected thumb, and the entire skeletal ray is hypoplastic in polydactylies proximal to the MP joint.

Musculotendinous abnormalities are common with the extrinsic extensor almost universally shared. Indeed, nearly half of the patients presented in papers on pollex abductus involve duplicate thumbs.[40,43] Deviation of the partners toward each other indicates abnormal insertions of the extrinsic tendons into the distal phalanges, and connections between the extrinsic flexors and extensors are not unusual. These tendinous interconnections will limit function and cause digital angulations. The first web is usually unaffected in polydactylies involving the distal phalanx, but as the level of arborization lies more proximally, the first web space becomes increasingly deficient and tight.

Type X: syndromic short skeletal thumb ray

Deficiencies of the osteoarticular column of the thumb may result in a short, hypoplastic thumb *(Fig. 27.13)*. Bony abnormalities can occur as isolated bone (brachymetacarpia, brachyphalangia), all bones in combination, or as part of a generalized syndrome, such as the acrocephalosyndactyly (e.g., Apert, Pfeiffer, Carpenter, etc.) syndromes or the Rubinstein–Tabyi syndrome. Joint function is usually impaired on either side of the abnormal bone(s). In patients with anomalies of a single bone, brachymetacarpia or brachyphalangia, the remaining components of the thumb tend to be unaffected, and in patients with generalized syndromes, other abnormalities of the thumb components are common. In the acrocephalosyndactyly (ACS) syndromes, delta phalanges are common. They usually involve the proximal phalanx with a longitudinal epiphyseal bracket on the radial side. This abnormal growth plate checks growth on the radial side and results in a radial clinodactyly of the thumb, which becomes more severe over time. The metacarpal is usually short and the distal phalanx is short and broad. Incidentally, many feel that the abnormal proximal phalanx and broad distal phalanx are variations of a polydactyly. Musculotendinous anomalies are associated with poor joint function but are not as common as those with type IIIA thumbs. Deficiencies of the first web are most common, occurring along a spectrum of mild adduction contracture to complex syndactyly involving the first two rays. ⊗ FIG 27.13 APPEARS ONLINE ONLY

The whole spectrum of patients with metabolic bone diseases, skeletal dysplasias, benign skeletal tumors and many syndromes may include thumb hypoplasia. In general, very little surgical correction is required for these youngsters. The need for surgical improvement is determined by very critical observation of these children at play.

Patient selection

General considerations

The child with thumb hypoplasia may present many unique problems with both pinch (precision, pulp, key) and grasp (precision, span, power), despite his/her ability to adapt remarkably to the functional deficiency.[23] The ideal prerequisites for reconstruction of a functional thumb include[55]:

1. A mobile, stable CMC joint with an intact metacarpal
2. A scar-free first web space of adequate width and depth lined with full thickness skin
3. Mobility in at least two of its three joints (CMC, MP, IP)
4. MP joint stability, particularly of the ulnar collateral ligament
5. Adequate motors for strong MP or IP flexion and extension
6. Capacity to be placed in a palmar abducted (i.e., opposition) position for pinch and grasp maneuvers.

All six of these components should be considered in any detailed analysis of the thumb.

Timing

As researchers and clinicians struggle with the possibilities of fetal surgery, many surgeons wonder if they should wait rather than performing reconstructive procedures of the congenitally different hand as soon as possible *(Fig. 27.14)*. Early reconstruction of the hypoplastic or absent thumb is certainly attractive in an effort to allow the infant to adapt more rapidly with optimal cortical representation. This ideal needs to be tempered with the knowledge that a congenital hand difference is, in itself, not a life-threatening condition (but may be associated with one), and the surgeon can use time to allow the affected part to grow, to observe development, and to assess the functional needs. The construction of the thumb with a stable osteoarticular column of adequate length, mobile joints, growth potential, scar-free first web, and gliding muscle tendon units is not easily accomplished in very small hands – despite our refined microvascular instruments and skills.

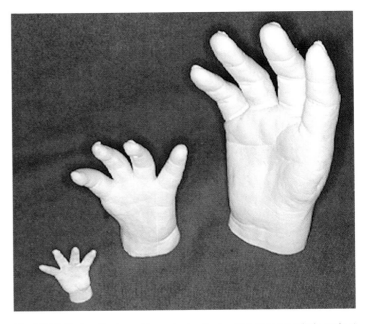

Fig. 27.14 Timing. Plaster molds made of patients with type V hypoplasia made at ages (left to right): 32 weeks' gestation, 12 months and 8 years of age demonstrate the tremendous growth difference. Despite their discrepant sizes, the anatomy of these hands was remarkably similar with normal index active and passive range of motion. Any surgery on the hand on the left would be quite challenging.

However, the arguments that are forwarded by the proponents of the early surgery persist. Among the most powerful points include anatomic, cognitive, and psychological factors. Anatomically, the release of tethered musculotendinous units and joint contractures will allow unrestricted growth, and physiological adaptation of the reconstructed thumb will occur secondary to growth and functional use.[55] On a cognitive level, early surgery will allow the development of the child with a reconstructed thumb to occur prior to thumb corticalization, which takes place at around 18 months of age. Psychologically, correction will alleviate anxiety in the parents and, therefore, in the child.

These purported advantages should be weighed against risks which include: (1) growth-related complications; (2) functional need assessment, and (3) patient cooperation. In slightly older patients, the affected thumb is larger so potential problems with osteotomies, alteration of growth, skeletal fixation, joint reconstruction and potential for compromise of blood supply are reduced. Also with an older patient, the surgeon is better able to accurately assess the functional needs of the child according to his or her interests, current adaptations, and lifestyle. Finally, and perhaps most importantly, an older child is potentially a more cooperative patient.

In the absence of other organ system complications, we try to reconstruct these problems when the child is between 10 and 18 months of age. Pollicization at 1 year is often preceded by centralization of the hand and wrist between 5 and 8 months of age in those with radial deficiency. The timing for correction of type IIIB deformities may be problematic. Though pollicization is the procedure of choice, some parents and families simply will not allow it. We agree with other surgeons that the alternatives involve difficult reconstructions, often including one or more stages, and are wisely deferred until the child is aged 4–5 years, a time when the hand is larger and the patient may be more cooperative with the postoperative therapy regimen.[5,23,31]

Surgical correction of the hypoplastic or absent thumb must be individualized. As these children may have other congenital anomalies, an early assessment of the upper limb deficiencies and a coordinated management plan can be formulated and instituted. Perhaps the most important and least emphasized variables are the confidence, surgical skill and experience of the surgeon and his/her team.

Treatment

This section on treatment is divided into two parts: in the first part, treatment considerations will be outlined for each type of thumb hypoplasia, and in the second part, surgical techniques will be outlined in detail for each particular clinical problem.

Treatment considerations for thumb hypoplasia (types I–V)

Type I: mild hypoplasia

These children are not usually functionally impaired (*Fig. 27.2*). In fact, many type I thumb hypoplasia patients, along with their parents, do not recognize anything abnormal about these hands. These thumbs are commonly found in patients who have a more severe radial dysplasia in the opposite upper limb. However, in this stronger limb, they have very little or no difficulty with key pinch, pulp to pulp pinch, opposition and grasping activities. Since functional problems are rare, surgical correction is not often needed. Occasionally, a child with a type I hypoplastic thumb will require a release of a mildly contracted web (see Type II management). All web releases involve more than simple skin incisions. Careful[56] attention must be directed to tight fascial bands within the web space, anomalous tendon and muscle anatomy and joint ankylosis. Of all the methods available, the 4-flap Z-plasty provides the best contour and appearance (*Fig. 27.15*). Dorsal transposition flaps from the index finger[34] and rotation flaps[56,57] are effective but require skin grafting on the visible dorsal surface of the hand. Of course, any method must be carefully individualized to the patient.

Type II: moderate hypoplasia

Five specific problems in the type II thumbs must be addressed individually: (1) narrowed first web space; (2) instability of the MP joint; (3) poor palmar abduction (opposition) for pinching and grasping; (4) lack of IP joint flexion, and (5) abduction posturing of the thumb ("pollex abductus") (*Figs 27.3, 27.4*). Usually, all that is needed to correct these thumbs is a release of the first web space and stabilization of the MP joint, with or without a transfer for palmar abduction or opposition. When the surgeon encounters a pollex abductus deformity, she/he should next look for abnormalities of the flexor pollicis longus (FPL) muscle. A more detailed description of treatment options is presented later in this chapter.

Type IIIA: severe hypoplasia

Most hand surgeons agree that this variation should be reconstructed surgically (*Fig. 27.5*). The five individual problems are the same as listed in type II, and the options and preferred solutions are listed below. Most authors opt to complete all necessary procedures including widening of the first web space, stabilization of the MP joint, and some type of opposition transfer at one time. The major variable becomes the status of the flexor mechanism, which may require a staged approach. After 35 years of experience, our preference has been to replace the very anomalous flexor mechanism with a tendon transfer in the presence of at least one good pulley at the level of the metacarpal head. The treatment of the more deficient type IIIB and IIIC varieties constitutes one of the more interesting ongoing controversies in hand surgery.

Type IIIB, type IIIC: severe hypoplasia

For most hand surgeons in Europe, North America and South America, pollicization is the treatment of choice because a well-performed pollicization provides a much better and more predictable outcome than any alternative types of staged reconstruction (*Fig. 27.6*).

However, cultural and parental beliefs may demand one of two alternatives – staged reconstructions with[58–61] and without[62] a microvascular joint transfer, which have both become popular in the Asian countries. Osteoplastic thumb reconstruction has a long history.[6,63–65] The osteoarticular

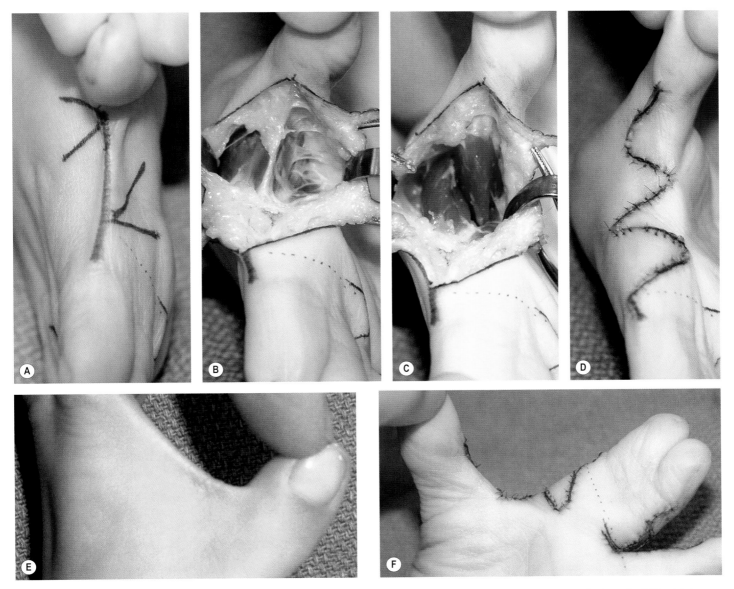

Fig. 27.15 1st web space release. **(A)** The skin markings have been made for a four-flap Z-plasty, which include two 90° incisions perpendicular to the tight web between the thumb and index finger. Each is then bisected at a 45° angle. **(B)** After the four separate flaps have been mobilized, reflected dense septal bands may be identified between the skin and muscle fascia, and larger fascial bands between the intrinsic muscle groups. **(C)** Incision and excision of these bands may require dissection to the CMC joint level. **(D)** Trimming and minor flap adjustments are always needed with the proper inset of the more mobile dorsal flaps with the more rigid palmar flaps. A skin redundancy on the radial side of the index finger has been eliminated with a straight extension. **(E)** The preoperative appearance is seen with a dorsal view. **(F)** The postoperative contour is shown from the palmar surface. This technique provides the best contour of all available methods of first web release.

column is connected with an intercalated bone graft between the index and hypoplastic thumb metacarpal *(Fig. 27.16)*. Multiple stages are then needed to first stabilize MP and IP joints and construct pulleys. At that point, tendon transfers are performed for opposition as well as IP flexion and extension. The major disadvantages of this procedure include the lack of CMC mobility, lack of growth, poor motion and the multiple stages required. Insensate abdominal pedicle flaps have been used to provide tissue for an adequate first web space. 🔄 FIG **27.16** APPEARS ONLINE ONLY

Another alternative is to transfer either the second[62,66–69] or third[70] or first metatarsophalangeal joint in a hyperextended position to create a new CMC joint and proximal metacarpal.

This composite joint must be harvested with a large dorsalis pedis pedicle, which provides venous drainage and adds bulk to the deficient thenar region. Tendon transfers are then performed to provide motion at either the MP or IP joints.

The management of these thumbs remains controversial. Without exception, experienced hand surgeons prefer a well-performed pollicization over a staged reconstruction to salvage these deficient thumbs. Any reconstruction will require: (1) stabilization of the thumb metacarpal with first web release; (2) MP joint stabilization and opponensplasty, and (3) staged extrinsic tendon transfers – FDS-ring to FPL for thumb flexion and EIP to EPL for thumb extension. Additional transfers for adduction may also be required. The size of these thumbs at birth make reconstruction appear attractive to many parents who are often reluctant, some strongly insistent, about considering any other option. Observation of the child at play will usually direct the surgeon and family towards the best course of management. For instance, a child who bypasses the hypoplastic thumb before reconstruction will usually continue to do so following reconstruction. Most undecided parents usually make up their minds after observing other patients with their new pollicized thumbs.

Type IV: floating thumb

Index finger pollicization is the treatment of choice *(Fig. 27.7)* unless there are too many cultural or parental concerns to consider the alternatives outlined above for alternative staged reconstructions.

Type V: aplasia

Index finger pollicization is the treatment of choice *(Fig. 27.8)*. Osteoplastic reconstructions and microvascular transfers are not. The technique is described in detail in the next section.

Clinical conditions and surgical treatment (types I–V)

Deficient first web space

The correction and widening of the first web space is the most effective single procedure performed for congenital hand differences. A scar-free web line, created by full thickness flaps, is essential for thumb mobility and growth. The many options include: (1) local transposition flaps;[71–73] (2) local rotational or sliding flaps with or without skin grafts;[34,57,74] (3) regional vascular island flaps;[75] (4) free fasciocutaneous tissue transfer;[76] (5) distant pedicled flaps,[24,63,77] and (6) the use of skin expansion.[17,55]

For all type II thumbs, local flaps are all that are necessary. Each of the techniques utilizes the same principle, lengthening the contractual limb of the Z-plasty by transposing tissue perpendicular to it. In general, the four-flap Z-plasty[72] is preferred because it provides the most predictable contour and release *(Fig. 27.15)*. The five-flap ("jumping man") technique[73] is equally effective but usually involves small flaps with vulnerable tips. A simple Z-plasty, on the other hand, does not give the proper contour and usually creates a central depression at the base of the web space.[78] The surgeon should learn and refine one technique. The use of local flaps with skin grafts, either on the dorsum of the hand or on the index ray, are popular[34,57] but not preferred due to the conspicuous appearance of the dorsal grafts and the associated contracture when harvested along the radial side of the index finger. If the hand requires repeated operations, such as those needed in the Apert hand, dorsal advancement or sliding flaps may be effective because with each procedure the dorsal tissue is re-advanced to create a broader web space.[55,79] The most frequent error in the treatment of these hands is the tendency to use local tissue when the deficit requires more tissue to be moved into the web space.

Additional methods must be considered with more severe narrowing of the first web space seen with type II and type IIIA thumbs. Distally based radial artery or dorsal interosseous arterial flaps can provide more than enough tissue to line the first web space and allow primary closure of the donor site.[55,75] The preferred donor is the radial artery. Preoperative Allen's testing must demonstrate an intact palmar arch. We do not hesitate to obtain either a MRA (magnetic resonance angiography) or an angiogram if there is any question. Predictably, the dorsal interosseous flaps are nourished by the abundant rete network of the carpal region. We would not use an ulnar artery distally based flap unless this artery, the major conduit to the hand, is revascularized with a reversed vein graft. Free groin flaps are very effective with minimal donor site morbidity. The major disadvantages are the anomalous vascular anatomy and the specialized training necessary for pediatric microsurgery. Distant pedicle flaps are not indicated and should be considered only under very special circumstances.

Technique of first web release with four flap Z-plasty

The contractual limb of the Z-plasty is marked first along the leading edge of the web with the thumb and index finger abducted as much as possible *(Fig. 27.15)*. The length of this limb determines the lengths of each of the four flaps. At each end of this line, two lines of the same length are drawn at right angles (90°), with the most radial line passing along the dorsal side of the web (parallel to the thumb metacarpal), and the most ulnar border passing on the palmar side of the web, which is usually very close to the thenar flexion crease. These two right angles are then bisected, creating four flaps (two palmar, two dorsal), each with a tip angle of 45°. The less mobile glabrous skin on the palmar surface is incised first as minor adjustments are often necessary and more easily accomplished with the mobile dorsal skin. Dorsal veins and nerves are protected with spreading dissection, and all four flaps are retracted as the web space is inspected. The radial neurovascular bundle to the index finger is protected. Often an arborization of the ulnar digital artery on the thumb side runs along the distal edge of the adductor pollicis muscle.

Skin incisions alone are usually inadequate for a full release of this web space. Tight fascial investments of the thenar muscles and intermetacarpal bands must be excised before a dramatic release is obtained *(Fig. 27.15B,C)*. If necessary, these explorations extend to the level of the CMC joint, where branches of the princeps pollicis artery should be protected. The origin of the first dorsal interosseous (1st DI) on the thumb metacarpal is next inspected and partially recessed if necessary. Release of the AddP from the third metacarpal carries a potential loss of important pinch strength. Although the 1st DI and AddP rarely require release with type II thumbs, they are frequently the tightest deforming force in severe contractures associated with type IIIA thumbs. When myotomies are performed as part of the web release, a 0.35 mm C-wire is passed between the thumb and index metacarpals to hold this position for 3 weeks postoperatively. If the radial digital artery (arteria radialis indicis) to the index finger remains as the tightest structure, it can be ligated when there is a common digital artery to the second web space.

Occasionally in type II thumbs, anomalous muscles acting as adductors may be encountered passing from the flexor surface of the thumb to the extensor surface of the index finger.[40] These muscles are excised. Additional MP joint stabilization procedures or tendon transfers are performed before the flaps are closed with 6–0 mild chromic sutures. When the correct incisions have been made, these flaps will naturally fall into place.

Metacarpophalangeal joint instability

Often the release of a moderate or severe first web space contracture will unmask a lax ulnar collateral ligament at the MP joint level. Stabilization of this lax joint in type II and III-A thumbs can be accomplished with a number of procedures: (1) tightening of the existing ligament and capsule;[31] (2) free tendon graft reconstruction;[48] (3) arthrodesis, or chondrodesis,[9] and (4) ligament reconstruction using the end of a tendon used to improve palmar abduction (opposition).[23] In the growing child, all must be performed without injury to the epiphysis.[41] Simple imbrication of the attenuated collateral ligament on one or both sides of the MP joint is advocated by some[31] for type II and IIIA thumbs but has not been permanent in our series. Reefing of the attenuated ulnar collateral ligament and joint capsule can be addressed by either plication or incision and closure of the lax structures with a "pants over vest" repair. The extensor mechanism, with its attenuated shroud fibers, is usually displaced radially and needs to be identified and mobilized from the dorsal joint capsule. A free palmaris or extensor digiti quinti tendon graft passed either through subperiosteal tunnels in the young child or through drill holes in the older youngster is more predictable. One portion of the graft must be palmar enough to reconstruct the volar accessory portion of the ligament. Both radial and ulnar sides of the joint require reconstruction in most type IIIA thumbs. When a FDS is used simultaneously for palmar abduction (opposition), one slip is passed through the metacarpal to be used on the ulnar side and the other slip for the radial side of the joint (*Fig. 27.17C*). Excess tendon on either side may be used for pulley reconstruction if needed.[80]

In type IIIA thumbs with flail joints and poor or absent extrinsic motors, stability of the MP joint is much more critical than motion. Here a chondrodesis in the young child or arthrodesis in the adolescent is indicated. In the young child, the metacarpal head can be shaved without injury to the growth plate and then fused to the epiphysis of the proximal phalanx.[9,41] Thumbs that have grown in an abducted position and have an asymmetrical joint can only be stabilized by fusion.[55] These stabilization procedures must be held with small C wires with the joint in slight (20°) of flexion. Unless held rigidly, these thumbs can easily drift into hyperextension with minimal cast motion.

Technique of tendon graft stabilization

A palmaris or another common tendon donor site is harvested and the MP joint adequately exposed. An extension of the most radial limb of a 4-flap Z-plasty provides good exposure for both sides of the joint (*Fig. 27.17*). After inspection of the extrinsic flexor and extensor tendons with or without intratendinous fibrous connections, joint capsule and collateral ligaments are inspected and imbricated if present. A subperiosteal vertical tunnel is made distal to the growth plate along

the metaphysis of the proximal phalanx, and a transverse gauge hole proximal to the metacarpal head will provide the bone fixation for the graft. The tendon is then passed from the metacarpal fixation point, beneath the extensor shroud, through the periosteal tunnel from dorsal to palmar. It is then passed below the adductor aponeurosis and shroud to the metacarpal. At this point, it is important that the upper portion of this graft mimic the cord (upper) portion of the collateral ligament and the lower portion provide stability similar to that of the volar accessory portion of the collateral ligament. If this lower portion is fixed at or dorsal to the axis of joint rotation, an MP joint extension contracture will predictably result. The graft is tightened with nonabsorbable sutures in 10–15° of flexion and in neutral between radial and ulnar deviation. Pin fixation should not be necessary.

When the ring FDS transfer is performed for palmar abduction (opposition), either bifurcation of the tendon is of adequate length for radial and ulnar collateral ligament reconstructions. Most type IIIA and some type II thumbs need both sides of the joint stabilized. In the past, many surgeons have neglected a lax radial side of the joint in their enthusiasm to correct the obviously deficient ulnar collateral ligament responsible for the abduction of the floppy thumb.

Poor/absent palmar abduction (opposition)

The degree of first web space contracture is a good clinical indication of the degree of hypoplasia of thumb abductors, and the need for opposition transfers can be determined both by thenar muscle examination and assessment of the thumb position during play activities. Often the child tends to use key pinching maneuvers because he or she cannot abduct the thumb adequately to obtain a pulp-to-pulp pinch or grasp and will use a two-handed grasp for holding larger objects. Substitution for the missing or hypoplastic thenar intrinsic muscles is not effective without a mobile CMC joint, adequate first web space, and stabile MP joint. Most commonly, adequate palmar abduction (opposition) of the thumb is created by transfer of either the abductor digiti quinti minimi (ADQM)[81–84] or the flexor digitorum superficialis of the long or ring finger (*Figs 27.17, 27.18*).[25,49,80,85]

Technique of ADQM transfer

The muscle is raised from an incision extending from the pisoform proximally to the mid-axial line of the proximal phalanx (*Fig. 27.18*). A skin island can be taken with the muscle,[86] which is then detached from its distal extensor and bone insertions. If there are difficulties separating the abductor digiti quinti minimi muscle (ADQM) from the flexor digiti quinti minimi muscle (FDQM), both muscles must be raised as a single unit.[82] A distal nutrient artery from the ulnar digital artery to the fifth finger must be ligated if present.[87] Additional length can be obtained with detachment from the pisiform[81] and retention on the flexor carpi ulnaris tendon. During this extra mobilization, the proximal axial pedicle to the muscle must be inspected carefully. The muscle is then passed through a very generous subcutaneous tunnel made between the skin and palmar fascia and then attached to the metacarpal, the radial collateral ligament at the MP joint, or the abductor aponeurosis. Insertion to the proximal phalanx or extensor

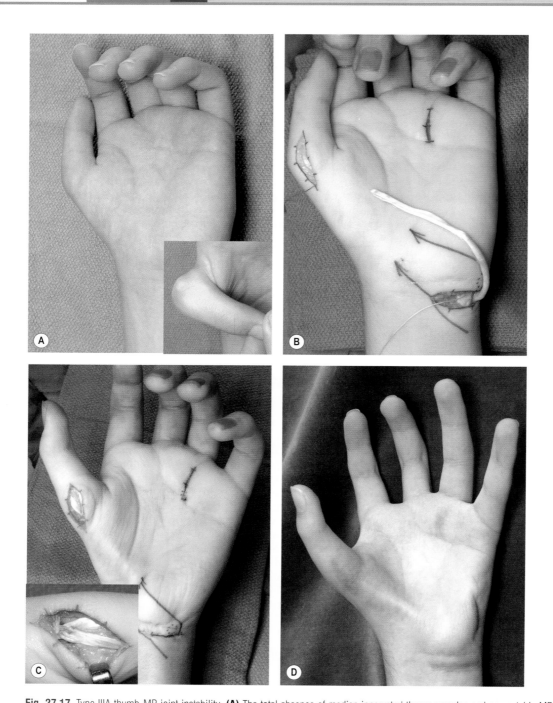

Fig. 27.17 Type IIIA thumb-MP joint instability. **(A)** The total absence of median innervated thenar muscles and an unstable MP joint are characteristic of a type IIIA hypoplastic thumb (inset). **(B)** The superficial flexor tendon to the ring finger has been looped around the flexor carpi ulnaris and passed through Guyon's canal toward the thumb. **(C)** The transfer is secured tightly and both free ends are used to reconstruct the absent collateral ligaments. The inset shows the upper (cord) and lower (volar accessory) portions of the new radial collateral ligament. **(D)** Three months postoperatively, the transfer is strong and the MP joint stable on both ulnar and radial sides.

mechanism should not be performed with any laxity of the ulnar collateral ligament.

Technique of FDS transfer

Harvest of the FDS tendon to the ring finger is done through a longitudinal incision at the base of the ring finger *(Fig. 27.17)*. The A1 pulley is released, the finger flexed, and both slips of the FDS pulled into the wound and cut as far distally as possible. The tendon is then delivered through an incision over the flexor carpi ulnaris (FCU) and then passed through a subcutaneous tunnel to the radial side of the thumb where the insertion options are the same as AbDQ. The pivot point for the transfer is either through Guyon's canal[55] or around the FCU. Note that we no longer make a loop from a slip of the FCU through which the tendon pivots. The thumb is placed in 45° of palmar abduction and held with

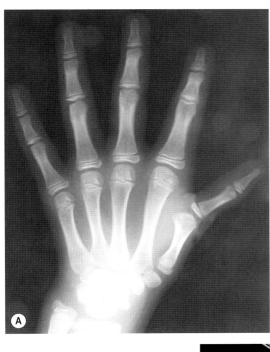

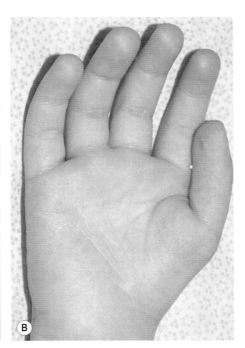

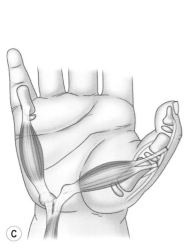

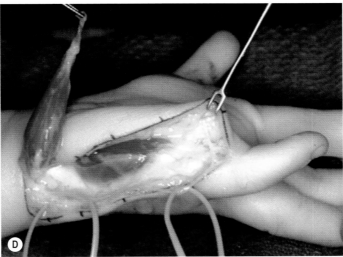

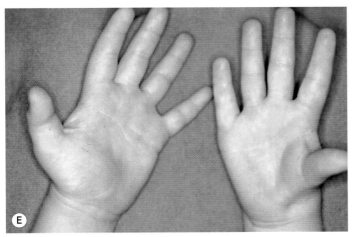

Fig. 27.18 ADQM transfer for opposition. **(A)** The radiograph of this type IIIA thumb shows a small web space and tightly adducted first metacarpal. **(B)** The clinical photo shows a marked deficiency of the median innervated thenar muscles. The radial and ulnar collateral ligaments are stable. **(C, D)** The abductor digiti quinti muscle is isolated on its origin from the pisiform and passed through a subcutaneous tunnel above the palmar fascia to the radial side of the thumb. If two distal tendons can be dissected, separate insertions into the thumb are performed. If one tendon is present, the preferred insertion is into the radial collateral ligament region. When a proximal dissection of the muscle is performed, its neurovascular bundle must be preserved. **(E)** The patient shown in A is seen 16 years later with functional palmar abduction from the muscle transfer.

a transverse C-wire through the thumb and index metacarpals. One slip of the FDS tendon is passed through a transverse drill hole near the metacarpal neck and secured. The two slips of the ring FDS are then used for reconstruction of the radial and ulnar collateral ligaments as described *(Fig. 27.17)*. At the same time, the existing ligament and capsule are tightened.

Lack of IP joint motion

The most difficult function to reconstruct in type II and IIIA thumbs is IP joint motion. Dorsal capsulotomy and tendon recentralization will improve the minimal deformities. In the pollex abductus anomaly, flexors and extensors with good proximal excursion need to be centralized with pulley construction. In cases of poor motion, tendon transfers are needed as a second stage. An available ring FDS is the most appropriate for IP flexion and an EIP for IP joint extension. Secondary transfers for extension include brachioradialis (BR) or extensor carpi radialis longus (ECRL) plus a tendon graft to the EPL.[48]

Pollex abductus

The clinical presentation of thumb abduction with limited IP motion is indicative of this anomaly *(Fig. 27.4)*.[40,88] Both the flexor and extensor tendons are exposed through a radial incision or the retracted flap of the web space release. Exploration and traction on the extrinsic tendons will give an estimation of distal IP motion and proximal muscle belly excursion. The interconnecting bands are divided and excised along the radial side of the MP joint and proximal phalanx.[40] The reconstruction here depends upon the degree of anomalous anatomy. Absence of both the short and long thumb flexors (FPB and FPL) will severely impair both pinch and grip functions. In those without a pollex abductus, the FPL is usually satisfactory and the pulley system can be strengthened by a slip of tendon – usually taken from the end of an FDS transfer. A piece of extensor retinaculum will also make a good pulley.[89] The FPL in the pollex abductus has a poor proximal excursion and can be transferred to the base of the thumb to act as an abductor pollicis longus (AbPL). Transfer of these abnormal aberrant tendons into a normal position as IP motors is not effective.

Following release of the extrinsic tendons and excision of anomalous muscles, a difficult decision must be made with regard to construction of the terminal flexor and at least one strategic pulley. Interphalangeal joint flexion can be created by transfer of an unscarred FDS tendon (ring or long) at the same time that palmar abduction (opposition) is restored by an ADQM (Huber) transfer.

Technique of pollicization

Even though pollicization greatly enhances the function of these hands, it is important to remember that the index finger is only placed in a more strategic position to simulate a thumb. The newly created CMC joint was the index MCP joint and, therefore, does not have the same degree of freedom as the normal CMC joint of the thumb *(Figs 27.19, 27.20)*. Since the normal cone of thenar intrinsic muscles are absent, the strength and stability of these thumbs in both pinch and grasp maneuvers does not approach normal.

Principles

The principles of this procedure, the most elegant in hand surgery, include: (1) transposition of the index digit as a vascular island; (2) a rotation and recession shortening of the ray; (3) a rebalancing of muscles and tendons, and (4) incisions to create a normal first web. The operation itself is divided into a number of steps.

Incisions and plan

A number of different incisions have been used over the past three decades *(Fig. 27.20A)*.[1,14,75,90–95] Although the markings of Buck-Gramcko[14,96] are used most frequently, we prefer a modification of the Littler incisions, which permit much greater flexibility for construction of a broad thumb-index web space.[48,97] A racquet-shaped incision is made around the base of the index ray along the MP flexion crease and extends down the radial border of the hand. The site of the new thenar flexion crease is made in the palm, and the distal portion of the incision is connected to the incision around the index ray. It is best to plan these incisions as though no thumb or thumb remnant was present and to incorporate this extra tissue into the flap designs only if appropriate. If a type IIIB, C or type IV thumb is present, the skeleton is filleted from its soft tissue envelope and intrinsic muscles transferred to the new thumb. In certain deficient hands, the soft tissue of the extraneous digit can be isolated on a vascular pedicle, as a vascularized adipofascial flap, and placed in the thenar area to augment the deficiency.[98]

Dissection and exposure

The dorsal flap is raised in the subcutaneous fat plane above the large dorsal veins, nerves, and lymphatics – all of which are preserved in a single layer of fat and areolar tissue above the extensor mechanism. Usually one large vein is present on either side of the dorsum of the digit. The neurovascular structures are dissected, and the palmar flap is raised above the level of the palmar aponeurosis, exposing the superficial palmar arch. The common digital bundle to the index-long web space and the floating thumb (if present) are exposed but individually dissected. Arterial loops around the nerve are present in less than 10% of our cases; however, neural loops around the artery are more common and are opened by spreading the nerve back to the level of the superficial arch. We have not commonly seen the arterial anomalies previously described[99] and do not feel preoperative angiography is necessary. The radial bundle to the index digit is usually hypoplastic but rarely absent. In the presence of a thumb, a common bundle gives one artery to the thumb and one to the index ray. With clear retraction of the neurovascular structures and skeletal and extensor origins of the volar interosseous, first dorsal interosseous and adductor pollicis (if a thumb is present) are detached and the muscles dissected back to their periosteal origin. The index extrinsic flexors are not altered and its lumbrical is left intact. Then the A1 pulley is decompressed. On the dorsal side, the extrinsic extensor digitorum communis and extrinsic indicis proprius to the index are isolated and divided at the level of the MP joint. The lateral bands are gently separated from the common extensor at over the proximal phalanx, which will soon become the new thumb metacarpal.

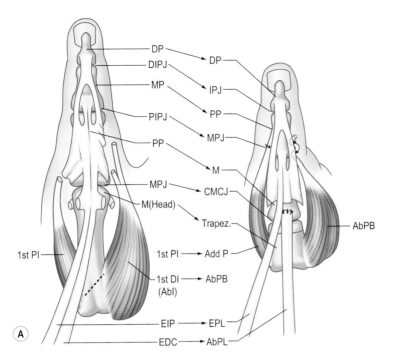

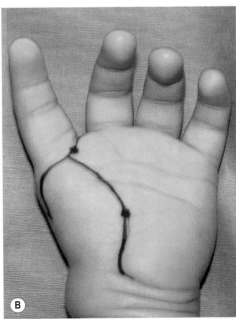

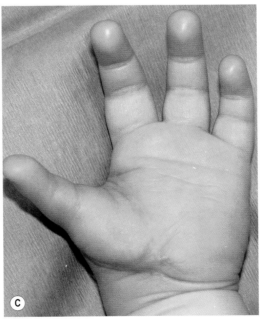

Fig. 27.19 Pollicization. **(A)** Rebalancing of the extrinsic and intrinsic muscles from a left index finger to the new left thumb (right). DP, distal phalanx; MP, middle phalanx; PP, proximal phalanx; M, metacarpal; DIPJ, distal interphalangeal joint; PIPJ, proximal interphalangeal joint; MPJ, metacarpophalangeal joint; CMCJ, carpometacarpal joint; EDC, extensor digitorum cominus tendon; EIP, extensor indicis proprius tendon; EPL, extensor pollicis longus; 1st PI, first palmar interosseous (ulnar interosseous) muscle; 1st DI, first dorsal interosseous muscle (radial interosseous; abductor indicis); AbPB, abductor pollicis brevis muscle; AddP, adductor pollicis muscle; FPB, flexor pollicis brevis muscle; AbPL, abductor pollicis longus tendon(s). **(B)** The preoperative markings are compared to the **(C)** clinical appearance 6 months following pollicization. The dot in the mid palmar aspect of the index finger is relocated the mid-portion of the thenar flexion crease in the postoperative state.

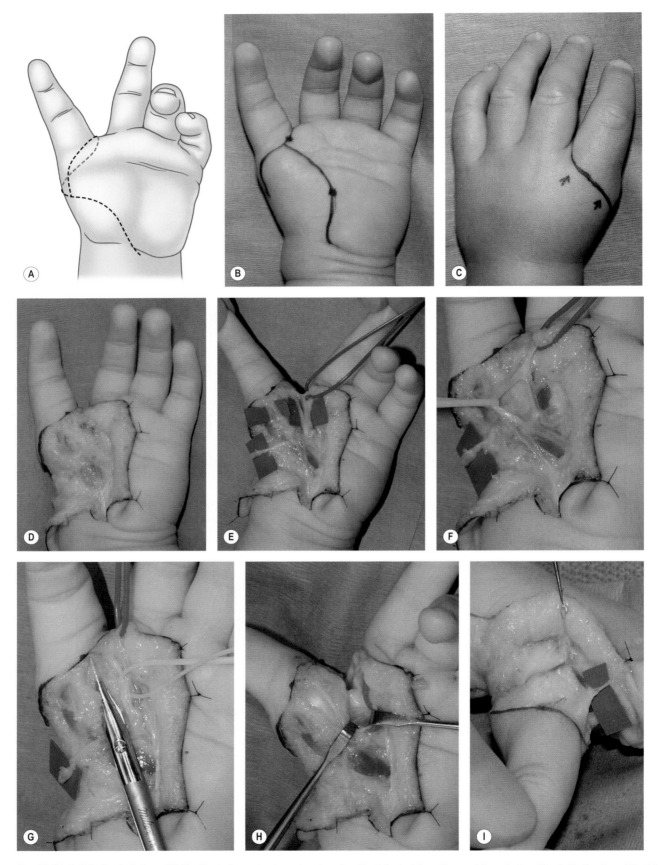

Fig. 27.20 Pollicization technique. **(A)** The illustration and palmar view show the site of the incisions. The most important marking is the location of the future thenar flexion crease within the palm. **(B)** The volar base of the index finger will be the mid-portion of this flexion crease. **(C)** The dorsal marking is made and the visible dorsal draining veins marked by arrows. **(D)** The palmar flaps are elevated above the palmar aponeurosis. **(E)** The common digital bundle to the index-long web space is isolated. The arborization to the radial side of the long finger (red loop) will be ligated. Note the neuroma in the dissected sensory nerve to the "floating thumb," which was ligated in the newborn nursery. **(F)** A neural loop around the common vessels to the web space must be carefully teased apart back to the level of the palmar arch. **(G)** A full release of the first **(A-1)** annular pulley is completed. **(H)** The transverse metacarpal ligament is exposed before its transection, which then provides increased mobility of the ray for the intrinsic muscle dissection. **(I)** The dorsal venous system is easily exposed by scissor dissection between the two layers of dorsal fat/areolar tissue.

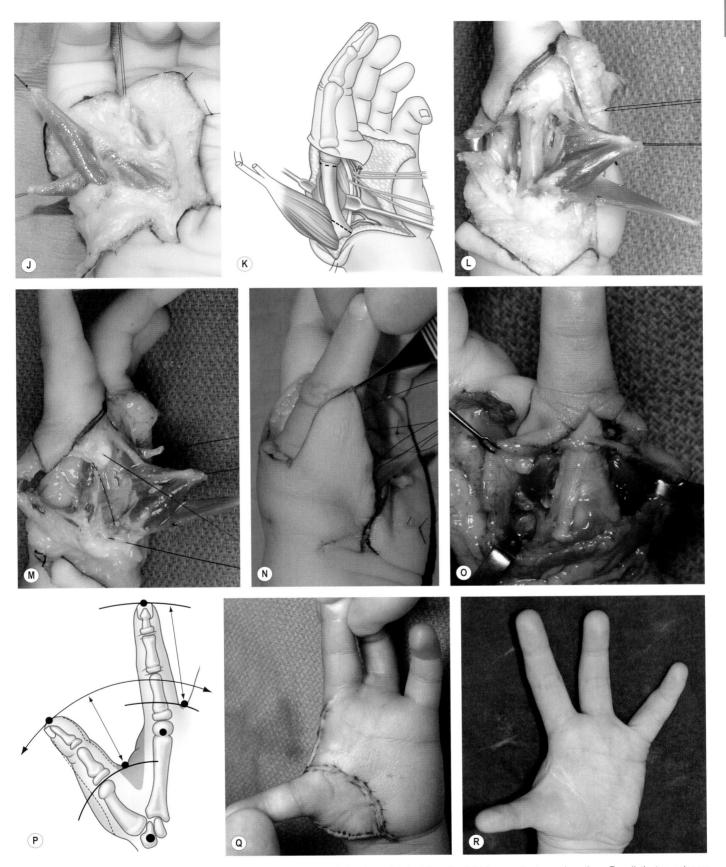

Fig. 27.20, cont'd **(J)** The first dorsal interosseous (abductor indicis) muscle has been detached from its distal bone and extensor insertions. Two distinct muscles are often found. **(K)** The illustration and **(L)** clinical picture show that the muscles are attached to their periosteal origin, which has been elevated off the metacarpal. The distal osteotomy is through the epiphysis and the proximal cut leaves the dorsal cortex of the metacarpal base. **(M)** The metacarpal head becomes the new thumb trapezium and is placed in a hyperextended position in front of the metacarpal base. Interosseous suture fixation is preferred to C wires, which can cause problems in young children. **(N)** With the thumb in its new position, the available skin is then draped over the dorsal surface before the cut-back incision is made. This maneuver makes maximal use of the all available tissue. **(O)** The extrinsic tendons have been shorted and reattached, and the intrinsic muscles have been attached distally either to bone or the extensor mechanism via the lateral bands. **(P)** The normal appearing first web space is a gentle curve between the MP joint of the thumb and that of the long finger. The shaded area represents the area covered by the additional flaps rotated to create this web. **(Q)** After closure, a broad web allowing maximal abduction should be present. **(R)** The same hand is seen 5 years later.

Skeletal shortening

From both dorsal and palmar approaches, a subperiosteal dissection of the metacarpal is completed and osteotomy sites marked (*Fig. 27.21*). The intrinsic muscle origins are carefully protected during this dissection, which extends anterior to the index metacarpal to the level of the CMC joint. The proximal osteotomy site is marked and an oblique cut made through the metacarpal, leaving a small post of dorsal cortex to which the metacarpal head will be attached. Here, we have left the entire shaft intact and fixed the metacarpal head to the anterior cortex. The distal metacarpal osteotomy is made through the epiphysis in order to arrest the growth of the metacarpal head, which becomes the new thumb trapezium. The index finger is now "recessed and rotated"[100] and secured anterior to the base of the index metacarpal with one or more interosseous sutures.[48,89,101] In this position, the MP joint must be in a hyperextended position[102,103] of >60 and <80 degrees, a position which permits only a few degrees of additional extension of the new CMC joint. Nonabsorbable sutures are preferred to C wires, which can become problematic in young children. This difficult fixation is facilitated by optimal assistance and retraction. At this point in the operation, the tourniquet is deflated for a minimum of 30 minutes. ⊛ FIG 27.21 APPEARS ONLINE ONLY

Tendon and intrinsic muscle rebalancing

The dorsal flap is first draped over the repositioned index finger, which is held in 45° of palmar abduction, and the dorsal cutback incision is made (*Fig. 27.20O*). This incision is intentionally delayed because optimal use of all available skin can be crucial for creation of a broad web space. Once made, wide exposure to the new thumb is provided. The EDC is advanced and sutured to the ulnar base of the index proximal phalanx (now the thumb metacarpal), so that it provides both extension and pronation. The independent EIP is advanced, a portion resected and sutured to the side-by-side to the extensor hood with the new thumb held in no more than 10° of MP and IP flexion. Recently, we have accomplished this by simple plication.[13] In rare instances when there is only one extensor on the index finger, this should be used as the EPL.[96]

The intrinsic muscle rebalancing is critical to the resting posture of the thumb. The small 1st VI (volar interosseous), which becomes the new AddP, is attached either to the ulnar collateral ligament at the MP joint or into the wing tendon of the extensor mechanism.[13,104] Preferably, the much larger 1st DI (or abductor indicis), which becomes the new AbPB, is inserted into the radial collateral ligament or the radial base of the new proximal phalanx. When two separate muscles are dissected, one is inserted into bone and the other into the wing tendon on the radial side of the extensor mechanism. Nothing is done with the lumbrical attached to the index FDP. Additional muscles may be found and used when a hypoplastic thumb is present[13,75] to increase the bulk of the thenar portion of the hand. In those cases, where the 1st DI (abductor indicis) is absent,[44,100,105] the EDC can be transferred to the palmar surface of the new thumb metacarpal (formerly index proximal phalanx).

The final position of the new thumb is in extension (not hyperextension), which will be properly balanced within 3–5 months when the extrinsic flexors tighten. Primary shortening of the new extrinsic flexor can be performed initially, especially with the stiff index finger.[106]

Skin closure and web construction

Following skeletal rotation and recession and reattachment of all available musculotendinous parts, one of the most challenging portions of this procedure, the tension-free closure, begins (*Fig. 27.20P,Q*). Each hand has a different amount of tissue with which to create a normal appearing, broad thumb index web space. First, the new thumb thenar flexion crease is sutured with the thumb in the appropriate amount of pronation in the palmar abducted position. In this position, the dorsal flap of the hand is advanced over the new thumb, and the dorsoradial flap of the index finger is advanced toward the MP joint of the long finger to create a normal appearing web space.[107] This may require additional mobilization and trimming of flaps. As a rule, we try to avoid a straight-line closure dorsally. Finally, the flaps on the radial side of the thumb are trimmed and closed. This skin closure provides a remarkable amount of stability to the new thumb's position. While many different incisions have been proposed,[5,75,91,92,108,109] this particular one is a modification of the Littler and Buck-Gramcko approaches.[55,75] The major differences are that the position of the new thenar crease is the most important point to be determined and the cutback incision into the index is delayed until the available skin can be draped over the index.

Treatment of other types of thumb hypoplasia (types VI–X)

Type VI: central deficiencies: cleft hand and symbrachydactyly thumb

Cleft hand

In treating a patient with the cleft hand anomaly, the following principles should be followed:

1. Release the first web syndactyly and contracture
2. Maintain maximal thumb mobility
3. Complete ulnar transposition of the index digit
4. Preserve the adductor pollicis, if present
5. Rotate full thickness skin flaps into the first web space
6. Release any syndactyly involving the two ulnar digits
7. Create an intermetacarpal ligament between index and ring fingers
8. Treat the thumb polydactyly in a standard fashion.

Several procedures and modifications have been described to accomplish these principles for the management of this condition.[28,52,71,110–114] Flaps of the cleft skin based on either the volar or dorsal surface have been used. Unfortunately, both of these designs suffer from the same anatomical problem: The skin flap from the cleft is a random pattern flap, and the viability of the distal portion of the flap can be suspect. More recently, Tajima has described closure of the newly created first web with a dorsal sliding flap.[115] Undoubtedly, this design poses less risk to the blood supply of the skin flap.

Our preferred method of thumb correction utilizes incisions much like those designed for a pollicization. An incision is made on the ulnar side of the index ray, which is then transposed as a vascular island to the long position. The metacarpal is usually disarticulated and transposed at the CMC joint level. Dorsal and palmar flaps are raised and sutured directly to the skin flaps created by incision of the ulnar side of the cleft. Simple or complex Z-plasties can then be performed on either side of the thumb-index web space as deemed necessary for contour improvement *(Fig. 27.21)*.

When these thumbs are triphalangeal, one of two options is preferred. A stable, well-aligned, mobile but long thumb is usually left uncorrected, and these longer thumbs function very well. However, the longer, flexed, or deviated triphalangeal thumbs should be treated. Shortening the thumb may require excision of the extra phalanx or osteotomies; the former approach invariably leads to stiffness. Improving alignment in the flexed or deviated triphalangeal thumb can also be challenging as the anomalous phalanx can be small. Excision of this phalanx may lead to stiffness and closing wedge osteotomies can be technically difficult. If the extra phalanx is small, the best option is to perform a closing wedge osteotomy and fuse it on its distal or proximal side to the neighboring phalanx.

A number of autosomal dominant cleft hand and foot syndromes exist. In these patients, a transverse failure of formation of the thumb may be present at the metacarpal or phalangeal level. When no phalangeal segments are present, vascularized toe to thumb transfer using the distal portion of the great toe (if present) is preferred for thumb reconstruction. Distraction lengthening is another alternative.[48,116,117] Motion in these thumbs is poor, but sensation is good, and function is very gratifying because the deformities are always bilateral. Secondary procedures for correction of intrinsic joint laxity or deviation are common.

Symbrachydactyly thumb

Observation of these children at play will provide insight into the need for any thumb reconstruction. Children with symbrachydactyly tend to be among the most functional as virtually all can oppose (not touch) the thumb to the small finger. They all have the components of a basic hand: a mobile radial ray, a cleft, and an additional ray or post on the opposite side of the hand for pinching and grasping functions. Even those with no phalangeal components can effectively grasp or pinch using only their metacarpal motion. Consequently, most of these children will not require any operative intervention, and to do so may be quite meddlesome. A hypoplastic thumb with good MP motion, stable joints, and present thenar intrinsics should be left alone.

Excision of nonfunctional nubbins will improve the shape of the cleft and provide a deeper web space for grip. Some patients with this anomaly have a thumb deficient in length and unable to oppose to the highly mobile ulnar border digit. Distraction lengthening can improve both function and appearance. These patients may also lack pulp-to-pulp pinch due to poor pronation of the thumb during pinch maneuvers. Rotational osteotomies at the metacarpal level will resolve this problem by placing the digits in a more favorable position. The severely hypoplastic thumb, with an absent or diminutive proximal phalanx and a flail MP joint, is best treated with a nonvascularized toe phalangeal transfer into the proximal phalangeal level *(Fig. 27.22)*. Although motion is not restored, the thumb becomes a more stable, functional post. These transfers are more likely to grow if performed before 1 year of age. Ablation of the small distal phalanx and

second toe microvascular transfer is an option best performed between 2 and 4 years of age. ⊕ FIG **27.22** APPEARS ONLINE ONLY

The ulnar digit in symbrachydactyly will often have an unstable MP joint and radial clinodactyly due to its asymmetrical proximal phalanx. The flexor tendons are usually strong and the extensors present but unbalanced. Stabilizations of MP joints with chondrodesis, bone grafts, and nonvascularized toe phalanges have all been performed with varying degrees of success. When positioned as stable posts, these fifth rays function quite well for hooking and balancing maneuvers. With time and growth, most of these fifth rays are lengthened with distraction techniques.

Type VII: constriction ring syndrome

The following principles apply to the management of these thumbs:

1. Immediate treatment of emergency conditions such as vascular compromise and progressive lymphedema
2. Early liberation of the thumb ray from an acrosyndactylous complex
3. Release of adduction contractures within the first web space when present and resurfacing with full thickness tissue if needed prior to any augmentation of thumb length.

Following release of the first ray, the functional requirements of the patient need to be accurately determined and the tissue(s) available carefully assessed. In those with distal amputations at the phalangeal level at or beyond the interphalangeal joint, no operative intervention may be the best course of action. Often all that needs to be corrected is a proximal constriction ring. Although the nail and palmar pulp may be atrophic, these thumbs are quite functional. Instability at the IP joint is easily corrected with a collateral ligament reconstruction using either a tendon graft or local tissues. Thumb length can be augmented utilizing one of three methods:

1. Distraction lengthening at the metacarpal level
2. Nonvascularized toe phalangeal transfer
3. Composite vascularized toe-to-thumb transfer.

Distraction lengthening[48,116,117] is best performed at the metacarpal level when satisfactory bone stock is present. The metacarpal can be easily – but slowly – lengthened up to 100% of its length as a two-staged procedure that includes application of distraction apparatus and osteotomy followed by bone grafting of the intercalated gap and internal fixation *(Fig. 27.23)*. Lengthening of deficient, terminal, and narrowed phalanges in this condition is not as predictable and the resulting digits are often stiff and thin. Distal nonunions and exposure of phalanges or hardware used for internal fixation are common complications. Therefore, second-toe composite vascularized transfers are preferred to distraction at the phalangeal level. ⊕ FIG **27.23** APPEARS ONLINE ONLY

Transfer of nonvascularized toe phalanges[118–120] is an excellent way to provide length and growth potential to an empty, redundant soft tissue envelope – occasionally seen distal to the level of amputation in this condition. Extraperiosteal harvest and transfer of the third or fourth toe proximal phalanx will result in survival and growth of the phalanx in

90% of patients under two years of age *(Fig. 27.24)*.[118] Our own experience has not been as successful since only 70% of these phalanges transferred early in life have retained normal growth potential. Survival and growth will occur in patients over 2 years of age but at a less predictable rate. The second toe is spared so that the entire toe is available for vascularized composite transfer if required. Secondary distraction lengthening of the transferred phalanx can be performed if further length is required. ⊛ FIG **27.24** APPEARS ONLINE ONLY

In patients with a congenital amputation through the proximal phalanx or metacarpal, composite microvascular transfer of a second toe has been our procedure of choice. The great toe can be transferred either as a complete or as a modified unit *(Fig. 27.25)*, but this option has been reserved for uncorrected thumb deformities, which present later in childhood. Since there is normal anatomy proximal to the level of amputation or band and there is an intact CMC joint, an excellent functional and aesthetic result of the "thoe" can be obtained. The presence of functional thenar intrinsics will also enhance the result *(Fig. 27.25)*. In several children, we have first lengthened a deficient metacarpal with an intact CMC joint in order to provide a good foundation for second toe transfer. The keys to the distraction procedure are to proceed slowly, to minimize soft tissue dissection, and to avoid injury to growth centers. The major problem with any toe transfer is the availability of toes, which, like the fingers, may be hypoplastic or aplastic in the CRS. ⊛ FIG **27.25** APPEARS ONLINE ONLY

Various types of on-top plasties have been described in the hand literature, and most consist of transfer and distal advancement of composite soft tissue and bone segments from adjacent fingers. We prefer free transfers to these local transfers, which tend to require extensive dissection and secondary contractures within the first web space. However, local ray transfers as pollicization procedures can be very effective, especially when the index ray is transferred to augment the thumb. A careful surgeon should avoid injury to the median and ulnar innervated thenar intrinsic muscles, including the adductor pollicis and its origin from the third metacarpal.

Type VIII: five-fingered hand

The optimal management of these patients is to pollicize the radial digit. The technique employed is similar to that for thumb aplasia (type V). Rebalancing of the intrinsic musculature is paramount to the success of the procedure. In the five-fingered hand anomaly, the dorsal interosseous to the radial digit is only unipennate, and secondary opponensplasty with an ADQM or ring FDS transfer is occasionally necessary. The most important procedure is the creation of a broad first web space with unscarred flap tissue.

When seen later in childhood or during adolescence, two other options are available: (1) the construction of a first web space with a forearm flap plus arthrodesis of the PIP joint or (2) a rotational recession osteotomy of the first metacarpal with pollicization and intrinsic rebalancing *(Fig. 27.26)*. This condition should not be confused with a triphalangeal thumb, in which the thumb is somewhat shorter than the other digits. Although an extra phalanx is present by definition, extrinsic and intrinsic muscle anatomy mimics a thumb more than a finger. The extra phalanx is often angulated and is commonly associated with radial polydactyly. ⊛ FIG **27.26** APPEARS ONLINE ONLY

Type IX: radial polydactyly

The management of patients with radial polydactyly will vary for the level of duplication and are discussed in more detail elsewhere in this book. In general, the surgeon should use the best parts of each thumb to construct the finest thumb possible. Distal polydactylies (types I and II) are usually managed by preservation of the ulnar duplicate, with extra soft tissue provided from the radial thumb. The resulting nail is smaller than the one on the normal side. The Bilhaut procedure is avoided if possible due to the predictable problems of nail ridging and diminished IP joint motion. The results can, however, be excellent with the more distal level polydactylies. In addition, polydactylies at the proximal phalangeal level (types III and IV) are commonly managed with ablation of the radial partner and closure with tissue from this thumb. Musculotendinous abnormalities need to be addressed with the division of interconnections and centralization of insertions. Advancement of the detached thenar intrinsics into the retained extensor mechanism is mandatory, and collateral ligament preservation and reattachment is key to providing a stable MP joint. The metacarpal head will be broad in these patients and requires trimming on the redundant radial side. Closing wedge osteotomy of the metacarpal may also be required to realign the newly constructed thumb. Appropriate trimming of excess skin should result in wound closure, which should be positioned in the high mid-axial position. Polydactylies in the metacarpal shaft (type V) can often be managed by simple ablation of the radial partner and concomitant four flap Z-plasty for any first web deficiency. Polydactylies at the CMC joint level (type VI) and triphalangeal varieties all need to be dealt with on their merit. Digital transposition of the ulnar thumb onto the retained base of the radial partner is not unusual. Skeletal realignment, tendon repositioning and first web releases can usually be completed in a single stage.

Type X: syndromic short skeletal thumb ray

Many patients with short thumbs do not require any treatment as the length deficiency is mild. In those who do have an obvious length deficiency, distraction lengthening with a secondary bone graft to the subsequent bony defect at the metacarpal level is possible.

Patients with generalized syndromes require a multidisciplinary approach to their management, and hand procedures can be coordinated with other required treatments. Children with complex hand anomalies, such as those with Apert syndrome, require special attention so that the function of these thumbs and hands can be optimized.

First web syndactyly needs to be managed in the first 3–6 months of life so that the child can develop prehension without interference. The same options for treatment are outlined in the previous section of this chapter. The deficiency of the first web in the majority of the children with craniosynostoses can be adequately treated with a four flap Z-plasty. In the more complex type II and type III hand anomalies[48] in Apert syndrome, where there is complete syndactyly of the first web, we have found tissue expansion of the first web to be a very satisfactory means of producing a long lasting release of the first web.[55] The deficiencies of length and angulation in these complex anomalies, which are osteotomy and an iliac crest bone graft *(Fig. 27.27)*. As these bones are quite small, this procedure is usually delayed until 4 or 5 years of age. ⊛ FIG 27.27 APPEARS ONLINE ONLY

Postoperative care

For nearly all of the aforementioned operations, immobilization in a well-padded long arm cast is required for at least 3–4 weeks. We prefer to remove the cast under light general anesthesia to minimize the traumatic experience for the child and to inspect and clean the wounds.

Once the cast is removed, for the next 6–8 weeks the hand is wrapped in Coban at night to reduce swelling. A thumb-spica thermoplast splint is worn at night and outside the house for additional protection during this period of time as well. After pollicization, the child works with the parents using special play activities, during which time the long and ring digits are buddy taped to encourage key pinch and grasp using the new thumb. It comes as no surprise that we have seen a positive correlation between good functional results and involved, attentive parents. Other than monthly evaluations by an occupational therapist, no additional therapy is necessary. Some children start to use the reconstructed or new thumb quite early; whereas, others are hesitant. Nevertheless, by 3–6 months, all children will have actively integrated the thumb into the activities of daily living.

Outcomes, prognosis, and complications

Type I

There are no difficulties with key pulp or nail pinch, grasp, or precision pinch that requires palmar abduction of the thumb. However, the recorded strengths may not reach normal levels. The motion depends upon the pre operative condition of the joints and strength of key pinch and chuck pinch are directly related to the existing thenar musculature.

Type II

Although these are not normal thumbs, functional restoration following early surgery is quite good.[5,9,31,80] Although motion of the MP joint is decreased following ligament stabilization or chondrodesis, good mobility of the CMC and IP joints will provide excellent function. Attempts to stabilize through chondrodesis often result in a nonunion. In these thumbs, flexion at the IP joint level is diminished and pinch strength reduced not because of a poor adductor pollicis (AddP) muscle but due to the weak flexor pollicis longus, which is usually quite malformed. Precision and power grasp between the thumb and three opposing digits is much less than normal. The amount and degree of loss is proportional to the anatomical variations encountered, including the pollex abductus abnormality, deficient flexor muscle mass, and the amount of surgery required for correction. Stiff thumbs with poor mobility are much more common when there is a partial or complete loss of the radius in the same forearm.

Type IIIA

The type IIIA reconstructed thumbs are short, slender, less mobile than the type II thumbs, and functional use is highly individual. The only certainty is that these thumbs are never normal. Many studies have correlated the outcome with the degree of anatomical abnormality and the amount surgery required.[31,80,107] Following MP joint stabilization, motion is diminished; following web release, the first ray is much more mobile and grasp is markedly improved; and following opposition transfers, palmar abduction is maintained if the muscle or tendon transfer is functional.[82] Chondrodesis in young children frequently fail a need to be repeated as arthrodesis when they are older. Thumb IP joint flexion is rarely normal and, in fact, the chance of obtaining good functional flexion in a child born without a flexion crease is very poor despite one recent optimistic report.[31] With a pollex abductus anomaly and a lax or flail MP joint, both MP and IP joint motion will be significantly reduced following reconstruction. The average IP motion in Lister's series was 21° following one or two-staged reconstruction of the flexor mechanism in the presence of multiple musculotendinous anomalies.[80] Children receiving flexor reconstruction also require joint stabilization at either the MP or IP joints. Efforts to release anomalous flexor tendons, interconnections, and/or muscles and use these parts to salvage IP joint motion can be very frustrating, particularly if one watches these children grow beyond adolescence.

Types IIIB, IIIC, and IV

The clinical outcomes following pollicization are not controversial and will be discussed with the type V thumbs. If pollicization is not undertaken, staged reconstructions following intercalated bone graft and/or tendon graft stabilization are predictable. The web space remains deficient. The thumbs are rigid with poor MP or IP joint motion, and the collateral ligament reconstruction at the MP joint level becomes lax with time. Outcome studies[121] indicate that these reconstructed thumbs are short, slender, and relatively immobile. There is no metacarpal growth, and as teenagers these children often express dissatisfaction with the thumb "they do not use." However, long-term follow-up interviews with a number of these children, now adults, reveal that some of these patients and their families are very attached to and enthusiastic about their small and stiff thumbs.

Some surgeons feel that the functional pinch and appearance is well worth the effort involved in complicated microvascular reconstructions.[67,68,115,122] However, the potential lack of growth and immobility are major deterrents.[1,6,65,85,109,123,124] The advantage of the microvascular procedures to stabilize the metacarpal base and augment soft tissue is that of growth and restoration of an adequate first web space. The functional results of a number of small series[62,66–68,70,115,125] verify that stability can be achieved but motion is severely impaired. These thumbs are small and have a rudimentary nail complex and scarred web space, which is generally less aesthetically acceptable than a well executed index pollicization *(Fig. 27.28)*. The technical difficulties and risks of any free tissue transfer in young children may also be significant. ⊛ FIG **27.28** APPEARS ONLINE ONLY

When a staged reconstruction for a floating thumb (type IV) is chosen, the first ray is small, narrow and stiff. The thumb does not grow at the metacarpal level if a bone graft has been used *(Fig. 27.29)*, but will grow and have some CMC joint stability if a vascularized joint has been transferred. Most of these transfers have taken place in Asian countries due to cultural restraints. The results are not as successful as index pollicization.[121,126] ⊛ FIG **27.29** APPEARS ONLINE ONLY

Types IIIB, IIIC, IV, and V: pollicization

Our experience with more than 300 pollicization procedures is similar to that of Buck-Gramcko, who has performed over twice this number.[96,103] It is critical to understand that the new thumb will never be normal. The adequacy of the functional and aesthetic postoperative result depends entirely upon the pre operative condition of the index finger.

A child with normal skin, bones, joints, tendons and muscles will achieve an excellent outcome from a *properly performed* pollicization. A youngster with a stiff, partially mobile digit associated with a radial club hand due to a radial absence will have a less functional outcome (see below). In such a hand, it is important to accurately position the new thumb in greater opposition to the other digits avoid too much CMC extension, which would position the thumb in a very vulnerable posture. Although assessment of these procedures is difficult, there is no paucity of outcome reports.[8,44,92,96,106,127–136] Most corroborate that preoperative condition determines postoperative result.

The most thorough study of this is the report of Manske *et al.*[45] When considered as a single group of patients, total active range of motion averaged 50% of normal, standard grip strength 21%, lateral pinch 22%, and use in normal activities 84% of normal. Interestingly, these results are not significantly altered by the age of the patient at the time of operation.[8] Furthermore, studies have documented that the function and strength of these neo-thumbs improve as the children grow.[137]

The appearance of a pollicized digit is much more difficult to determine due to the subjective interpretation required. Some have tried to quantify appearance by measuring the length of the digit relative to the PIP flexion crease, the resting posture of the new thumb, and rotation relative to the other digits.[128,134] Meanwhile, others have emphasized the creation of a web across the first web space, which avoids the appearance of a finger positioned on the side of the hand.[45,97] We have observed that the parents and grandparents are almost uniformly pleased with the post operative appearance of pollicization and that the young patients do not express much of an opinion until they are teenagers, at which time many will let you know whether they like their thumbs or not. Just ask!

The influence of the age at the time of pollicization is always debated. As stated earlier, many surgeons postulate that under ideal circumstances this operation should be completed within the first year of life[14,45,80,134] in order to improve an earlier cortical awareness of the new "thumb." Developmental scientists have demonstrated that the child is aware of the thumb as a radial post by 1 year of age.[138] Some argue that since there is no thumb, the index digit is the radial substitute and that pollicization represents a repositioning

of the radial post. Manske's data[45] does not support early pollicization for functional reasons. We feel that the size of the hand and the experience, knowledge and confidence of the surgeon are more important considerations because the surgeon has only one chance to get a pollicization right.

When considering complications, the major learning curve relates to the incisions, muscle rebalancing and the creation of a normal first web space. It has been well-documented that complications rates are low in experienced hands.[139] Devascularization due to injury to the neurovascular pedicle can occur, particularly in patients with clubbed hands and no radial digital artery. This potential problem is avoided by microvascular repair and vein grafting if needed. Invariably, flap losses and their resulting contractures and disfigurement are related to technical problems during surgery. We have never seen venous compromise in our practice, but this has been reported,[139] and may be due to excessive dissection of the dorsal veins, kinking, tight dressings, or abnormal anatomy. Injury to the innervation of intrinsic muscles may go unrecognized during dissection and can be reconstructed with later transfers. To avoid this problem, these muscles are left attached to the periosteum and are not dissected proximal to the level of the palmar arch. Adduction contractures of the new thumb are the result of either poor positioning and immobilization of the skeletal ray or tight first volar interosseous muscle pull. Aseptic necrosis of the new trapezium (formally the metacarpal head) has not been a problem in our cases but has been seen. A fibrous union will function very well as the new CMC joint. Ossification of the periosteal tissue is common due to the periosteum left behind with the intrinsic muscles. Symptomatic spicules are simply excised.

Other types of thumb hypoplasia (types VI–X)

Type VI: central deficiencies – cleft hand and symbrachydactyly thumb

Cleft hand

Since most of these thumbs would fall into the Blauth type I or II categories, the results are similar. The major considerations for function relate to the adequacy of the web space construction and the integrity of the first DI and AddP muscles that are so important in all types of pinch. Strength will be lost from the thumb when the 1st DI is either recessed or detached during the index transposition. Every effort should be made to preserve what AddP muscle is present and its periosteal origin. When the index is transposed into the long position, this periosteum is reattached to the index metacarpal. Grip strength is more dependent on the ulnar three digits and not on the thumb.

Symbrachydactyly thumb

This thumb is universally smaller than the normal thumb on the contralateral hand. Once stabilized, it provides a mobile radial ray for the rest of the hand, and interphalangeal (IP) joint motion is either diminished or absent. When the IP flexion crease is absent at birth, attempts to restore motion with joint releases and extrinsic tendon reconstructions are dismal. Flexor tendon grafts are also disappointing due to the malformed motors in the forearm. If attempted, wrist flexors or extensors should be used.

Type VII: constriction ring syndrome

The functional outcome of a thumb with a congenital amputation at the interphalangeal joint level is excellent, provided there is a broad, unscarred web space between the thumb and the next digit. Thumbs lengthened with non-vascularized toe phalangeal transfers have the advantage of increased length with little mobility at the MP joint level. Thumbs lengthened with a vascularized toe transfers have the advantages of normal length, normal sensation if performed in young children, and the disadvantage of less than normal motion.[76] The functional results of these transfers in this group are superior due to the normal anatomical motors in the forearm.

Type VIII: five-fingered hand

The results are similar to those described for index pollicization without radial dysplasia. Similar outcomes have been achieved in those who had forearm flaps followed by rotation-recession osteotomies at the metacarpal level. These thumbs are all well positioned in palmar abduction but lack forceful adduction, power pinch, and grasp. The thumbs are long and slender and do not have normal or close to normal key pinch and thumb-to-index grasping strength.

Type IX: radial polydactyly

Refer to Chapter 28 in this volume.

Type X: syndromic short skeletal ray thumb

Results must be individualized to the specific thumb condition. For those with the Apert syndrome, the thumb is longer, motion is present at the MP and CMC joints, and the degree of independent function depends more upon the quality of the first web space.

Thumbs that have been lengthened with distraction techniques are longer, thinner at the phalangeal level, and stiffer at joints distal to the distraction. If distracted slowly, at approximately 0.5 mm/day, damage to the intrinsic muscles is minimized.

Secondary procedures

Additional procedures have been unusual in our experience. The most common has been opposition transfers for patients with a partial or complete absence of the radius and inadequate median innervated thenar muscles. In all of these patients, this procedure was discussed as part of the initial "game plan" prior to pollicization. In eight of our over 300 pollicizations, an osteotomy was necessary to correct the CMC hyperextension, and in seven patients (treated early in the series), it was necessary to stop persistent growth of the metacarpal. Eleven children have come back as adults to have symptomatic bone spicules from retained periosteum removed. Extensor tendon tenolysis or shortening was necessary in only ten hands. It is expected that the revision rate would be higher if our patient population were less mobile and diligent about long-term follow-up.

Many revisions have been performed on patients whose pollicization was performed by another surgeon. The most common problems were: (1) poor position of the skeletal ray; (2) excessive scarring from initial skin loss; (3) adherent extensor tendons, and (4) lack of palmar abduction (opposition). Ten patients have come back as adults: five to have a carpal tunnel release and five to have a painful, dysplastic carpal bone removed. Symptoms were related to repetitive activities at work and/or pregnancy, and all patients were between 20 and 35 years of age.

The inadequate index finger

The inadequate index finger deserves special attention because in many clinical cases, a less than normal (i.e., stiff) index finger is available for potential pollicization (*Fig. 27.30*). These cases include: ⊕ FIG **27.30** APPEARS ONLINE ONLY

1. A syndactylized index ray in a child with Holt–Oram syndrome
2. An index joined to the long finger with a complete simple syndactyly (i.e., typical cleft hand, index-long syndactyly with absent or hypoplastic thumb)
3. A stiff index finger associated with a complete or partial absence of the radius
4. A stiff index ray with a fixed proximal interphalangeal joint flexion contracture with or without a complete or partial absence of the radius
5. The mirror hand (ulnar dimelia)
6. The five-fingered hand.

In all of these cases, the clinical deficiencies of the index ray are obvious on physical examination, and the major question is whether anything can be accomplished surgically to improve either the clinical function or appearance of the hand. The absence of flexion creases indicates that there has been very little if any motion in utero and that there are deficient joints, muscles, and/or tendinous structures. At surgery, fibrous bands are present between the phalanges, which may not appear joined on radiographs. Flexion contractures (camptodactyly) may be present in the index or all digits with decreasing degrees of severity from the radial to the ulnar digits. These clinical situations do not present frequently but occur more often than anticipated. In our experience, one of these clinical scenarios is present at least 15% of the time.[97]

There are no standard guidelines for treatment in the literature and surgical recommendations are more dependent upon a given surgeon's experience than on practical reasoning. Most recommendations have been overwhelmingly conservative.[8,45,92,96,97,103,129,130,134,140–146] Options for reconstruction include: (1) no surgical treatment; (2) rotation recession osteotomy of the index ray;[147] (3) formal pollicization of the index ray, or (4) pollicization of the fifth finger.[140]

The determination of what to do and how to do it can be made much easier by an analysis of larger series of pollicizations.[8,45,92,96,103,129,140–143] Logically, the quality of the result depends predominantly upon the preoperative condition of the index ray.

For those with syndromic associations, which include major central neurologic deficits, no surgical treatment is indicated. Pollicization alone for the stiff index digit is considered by some for aesthetic reasons alone. Often, a more mobile index has been moved to the thumb position on the opposite hand. It is important to place the stiffer thumb in a more adducted position. Proper length and the creation of a normal web that extends to the index PIP joint in the thumb position are both crucial to a good appearance.

The position of the pollicized index finger is crucial for a pinch to the long finger and a grasp to the fifth finger (*Fig. 27.30*).[96,103] Usually, the new thumb will have diminished extrinsic motion, particularly in extension, because the muscles originating on the radial side of the forearm are either abnormal or absent. It is most important that this thumb be positioned for good opposition to the fifth finger, a posture that places it in less abduction than normal. If placed in too much palmar abduction and extension, this immobile post will become caught on objects or within pockets.

One alternative, rarely chosen for these patients, is the rotation-recession osteotomy in lieu of a formal pollicization.[147] We have preferred this procedure in older children, teenagers and adults with a stiff, flexed index finger, those with scarring from previous procedures, mirror hands, the five-fingered hand, and the very stiff index ray associated with a radial club hand. The principles of treatment are the same, but the ray is not shortened to the full extent of a formal pollicization. Any intrinsic muscles that are present are reattached and the extrinsic flexors and extensor tendons are shortened as appropriate. The position of the new thumb must be very carefully chosen for optimal pinch. Many radial club hand patients are born with a camptodactyly involving all proximal interphalangeal joints, which becomes progressively more severe in the most radial index and long digits. In these contracted digits, we also perform full releases with Z-plasties or full thickness skin grafts if needed. Then we consider a rotation recession osteotomy instead of a classic pollicization.

The possible combination of deformities with congenital hand differences is almost infinite, and there are many instances in which it is possible to pollicize an index digit after a number of previous procedures involving this ray have been completed. Most examples involve either a syndactylized index finger within a mitten hand or a typical cleft hand in which the index and long fingers are joined within a simple syndactyly.[148,149] In either case, the syndactyly is released before formal repositioning of the index digit.

Access the bonus content for this chapter online at **http://www.expertconsult.com**

Fig. 27.9 Thumb in typical cleft hand. **(A)** Three layers of median innervated intrinsic muscles are present in most typical cleft hands. Commonly, the index ray is joined to the thumb by a simple syndactyly. All degrees of absence of the long rays may present. The first dorsal interosseous is present and tight, and the degree of adductor pollicis hypoplasia is proportional to the amount of the third metacarpal present. A very small adductor pollicis is illustrated here. **(B)** A sampling of molds shows the wide variation in the size and depth of the central clefting. The thumbs are smaller than normal, and the longer thumbs with flexion contractures are triphalangeal.

Fig. 27.10 Symbrachydactyly thumb (atypical cleft). **(A)** The border thumb and fifth rays are the most complete in the hand. Thenar and hypothenar muscles are present and often small. Central digits are represented by hypoplastic nubbins. There are all degrees of metacarpal hypoplasia within the central three rays of the hand. Extrinsic flexors and extensors are present but abnormal. **(B)** A very wide range of variation is present in these hands.

Fig. 27.11 Constriction ring syndrome thumbs. **(A)** The thumb in these hands may present with a shallow or deep constriction ring or an amputation at any level along the skeletal ray. The phalanges at the level of loss are characteristically narrow and taper to the distal stump. **(B)** The intrinsic muscles are all present up to the level of the amputation. The proximal anatomy in this condition is normal. **(C)** The thumb is absent on the left and shows increasing length in these molds. No two hands are identical. There is great variation in the depth and location of constriction rings along the digits.

Fig. 27.12 Five fingered hand. **(A)** In the five fingered hand, the normal complement of median innervated thenar intrinsic muscles are absent. First dorsal interosseous, volar interosseous and lumbrical muscles are present in this ray, which anatomically is a digit, not a thumb. **(B)** The clinical appearance (preoperative) on the left shows that the patient has tried to flex and autopronate this ray to become a thumb.

Fig. 27.13 Type X-short skeletal ray. **(A)** A short thumb with or without radial clinodactyly is seen in many syndromes. The primary osseous abnormalities are usually seen at the proximal phalangeal joint level. The median and ulnar innervated intrinsic muscles are all present and very hypertrophied. Extrinsic and intrinsic flexors and extensors are normal up to the phalangeal level. **(B)** The left thumbs of children with four different syndromes all look similar. I: Rubinstein-Tabyii; II: Pfeiffer; III: Greig cephalopolysyndactyly; and IV: Apert acrocephalosyndactyly.

Fig. 27.16 Spectrum of metacarpal hypoplasia. **(A-D)** There is no arbitrary distinction between specific categories of thumb hypoplasia based on the skeletal appearance alone. These thumbs, which show varying degrees of hypoplasia with a presumably intact CMC joint, would be classified as type IIIA. **(E-H)** The smaller metacarpals in these examples would signify type IIIB thumbs. **(I-L)** These thumbs, with no skeletal connection, would be classified as "floating thumbs," type IV. When a syndactyly exists between the thumb and index digit, an associated congenital heart defect (the Holt–Oram syndrome) may be present.

Fig. 27.21 Cleft (typical) hand thumb. **(A)** The left hand and **(B)** radiograph of a young child

with an unusual cleft hand shows a triphalangeal thumb, a duplication at the metacarpal level, a short index ray with no distal two phalanges, and a transverse bone connecting the long and ring metacarpals at the MP joint level. The schematic illustration shows the proposed reconstruction. **(B-E)** In a first stage, the index ray (c) was transposed on top of the long metacarpal (f). Only the ulnar portion of the transverse bone (h) was saved because it articulated with the ring proximal phalanx. At the second stage, shown here, the thumb duplication (a, b) was transferred on top of the index ray to make a longer and more complete digit. Nerves and tendons were all joined. **(G-I)** The patient developed a very functional pinch between the long (and untouched) triphalangeal thumb and the index finger. At skeletal maturity, her hand and radiograph are seen. The patient has become a very confident young lady and, in fact, has won regional New England piano competitions.

Fig. 27.22 Symbrachydactyly (atypical cleft) thumbs. **(A, B)** The left hand of this child with the Moebius syndrome was reconstructed with a second toe transfer at age 18 months and is seen on the right at age 5 years during the distraction lengthening of the fifth metacarpal. The distraction was done in two stages: (1) osteotomy and application of distractor and (2) bone grafting. **(C, D)** Ten years later, the second toe transfer continued to grow in comparison to the ulnar metacarpal post. **(E, F)** The left hand and radiograph of another patient with generous soft tissue nubbins, which represent the thumb and digits. **(G, H)** He was an ideal candidate for nonvascularized toe phalangeal transfer to the thumb and index rays. The first web space was also deepened and widened with local flaps. Despite the limited mobility, this reconstruction was very functional. Despite the limited mobility of the hand, he had very functional use of this hand as a helper hand.

Fig. 27.23 CRS thumb treated with distraction lengthening. **(A)** The radiograph of a young girl with a congenital amputation at the thumb interphalangeal joint level with a tight first web space. Note the tapered appearance of the proximal phalanx. **(B)** A distraction apparatus in place is pulling one end of the metacarpal away from the osteotomy site at mid diaphyseal level. One clockwise turn of the screw equaled a 1.0 mm gain. **(C)** The new bone regenerate (callotasis) advances toward the mid portion of the gap created. The stretching injury to soft tissue is impressive! All vessels, nerves and tendons are intact. **(D)** This thumb metacarpal is now as long as the index. **(E)** Five years later both metacarpals are growing but the index is now longer. **(F)** The first web space was deepened to increase thumb mobility and increase its span. **(G)** Although shorter than normal, this thumb has functioned very well on her dominant hand.

Fig. 27.24 CRS thumb treated with toe phalanx. **(A-D)** This child with CRS acrosyndactyly had the fibrous connections holding all fingertips released in the newborn nursery. The thumb ends at the metaphysis of the proximal phalanx and the index finger at the middle phalanx. Nonvascularized toe phalanges from the third and fourth toes were transferred on top of the index and thumb. **(D)** The periosteum is intact, and the collateral ligaments and volar plate are attached to the skeletal part at the amputation stump. Joint motion was preserved in this child. **(E, F)** A four-flap Z-plasty deepened the first web space and improved her grasping ability. She is now 20 years of age and has had normal growth of the transferred phalanges. No further reconstruction has been performed.

Fig. 27.25 CRS thumb treated with microvascular toe transfer. **(A-C)** This boy, born with acrosyndactyly, demonstrated thumb loss at the interphalangeal joint level, no first web space, and congenital amputations of the index and long digits at the phalangeal level. Connecting bands

present at birth were released in the newborn nursery. His first surgery was a distally based radial forearm fasciocutaneous flap to the first webspace and release of the camptodactyly of the ring finger. **(D-F)** Thumb length was augmented with a modified great toe transfer. A methylmethacrylate mold of the opposite normal thumb is used to measure and contour the larger great toe at the time of operation. The incision markings are shown on the ipsilateral great toe, and the specimen is seen in transit to the recipient left thumb. **(G, H)** The thumb is seen 4 years later. Sensation is normal, and motion measures 30° at the IP joint and 50° at the MP joint. The contour has been excellent. No revisions have been performed.

Fig. 27.26 Five fingered hand. **(A, D)** The right hand of a child with bilateral five fingered hands is shown. She has auto-rotated the most radial digit into a pseudo thumb position in an effort to functional more effectively. **(B, E)** In one procedure, the thumb was shortened and fused at the proximal interphalangeal joint and a first web space created with a radial forearm fasciocutaneous flap, which is seen below before, during, and 5 years after the procedure. A superficial flexor tendon was transferred to improve palmar abduction (opposition). **(C, F)** There was been no contracture or diminution of this web space, which was lined with full thickness flap tissue.

Fig. 27.27 Type X-short skeletal ray. **(A)** The preoperative appearance and thumb radiographs of a young boy with bilateral radial clinodactyly of the thumbs ("hitchhiker thumbs") associated with the Rubenstein–Tabyii syndrome. **(B)** The soft tissue was lengthened on the radial side with a large Z-plasty, and a composite graft and the bone seen lengthened here with an opening wedge osteotomy and corticocancellous bone graft held with two C-wires. **(C)** The same thumbs are seen 7 years later. The right side has grown normally, and on the left side, the deformity has recurred because of the premature closure of the most radial border of the physis.

Fig. 27.28 Type IIIB microvascular reconstruction. **(A, B)** The radiograph and clinical picture

show a type IIIB thumb in which there is no proximal metacarpal or CMC joint. This thumb has no skeletal attachment to the rest of the hand. **(C, D)** A second-toe metatarsophalangeal joint, with covering soft tissue flap, has been transferred to provide the skeletal connection and stability. The picture shown is at skeletal maturity. Tendon transfers were needed to provide extrinsic flexion and extension to the thumb, and the skin flap helped build up the thenar region. (Case provided by G. Foucher, MD)

Fig. 27.29 Type IIIB staged reconstruction. **(A, B)** The preoperative radiograph and clinical appearance of a type IV thumb in a child whose parents insisted upon saving it. **(C, D)** A bridging iliac corticocancellous bone graft was used to stabilize the thumb, which became an immobile post and did not grow commensurately with the child. At age 14 years, the same child came to the authors' clinic and asked when she would be given her a "normal" thumb.

Fig. 27.30 Inadequate index finger. **(A)** This 7-year-old boy with bilateral absence of the radius shows his pectoralis major muscle transfer, which is now working as an elbow flexor. After preliminary distraction, the hand and wrist were centralized over the distal ulna. **(B)** The characteristic widening of the distal ulna is seen. From ulnar to radial, the PIP joints of the digits had increasing fixed flexion contractures to the extent that the index finger was flexed 100° degrees and was useless. After a successful pollicization on his other hand, the patient asked for improvement of this hand. **(C)** First, the proximal and middle phalanges were shortened, and an arthrodesis was performed at the PIP joint level. **(D)** Next, a rotation-recession osteotomy placed the new thumb in enough palmar abduction to allow pulp to pulp pinch with the long finger and grasping of small objects. This position purposefully keeps the thumb from becoming caught in pants pockets and other objects. **(E)** Internal plate and screw fixation was used. Motion was present only at the MP joint. Within weeks of the operation, he began to use this previously ignored digit.

Access the complete references list online at **http://www.expertconsult.com**

6. Blauth W. The hypoplastic thumb. *Arch Orthop Unfallchir.* 1967;62(3):225–246.

   This article presents early classification of thumb hypoplasia that has become the "gold standard" of diagnosis. Despite minor modifications, today's well-accepted classification system still bears Blauth's name.

9. Manske PR, McCarroll Jr HR, James M. Type III-A hypoplastic thumb. *J Hand Surg Am.* 1995;20(2):246–253.

   This article clearly defines the anatomical and functional differences between type IIIA and IIIB thumbs. They conclude that CMC joint stability and extrinsic tendon abnormalities allow differentiation between these two types of thumb hypoplasia. They recommend reconstruction for IIIA thumbs and ablation with pollicization for IIIB thumbs.

13. Littler J. The neurovascular pedicle method of digital transposition for reconstruction of the thumb. *Plast Reconstr Surg.* 1953;12:303–319.

   This is a classic article on the technique of digital transposition by a master hand surgeon. He refined the techniques for traumatic thumb loss developed by Bunnell and others after the Second World War and applied them to congenital cases.

14. Buck-Gramcko D. Pollicization of the index finger. Method and results in aplasia and hypoplasia of the thumb. *J Bone Joint Surg Am.* 1971;53(8):1605–1617.

    Buck-Gramcko obtained a large experience with pollicization after the thalidomide crisis in Europe. This seminal paper describes the classic technique that he developed, which remains the present-day standard for pollicization.

45. Manske PR, Rotman MB, Dailey LA. Long-term functional results after pollicization for the congenitally deficient thumb. *J Hand Surg Am.* 1992;17(6):1064–1072.

    This is a well-documented study on the long-term outcomes of pollicization. The results show that the pollicized digit is quite functional, albeit it never achieve as much strength or mobility as a normal thumb. Outcomes fell into two categories depending on the preoperative state of the index finger. They found no difference in outcome between patients who underwent pollicization very early in life and others who underwent pollicization in early childhood.

68. Foucher G, Medina J, Navarro R. Microsurgical reconstruction of the hypoplastic thumb, type IIIB. *J Reconstr Microsurg.* 2001;17(1):9–15.

72. Woolf R, Broadbent T. The four-flap Z-plasty. *Plast Reconstr Surg.* 1972;49:48–51.

98. Upton J, Sharma S, Taghinia AH. Vascularized adipofascial island flap for thenar augmentation in pollicization. *Plast Reconstr Surg.* 2008;122(4):1089–1094.

106. Bartlett GR, Coombs CJ, Johnstone BR. Primary shortening of the pollicized long flexor tendon in congenital pollicization. *J Hand Surg Am.* 2001;26(4):595–598.

136. Clark DI, Chell J, Davis TR. Pollicisation of the index finger. A 27-year follow-up study. *J Bone Joint Surg.* 1998;80(4):631–635.

28

Congenital hand IV: Disorders of differentiation and duplication

Steven E. R. Hovius

SYNOPSIS

- Syndactyly is one of the most common congenital differences in the upper extremity and can be classified as incomplete (soft tissue only, not extending to the tip), complete (soft tissue only, extending to the tip), complex (with distal bony union) or complicated (with more than only distal bone fusion).

- Timing of surgery depends on the fingers involved and whether the syndactyly is cutaneous or not. In the simple digit 3–4 syndactyly there is no hurry, while in the simple thumb-index syndactyly release is undertaken early. When bony fusion accompanies syndactyly (complex/complicated), these fusions should be separated early to prevent asymmetric growth if the fused fingers have different lengths.

- Creating a web and nail fold and adding skin to the inner borders of the digits in complete syndactyly are the three key elements in separating the digits.

- Poland syndrome is characterized by unilateral absence of the sternocostal head of the pectoralis muscle combined with ipsilateral short and webbed fingers. The central three digits are most affected. It can vary from a smaller hand, simple syndactyly to symbrachydactyly, up to more severe hypoplasia of the entire arm.

- Apert syndrome (acrocephalosyndactyly) is characterized by craniosynostosis with complex acrosyndactyly of both hands and feet. Common features of both hands in Apert Syndrome are: brachy-clinodactyly of the thumb, complex syndactyly of index/long/ring finger, symbrachyphalangism and simple syndactyly of the fourth web. Three different types of hand malformations can be recognized: the flat, "spade" hand (type I), the constricted cupped, "mitten" hand (type II) and the coalesced "rosebud" hand (type III).

- The surgical sequence in correction of Apert syndrome is release of thumb and index or deepening of the first web and separation of digit 4 and 5, followed by separation of the other digits and correction of clinodactyly of the thumb. If present, 4–5 metacarpal synostoses can be separated.

- Symphalangism is a longitudinal bony fusion of the finger and/or toe joints. In hereditary symphalangism, the PIPJ is mostly involved.

- In metacarpal synostosis, curvature of the epiphysis, discrepancy in length between the two involved metacarpals, and the shape of the bones, will direct the choice of treatment. Surgical treatment in metacarpal synostosis is functional and aesthetic. Consultations are necessary until skeletal maturity because of angulation, length discrepancies and rotation that can occur due to growth.

- Congenital radioulnar synostosis is less common than the post-traumatic version. In most cases of radioulnar synostosis, the proximal third is involved, with bilateral involvement in 60%. It is common in craniofacial hand disorders. Treatment is recommended in patients with a fixed pronation of more than 60° and complaints of disability in daily life.

- Polydactyly of the hand can be divided into radial, central (digit 2, 3, and 4), and ulnar polydactyly, referring to the region of the extra digit or part of a digit. It can occur isolated or syndromic. Syndromes are more associated with ulnar polydactyly than radial polydactyly. The most commonly used classification for radial polydactyly is the Wassel classification (also known as the Iowa system). Ulnar polydactyly is either classified into two or three types.

- Timing of surgery is arbitrary. Surgery is recommended in the first year of life by many authors, and depends on the severity of the condition. Floating little fingers are often removed early. At the first operation as much correction as possible is performed on both soft tissues and bones. Correct alignment and balancing forces on the joints and bones is crucial. Growth will make insufficiently corrected tissue worse.

- Inadequate correction in proximal radial polydactyly leads to complications such as S- and Z-deformities mostly due to imbalance. In distal polydactyly it can lead to nail deformities and broadness of the distal end of the thumb.

- Triphalangeal thumb can vary from a longer thumb with deviation due to the extra phalanx to a nonopposable thumb with an inadequate first web and aberrant muscles and tendons, with the thumb in the same plane as the hand, resembling a five fingered hand. Triphalangeal thumb can be associated with polydactyly, syndactyly, cleft hand and longitudinal ray deficiency (e.g., Holt–Oram syndrome). It occurs isolated or as an autosomal dominant trait.

- In less complex opposable triphalangeal thumbs, primary surgical strategies are focused on the distal two joints of the "thumb" comprising correction of deviation, reduction of additional length and joint stabilization. In more complex nonopposable triphalangeal thumbs, treatment not only is concentrated on the middle and distal phalanx but also on balancing of the MCPJ and CMCJ, together with reduction of metacarpal length up to formal pollicization. Additional polydactyly and syndactyly, if present, will also need attention.

- Camptodactyly is a contracture of the PIPJ in the antero-posterior direction (campylo = arched and dactylos = finger). Camptodactyly is mostly sporadic without obvious family history. The most involved finger is the little finger, followed by the ring finger. All fingers can be involved. It can occur in the first year of life and progress further or present during adolescence. Conservative treatment is mostly advocated. Multiple surgical treatment regimens have been proposed varying from full release, tendon transfers and skin grafts to correction osteotomy, arthroplasty and arthrodesis. All techniques have relative merit.

- Clinodactyly is derived from "*klineia*" (to bend, incline or slope) and "*dactylos*" (finger, toe) and is used for a deviated finger in a radio-ulnar direction. The deviation is caused by an abnormally shaped bone. The middle phalanx of the little finger and the proximal phalanx of the thumb are the most frequently involved. Treatment can be a closed wedge osteotomy, reversed wedge osteotomy or an opening wedge osteotomy, with or without bone graft or a physiolysis.

 Access the Historical Perspective sections online at
http://www.expertconsult.com

Syndactyly

Introduction

The distal end of the 'normal' web lies on the palmar side roughly at the mid-level of the proximal phalanx.[1] A more distal web is called syndactyly. Syndactyly is one of the most common congenital hand malformations with an incidence of 1 in 2000 live births. Familial syndactyly is reported in 15–40% of syndactylies.[2,3] They are more common in Caucasians than in people from African descent. About 50% of patients have bilateral involvement. Males are more affected than females varying from 46–84%. The incidence of ray involvement in syndactyly is in digit 3–4: 50%; digit 4–5: 30%; digit 2–3: 15% and digit 1–2: 5%.[1,2] It can appear isolated or in association with other deformities in the upper or lower extremity or as part of a syndrome (like Poland Syndrome or Apert Syndrome). Syndactyly can be associated with polydactyly and/ or clefting (like in synpolydactyly, Greig syndrome, Oculodentodigital syndrome and cleft hand).

Syndactyly can be classified as incomplete (soft tissue only, not extending to the tip), complete (soft tissue only, extending to the tip), complex (with distal bone union) or complicated (with more than only distal bone fusion) *(Fig. 28.1)*.[2] For the first web the terms simple, complex and complicated are used most.

Basic science/disease process

In the developing limb bud, fingers become apparent at day 41–43 and are fully separated at day 53.[5–7] Apoptosis is needed for separation of the fingers. This process is mediated by BMP-4 (bone morphogenic protein).[8] Current understanding relates these anomalies to differentiation disturbances in the developing hand plate.[9]

Diagnosis/patient presentation

Syndactyly can be present in a large variety of forms as it is only a descriptive term. The fingers can be normal or anomalous; the number of affected fingers can differ, as well as the nature of involvement *(Fig. 28.2)*.

In the patient with cutaneous syndactyly, only the soft tissues between the fingers are attached. These skin bridges can vary from supple to tight, influencing surgery. In the incomplete form, the attachment usually ends just before the proximal interphalangeal joint (PIPJ). In the complete form the nails can be separated with full pulps of the affected fingers to conjoined nails with ridges and insufficient pulp on the attached sides. If the involved fingers have normal bone structure, the joints and tendons are mostly normal. If not, like in symbrachydactyly, the tendons and joints will be affected as well as the neurovascular bundles which can divide more distally. When fingers are of unequal length the longest finger will tend to bend more during growth especially if the distal ends are fused.

Complex syndactyly with distal bone fusion involving only two fingers can be recognized by a tapered distal end with inward rotation of the fingers and abnormally ridged or confluent nails. When more fingers are distally fused they can be flat to very cupped with anomalous nails; abnormal bones with different lengths and abnormal located insufficient developed joints.

Complicated syndactyly is characterized by an abnormal bone structure inside the syndactyly with fusions, rudimentary bones, missing bones, abnormal joints and sometimes cross bones.[5,10]

Patient selection

Timing of surgery depends on the fingers involved and whether the syndactyly is cutaneous or not.

Early indications for surgery are syndactylies between fingers of unequal length; with distal bone fusions; and in complex or complicated acrosyndactyly especially if the thumb is involved. These early indications are to prevent asymmetric growth and/or to create a possibility to grasp.[11] In the simple digit 3–4 syndactyly, there is no hurry.

Simple syndactyly release can be performed from 6 months onwards. Most surgeons will operate on these children between 1–2 years to prevent anesthesia problems.[12]

In complicated syndactylies for some affected rays, the support for the individual fingers is often not enough to let them function well following separation, although parents or children often request to separate these fingers. Careful assessment of the maturity of each individual finger is necessary before release of syndactyly is undertaken. Especially in

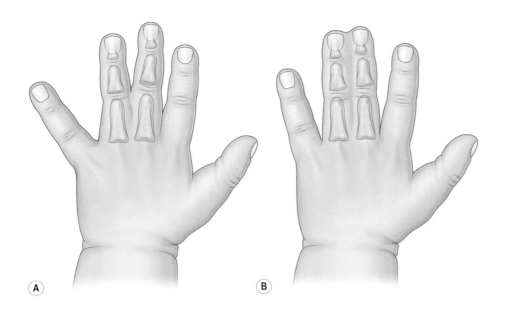

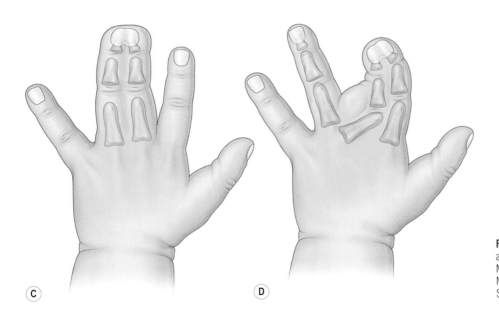

Fig. 28.1 (A) Incomplete, **(B)** complete, **(C)** complex and **(D)** complicated syndactyly. (Redrawn after Upton J. Management of disorders of separation – syndactyly. In: Mathes SJ, ed. Plastic surgery, Vol. 8. Philadelphia: Saunders Elsevier; 2006:140.)

symbrachydactyly the choice to separate can be extremely difficult.

Treatment/surgical technique

Treatment of syndactyly should not only address the key points of adequate release but also in the least number of operations while minimizing complications.[12] Release of syndactyly implicates separation of conjoined skin and subcutaneous tissue preserving integrity of the neurovascular bundles. Furthermore, conjoined ligaments and bands and existing sites of osseous union are divided. On the dorsal side subcutaneous fat can be removed but care has to be taken to prevent damage to the neurovascular bundle. For safety reasons two adjacent complete syndactylous fingers are not separated at

the same time as vascular anatomy can be different. In short multiple syndactylous fingers, for instance, dominant digital vessels can only exist on the lateral sides of the conjoined fingers. Sometimes it is necessary to sacrifice one of the vessels in a distal bifurcation. The nerves in these cases can mostly be dissected more proximally. In young children bone or cartilaginous fusions can be separated by knife or osteotome.[11]

Hints and tips[11,13,14]

Key points in syndactyly release are:
- Creation of a web
- Treating the lateral soft tissue defects
- Separation of the fingertips

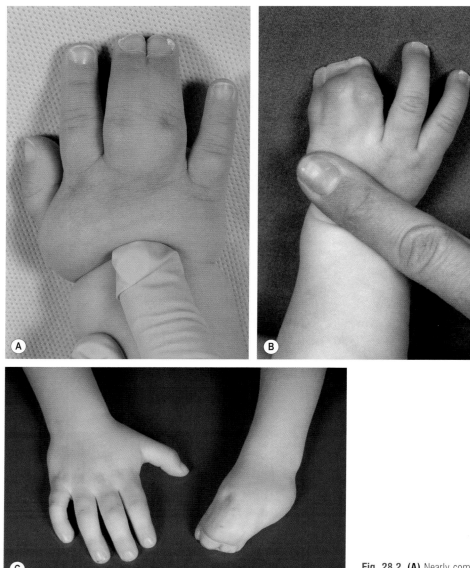

Fig. 28.2 (A) Nearly complete syndactyly, **(B)** complex syndactyly radial side and **(C)** complicated syndactyly.

Creation of a web

The web in syndactyly can basically be created by a dorsal flap; a palmar flap or a combination of both. These techniques have already been practised in the second half of the 19th century and are still used today. To these techniques have been added flaps with slightly different design or flaps more proximal from the dorsum of the hand.[14–19] I use a dorsal clover leaf flap because the wings will cover partly the lateral side of the proximal phalanx and the tip is interdigitated on the palmar side preventing linear scars in the web itself as well as palmarly. In an effort to prevent skin grafts, dorsal metacarpal flaps have been used to create the web, followed by primary closure of the fingers *(Fig. 28.3)*.[18–20]

For the first web, different kinds of Z-flaps (four flap, double, double opposing, five flap) transposition flaps from the dorsum of the hand and index or thumb are used depending on the width and deepness of the created defect following release. Also pedicled flaps and free flaps have been advocated for the larger defects.[21] In the first web, the release of the tight fascia on the first dorsal interosseous muscle in combination with the fascia on the adductor muscle is essential to create a deeper web. Sometimes even the insertion of the adductor muscle is shifted more proximally to open the web.

Upton has published an excellent overview of all the different flaps for web reconstruction.[5] For incomplete syndactyly many variations of rotating Z-flaps have been described for web reconstruction *(Fig. 28.4)*.[22]

Treating the lateral soft tissue defects

In syndactyly, the shortage of skin is very often underestimated. In the regular simple syndactyly, skin shortage is at least 36% of the circumference of the finger which is

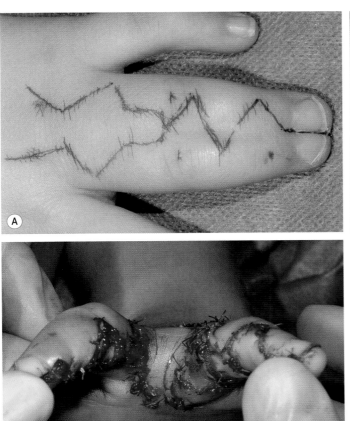

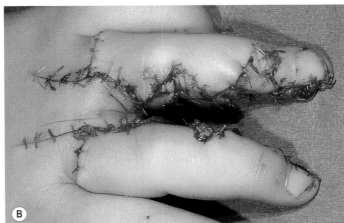

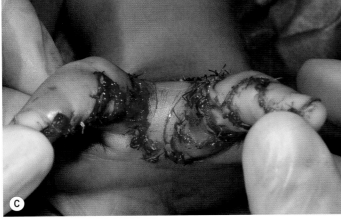

Fig. 28.3 Release of complete syndactyly with dorsal clover leaf flap. **(A)** Proximal dorsal triangles can be closed primarily. **(B)** Interdigital flaps are approximated, additional skin grafts applied and direct closure at the nail wall is performed. **(C)** Note web flap.

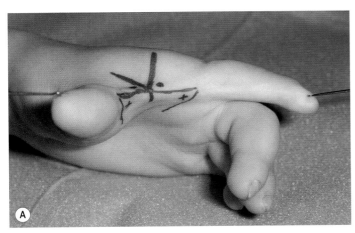

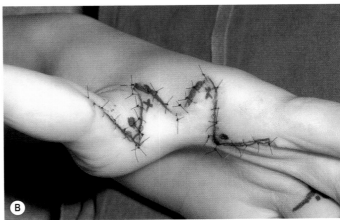

Fig. 28.4 (A,B) Incomplete 1st web release with 5-Z plasty.

separated. Cronin has popularized the zig-zag skin separation distal to the flap for web reconstruction.[23] The created triangular flaps provide coverage at the PIPJ. The triangular flaps can either be fully or partially interdigitated depending on the extent of the skin shortage. In this way the areas for skin grafting can be diminished and placed on less demanding parts of the fingers. Full thickness skin grafts (FTSG) are mostly used to cover the defects *(Fig. 28.5)*. They can be taken from the groin more laterally to prevent later hair growth on the grafts or from other sites like the inner side of the upper arm or from the cubital fossa. Also thicker split thickness skin grafts (STSG) can be taken from the nonweight bearing part of the sole of the foot. Withey *et al.* used only STSGs at the proximal base of the inner sides of the released fingers together with a large number of triangular flaps. The remaining defects were left open resulting in good scars.[24]

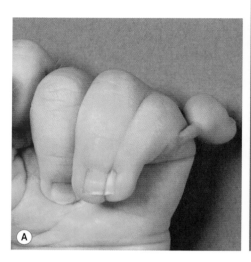
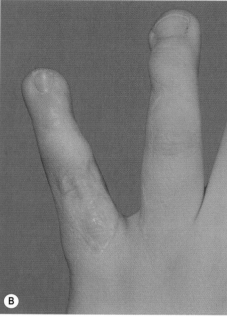
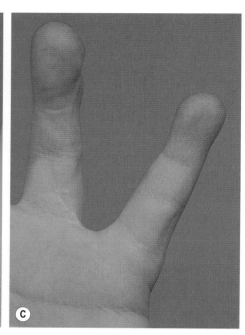

Fig. 28.5 Release of complex syndactyly of digit 4 and 5 (**A,** note also ulnar polydactyly); (**B,C**) with 10-year follow-up.

Separation of the fingertips

If the nails are separately developed in complete syndactyly, the pulp can be separated and the skin advanced to the rim. If the nails are partly fused with a deep furrow and indentation on the pulp side than simple separation and primary closure is often still possible. If the nails are conjoined, with hardly or no ridge than nail wall reconstruction with flaps is necessary. Buck-Gramcko has introduced the pedicled pulp flaps for nail wall reconstruction from the adjacent finger pulp.[25] The disadvantage of these flaps is the sometimes thinner finger tips. Alternatives are the use of a thenar flap, but this has the disadvantage that the finger has to be supple to reach the thenar easily and it is a two-stage procedure.[26]

Hints and tips

Incomplete syndactyly
- Web reconstruction – opposing Z-plasties
- Skin defects – full thickness skin grafts (not always)

Complete and complex syndactyly
- Web reconstruction – dorsal clover leaf flap
- Nail wall reconstruction
  - separate nails or nail with ridge: separation and skin closure
  - confluent nail: use of adjacent pulp flaps
- Bone separation if necessary
- Skin defects – full thickness skin grafts

Postoperative care

Perioperative paraffin gauze is applied on the wounds and grafts, followed by moist dressings, synthetic cotton, and an elastic bandage. The elbow, forearm and hand are subsequently covered with a longitudinal adhesive bandage to prevent removing the dressing. The general concept among most authors is to perform wound inspection in the first 2 weeks after operation.[14,25]

One week postoperatively, wound inspection is performed and a brace is applied as a boxing glove until wound healing is adequate. Further immobilization is dependent on surgery for associated malformations.

Outcomes, prognosis, and complications

Outcome can be related to web creep, scarring, graft take, rotation, deviation and loss of function.

Early complications can be skin slough, flap necrosis, infection, up to nearly complete adhesion of fingers.

Web creep has been reported to be from 0% to 12% depending on the used techniques, the long-term follow-up, and the variety of included patients. Reoperations have been performed for web creep in up to 8% of patients.[20,27–30]

With regard to skin grafts, FTSGs have a better skin quality than STSGs; they can also create problems such as graft loss; skin contracture; web creep; hair growth; hyperpigmentation, and hypertrophic scarring.[19,25,31–35]

Skin contractures in using STSGs are reported to occur in 40%, while this was only 22% when using FTSGs.[33] Flexion contractures are reported in a series with long-term follow-up to be 13% and rotation and lateral deviation in 12%.[36] Hair growth when using FTSGs from the groin is reported as being 71%.[30] Leaving small areas open between numerous triangular flaps seems to result in less scarring and there is no difference in web creep versus the classical approach.[24]

In a group treated with dorsal metacarpal flaps or extended dorsal interdigital flaps and primary closure,

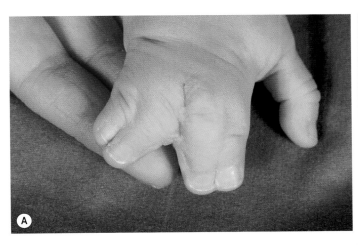
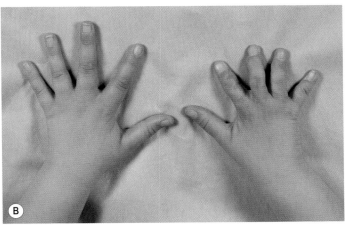

Fig. 28.6 Re-syndactyly following separation. Note initial operation with separation 3–4 instead of starting with 2–3 and 4–5 at **(A)** the first operation and **(B)** long-term follow-up following re-separation.

results were better, avoiding all the problems with skin grafts.[18–20]

In complex and complicated syndactylies following separation, rotated and deviated fingers can occur as well as insufficient functioning of the individual separated fingers. Joint instabilities are also possible and may be underestimated. This is however a consequence of the initial deformity and is difficult to treat.

Patients should be followed till the end of growth to detect later problems, such as web creep and scar contractures. Redo releases of residual syndactyly is often undertaken, especially at the first web in more complex cases *(Fig. 28.6)*.

Secondary procedures

Secondary procedures are: scar contracture release and re-deepening of webs with or without flaps. In complicated syndactylies, ligament reconstructions, osteotomies, chondrodesis and arthrodeses can be necessary.

Poland syndrome

Introduction

The reported incidence of Poland syndrome is approximately 1 in 7000–100 000. There is a male predominance, especially in sporadic cases, and the right side is involved in 60–75% of the cases. In females however, the left and right side occurrence is almost equal. In familial Poland syndrome, the male:female ratio and side predominance is the same.

Basic science/disease process

Several mechanisms in the pathogenesis of Poland syndrome have been described. Despite some familial occurrence, no inheritance patterns have been determined. The most prevailing theory focuses on the interruption of blood supply to the limb bud in the 6th week of gestation. The interruption

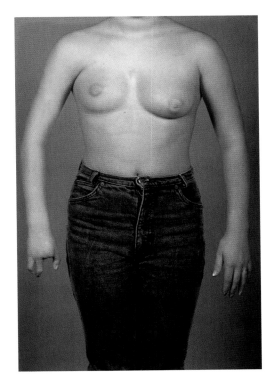

Fig. 28.7 Symbrachydactyly and pectoralis major anomaly and smaller breast on the right side.

will cause hypoplasia to the ipsilateral subclavian artery or one of the branches[39,40] determining the diversity of the defect.

Diagnosis/patient presentation

In Poland syndrome, patients present with a broad range of ipsilateral trunk, upper limb and hand anomalies. The classical presentation comprises a combination of absence of the sternocostal portion of the pectoral major muscle, hypoplastic arm and a hypoplastic hand with a simple syndactyly usually of all web spaces *(Fig. 28.7)*. The thoracic deformities might range from the classical absence to complete hypoplastic shoulder girdle with involvement of the ribs and nipple, scoliosis, and seldom dextrocardia.[41,42] Furthermore, Poland syndrome can be associated with multiple other malformations, ranging from craniofacial, internal organs to the lower extremity.[43,44]

Patient selection

Because of the variety in clinical presentation in Poland syndrome, each treatment is individualized, based on the functional and aesthetic possibilities.

Treatment/surgical technique

Because of the wide scope in presentation of the syndactyly and symbrachydactyly, several treatment options are possible (see Chapters 27 and 29). Reconstruction of the breast, deficient muscle contour or chest wall deformity is beyond the scope of this chapter.

Postoperative care

See Chapter 27.

Outcomes, prognosis, and complications

Outcome is very much related to the original defect and the reconstruction used.

In syndactylous hypoplastic fingers, the separated individual fingers can be less functional than before the operation, resulting in poor outcome. Normally, similar outcome and complications occur as in syndactyly and symbrachydactyly. For prognosis and complications on nonvascularized and vascularized toe transfers, see Chapters 14 and 27.

Secondary procedures

The secondary procedures relate to the broad variety of treatment options available for the treatment of the hand in Poland syndrome. Secondary procedures are mostly re-deepening of scarred webs. If tightened ligaments become lax, arthrodesis of the unstable joint can be done, after the growth plate is closed.

Apert syndrome

Introduction

Acrocephalosyndactyly syndrome is characterized by craniosynostosis combined with acrosyndactyly (distal part of the fingers fused) and symphalangism (congenital ankylosis of the proximal phalangeal joints) of the index, long and ring fingers of both hands and a radial clinodactyly of the thumb in a symmetrical way. The little finger is usually the best finger with a simple syndactyly at the fourth web. Both feet are also affected.

The birth prevalence of Apert syndrome ranges from 7.6 to 22.3 per million live births, the lowest incidence being in Hispanics and the highest in Asians. Males and females are equally affected.[45] In the author's series, the male to female ratio was 1.5:1.

The craniofacial features in Apert syndrome consist of a variety of skull deformities originating from premature closure of the coronal and often lamboid sutures of the skull, and a midface hypoplasia. These deformities can lead to a high incidence of intracranial pressure and obstructive sleep apnea. Craniofacial operations include early cranial vault expansion and if indicated, midface advancement is performed later in life. Other differences are an oily skin, hyperhydrosis, decreased eyesight and hearing, and increased strabismus. Children often display impaired language development and motor skills.

In the lower extremity, the hips become increasingly stiff over time. The knees demonstrate mild to moderate genu valgum. The feet have simple and complete syndactyly. No acrosyndactyly of feet was encountered in contrast to the hand. If present, medial polydactyly is mostly at the base of the first metatarsal. The foot deformity causes shoe fitting problems and abnormal gait, and possible pain due to callouses over the prominent fifth and third metatarsal heads.

Basic science/disease process

Apert syndrome is caused by a mutation in the gene encoding fibroblast growth factor receptor-2 (FGFR 2). The gene map locus is 10q26. Two mutations are well recognized and are related to substitutions at two amino acid positions P253R and S252W in FGFR 2. The more severe type of Apert hand is mostly related to the P253R mutation. In our series, nearly all type III Apert hands were attributed to this mutation. Most cases are sporadic, but autosomal dominant inheritance has been reported.[48,49]

Diagnosis/patient presentation

In the Apert syndrome child, the level of function depends more on their intellectual capacities than the severity of extremity involvement. Most Apert children are capable of self-care over 5 years of age. Regarding the upper extremity, motion of the shoulder is not normal and decreases with age. In the older Apert patient, a marked deltoid muscular atrophy is often encountered. They appear to have anterior subluxation of the humeral head.[50] The elbow deformities can differ more extensively between these patients than at the shoulder. Elbow function can be slightly decreased but mostly do not worsen over the years.[50]

Upton has classified the Apert syndrome hand into type I, II, and III for ease of clinical decision-making (Table 28.1). In the type I hand ("spade" hand), there is a radially deviated small thumb with a shallow first web. The index, long, and ring fingers display complete or complex syndactyly. The little finger is attached by a simple complete or incomplete syndactyly and can mostly move at the DIPJ. The MPJs have adequate range of motion. In the type II hand ("mitten" or "spoon" hand), the thumb is radially deviated and has an incomplete or complete simple syndactyly with the index. The index, long, and ring fingers are distally fused, creating a curve in the palm with divergent metacarpals. The little finger is attached to the ring with a mostly complete but simple syndactyly.

Table 28.1 Apert syndrome: common features of hands in Apert syndrome

	Thumb	Digit 2, 3, 4	Digit 5
Type I	Brachyclinodactyly Incomplete 1st-web syndactyly	Symphalangism Complex syndactyly	Simple (incomplete) syndactyly of 4th web or separate digit MC 4–5 synostosis possible
Type II	Brachyclinodactyly Simple (incomplete) syndactyly	Symphalangism Complex syndactyly	Complete syndactyly Duplication P3 possible MC 4–5 synostosis possible
Type III	Brachydactyly Complex syndactyly Paronychial infections Skin maceration	Symphalangism Complex syndactyly paronychial infections Skin maceration	Complete syndactyly Duplication P3 possible MC 4–5 synostosis possible

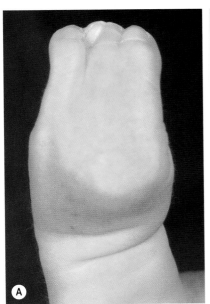
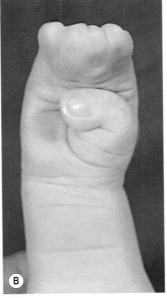
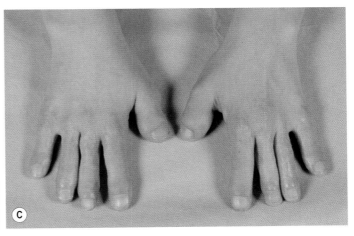

Fig. 28.8 **(A)** Apert hand left dorsal view. **(B)** Right hand palmar view and **(C)** postoperative result at 18 years of age.

In the type III hand ('rosebud' hand) the thumb, index, long, and ring are distally fused either cartilaginous or bony attachments. The thumb can be very difficult to identify separately from the index. The little finger is united to the ring by simple complete syndactyly. The nails can be confluent or have ridges indicating the distal finger underneath. Proximal synostosis at the base of the fourth to fifth metacarpal can be present, as well as carpal fusions.[51] In our series of 66 patients the ratio of type III:type II:type I hand was 4:3:3; although Upton reports that type III is the most uncommon.

Up to 7% ulnar polydactyly has been reported.[52] In the author's series, there is one case of a duplicated distal phalanx of the index and two cases of duplication at the little finger (5%). In the type III hand, finger nails growing through surrounding skin causing frequent paronychial infections is frequently seen.

The flexion creases are often absent. Dimples on the dorsum indicate the metacarpophalangeal joints (MPJs). Distal to the MPJs, neurovascular structures can vary considerably in branching, or are absent. Distal in the hand, tendons can have a different shape and course. Regarding the thumb, adduction, palmar abduction, and flexion are always present. The first dorsal interosseous is hypertrophic and fan shaped extending to the delta phalanx of the thumb in the more severe types. The abductor pollicis brevis muscle (APB) is anomalous as it inserts into the radial aspect of the distal phalanx of the thumb causing radial deviation.[53] Lumbricals if present act as MPJ flexors. The hypothenar muscles are present and normal.

The proximal phalanx of the thumb is abnormal and triangular shaped. The IPJ and the CMCJ have little motion, while the MPJ is mobile. With skeletal maturity the IPJ fuses after first being segmented. The distal phalanx and nail matrix are broad.[54,55]

Symphalangism at the proximal interphalangeal joints of the index, long, and ring finger is a persistent finding. In border digits (the index and the fifth), the epiphyseal growth plate can be aberrant at the MPJ causing lateral deviation following separation.

Table 28.2 Preferred treatments in Apert syndrome

	Zuker et al.[56]	Upton[51]	Fearon[57]	Guero[54]	Chang et al.[58]

First stage	Bilateral
	3 months of age
	  1st-web 4 flap
	  Z-plasty or dorsal
	    skin flap web-index
	  2nd and 4th-web
	    space with dorsal
	    flap
		Bilateral
		1–6 months of age
		  1st-web space with
		    dorsal skin flap
		  Resection index
		  4th-web release
		  Incision of nailfold/
		    macerations
			Both hands and feet
			9–12 months of age
			  Deepening of
			    1st-web and
			    3rd-web one hand
			  Release of 2nd and
			    4th-web on other
			    hand
			  Similar releases on
			    feet
				Bilateral
				9–10 months of age
				  1st-web release
				    with Buck-Gramcko
				    flap
				  Release APB
				  Release of 4th-web
				    for a 3 fingered
				    hand
				  Release of 3rd-web
				    for a 4 fingered
				    hand
					Bilateral
					6–15 months of age
					  Release of border
					    digits

Second stage	Unilateral
	Before age 3
	
	Groin flap in
	  3rd-web if
	  necessary
		Within 6 months of
		  1st stage
		Unilateral
		Before 3 years of age
		  Long-ring release
		  Re-deepening
		  1st-web
			3 months after 1st
			  stage
			
			Release of the
			  remaining webs on
			  both feet and
			  hands
				Unilateral;
				6 months between
				  unilateral stages
				
				In 4 fingered hand:
				  release of 4th-web
				In 3 fingered hand:
				  release of 2nd-web,
				  removal of 4th ray
					Unilateral
					Before age 2;
					3 months between
					  unilateral stages
					  Release of middle
					    digit mass
					  Excision of bone,
					    leaving 3 digits
					  Opening wedge
					    osteotomy thumb
					    clinodactyly

Goal	Four fingers and
	  thumb
			Two-stage syndactyly
			  release of all fingers
			  and toes
				Three/four fingers and
				  thumb
					Three/four fingers
					  and thumb

Additional		4–6 years
		  Metacarpal
		    synostosis
		    correction
		  Thumb clinodactyly
		    correction
		  Re-deepening
		    1st-web
			9–12 years
			  Dorsal osteotomies
			    at "PIP" for
			    anatomic position
			  Correction radial
			    clinodactyly
			  Addressing foot
			    disorders if present		

Patient selection

Many articles have been published on treatment timing in Apert syndrome.[51,54,56–58] Most philosophies try to diminish the number of operations by releasing as many fingers as possible in one session. The way this is accomplished varies among authors (*Table 28.2*).

Treatment/surgical technique

Separation of thumb and fingers, correction of thumbs and mobilization of the little finger in as few operations as possible is the surgical goal. The author's preferred method is illustrated in *Table 28.3* and *Figures 28.8 and 28.9*.

Separation of fingers

Mostly dorsal flaps are used to create webs. For the remaining distal syndactyly, fingers can be separated by zig-zag, or straight incisions in the fingers with symphalangism. Nail walls can be reconstructed with flaps from the adjacent finger pulp.

The residual defects are covered with skin grafts. Chang only used local flaps and skin grafts, while Zuker et al. and Kay use groin flaps for the central digits and the first web, respectively.[21,56,58] Often further corrections are necessary to deepen webs.

Habenicht uses small external fixators to transversely distract the complicated and complex syndactyly of the central fingers, with separation of the distal bone fusions. The created skin is used for coverage of the defects instead of skin grafts. Other methods such as silastic sheets and tissue expanders to separate fingers have been discarded.[59]

Thumb and first web

A well separated thumb is crucial in these hands. In a shallow first web (in the type I hand), a 4- or 5-flap Z-plasty can be utilized. In a complete or nearly complete syndactyly (in the type II hand), a large dorsal flap is used to create a first web.[60]

Table 28.3 Apert syndrome – author's preferred treatment

Stage	Age	Procedures	Types
First	3 months	Both hands	All types
		Thumb separation with dorsal cloverleaf flap with straight line incision distally	Type II and III
		1st-web deepening with double-opposing Z-plasty	Type I
		Index amputation if necessary	Only severe type III
		4th-web separation with cloverleaf flap with straight line incision distally	All types
		2nd, 3rd, 4th distal digit separation with modified Buck-Gramcko flaps	Only type III
		2nd-web separation with cloverleaf flap with straight line incision distally	Type I and II
Second	12 months	One hand	In all types
		Separation of 3rd-web with cloverleaf flap with straight line incision distally	In type I, II, and if amputation index in III
		Separation of 2nd-web with cloverleaf flap with straight line incision distally	If no amputation in type III
		Re-deepening of the 1st-web	If necessary in all types
		Skin release radial side thumb with Z-plasty and release of APB	Type I and II
		Open or reversed wedge osteotomy of clinodactyly of thumb	Type I and II
		Synostosis MC4–5 (excised bone can be used for the wedge osteotomy of thumb	If present
Third	<24 months	Same as second stage, on contralateral side	

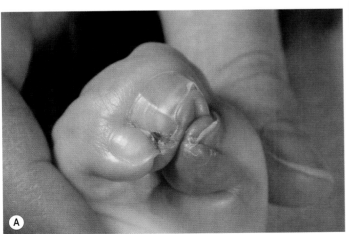
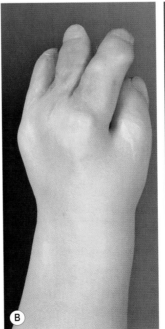
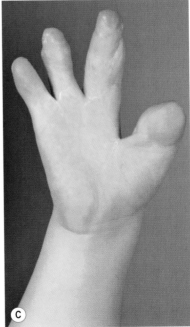

Fig. 28.9 (A) Apert type III hand left. **(B)** Long term follow-up left hand dorsal view and **(C)** right hand palmar view.

Tight fascia around the adductor muscle is released to open up the first web.

Preferably, a hand with four fingers and a thumb is created. In the type III hand however, it can be necessary to sacrifice the index to create a useful first web with a dorsal flap.[61,62]

Clinodactyly of the thumb is often corrected in the second stage because of more skeletal maturity. The tight skin on the radial side at IPJ level can be released with a Z-plasty. The APB is released from the distal phalanx. The triangular bone is treated as in clinodactyly (see below).

Dao *et al.* considered the abnormal radiodistal insertion of the APB responsible for the deviation of the thumb, and released the APB muscle and tendon distally without performing a corrective osteotomy.[53] In the type III hand, the thumb is short and has less bone volume distally.

Additional procedures

Synostosis, if present, at the proximal 4th–5th metacarpal should be separated early to improve function of the fifth ray in this rather stiff hand. Aberrant growth plates at the index and little finger can cause clinodactyly after separation. Wedge osteotomies may be needed secondarily to correct this deviation. Even without aberrant growth plates, the border digits tend to laterally deviate.

Postoperative care

Postoperatively, the hand is carefully dressed and covered by a small plaster splint. Over this plaster, a completely covering adhesive bandage is applied preventing elbow extension. At the outpatient clinic a week later the wound is inspected and a brace fully covering the hand is applied, until wound healing is achieved.

Outcomes, prognosis, and complications

The hand function is improved the most if the thumb is separated together with separation of the little finger, as it is the best finger. In this way, the thumb can adduct powerfully with the ulnar proximal part of the thumb. Also, a sort of tripod pinch with the more mobile little finger is ensured. Movement of the fingers, except the little finger is only at the MPJ. Lengthening of the thumb and separation of the remaining fused fingers does not improve function considerably, however it is requested to improve the appearance.

Complications

The hyperhidrosis and oily skin makes the skin grafts prone to maceration, skin slough and even infection. Barot and Caplan reported a 22% partial skin graft loss.[63] Guero operates on these children in winter, to diminish sweltering bandages and casts.[54] Secondary procedures for web contractures are therefore common. The revision rate for secondary web contracture varies among authors from 3–18%.[54,57,58,63] In the author's series, there has been 13% secondary contracture release. Revising web contractures depends very much on the surgeon's idea of contracture. Patients rarely complain of web contractures. The author tends to deepen the first web extra if a syndactyly release of fingers is planned. Other described interventions are amputation of a finger due to limited opening of the first web space or because of ankylosis.[54]

Secondary procedures

Secondary operations include:
- Web deepening with advancing of the primary flap or skin grafting the newly created defect

- Wedge osteotomies of the border digits as necessary to correct the deviation following separation due to partial closure of the epiphyseal plate
- Extra thumb lengthening is sometimes requested in very short thumbs in type III hands.

Synostosis

Introduction

Synostosis is derived from the Greek; *syn* = together and *osteon* = bone, and is defined as a union of two or more adjacent bones. Abnormalities in union of the bones of the upper extremity occur at all levels because of a failure of segmentation. Fusions may occur at more than one level. For instance in Apert's syndrome, symphalangism in conjunction with metacarpal synostosis and carpal fusion may also occur. Most synostotic differences present with another condition. The presence of a synostotic anomaly does not necessitate surgical treatment, but is dictated by functional discomfort and aesthetics.

Symphalangism was first described by Cushing as an autosomal dominant genetic skeletal disorder[64] and is characterized by longitudinal bone fusions along the finger and toe joints. Most commonly, the PIPJ is fused. Associated bone fusions are carpal or tarsal synostosis, and stapes fixation resulting in conductive deafness. Flatt and Wood[65] classified the congenital difference as true symphalangism with normal length of digits; with symphalangism in symbrachydactyly; or associated with other anomalies (i.e., Apert or Poland). The incidence of true symphalangism is 0.03–4%.[60] Because of the conjunction with other conditions, the general incidence of all types of symphalangism is not known.

Metacarpal synostosis is a rare congenital anomaly, with wide anatomical variations. The fourth and fifth metacarpals are usually affected. The synostosis is more common in patients with a craniofacial and hand difference. Incidences in a large group of congenital hand anomalies range from 0.02%[66] to 0.07%.[67] Buck-Gramcko and Wood distinguished three groups based on the length of fusion: type I, fusion at the base; type II, fusion of about half; type III, more than half; IIIa separated MCPJ, and IIIb common MCPJ.[67] A classification, useful for treatment, has been proposed by Foucher *et al.*[68] It comprises the shape of the synostosis, the growth direction of the epiphysis, the deformity of the finger distal from the synostosis, the webbing, and the hypoplasia of the metacarpal bone.

Carpal coalitions are reported rarely, and often go unnoticed. All combinations of carpal fusions have been mentioned, with the most frequent synostosis being between the triquetrum and lunate, and the hamate and capitate.[69,70] In a predominantly white population, an incidence with a range of 0.07–0.1% has been mentioned,[71,72] compared with 8% in a Nigerian population. Despite the fact that coalition will theoretically impair the movement of the wrist, no disabilities have been described.

Radioulnar synostosis is a rare upper limb malformation and is defined as a fusion of the proximal ends of the radius and ulna, which will prohibit normal rotational movement of the radius around the ulna. Radioulnar synostosis can be unilateral or bilateral (60%), of autosomal dominant inheritance, or associated with other congenital differences. In one-third of cases syndromes and anomalies are listed.[5,73,74]

Basic science/disease process

Mutations in genes involved in limb development and mutations in the Noggin gene (NOG) have been associated with synostosis. An interruption of apoptosis responsible for the segmentation is believed to be the most common cause for synostosis. The gene responsible for the hereditary form of symphalangism (SYM or SYM1) is the NOG, which maps to human chromosome 17 (17q21–q22).[77] Mutations in HOXA11 are associated with radioulnar synostosis.

Diagnosis/patient presentation

In hereditary symphalangism, the PIPJ is the most commonly involved joint with a compensatory movement in the DIPJ and normal movement of the MPJ. The DIPJ is involved in symbrachydactyly. At physical examination, the fingers are slender, with atrophic skin, and the flexion creases are absent at the involved joints. The anomaly presents at one or more fingers, from ulnar to radial. The thumb is seldom involved. In radiographic examination of the child's hand, a pseudo joint can be visible, represented by the cartilaginous bar between the two bones. Later in life, radiographs will show a minimal joint space due to full coalition at the joint.

In metacarpal synostosis, the most common fusion is between the fourth and fifth metacarpals *(Fig. 28.10A)*. A short and abducted little finger is seen in these cases. However, the extent of deformity is dependent on the plane of the joint space and the configuration of the epiphysis of the involved metacarpal heads. A radiograph will give insight into the skeletal abnormality and will guide in the abnormalities of soft tissue alignment.

Patients with radioulnar synostosis *(Fig. 28.10B)* will present within the first 3 years of life because of the inability to perform tasks in daily life, as holding objects two-handed. In severe cases, they will hyperabduct their shoulder, and compensate with a hypermobility of the wrist for the excessive pronation.

Patient selection/treatment/surgical technique

The treatment of symphalangism is mostly conservative. Because of anomalies of the flexor and extensor tendons, early surgical intervention is not successful. In well-segmented joints only, exploration and release of the collateral ligaments and dorsal capsule may improve function; however, results are not predictable. Arthrodesis in a more functional position of the involved joints at skeletal maturity will improve function and grip. Distraction lengthening of the stiff fingers in symbrachydactyly may improve the pinch between the thumb and a short index finger. It can lead to possible better aesthetics, however, the treated fingers can become thin and stiff.

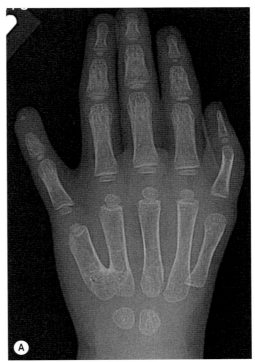

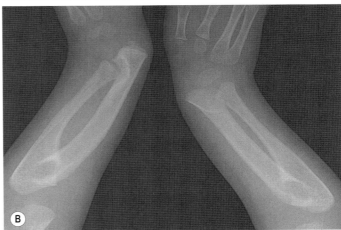

Fig. 28.10 (A) X-ray of metacarpal 4–5 synostosis. **(B)** X-ray of bilateral carpal and radioulnar. synostosis.

The indications for treatment of a metacarpal synostosis are both functional and aesthetic, and depend on the type of fusion. The abducted little finger may get caught in pockets and therefore be a problem. The goal of treatment will be a longitudinal, axially oriented ray with the MCP joint in line with the other joints, preserving its motion and joint surface, and correction of angulation and rotation. Less functional digits should be positioned out of the way of the thumb to little finger prehension.[5] Several operative treatments have been advocated, depending on the type of synostosis[5,68] ranging from osteotomy alone[68,78] to lengthening with bone graft or callodistraction[5,68,79] and longitudinal splitting combined with an interposition bone graft.[5]

Carpal synostosis will only need treatment in painful fibrocartilaginous coalition. If this is the case, it is advised to fuse the involved carpal bones.

In radio-ulnar synostosis, only few patients will need surgery because patients will compensate with wrist and shoulder movement. Treatment is recommended when a patient is compromised in daily actions with a fixed pronation of 60° or more in unilateral and bilateral cases.

To restore movement, longitudinal osteotomy at the fusion site in combination with a vascularized adipofascial flap and alignment of the radial head[80] has been performed. Several types of osteotomies have been described. Only resection of the synostosis is disappointing with rapid re-fusion as a result. To prevent re-fusion, the anconeus muscle has been used, as well as pedicled and free vascularized fat flaps.[80,81] Derotational osteotomies are performed just distal to the fusion,[82] or at the proximal radius and distal ulna.[83,84]

Postoperative care

In symphalangism, postoperative treatment consists of passive movement of the released joints. When an osteotomy is performed, treatment should be focussed on the type of fixation. If a metacarpophalangeal joint is released, with or without additional tendon transfers, these should be addressed accordingly.

Outcomes, prognosis, and complications

In most of the cases, metacarpal synostosis will not need treatment. If treating metacarpal synostosis, early problems are the diminished metacarpophalangeal movement, mostly present preoperatively, and insufficient alignment of the involved digits in metacarpal synostosis. Late problems may be a recurrent abduction of the little finger, and a re-ankylosis at the osteotomy site, despite interposition.

In radioulnar synostosis, improved function and decreased musculoskeletal discomfort in adjacent joints are reported with up to 80% having good to excellent results.[80] As mentioned earlier, even with an interposition graft, re-ankylosis is possible with increased pronation. Neurologic and vascular compromise, and Volkmann ischemic contracture have been reported,[85] especially in cases of longitudinal osteotomy at the fusion site. This should be avoided by monitoring the degree of rotation and removing a segment at the osteotomy site.[5]

Secondary procedures

Secondary procedures performed on metacarpal synostosis and radioulnar synostosis are reoperations because of incomplete correction, re-ankylosis, or loss of motion. Because of the influence of growth, children should be observed until skeletal maturity, especially in metacarpal synostosis. Less motion in the metacarpophalangeal joint should also be addressed.

Polydactyly

Introduction

Polydactyly (*poly* = more; *dactylos* = finger) refers to the disorder in which patients have more than five digits on at least one extremity. Together with syndactyly and camptodactyly, it is the most common congenital upper extremity difference.

The disorder is easily detected leading to cosmetic concern with the parents and if not treated, to cosmetic concern of the affected child. Additionally, depending on the level of the duplication, it can cause functional impairment. Polydactyly of the hand can be divided into radial, central and ulnar polydactyly, referring to the region of the extra digit or part of a digit. The International Federation of Societies for Surgery of the Hand classified these malformations in group III.[86]

The incidence of polydactyly varies depending on the studied population. Region, race and combined numbers of all polydactylies, or only radial or ulnar sided polydactyly, provide very different incidences in published series. The incidence can range from 2% to 30% when considering all types of polydactylies and up to 40% in the Chinese population. The prevalence of polydactylies is 10.7 of 1000 live births in people with an African descent compared with 2.5 of 1000 live births in Chinese people and 1.6 of 1000 live births in Caucasians. Ulnar polydactyly is 10 times more common in those of African descent and twice as common in males, whereas radial polydactyly is more common in Asians. Central polydactyly is extremely rare in all published studies.

At the author's center, out of 200 new patients per year with congenital hand deformities, about 15% have polydactyly, including 50% with radial polydactyly, 9% with central polydactyly, and 33% with ulnar polydactyly (some in combination). In the author's series, 42% of polydactylies are bilateral.

Radial polydactyly is mostly isolated, whereas syndromic association is more common in ulnar polydactyly. Furthermore, ulnar polydactyly is mostly bilateral and can be associated with syndactyly and polydactyly of the feet. Children born to parents with nubbins or floating little fingers inherit the same type of polydactyly. Children born to parents with more developed extra little fingers can present with all types of polydactyly.[87]

Many syndromes have been described in combination with different kinds of polydactyly. Already, 97 genetic syndromes have been associated with polydactyly.[88] In syndromes, there may be anomalies of the hands and feet. Moreover, combinations of polydactyly in the hand can occur, such as radial with ulnar, and central with ulnar. In the Greig syndrome (cephalopolysyndactyly), polydactyly can occur in any combination. For common syndromes associated with polydactyly, see *Table 28.4*.

A separate entity is the mirror hand or ulnar dimelia. In the forearm, two ulnae exist without a radius. Because the medial side is a mirror image of the lateral side, the term mirror hand became popular. It is extremely rare.[75] The classic mirror hand is unilateral, usually with 7–8 fingers without a thumb, and is not combined with other anomalies. The etiology is unknown. The inheritance pattern has not been found. Geneticists believe it to be a spontaneous mutation.

Basic science/disease process

Genetic aspects

In the patient with isolated radial polydactyly, a diminished genetic penetrance exists, with a variable expression. Furthermore, in numerous families with inherited isolated dominant radial polydactyly and triphalangeal thumb, a connection with chromosome 7q36 is demonstrated. In this particular

Table 28.4 Common syndromes associated with polydactyly

Syndrome	Hand difference	Concurrent symptoms
Radial polydactyly		
Holt–Oram	Hypoplastic thumb to bifid thumb Different anomalies of the upper limb, unilateral or bilateral	Cardial abnormalities
Fanconi anemia	Variety of radial differences of the hand Radial dysplasia	Pancytopenia, abnormalities of heart, lungs, kidney's and digestive tract, deafness, eye/eyelid problems, short stature
Townes–Brocks	Polydactyly	Imperforate anus, abnormal shaped ears, kidney abnormalities, hearing loss, heart defects, genital malformations
Ulnar polydactyly		
Bardet–Biedl	Ulnar polydactyly in majority of cases, might be in combination with syndactyly	Poor vision, reduces or loss of smell, cardiovascular disease, urogenital disease, mental and growth retardation, obesity
Smith–Lemli–Opitz	Polydactyly Syndactyly of second and third toe	Microcephaly, mental retardation, malformations of the heart, kidneys, gastrointestinal tract and genitalia
Trisomy 13	Polydactyly Abnormal palm pattern, overlapping fingers over thumb	Microcephaly, mentally and motor challenged, eye defects, meningomyelocele, rocker-bottom feet, cutis aplasia, cleft palate, urogenital defects, heart defects
Combined polydactyly		
Greig syndrome	Variety of polydactyly with or without syndactyly, broad thumbs	Ocular hypertelorism, macrocephaly Polydactyly of the feet (medial and/or lateral)

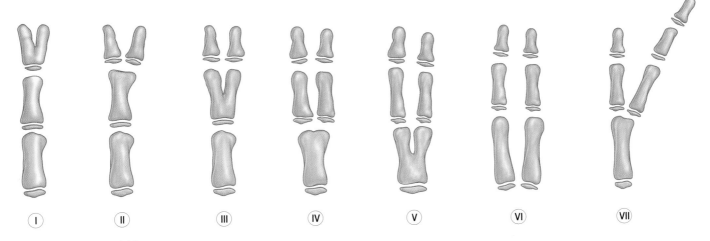

Fig. 28.11 Wassel type I–VII.

chromosome lies the regulatory element of the SHH protein. In isolated ulnar polydactyly an autosomal dominant inheritance pattern occurs, with a diminished genetic penetrance and a variable expression. It is genetically heterogeneous, implying that the cause lies in mutations in various genes.

Diagnosis/patient presentation

Radial polydactyly

In radial (pre-axial) polydactyly, the most commonly used classification is the Wassel classification.

The Wassel classification *(Fig. 28.11)*[89] is based on radiology and is easy to remember. The levels of duplication of the different types are: type I at the distal phalanx; type II at the IPJ; type III at the proximal phalanx; type IV at the MCPJ; type V at the metacarpal and type VI at the CMCJ. Thumbs of which at least one is triphalangeal are type VII, this can be either at the MCPJ or at the CMCJ.

In most series, the three most common Wassel types are, respectively, Wassel IV (about 50%); Wassel II (about 20%), and Wassel VII (about 12%). The percentages are variable in the different reported series.[90–92] As 31% in our polydactyl series could not be well classified, we modified the classification system.[92] The essence lies in keeping the Wassel classification but naming the differences such as deviation and triphalangism (see below).

At first consultation, following medical history and general physical examination, both upper limbs are examined. If the index to little finger is normal, with normal hand and finger creases, and a normal hypothenar region, the examination is concentrated on the radial side of the hand. In my experience it is worthwhile to perform this systematically, as quite often more anomalies are present than only an extra thumb.

The examination is performed from proximal to distal, starting with examination of the thenar muscles. The thenar musculature varies widely from normal to severely hypoplastic. In the Wassel I and II, the thenar musculature is mostly normal, in contrast to the Wassel V, VI, and VII. Hypermobile joints should always be related to the other joints in the hands. It is important to look for creases both dorsally and palmarly. If creases are present, then a movement in that particular joint can be expected.

The CMCJ in polydactyly can be normal, stiff or hypermobile. If abnormalities in the CMCJ are present, they are mostly encountered in the more proximal polydactylies. If polydactyly is situated at the CMCJ, the MCPJ in the best thumb can be near normal. In these cases, the movement is dependent on the presence of a syndactyly between the duplication.

Depending on the location of the polydactyly, the MCPJ can be stiff, normal moving or hypermobile and hypoplastic. For instance in a polydactyly involving the MCPJ, quite often the duplication moves as a block. In most of these cases, the radial sided thumb is hypoplastic and stiff, and the ulnar thumb is the better one, often moving well at the IPJ. Finally, the IPJ can present with normal movement, stiffness or hypermobility. If the duplication is at the IPJ, both parts can move as a block. The range of motion in those cases is typically less than in a normal IPJ. In an asymmetric duplication at the IPJ, the best developed part usually moves better.

Normal examination includes extrinsic and intrinsic movement. In a newborn it is often difficult to distinguish between these movements. However, flexion and extension can be evaluated, as well as the presence of palmar abduction. In duplicated thumbs, the flexor pollicis longus is Y-shaped in the majority of cases, with a less developed tendon to the most hypoplastic thumb. Therefore, flexion can be seen simultaneously in both thumbs. The extensor apparatus is usually less developed or absent in the more hypoplastic thumb. It can be Y-shaped as in the flexor and asymmetrically attached, therefore, deviating the distal part. The fingertips can be either normal or asymmetric. The asymmetric side is typically found on the opposing sides of the two thumbs. The nails are smaller and asymmetrical in most cases. The first web is nearly always normal in the distal duplications. In more proximal polydactylies the first web can be narrower than the normal contralateral side.

Ulnar polydactyly

In ulnar (post-axial) polydactyly classifications include either two or three types. In the two-stage classification according to Temtamy and McKusick, type A comprises an extra little finger at the MCPJ, or more proximal including the CMCJ. The little finger can be hypoplastic or fully developed. Type B varies from a nubbin to an extra, nonfunctional little finger part on a pedicle. In the three-type classification, type I includes nubbins or floating little fingers, type II includes duplications at the MCPJ, and type III includes duplications of the entire ray.[90,93,94]

The most common presentation of ulnar polydactyly is a small appendix on a skin pedicle, in which a neurovascular bundle is present. The appendix, in most cases attached at the ulnar border of the proximal phalanx, has mostly a small nail and thus a distal phalanx, and is non functional. Sometimes two bones are present. If the extra little finger is more developed, the more common site of duplication is at the MCPJ. In these cases, the fifth metacarpal is broad. Depending on the extent of development and the attachment at the MCPJ, the extra little finger flexes and extends well. Full motion of the MCPJ of the normal fifth finger can be affected. Flexor tendons and extensor tendons are usually Y-shaped and asymmetrical, as in the duplicated thumb. The extra finger is usually abducted at the MCPJ and radially deviated at the PIPJ.

If the extra little finger is at the base of the metacarpal or at the CMC, the joint of the finger is usually well developed. Physical examination of ulnar polydactyly depends on the development of the extra little finger. Nevertheless, the same rules apply, as described in the examination of radial polydactyly.

Central polydactyly

In central polydactyly, the second, third and/or fourth digit can be involved in the duplication. Fully developed extra independent fingers are rare. In order of appearance, the most frequently affected is the ring finger, followed by the long finger, and ultimately the index finger. Frequently, the duplication of the fourth finger is partial and hidden by a syndactyly, typically to the third finger. A number of varieties are possible because the duplication often is not confined to one finger. In addition to the bony deformity and aberrant growth plates, anomalies of the flexor and extensor tendons and neurovascular structures are present.

In ulnar dimelia (mirror hand) the hand looks very peculiar and is restricted in function due to the lack of a thumb and the presence of multiple digits. Seven to eight fingers are present without a thumb. Syndactyly can occur. The wrist is broad and mostly flexed. The arm is shorter with a broad elbow; an extension deficit and restricted forearm rotation and shoulder movement.

Patient selection

Polydactylies are usually treated surgically. Functional impairment can vary from slight to severe, depending on the extent of the deformity. Polydactylies can be a nuisance in, for example, shaking hands, putting hands in pockets or narrow spaces and in wearing gloves. However, most parents visit the outpatient clinic with their child for aesthetic and social reasons. In patients with a syndrome with serious concomitant disease, surgery can be delayed or even be avoided.

Treatment/surgical technique

The timing of surgery is arbitrary. Surgery is recommended at the end of the first year of life by many authors, as it is important to be able to identify the structures properly and to minimize the anesthetic risks. Floating little fingers are often removed early in the newborn nursery under local anesthesia.

Knowledge of patho-embryology and patho-anatomy is essential to obtain long-term good results. Try to visualize aberrant anatomy without too much dissection!

Radial polydactyly

Hints and tips

Principles in treatment of radial polydactyly are:

- "Make one thumb from two, do not simply excise one."
- Decide which thumb should be kept.
- Do not just excise the most hypoplastic thumb but preserve tendons, ligaments and skin to align, balance and augment the residual thumb.
- At the first operation as much correction as possible is performed on both soft tissues and bones.
- Always be aware and search for less obvious anatomical anomalies, besides the extra digit.
- Align articular surfaces as axial and as congruent as possible by transverse and longitudinal osteotomies.
- Perform ligament reconstructions or releases.
- Balance tendon insertions.
- Adjust skin cover as accurately as possible.
- Postoperative dressings should be meticulously applied and resistant to removal by the child.

The surgical technique of Wassel type II and type IV will be discussed further, as they are the most frequent types.

Radial polydactyly at the IPJ (Wassel type II)

Wassel type II normally has a broad proximal phalanx with two (partial) distal phalanges with varying degrees of fusion of the bones or epiphyses *(Fig. 28.12)*. In the case of an unequal duplication, it is straightforward to select the smaller thumb to be excised. The incision can be made dorsally in a zig-zag manner for good exposure. I prefer a more lateral incision because it leaves less conspicuous scars. First the nail and nail bed of the smaller thumb is excised and then the skin over the extensor tendon is developed, if present. At the lateral side distal to the IPJ, the collateral ligament with periosteum or a small piece of cartilage is dissected proximally. The IPJ is then opened and inspected. The flexor tendon, if present, is identified and preserved and released distally. In excising the extra phalanx, the cartilage can be cut intra-articularly at the junction, corresponding to the former two thumbs. This leaves a surplus of skin, a proximally attached ligament, either (or not) an extensor and flexor tendon and a broad proximal phalanx. On the side of the excised distal phalanx a longitudinal wedge of bone from the articular surface of the proximal phalanx is removed, taking care not to remove the collateral ligament. If necessary, a transverse wedge is removed distally leaving the IPJ surface intact and subsequently placing the IPJ perpendicular to the axis of the proximal phalanx. Then the extensor and flexor of the remaining distal thumb are inspected. Mostly, the smaller part of the flexor will be excised at the border of the remaining flexor tendon. The smaller extensor tendon can be used to augment the extensor tendon of the remaining thumb. If the extensor tendon is used to reinforce the collateral ligament, it could influence extension of the remaining thumb. The collateral ligament is attached to the remaining distal phalanx. The remaining skin is carefully inserted on the lateral side, taking care to augment the deficient pulp on that side and bulkiness of skin should be prevented. Excess skin will stay visible and will not be cosmetically pleasing.

In the event of two equal hypoplastic distal thumbs, which are fortunately less frequent, the two outer halves can be joined after excising the two inner halves longitudinally, in the Bilhaut–Cloquet operation.[95] The author prefers a good smaller nail than a larger nail with a broad ridge which draws attention. Therefore he removes one nail and nail bed in nearly all cases and try to augment the usually insufficient pulp.

Radial polydactyly at the MCPJ (Wassel type IV)

Wassel type IV often demonstrates a hypoplastic or smaller extra thumb on the radial side. The operative technique has great similarities with the operation at the IPJ *(Fig. 28.13)*. The radial thumb is excised preserving the radial collateral ligament with some cartilage and after dissecting the extensor and flexor tendons the joint is inspected. The broad distal metacarpal is treated in the same way as the proximal phalanx in the IPJ in the Wassel type II, by excising a portion. The proximal phalanx is then aligned after exploring the flexor and extensor tendons of the remaining thumb. The flexor tendon can be asymmetrically situated without pulleys. Asymmetric tendons should be realigned in the 'ulnar' thumb. If deviation at the IPJ is present, it should also be corrected with a transverse wedge osteotomy at the distal end of the proximal phalanx, as it will not adjust spontaneously during growth. In diamond-shaped polydactylies, IPJ corrections are always necessary. In equal sized thumbs, the ulnar thumb is usually preserved as the ulnar collateral ligament is more important. The radial collateral ligament is subsequently reconstructed providing stability on the new radial side of the MCPJ. With the radial collateral ligament the thenar musculature is also reattached. Again skin coverage of the radial side should be meticulously adjusted to the residual defect. Adjustment of the first web is rarely necessary in Wassel type II and IV.

Ulnar polydactyly

In the floating little finger type, the pedicle is excised at its base and the neurovascular bundle is buried to prevent painful neuromas in the scar *(Fig. 28.14)*. It can be performed in the newborn nursery under local anesthesia. Care should be taken no avoid residual at the base as this can occur when a ligature is used around the pedicle. Revisions may be necessary later in life. If a more developed extra

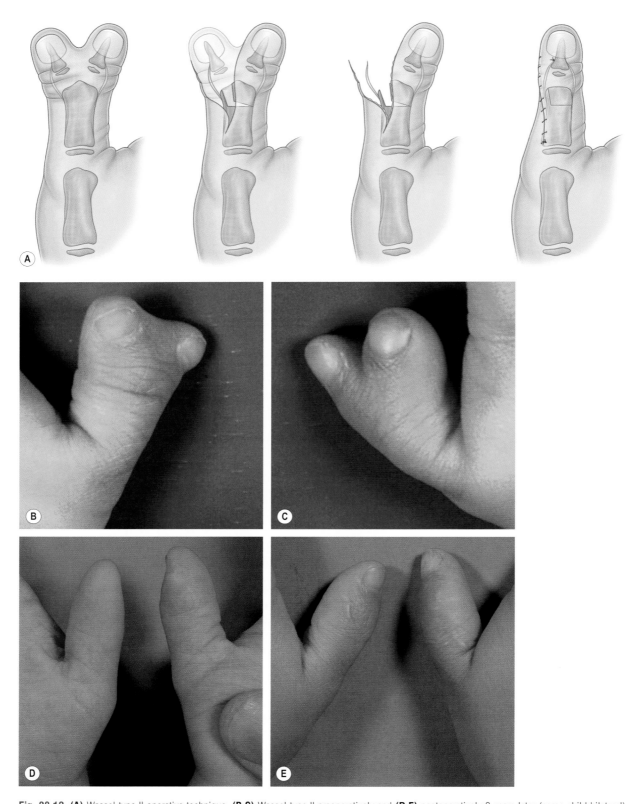

Fig. 28.12 **(A)** Wassel type II operative technique. **(B,C)** Wassel type II preoperatively and **(D,E)** postoperatively 2 years later (same child bilateral).

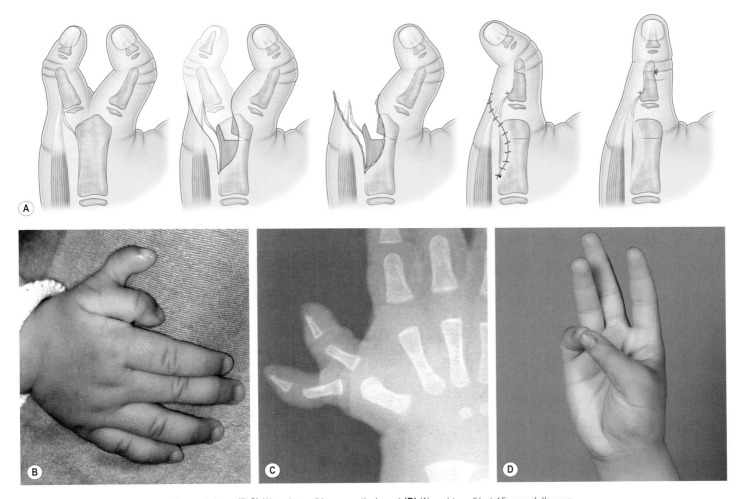

Fig. 28.13 **(A)** Wassel type IV operative technique. **(B,C)** Wassel type IV preoperatively and **(D)** Wassel type IV, at 15 years follow-up.

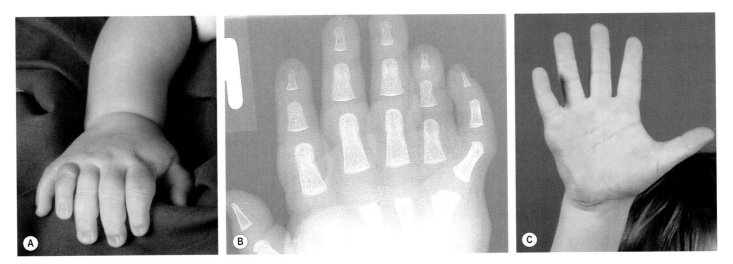

Fig. 28.14 **(A,B)** Ulnar polydactyly at MCPJ, preoperatively with X-ray and **(C)** at 4 years follow-up.

little finger exists the same principles apply as for radial polydactyly.

Central polydactyly

The basic problem in central polydactyly, in the majority of cases, is the often bizarre configuration of the skeleton with duplication and aberrant bones hidden by syndactyly. As the variety in presentation is extensive, basic rules should be followed (alignment of bones and articular surfaces) and, if possible, balanced by available tendons. However, involved fingers are insufficient or hypoplastic, and the joints are stiff. Syndactyly releases should be performed only if the fingers will obtain sufficient support *(Fig. 28.15)*.

Mirror hand

Reconstruction in the very rare mirror hand can include elbow correction, osteotomies at the forearm to improve supination and correction of flexion deformities at the wrist. The hand mostly involves resecting two or three fingers on the lateral side making a thumb of the best finger (usually the extra long finger) and creating a sufficient first web.[90]

Postoperative care

The reconstructed hand following polydactyly is immobilized for 6 weeks, allowing finger movement in the bandage. Following the initial 6 weeks, and depending on the level and complexity of the reconstruction, further treatment consists of uninhibited full motion to a removable splint for several weeks. Hand exercises under supervision are seldom necessary. In the simple ulnar polydactyly, a bandage is given for 2 days, as in regular wound care.

Outcomes, prognosis, and complications

When reconstruction in a congenital hand is performed, definitive outcome can only be assessed after growth has been completed. Therefore, it is advisable to check children several times during growth. At the outpatient clinic, examination is performed as described *(Table 28.5)*. Specific attention should be paid to nail deformities, movement and stability of joints, active range of motion, and appearance, broadness and malalignment of the skin. Older children and parents hardly complain of lack of function even though joints can be stiff. Painful thumbs are very rare. However, they do complain about appearance, often masked by an insignificant functional

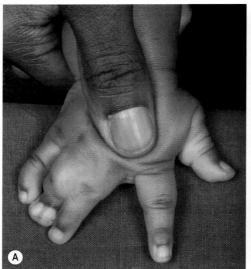
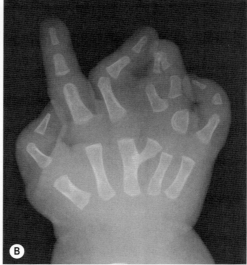
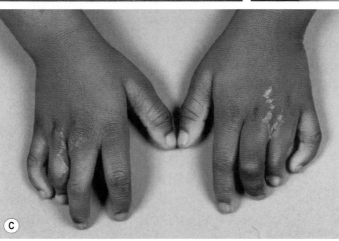

Fig. 28.15 (A,B) Bilateral central polydactyly with syndactyly (synpolydactyly); preoperative right hand and X-ray and **(C)** at 6 years follow-up, of both hands.

Table 28.5 Polydactyly: sequence of examination of the first ray

	To be noted
Aspect	
Appearance	Normal/hypoplastic
Alignment	Straight/deviated
Position	Flexed/extended
Skin	
Creases	Normal/absent at joint(s)
Fingertip	Normal/asymmetric pulp
Syndactyly	Complete/incomplete
1st-web	Normal/narrow
Nails	
	Normal/asymmetric/broad/small
Joints	
CMC, MP, IP	Stable/hypermobile/unstable
	Normal/impaired movement/stiff
Bones	
MC, P1, P2, (P3)	Normal/broad/slender
Muscle/tendon	
Thenar	Normal/hypoplastic
Extension	Present/absent/aberrant
Flexion	Present/absent/aberrant
Adduction	Present/absent/aberrant
Palmar abduction	Present/absent/aberrant
Radial abduction	Present/absent/aberrant

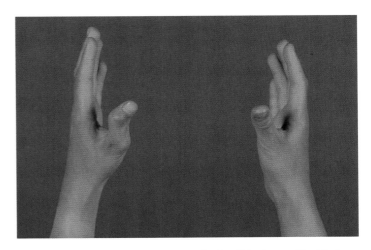

Fig. 28.16 Z-deformity following resection of only radial extra ray without further correction in unilateral Wassel type IV.

complaint. At teenagers often visit the outpatient clinic wanting the aesthetic outcome to be improved.

Outcome can be divided into unavoidable and avoidable results. In the unavoidable outcome in Wassel type II, the distal part of the thumb can be from nearly normal to hypoplastic, depending on the initial presentation. Insufficient pulp, smaller nails, and less developed IPJs are inevitable. In nail bed reconstructions, the nail will never be completely normal.

Avoidable outcomes in Wassel type II relate to inappropriate alignment, resulting in nail deformities, scarring at the nail wall, and extra nail development. If the collateral ligament is constructed with cartilage or a small piece of bone from the excised phalanx, new formation of bone can be the result. At the IPJ, incongruent alignment causes deviation, instability or stiffness. Too much resection at the base of the distal phalanx damages growth of the remaining distal phalanx.

In the unavoidable outcome in Wassel type IV, the residual thumb is always lesser developed than the normal contralateral thumb.[1] The pulp is often less developed, the nail is usually smaller, and motion can vary from nearly normal to stiff, especially at the IPJ.[96,97] Goldfarb found only a difference in nail width; however, motion was not taken into account in this study. But even though the thumb appears smaller, patients are satisfied as long as it is well-shaped.[97,98]

Avoidable outcomes in Wassel type IV also relate to inappropriate alignment. IPJ and MCPJ angulation decreases the aesthetic outcome.[96,97] Deviations at either the IP or MP joint can mostly be prevented at initial operation by aligning the articular surfaces and balancing the thumb properly. Too much resection at the MP joint results in growth disturbances at the proximal phalanx of the remaining thumb. In late S- and zig-zag deformities **(Fig. 28.16)**, proper initial alignment has not been accomplished. Residual unstable IP- or MCPJs can develop following improper ligamentous reconstruction at the initial stage.

In ulnar polydactyly a small painful mass can remain following ligation or inadequate resection of the pedicle of the extra floating little finger. If the extra finger originates at the MCP joint, full flexion at the MCP joint is mostly not possible as the joint is not normally developed.

Secondary procedures

Growth can make secondary interventions advisable without really being complications. Possible secondary procedures either or not in combination can include:

- Ligament reconstruction
- Tenolysis
- Tendon re-balancing
- Opposition transfers (sometimes in the more proximal Wassel types)
- Nail deformity correction
- Osteotomy and alignment of articular surfaces
- Neurolysis and neuroma treatment in adult patients
- Arthrodesis of IPJ or MCPJ
- Scar revision.

Triphalangeal thumb

Introduction

The general incidence is estimated by Lapidus as being 1 in 25 000 live births.[99] Of all patients with a triphalangeal thumb (TPT), two-thirds have a family history of thumb abnormalities. They mostly have bilateral deformities and have nonopposable thumbs.[3] TPT can be inherited as an autosomal dominant trait.[100] Sporadic cases are mostly unilateral and supposed to be opposable. In our series, which comprised many inherited cases, thenar muscle deficiency varied considerably. This muscle deficiency is related to the degree of opposability of the thumb.[101] In the Netherlands, the incidence of TPT is probably higher than stated in most reports, due to a number of families with an autosomal dominant trait.

Basic science/disease process

By combining family pedigrees. the inheritance pattern of TPT is as an autosomal dominant trait.[100] The location of the gene has been discovered on chromosome 7q36 in 1994.[103] The exact location in terms of base pairs has not yet been identified.

Diagnosis/patient presentation

A wide variety of phenotypes can occur with TPT. Anatomical differences are not only restricted to the extra phalanx, therefore a thorough examination should be performed of both upper extremities.

The extra middle phalanx is a constant finding in TPT. Its shape can vary from a very small wedge shaped extra phalanx resulting in a deviation at the IPJ to a fully developed extra phalanx resulting in a long thumb. Other features can be a near normal to very hypoplastic thenar musculature; a near normal to contracted and less deep first web and an extra partial or fully developed ray. The thumb can be in the same plane as the other fingers with a finger like appearance, hence the name of five fingered hand in some of these cases.

In TPT, both IPJs are mobile. In the small wedge shaped middle phalanx, no clinical distinction can be made in movement at the proximal or distal IPJ. When the middle phalanx is trapezoidal or rectangular often active movement is possible at both joints.

The MPJ can be stable to very unstable; hyperextension at this joint is common. The CMCJ can vary from hypoplastic to malformed, resulting in variations from a less mobile to an unstable joint. The CMCJ can also be absent. Also the trapezium and scaphoid can be hypoplastic, malformed or absent.

In inherited cases, differences are often bilateral. An extra ray is common in these patients, and triplications may occur. The ulnar thumb is nearly always the best developed in cases of two thumbs.

In TPT, other malformations can also occur such as syndactyly; ulnar polydactyly; cleft hand; longitudinal radial deficiency; differences of the lower extremities and as part of a syndrome with abnormalities in one or more of the other systems.[104–106]

The aforementioned makes classification of TPT difficult. Wood[107,108] classified TPT on the shape of the extra phalanx, distinguishing three types of an extra middle phalanx in the thumb: delta type, trapezoid type and full rectangular type.

Buck-Gramcko created a classification with six types, based on treatment options, including joint mobility, web space, intrinsic and extrinsic muscle abnormalities. If TPT is combined with polydactyly further classifications are possible. Wassel classified all possible combinations into Wassel VII. Our group has developed a classification for TPT combined with duplication or triplication, based on the Wassel classification in which TPT is classified according to the joint (Fig. 28.17).

Patient selection

In TPT, the patient's precision grip is impaired as a result of diminished opposition, joint instability or additional length; leading to alternative, compensating maneuvers. If syndactyly or an extra thumb is also present proper use of the hand is further decreased. Children may compensate easily for these drawbacks. Parents of young patients and older children with TPT however often want the anomaly corrected for appearance and very rarely for functional deficits. Timing of operation is not always clear in minor defects, such as small triangular phalanges.

The author's series includes a high number of dominant hereditary triphalangeal thumbs, with or without polydactyly. The affected parent was often intensively teased at school and therefore wished their child to be operated before going to school.

Because of the presence of cortical representation of a thumb, a hard indication to operate very early is not present, as a new learning process is not necessary. In only rare cases is a scissors grip between index and middle finger used. It is advisable to operate on these patients before the age of 2 years for early adaptation of the cortex to the newly created thumb.

Treatment/surgical technique

Bunnell[109,110] advised not to operate on TPTs. Beatson[111] and Milch,[112] among others[113,114] proposed removal of the abnormal phalanx to reduce length and to correct deviation. After removal of the extra phalanx, the risk of an angulated joint as end result exists.[115,116] Buck-Gramcko[117] stated that resection of the delta type extra phalanx and ligament reconstruction in the young child gives adequate results in a single procedure.

For patients with a trapezoidal or rectangular extra middle phalanx several types of osteotomies are described such as resection of the distal joint and part of the distal phalanx followed by arthrodesis[116] to excision of the proximal interphalangeal joint (PIPJ).[2] Buck-Gramcko[117] added an osteotomy of the first metacarpal with reinsertion of the intrinsic muscles and widening of the first web. If necessary an opposition transfer was also performed.

In the "five fingered" hand, pollicization is advised.[118] If the first web needs only minimal deepening, a four-flap Z-plasty[119] can be used. Foucher[120] described a W-transposition flap in which skin and subcutaneous tissue is used from the dorso-radial side of the proximal phalanx of the index to provide skin for the first web. A large rotation flap of the dorsum of the hand can be used in a nonopposable TPT where, in addition to deepening, lengthening of the first web is required.[117,121] In larger deficiencies of the first web, where the ray is placed

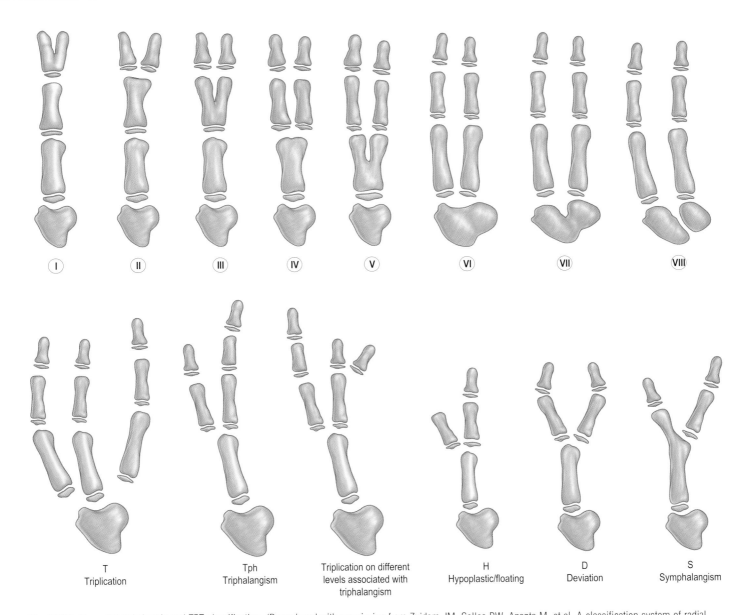

Fig. 28.17 Our radial polydactyly and TPT classification. (Reproduced with permission from Zuidam JM, Selles RW, Ananta M, et al. A classification system of radial polydactyly: inclusion of triphalangeal thumb and triplication. *J Hand Surg Am.* 2008;33(3):373–377.)

in palmar abduction (such as in patients with a five fingered hand), Upton[122] favors a distally based radial forearm fasciocutaneous flap.

An opposition transfer can be performed if hypothenar muscle deficiency exists. The most used tendon transfers for opposition transfer are the abductor digiti minimi muscle (Huber technique[123]), the superficial flexor of the ring finger[114] and the flexor carpi ulnaris.[124]

When TPT is accompanied by radial polydactyly Wassel[89] and Wood[115] advised extirpation of the TPT even if the other biphalangeal thumb is more rudimentary. Wood transposed the rudimentary biphalangeal thumb to the base of the metacarpal of the TPT, creating a shorter thumb. This transposition can be combined with a metacarpal osteotomy. Upton,[125] on the other hand, excises the rudimentary biphalangeal thumb, retains the triphalangeal thumb, and corrects the TPT. No

clear evidence exists regarding the best technique as most published series are small.

Timing of operation differs not only for the several types of TPT but also among various authors. Buck-Gramcko[117] excises the short middle phalanx before the age of 6 years, because if the child is older the joint does not remodel anymore. Wood[108] on the other hand operates between 6 months and 2 years of age.

Author's preferred method of treatment[126]

Delta middle phalanx

In children <6 years, resection of the extra phalanx is performed under fluoroscopy control *(Figs 28.18, 28.19)*. Subsequently the radial collateral ligament at the new IPJ is

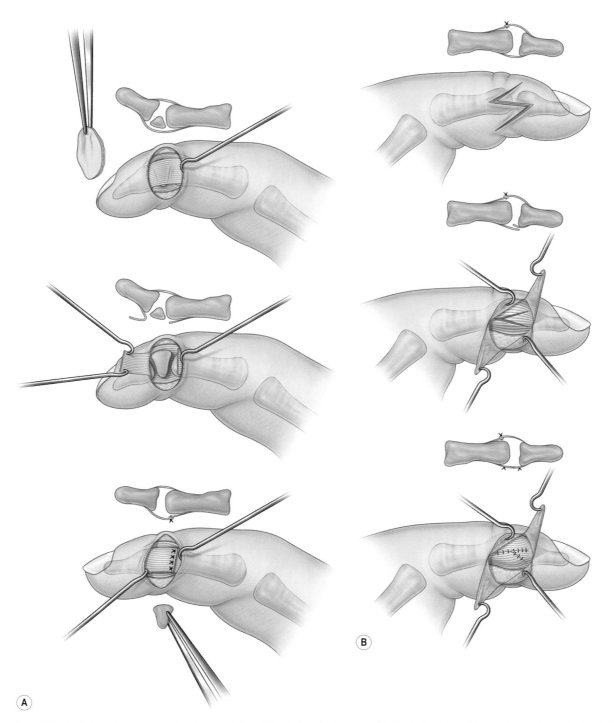

Fig. 28.18 (A,B) Operative technique of extirpation of the middle phalanx in the young child (note the skin and ligament correction on both sides).

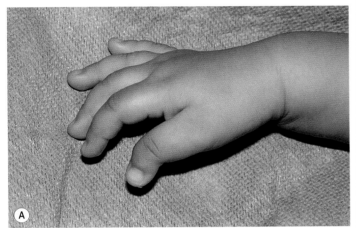
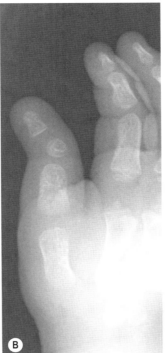
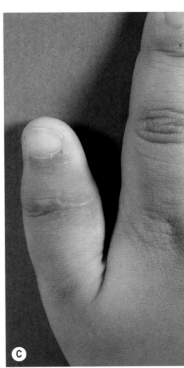

Fig. 28.19 (A,B) Preoperative TPT with delta phalanx and **(C)** postoperative result following resection of the middle phalanx of the thumb and ligament reconstruction; note the reduction in length.

released and the ulnar collateral ligament tightened. The skin is released on the radial side with a Z-plasty and adjusted on the ulnar side by excision of skin. When the child is older, a corrective osteotomy with arthrodesis at the DIP-joint is advised. This latter technique can be also performed in the trapezoidal middle phalanx.

Rectangular middle phalanx and five fingered hand

Via a Y-shaped incision dorsally a reduction osteotomy of the middle phalanx is made followed by arthrodesis of the distal interphalangeal joint. In this method a 1–1.5 cm shortening is achieved. The skin is then closed as a V. As the shortening is not enough, this procedure is combined with a shortening, rotation and palmar abduction corrective osteotomy at the metacarpal level to correct for position and length of the thumb (1–1.5 cm extra shortening). Furthermore, the extensor tendons as well as the intrinsics, are shortened. In recent years, a volar plate tightening at the MCPJ was added to prevent hyperextension. Basically, this procedure resembles a pollicization. The original CMC1J, even though it is not optimal, is better and more stable than a reconstructed CMCJ in a formal pollicization. For this reason, the author does not use a formal pollicization in the five fingered hand.

First web deficiency

Correction can mostly be performed with a simple 4 or 5 flap Z-plasty. When more skin is needed, a flap from the dorsora-dial side of the index is used as described above. In case of polydactyly, the extra skin from the radial discarded extra thumb can be used to shift to the ulnar thumb, while the skin of the ulnar thumb is used for the first web *(Fig. 28.20)*.

Postoperative care

For postoperative care, see the section on radial polydactyly, above.

Outcomes, prognosis, and complications

The author's group performed a long-term follow-up of operated (40 patients, 68 hands) and nonoperated patients (15 patients, 29 hands). Patients scored their function and appearance. The improvement in appearance was significant in the operated group; the improvement in function was higher but not significant. There was a trend towards a stronger thumb in the operated group; however, no opposition transfer had been performed.

Treatment of patients with TPT is not easy and often underestimated due to a lack of knowledge of possible deformities which may occur, therefore leaving these uncorrected. Skin problems, infection, and mal-union or nonunion are very rare. In our experience, treating patients with TPTs, one of the problems was unpredictable growth of the thumb, especially of the first metacarpal after initial shortening. They resulted in longer thumbs than intended (method of measuring: thumb tip is distal to the PIPJ of the index.[127] Parents and older children should therefore be informed. Furthermore, the arthrodesis of the distal IPJ can give a nail deformity. The V-Y approach can avoid this when performed with caution in relation to the nail bed.

Secondary procedures

Secondary procedures which are not directly related to complications are opposition transfer to improve opposition

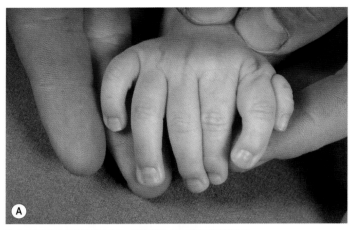

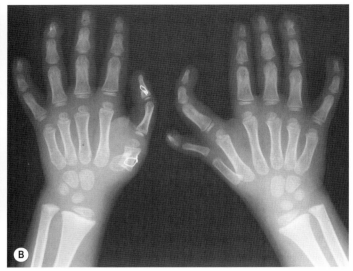

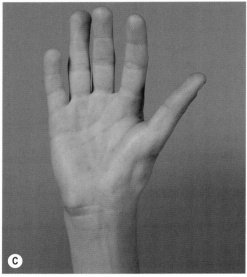

Fig. 28.20 (A) Right hand preoperatively in bilateral polydactyly with TPT. **(B)** X ray with one side operated following reduction-arthrodesis at the DIPJ and reduction-rotation and abduction osteotomy at the first metacarpal with shortening of the intrinsic and resection of the radial ray. **(C)** Long-term follow-up of correction on right side.

strength. Not many patients feel this operation is necessary. Thumb length corrections can be performed using epiphysiodesis or shortening osteotomies when growth has stopped. Occasionally, volar plate tightening procedures are offered for hypermobile MCPJs.

Camptodactyly

Introduction

Camptodactyly is a contracture of the PIPJ in the anteroposterior direction (*campylo* = arched and *dactylos* = finger). It occurs as consequence of an anatomical imbalance of the extrinsics and anomalous insertion of intrinsics to the affected finger(s). Camptodactyly can be sporadic without previous family history. Familial cases can inherit in an autosomal dominant pattern. In about 30% of cases camptodactyly has a familial background. This condition can furthermore be present in many syndromes such as Holt–Oram syndrome and Poland syndrome. Prevalence can vary considerable from 1–24%.[128] Camptodactyly usually stops being progressive with skeletal maturity.

Basic science/disease process

As a consequence of the imbalance of flexors and extensors, flexion at the PIPJ occurs; this can lead to deformation of the intra-articular bone ends with a stiff joint as a result, and deficient skin on the palmar side. With increasing age, the extensor mechanism becomes more insufficient leading to a further extension lag. Other mechanisms have also been described, such as circulatory disturbance, skin shortness, subcutaneous bands, lumbrical abnormality, short flexor superficialis, shortness of the flexor profundus and retraction of the collateral ligaments and volar plate.

Diagnosis/patient presentation

The functional defect is mostly limited and therefore appearance is mainly the concern. In severe forms however, functional deficit can be substantial especially when more fingers are affected. The fifth finger is the most affected (>70%), followed by the fourth finger (<20%). The other fingers are involved in less than 10% of patients with camptodactyly.

Patients with camptodactyly can be divided into three groups:

1. The newborn male or female patient with camptodactyly of mostly the fifth and/or fourth finger and sometimes all fingers
2. The adolescent mostly female with sudden onset or increasing camptodactyly of mostly only the fifth finger following growth spurts
3. Severe camptodactyly associated with other malformations.[138,139] However, it is disputed by others if this group should be diagnosed as camptodactyly.[132]

Foucher *et al.*[140] recognized four conditions: (Ia) The early and stiff; (Ib) the early and correctable camptodactylies; (IIa) the late and stiff; (IIb) the late and correctable deformities. Tests to assess degree of severity of camptodactyly are as follows[140]:

1. Can the PIPJ be actively extended while the wrist is held in a neutral position?
2. Does skin blanching appear while extending the finger as much as possible at both the MP- and PIPJ?
3. Does the PIPJ flex when the wrist and MCPJ are extended (the superficial flexor tenodesis test)?
4. Can the PIPJ extend passively by tenodesis effect while the MCPJ and wrist are held in flexion (central band or Smith test)?
5. Can the PIPJ actively extend while the MCPJ is held in slight flexion (the Bouvier maneuver)?
6. Is the flexor digitorum superficialis (FDS) of the little finger independently working from the fourth finger?

Patient selection

The best patient to operate is the patient who has a supple PIPJ but cannot actively extend the PIPJ well. Furthermore, patients should be selected on the basis of expected compliance to hand therapy.

The older patient with a stiff PIPJ is a bad candidate for release of the PIPJ with the intention to obtain a reasonable moving PIPJ.

Treatment/surgical technique

A splint is applied for all patients with camptodactyly in which the PIPJ is not supple *(Fig. 28.21)*. The splint stresses the PIPJ gradually to as much extension as possible. The MCPJ is in flexion in a forearm splint. A reduction to <30° extension lag is considered good enough to refrain from surgery.

The duration of splinting therapy before further surgical treatment varies from 3 to 12 months. Some authors consider an extension lag of 60° as an indication for surgery.[132]

If the splinting programme demonstrates a passively improved joint without improved active extension or if the joint movement is not improved, surgery can be indicated. In the older patient, one should think twice before surgery is performed, especially when joint movement is not improved. In noncompliant patients or parents, surgery is not recommended.

A variety of operations has been proposed as the etiology is unclear. Operations range from skin plasties, arthrolysis, tenotomies, tendon transfers, and osteotomies to arthrodesis. The author's preferred technique is based on the algorithm and description of the operative technique by Foucher.[132,140]

In the correctable PIPJ, mostly skin and fibrous bands release are performed, with exploration of the lumbrical muscle, interosseus muscles, FDS and FDP. Very often the lumbrical is anomalous together with the FDS *(Fig. 28.22)*. If the FDS is usable, and pulling on the lateral band gives extension to the PIPJ an FDS tendon transfer to the lateral band will be performed.

In the noncorrectable PIPJ, which improves after splinting, an extensive skin release is performed with a Malek flap (proximally based palmar homodigital flap). Subsequently, the flexor sheath just proximal from the PIPJ is opened

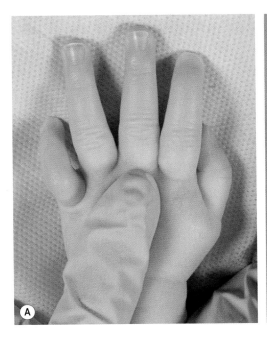

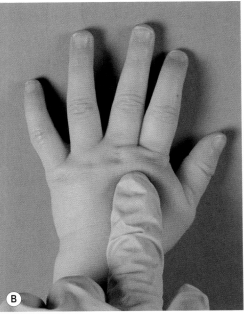

Fig. 28.21 (A) Note the flexed PIP joint of digit 5 and less of digit 4 before splinting. **(B)** After long-term night splinting.

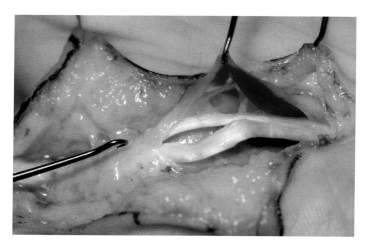

Fig. 28.22 The lumbrical muscle inserts into the FDS at the A1 pulley.

transversely and the checkreins, accessory ligament and if necessary the palmar plate is released creating passive extension. The intrinsics and extrinsics of the operated finger are explored and released if an anomaly is present. An FDS tendon transfer is used from the same or otherwise adjacent finger to restore active extension. The transfer is attached to either the lateral band if sufficient or to the central band if the lateral band is not sufficient.[132,140]

Postoperative care

Postoperative care consists of a splint of which the duration depends on the technique used. A K-wire for 2 weeks can be used for the PIPJ following release of the joint. Compliance to hand therapy is essential.

Outcomes, prognosis, and complications

In the young child, splinting of the stiff PIPJ results in a good outcome, with an 80–92% improvement rate after long-term splinting.[141,142] In the Caucasian hand, these good results could not be achieved in the same way. Young children with stiff joints do react well with splinting, resulting in a mean improvement of 40° following 19 months of splinting.[139,140] The variety of operations which has been proposed inevitably results in various outcomes ranging from 14% to 35% improvement.[132,143] Because of this insufficient outcome, and even sometimes worsening of the contracture, some authors prefer to rely only on splinting.

Foucher created an algorithm in which patients presenting late with a stiff joint are not operated. In all other patients, splints were applied. If no satisfactory improvement in extension was present, surgery was performed resulting in improvement rates from 68% to 88% depending upon whether or not the joint was passively correctable.[140] Complications can include: insufficient possibility to extend the PIPJ after surgical treatment; osteoarthritis; recurrence of contracture; stiffness and pain.

Secondary procedures

Secondary procedures include: re-release of capsular contracture, corrective osteotomy, or formal PIPJ arthrodesis.

Clinodactyly

Introduction

Clinodactyly is reserved for radio-ulnar deviations in the hand and latero-medial deviations in the foot. The angle of deviation defining clinodactyly varies among authors from >8° to >15°.[144,145] Clinodactyly is a symptom and not a disease. It may be isolated or may be associated with other congenital malformations, such as in Down syndrome or Apert syndrome. Burke described 25 syndromes associated with clinodactyly.[146] The incidence varies from 1–19.5%, depending on the degree of angulation used to determine clinodactyly.[147] Depending on the inclusion criteria, different groups can be distinguished: familial clinodactyly usually without associated differences (brachymesophalangism); clinodactyly with associated malformations; asymmetric injury to the growth plate, and triphalangeal thumb.

Brachymesophalangism is the most frequently encountered form of clinodactyly. It is a result of the articular surface which is not perpendicular to the longitudinal axis due to the abnormally shaped bone. The phalanx looks like a delta phalanx without the osseous rim as in the delta phalanx with a C-shaped epiphysis. The middle to distal phalanx ratio is 1:1, compared with 1.3:1 in normal fingers.[148]

Second, an aberrant growth plate surrounding one side of the delta phalanx in a C-shape results in deviation at the involved joint(s). Other names for delta phalanx are triangular bone and longitudinally bracketed diaphysis.[149–151] Reports suggest that anomalies with a delta phalanx should be clearly distinguished from the classical clinodactyly.[152] As it is not clear, the author would reserve clinodactyly for a congenital difference with or without a C-shaped epiphysis. Angulations after injury to the growth plate in an otherwise normal finger or a deviation in a joint following syndactyly release are secondary conditions.

Basic science/disease process

Clinodactyly is considered to be a congenital deformity at the phalangeal level. The mode of inheritance of clinodactyly is as an autosomal dominant trait with incomplete penetrance.[154] The middle phalanx is ossified later in embryonic development than the other phalanges, and latest in the little finger. Brachyphalangism therefore appears most in the little finger.[155] In proximal phalanges however, also aberrant growth plates also occur resulting in clinodactyly and brachyphalangism, and often in selective fingers. The exact etiology is still unknown.

Diagnosis/patient presentation

The most common form of clinodactyly is seen in the middle phalanx of the little finger presenting with an inward deviation of more than 10°. A positive family history in these patients is frequent. These little fingers mostly do not scissor over or under the ring finger, making this deformity more an aesthetic than a functional problem. Scissoring can also be prevented by abducting the little finger in the MCPJ. The deviation is clinically not only visible at the PIPJ but also at the DIPJ.

The thumb is next in-line in frequency of occurrence *(Fig. 28.23)*. The thumb can be an isolated occurrence or as part of a syndrome. The angle of deviation can amount to 70°. In Apert's syndrome, the thumb can be severely deviated. The fingers are less involved and in most series, the least affected is the long finger. More than one digit can be affected. Over half of the patients present with a delta phalanx. As a considerable number of patients present with clinodactyly after epiphyseal closure, the presence of a delta phalanx is difficult to assess radiologically. X-rays of both hands and affected fingers in two directions are a prerequisite in making the diagnosis.

Patient selection

Clinodactyly in the little finger without scissoring is not often treated operatively because of the risk of impairing joint motion in a normal functioning finger. In those patients where function is impaired, an indication to operate can exist. In a more severe deviation with a longitudinally bracketed epiphysis, age of surgery depends on the technique. Resection of the lateral physis with interposition of fat is performed at a younger age than a formal wedge osteotomy with or without bone graft. In syndromic clinodactyly correction of clinodactyly depends very much on the associated abnormalities.

Treatment/surgical technique

Treatment for clinodactyly can be divided into the following procedures:

- Opening wedge osteotomy with or without bone graft
- Closing wedge osteotomy
- Reversed wedge osteotomy
- Release of soft tissues on the concave side
- Tightening of soft tissues on the convex side
- Physiolysis.

Although a closing wedge osteotomy is advised for moderate and severe deviations (>30°)[156] the author is not in favour of using this technique, as the affected finger will be further shortened.[157] An open wedge osteotomy lengthens the digit the most and is preferred. In the more severe deviations however, bone correction only will not be enough. Release of soft tissue (collateral ligaments and the skin) on the contracted side is also necessary. The thenar musculature at its insertion

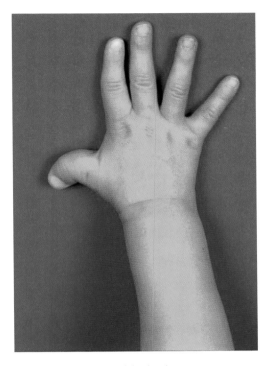

Fig. 28.23 Clinodactyly of the thumb.

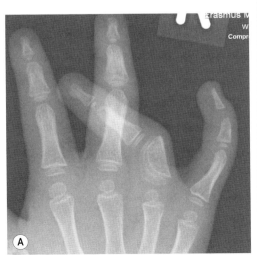
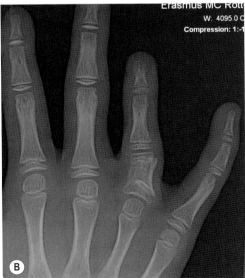

Fig. 28.24 (A) Reversed wedge osteotomy of the ring finger preoperatively and **(B)** postoperatively, the wedge is placed at the radial side of the proximal phalanx.

in the radially deviated thumb should also be released; otherwise a recurrence will be inevitable. Tightening of soft tissue structures, especially collateral ligaments on the convex side can also be useful.

In the less severe deviations a reverse wedge osteotomy works well but is technically more demanding *(Fig. 28.24)*. The advantage of the reverse wedge is that no other donor site is necessary. In the open wedge technique and in the reverse wedge technique, the graft is transfixed with a percutaneous K-wire either or with a suture to hold the bone graft in position.

In 1987, Vickers described a new technique by excising the continuous region of the physis and diaphysis in the isthmic region of the middle phalanx via a lateral incision. The bone is further removed in this region with a burr or curette. The remaining cavity is filled with a fat graft. This operation is called physiolysis and works well in younger children (under the age of 6 years), with less severe clinodactyly and a trapezoidal phalanx.[158,159]

Postoperative care

In the physiolysis technique, the operated finger can be taped to the adjacent finger for approximately 2 weeks. In the closing wedge technique, 3 weeks of immobilization is enough. In the reverse and open wedge osteotomies, also depending on the soft tissue correction, 4–6 weeks immobilization is often carried out.

Outcomes, prognosis, and complications

Reversed wedge osteotomies normally heal well. Slight angulations in the dorsal-palmar plane following surgery mostly disappear during growth. In open wedge osteotomies, skin and ligament release can be insufficient, leading to skin tightness and recurrence of angulation. In physiolysis, results in children over 5 years are not as good as in younger children. Furthermore, it works well in less severe clinodactylies.

Complications of the bone can be malunion or malrotation. Nonunion in children is very rare. Even if the X-ray demonstrates a nonconsolidated osteotomy, the fibrous tissue bridging the two parts can prevent movement, and will have no clinical implications. Furthermore, extensor tendon adhesions can result in a mallet like deformity. In some cases stiffness of joints can occur. Pain is rarely an issue.

Secondary procedures

Secondary procedures mainly address recurrence of the deviation either by insufficient release or excision of the physis or by inadequate soft tissue release. A new osteotomy and soft tissue release can be performed.

Acknowledgments

Christianne van Nieuwenhoven, MD, PhD has helped tremendously throughout all the chapters.

Access the complete references list online at **http://www.expertconsult.com**

1. Dobyns JH, Doyle JR, Von Gillern TL, et al. Congenital anomalies of the upper extremity. *Hand Clin.* 1989;5(3): 321–342.

9. Ogino T. Teratogenic relationship between polydactyly, syndactyly and cleft hand. *J Hand Surg Br.* 1990;15(2): 201–209.

13. Tonkin MA. Failure of differentiation part I: Syndactyly. *Hand Clin.* 2009;25(2):171–193.

   This is a review of the classification, incidence, indication, and review of surgical techniques and complications in syndactyly in different hand anomalies associated with syndactyly.

16. Niranjan NS, Azad SM, Fleming AN, et al. Long-term results of primary syndactyly correction by the trilobed flap technique. *Br J Plast Surg.* 2005;58(1):14–21.

51. Upton J. Apert syndrome. Classification and pathologic anatomy of limb anomalies. *Clin Plast Surg.* 1991;18(2): 321–355.

   An excellent overview of Apert syndrome concerning limb anomalies.

56. Zuker RM, Cleland HJ, Haswell T. Syndactyly correction of the hand in Apert syndrome. *Clin Plast Surg.* 1991;18(2):357–364.

57. Fearon JA. Treatment of the hands and feet in Apert syndrome: an evolution in management. *Plast Reconstr Surg.* 2003;112(1):1–19.

68. Foucher G, Navarro R, Medina J, et al. Metacarpal synostosis: a simple classification and a new treatment technique. *Plast Reconstr Surg.* 2001;108(5):1225–1234.

89. Wassel HD. The results of surgery for polydactyly of the thumb. *Clin Orthop Relat Res.* 1969;64:175–193.

96. Ogino T, Ishii S, Takahata S, et al. Long-term results of surgical treatment of thumb polydactyly. *J Hand Surg Am.* 1996;21(3):478–486.

   Some 113 hands with reconstruction of radial polydactyly and an average follow-up of 4 years were evaluated. According to Tada's evaluation, 97 hands were classified as good, 12 hands as fair, and 4 hands as poor. The type of deformity, type of procedure, and skill of the surgeon influenced the outcome. Wassel type III, V, and VI and triphalangeal thumb polydactyly have a higher incidence of unsatisfactory results.

97. Goldfarb CA, Patterson JM, Maender A, et al. Thumb size and appearance following reconstruction of radial polydactyly. *J Hand Surg Am.* 2008;33(8): 1348–1353.

126. Hovius SE, Zuidam JM, de Wit T. Treatment of the triphalangeal thumb. *Tech Hand Up Extrem Surg.* 2004;8(4):247–256.

   In the triphalangeal thumb (TPT), the extra phalanx can have different shapes, from wedge to rectangular. Furthermore, the involved joints, ligaments, muscles and tendons of the first ray, from distal interphalangeal joint (DIP) to radio-carpal joint can be hypoplastic, malformed or absent with varying degrees of stiffness or instability. Also, the first web can be insufficient and radial polydactyly as well as other hand deformities can be present. In this series depending on the malformation, operations varied from removal of the delta phalanx with ligament reconstruction to multiple osteotomies and rebalancing as well as pollicization.

140. Foucher G, Lorea P, Khouri RK, et al. Camptodactyly as a spectrum of congenital deficiencies: a treatment algorithm based on clinical examination. *Plast Reconstr Surg.* 2006;117(6):1897–1905.

Camptodactyly is classified into four groups. Camptodactyly can be correctible or noncorrectible and can be moderate or severe. Careful assessment with clinical tests can distinguish the possible treatment varying from splinting, the lasso procedure with or without lumbrical repositioning and tendon transfer of the FDS of the fourth or fifth finger.

150. Wood VE, Flatt AE. Congenital triangular bones in the hand. *J Hand Surg Am.* 1977;2(3):179–193.

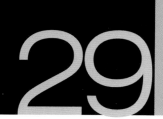

Congenital hand V: Disorders of overgrowth, undergrowth, and generalized skeletal deformities

Leung Kim Hung, Ping Chung Leung, and Takayuki Miura (Addendum by Michael Tonkin)

SYNOPSIS

- Macrodactyly presents with widely variable clinical pictures, often accompanied with unilateral enlargement, lateral deviations and joint problems. Corrections are difficult and partial. Repeated surgery is often required.
- Brachydactyly is characterized by complex shortening of the digits. The finger shortening ranges from simple undergrowth to total absence of some phalanges. Functional impairment ranges from minimal to severe, when brachydactyly is associated with fusion.
- Constriction band syndrome presents as simple embryonic amputations of digits or soft tissue constricting rings around the fingers or limb. Timely surgical correction is indicated for the simple solitary presentations. Extensive digital losses require special considerations for reconstruction.
- Generalized skeletal abnormalities associated with hand anomalies occur under the categories of a large variety of syndromes, some of which are extremely rare. The management plan depends on the overall clinical picture: decisions should not be made based on the affected hand alone.

Introduction

Macrodactyly, brachydactyly, constriction band syndrome, and general skeletal deformities are rare anomalies of the hand. While other anomalies such as polydactyly and syndactyly present with rather uniform clinical pictures, the categories of anomaly in this chapter present with divergent pictures, i.e., none of the affected individuals presents with a similar morphological picture. Functional impairment follows morphological abnormalities. Hence, one may find affected individuals suffering from major functional impairments, or no impairment at all.

The diagnosis of structural anomalies should be straightforward. However, in the category of brachydactyly, a mixture of abnormalities may co-exist, such as extra digits and fusion. Constriction band syndrome may be mistaken

with undergrowth. Awareness of the special circumstances will help with the diagnosis and subsequently the plan of management.

Macrodactyly

Macrodactyly is a rare condition in the hand. In Swanson's classification of congenital deformities of the hand, macrodactyly is labelled as "overgrowth", in contrast to "undergrowth", which is also known as hypoplasia.[1,2]

In a survey done in the 1980s, in Hong Kong, on 326 patients presenting with congenital abnormalities of the hand, only two cases were found, comprising only 0.5% of the entire series *(Table 29.1)*.[3] The incidence per 10 000 births was estimated to be around 0.2, including all disorders of overgrowth,[4] and at the turn of the last century a total of 165 cases of macrodactyly had been reported in the English literature.[5] More than one digit was involved in two-thirds of cases and most often, the index and middle fingers were affected simultaneously.

"Overgrowth" or "macrodactyly" is a misleading term. While hypoplasia of the hand has demonstrable undergrowth of the whole hand or component segments of the hand, macrodactyly has a bizarre involvement of segments of the hand unrelated to the anatomical units. In fact, if a finger or a thumb is considered an anatomical unit, macrodactyly does not involve one single unit. Macrodactyly affects either half of the unit, one and a half, or two and a half units. The overgrowth components are the soft tissues. Bone and joint changes, and adjacent tendon and ligament hypertrophies, are secondary effects.[6]

Surgical dissections have indicated that the major pathology involves hypertrophied digital nerves and their adjacent soft tissues. Histologically, the hypertrophied tissues appear like benign neurofibromas. The correct terminology for "macrodactyly" therefore, might be "digital-nerve orientated benign neurofibroma."[7]

Table 29.1 Survey on congenital anomalies of the hand in Hong Kong 1981–1982

	Diagnosis	Patients (n)	Limbs (n)	Involved limbs (%)
I	Failure of formation	39	44	11.1
II	Failure of differentiation	99	119	30.0
III	Duplication	143	158	39.9
IV	Overgrowth	2	2	0.5
V	Undergrowth (pure hypoplasia)	6	8	2.0
VI	Constriction band syndrome	13	18	4.5
VII	Generalized skeletal disorder	24	47	11.9
Total		326	396	100.0

Reproduced with permission from Leung PC, Chan KM, Cheng CY. Congenital anomalies of upper limb in a Chinese population. *J Hand Surgery* 1982;7(6):563–565.

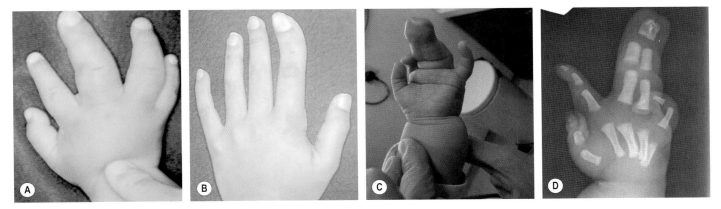

Fig. 29.1 (A) Macrodactyly of middle fingers and ring finger. **(B)** Macrodactyly of the index finger. **(C)** Syndactyly and macrodactyly may co-exist. **(D)** Radiograph of syndactylized macrodactyly.

If only one digital nerve along one side of a finger is affected, the hypertrophy (macrodactyly) will be confined to that side which will push the un-hypertrophied side away from the mid-line of the finger, causing a severe, whole finger clinodactyly. If the hypertrophy affects the common digital nerve before it divides into digital branches on the adjacent sides of two fingers, both sides of the fingers will be affected, causing divergent clinodactyly.[8]

The pathology exists since birth and grows rapidly as the child grows, leading to severe deformities, whereby aggressive correction may become necessary **(Fig. 29.1A,B)**. Very rarely, syndactyly occurs together with enlargement **(Fig. 29.1C,D)**, which could be a manifestation of Proteus syndrome (see below).

Surgical correction is complicated and difficult because of the extensive involvement. The policy to be adopted is one of ablation of the abnormal tissues, and reduction or control of the abnormal growth potential of the involved limb. Surgical treatment consists of radical excision of the soft tissues around the digital nerves which might need to be longitudinally split so that only a portion is left intact while the rest is to be ablated together with the soft tissues. Excision of the entire involved nerve has also been performed. When the bones and joints have undergone secondary hyperplasia, shortening with or without excision of one growth plate or fusion of the joint or wedging may have to be done. In the worst case, sacrifice of some digital segment might be necessary. Unless in extreme situations, the involved digit may not need to be sacrificed **(Fig. 29.2)**.[8]

Macrodactyly and proteus syndrome

There is an unusual form of macrodactyly where there is lipofibromatous hypertrophy of subcutaneous tissues, and the peripheral nerves are not directly involved. The macrodactyly could be localized, but different parts of the body may be more diffusely and asymmetrically involved as in the Proteus syndrome.[9] Wiedemann *et al.* were the first to group the various presentations, naming this Proteus syndrome.[10] The genetic cause of Proteus syndrome is still uncertain and debated. It may be a form of genetic mosaicism. It is progressive and is associated with skeletal and vascular changes as well as joint stiffness.[11]

Brachydactyly

Under Swanson's classification[1] for congenital deformities of the upper limb, Brachydactyly is put under the fifth category

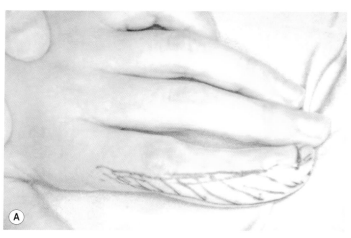
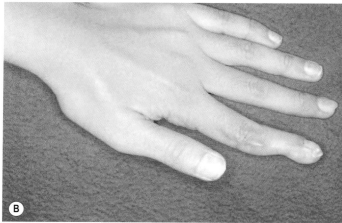

Fig. 29.2 (A) Surgical planning for macrodactyly correction. **(B)** Useful finger after correction.

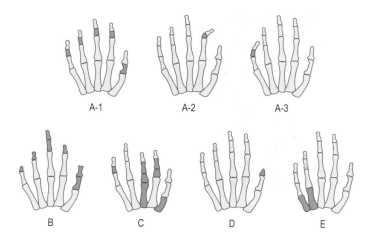

A-1   A-2   A-3

B   C   D   E

Fig. 29.3 Bell's classification of brachydactyly. (Redrawn after Bell J. *On Brachydactyly and symphalangism*. Cambridge: Cambridge University Press; 1951:1–31.)

of "undergrowth" (hypoplasia). One might have a simple impression that this type of congenital malformation is straightforward under-development. On the contrary, brachydactyly might be the most complicated group of congenital anomalies of the hand. If the undergrowth involves the whole hand evenly, or the entire structure of its major components, e.g., one digit, it would be quite straightforward. However, undergrowth is often affecting only some structures of a digital unit, and moreover, the undergrowth is not infrequently associated with other groups of congenital deformity such as failure to differentiate, failure to form, and duplication. Such complexity may even reach such a stage that classification becomes difficult and priority needs to be subjectively set for proper identification.

In 1951, Bell attempted to classify brachydactyly by distinguishing five main types, which he labeled A, B, C, D, and E *(Fig. 29.3)*.[11]

A. Brachymesophalangy
  A1. Where all middle phalanges are shortened
  A2. Where only the index finger middle phalanx is shortened

A3. Where only the little finger middle phalanx is shortened.
B. Apical dystrophy, where there are no nails in the fingers and the thumb is of normal length but broad.
C. "Drinkwater" type, where shortening mainly involves the proximal and middle phalanges of the index and middle fingers.
D. Brachymegalodactyly or stub thumb, where the distal phalanx of the thumb is short and broad.
E. Brachymetacarpia, where some metacarpal bones are short.

Miura[12] reviewed 149 cases of brachydactyly of different types in Japan and simplified Bell's classification by describing them as:
- Brachymesophalangy 5 (that involves the little finger, with 72 cases and was the most common type)
- Brachymesophalangy 2 (that involves the index finger, 19 cases and 7 cases were combined with Brachymesophalangy 5)
- Brachytelephalangy 1 (that involves the distal phalanx of the thumb, 14 cases, and 7 cases were combined with Brachymesophalangy 5)
- Brachymetacarpia (with short metacarpal of different rays, 44 cases, and 36 cases were combined with different types of brachyphalangy).[6]

When there is brachymetacarpia and brachyphalangy, the condition is usually bilateral and a high proportion of subjects have involvement of their feet as well *(Fig. 29.4)*.

Brachydactyly could also be related with clinodactyly, i.e., congenital deviation of one finger *(Fig. 29.5)*. The condition frequently affects the middle phalanx of the little finger and is inherited as autosomal dominant. In other situations, the deviation could be the result of a delta shaped middle phalanx. When the index finger is involved, the deviation may be towards the radial side and the condition would be one of Mohr–Wriedt syndrome which is an autosomal dominant congenital anomaly affecting also the feet with clinodactyly or syndactyly *(Fig. 29.6)*.

A delta-phalanx may occur in all digits resulting in the most serious types of brachydactyly and clinodactyly giving functional disabilities *(Fig. 29.7)*.

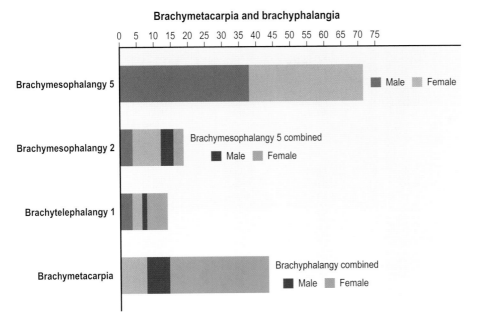

Brachymetacarpia and brachyphalangia

Fig. 29.4 Incidence of different types of brachydactyly. (Redrawn after Miura T. A clinical study of congenital anomalies of the hand. *Hand* 1981;13:59–68.)

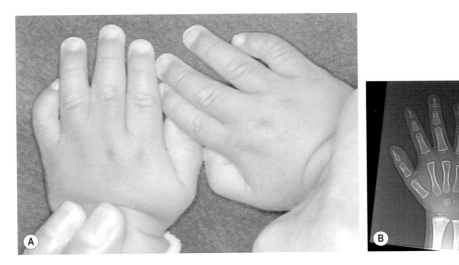

Fig. 29.5 **(A)** Brachymesophalangy and clinodactyly of small fingers. **(B)** Radiograph of the same patient's left hand.

Other causes of brachydactyly

Shortening of the distal phalanx (usually of the thumb) or shortening of the metacarpals (Brachymetacarpia), unless very severely affected, should not give functional impairments apart from varying degrees of cosmetic concern *(Fig. 29.8)*. Complete absence of the metacarpal, usually the fifth, will cause a grossly deviated little finger and creates a cosmetic and functional problem.

Sometimes the distal phalanx of the little finger is affected. The short distal phalanx then gives a unique palmar-radial curve which has been described as Kirner's deformity *(Fig. 29.9)*. Brachydactyly is made more complicated when it is associated with syndactyly *(Fig. 29.10)* and may even be combined with polydactyly *(Fig. 29.11)*.

The combinations of anomalies could be so complicated that undergrowth, failure of formation, failure of differentiation and duplication all co-exist and suggest that a new concept is needed to explain the mechanisms of these deformities. The Japanese Society for Surgery of the Hand, therefore introduced the concept of 'failure of induction during fetal hand development' and added a new subgroup to the Swanson classification.[1] The description of "brachysyndactyly (or symbrachydactyly)" is included for cases of failure of formation or undergrowth *(Fig. 29.12)*.[13,14]

Treatment considerations

As brachydactyly may range from the least conspicuous cosmetic visual abnormality to the most disturbing anomaly with serious functional impairments, planning for treatment and advice to parents varies greatly.

Minor deformities affecting mild shortenings of the metacarpals or middle phalanges may not deserve any surgical correction. While functional ability is well maintained, the

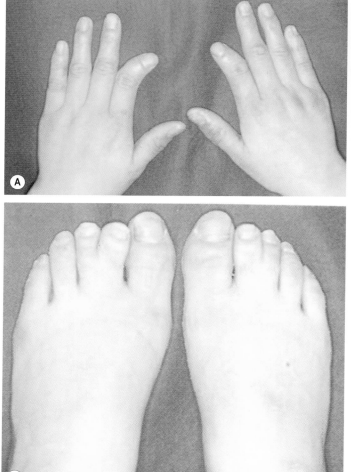

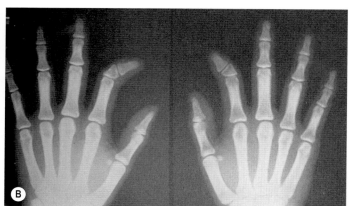

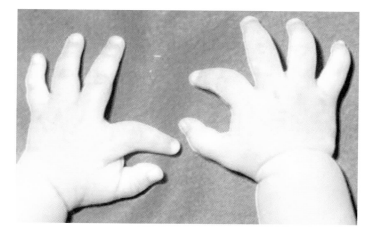

Fig. 29.6 (A) Mohr–Wriedt syndrome. **(B)** Radiographs. **(C)** Feet of child with Mohr–Wriedt syndrome.

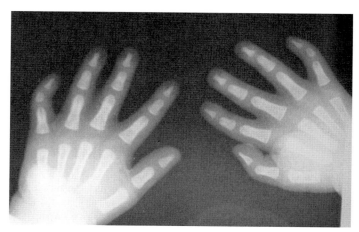

Fig. 29.7 Brachydactyly and clinodactyly.

Fig. 29.8 Mildest type of brachydactyly with short metacarpals.

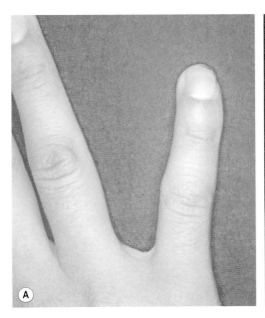

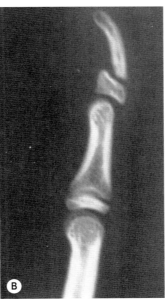

Fig. 29.9 (A) Kirner's deformity: clinical picture. **(B)** Radiograph of Kirner's deformity.

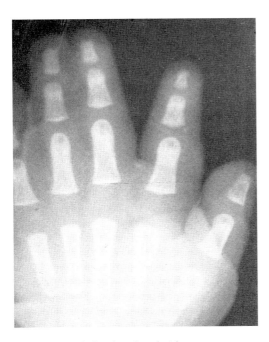

Fig. 29.10 Brachydactyly and syndactyly.

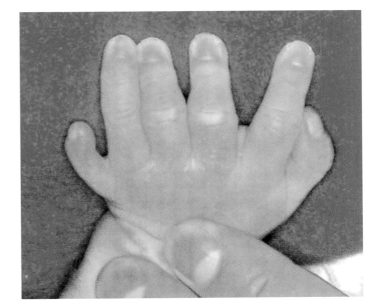

Fig. 29.11 Brachydactyly and syndactyly and polydactyly.

moderately obvious shortenings that could be improved surgically may best be deferred to until at pre-school age to allow better maturation of soft tissues.

With such a complicated mixture of anomalies, planning needs to be proactive because surgical correction might often require multiple procedures. Discussions will be done under the following headings:

- Brachymesophalangy
- Brachymetacarpia
- Clinodactyly with brachydactyly
- Symbrachydactyly.

Brachymesophalangy

Simple shortening of the middle phalanges does not give rise to functional disturbances. There might be two situations under which surgical correction might have to be considered: (1) when shortening is producing a lateral decline of the digit (i.e., clinodactyly), and (2) when the distal phalanx is affected, giving an expanded, unattractive distal end of the finger or thumb with a broad nail.

For the short phalanx, which gives rise to a bent finger, either a ligament reconstruction when the phalanx appears to

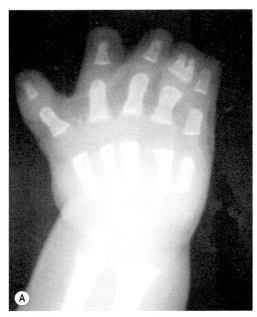

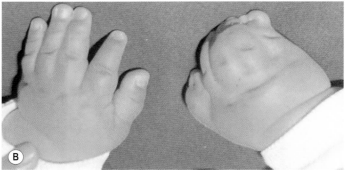

Fig. 29.12 (A,B) Different types of symbrachydactyly.

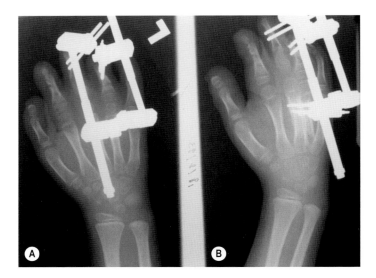

Fig. 29.13 (A,B) Elongating short proximal phalanges.

Complete absence of the metacarpal bone may occur and usually affects the fifth metacarpal. The little finger is dangling over the adjacent metacarpophalangeal joint with gross ulnar deviation at the metacarpophalangeal joint. Movements of the little finger are compromised because of absence of the intrinsic muscles, and movement of the little finger may be affected because of "forking" of the tendons. The little finger may need to be removed, but an alternative approach is to create a synostosis between the proximal phalanges after soft tissue release.

Clinodactyly with brachydactyly

When brachydactyly is associated with a delta phalanx, commonly occurring in the index finger which is free to bend radially, severe clinodactyly is the result. Apart from an abnormal appearance, functional pinch is also affected. When the shortening is not severe, correction of the clinodactyly is the priority, even at the expense of further sacrificing a slight amount of length. Surgical treatment of the delta phalanx is undertaken. A delta phalanx may be corrected by removing the delta bone when it is small, followed by careful tightening of the joint capsule. When the delta bone is longer than 1 cm, it should be corrected by a wedge osteotomy on the wide side, followed by capsular tightening on the same side. A K-wire fixation might be necessary. The abnormal phalanx may be excised after which the extensor tendon hood needs to be shortened, while the convex side of interphalangeal joint needs to be augmented and strengthened with adjacent fibrous bands. If necessary, part of the extensor tendon hood could be shifted to help strengthen the lax collateral ligament.

Symbrachydactyly

In symbrachydactyly, there is the presence of webbed fingers or syndactyly. Occasionally the fingers are very hypoplastic or are absent resulting in just a single digit or a claw like pincer. The procedures for syndactyly release in symbrachy-dacty are the same as for simple syndactyly. Because the digits

have no other abnormality except shortening; or an osteotomy on the affected phalanx to bring its proximal and distal interphalangeal joints parallel, will be indicated.

Brachymetacarpia

Short metacarpals do not give rise to functional impairment. In some cases, when the shortening occurs in the central digits, the disfigurement becomes striking and parents and child may want correction. If the shortening is mild, elongation may be achieved by a block bone graft in a single operation.[15] Elongation for more major deficiency is achieved through the bone transport using a mini-bone distractor.[16] Application of this device is awkward because the only site to allow the pins to go into the short metacarpal is the dorsum of the hand. Leaving the distractor in the child's hand for a few months is not a pleasant experience for any child. The small size of the metacarpal further jeopardizes the lengthening procedures. Family support and persistent counseling will be the key issues to maintain good compliance. Excellent results are not easy to be achieved *(Fig. 29.13)*. The most common problem that could arise from lengthening is loss of motion in the metacarpophalangeal joint.

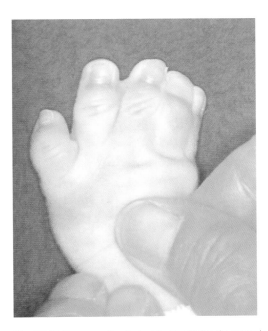

Fig. 29.14 Severe symbrachydactyly. Sacrificing the second ray to give a broad first web could be considered.

are short, the interdigital spaces should be made deeper than usual in order to gain more functional length.[17] This is particularly helpful for the first web. The adductor pollicis muscle and the first dorsal interosseous muscle could be released with their insertions and reset to a more proximal site. A dorsal transposition skin flap is frequently required to cover the web and gives good results.[18]

In severe symbrachydactyly, the middle rays could be rudimentary when the first interdigital space is extremely narrow. In such case, even the most radical web widening procedure might not achieve the purpose of creating a reasonable grip. Consideration should then be given to sacrifice the index ray with ablation *(Fig. 29.14)*.

Bone transplantation using a toe phalanx has been useful to provide length or to stabilize the hypoplastic digits.[19] These procedures should be carried out before 2 years of age to avoid resorption of the transplanted bone segments. The middle phalanx from the second to fifth toes can be used. This is placed into a skin pocket developed in the finger, and the bone transplanted is stabilized with closure of any available surrounding tendon. Alternatively, a part of the distal metatarsal with a part of the epiphysis could be fashioned and used as a graft. This "match-stick" type of graft could be more easily tailored to need. It carries a physis and the donor defect can heal itself without residual problems. It has the potential to grow and lengthen with growth of the hand. For the most severe type with absence of any digit, microsurgical toe transplantation will provide a useful pincer function.[20] The degree of mobility in the transplanted toe will vary, but a stiff digit does not limit the usefulness of the transplant or the function of the hand.

For symbrachydactyly, distraction lengthening may also be applied to improve the length of the digits. However in most cases the digits are very hypoplastic making the application of the apparatus impossible in the young child. The lengthening duration is likely to be further drawn out and complicated since the healing potential in the bone is poor. It may be more advisable to bone graft the hypoplastic digits first to provide initial stabilization and improvement in length and in a later stage to try lengthening if necessary. *Figure 29.14* illustrates a hand with symbrachydactyly and short digits which could be selectively lengthened subsequent to the creation of a wider first web.

Constriction band syndrome

Constriction band syndrome is a condition quite common among the varieties of congenital hand anomalies. In an earlier survey done in Hong Kong, 4.5% of the 326 cases of congenital abnormalities belonged to the constriction ring category.[3]

Though it is generally accepted that the cause of the constriction band is intrauterine strips of amniotic membrane circling around the extremities, there is yet no absolute proof to the theory. Controversies exist when the constriction ring covers only part of the circumference of the digit or extremity and the co-existing presence of absent digits and syndactyly. In the former case, although a tight constriction may produce amputation of the distal part, the bizarre nature of the absent parts is not easy to explain. The syndactyly co-existing with constriction rings is hallmarked by a proximal sinus over the un-separated pair of fingers, producing the so-called "fenestrated syndactyly." This morphological appearance can hardly be explained well by an intrauterine strip of amniotic membrane.[21] Moreover, constriction ring syndrome is also related to other congenital skeletal anomalies such as talipes equinovarus. On the other hand, patients having short fingers with different degrees of hypoplasia, different missing segments of the digit, and odd positioning of the deficient parts may be better grouped under symbrachydactyly. The true form of transverse growth arrest would be more or less congenital amputation with absence of the terminal parts and yet with relatively normal proximal parts *(Fig. 29.15)*.

Surgical treatment

If the constriction is very mild, it is not necessary to release the constriction. If the constriction is serious and is complicated with edema distally, it should be released as soon as possible. Urgent release may be performed under local anaesthesia with a direct perpendicular incision over the constriction site. This would be left dressed openly for 2 days to allow the distal edema fluid to subside before properly fashioning a local Z-plasty to close the defect *(Fig. 29.16)*.

Release of the constrictions, separation of the fenestrated syndactyly and treatment of the amputated digits are standard procedures for constriction band syndrome. The timing of separation of the fenestrated syndactyly differs from case to case, especially in cases where the interdigital spaces are shallow. The timing of operation should be postponed if the deepening of the shallow interdigital space is planned as a primary procedure at the same time as separation of the fenestrated syndactyly.

If the fusion of the digits is partial, separation of the digital rays should be performed as early as possible to prevent the deformity from further growth and deviation. If the deformity

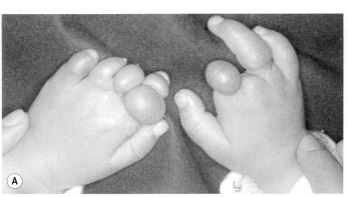
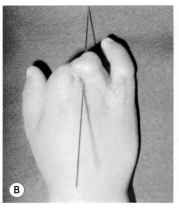
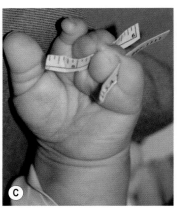

Fig. 29.15 (A) Constriction band syndrome. **(B)** Sinuses between adjacent fingers affected by constriction bands are diagnostic of the condition (ruling out congenital absence of parts). **(C)** Note the hollow spaces between the short fingers resulting from construction right syndrome.

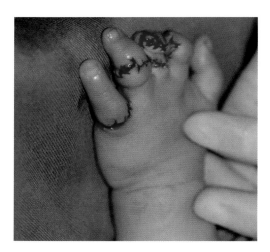

Fig. 29.16 Z-plasties to release tight rings.

caused by fusion of the digits is severe, the fenestrated fusion of the digits should be separated as early as possible; reconstruction of the interdigital spaces can be postponed to a secondary procedure.

Often, fusion distal to the fenestration can be simply separated and a full thickness skin graft is used. The surgical correction for the interdigital space, whether it is primary or secondary, is the same as the procedures used in syndactyly. However, if the digits are short (amputated), the inter-digital spaces are made deeper,[17] as in the case of symbrachydactyly **(Fig. 29.17)**.

Surgical procedures for the absent digits, except the thumb, are not usually required. If the thumb is partially amputated, the first web could be deepened and the thumb length should be proportionally extended. Alternatively, the thumb could be reconstructed by elongation or digital transfer in the so-called "on-top" plasty, usually from the index digit.[21,22]

Bone grafting, lengthening, and toe transplantation

Unlike symbrachydactyly, hands suffering from constriction band syndrome are seldom as severely involved. The

remaining digits are seldom as hypoplastic. Therefore many of the hands remain functional despite the short or absent digits. If necessary, interpositional bone grafting using toe phalanx or segment of metatarsal bone (with epiphysis) may be performed. However the skin is usually tight and would limit the amount of lengthening that could be achieved in a single stage. Partial toe transplantation may also be considered for improving pincer function in the hand. However, since toes are commonly also affected in constriction band syndrome there can be a problem with their availability for transplantation. It is also difficult to correctly estimate the growth potential of the transplanted toe, making it either too short or too long several years after transplantation necessitating further surgical interventions **(Fig. 29.18)**.

Distraction lengthening of the digit is a good alternative for constriction band syndrome.[23] Technically, it could performed easily. However, since the skin is tight, the process of lengthening may be quite painful and takes longer time to complete in order to stretch out the soft tissues and skin. The distraction frame can be quite difficult to maintain in young children.

Generalized skeletal abnormalities

The most common generalized skeletal abnormality is multiple exostoses **(Figs 29.19, 29.20)**. The genetic mutations have been shown to be the EXT1 and 2 genes,[24] although many isolated cases with incomplete genetic alterations or presentations are seen in clinical practice. There is a 10-fold increase in the likelihood for malignant changes for multiple exostoses simply because of the high number of chondroid lesions that occur simultaneously in the single person.

Usually one or two small bony bumps or deformities present themselves at an early age but the degree of generalized skeletal involvement will only gradually manifest itself as the child grows. The bony bump is located in the metaphyseal region and is typically described as "overhanging", especially around the knees. It may cause discomfort with the soft tissues for example when it occurs deep to the scapula. In the fingers, they tend to cause stiffness in the joints. However, shortening of the bone may occur. The mechanism why the physis should be affected is poorly understood. This

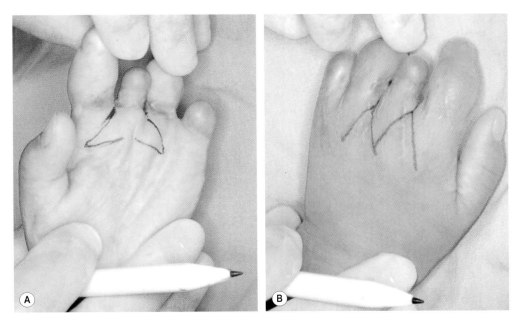

Fig. 29.17 (A,B) Deepening webs in congenital constriction band syndrome.

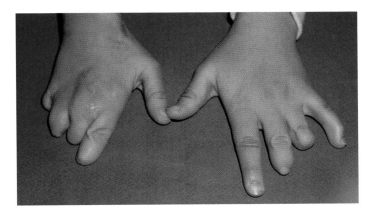

Fig. 29.18 Partial toe transplant 5 years after surgery. Length still the issue.

frequently affects the ulna and can result in significant deformity of the forearm.

Exostoses in the forearm bones frequently become formed in the interval between the radius and ulna. This may block rotation in the forearm, and may result in bowing of the bones. When it occurs around the wrist, it may cause instability of the distal radioulnar joint, stiffness, or deformity of the wrist similar to Madelung's deformity. When it occurs around the proximal radioulnar joint, it readily presents with pain and limited movements because of the constraint of space. Masada has described three types of forearm deformities in multiple exostosis[25]:

Type I: Shortness of ulna and bowing of the radius, no dislocation of radial head

Type II: Dislocation of the radial head

    IIa osteochondroma at the proximal metaphysis of radius

    IIb no such osteochondroma

Type III: Shortness of the radius.

The incidence was reported to be type I (61%); type IIa (6%); type IIb (14%); and type III (19%).

Deformity of the wrist in exostosis results in a deformity similar to Madelung's deformity. It consists of failure of growth of the ulnar aspect of the distal radial epiphysis, increase in radial inclination, and may be associated with bowing of the distal radius, hypoplasia of the distal ulnar epiphysis, and dislocation of the distal radioulnar joint. These changes cannot be simply explained alone by the mechanical compression effects of the exostosis.

Management of exostosis has three aspects. Symptomatic exostoses are removed by surgical excision. There is also the need for monitoring of any malignant developments in the exostoses (and their subsequent surgical treatment), and third is the management of forearm deformities.

Surgical removal of exostosis is not without complications. There is a potential risk for bleeding if a large bony defect is created. Another concern with multiple exostoses is the possibility for malignant changes. The type of malignancy is usually chondrosarcoma arising from the cartilage cap of the exostosis. Therefore any exostosis that has a rapid increase in size or inexplicable pain may signify malignant change and should be surgically removed. With the general availability of MRI scans, patients should be screened on a regular basis to detect early changes in the lesions.[26] This is likely more important for deep exostoses hidden from palpation such as those arising from the pelvic girdle or the deeper aspects of the ribs. Some pelvic exostoses may grow to a large size to affect child bearing and deserve treatment even before any symptoms appear.

Treatment of forearm deformities in multiple exostoses has been highly controversial. Classic studies have suggested that many of these patients when they reach adulthood could cope with their daily activities and seldom complain about their upper limb functions.[27] On the other hand, surgical procedures to reduce the degree of bone bowing, to reduce the difference in length between the forearm bones (usually by

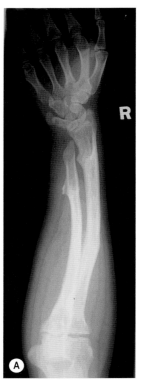

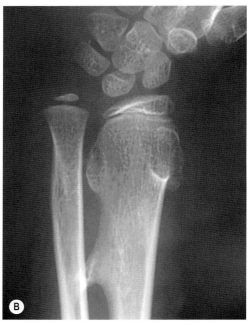

Fig. 29.19 (A,B) Multiple exostoses.

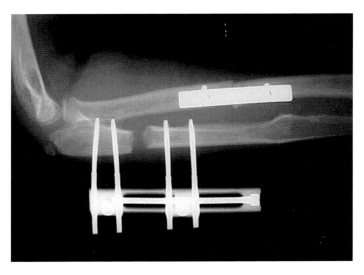

Fig. 29.20 Multiple exostoses treated with ulnar lengthening and radial shortening.

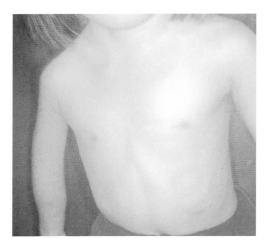

Fig. 29.21 Poland syndrome.

Other skeletal anomalies

Other congenital anomalies affect different internal organs while at the same time present with skeletal and hand deformities. Some examples of the relatively common anomalies include the following:

Poland syndrome

There is either total or partial absence of the pectoralis major muscle together with hand abnormality. Congenital heart problems may co-exist *(Fig. 29.21)*. The most common associated hand anomaly is symbrachydactyly.[30] See Chapter 28.

Apert syndrome

This is also known as acrocephalosyndactyly which presents as cranio-maxillary facial deformities, dyschondroplasia and complex syndactyly *(Fig. 29.22)*. The complex osseous-syndactyly of Apert syndrome represents the most severe type of fused fingers. In the worst case, the hand has no suggestion of finger webs. The principle of treatment should be

distraction lengthening), and to relocate the radioulnar joints have been shown to be useful to prevent further progression of the deformities, and to provide the patients with a cosmetically more acceptable upper limb with balanced joints and preserved hand and forearm functions.[28,29]

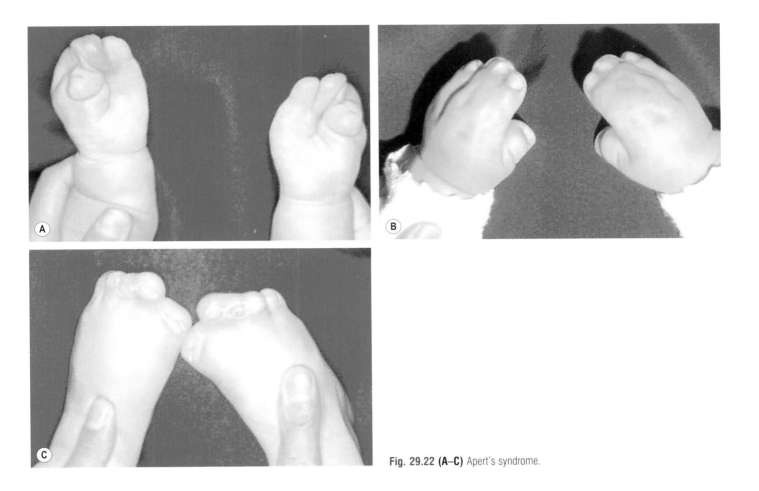

Fig. 29.22 (A–C) Apert's syndrome.

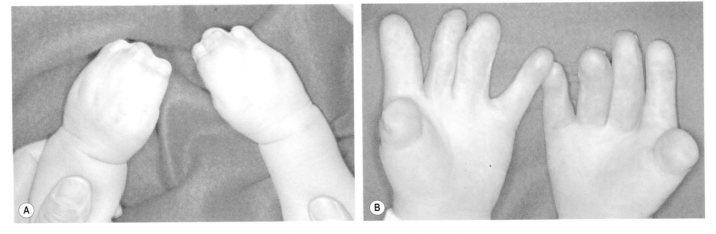

Fig. 29.23 (A) Symbrachydactyly in Apert's syndrome. **(B)** Symbrachydactyly after repeated surgical separations.

the creation of a more useful extremity with a number of digits to provide a grip or pincer.[8,18] In the most severe cases, sacrifice of one or two rays may be necessary so that deep webs could be created, and more soft tissues and skin could be made available to cover the preserved rays. However, more recent attempts have been towards early separation of the synostosis that allow growth of the bony skeleton and movement of the digits and subsequent staged separation of the

fingers.[31] Skin grafting is always required. The risk of circulatory hazard is real and therefore, staged reconstruction is advisable *(Fig. 29.23)*.

Haas syndrome

This resembles Apert syndrome but presents with the characteristics of six metacarpals, hypoplastic thenar muscles, more than five digits, all of which have three phalanges and different degrees of fused rays *(Fig. 29.24).*[32]

Congenital alopecia

Patchy absence of hair over the scalp is associated with short fingers and in particular, hypoplastic thumbs.

Pierre–Robin syndrome

This presents with severe maxillofacial anomalies with cleft palate, cleft lip, micrognathia, and clasped thumbs. At times, other hand abnormalities are associated. Glossoptosis is also present, and when associated with absent gag reflex, may present with airway risks during operation *(Fig. 29.25).*

Freeman–Sheldon syndrome

This is also known as cranio-carpo-tarsal dystrophy. Craniofacial abnormalities are associated with metacarpal

bone shortening and metatarsal shortenings which affect mainly the ulnar side in the hand and lateral side in the foot.[33] The result in the hand is the so-called "wind-blown" hand, which refers to hyperflexion of the thumb and fingers at the M-P joints which are also deviated severely ulnar-ward *(Fig. 29.26).*

Mohr–Wriedt syndrome

This syndrome presents with hand and foot abnormalities. Middle phalangeal shortening and co-existing slanting articular surfaces produce clinodactyly. The other fingers are typically normal.[34] In the foot, the second toe is often shortened, deviated towards the big toe, while the web between the second and third toe is syndactylized.

Madelung's deformity

This syndrome presents with radial deviation of the hand secondary to the overgrowth of the distal ulna. The actual

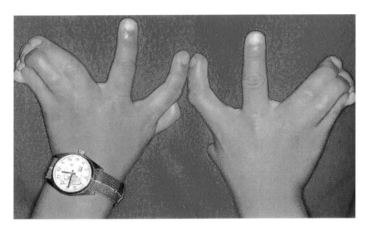

Fig. 29.24 Haas syndrome.

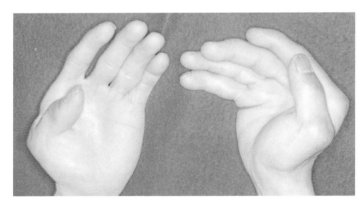

Fig. 29.26 "Wind-blown hand" in Freeman–Sheldon syndrome.

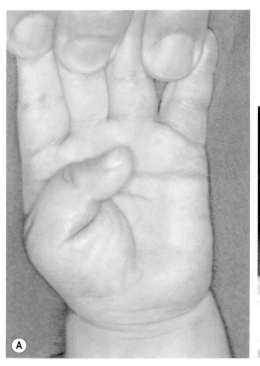

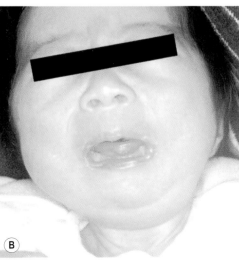

(A) **(B)**

Fig. 29.25 (A,B) Pierre–Robin syndrome with clasped thumb.

cause of the relative shortening of the distal radius is due to the early growth arrest of the ulnar half of the distal radial epiphysis which produces the so-called carpus curves with shortening *(Fig. 29.27)*.[33] The carpal bones appear to be arranged in a triangular shape with the lunate at the apex. Madelung's deformity is a typical presenting feature of dyschondrosteosis but many cases of Madelung's deformity are sporadic occurrences.

The child suffering from this deformity has variable presentations but predominantly with stiffness and curved and "bayonet appearance" of the forearm. The wrist is usually central but with a prominent ulnar head limiting pronation.[35] At an early stage, the true nature of Madelung's deformity may not be fully realized and treatment may be started with the form of wrist splinting to prevent ulnar deviation. Splinting is likely to fail with further growth of the child when the ulna begins to overtake the radius, and gradually the typical Madelung's deformity becomes obvious.

The timing of surgical treatment depends on the speed of development of the deformity. Vickers has proposed to use the Langenskiöld procedure by resection of the fused ulnar part of the distal radial physis and filling it with fat, together with resection of a tethering ligament between the lunate to the radius.[36] However, long-term results of this procedure are not known. The usual treatment plan is to wait as long as possible so that one adequate correction would satisfy the need of centralizing the wrist. Since the deformity is a growth related problem, intervention that is too early may require a second operation. The full-blown deformity involves a protruding distal ulna and an ulnarly deviated distal radial articular facet, together with a wedged carpus. Shortening the ulnar bone alone does not solve the problem well.[8,37] Correction of the radial inclination requires a radial osteotomy. However, the radial inclination should not be "normalized" completely as this might limit future ulnar movements of the carpus. The complete procedure thus involves a radial wedge osteotomy of the distal radius above the epiphysis, and shortening osteotomy of the ulnar bone with or without radial wedging *(Fig. 29.28)*.

Conclusions

Diagnosis of the specific anomaly is the important first step towards the planning of management for the four different types of hand anomalies discussed under this chapter.

Only constriction band syndrome may present as a surgical emergency if a tight band constricts the digit or limb, so much so that circulation is compromised. Immediate release to restore circulation is therefore mandatory. Surgery should include multiple surface Z-plasties, and soft tissue constriction ring removal on a deeper level.

The timing for surgical correction should be planned according to school considerations. The initial surgical correction could be pre-school. Then, when multiple repeated corrections are required, vacations should be considered as optimal times. The general guidelines include: function first; cosmetics second; preservation of circulation and avoidance of excessive skin removal; and functional gain to be achieved at the expense of limited loss.

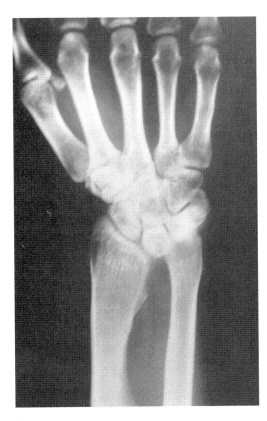

Fig. 29.27 Madelung's deformity.

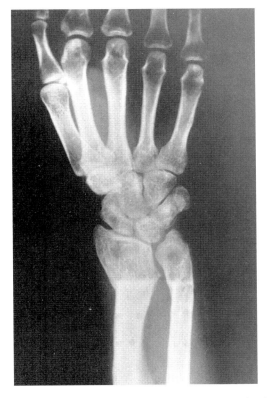

Fig. 29.28 Osteotomy on the radius and shortening on the ulnar.

Patients and parents should be thoroughly warned of the limitations of surgery before any surgical attempt. Over-optimistic promises should not be given. Patients and parents should be aware the frequent need of repeated surgery.

Although functional restoration may not be perfect, the outcome, even before the surgical correction, should be predictable to the surgeon and be explained to the patient and parents. In some of these anomalies, cosmetic considerations could be a major concern and an indication for surgical correction. Patients and parent should be discouraged to adopt unrealistic expectations.

Addendum: Congential trigger thumb
Michael Tonkin

Although congenital trigger thumb does not fit well into any classification scheme for congenital hand anomalies, it is one of the most common pediatric hand problems in practice.

Etiology

Pediatric trigger thumb is a stenosing tenovaginitis of the flexor pollicis longus tendon within its fibro-osseous tunnel, with the obstruction to tendon glide occurring at the A1 pulley. Controversy continues as to whether this is a true congenital condition or whether it is an acquired condition. The distinction between the two would appear to rely on whether or not the condition is present at birth. Although many authors have described presence at birth, the majority of these studies depend upon a retrospective history from the parents. The presence of trigger thumb in twins, the frequent bilateral nature of trigger thumb and the association of trigger thumb with Trisomy 13 are factors which have been used to support the theory of a congenital cause.[38–42] However, several investigators have performed assessments within the early postnatal period, finding an absence of trigger thumbs in a combined number of 9000 neonates.[43–45] The study of Kikuchi and Ogino examined 1116 babies within 14 days of birth.[46] None presented with trigger thumbs. Of 601 children assessed by a questionnaire at 12 months of age, only two had developed trigger thumbs within that period, an incidence of 3.3 per 1000 live births. Three other children subsequently developed trigger thumbs, one bilateral, after the age of 12 months. Although response to the 12-month questionnaire was only obtained from 53% of patients and, the true prevalence of trigger thumb after 12 months in this cohort of patients cannot be established, this study does tend to suggest that trigger thumb deformity is an acquired condition and is not present at birth. However, if the incidence of one patient per 2000 live births, described by Ger et al., is accurate, the number of children required to establish an absence of trigger thumb at birth would need to be far greater than those examined in the study.[47]

Trauma has been incriminated as a possible cause of acquired trigger thumb. However, the absence of this history is more usual than not. Furthermore, the definition of what is a traumatic incident and what is not in a two year old is unclear.

Notta described a node affecting the flexor tendons of digits which impeded their movement.[48] Notta's node is palpable proximal to the A1 pulley in children with a locked flexion deformity. If the deformity is correctable, either actively or by the examiner's passive extension of the digit, the node can be felt to click as it passes beneath the A1 pulley. Some consider the node to be primary, preventing passage of the tendon past the edge of the obstructing A1 pulley. Most believe that this is a secondary phenomenon consequent upon the bunching of the tendon as its passage is impeded. It seems to disappear following surgical release, which supports the latter theory.

Two other observations are interesting. The first is that there is a percentage of "trigger thumbs" that present with the digit locked in extension. In this instance, the failure to glide through the A1 pulley is from distal to proximal when Notta's node presumably abuts against the distal end of the A1 pulley. The literature does not provide us with an incidence of triggering in extension, indeed some may have interpreted this as a spontaneous resolution of triggering in a digit previously locked in flexion.

The second observation is that many children with a trigger thumb have hyperextensibility of the metacarpophalangeal joint. Ligamentous laxity is greater in children. No study has made a comparison of the incidence and degree of metacarpophalangeal joint hyperextension in children with and without trigger thumbs. However, it is logical to propose that the diameter of the A1 pulley, which is attached to the palmar plate of the metacarpophalangeal joint, decreases during hyperextension of the metacarpophalangeal joint, potentially restricting gliding of the tendon.

The current evidence suggests that the appearance of trigger thumb is more likely to be after birth. There is no real evidence of a primary pathological process other than a mismatch in size between the flexor tendon and the pulley.

Management

The rate of spontaneous resolution following observation and the rate of resolution following a combination of observation, manipulation and splinting, vary. Ger et al. found no cases of resolution in 53 thumbs diagnosed before the age of 6 months, following 40 months of nonoperative therapy.[47] Steenwerckx et al. reported similar findings in 57 thumbs after 6 months.[49] Other reports document high rates of spontaneous resolution,[49–55] up to 96% for those thumbs that trigger during active extension with a lesser resolution rate for those with a fixed flexion posture.[50] Dinham and Meggitt observed a spontaneous recovery rate of 30% in those children presenting with trigger thumb prior to the age of 6 months and a rate of 12% for those presenting between 6 and 30 months.[41] They advised treatment guidelines accordingly, advising that trigger deformities present in the early postnatal period should be observed for 12 months; those presenting between the ages of 6 and 30 months should be observed for 6 months; and that operative treatment should be performed before the age of 4 years to prevent the creation of residual flexion deformities. Although there has been an occasional report of interphalangeal joint radial deviation and a rotational deformity of the IP joint in older children,[56] there are no reported instances of persistent deformity if the condition is corrected surgically by the age of 3 years, or even later, according to some authors.[57]

Recently Baek *et al.* found a 63% rate of spontaneous resolution in 71 trigger thumbs.[58] No treatment was instituted in these children who were assessed 6-monthly for a minimum period of 2 years. They found that the flexion deformity can be expected to improve even in those patients who did not have complete resolution. The general trend in the literature pertaining to children of Asian descent is to recommend a prolonged period of observation with or without splinting and passive exercises.

From the above it can be seen that the necessity for and timing of surgery for pediatric trigger thumbs are open to debate. Most would advise surgery for persistent painful episodes of triggering. Intermittent, nonpainful triggering may be safely observed for a prolonged period of time, with or without the addition of night splinting in extension, without fear of the complication of joint deformity. It is questionable as to whether or not treatment with night splints for an extended period of time (up to 5 years or longer) is a greater imposition on child and parents than a surgical procedure. It is the author's (MT) practice to offer the parents surgical release if there is a persistent flexion or extension contracture for longer than 3 months and/or if there is accurate documentation by the parents of an uncorrectable flexion contracture for 12 months. However, this advice is offered along with the information that spontaneous resolution may well occur, even in these circumstances.

Video 1

The surgical procedure is performed as day-only surgery under general anesthesia and with an arm tourniquet. The incision is transverse at the base of the thumb (metacarpophalangeal joint level). This incision is not easily extensile and therefore its position is important if one is to obtain an optimal view of the A1 pulley. If Notta's node is easily palpable, an incision centered on this node provides very adequate access. Often, this leads the surgeon to an incision halfway between the two basal thumb creases that are present in most hands. The neurovascular bundles of the thumb lie more anteriorly than those of the digits. The A1 pulley should be visualized and palpated with the tip of forceps to identify its proximal and distal edges. The surgeon or assistant should not attempt to passively correct the flexion deformity manually prior to incision of the A1 pulley. Full and easy correction following pulley release provides evidence of a complete release. The incision should be made in the midline of the pulley or erring to its radial side. This avoids continuing the incision through the fibres of the oblique pulley, whose origin on the ulnar side abuts the distal end of the A1 pulley. Occasionally, there are further transverse fibres just distal to, but separate from the A1 pulley, which deserve release.

With careful attention to detail, complications should be minimal to nil. Absorbable 6/0 Vicryl Rapide sutures avoid the necessity for suture removal. Bathing and massage can begin at about 7–10 days postoperatively. Although Michifuri *et al.*[59] reported a complication rate of 15%, including digital nerve injury, this is not the author's (MT) experience. There may be some inflammatory response during wound healing but this settles once the sutures have dissolved or are rubbed out with massage.

Access the complete references list online at **http://www.expertconsult.com**

2. Leung PC, Chan KM, Cheng CY. Congenital anomalies of upper limb in a Chinese population. *J Hand Surg.* 1982;7(6):563–565.

   This paper offers an excellent description of macrodactyly in addition to descriptions of other congenital anomalies of the hand.

3. Miura T. A clinical study of congenital anomalies of the hand. *Hand.* 1981;13:59–68.

11. Bell J. *On brachydactyly and symphalangism.* Cambridge: Cambridge University Press; 1951:1–31.

    This paper by Bell presents an excellent timeless description of brachydactyly and symphalangism.

12. Miura T. Clinical differences between typical and atypical cleft hand. *J Hand Surg Br.* 1984;9:311–315.

13. Miura T. *Atlas of congenital hand anomalies.* Nagoya: Kanehara; 1993.

14. Saito H, Koizumi M, Takahashi Y, et al. One-stage elongation of the third or fourth brachymetacarpia through the palmar approach. *J Hand Surg Am.* 2001;26(3):518–524.

15. Ogino T, Kato H, Ishii S, et al. Digital lengthening in congenital hand deformities. *J Hand Surg.* 1994;19: 120–129.

This paper by Japanese colleagues offers an excellent description of digital lengthening in congenital hand deformities.

19. Kay SP, Wiberg M. Toe to hand transfer in children. Part 1: technical aspects. *J Hand Surg.* 1996;21(6): 723–734.

    The Leeds group discusses thoroughly toe-transplantation in children with details on indications, surgical techniques, and outcomes.

20. Miura T. Congenital constriction band syndrome. *J Hand Surg Am.* 1984;9:82–88.

21. Nakamura R, Miura T. Use of paired flaps to simultaneously cover the dorsal and volar surface of a raw finger. *Plast Reconstr Surg.* 1974;54:286–289.

28. Akita S, Murase T, Yonenobu K, et al. Long-term results of surgery for forearm deformities in patients with multiple cartilaginous exostoses. *J Bone Joint Surg Am.* 2007;89:1993–1999.

29. Peterson HA. Deformities and problems of the forearm in children with multiple hereditary osteochondromata. *J Pediatr Orthop.* 1994;14:92–100.

    This article gives an in-depth discussion on wrist and forearm congenital deformities related to osteochondromas.

46. Kikuchi N, Ogino T. Incidence and development of trigger thumb in children. *J Hand Surg Am.* 2006;31:541–543.

47. Ger E, Kupcha P, Ger D. The management of trigger thumb in children. *J Hand Surg Am.* 1991;16:944–947.

48. Notta A. Recherches sur une affection particulière des gaines tendineuses de la main, caractérisée par le development d'une nodosité sur le trajet des tendons fléchisseurs des doigts et par l'empechement de leurs mouvements. *Arch Gen Med.* 1850;24:142–161.

30

Growth considerations in pediatric upper extremity trauma and reconstruction

Marco Innocenti and Carla Baldrighi

SYNOPSIS

- Skeletal growth is possible because of the presence of an active physis.
- The physis is physiologically regulated by several factors and can be hindered by congenital conditions (chondrodysplasias), direct damage, or interruption of its blood supply.
- When the physis is damaged, therapeutic options include completion of epiphyseal arrest, resection of epiphyseal bar, and epiphyseal distraction.
- Where there is involvement of the whole epiphysis, autologous epiphyseal transfer may achieve the dual goals of restoring joint function and growth potential.

 Access the Historical Perspective section online at
http://www.expertconsult.com

Introduction

- The growth plate is a temporary anatomical entity, which allows axial growth in long bones. Once skeletal maturity is approached, the function of the growth plate gradually decreases and eventually stops.
- Trauma, infection, irradiation, thermal injury, tumor, and congenital disorders may affect the growth plate and interfere with the growth process.
- Any damage to the growth plate in a skeletally immature individual leads to growth disturbance with deformity and/or length discrepancy.
- Goals of the surgical treatment should be restoration of the physiological growth, prevention of angular deformities, and correction of established deviation of bones and joints.

Basic science/disease process

Anatomy and physiology of the epiphyseal growth plate

The physis (also known as growth plate, epiphyseal plate, epiphyseal growth plate, epiphyseal cartilage) is a highly specialized and organized cartilaginous structure derived from the mesoderm. It develops in the bone bud, secondary to the primary ossification centers (metaphysis) and is responsible for longitudinal and circumferential bone growth.[1] The physis must be distinguished from the epiphysis, or secondary ossification center *(Fig. 30.1)*.

The physis consists of proliferating chondrocytes surrounded by synthesized extracellular matrix. The extracellular matrix is composed of water, collagen fibrils (mainly types II, IX, X, and XI) and proteoglycans (aggrecan, decorin, annexin II, V, and VI) arranged to form a sort of sponge with very small pores.[2] This arrangement confers peculiar mechanical properties that permit the physis to be "hard" when an axial load is applied rapidly (a jumping child) or "soft" when deformed slowly (when chondrocytes secrete new extracellular matrix).[3]

The physis is traditionally divided into horizontal zones of chondrocytes at different stages of maturation *(Fig. 30.1)*. The resting zone (reserve zone or germinal matrix), immediately adjacent to the epiphysis, contains small, uniform, irregularly scattered chondrocytes, also referred to as stem cells, with low rates of proliferation but rich in storage materials (lipids and cytoplasmic vacuoles) for later growth.[4,5] The resting zone is responsible for protein synthesis and for maintaining a germinal structure. Injury to this layer results in cessation of growth.

When chondrocytes enter into the proliferative zone they undergo rapid duplication, increase the synthesis of collagen,

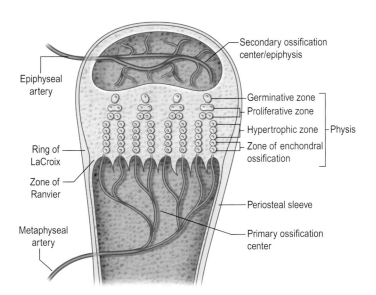

Fig. 30.1 Cross-sectional anatomy of the physis.

in particular types II and XI,[4] and become flat and well organized into longitudinal columns. Mitotic activity is present only at the base of these columns. This layer is responsible for longitudinal growth of the bone via active cell division. These first two zones have an abundant extracellular matrix that confers a great deal of mechanical strength, in particular in response to shear forces.

Further morphological changes – maturation, degeneration, and provisional calcification, – take place in the transformation (or hypertrophic) zone, divided into upper and lower hypertrophic zones.

The presence of provisional calcification[4–6] confers shear resistance to the lower hypertrophic zone. In contrast, the upper hypertrophic zone containing scant extracellular matrix is the weakest portion of the physis and it is here that most injury or alteration to the physis occurs.[7–9]

In continuity with the metaphysis is the zone of enchondral calcification where the mineralization process of the matrix becomes more intensive.

The periphysis is a fibrochondroosseous structure that surrounds the physis of tubular bones and plays an important role in skeletal development[10] *(Fig. 30.1)*: (1) it allows gradual circumferential growth of the physis; (2) it continues to maintain its transverse diameter[11]; and (3) it is critical to the overall stability of the growth plate and to support for the physis bone–cartilage junction.[11–13]

The part of the periphysis adjacent to the epiphysis is a wedge-shaped group of germinal cells known as the zone of Ranvier; while the part adjacent to the metaphysis is known as the ring of LaCroix. Histologically, the Ranvier and LaCroix zones are a single structure *(Fig. 30.1)*.

Chondrocyte proliferation and differentiation in the physis, and therefore longitudinal skeletal growth, are regulated on both a systemic and local level.[14] A number of endocrine, paracrine, and autocrine factors and their respective receptors are involved in this process. Amongst these, the parathyroid hormone-related protein (PTHrP) and the Indian hedgehog (Ihh) play a prominent role in skeletal maturation.[1,15,16] There

is also mechanical control of growth, which is important in pediatric orthopedic surgery because it is the basis of the widely used epiphysiodesis and epiphyseal distraction procedures.[3]

Vascular anatomy of the growth plate

The epiphyseal and physeal cartilage vascular anatomy in newborn and early postnatal life is integral to long-bone development and differs from later postnatal periods. In late fetal and early postnatal life epiphyseal cartilage canals (or transphyseal vessels) are seen passing through the physeal cartilage and communicating with the metaphyseal marrow. Such vessels play an active role in forming the secondary ossification centers[17,18] but their primary earlier function is to provide nutrition by diffusion to epiphyseal chondrocytes.

The transphyseal vessels are constantly obliterated several months after birth. Once the obliteration has occurred, the physeal cartilage becomes an avascular structure supplied by the epiphyseal vessels, by diffusion, and by the metaphyseal vessels invading the lowermost regions of the hypertrophic zone.[19,20]

The main vascular supply to the germinal zone is from the epiphyseal vessels. Two types of epiphyseal vascularization are described.[21] Type A epiphyses are almost entirely covered by articular cartilage, and the epiphyseal vessels enter the epiphysis after traversing the perichondrium. With this anatomical configuration, the blood supply to the epiphysis, and consequently to the germinal zone, is susceptible to damage if the epiphysis is separated from metaphysis. Type B epiphyses are only partially covered by articular cartilage. Their blood supply enters from the epiphyseal side and is protected from vascular injury during separation. The proximal femur and proximal radius are the only two examples of type A epiphyses.

Growth plate closure and skeletal age assessment during puberty

It is generally assumed that long-bone physes close at 14 years of skeletal age in females and at 16 years in males while the axial skeleton completes its development later.[22–24] In 50% of normal children and adolescents, skeletal age does not differ from chronological age.[25] Prediction of limb length discrepancy and final standing height as well as decisions regarding when to perform an epiphysiodesis are first subjected to determination of skeletal age.

A complication unique to physeal injuries is growth disturbance. Once damage to the physis has occurred, the predicted amount of growth remaining from that specific physis must be determined to plan the treatment. This can be accomplished by determining the skeletal age of the patient and then using information on physeal growth rates and patterns assembled by Green and Anderson.[26–30]

Treatment decisions are often made during puberty. Puberty is the period of time in the growing individual characterized by a significant increase in growth rate.[31,32] In girls, puberty starts at 11 years and ends at 13 years of skeletal age; in boys, it starts and ends 2 years later (13 years and 15 years of skeletal age).[25] Peak height growth and Tanner stage 2[33] signal the beginning of puberty. The 2 years of pubertal growth spurt are known as acceleration phase followed by a deceleration phase that continues until skeletal maturity.

The radiographic markers currently used to assess skeletal age are all based on the appearance of ossification centers in specific skeletal segments at specific times. Several age assessment methods are based on the use of anteroposterior radiographs of the left hand and wrist.[34–37] Other methods use left elbow radiographs.[25,38] The axial skeleton can also be used to determine the skeletal age: Risser sign[39] is based on the appearance of the left iliac apophysis of the pelvis. However, other radiographs can be used to assess skeletal age.[25]

Different assessment methods become helpful at different ages. The Greulich and Pyle atlas[34] is probably the most common and widely used method to assess skeletal age. This technique, however, has some limitations, especially during puberty because it does not make it possible to assess skeletal age at 6-month intervals during the 2 years of peak growth rate.[25] On the other hand, during the pubertal acceleration phase, the elbow, at the level of the distal epiphysis ossification centers and the olecranon apophysis, undergoes peculiar and identifiable morphological changes every 6 months[25,38] *(Figs 30.2 and 30.3)*. Elbow ossification centers always appear in a determined sequence (the mnemonic is CRITOE: capitellum, radial head, internal (medial) epicondyle, trochlea, olecranon, external (lateral) epicondyle). The ages of appearance as a general guide, are 1–3–5–7–9–11 years.

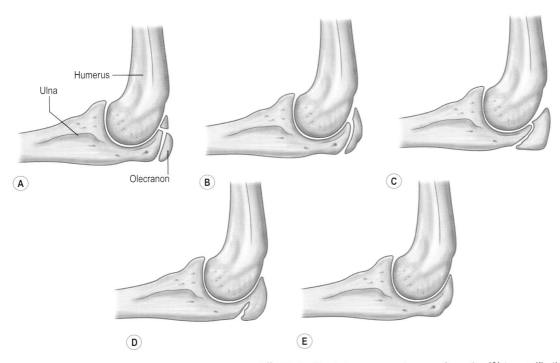

Fig. 30.2 Olecranon maturation according to Dimeglio *et al.*,[35] with significant changes occurring every 6 months. **(A)** two ossification centers (girls 11 years; boys 13 years); **(B)** half-moon shape (girls 11.5 years; boys 13.5 years); **(C)** rectangular shape (girls 12 years; boys 14 years); **(D)** beginning of fusion (girls 12.5 years; boys 14.5 years); and **(E)** complete fusion (girls 13 years; boys 15 years).

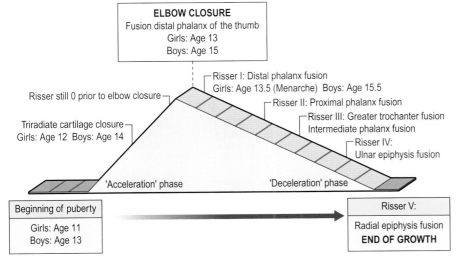

Fig. 30.3 Pubertal diagram. Acceleration phase, between skeletal age of 11 and 13 years in girls and 13 and 15 years in boys; Risser sign is 0. End of the acceleration phase, complete elbow and distal phalanx of the thumb closure; Risser sign is still 0.

During the acceleration phase, the skeletal age is best assessed with X-rays of the left hand and left elbow.[40–43] In the deceleration phase, the growth rate decreases significantly. The remaining growth in both boys and girls is around 6 cm, of which 4.5 cm belong to the trunk and skull. During this phase, the most useful tools for skeletal age assessment are again the left hand and the Risser stage.

Regardless of the assessment method used, skeletal age alone is not enough and it should be related to other clinical and radiological findings such as standing and sitting height, Tanner stage, and annual growth rate.

Diagnosis/patient presentation

Conditions affecting the growth plate

A complication unique to physeal injuries is growth disturbance. Trauma is the most common cause of physeal injury and growth disturbance, but physeal growth arrest may as well occur after infection, tumor, irradiation, thermal injury, laser beam exposure, and sequelae of Blount's disease (growth disorder with bowing of the tibia).[44–47]

Trauma

Incidence and distribution in the upper extremity

Physeal injuries represent 15–30% of all fracture in children[48–52] and frequently involve the upper extremities.[51,53] The incidence varies with age, with a peak in adolescence.[51,53,54] The upper hypertrophic zone, just above the area of provisional calcification, is the weakest layer of the physis and where most injuries to the physis occur.[7–9] This observation implies that, after most injuries, the germinal layer of the physis remains intact and attached to the epiphysis. Consequent normal growth should resume unless insult to the blood supply of the germinal layer or development of a "bony bridge" across the injured physis occur.

Classification of physeal fractures

Several classification systems for physeal injuries have been described.[55–61] The Salter and Harris classification (*Fig. 30.4*)[62] is by far the most widely used system. This classification helps to distinguish different types of fractures and provides prognostic information as well. In Salter–Harris type I (*Fig. 30.4*), the injury is a separation of the epiphysis from the metaphysis. It occurs entirely through the physis and therefore the surrounding bone is not involved. It is rare and tends to be seen in infants or pathologic fractures, such those secondary to rickets or scurvy. Because the germinal layer remains with the epiphysis, growth is not hindered unless blood supply is interrupted (traumatic separation of the proximal femoral epiphysis). Often, X-rays of a child with a type 1 Salter–Harris fracture will appear normal. Healing of type I fractures tends to be rapid and complications are rare.

In Salter–Harris type II injury (*Fig. 30.4*), the fracture extends along the hypertrophic zone of the physis but then it continues and exits through the metaphysis. This is the most common type of growth plate fracture, and tends to occur in older children. The epiphyseal fragment contains the entire germinal layer as well as a metaphyseal fragment, known as Thurston Holland's sign. The periosteum on the side of the metaphyseal fragment is usually intact and provides stability after reduction. Growth disturbance is uncommon because the germinal layer remains intact.

In Salter–Harris type III injury (*Fig. 30.4*), the fracture starts through the hypertrophic zone and exits through the epiphysis. These injuries also tend to affect older children. By definition, type III fractures cross the germinal layer and are usually intra-articular. Consequently they raise concerns about growth and, when displaced, they require anatomic, and often open, reduction.

In Salter–Harris type IV injury (*Fig. 30.4*), the fracture starts from the metaphysis and then extends through the physis and into the epiphysis. By definition these fractures disturb the germinal layer and are usually intra-articular. Consequently, these injuries may impair normal growth and affect articular congruency. In type IV injuries, an anatomic reduction is mandatory in order to prevent osseous bridging across the physis and to restore the articular surface.

A Salter–Harris type V injury (*Fig. 30.4*) occurs when the physis is crushed from a pure compression force. It is so rare that some authors question whether such an injury exists.[63] For those authors who have reported on this injury,[62,64] it carries the most concerning prognosis as the growth disturbance is almost a rule. It often requires later surgical treatment to restore limb length and alignment.

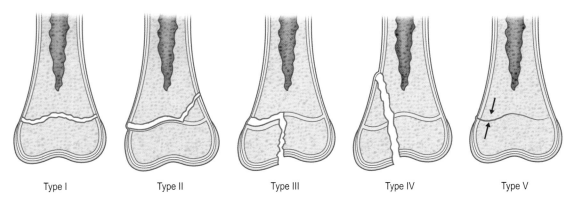

Type I   Type II   Type III   Type IV   Type V

Fig. 30.4 Salter–Harris classification of physeal fractures. (Redrawn after Salter RB, Harris R. Injuries involving the epiphyseal plate. *J Bone Joint Surg Am.* 1963;45:587–621.)

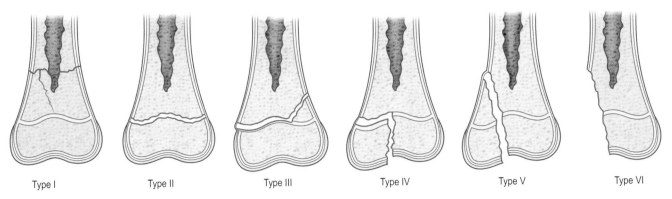

Type I   Type II   Type III   Type IV   Type V   Type VI

Fig. 30.5 Peterson classification of physeal fractures. Type VI injuries are open and associated with loss of the physis. (Redrawn after Peterson HA. Physeal fractures: part 3. Classification. *J Pediatr. Orthop.* 1994;14:439.)

Despite being widely used, the Salter–Harris classification excludes few physeal injuries: the Rang's type VI epiphyseal injury[59,60] which represents an injury to the perichondral ring; and two additional injuries described in the Peterson classification system *(Fig. 30.5),*[54] which is very similar to the Salter–Harris scheme. The Peterson type I fracture is a transverse fracture of the metaphysis that extends longitudinally into the physis. Clinically this type of fracture is commonly seen in the distal radius. The Peterson VI fracture is an open injury associated with loss of the physis.

Treatment of physeal fractures

Growth plate injuries that are less severe, and occur closer to the time of closure of the growth plate, carry the best prognosis. More severe injuries occurring in younger patients require observation and possibly treatment to prevent problems. The principles of treatment of physeal fractures are the same as those involved in the treatment of all fractures, with a few important considerations.

The goal in the treatment of physeal injuries is to obtain and maintain an acceptable reduction while avoiding any further damage to the germinal layer of the physis during reduction. Thus the most important goal and the most subjective one is to establish the limits of acceptable reduction.

The age of the patient, the location and displacement of the fracture, and the time elapsed since the injury must be all taken into consideration when assessing a nonanatomic reduction. Although animal studies have not shown that delay in reduction produces a growth disturbance,[65] the recommendation is to accept any displacement in type I and II injuries after 7–10 days[9,66] and rather plan an osteotomy later. As a general rule the remodeling potential is inversely proportionate to the age of the patient and is also related to the location and type of injury. Consequently, a greater deformity can be accepted in younger children.

Because type III and IV injuries are by definition intra-articular, the focus must be on achieving an anatomic reduction regardless of the age of the patient and the time that has elapsed since the injury. Once the physeal fracture has been reduced, the reduction can be maintained with cast, pins, internal fixation, or combinations of these three.

Tumor

Bone sarcoma involving the epiphysis

Most of the common primary malignant bone tumors occur in patients aged under 30 years.[67] Typically osteosarcoma and Ewing sarcoma are found in adolescents and young adults, but they may also be diagnosed during infancy. The current approach to systemic therapy[67] includes preoperative (neoadjuvant) chemotherapy and postoperative (adjuvant) chemotherapy for both osteosarcoma and Ewing sarcoma. Radiotherapy is indicated only in Ewing sarcoma and it may be the only local treatment in cases of tumor in unfavorable locations, such as spine and pelvis, and in all cases where radical surgery is unlikely to be successful. Postoperative radiotherapy is indicated in all cases of intralesional resections with the aim of reducing the risk of local recurrence.

With advances in bone reconstruction, the role of surgery has become predominant in the treatment of primary bone tumor, and the percentage of limb salvage versus amputation has significantly increased. In the upper limb, bone sarcomas are more frequently located in the distal radius and proximal humerus. Although the tumor is usually initially located at the metaphyseal level, the growth plate and the physis are always to be considered as a possible target of sarcoma invasion. From a functional standpoint, it is critical to know whether the surgical resection may spare the epiphysis or not.

In the past, the growth plate was thought to be a biologic barrier to bone tumor invasion[68–70]; unfortunately this theory has not proven to be valid[71–73] *(Fig. 30.6)*. The current view is that invasion of the physis must always be suspected when the tumor is located in the proximity of the growth plate and all patients should be investigated with magnetic resonance imaging (MRI). In the event of epiphyseal involvement, the oncological resection must include the epiphysis and the only possible reconstructive option for such a defect in the pediatric age is autologous epiphyseal transplant.

Congenital chondrodysplasia

Chondrocyte proliferation and differentiation in the physis, and therefore skeletal growth, are regulated by various endocrine, paracrine, and autocrine factors. Any disturbance of the epiphyseal growth plate physiology and development results in various skeletal abnormalities known as dysplasia or chondrodysplasia. These cases may also require reconstruction to maintain growth.

Patient selection

When the physis is damaged and deformity results or is foreseen, several treatment options are available. The best treatment for a growth plate injury depends on the individual situation. Although physeal injuries are common, problems arising are rare, occurring in only 1–10% of all physeal fractures.[9,51,54] Comminuted fractures, high-energy injuries, and physeal injuries that cross the germinal layer are more prone to result in physeal arrest with subsequent growth disturbance. Physeal injuries are most common in adolescents close to skeletal maturity. In these individuals, the remaining

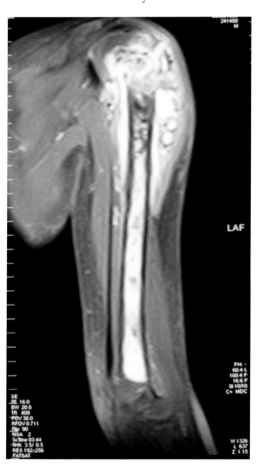

Fig. 30.6 Osteosarcoma involving the proximal epiphysis and the adjoining diaphysis in a 6-year-old child.

growth is limited.[9,51,54] Consequently, even when it occurs, physeal arrest will produce minimal or no length discrepancy or angular deviation and will seldom require treatment.

Growth disturbance resulting from a physeal fracture is usually evident 2–6 months after the injury, but it may take up to a year to manifest.[9] This information is important both to warn the parents about possible complications and to anticipate close long-term follow-up. In fact the management of a posttraumatic growth disturbance is easier when directed exclusively towards treating the arrest rather than tackling both the arrest and the acquired deformity.

Growth disturbance is usually a consequence of the development of a bony bridge, or bar, across the physis. However, when the injury only reduces rather than stops the growth rate of a portion of the physis, it may still produce asymmetric growth and angular deformity with no development of bony bridge.[74] If the bony bar involves a large portion of the physis, it may stop the physeal growth completely. However, in most cases the bony bar is confined to a rather small portion of the physis and the growth stops only at that point. The remaining healthy physis continues to grow, creating a tethering effect which may produce either a shortening or a progressive significant angular deformity, or both.

The extent and location of the bar, the skeletal age of the patient, and the amount of growth remaining from the physis must all be determined to plan the treatment of a physeal bar appropriately. Plain radiography, tomography, computed tomography (CT), or MRI[44,75–78] may all be used to assess the anatomy of a physeal bar. MRI is by far the preferred method currently used to investigate physeal anatomy.[79–82] In particular, fat-suppressed, three-dimensional, gradient-recalled echo sequences can provide an accurate three-dimensional reconstruction of the physis and estimate the percentage of physeal arrest.[82] The classification of partial physeal arrests is based on their location within the physis *(Fig. 30.7)*: peripheral (type A) or central (type B or C). In type B, the bar develops in the center of the physis and is surrounded by a perimeter of healthy physis. This may create a tethering effect that "tents" the epiphysis, leading to joint deformity. In type C (central) the bar traverses the entire physis (front to back or side to side) while the physis on both sides of the bar is normal.

Treatment/surgical technique

Treatment of physeal arrest

Different treatment options are available for the management of physeal arrests. These options include observation, completion of a partial physeal arrest, epiphysiodesis, physeal bar resection, or physeal distraction.

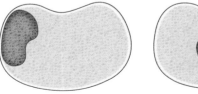
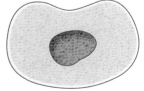
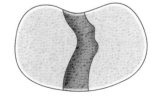

Type A   Type B   Type C

Fig. 30.7 Classification of physeal bars. Type A, peripheral; type B, central, surrounded by normal physis; type C, central, traversing the physis.

Observation

Observation may be the best option when the physeal bar involves the entire physis with complete growth arrest, existing limb length inequality and/or angular deformity is acceptable, or the individual is close to skeletal maturity with little longitudinal growth remaining.

Completion of a partial physeal arrest and epiphysiodesis

Completion of a partial physeal arrest may be indicated if there is an acceptable existing angular deformity that may become clinically unacceptable if left untreated. To avoid significant limb shortening of the upper extremity, the surgeon must evaluate the predicted remaining growth and foresee a lengthening procedure if necessary. In the upper extremity limb, length discrepancy is a relative issue but the asynchronous rate of longitudinal growth between two bones in an anatomic region where the two bones are paired in close longitudinal relationship, as in the forearm, or asynchronous growth in an anatomic region where the harmonic activity of several physes contributes to the final size and shape of the bone, such as the distal humerus, might lead to a great risk of anatomic distortion. If the likelihood of length inequality is high, epiphysiodesis of a noninjured physis should be performed at the time of completion of the physeal arrest.

Epiphysiodesis is an established method of limb length equalization or angular deformity correction in children and adolescents with projected limb length discrepancies at maturity as great as 5 or 6 cm. It consists of temporarily stopping or permanently destroying the activity of the whole or just a part (hemiepiphysiodesis) of the growth plate. First introduced by Phemister in 1933,[83] epiphysiodesis has evolved into various reversible or irreversible, open or percutaneous techniques with and without instrumentation. The ideal tool should be minimally invasive, have minimal morbidity, and be reliably reversible. Pitfalls include errors in the prediction of growth and planning of the surgery. In particular with nonreversible techniques, timing must be precise. Overcompensation for limb length discrepancy or creation of an opposite angular deformity can be very distressing for the patient, family, and surgeon. Although many different techniques have proven their efficacy, percutaneous epiphysiodesis using transphyseal screws combines the minimal invasiveness of a percutaneous technique with reversibility.[84]

Physeal distraction

Physeal distraction is an alternative treatment for partial physeal arrest. Physeal distraction uses the growth plate as a zone of least resistance. It involves the damaged physis and therefore acts at the site of the deformity. It requires a force to be applied longitudinally across the physis, permitting both lengthening and angular correction on multiple planes, with external control of the correction until consolidation. Prior resection of the bony bar is not necessary.

A distinction must be made between distractional epiphysiolysis and chondrodiastasis,[85,86] chondrodiatasis,[87] and hemichondrodiatasis.[88]

The chondrodiastasis technique employs large forces or rapid rate of distraction (>1 mm/day) or both.[89] This provokes a distraction and opening of the physis that provides a rapid *in situ* correction from the bony bar without prior bar resection, but almost invariably it produces a premature physeal fusion.[89,90] This notion limits the indications to patients nearing skeletal maturity and preventive lengthening according to predicted limb length discrepancy.[91,92] In the literature, physeal distraction techniques are mostly reported for the treatment of lower-limb deformities and little is known about their application in the upper limb.

Bar resection

If a portion of the physis has prematurely closed, but the reminder of the physis is healthy and there is substantial growth remaining, resection of the physeal bar and insertion of interposition materials are indicated. This technique in fact preserves longitudinal bone growth ability.[93,94] The procedure was first introduced by Langenskiold and has been documented in both human and animal models.[45,76,93,95–98]

The surgical technique of bar resection consists in removing the bone bridge along with the neighboring portions of metaphysis and epiphysis and filling the cavity with an inert material that will prevent recurrence of physeal bar formation *(Figs 30.8 and 30.9)*.

Type A peripheral bars can be removed under direct vision, taking care to resect a wide cuff of periosteum. Type B and C central bars need to be approached through a window in the metaphysis or through an osteotomy *(Fig. 30.8)*. Their resection may be facilitated by the use of fluoroscopy, fiberoptic

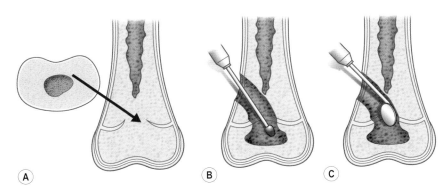

Fig. 30.8 (A) Central bar. **(B)** Bar resection through metaphyseal approach. **(C)** Assessing the resection.

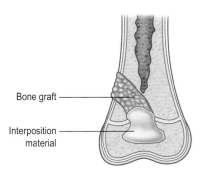

Fig. 30.9 Interposition material is positioned accurately to prevent bleeding and dislodgment. Bone graft is used to fill the tunnel in the metaphysis.

lighting, and dental mirrors as well as magnifying loupes *(Fig. 30.9)*.

Physeal bar resection is recommended when all the following conditions are present: the remaining physis must be undamaged and must be large enough to permit growth to continue; and there should be a significant amount of growth remaining in that physis before physiologic physeal closure. Bars involving more than 50% of the physeal surface are unlikely to respond to surgical treatment.[46,59,76,93,94,95,97] Despite the acceptance that younger patients, with higher growth potential, will benefit from physeal bar resection, there is still no agreement in quantifying the amount of this growth potential.[76,95,98]

According to Bright,[99] indications for a bone bridge resection are as follows: there must be more than 50% of remaining healthy physis; the expected physeal growth must last for 2 years or more; there must be good soft-tissue coverage of the lesion; and, in the case of growth arrest due to infection, the infection must have been absent for more than 1 year.

Once the bar is completely resected, various interpositional materials can be used to fill the void and prevent transphyseal bone bridge formation.[59,76,95] Of the interposition materials described, fat is the most commonly used.[93,100] It has the advantage of being autologous and immediately available. Failure to prevent reformation of the physeal bridge[101,102] may be due to the fact that fat may not provide adequate hemostasis of the cavity and may migrate.[94,103]

Silicone (Silastic) has been experimentally used in both human and animal studies with good results[99,104] but Silastic has been withdrawn from the market.[96] Methylmethacrylate, commercially known as Cranioplast, is a material used to fill partial defects of the skull, is radiolucent, and is thermally nonconductive. The advantage as interposition material[94] is that its solid structure may help to support an epiphysis if a large metaphyseal defect has been created.[103] It may, however, damage the healthy physis because of heat produced by exothermic reaction during the solidifying phase.[105] It may also be problematic to remove if further reconstructive procedures are required. Rarely it can migrate from the physis into the diaphysis, and cause a pathological fracture.[106]

Expanded polytetrafluoroethylene (EPTFE) membrane (Gore-Tex® dura substitute; WL Gore, Flagstaff, AZ, US) is generally used as an artificial dura substitute. The advantages of EPTFE membrane are that it is inert, nonreactive, and

unaffected by long-term exposure within the body,[107] easy to handle, and provides good hemostasis. The disadvantage is that, being a soft material, it does not provide sufficient mechanical support and it is therefore only recommended when the resected area is at most 30% of the cross-section of the physis.[108]

Bone wax is readily available and commonly used in medical applications to control bleeding. It has been successfully used as interposition material with the advantages of being inexpensive and permitting good hemostasis. It is not associated with excessive complications.[109] The disadvantage is that it does not offer a good mechanical support to the physis after bar resection.

Regardless of which interposition material is selected, the purpose is to fill the cavity created in the physis with the material so that bar formation is prevented. After bar resection, radiographic markers should be placed on each side of the physis to assess growth resumption.

Results after bar resection are variable. Even with appropriate patient selection and standardized operative technique, failure may result. Graft dislocation out of the cavity is one of the causes of failure.[110] It is therefore recommended to anchor the interposition material so that it will not dislodge, allowing bleeding into the cavity.[94] It is important that, even when growth resumes, premature closure of the physis is to be expected.[54,76,95,103,110]

Physeal bar resection with interposition of certain materials plays a role in the treatment of partial physeal arrest; however, its results are relatively modest.

Corrective osteotomies, lengthening or shortening

Epiphysiodesis and resection of the bone bridge with the insertion of interposition materials[93,94] are the two main methods to treat partial physeal arrest that also prevent further progression of angular deformity. In addition, for mild deformities of less than 20°, we can expect spontaneous remodeling after bar resection,[93,94,111] although this has not been universally reported.[74] When an angular deformity is already evident, corrective osteotomy is indicated because remodeling sufficient to correct the deformity cannot be expected. Corrective osteotomy should be considered for any angular deformity that is judged to be "clinically unacceptable."[76,95,94,103]

It is well known that the physeal growth rate responds to the force applied on the physis itself: growth is stimulated by both mild tension and mild compression.[112] However, according to the Hueter–Volkmann principle,[113] when compression on the growth plate exceeds a certain level, growth is indeed suppressed.[112] If the compression is applied only on one side of the physis, worsening of the deformity may ensue. Improved alignment may therefore facilitate more normal growth.

Bone lengthening involves the principle of distraction-induced osteogenesis and the use of an external fixator. Because of the nonweight-bearing status of the upper extremity, limb length discrepancy of the upper limbs is better tolerated and of less functional and cosmetic significance than their counterparts in the lower extremity. For these reasons, along with the incumbent risks associated with the surgery, indications for bone-lengthening procedures in the upper extremities are confined to selected cases.[101,114–125]

Reported complications of upper limb lengthening include pin tract infections, complications related to callus stability and formation (callus deformities after fixator removal, refractures, and malunions), diminished range of motion, elbow flexion contractures, pin-related nerve injuries, temporary radial nerve paresis as a complication of humeral lengthening, and sympathetic dystrophy.[126–130] Considerable morbidity results from nerve injury secondary to the transfixing wires.[129,130] In addition, in distraction lengthening of the upper limb, the bone formation takes longer compared to the lower limb because of the lack of weight-bearing. Therefore the external fixator must be kept on for several months. The length of treatment further decreases patient compliance and can be a major issue in young children and adolescents.

Epiphyseal transfer of the proximal fibular epiphysis

Indications

The main indications for epiphyseal reconstruction are loss of an epiphysis following trauma, tumor resection, or infection in children. Vascularized epiphyseal transfer is a procedure that can simultaneously achieve the double goal of reconstructing a lost joint and maintaining growth potential. Because of its biological and morphological characteristics, the proximal fibula is by far the best donor site for reconstruction of large bone defects of the upper extremity. In fact, unlike other bone segments suggested for vascularized epiphyseal reconstruction,[155,156] the proximal end of the fibula contains a true epiphysis with a growth plate that, if properly revascularized, maintains its growth potential at the recipient site. In addition, the fibula is a tubular bone with a long expendable diaphysis that is perfectly suited for upper limb reconstruction, allowing safe and stable bone fixation.

The two most common locations of bone sarcomas of the upper extremity in the pediatric age are the distal metaepiphysis of the radius and the proximal humerus, with a slightly higher incidence for the latter. Due to morphological and dimensional similarities, the proximal fibula is ideal for distal radius reconstruction.[151] In addition, under the influence of a new biomechanical environment, the plasticity of the immature bone allows remarkable remodeling of the epiphysis after its transfer into the new anatomic location. Since the forearm is a two-bone segment and severe wrist deformity may result from asymmetrical growth of radius and ulna, the younger the patient, the greater is the indication for epiphyseal transfer in this location.

Despite the anatomic mismatch between the fibular head and the glenoid fossa and the difference in transverse diameter of the shafts between the humerus and the fibula,[148] autologous proximal fibular transplant remains the best option for autogenous reconstruction of the proximal humerus *(Fig. 30.10)*. Over time, the fibular diaphysis undergoes hypertrophy, which minimizes the size discrepancy. Moreover, remodeling of the fibular head, although less impressive than in distal radius reconstruction, is expected, leading to more than acceptable shoulder joint stability and function *(Fig. 30.11)*.

Proximal fibula epiphyseal transfer has proven to be an excellent option in limb salvage surgery in pediatric oncologic

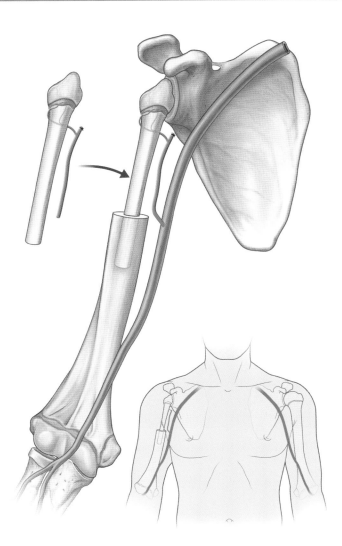

Fig. 30.10 In proximal humerus reconstruction the smaller fibula is usually inserted inside the humeral medullar canal with a periosteal flap overlapping the bony junction. This type of assemblage improves stability and ability to heal. Vascular anastomoses are usually performed end to end to the deep humeral vessels.

cases. Congenital differences of the upper limb, such as radial dysplasia, may also benefit from this surgical procedure. These cases, though, raise the following concerns and considerations: the new radius may be expected to grow more than the native ulna, which usually is hypoplastic, thus developing wrist instability and ulnar deviation. Ideal timing for reconstruction occurs in a period when the child is learning to walk, and harvesting the fibula may temporary affect the donor site, delaying this milestone. Very poor literature is available at the moment on epiphyseal transfer for radial dysplasia and there is no report on medium- or long-term outcomes which could help to validate the technique.[146,150,157]

Vascularized epiphyseal transplant based on the anterior tibial vascular system is a long and demanding procedure with high rate of complications, although transient, at the donor site. For these reasons, the cost-effectiveness ratio

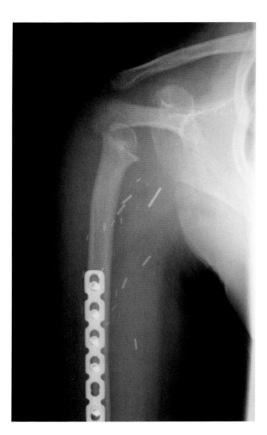

Fig. 30.11 Reconstruction of the proximal humerus at 5-year follow-up. The transferred proximal fibula underwent significant remodeling and hypertrophy as well as enough longitudinal growth to prevent limb length discrepancy.

should be carefully evaluated. From a personal experience of 30 cases, we have concluded that distal radius reconstruction is indicated up to 13 years of age because the radius and ulna require symmetrical growth until skeletal maturity. On the other hand, the humerus tolerates well a length discrepancy from both functional and cosmetic standpoints, setting the age limit for such a procedure around 10 years of age.

Vascular supply of the proximal fibular epiphysis

In the past 30 years, the vascular anatomy of the proximal fibular epiphysis has been extensively investigated in order to define the best pedicle supplying both the epiphysis and the diaphysis of such a graft. There is general agreement that the proximal epiphysis of the fibula is supplied by two vascular sources: (1) the lateral inferior genicular artery; and (2) the recurrent branches of the anterior tibial artery. The role of the two systems is differently emphasized according to different authors,[158–162] but the majority of reports confirm that the anterior tibial artery provides the major contribution to the blood supply of the proximal fibular growth plate. Summarizing the data available in the literature, the lateral inferior geniculate artery mostly supplies the capsule of the proximal tibiofibular joint, the anterior and posterior recurrent branches of the anterior tibial artery supply the epiphysis, and the peroneal artery supplies the fibular shaft. It has also been experimentally demonstrated[160,161] that the anterior

tibial artery is able to vascularize the proximal two-thirds of the fibular diaphysis through tiny musculoperiosteal perforators which distribute to the periosteum of the shaft.

Almost all possible vascular pedicle combinations have been described in use in clinical practice. Pho *et al.* reported on 3 cases[145] where the peroneal artery was used as the pedicle, postulating that the presence of intercommunicating branches between the metaphyseal and epiphyseal systems allowed for acceptable blood supply to the growth plate based solely on the peroneal artery. Although this is probably anatomically possible, if enough soft tissue is left around the fibular neck, further experiences[148,153] have had disappointing results on the growth rate of grafts supplied by the peroneal artery alone.

The use of a bipedicled graft has been suggested,[144,146,148] with the purpose of providing two separate blood supplies to the epiphysis and the diaphysis. This option, however, is technically demanding, time-consuming, and requires two anastomoses at the recipient site. In addition, the physis is very susceptible to ischemia, and normal growth can be expected only if ischemia time is less than 3 hours.[163] For these reasons, a single pedicled graft is definitely a better choice.

The anterior tibial system has proven to be adequate in supplying both the epiphysis and the shaft and it is therefore the preferred pedicle for such a graft *(Fig. 30.12)*. A potential disadvantage to the use of the anterior tibial vascular system is that the pedicle is very short (the distance between the division of the popliteal artery and the origin of the recurrent branch at the fibular neck). To overcome this issue, it has been suggested to use a reverse-flow pedicle.[148,151,157] In this way, long vessels are provided, allowing comfortable anastomosis at the recipient site.

Harvest technique of the proximal fibula based on the tibialis anterior artery (video)

The flap includes the proximal fibular epiphysis and a variable amount of the adjoining diaphysis. The epiphyseal articular surface is oriented upward and medially to form the proximal tibiofibular joint. The biceps femoris tendon and the lateral collateral ligament are inserted in the lateral and proximal aspect of the epiphysis, which is also where the origins of the peroneus longus and extensor digitorum longus muscles are located. The common peroneal nerve crosses the fibular neck, moving toward the anterior compartment of the leg. The superficial branch is located in the space between the extensor digitorum longus and peroneus longus muscles, while the deep branch reaches the interosseous membrane and joins the anterior tibial vessels, giving several motor branches to the surrounding muscles. Proceeding proximally, the dissection of the vascular pedicle with preservation of the motor branches becomes increasingly demanding because of the increasing number of motor branches surrounding the vessels.

The harvest technique has been refined over the years and has been finally described in detail[164,165] with the purpose of standardizing it and making it reproducible. The aim of the procedure is to harvest the proximal fibula, preserving the blood supply to both the epiphysis and diaphysis with the least possible local morbidity. The following step-by-step description is the optimal surgical sequence according to the experience of the senior author.

Video
1

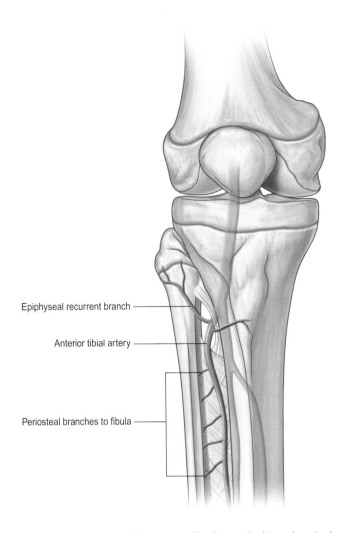

Fig. 30.12 The anterior tibial artery supplies the growth plate and proximal epiphysis by means of a recurrent epiphyseal branch and the proximal two-thirds of the diaphysis by means of musculoperiosteal perforator branches.

Epiphyseal recurrent branch

Anterior tibial artery

Periosteal branches to fibula

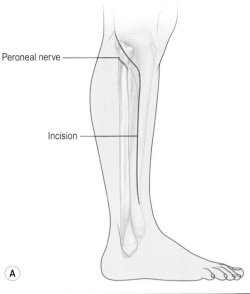

Peroneal nerve

Incision

(A)

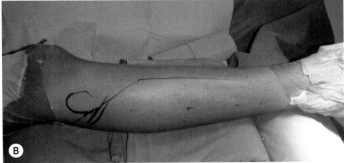

(B)

Fig. 30.13 An anterolateral approach is used for the harvest of the proximal fibula based on the anterior tibial vascular system. The skin incision is on the projection of the intermuscular space between the tibialis anterior and extensor digitorum longus muscles. The incision is prolonged proximally and posteriorly over the tendon of biceps femoris muscle.

Skin incision

The surgical approach is developed in the plane between tibialis anterior and extensor digitorum longus muscles because this allows for direct visualization of the neurovascular bundle. The skin incision is therefore located in the anterolateral aspect of the leg and is extended proximally up to the neck of the fibula where it proceeds posteriorly and proximally over the biceps femoris tendon *(Fig. 30.13)*.

Exposure of the anterior tibial pedicle

The anterior tibial artery and veins lie on the interosseous membrane. The peroneal nerve surrounds the vessel according to a very intricate tridimensional pattern and delivers several motor branches to the muscles of the anterior compartment of the leg *(Fig. 30.14)*. These motor branches are more numerous in the proximal part of the leg and it is therefore recommended to start the dissection distally and proceed proximally, maintaining the same plane to the fibular neck.

Great care should be taken not only in dissecting the nerve from the vessels but also in preserving the small perforator branches of the anterior tibial artery which pierce the extensor digitorum longus and peroneus longus muscles, interposed between the vascular pedicle and the fibular shaft, supplying the periosteum of the proximal two-thirds of the diaphysis.

Dissection of the peroneal nerve at the fibular neck

The point where the peroneal nerve approaches the fibular neck is an important anatomic landmark. The nerve is in close contact with the bone and is covered by the proximal portion of extensor digitorum longus and peroneus longus muscles, which must be sharply divided in order to expose and protect the nerve and its motor branches *(Fig. 30.15)*. Medially, at the same level, the recurrent epiphyseal branch of the anterior tibial artery rises from the main artery and pierces the muscular cuff and feeds the epiphysis. Its direct dissection is unnecessary and potentially dangerous; it is therefore

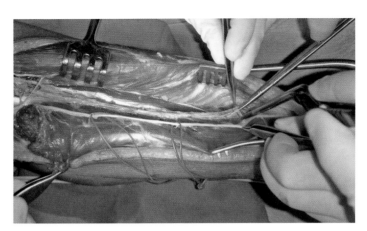

Fig. 30.14 During the diaphyseal dissection of the pedicle, great care must be paid to isolating the peroneal nerve and its motor branches to the muscles of the anterior compartment.

recommended to preserve the proximal insertion of the muscles attached to the proximal epiphysis in order to protect the fragile epiphyseal vascular network.

Section of the interosseous membrane and distal osteotomy

The interosseous membrane must be sharply detached from the tibia, and all the soft tissue interposed between it and the vascular bundle must be carefully protected *(Fig. 30.16)*. The perforator vessels to the shaft of the fibula branches off laterally and pierces the of extensor digitorum longus and peroneus longus muscle bellies. In order to maintain the vascular connection between the artery and bone, a longitudinal strip of muscle approximately 1 cm wide should be preserved around the harvested fibula *(Fig. 30.17)*. The fibula is cut distally at the desired length, and an extra portion of periosteum is left in order improve healing capacity at the recipient site. The anterior tibial artery and veins are ligated as distally as possible to obtain a long reverse-flow pedicle.

Harvest of the biceps femoris tendon and capsulotomy of the proximal tibiofibular joint

The insertions of the biceps femoris tendon and the lateral collateral ligaments are almost at the same point at the apex of the fibula. The tendon should be divided in two strips *(Fig. 30.18)*: the posterior portion is harvested with the fibula to provide additional soft tissue useful for stabilization of the recipient joint. The anterior half is used to reinforce the lateral collateral ligament after its reinsertion on the lateral aspect of tibial metaphysis by means of staples or transosseous sutures. Gentle external rotation of the fibula allows for the division of the medial and posterior capsule of the proximal tibiofibular joint after coagulation of the lateral inferior genicular artery.

Final dissection of the proximal portion of the vascular pedicle

The anterior tibial artery should be dissected up to the division of the popliteal artery *(Fig. 30.19)*. The recurrent branch

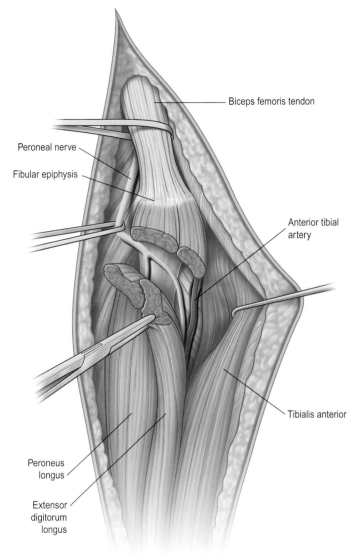

Biceps femoris tendon

Peroneal nerve

Fibular epiphysis

Anterior tibial artery

Tibialis anterior

Peroneus longus

Extensor digitorum longus

Ⓐ

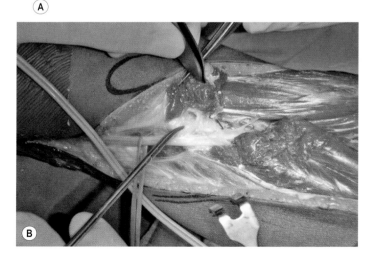

Ⓑ

Fig. 30.15 (A, B) The peroneal nerve is an important landmark in proximal dissection. The nerve is exposed in its intramuscular portion by means of sharp section of the extensor digitorum longus and peroneus longus muscles. The muscular cuff proximal to the section must be left intact because it protects the recurrent branch to the growth plate of the anterior tibial artery.

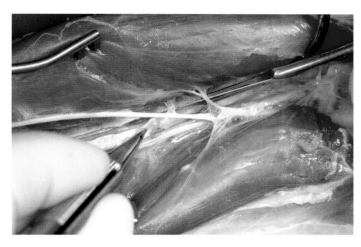

Fig. 30.16 Sharp detachment of the interosseous membrane from the tibia. Note the location of the vascular pedicle and its relationship to the peroneal nerve.

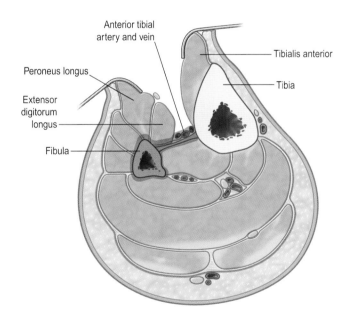

Fig. 30.17 The perforator branches to the diaphysis are too small and fragile to allow a direct intramuscular dissection. It is therefore suggested that a strip of muscle containing the perforators be left intact between the vascular pedicle and the bone.

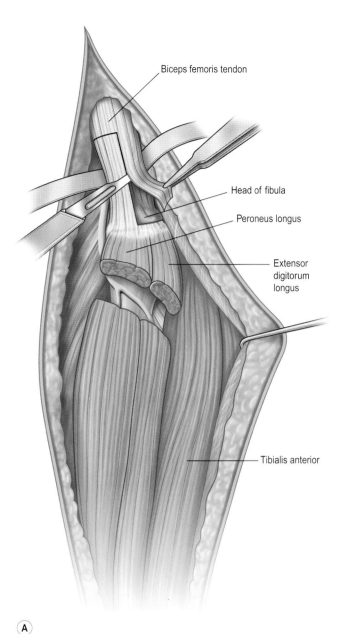

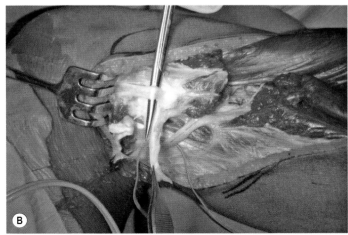

Fig. 30.18 (A, B) The biceps femoris tendon is longitudinally divided in two strips. One is harvested with the bone flap and may be used to improve the stability of the joint after the transfer. The second one is fixed to the lateral aspect of the tibia to reinforce the lateral collateral ligament.

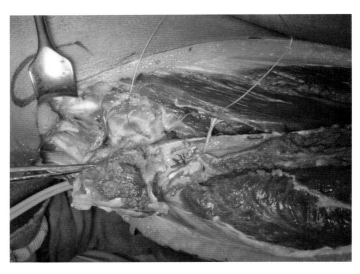

Fig. 30.19 After release of tourniquet and 20–30 minutes of reperfusion of the flap, the tibialis anterior artery is ligated and severed just distal to its emergence from the popliteal artery.

rises from the anterior tibial artery approximately 2 cm distal to its origin, and is often difficult to identify. For this reason, it is advisable to preserve all the small vessels which pierce the muscular cuff toward the fibular epiphysis. After release of the tourniquet, the muscular cuff surrounding the epiphysis, the diaphyseal periosteum, and the medullary canal are carefully inspected. After a few seconds, bleeding should be observed at the three levels, confirming the successful harvest of the proximal fibula, based on the anterior tibial artery pedicle *(Fig. 30.20)*. Due to low tolerance to ischemia, it is suggested to wait 20–30 minutes before clipping and dividing the proximal pedicle.

Postoperative care

Donor site

In order to protect the reconstructed lateral collateral ligament a cast at 30° flexion of knee and neutral ankle position is applied. In children below the age of 8 years old the cast is maintained for 4 weeks; in elder and compliant children the cast may be substituted after 2 weeks with a brace of appropriate size, for a total of 4 weeks of immobilization. The rehabilitation program is started at 1 month postoperatively with the aim of recovering full motion of the knee without compromising stability. A transient palsy of the peroneal nerve occurs in almost all cases. These patients are managed with splinting and passive mobilization to avoid equinus deformity. Full weight-bearing is usually possible at 2 months after surgery.

Recipient site

A long spica cast or a shoulder brace is applied for 4 weeks respectively after distal radius and proximal humerus

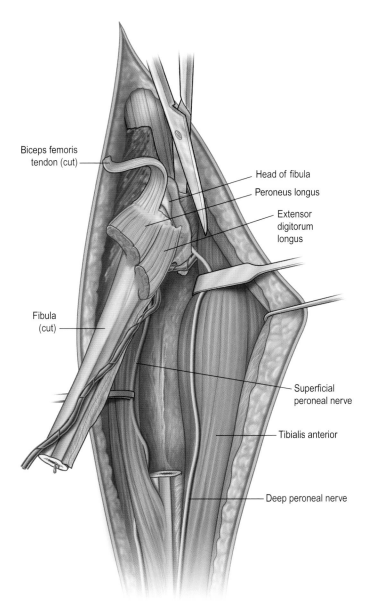

Biceps femoris tendon (cut)

Head of fibula

Peroneus longus

Extensor digitorum longus

Fibula (cut)

Superficial peroneal nerve

Tibialis anterior

Deep peroneal nerve

Fig. 30.20 At the end of the dissection, before severing the vascular pedicle, the tourniquet is released to reset the ischemia time. Bleeding should be observed from both the epiphysis and the medullar canal after a few minutes. 1, posterior articular capsule is severed; 2, bleeding from the bone is observed.

reconstruction. The rehabilitation program follows the immobilization period and must take into account different variables such as type and stability of bone fixation, amount of muscles excised during the resection, and age and compliance of the patient.

Outcomes, prognosis, and complications

Analysis of the results takes into account the survival of the grafts, as well as their consolidation, longitudinal growth, and remodeling. In a personal series of 27 cases of upper limb skeletal reconstruction after bone sarcoma resection with epiphyseal transplant, all the transferred bones except one survived and healed with the recipient bone in a period of time ranging from 1 to 2 months. This variability depended on the age of the child and the length of the reconstructed segment. In some cases, the viability of the transplant was confirmed by bone scan.

Significant axial growth, calculated by the progressive increase in the distance between the tip of the metal plate used for bone fixation and the apex of the epiphysis of the transferred fibula, has been observed in approximately 70% of cases monitored. Its extent was variable depending on factors that are only partially known, amongst which the patient's age was predominant. The annual growth trend varied between 0.7 and 1.35 cm *(Fig. 30.21)*, and in all cases there was prevention of future length discrepancy with the opposite limb. As far as the radius is concerned, symmetrical growth was observed in the neoradius in all cases, not only with respect to the opposite limb, but also to the adjacent ulna, which confirms the integration of the fibula into its new anatomical site. The average flexion of the wrist was 75°, while the average extension was 63°. The overall range of movement was equal to on average 70% of the opposite hand, which allowed for excellent functional recovery. The prosupination range was also restored.

In cases of humeral reconstruction, the functional outcomes were not as positive. The morphological and dimensional discrepancy between the fibular head and the glenoid fossa may lead to proximal migration of the fibular epiphysis and, in some cases, subacromial displacement. Moreover, the extent of soft tissue involved in the neoplasia and consequently removed further hinders functional recovery. In all monitored cases, however, shoulder abduction between 70° and 100° was observed.

Premature ossification of the growth plate and consequent end of growth were observed in 5 cases of humeral reconstruction. Two of these transplants were based on peroneal vessels which, in our opinion, are not as reliable in ensuring correct epiphyseal perfusion. In the other 3 cases, the epiphyseal artery was probably damaged during stabilization in the glenohumeral joint. Five fractures of the neohumerus and two of the neoradius were observed. All the fractures but one healed conservatively in due time. Replacement of an inadequate fixation was performed in 1 case.

In 4 cases of proximal humerus reconstruction, incorrect alignment between the fibula head and glenoid fossa was observed. In these cases, the epiphysis migrated subacromially. The reasons for this complication are the anatomical mismatching between fibular head and glenoid fossa and the extensive oncological excision of muscles and ligaments with consequent joint stability. All the 4 cases, however, recovered an acceptable range of motion.

With transosseous suture of the lateral collateral ligament at the donor site, no residual instability of the knee was ever observed. Neuropraxia of the peroneal nerve occurred in approximately two-thirds of cases. This was probably caused by stretching of small motor branches during the dissection. This deficit resolved spontaneously within 1 year in all but two cases. One of the patients had a permanent residual paralysis of the tibialis anterior and one of the extensor digitorum longus muscles.

Secondary procedures

Secondary procedures may be necessary at both the donor and the recipient site.

Donor site

In case of permanent palsy of the peroneal nerve a tendon transfer is indicated to restore the function of the tibialis anterior muscle. In our series we observed no cases of knee joint instability.

Recipient site

A feared complication is the total loss of the graft due to failure to restore its blood supply. We did not observe this complication but its treatment would require the use of a massive frozen allograft as salvage procedure. In the majority of cases the fate of an osteoarticular allograft in the medium/long term is a massive resorption of the articular cartilage which should be treated with a prosthetic replacement of the allogenic humeral head.

In our experience we have observed premature growth arrest, probably due to vascular damage to the physis, in 5 cases of proximal humerus reconstruction. Despite the limb length discrepancy all patients have an acceptable function and no further surgery was required.

A relatively frequent complication is graft fracture in proximal humerus reconstruction. In our series this event was usually successfully treated conservatively with immobilization in a cast. Nonetheless, revision of the hardware and cancellous bone grafting may be considered in cases of displaced fractures.

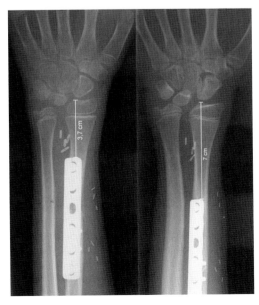

Fig. 30.21 Postoperative radiograph and 4-year follow-up of one case of distal radius reconstruction. In this case the average growth per year was 0.9 cm.

Access the complete references list online at **http://www.expertconsult.com**

3. Rauch F. Bone Growth in Length and Width: The Yin and Yang of Bone Stability. *J Musculoskelet Neuronal Interact*. 2005;5:194–201.

This entertaining article presents in a very approachable manner the morphophysiology of the growth plate and the mechanisms that regulate bone growth.

25. Canavese F, Charles YP, Dimeglio A. Skeletal age assessment from elbow radiographs. Review of the literature. *Chir Organ Mov*. 2008;92:1–6.

A useful method to assess skeletal age during puberty is presented in this article. The paper also offers an accurate description of growth during puberty and contains a review of the literature of other methods used for skeletal age assessment in growing individuals.

82. Sailhan F, Chotel F, Guibal AL, et al. Three-dimensional MRI imaging in the assessment of physeal growth arrest. *Eur Radiol*. 2004;14:1600.

95. Birch JG. Surgical technique of physeal bar resection. *Instr Course Lect*. 1992;41:445.

144. Tsai TM, Ludwig L, Tonkin M. Vascularized fibular epiphyseal transfer: a clinical study. *Clin Orthop*. 1986;210:228–234.

In this article, a clinical series of eight pediatric patients who underwent joint reconstruction by means of fibular epiphyseal transplant is reported. Four of the patients showed continued growth of the transplanted bone. A double-pedicled flap was described for the first time in this pioneering report.

145. Pho RW, Patterson MH, Kour AK, et al. Free vascularised epiphyseal transplantation in upper extremity reconstruction. *J Hand Surg (Am)*. 1988;13:440–447.

153. Innocenti M, Delcroix L, Romano GF, et al. Vascularized epiphyseal transplant. *Orthop Clin North Am*. 2007;38:95–101.

160. Taylor GI, Wilson KR, Rees MD, et al. The anterior tibial vessels and their role in epiphyseal and diaphyseal transfer of the fibula: experimental study and clinical applications. *Br J Plast Surg*. 1988;41:451–469.

This is the first article reporting both an experimental and clinical experience in proximal fibular epiphyseal transfer based on the anterior tibial vascular system. The most remarkable finding consisted of assessing the ability of the anterior tibial artery to supply not only the proximal growth plate but also a considerable amount of fibular shaft. This improvement in the knowledge of the vascularity of the proximal fibula allowed reliable use of a fibula flap with a single pedicle.

165. Innocenti M, Delcroix L, Manfrini M, et al. Vascularized proximal fibular epiphyseal transfer for distal radial reconstruction. *J Bone Joint Surg Am*. 2005;87(suppl 1):237–246.

In this article, the operative technique for harvesting the proximal fibula supplied by the anterior tibial vascular system is reported in detail. A step-by-step description of the procedure is provided and supported by anatomical drawings and related clinical pictures. Recommendations and pitfalls may help the reader in approaching this reconstructive technique.

31

Vascular anomalies of the upper extremity

Joseph Upton III

SYNOPSIS

- Vascular anomalies of the upper limb are divided into tumors (including hemangiomas) and malformations.
- Hemangiomas have a biphasic growth phase consisting of proliferation and spontaneous involution; malformations are quiescent, do not involute and grow commensurately with the patient.
- Hemangiomas are usually treated conservatively.
- Vascular malformations can be managed by observation, sclerotherapy, embolization, or surgical resection.
- Surgical resections can be predictably performed if basic principles are followed; VMs, LMs and combined lesions are most amenable; technical refinements have made these operations safer and more predictable.
- Fast flow lesions with or without AVF comprise the most difficult group of lesions; their natural history is one of gradual progression.
- Large, diffuse vascular malformations of the upper limb are no longer hopeless clinical problems; surgical treatment must be individualized to each patient.

Introduction

During the past four decades, there has been a steady, almost exponential increase in our knowledge of vascular anomalies. A biological classification system has evolved and is under constant refinement.[1] A careful physical examination augmented with advanced imaging will yield an accurate diagnosis from the vast myriad of possibilities. A multidisciplinary team can offer individualized treatment with some degree of predictability. In less than 40% of these lesions, one option is surgery, which is fraught with potential complications and poor outcomes. However, in many patients surgical treatment is often the best remedy and should not be viewed as the last resort. A carefully planned and well-orchestrated procedure and rehabilitation can yield remarkable outcomes.[2]

History and classification

The etiology of vascular birthmarks has long stimulated the fertile imagination of man. At any point in time, classification systems have reflected a balance between folklore and science. Well into the 19th century, the doctrine of maternal impressions dictated that a gravid mother's craving for strawberries, sight of an accident, or emotional longing could imprint a vascular blemish, a naevus maternus, on her unborn child.[3] With the development of the microscope a vast number of histological terms have been introduced and to this day, most of these lesions are inaccurately labeled as hemangiomas. Study of the histopathology and natural history of these lesions spurred intriguing embryological classifications,[4,5] which seemed logical at the time but failed to distinguish involuting from noninvoluting lesions and offered little guidance in management. In the late 1970s, Mulliken and Folkman proposed a working hypothesis that these cells could be distinguished by their cellular characteristics and subsequently surgical specimens were analyzed by selected histological stains, electron microscopy and autoradiography (uptake of tritiated thymidine into DNA). On the basis of these studies two types of lesions were present: those, which showed endothelial hyperplasia designated as *hemangiomas*, and those, which did not, called *malformations*. A binary schema based on biologic activity was proposed[1] and accepted by the International Society for the Study of Vascular Anomalies (ISSVA) in 1996.[6] This system has been corroborated by radiological studies[7,8] and immunohistological staining.[9] However, "no system is carved in stone and must be written on recyclable paper" and is in a constant state of revision. For example, the initial category of hemangiomas has been changed to vascular tumors to include all vascular tumors in all age groups. A particular vascular lesion may be moved from one category to another or may be discarded completely with our expansion of clinical experience and basic science investigation. For the past 30 years, this system has been very helpful to the upper limb surgeon in the proper diagnosis and management of these lesions *(Table 31.1)*.[2] Most frustrating are the large number of eponyms with and without abbreviations, which have been attached to these lesions. These terms are often used indiscriminately without specific reference to cell type, flow characteristics and growth. Adding to the confusion is the common association of growth disturbances. Both overgrowth and undergrowth with and without dysplastic fat deposition may accompany vascular anomalies. The summary

Table 31.1 ISSVA classification of vascular anomalies	
Vascular tumors	**Vascular malformations**
Slow-flow vascular malformations	
Hemangioma	Capillary malformations CM)
Infantile hemangioma (IH)	Port-wine stain
Congenital (CH)	Telangiectasias
Noninvoluting congenital hemangioma (NICH)	Angiokeratoma
Rapidly involuting congenital hemangioma (RICH)	Venous malformations (VM)
Hemangiomatosis	Common sporadic VM (VM)
Pyogenic granuloma	Blue rubber bleb syndrome (BRBS) or Bean syndrome
Kaposiform hemangioendothelioma KHE)	Glomuvenous malformation (GVM)
Rare tumors:	Familial cutaneous and mucosal venous malformation (VMCM)
Hemangioendothelioma	Maffucci syndrome
Infantile fibrosarcoma	Diffuse VM (Bockenheimer)
Hemangiopericytoma	Lymphatic malformations (LM)
Giant cell angioblastoma	Common lymphatic malformation (LM) Lymphangiomatosis Gorham-Stout syndrome
Fast-flow vascular malformations	
	Arterial malformation (AM)
	Arteriovenous malformation (AVM)
	Arteriovenous fistula (AVF)
	Complex-combined vascular malformations
	CVM, CLM, LVM, CLVM (Klippel–Trenaunay),
	CAVM (Parkes–Weber), AVM-LM,CM-AVM
	Proteus, hemihypertrophy, capillary-lymphatic-overgrowth-vascular-epidermal nevus (CLOVE)

in *Table 31.2* helps delineate our present state of knowledge of this nosologic quagmire. ⊛ TABLE **31.2** APPEARS ONLINE ONLY

A correct diagnosis impacts directly upon appropriate treatment and an incorrect diagnosis may result in unnecessary or harmful remedies. Most upper limb surgeons designate all fast flow anomalies with or without arteriovenous fistulae as Parkes–Weber syndrome (PWS). However, PWS patients comprise a very small percentage of the fast flow group, which comprises about 15% of upper extremity fast-flow malformations.[10] Not all slow flow combined malformations should be called Klippel–Trenaunay syndrome (KTS), an eponym we reserve for combined CLVM lesions. The VMs collectively comprise the largest clinical group of patients evaluated by the hand surgeon. The majority are small or large lesions involving all portions of the upper limb and/or ipsilateral chest wall. Other subgroups have emerged. The diffuse VMs involving all structures within the upper limb including bone have been designated Bockenheimer lesions,[11] originally described as "diffuse genuine phlebectasias", and are not amenable to surgery with the exception of pathologic fractures and localized areas of symptomatic thromboses. Maffucci patients are commonly associated with skeletal enchondromas but many of the skeletal lucencies may be clusters of VMs, which are also found in abundance within the soft tissue planes.[12] The glomuvenous (GVM) lesions occur in clusters with a characteristic appearance, are painful, have been localized to chromosome 1p21–22, and in the past were called glomus tumors or glomangiomas.[13] They have been renamed to stress the fact that they are malformations and not tumors as suggested by the suffix "-oma." The VMs seen in the blue rubber bleb nevus syndrome (BRBN) also have a characteristic cutaneous appearance, are also familial and often confused with GVM, Maffucci and CM-VM.[14] The associated gastrointestinal lesions, often localized to the small bowel, are often the cause of anemia and iron deficiencies (see *Table 31.7*).[14,15]

Lymphatic malformations often occur in combination with other vascular elements but the most common varieties are either isolated or diffuse LMs, which may involve any portion of the upper limb and/or ipsilateral chest wall.[10] Lymphangiomatosis conditions are not of primary concern to the upper limb surgeon as they involve visceral organs and/or the lungs and in the long run are life endangering. LMs in the Gorham–Stout syndrome involve skeletal structure including the humerus, radius, ulna and tubular bones of the hand.[16] Pathologic fractures can occur.

There are many conditions in which vascular anomalies, *overgrowth* or *undergrowth* co-exist and with our present state of knowledge, it is difficult to draw clear lines due to the increasing amounts of growth factors found in the omnipresent dysplastic fat tissue within these extremities. Often at their vascular clinic reviews, the authors encounter lesions that do not fit into any specific category and are designated as "PUVA", provisionally unique vascular anomalies. With time, this large group of "unknowns" will become more precisely defined. The emergence of the CLOVES syndrome is a good example, important to the hand surgeon. Children with this present with condition large extremity and truncal CMs, moderate to marked overgrowth, large fat accumulation within all tissue planes, either LMs or VMs and epidermal nevi.[17,18] Previously, most had been called "macrodactylies", "gigantism" or Proteus and did not fit the criteria for the Proteus syndrome *(Table 31.2)*.[19]

Another group of confusing lesions can be found in the fast-flow group where all lesions should not be called Parkes-Weber anomalies. Most fast-flow lesions are easily diagnosed by their clinical characteristics, palpable bruits, shunts and progressive growth. A small group of these children seen by the extremity surgeon may have mild hypotonia, lipomas in any subcutaneous location, fast flow deeper lesions and frontal bossing. Males have a nevus on the glans of the penis. In the past they were placed in the Bannayan-Riley-Ruvalcaba (BRR) syndrome or the Cowdan syndrome. Genetic testing is diagnostic and they are now called the PTEN hamartoma-tumor syndrome (PHTS) (see *Table 31.8*).[20,21] The hand surgeon may also see the capillary malformation-arteriovenous malformation (CM-AVM) syndrome, which initially appears to be an innocent CM, which are pinkish red and surrounded by a small halo. One-third of these patients may have an existing AVM and 12% may evolve into a Parkes–Weber syndrome (PWS) and intracranial AVMs should be considered. This condition is hereditary and results in a mutation in RASA1.[22] The PWS describes a diffuse AVM of an overgrown extremity with an overlying CM.[2,23,24] In contrast to lesions with direct arterio-to-venous shunting (AVMs with AVFs), PWS lesions show diffuse involvement of all soft tissue structures with fast flow arterioles in the initial absence of large draining veins. Large shunts develop secondarily. The lower extremity is involved much more frequently than the upper.

Diagnosis/patient presentation

Evaluation begins with a detailed history and physical examination. In contrast to the rapid growth and slow involution that characterize infantile hemangioma (IH), vascular malformations expand commensurately with the child. Although vascular malformations are by definition present at birth, many are inconspicuous and some do not appear until late childhood. Dermal ectasias, such as the relatively common capillary malformation ("port-wine stain"), are usually noted in the newborn nursery. Rarely, later in life will it become obvious that some of these capillary stains overlie a slow-flow (venous or lymphatic) anomaly or a fast-flow (arteriovenous) malformation. Venous and lymphatic malformations often co-exist and may be quite insidious in their initial presentation. Venous malformations may not manifest until late childhood or adolescence; large lesions are usually obvious within the first 4–8 years of life. Fortunately, the vast majority of vascular malformations are correctly diagnosed by clinical examination alone.[3,25,26] It is important to obtain baseline functional data including length and circumference measurement of the lower limbs early in life and to follow these children as they grow. The clinical characteristics of the more common malformations will be described with the individual case presentations.

The diagnostic work-up varies for each type of vascular anomaly *(Table 31.3)*. Ultrasonography, sometimes with Doppler scans, confirms the initial distinction between a vascular tumor and vascular malformation.[27] These studies are easily performed in the clinic. This diagnostic tool not only pinpoints the location of the lesion but also enables its identification as either slow-flow or fast-flow. Expensive diagnostic studies are unnecessary in the case of a diffuse or localized, asymptomatic slow-flow malformation or a small fast-flow lesion amenable to simple excision and closure. When a patient is symptomatic or if an operation is being considered for a large vascular anomaly, one should learn as much as possible about the size, extent, depth, and three-dimensional characteristics and obtain specific information about the location, caliber, and flow characteristics. Magnetic resonance imaging (MRI) with contrast (gadolinium) is the "gold standard." Fat suppressed T-1 weighted sequences with contrast will differentiate between a vascular tumor and malformation.[28] Computed tomography (CT) can be used to detect interosseous involvement or skeletal distortion, caused by a vascular malformation, and help delineate soft tissue planes. Large cystic cavities in an LM are clearly depicted. New three-dimensional rendering of both fast-flow and slow-flow malformations using CT technology provides very impressive views of the entire malformation and its relationship to neighboring soft tissue and skeletal structures. Nevertheless, it is questionable whether CT angiography (CTA) is really useful in planning therapy. However, formatted three-dimensional rendering of CTA can be invaluable preoperatively. Plain radiology of the affected region provides very little information other than showing the presence of phleboliths and interosseous involvement or other skeletal distortions. Angiography has very little use in the diagnosis of slow-flow malformations, although it is indispensable in the diagnosis and assessment of fast-flow lesions.[2,10] The angio-architecture and three-dimensional anatomy of the malformation can be precisely determined and the arterial suppliers and draining veins clearly identified. Indirect and direct phlebography techniques are sometimes used for diagnostic and therapeutic purposes for VM in the extremity.

Treatment/surgical technique

Video 1

Surgical treatment of vascular anomalies is neither for the timid nor arrogant. A well-balanced approach that incorporates calculated risk and cautious execution is necessary – one that can only be cultivated with experience. The surgeon who devotes a practice to the treatment of these lesions is obligated to document meticulously and analyze critically; habits that will serve one well for life-long learning, most lesions can never be absolutely eradicated. Recurrence is the rule, despite significant extirpative operations. This is an important consideration in preoperative planning and future interventions.

Surgical principles gain acceptance with time and must be periodically reassessed and refined, particularly in this rapidly advancing field. Principles should not be confused with surgical techniques that change frequently, and are modulated to a great extent by technology. Many of the following principles have evolved from the early operative experience with vascular malformations (especially the fast flow types), which was punctuated with complications *(Table 31.4)*.[2,3]

1. *Preoperative planning* should include correlation of the size, extent, and involvement of structures with physical examination, MRI scans, radiographs, and angiograms. All studies should be reviewed preoperatively; serial

Table 31.3 Vascular anomalies and overgrowth conditions

	Hemangioma	CM	VM
Physical examination	++++	++++	++++
Ultrasound	+++	−	+
MRI, MRV, MRA	++	−	+++
Radiographs	−	−	++ phleboliths bone
CT	+	−	+
Angiography	−	−	−
Biopsy	+	−	+

	LM	Combined	AVM
Physical examination	++++	++++	++++
Ultrasound	+	+	+++
MRI, MRV, MRA	+++	+++	+++
Radiographs	+ bone	+ bone	+ bone
CT	+	+	+
Angiography	−	−	++
Biopsy	+	+	+

MRI, magnetic resonance imaging; MRA, magnetic resonance angiography; MRV, magnetic resonance venography; CT, computed tomography; CM, capillary malformation; VM, venous malformation; LM, lymphatic malformation; AVM, arteriovenous malformation.

studies of growing children are often invaluable in demonstrating the true extent of involvement of the extremity. A thorough explanation of all potential complications must be given to the patient and/or parents.

2. The surgeon should mentally *outline the extent of the resection and abide by it*. Use of the pneumatic tourniquet and complete exsanguination is necessary to visualize normal and abnormal structures clearly, regardless of the size of the malformation. Once the operative field becomes bloodstained, the identification of nerves,

tendons, intrinsic muscles, and other structures is more difficult.

3. *Placement of incisions* is important – particularly in children. A high mid-axial incision in the digit is preferred, as it can be used again and is hidden. With growth, palmar scars within or near the palm can lead to contracture. If a palmar approach is chosen, a zig-zag incision is preferred, utilizing existing skin creases. If multiple debulking procedures are contemplated in the upper arm or forearm, each incision should be planned carefully to avoid unnecessary scarring. The medial

Table 31.4 Principles of management

1. Clear explanation of surgery and complications. Give parents time to make decisions
2. Carefully planned and thorough dissection within a well-defined region
3. Meticulous hemostasis under tourniquet control, bloodless field
4. Fine instruments, magnification, good assistance
5. Judicious incision placement. Avoid dorsum of hand or digit
6. Identification of all structures, preservation tendons, joints and nerves
7. Dissect no more than half of a digit or limb at a time
8. Avoid vascular compromise. One side at a time. One vessel intact
9. Avoidance intraneural dissections. Neuromas are a nemesis
10. Quick operating rehearsed with assistance if possible
11. Resect marginal skin. Tension free closures. Good tissue coverage
12. Thoughtful, meticulous closures. Subcuticular techniques best
13. Liberal use of drains, tissue sealants and delayed closures
14. Appropriate early immobilization and subsequent early joint ROM
15. Aggressive treatment of complications. Amputation of functionless extremities
16. Conscientious, regular follow-up for those with significant malformations
17. A full explanation of potential complications to parents and patients

surface of the arm, elbow and forearm is the least conspicuous. Incisions in the weight-bearing plantar surfaces of the foot should be avoided. The placement of incisions in the medial arch, along the borders of the foot, and on the dorsal surfaces is safe. Scars in the web spaces or along eponychial and/or paronychial folds will contract and are likely to become problematic.

4. *Magnification*, either loupe or microscopic, makes a tremendous difference in the identification and preservation of normal neurovascular structures. Small vessels, such as vincular pedicles to the flexor tendons and nutrient vessels to the carpal bones, should be saved if uninvolved. Often, vascular anomalies will displace, but not typically invade, neighboring soft tissues.

5. *Thorough dissection* limited to a specified area should be performed so that subsequent re-entry into a densely scarred bed will be unnecessary. Often, the malformation extends well beyond its anticipated limits. In certain regions, limited staged excisions are better than one extensive and protracted dissection that leaves behind tissue containing abnormal vasculature. For example, the digits (including the thumb) should be debulked in stages. A single procedure is usually best for the dorsum of the hand, wrist, and palmar surface of the same in a patient with a diffuse LM or VM.

6. *Avoid vascular compromise*. Only one-half of a digit should be dissected at a time (see *Table 31.6*). If possible, at least one or two large dorsal veins per finger should be preserved to enhance venous drainage, especially when excising a diffuse lymphatic lesion in the hand or foot. The superficial venous system should not be resected unless a deep system has been identified. When a critical arterial segment to a digit, hand or foot is removed, this segment should be reconstructed with a vein graft so that at least one digital artery is preserved per digit and one major artery supplies the hand or foot with a functional intact palmar or plantar arch.

7. *Avoid intraneural dissection* whenever possible, despite gross involvement. Although many vascular malformations, particularly the venous type, are entangled in nerves, dissection often leaves in-continuity neuromas with partial or complete loss of distal sensory or motor function. The symptoms are usually much worse than the initial ones.

8. *Avoid partial dissections within large muscle groups*. Removal of the entire muscle en bloc is preferred to avoid a secondary contracture of the entire musculotendinous unit. If more than half of a skeletal muscle is excised piecemeal, a secondary contracture is likely. VMs, mixed CLVMs, CAVMs and LVMs are the most problematic lesions. Pure LMs may extend beneath the muscular fascia but expand along fascial planes and usually do not penetrate the muscles themselves.

9. Cutaneous *flaps should not be inset under tension* and nonviable skin should be replaced with a skin graft or a flap. Tissue with questionable viability can be observed and resected later, if necessary. It is usually best to remove and replace skin that is heavily scarred from a previous procedure, chronically infected and ulcerated, populated by coalesced lymphatic vesicles or deprived by a proximal steal phenomenon.

10. *Drains* should be used liberally, and delayed primary closure of the wound should be considered. Persistent postoperative bleeding is usually best treated with direct pressure, elevation, and immobilization, rather than by re-exploration. Baseline coagulation studies should be performed for large/diffuse VM and LVM. Liberal use of tissue sealant products is encouraged.

11. *Immobilize the operated extremity* in a young child or adolescent. In the treatment of children with vascular anomalies, the postoperative lack or loss of immobilization is the single most important cause of wound dehiscence, maceration, and chronic infection.

12. The surgeon who has the courage to treat difficult fast-flow lesions should also *be prepared to amputate a symptomatic nonfunctional or painful digit, hand, leg or foot* following unsuccessful attempts at palliation. The reconstructive surgeon need not view amputation as a failure.

13. *Follow-up evaluation* should be performed compulsively at yearly intervals, regardless of the particular type of malformation, size, and hemodynamic activity. The true extent of the lesion can never be absolutely eradicated short of an amputation. Early childhood, adolescence, and pregnancy are times when change may occur in vascular malformations due to hormonal influences. These patients and parents often have questions that are not easily answered by their family physician owing to the paucity of information available in the medical literature. Both slow-and fast-flow lesions may expand

Table 31.5 Caveats of palmar dissections

1. Anatomy complex. Have three-dimensional perspective
2. Compulsive hemostasis under tourniquet. Avoid inkwell phenomenon
3. Proximal to distal dissection of nerves. Look for epineural fat and follow epineural connective tissue plane
4. Identify deep motor branch of ulnar nerve in Guyon's canal and mid palm
5. Median and ulnar nerves often involved. Take your time
6. Although displaced, arterial is anatomy normal. Follow adventitial connective tissue plane. Save palmar arches
7. Completely resect involved intrinsics to avoid contracture
8. Try to preserve 1st DI and AddP muscles
9. Simple muscle splitting for localized calcified thrombi
10. Tissue sealants and drains to avoid bleeding
11. Postoperative compression of thumb and digits easy with Coban
12. Postoperative compression of palm difficult. Wrapping ineffective. Uniform pressure with VAC or dorsal/palmar splints
13. Stay within a well-defined region. Tendency to be too aggressive
14. Resect and replace marginal skin

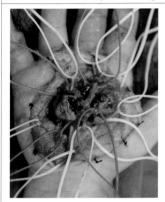 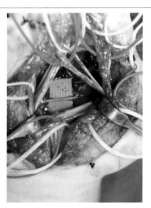 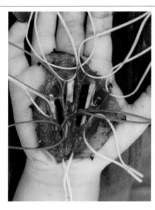

Diffuse VM palm   Motor branch of the ulnar nerve   Dissection complete

dramatically during pregnancy, with use of high estrogen anti-ovulation medication, or following trauma. Large AVMs, LMs or mixed lesions may be well tolerated by young children only to become burdensome to teenagers due to their expansion, bulk, ulceration, and appearance or steal symptoms.

14. *Give the patient and parents adequate time to make their decision.* The diagnosis and treatment of vascular anomalies is a rapidly changing field. It is important to keep both parents and patients at the appropriate age clearly informed about the natural history of their particular malformation, options for treatment and new types of therapies. It is axiomatic that the surgeon provide a *clear explanation of all potential complications* and expected short and long term outcomes prior to any surgical treatment.

Caveats of palmar dissections. Multiple technical refinements have made these dissections, once considered impossible, both predictable and safe. These are summarized in **Table 31.5**.

Caveats of thumb/digital dissections. Surgical approaches to the thumb and digit are similar to those summarized above and have become much safer with microvascular techniques. These are summarized in **Table 31.6**.

Vascular tumors

Infantile hemangioma (IH)

Basic science/disease process

IH is usually single and involves the upper limb in 15% of cases. The median appearance is at age 2 weeks. When dermis is involved, the skin appears pink. Deeper lesions may cause a pale, bluish discoloration **(Fig. 31.1)**. It grows very fast during the first 9 months (proliferating phase), begins to shrink and fade by 12 months (involuting phase), and involution is complete by 5 years (involution phase) leaving residual telangiectasias, fibrofatty residuum and redundant, atrophied skin.[25,29,30]

Diagnosis/patient presentation

Some 90% of IH diagnoses are made by history and physical examination. Hand-held Doppler shows fast flow. Ultrasonography shows fast flow, increased resistance and increased venous drainage.[27] On MRI scans, hemangiomas are isointense on T1, hyperintense on T2, and enhance during

Table 31.6 Caveats of thumb/digital dissections

1. Anatomy much easier than palm; outline region to be debulked *before* exsanguination
2. Incisions: mid-axial or mid-lateral, avoid zig-zag incisions in glabrous skin to avoid hypertrophic scars; utilize dorsal extension creases if necessary
3. Tourniquet control: digital for distal half and regular proximal digit and thumb
4. Subdermal flap elevation 1st, deeper dissection later
5. Decompress Grayson and Cleland ligaments to identify n-vb bundle; these structures distorted but always present
6. One side of digit (palmar and dorsal at a time; leave one bundle untouched and do not dissect more than 270° around digit
7. Identify and dissect along paratenon of extensor; remove malformation between extensor and bone
8. Preserve vincular vessels at joint space level and dorsal sensory branches of digital nerves: dissect along adventitial planes (arteries) and epineural plane (nerves); keep n-v bundle intact
9. Complete excision of malformation; extend along vincular vessels if necessary
10. Palmar dissection restricted to ipsilateral side of digit or thumb
11. Palmar pulp dissection: "berry pick" VM, LM or LVM out of septal pockets and keep nerve attachments to skin intact
12. Extend dissection into palm to level of MP joint and distal palmar flexion crease
13. Tissue sealants and drains to avoid bleeding
14. Drape redundant skin over digit and release tourniquet before resection; tension free closure
15. Postoperative compression dressing held with Coban

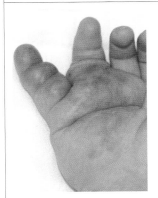

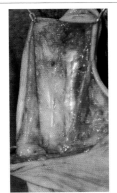

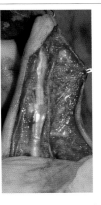

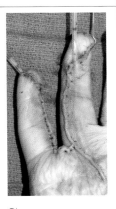

| Diffuse VM | Ulnar neurovascular bundle | Radial neurovascular bundle | Closure |

proliferating phase. Rarely, is biopsy needed. Immunostaining for GLUT1, a glucose transporter specific to IH, will differentiate this lesion.[31]

The majority of IH involve the head and neck, lumbosacral region, and liver. The PHACES association includes IH on the face with at least one of the following: posterior fossa brain malformation, hemangioma, arterial cerebrovascular anomaly, coarctation of the aorta and cardiac defects, eye/endocrine abnormalities, and sternal clefting or a supraumbilical raphe. These children need the appropriate specialty consultations.

Treatment/surgical technique

Most IH are managed by observation because 90% are small, localized, and do not impair function. To protect against ulceration and/or maceration during the proliferating phase, topical antibiotic cream and a petrolatum gauze barrier may be used. Ulcerated wounds are treated with local wound care and rarely need biologic coverage such as skin grafts.

Problematic lesions too large to treat with intralesional corticosteroid injections are first managed with oral prednisone started at 3 mg/kg per day for 1 month and then tapered until it is discontinued 10–12 months later.[30] Complications of long-term corticosteroid therapy are well known and usually disappear with discontinuation of therapy. Recently, propranolol has been used but its efficacy and safety compared to corticosteroids has not been established.[32,33] Alternatively, the child may be switched to vincristine; interferon is no longer used in those under 12 months of age, due to spastic diplegia.

Surgery in the upper limb is indicated only for problematic ulcerations or large lesions interfering with function.[2] The particular child in *Figure 31.2* has a large lesion, enveloping all neurovascular structures and chronically ulcerated. Excision and neuroplasty through a high mid-axial incision both enabled functional use of the digit and avoided secondary contracture of the digit.

Congenital hemangioma (CH)

Basic science/disease process

The upper limb surgeon must be familiar with a variation known as CH, which in contrast to IH are rare lesions fully grown at birth and do not exhibit the proliferation and regression so typical of IH. These lesions appear different with a red-violaceous color, course telangiectasias, a central pallor

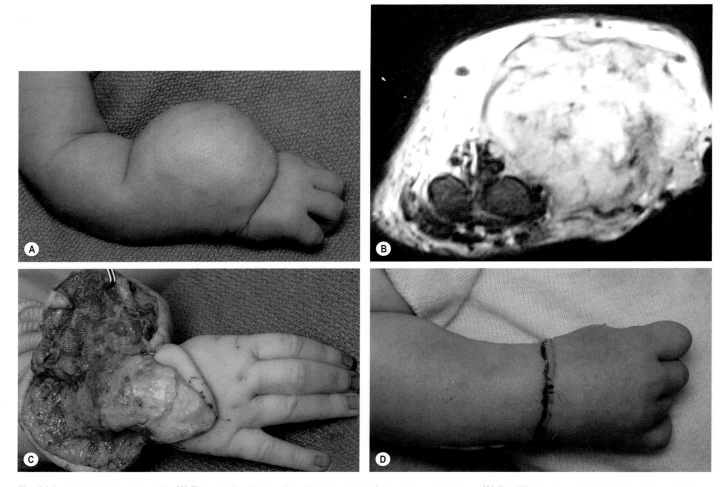

Fig. 31.1 Infantile hemangioma (IH). **(A)** This well-localized, solitary IH on the dorsal forearm has a bluish hue. **(B)** The MRI shows a multi-lobular, isointense lesion on T2-sequence. **(C)** Excision included extensive dorsal tenosynovectomy. **(D)** 2 weeks later active extension is initiated.

and a peripheral halo. There are two variations of CH: the rapid involuting congenital hemangioma (RICH) and the noninvoluting congenital hemangioma (NICH) *(Fig. 31.3)*. Both lesions are commonly seen in the extremities and have an equal sex distribution. RICH involutes rapidly after birth; 50% is gone by 7 months and are completely involuted by 14 months of age.[34,35,36] Fibrofatty deposits are not present. NICH does not regress and persists as raised, lumpy, plaque-like lesions with a characteristic peripheral halo. A persistent fast flow component remains unchanged.[37]

Diagnosis/patient presentation

Diagnosis is made by physical examination, clinical course and ultrasonography. CHs stain negative for GLUT1.

Treatment/surgical technique

RICH does not require operative management early in life, as it undergoes accelerated regression. Only large lesions in other parts of the body may need oral corticosteroid or second-line drug therapy. NICH may require intralesional corticosteroid injection in problematic regions of the upper

limb. Large, lumpy masses within the palm of the hand, interdigital web-spaces, or causing muscle or tendon impairment are best excised. Large lesions on the arm, forearm and within the antecubital fossa are excised later in childhood.

Pyogenic granuloma

Basic science/disease process

Pyogenic granuloma (PG) is a solitary red papule that grows rapidly, forming a stalk. It has been called a lobular capillary hemangioma.[37] It is small with an average diameter of 6.5 mm. The male:female ratio is 2:1. It commonly involves skin and in the upper extremity is most problematic on the glabrous surfaces of the digits, in nail folds *(Fig. 31.4)*, within web spaces and flexion creases. They appear as red papules growing on the end of a stalk. Persistent bleeding and constant ulceration are common. PG is distributed all over the body including the mucous membranes; cheeks, lips, oral cavity, eyelids and forehead are most common. Histological examination will differentiate PG from hemangiomas.[38]

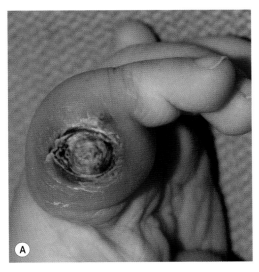

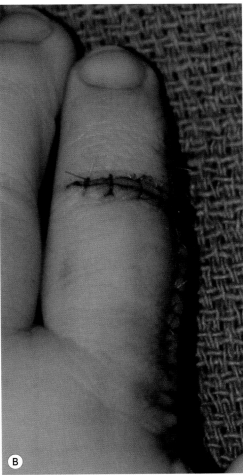

Fig. 31.2 Infantile hemangioma (IH). An expanding IH with chronic ulceration and bleeding in a 9-month-old child. Excision was performed through a high mid-axial incision and normal skin creases.

Diagnosis/patient presentation

Diagnosis is made by physical examination because the appearance is classic.

Treatment/surgical technique

Numerous treatments have been described for PG: curettage, shave excision, laser therapy, or excision. Complete excision is preferred in the hand and upper limb. Skin graft coverage may be necessary for large resulting defects.

Vascular malformations

Capillary malformations

Basic science/disease process

Capillary malformation (CM) consists of dilated capillaries in the superficial dermis. CM is most often solitary, but can be small or extensive and may occur in any region of the extremity *(Fig. 31.5A,B) (Fig. 31.5C–F)*. With time and aging, these pink lesions will often darken and develop some fibrovascular overgrowth. They can be associated with deeper vascular lesions both slow-flow (Klippel–Trenaunay, CLOVES) and fast-flow (Parkes-Weber, CM-AVM, PHTS) (see *Tables 31.2, 31.8*) and with skeletal and soft tissue hypertrophy. A CM on the face in the one or more of the trigeminal nerve distributions is indicative of the Sturge–Weber syndrome. These patients are at risk for seizures, retinal detachment, glaucoma and stroke. ⊕ FIG **31.5C–F** APPEARS ONLINE ONLY

Diagnosis/patient presentation

Diagnosis is made by physical examination. Deeper lesions must be studied with radiographs, scans and ultrasonography.

Treatment/surgical technique

No treatment is necessary for extremity CMs. Tunable pulsed-dye laser (585 mm) can effectively decrease the intensity of the cutaneous blush.[39,40] Patients including infants are often treated awake and with topical anesthesia. More dramatic outcomes are obtained in the head and neck region and face than in the trunk and extremities. Multiple treatments are necessary. Outcomes in younger children are better than adults; results are variable 90% lightening of lesions, 50–90% improvement, 20%, minimal change. Many will re-darken with time.[41] Surgery in these extremities is usually focused upon the deeper venous, lymphatic, combined or fast-flow lesions. Occasionally, a dark purple, overgrown extremity CM will be resected or replaced with a graft.

Lymphatic malformations

Basic science/disease process

Lymphatic malformation (LM) results from an error in the embryonic development of the lymphatic system. Since

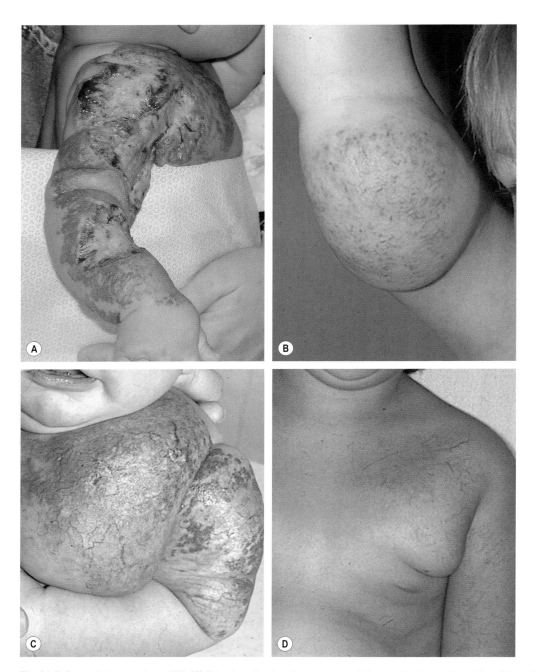

Fig. 31.3 Congenital hemangioma (CH) **(A)** Extensive skin ulceration may occur during proliferation and involution. CH requires local wound care. **(B)** A NICH shows course telangiectasias, hard nodules surrounded by a peripheral halo. **(C)** A RICH shows typical enlargement and course telangiectasias during infancy. **(D)** Several years later with no treatment.

lymphatic and venous systems have a common origin, combined lymphatico-venous malformations (LVM) frequently occur.[42,43] LM is characterized by the size of the malformed channels: microcystic, macrocystic, or combined. Most lymphatic lesions are noted at birth or within the first two years of life. Large macrocystic lesions may be slightly compressible and those with smaller channels are rubbery, a characteristic distinguishing feature. They do not decompress with overhead elevation. Overlying skin may appear normal, have

a bluish hue or contain clear or pink vesicles. Dermal involvement often overlies a large lymphatic lesion and this skin may be thick and exhibit cutaneous puckering much like the *"peau d'orange"* skin seen in lymphedema. These cutaneous vesicles may coalesce, drain clear fluid, bleed and lead to chronic wounds and sepsis.

LM may be located anywhere within the upper limb and is characteristically macrocystic in the cervicofacial and neck ("cystic hygroma"), mediastinum and axilla *(Figs 31.6, 31.7)* and microcystic in the distal forearm, wrist and hand. LMs are predominantly in the subcutaneous planes, in contrast to other vascular malformations. LMs may be accompanied by increased amounts of dysplastic fat adding to the bulk of the malformation. It is unusual for LMs to directly involve muscle tissue as they are primarily found within the subcutaneous tissue planes. Extensive LM in the arm, forearm and hand

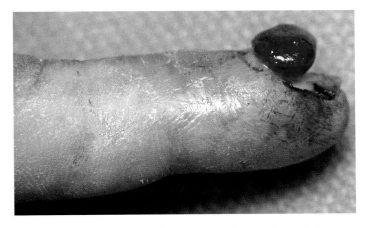

Fig. 31.4 Pyogenic granuloma (PG). A periungual PG with typical stalk will continue to bleed unless completely removed with curettage or excision. In the young child this must be differentiated from an unreduced Salter I injury of the distal phalanx.

extends along muscular fascial planes and along the major peripheral nerves. Despite the size and weight, the involved extremities can be quite functional. The most problematic regions are within intertriginous skin folds, interdigital web spaces, nail folds and within open wounds caused by vesicle leakage. An innocuous paronychial infection of a digit can rapidly progress to "wild-fire" cellulitis. When treated with the appropriate antibiotic, these infections resolve as rapidly as they appear.[2]

There is no characteristic pattern of skeletal involvement with LM. The long and tubular bones of the extremities and joints are rarely affected. The eponym Gorham disease is used for skeletal involvement.[44] Extensive LM may be associated with skeletal disuse atrophy. Smaller lesions confined to the distal extremities can present with overgrowth of the hand or foot. LMs and combined lesions containing lymphatic components (CLVM, LVM) can progress to gigantism. Joints are rarely affected but can become severely restricted by the bulky LM *(Table 31.2)*.

Diagnosis/patient presentation

Some 90% of LMs are diagnosed by history and physical examination. Small, superficial lesions do not require further diagnostic work-up.[25] Large or deep lesions may require MRI scans to confirm the diagnosis, define the three-dimensional characteristics of the LM and plan treatment. These scans show characteristic fluid-filled spaces with or without air-fluid levels, multiple septations of variable thickness,

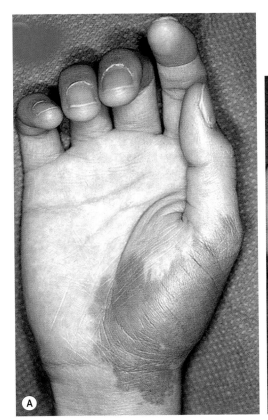

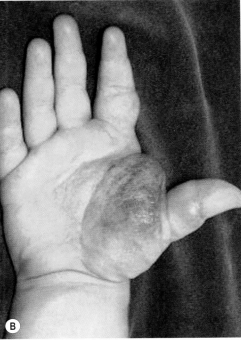

Fig. 31.5 Capillary malformation (CM) variations. **(A)** Solitary CM over the thenar region in a teenager; stain darkened during the adolescent growth spurt. **(B)** Localized CM plus large AVM with multiple AVFs in a young child with a palpable bruit.

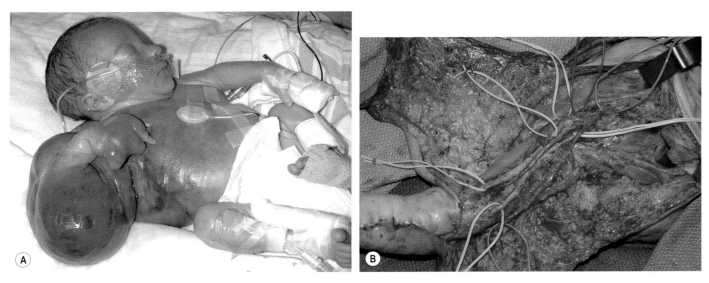

Fig. 31.6 Macrocystic axillary LM in a neonate. **(A)** This extensive LM diagnosed by prenatal ultrasonography; child born by caesarean section. Constant fluid shifts and intralesional bleeding complicated initial management. **(B)** At 6 months an aggressive debulking was performed with isolation and preservation of all neurovascular structures. Surgery took 6 hours with a blood loss of <100 cc. A dramatic result was preserved with compression wrapping.

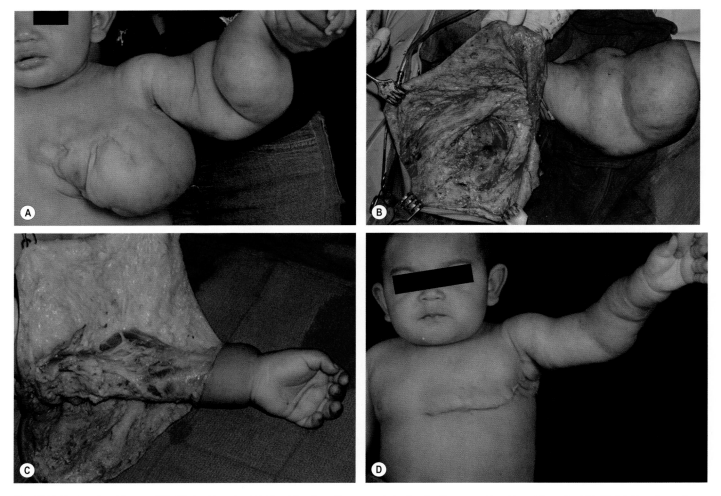

Fig. 31.7 Chest wall and forearm LM. **(A)** A rubbery hard LM involving the entire arm and chest wall with a normal hand in a 16-month child. **(B, C)** Staged resections started with the chest wall where pectoralis major, latissimus dorsi and serratus anterior muscles have been preserved. The forearm was debulked in two additional stages. **(D)** Three months postoperatively, following three operations.

hyperintense T-2 weighted sequences due to water content, and slight rim enhancement following contrast administration. Diffuse enhancement is not present. Direct puncture of macrocystic lesions further delineates the architecture of the lesion prior to sclerotherapy. Large venous channels are often present.[45] Ultrasonography (US) shows multiloculated macrocysts with "rim enhancement" and hypo-echoic microcystic lesions with little flow. US is commonly used to document intralesional bleeding. Histologic confirmation of LM is rarely necessary. LM characteristically shows abnormally walled channels willed with eosinophilic, protein rich fluid and collections of lymphocytes. Immunostaining with lymphatic markers D2–40 and LYVE-1 are positive.[46]

Treatment/surgical technique

LM is a benign condition, and intervention for small asymptomatic lesions is not necessary. More aggressive management is reserved for symptomatic lesions that cause pain, cellulitis, compression neuropathies, significant deformity or functional impairment. An infected LM within the extremity can be controlled with local wound care, oral antibiotics and occasionally, intravenous antimicrobial therapy. The rapidly advancing "wild fire" infections seen in these lesions can cause sepsis but will regress as rapidly as they progressed with appropriate treatment. Sclerotherapy is the first-line management for large, problematic macrocystic LMs. Several sclerosants have been used: doxycycline,[47] sodium tetradecyl sulfate (SDS), ethanol, bleomycin,[48] and OK-432.[49] SDS is most widely used. Ethanol has the highest complication rate and OK-432, though very effective, is not widely available. Multiple injection sessions are required for all but the smallest lesions. Swelling, compartment syndromes and skin extravasation are the most common complications encountered in the upper limb. Ethanol though effective has the highest complication rate and is particularly toxic to neurovascular structures (see *Fig. 31.14*). We prefer sclerotherapy for the macrocystic LMs primarily located in the head and neck, axilla and proximal portions of the upper extremity. Microcystic lesions are best treated surgically.

Resection is reserved for: (1) symptomatic LM causing bleeding or fluid loss, infection, bleeding, pain, or obstruction of function; (2) lesions (microcystic) which cannot be adequately treated with sclerotherapy, and (3) small, well-localized lesions which can be resected for cure. Surgical principles and technical caveats have been outlined. The neonate in *Figure 31.6* presented a good example. Despite sclerotherapy, bleeding, fluid shifts metabolic balance fluid shifts could not be adequately managed. Resection included a careful identification of all neurovascular structures within the beyond the brachial plexus and excision of large amounts of dysplastic adipose tissue. Characteristically, the LM in this baby was confined to the subcutaneous tissue planes and extended only between muscle groups. Staged debulking of large upper extremity LMs is much safer than large radical resections. We often start with the bulkiest chest wall, axillary and arm regions before extending more distal into the forearm and hand *(Fig. 31.7)*. Areas of involved skin are preferentially removed and only one side of a forearm, wrist, hand, or digit are debulked at one operation. Flap compromise, wound dehiscence and infection are early problems and tendon adherence, neuromas and joint stiffness may be encountered later. Compression neuropathies are often missed.

Because of its complex anatomy, the hand is the most difficult region to dissect for an LM or any other type of vascular malformation. There are very few natural fascial planes within the indurated lymphatic tissue, which may have been scarred by previous inflammation. However, smooth, areolar connective tissue planes can usually be found around both nerves and arteries and should be followed meticulously. Of all surgical principles outlined previously, limited and thorough dissection is most important for LM in the hand *(Table 31.4)*. In contrast to the digits and thumb, post-operative edema is almost impossible to control, and may affect joint mobility and tendon gliding. At this level all LMs are microcystic and are accompanied by a large amount of adipose tissue, with the consistency ranging from soft to hard rubber (see *Fig. 31.8B*). Resection in the hand is reserved for those instances where there is functional impairment. These procedures are lengthy and tedious. Technique must be meticulous, preserving all sensory and motor nerves, common digital arteries and the palmar arch. Incisions through glabrous skin must be well designed, as there is a tendency for hypertrophic scar formation, particularly when there is dermal involvement. With dorsal debulking, several large dorsal veins should be preserved in-continuity with the cephalic drainage system of the forearm. Nevertheless, removal of these veins does not predictably cause venous congestion *(Table 31.5)*.

LMs in the thumb and digits are common. Fortunately, these locations are the easiest in the limbs to debulk *(Table 31.6)*. Muscle is usually not involved, and the LM usually does not extend below or penetrate through flexor or extensor tendons. Outcomes following resection of LM of the thumb and digits are much better – similar to those for VMs. The entire dorsal area can be debulked, along with removal of one-half of the palmar side in one procedure. Liposuction, even with ultrasonic technique, is not a good option because of the firm, rubbery consistency of microcystic LM and potential for injury to neurovascular structures. Involved dorsal skin should be excised and replaced by thick split-thickness or full-thickness skin grafts. Multiple digits can be debulked during one operation, and the dorsum of the hand at another stage. Mid-axial incisions are always used *(Figs 31.8, 31.9A) (Fig. 31.9B,C)*. Microscopic dissection is always preferred. The large dorsal veins in the hand or digit are preserved. Vincular vessels at the joint space level are preserved whenever possible. Incisions through the glabrous surfaces of the palm or digit have a predilection for hypertrophic scarring. Intradigital commissures and web spaces must be closed in their normal configuration. Coban™ effectively controls postoperative edema with circumferential wrapping. FIG 31.9B, C APPEARS ONLINE ONLY

Outcomes, prognosis, and complications

The degree of functional gain and appearance is proportional to the extent of the malformation. The use of the pneumatic tourniquet in limb surgery significantly decreases the recurrence rate seen in the head and neck region.[50,51] Persistent drainage, wound dehiscence and skin loss are <8%; secondary neuromas and hypertrophic scarring are much more common (20%).[10] With appropriate postoperative therapy and splinting, joint stiffness can be minimized. The likelihood of decreased

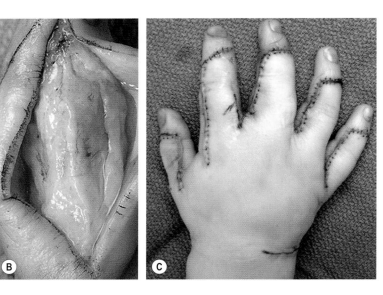

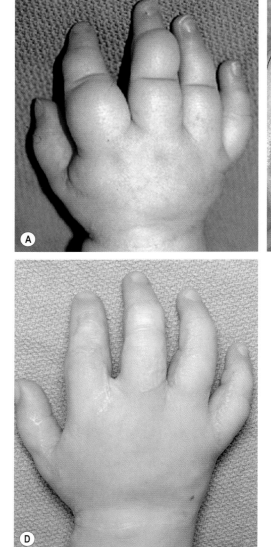

Fig. 31.8 LM hand. **(A)** A 4-year-old child presented with an extensive microcystic LM of the entire forearm, wrist, and hand. The dorsum was approached through an ulnar incision with preservation of dorsal venous system, nerves and extensor tendons. **(B)** The LM along the digits is microcystic, indurated and envelops all structures. Joint spaces are not involved. **(C)** Multiple digits and thumb are debulked during a single stage. **(D)** With continued compression wrapping and exercise, contour and function have been maintained 15 years later.

mobilization is age dependant. Upper extremities with large, heavy, edematous hands will always be "helping extremities" and digits with limited range of motion will never be normal due to the scar from pervious surgeries and residual LM within the remaining soft tissue. However, extremities with well-localized LM can be expected to function normally following well planned and executed surgery.

Venous malformation

Basic science/disease process

Venous malformation (VM) is the most common vascular anomaly. It is comprised of thin walls and abnormal smooth muscle cells, arranged in clumps instead of in a concentric orientation. This will result in gradual dilatation and expansion with time and growth.[3] Although VMs are present at birth, they are not always obvious. Within the first 5–6 years of life, all but the smallest or deepest lesions will become clinically evident. Less than 10% are clinically indolent until adolescence. Approximately, 40% of all VMs involve the extremities and more than half of these involve deeper structures including muscle, bone, nerve and connective tissue planes. They grow commensurately with the child, and slowly expand during the adolescent growth spurt. VM is typically sporadic and solitary and half have a somatic mutation in the endothelial receptor TIE2.[52]

VM may range from small, localized skin lesions to diffuse malformations involving all tissue planes including bones

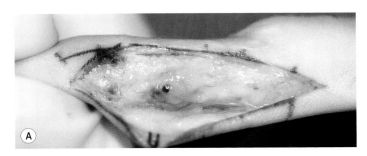

Fig. 31.9 LM digit. **(A)** LM along the side of a digit.

and joints. These lesions become engorged when the limb is in a dependent position and decompress (reduce in size) when the limb is held above the level of the heart *(Fig. 31.10)*. This particular patient has an extensive VM involving the entire hemithorax with a large stagnant venous collecting system in the axilla. Consequently, she is on long-term anti-coagulation. Most VMs are located in the subcutaneous plane superficial to the muscular fascia. They occur anywhere in an extremity, from the axilla to the fingertips and from the groin to the tips of the toes. In contrast to LM, VM may involve muscles directly.[53] The majority of VMs are solitary and asymptomatic. Often they are multi-loculated, incompletely decompressed with elevation and have palpable regions of scar from previous inflammation around intralesional thrombi, which feel like small peas in a sac.[2,10]

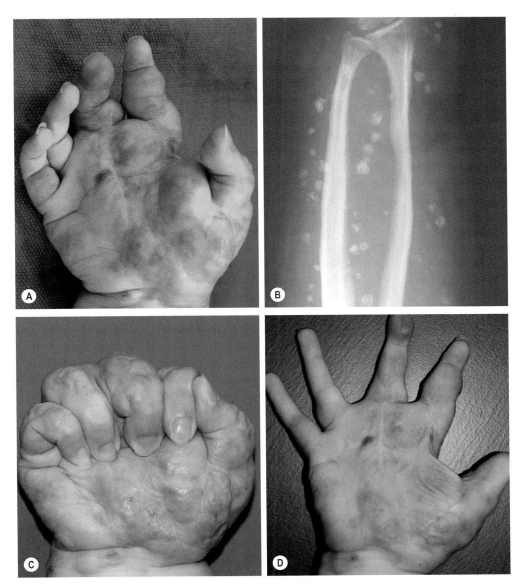

Fig. 31.10 VM hand. **(A)** In a dependant position of the hand with a diffuse VM becomes engorged a bulk and weight become a functional impediment. **(B)** Calcified phleboliths are often present. **(C)** Functional motion is impaired only by the malformation. **(D)** After elevation there is no pain, fullness or congestion.

The configuration, size and caliber of venous channels in VMs have no pattern, such as the characteristic microcystic and macrocystic cavities and channels of an LM. Large caliber veins may be located on a digit, foot, and leg or within the axilla. Extensive lesions, with and without lymphatic components, do not characteristically penetrate the pulmonary cavities but may encircle the structures within the mediastinal cavity. Often these large, dilated, redundant draining veins of extremities place the patient at risk for clot formation and subsequent pulmonary embolism.

VMs do not progress from a slow-flow to fast-flow state; they grow (expand) commensurately with the child. Any enlargement following a partial resection represents redirection of flow into adjacent anomalous channels. There is definitely a hormonal modulation in females with medium and large sized lesions. They often increase in size during the adolescence growth spurt, menses, while on anti-ovulant medication and during pregnancy. In women who experience an exacerbation of their symptoms during pregnancy, there is no postpartum reduction to the previous size. Patients must be followed carefully through adolescence and subsequent pregnancies.[10,26]

Functional problems are related to the size, weight and location of the VM. Pain and paresthesias are usually the result of local inflammation around intralesional thrombi or nerve compression, usually at the elbow, wrist, hand and/or tarsal tunnel of the foot. Areas of phlebothrombosis or local hemorrhage become swollen; firm and painful, especially when compressive garments are applied. Most symptoms are aggravated after exercise involving repetitive movements such as lifting, gripping, running, or kicking. Many VMs will be surprisingly large with minimal, if any, symptoms in young children.

Syndromes with VM

This is an emerging group of syndromes, which contain VM and which have become clinically distinct *(Table 31.7)*. Less than 20% of all VM patients will have a syndromic designation with a very specific pattern of malformation including glomuvenous malformation (GVM)[54,55] and capillary malformation venous malformation (CMVM).[56] In the blue rubber bleb nevus syndrome (BRBNS),[57,58] small blue nodules are present in isolation or with extensive connections. A small number of upper limb patients present with combined lymphatic-venous malformations with or without capillary staining: LVM, CLVM (Klippel–Trenaunay) Understandably, this group of lesions can be confusing but the management is similar. 🖳 TABLE **31.7** APPEARS ONLINE ONLY

Complications of untreated VMs include pain, swelling, bulk and contour deformity and psychosocial morbidity. Intralesional thromboses are the most frequent cause for pain.[10] VM can cause leg-length discrepancy, hypoplasia due to disuse atrophy, pathologic fracture, hemarthrosis, and degenerative arthritis. VM of muscle may result in pain, weakness, fibrosis leading to joint contracture and subsequent disability.[53] Phlebothromboses within large, stagnant venous channels in the arm, axilla and ipsilateral chest wall have been the focus for pulmonary embolism. A coagulation profile should be obtained in all patients with an extensive VM, with or without capillary or lymphatic components, particularly if there is any history of bleeding, ecchymosis or hemarthrosis. The salient findings are decreased fibrinogen and elevated D-dimers; prothrombin time may be increased, whereas platelet counts are usually in the normal range.

Diagnosis/patient presentation

At least 90% of VMs are diagnosed by history and physical examination. Dependant position of the anomaly will confirm the diagnosis: VM will enlarge due to reduced venous return in the extremity *(Fig. 31.10C,D)*. Small, superficial, asymptomatic lesions require no further work-up. However, larger and/or deeper lesions should be evaluated by MRI to: (1) confirm diagnosis; (2) define the three-dimensional extent of the lesion, and (3) plan long-term treatment. VM is hyperintense on T-2 weighted sequences. In contrast to LM, VM will enhance with contrast, show phleboliths as signal voids, and may involve muscle. US may be used for some localized lesions; characteristic findings show slow-flow anechoic-hypoechoic channels separated by more solid regions of variable echogenicity. Phleboliths are hyperechoic with acoustic shadowing. Magnetic resonance venography (MRV) is helpful for large lesions of the arm, forearm and chest wall. CT scans are used to assess skeletal VM.[28,45] Histological diagnosis of VM is rarely necessary, but may be indicated if there is a suspicion of malignancy or if the imaging is not confirmatory. Arteriography is not helpful *(Table 31.2)*.

Treatment/surgical technique

The treatment algorithm is similar to that outlined for LM.[2,10] Compression garments are the first-line of treatment and are used to reduce blood stagnation within the lesion and reduce the risk of expansion, to reduce the chance of localized intralesional coagulopathy (LIC), phlebolith formation, and to reduce pain. Those with pain and large lesions are given daily aspirin (81 mg) to prevent phlebothrombosis. Large lesions are at risk for the vicious cycle of blood stagnation, stimulation of thrombin, and conversion of fibrinogen to fibrin. Subsequent fibrinolysis results in LIC. A chronic coagulopathy can cause either thrombosis (phlebolith formation) or bleeding. Low molecular weight heparin (LMWH) is considered for those children and adults with significant LIC or at risk for disseminated intravascular coagulation (DIC). Those with large VMs and low fibrinogen levels pre-sclerosis are given LMWH 14 days before and after the procedure. Anticoagulation is held for 24 h perioperatively (12 h before and after the intervention) to prevent bleeding complications. Patients who develop a serious thrombotic problem, such as a pulmonary embolus, require long-term anticoagulation or a vena caval filter. Low dose aspirin (81 mg/day) is given to those with large lesions with pain and intralesional thrombus formation.

Sclerotherapy is the next treatment option for symptomatic lesions that cause pain, functional impairment, nerve compression, a mass effect, or major contour problems.[10,59] In the arm, elbow, and proximal forearm, sclerotherapy is safer and more effective than resection *(Fig. 31.11)*. Symptomatic regions must be specifically targeted. Although the sclerotherapy reduces the size of the malformation, it generates a tremendous amount of scar and does not remove the malformation. The VM usually re-expands, and multiple sessions are invariably needed, sometimes for a lifetime. Direct puncture sclerotherapy is used for VM. Our preferred sclerosants are STS and ethanol; STS is safer and more commonly used. Most patients are managed under anesthesia using US guidance. The most common complications are skin ulceration (10–15%), local extravasation, compartment syndrome in the arm or forearm and secondary contracture (see *Fig. 31.14A*).[10] OK-432 is reported to be safer and more effective but has limited availability.[49] Post-treatment monitoring is required for large lesions with an extremity surgeon on-call for problems. Large VMs of the axilla and arm contain anomalous veins too large

for sclerotherapy; these are embolized. Sclerotherapy is most effective for small and large VM in the axilla, arm, elbow and proximal forearm where muscle may be directly involved. Multiple sessions are required. The extremity surgeon and interventional radiologist must have a good working relationship; compartment syndromes can and do occur. Surgical resection is preferred in the distal forearm, wrist, thumb, and digits, where there is little muscle tissue *(Figs 31.12, 31.13)*. The secondary scar generated by sclerotherapy in these regions is detrimental to nerve function, tendon and muscle gliding and joint motion. Large vascular channels respond

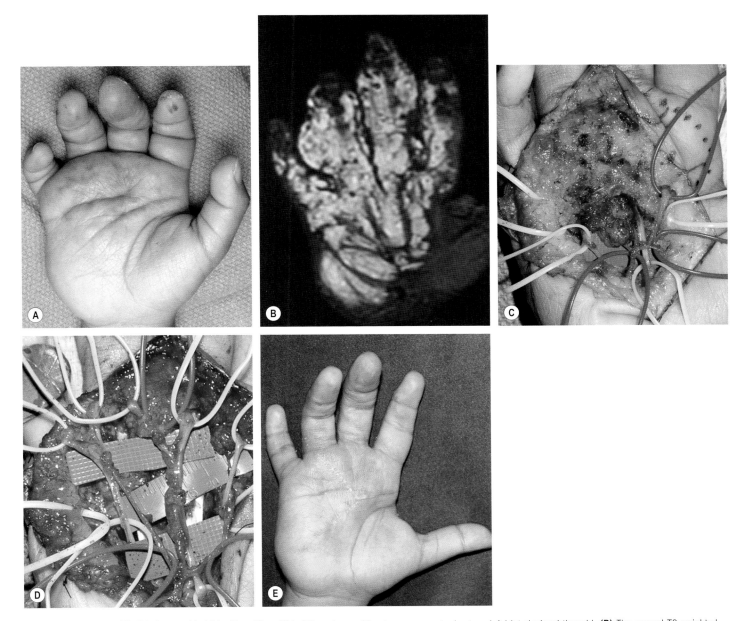

Fig. 31.13 VM palm. **(A)** This 6-year-old child with a diffuse VM of the palm could not wear garments due to painful intralesional thrombi. **(B)** The coronal T2-weighted show multiple signal voids within a diffuse, through-and-through VM. The mid palm was most symptomatic. **(C)** The dissection begins with identification of the palmar arch (red loops) and median and ulnar nerves (yellow loops). VM contains multiple thrombi admixed with dysplastic fat. **(D)** A complete proximal-to-distal resection was completed with preservation of all neurovascular structures, flexor tendons and lumbrical muscles, including their motor branches. **(E)** Five years later normal sensation and motion has been maintained. VM remains but is not symptomatic.

better to sclerotherapy than small nests or clusters of VM commonly seen in GVMs or Maffucci patients. Surgical resection is preferred. Routine sclerotherapy prior to surgical resection is preferred by many surgeons but is not as effective as that for fast-flow lesions with arteriovenous fistuli. ⊛ FIGS **31.11 and 31.12** APPEAR ONLINE ONLY

Resection is reserved for VMs that are well localized in a single muscle group (such as the intrinsic muscles of the hand), lesions with thromboses, and those causing neurologic impairment or compressive problems *(Table 31.5)*. In the distal extremity, resection of the entire involved muscle group is preferred, especially for a small muscle-tendon unit. Examples include the intrinsic muscles for which other muscles can substitute or the extrinsic flexors for which tendon transfers are possible. Partial resection of these small muscle-tendon units cannot be recommended; this fails to improve function. Flexion contractures followed by prolonged rehabilitation often occurs after subtotal resection of muscles. The indications for surgical resection are primarily functional, but can also be aesthetic.

Video 2

The principles of treatment are summarized in *Table 31.4*. The advantages of surgical resection in the upper extremity are: (1) a pneumatic tourniquet is used to provide a bloodless field; (2) all anatomic structures can be identified; (3) only the malformation is removed; (4) nerves, muscles, and tendons may be left injured, and (5) well-localized lesions can be completely removed. However, the recovery time is longer; the rehabilitation more difficult and there is always a chance of local VM re-expansion in adjacent regions.

The proximal forearm presents one of the most difficult operative fields for the extremity surgeon due to the high density of important anatomic structures in a compact space. Subcutaneous VMs are not problematic in this area. Intramuscular lesions are difficult to resect because the potential for damage to adjacent muscle and injury to the many small motor branches of the median nerve. Localized lesions deep within the flexor pronator region are difficult to approach without damage to the wrist flexors and deep digital and thumb flexors. Sclerotherapy is the first-line of treatment *(Fig. 31.11)*. On the dorsal surface, it is much easier to identify and decompress the radial nerve through the Arcade of Frohse; however, the risk for injury to extensively involved extensor muscle bellies is high. VMs in this region are usually diffuse and extend well beyond the fascial planes into the muscles. Commonly, VMs and other vascular anomalies involve the dorsal interosseous system along the entire length of the interosseous membrane and may extend into the volar compartments. Surgical decompression of the cubital tunnel, radial tunnel as well as the volar side of the median nerve usually relieves neurogenic pain, which may also be secondary to bleeding or thrombophlebitis within the VM, following multiple procedures or attempted sclerotherapy. Neural wrapping with acellular dermal matrix, autogenous vein, other alloplastic materials or local uninvolved tissue is a helpful adjunct to any neuroplasty in this region.

The distal forearm, wrist, palm, thumb and digits are regions more amenable to surgical extirpation because less muscle mass and more solid tendinous and neural structures occupy the region. Frequently, what appears to be a superficial lesion in the distal forearm and wrist extend deep to and through the interosseous membrane and involve the rete

system. Resections in this region must be thorough, and usually includes removal of the interosseous membrane. Denervation of both and anterior and posterior interosseous nerves will alleviate postoperative wrist pain *(Fig. 31.12)*. The median and ulnar nerves are frequently involved in this region, but intraneural dissection is indicated only when there are symptoms. Secondary neuromas within the main nerves or their sensory branches at the wrist level can be severely disabling for both children and adult patients. A deep palmar VM commonly enlarges within the first web space and extends along the adductor pollicis muscle beneath the first dorsal interosseous muscle. Both muscles are important in pinch and should be preserved if they are not extensively involved. Deep dissection beneath the palmar arch will often expose the deep motor branch of the ulnar nerve, which may or may not be displaced by the VM *(Fig. 31.13)*.

What appears to be localized VM in the palm and dorsum of the hand is always much more extensive than it appears clinically. The margins of many VMs may not be evident on MRI or MRV scans. Dissection in this region is difficult and general guidelines must be strictly observed *(Table 31.5)*. Sclerotherapy in this portion of the hand has many potential complications due to the high concentration of neurovascular structures, gliding tendons and delicate intrinsic muscles *(Fig. 31.14)*.

Outcomes, prognosis, and complications

Few outcome studies are available due to the extremely variable presentation of VMs within the upper extremity and ipsilateral chest wall, and the many syndromic designations and confusion in terminology. VMs can be resected with predictable results. Early complications often beget later problems and less than optimal outcomes. Problems occur in up to 20% of patients and are seen early (swelling, hematoma, delayed wound healing, skin necrosis) or late (neuroma, scar contracture, joint stiffness). Wrist and forearm flexion contractures following partial intermuscular resections are common for proximal forearm lesions. Symptomatic neuromas develop in 35% of those who have intraneural dissections.

Arteriovenous malformation

Arteriovenous malformation (AVM) results from an error in vascular development during embryogenesis in which an absent capillary bed causes shunting of blood directly from an artery into a venous system. This shunt occurs through a direct arteriovenous connection (fistula) or abnormal feeding vessels between an artery and a vein (nidus). This observation of Halsted in 1919 may explain why these AV connections are common in the central nervous system, where apoptosis is rare.[60,61] A number of genetic abnormalities have been described *(Table 31.8)*. These lesions are present at birth only in one-third of patients; 15% involve the extremities. Almost 80% become clinically evident before the termination of adolescence and the natural history is one of slow progressive growth and expansion. These malformations worsen with time and are staged by the Schobinger system *(Table 31.9)*. It is not unusual for a lesion to progress from quiescent through destructive phases. The timing of progression is not predictable when first seen. ⊛ TABLE **31.8** APPEARS ONLINE ONLY

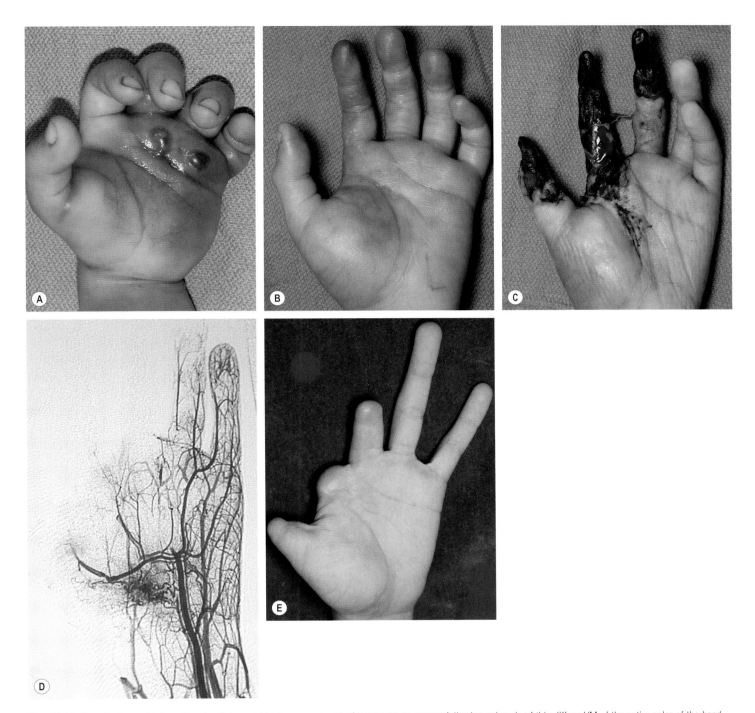

Fig. 31.14 Complications of interventional radiology. Intrinsic compartment releases were necessary following sclerosis of this diffuse VM of the entire palm of the hand. Ethanol was used to embolize this AVM with a nidus within the palm. The distal portions of the thumb, index, and long digits were lost.

Not all fast flow lesions in the upper limb should be labeled as Parkes–Weber syndrome (PWS). We have separated these lesions into four categories in which the arteriovenous flow is related to: (1) a direct AVM *(Fig. 31.15)*; (2) flow through a nidus *(Fig. 31.14B, see Fig. 31.19)*; (3) flow through a vascular tumor (see *Fig. 31.17*) and finally, (4) diffuse high flow vessels perfusing all tissue planes (see *Figs 31.18, 31.21*). PWS is rare and should be restricted to the last condition.

Basic science/disease process

The cardinal features of AVM in a limb are warmth, pain, paresthesias, hyperhydrosis, and compression neuropathy. A CM may be the only initial sign of an AVM, which may not become evident until later in childhood. Vascular thrills and bruits are not always marked. In some patients, a pulsating mass and accompanying thrill may be psychologically disturbing. Many patients seem to tolerate symptoms for a lifetime *(Fig. 31.15)*. AVM may be present at the dermal level. Cutaneous mottling and atrophy, progressing to ulceration, are secondary to the "steal phenomenon," i.e., blood is shunted to the proximal portion of the limb, resulting in peripheral vascular insufficiency, usually first evident in the finger, toes hands and feet *(Fig. 31.16)*. Chronic infection,

ulceration, recurrent bleeding, and intractable pain are the end-stage problems in these unfortunate patients. These malformations are regional and are rarely found with associated fast flow anomalies elsewhere in the body. Patients with an AVM involving the entire extremity and ipsilateral chest wall or those involving the entire lower extremity and pelvic region often demonstrate a positive Nicoladoni sign, a decrease in pulse rate with application of a pneumatic tourniquet to the affected extremity. A large AVM in an extremity can cause cardiopulmonary overload *(Fig. 31.17)* (see *Fig. 31.21*). Some children develop extraordinary postures to alleviate their pain *(Fig. 31.18)*. AVMs do not cause disseminated intravascular coagulopathy. Intralesional bleeding can cause compartment compression. Bony hypertrophy and elongation are present in more than half of these affected limbs. Skeletal involvement carries an unfavorable prognosis but is not an absolute contraindication to surgical intervention. ⊛ FIG **31.18** APPEARS ONLINE ONLY

Table 31.9 Schobinger clinical staging system

Stage I	Quiescent	AVM mimics a capillary malformation or involuting hemangioma
Stage II	Expansion	Lesion larger, warmer, throbbing with thrill or bruits
Stage III	Destruction	Stage II plus ulcers, hemorrhage, persistent pain, tissue necrosis and bone destruction
Stage IV	Decompensation	Stage III plus increased cardiac output and cardiac failure

Diagnosis/patient presentation

AVM can mimic other extremity malformations and there are many vascular conditions containing fast flow

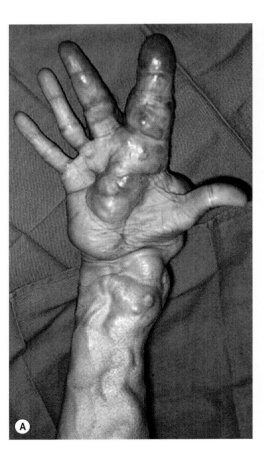
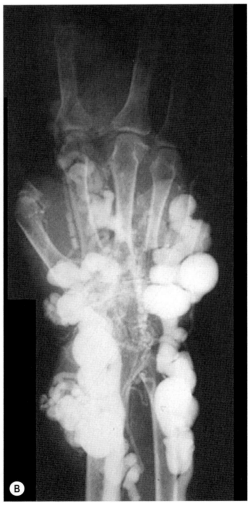

Fig. 31.15 Natural history of fast-flow AVM. **(A)** A 67-year-old adult executive complained of gradual swelling and pulsation in the hand since teenage years. Attempted surgical removal of symptomatic regions had been aborted due to excessive bleeding. **(B)** Early angiographic sequences showed large, tortuous macro-fistulous shunts involving radial and ulnar arterial systems and both palmar arches; very little flow to the distal digits.

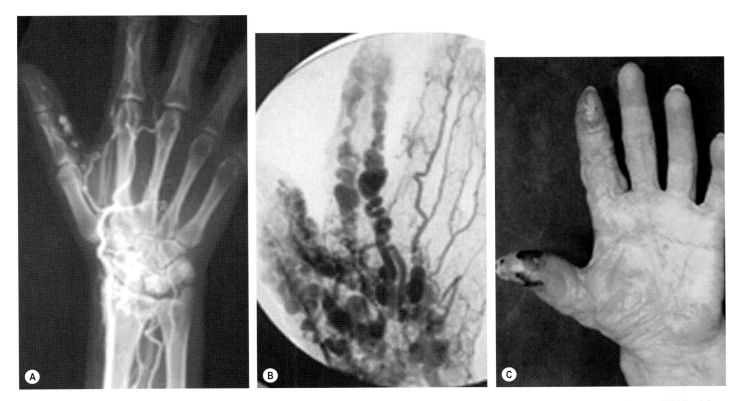

Fig. 31.16 Fast flow AVM with steal phenomenon. **(A)** Angiogram of a 21-year-old patient who presented with an asymptomatic bruit of the wrist shows an AVM involving the radial and interosseous systems. **(B)** Inverted arteriographic images taken 20 years later show large tortuous radial and interosseous vessels leading to large aneurysms with shunting in the distal metacarpal region. **(C)** Tip discoloration of the thumb and long digit caused by steal phenomenon. Distal ischemia of the thumb will ultimately progress to tissue necrosis.

malformations *(Table 31.8)*. Most lesions are diagnosed by history and physical examination, and fast-flow characteristics are confirmed by Doppler US in the clinic. MRI may be obtained to: (1) confirm the diagnosis; (2) outline the true extent of the lesion, and (3) plan management. The T2-weighted sequences show tortuous, dilated, arteries and large draining veins, enhancement, flow voids. The "nidus" is identified as a blush within the central portion of the lesion *(Fig. 31.17A, see Fig. 31.19B)*. MRA and CTA scans demonstrate the three-dimensional characteristics and are preferred over angiogram by mostinterventional radiologists.[62] Extremity surgeons prefer angiography to show the anatomic size, caliber, flow dynamics of the shunts prior to any surgery.[2,10] Anatomic abnormalities are common in the upper limb and include: giant feeding vessels; persistent interosseous vessels; corkscrew configuration of arteries; large median artery; duplicated brachial systems, and large draining veins. Palmar arches are often obliterated with active shunting, and muscle groups may be completely replaced by active AVFs. CT scans are indicated for skeletal involvement. Although critical in the evaluation of other malformations, histopathological diagnosis of AVM is rarely necessary but can be important to rule out rare malignancies such as infantile fibrosarcoma.

Treatment/surgical technique

The puzzling question with fast-flow lesions is their unpredictable natural history and rate of progression. Simple observation is the initial treatment in all but the most symptomatic AVMs. Compression garments may be of some help *(Fig. 31.18C)*. The goal of treatment is to control the progression of the malformation and to alleviate symptoms: pain, ulceration, bleeding, distal discoloration or functional problems. Management options include embolization, surgical resection or a combination *(Fig. 31.19)*. Surgical resection offers the best chance for long-term control, but re-expansion rate following extirpation is high and the deformity created by the resection may be significant. Radical extirpation may often create a deformity worse than the malformation itself. Amputation is the definitive cure, which may be achieved with functional limitations (see *Fig. 31.21*). Therefore, embolization is the first line of intervention for type A and B lesions[2] in the Schobinger I (quiescence) or II (expansion) stages. Well-localized lesions respond better than diffuse AVMs involving multiple tissue planes, but all lesions will re-expand to some degree especially if the central nidus has not been obliterated.

It is important that the extremity surgeon understand the rationale of embolization, which is often used as the primary treatment for these lesions. Inert substances are injected into the nidus to obliterate the abnormal vascular channels, promote ischemia and ultimate scarring of the malformation. Substances used for this process may be liquid (ethanol, n-butyl cyanoacrylate (n-BCA), onyx or solid (polyvinyl alcohol particles, PVA), or coils of many varieties. It is critical that these materials are delivered directly to the nidus of the AVM. Obstruction of the inflow vessels is the major

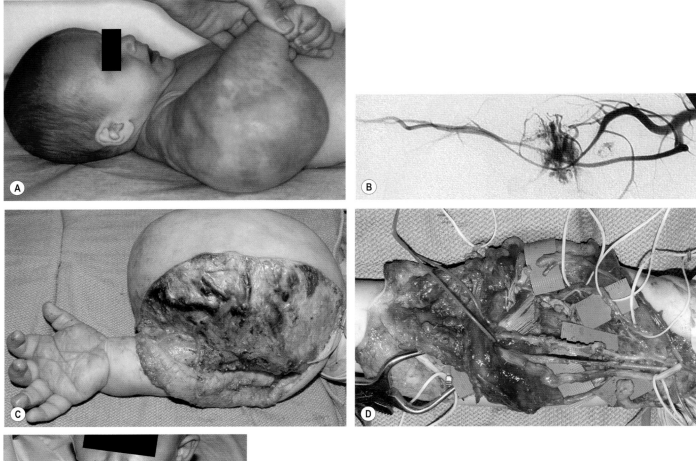

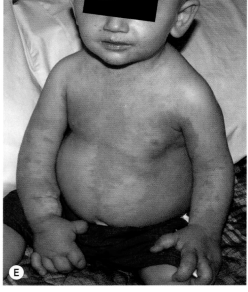

Fig. 31.17 CLOVES with AVM. **(A)** A 6-month-old baby was referred, with large AVM of right arm and forearm, failure to thrive, and refractory cardiac failure. Arm amputation was recommended by many consultants but refused by the family. **(B)** Angiography showed nidus located at level of elbow and forearm. **(C)** Massively enlarged draining veins were encountered. Dissection proceeded toward the center of the mass. **(D)** Individual branches of axillary and brachial artery were mapped and surgically ligated. The dysplastic radial artery (red loop) was replaced with a graft; median, ulnar and radial nerves (yellow loops) were preserved despite massive stretching. **(E)** Incision healed well and patient maintained full elbow flexion/extension and sensation. There were also truncal CMs, overgrowth of multiple limbs and epidermal nevi. He was later diagnosed as CLOVES.

problem with selective embolization and will result in: (1) collateralization of vessels; (2) expansion of the malformation; (3) aggravation of symptoms.[63] For temporary preoperative embolization, Gelfoam powder, PVA, and Embosphere are used instead of liquid agents. Over the past decade our interventional radiologists have preferred onyx, an ethylene-vinyl alcohol copolymer. At the time of resection the embolized tissue with its attendant inflammation will have a mass effect, which facilitates resection. Excision should be completed within 36–72 h post-embolization, before recanalization restores blood flow to the region of the lesion. The major complications to embolization are skin ulceration, local compartment syndrome, and rarely, distal ischemia *(Fig. 31.14B)*. Extremity surgeons must be available following these procedures in interventional radiology.

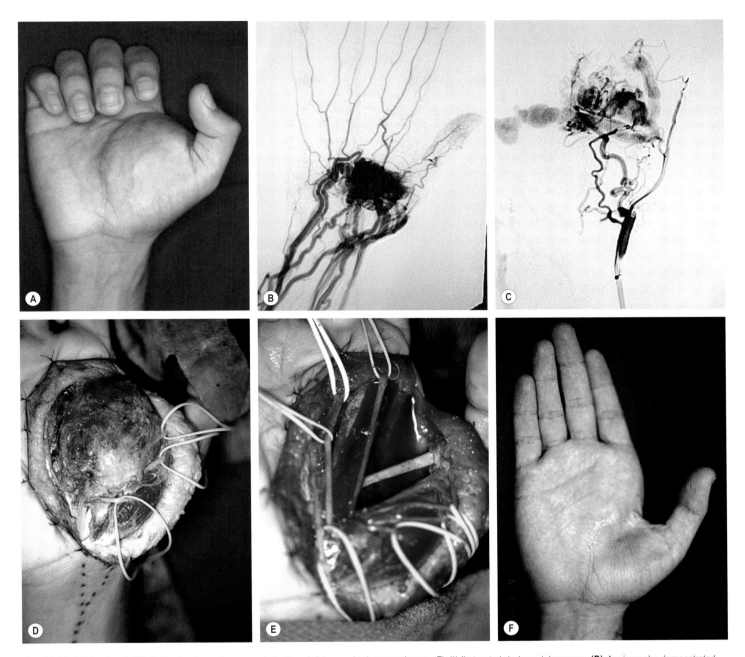

Fig. 31.19 AVM of hand. **(A)** Professional wrestler presented with painful mass in thenar eminence. Thrill first noted during adolescence. **(B)** Angiography demonstrated AVM nidus at superficial palmar arch, supplied by radial, interosseous and ulnar vessels. Distal digital and thumb arterial vaso-architecture was normal. Embolization performed with N-butylcyanoacrylate (NBCA). **(C)** Post-embolization study showed obliteration of most of AVM with residual large draining veins. **(D)** Two days after embolization, the mass was explored: yellow vessel loops mark recurrent motor branch and multiple sensory branches of the median nerve. **(E)** All nerves, flexor tendons and uninvolved thenar muscles were preserved during resection. **(F)** Five years later, he continues to demonstrate good function. Palmar abduction is present (abductor pollicis muscle), but key pinch is weak due to subtotal loss of the adductor pollicis muscle.

Resection is indicated whenever the AVM with or without AVFs leads to chronic ulceration or bleeding, compartment compression, nerve compression, uncontrolled CHF, gangrene, or unrelenting pain. The procedure must be tailored to the patient's needs. In all but the most localized lesions, resection for AVM in a limb is palliative. The surgeon who undertakes resection of an AVM in a limb must have specific objectives that can be accomplished during a safe tourniquet time. The general principles of treatment outlined earlier for slow-flow anomalies also apply to fast-flow anomalies *(Table 31.4)*. Problems arising during these procedures can get out of control; these are well known to all surgeons who have written about operating on these anomalies. Dramatic outcomes can be achieved with a well-planned and executed procedure *(Fig. 31.20)*. There is no predictable procedure that when performed in childhood will prevent subsequent expansion of an AVM, short of a limb amputation. In few other areas of hand surgery is careful explanation of potential complications so important. The patient with a diffuse AVM causing cardiopulmonary overload will probably not respond to any type of staged excision. In contrast, the patient with a more quiescent lesion that has been present for a long time may do well following resection. Incomplete resection cannot be recommended. Postoperative expansion may take many years following a thorough resection and is best managed by selective embolization. However, amputation of a very symptomatic, almost parasitic part is encouraged. Severe pain and bleeding are often the precipitating symptoms *(Fig. 31.21)*. ⊚ FIGS **31.20 and 31.21** APPEAR ONLINE ONLY

The same anatomic concerns outlined with the slow-flow malformations apply to this group of very dynamic lesions. Nerves and tendons should be preserved. Heavily involved muscle groups should be resected with high priority given to preservation of the adductor pollicis and first dorsal interosseous muscles in the hand and elbow flexors and extensors in the arm Revascularization of the hand, digit or thumb should be performed if both axial vessels have been excised. Similarly, marginal skin requires resection and appropriate resurfacing.

PTEN-associated vascular anomaly (PTEN-AVA)

Basic science/disease process

The PTEN (phosphatase and tensin homologue) gene encodes a tumor suppressor lipid phosphatase.[64] Children with these PTEN mutations have the PTEN hamartoma-tumor syndrome (PHTS). This is an autosomal dominant condition, which in the literature has previously been called the Cowden syndrome or the Bannayan--Riley–Ruvalcaba syndrome (BRRS).[65,66] The PTEN mutation is associated with multiple benign and malignant tumors which require surveillance.

Males and females are equally affected. The lower extremities, especially the thighs and calf musculature, are involved much more frequently than the upper extremities, where the arm and forearm regions are more involved than the wrist and hands. Half (54%) of these patients have fast flow malformations with arteriovenous shunting and are designated PTEN-AVA. These children have distinctive macrocephaly; males have penile freckling and these masses can be large and multiloculated. Large amounts of adipose tissue surround the shunts and the mass effect of the affected limb may result in functional compromise. The lesions directly involve the muscles, surround neurovascular tissues, and extend within intramuscular fascial planes. Bone is usually not involved. Lesions may grow to massive proportions.

Diagnosis/patient presentation

The diagnosis is made by physical examination and confirmed by histological and genetic analysis. Histology shows tortuous arteries with mural hyperplasia.

Treatment/surgical technique

Although sclerotherapy has been used to control large tortuous veins and isolated clusters, surgical resection is the definitive treatment of choice. Extirpation may be more difficult if prior sclerotherapy has been performed. Resections in the arm, forearm and hand often involve microvascular dissections of involved neurovascular structures.

Parkes–Weber syndrome (PWS)

PWS is an eponym denoting a fast flow malformation in association with soft tissue and/or skeletal overgrowth and overlying CM.[62] The term is incorrectly used in its association with KTS and should not be used to describe all fast flow lesions within the extremities.

Basic science/disease process

No genetic foci or mutations have been identified to date.

Diagnosis/patient presentation

The diagnosis is made by physical examination and ultrasound. The lower extremity is involved much more frequently than the upper. Diffuse or localized CMs are often present; other skin changes include pseudo Kaposi lesions, lymphedema and skin ulceration late in the progression of the malformation. Lymphedema is common. The angiograms in a classic PWS do not initially show specific AVFs with large draining veins. These early studies show diffuse high flow vessels infiltrating the involved soft tissue and skeletal structures without large draining veins so characteristic of shunts. The CM is often diffuse and irregular and covers the region of underlying hypervascularity *(Figs 31.18, 31.21)*. PWS should be distinguished from other fast flow lesions: PTEN-AVA, other vascular tumors, AVM with AVFs, and CM-AVM. MRI, MRA, ultrasound, and biopsy are warranted with an increase in symptoms. The clinical prognosis is one of progressive expansion and destructions.

Treatment/surgical technique

Management is identical with the indications and principles previously presented for fast flow lesions. Initial treatment is always conservative, but these children should be followed through adolescence and adulthood. Symptomatic regions respond to selective embolization. Cardiac compromise may be insidious; cardiologists must evaluate these children yearly. Regional resections are warranted for selective cases but must be carefully planned and executed with the realization that these lesions are often progressive. Amputation of nonfunctional digits, hands, and arms is usually delayed; pain is often the precipitating factor for an amputation. Experience has taught us that amputations of parasitic parts is often unnecessarily delayed either by the reluctant surgeons or anxious parents with unrealistic expectations.

Outcomes, prognosis, and complications

Children must be monitored both for cardiac symptoms and overgrowth issues. The progress may be slow and not predictable early in life. All patients had some degree of pain, swelling, overgrowth and nerve compression at some anatomic level. Selective embolization successfully controlled symptoms in 70% of patients. We have never documented regression of this type of malformation. Amputations have been performed in 30% of fast flow patients; not all of these have been followed through adolescence and early adulthood.

Capillary malformation-arteriovenous malformation (CM-AVM)

Basic science/disease process

This is an autosomal dominant condition caused by a loss-of-function mutation in the RASA1 gene.[62,67] Patients usually present with a positive family history of similar lesions.

Diagnosis/patient presentation

The CM is evident by physical examination and is distinguished by a faint halo around the lesion. We have seen these in the upper extremity. Almost 10% of patients have an underlying fast flow AVM involving the central nervous system, a very frequent location for AVMs. A full neurologic examination is indicated with a cranial MRI. Extracranial AVMs are rare in patients. Lesions are common in the lips or mouth.

Treatment/surgical technique

No treatment is necessary for the upper extremity CM. AVMs are followed symptomatically and treated as previously outlined.

Klippel–Trenaunay syndrome (KTS)

KTS is an eponym denoting a slow flow capillary-lymphaticovenous malformation designated as CLVM and is readily distinguished from PWS by the slow flow dynamics of the malformation.

Basic science/disease process

No positive genetic associations have been made.

Diagnosis/patient presentation

An accurate physical examination will determine the presence of both lymphatic and venous components, as the CM is obvious at birth. There is a wide range in clinical presentation.[68–70] There are no major hemodynamic alterations in the cardiovascular system. The lower extremities (95%) are involved much more frequently than the upper (5%) and the trunk and pelvis are rarely affected. The limb hypertrophy is not as profound as in patients with the Proteus syndrome, CLOVES syndrome, or in hemihypertrophy patients. However, upper limb involvement may be accompanied by massive soft tissue enlargement of not only the upper limb but also the chest wall. In 10% of these limbs, hypoplasia may be present. Kyphoscoliosis and pulmonary compromise often develop as the child grows. Leg length discrepancy is common. KTS patients are not at risk

for Wilms tumors and do not need to be screened with abdominal ultrasound examination.[71] The VM pattern is similar to phlebectasias with large draining veins in the arm and axilla. There are usually diffuse clusters of large veins and sinuses involving muscle, fascial planes and occasionally bone. All forms of LM may be present including skin vesicles, coalesced vesicles causing maceration and ulcers, macrocysts in the proximal portion of the upper limb and microcysts in the more distal regions. All lesions are accompanied by large amounts of adipose tissue. Occasionally, VM predominate; the upper limb equivalent of the lateral "vein of Servelle" is present and does communicate with the deep venous drainage system along the axial vessels to the limb. Because the GU and GI systems are commonly involved, these patients may be very symptomatic. Similar to the foot, massive enlargement of the wrist and hand with splaying of the digits with or without ulnar deviation may occur.

Treatment/surgical technique

Management is initially conservative and depends upon the predominance of the venous or lymphatic components. Management of the venous components is initially conservative. Epiphysiodesis to control bilateral growth symmetry is not as essential in the arm as it is in the lower extremity. Nerve compressions and lymphatic components respond very well to surgery. Surgical principles are the same. In the upper limb, resection is performed to improve function, relieve compression neuropathies, and restore motion and contour. Those with large lesions, chest wall involvement and those with large stagnant venous collecting systems in the arm and axilla are at risk for pulmonary embolus and are maintained on anticoagulants. Staged contour resections are difficult but well worth the effort.

Outcomes, prognosis, and complications

Clinical outcomes vary with the size and extent of the LVM and a similar to those for large isolated VMs and LMs. Outcome studies for upper limb KTS patients do not exist.

CLOVES syndrome

Congenital lipomatosis overgrowth, vascular malformations, epidermal nevi, and scoliosis syndrome (CLOVES) constitutes the components of a recently described overgrowth condition which also contains a fast-flow vascular malformation.[72,73]

Basic science/disease process

The upper extremity is involved. Previously, many of these children were diagnosed as Proteus patients but did not satisfy the criteria for inclusion. CLOVES patients do not have uncontrolled progressive skeletal overgrowth, and the soft tissue enlargement consists primarily of dysplastic adipose tissue. Truncal CMs are present in all patients. Patients may also have fast flow AVMs (*Fig. 31.17*). Overgrowth in the limb is similar to that seen with LMs. It may or may not be oriented along a nerve territory (*Table 31.2*).

Diagnosis/patient presentation

Diagnosis is similar to other conditions and starts with physical examination. Ultrasound shows the fast flow components, which can be further defined by MRA and MRI. Radiographs and MRI scans will delineate soft tissue and skeletal overgrowth. CT scans are usually not necessary.

Treatment/surgical technique

Resection of the lipomatous component, staged debulking and appropriate epiphysiodesis of the forearm and hand are predictable and useful for the individual patient. Skeletal angulation and rotation at all levels are corrected with osteotomies. Most families do not elect to have laser treatment of hand and upper limb CMs.

Access the bonus content for this chapter online at **http://www.expertconsult.com**

Fig. 31.5 (C) CM plus overgrowth of thumb, long and ring digits in a child with CLOVES. **(D)** Extensive CM plus lipomatous overgrowth, syndactyly and no skeletal overgrowth. **(E)** Limb of child with CM-AVM. **(F)** CM in an older man. Note variable effect of laser treatment on the dorsal forearm. CM darkened with cobblestone appearance during the adult years.

Fig. 31.9 (B) Lymphatic microcysts and small venous thromboses are studded within dysplastic adipose tissue. **(C)** The neurovascular bundle has been dissected with preservation vincular branches at the joint levels.

Fig. 31.11 Sclerotherapy. Radiographic studies of the vulnerable proximal third of the forearm show a VM, which is ideal for sclerotherapy: **(A)** Isointense to adjacent skeletal muscle on axial T1-sequence; **(B)** enhances on axial T1 plus gadolinium contrast; **(C)** shows signal voids on axial T2 representing phleboliths; **(D)** fills with direct puncture and injection of contrast; **(E)** shows small calcified phleboliths on radiographs; **(F)** has multilobulated structure with signal voids on sagittal T2 sequences

Fig. 31.12 VM distal forearm. **(A,B)** A middle-aged man presented with carpal tunnel symptoms. Coronal T1 (above) shows a lesion with signal voids and T2-sequences (below) demonstrate enhancement, both consistent

with VM. **(C,D)** Enhanced T1-weighted sequences show extension across the interosseous membrane. **(E)** Excision included the pronator quadratus muscle. **(F)** Full function returned 6 weeks postoperatively.

Fig. 31.18 Parkes–Weber syndrome (PWS). **(A)** A 6-year-old child with a CM of the wrist and hand a pulsatile mass of he distal forearm. Diagnosis of PWS was made and she was treated with a compression garment. Flexion contractures gradually developed in the wrist and all digits. **(B)** Angiogram at age 7 showed diffuse hypervascularity and multiple microfistuli without large draining veins. **(C)** Pain gradually increased as she grew. She learned to control this pain by dislocating her glenohumeral joint, a maneuver that compressed the massively enlarged subclavian artery and vein. She often slept in this position.

Fig. 31.20 AVM with AVFs of thumb. **(A)** A 60-year-old man presented with pulsatile bleeding from excoriated regions of his right thumb. He first noted swelling as a young child, and lived with periodic bleeding and ulceration his entire life. **(B)** Arteriography showed extensive macro-fistulous AVM involving radial side of his dominant hand. **(C)** Congenital absence of his left hand made him completely dependent on right upper limb. **(D)** Following resection of scarred and unstable pulp surface and debulking entire

thumb, resurfacing accomplished with neurovascular island flap from ulnar side of long finger. **(E)** Flap extended to nail plate distally and included entire working pulp surface of thumb. **(F)** This grateful patient has a stable functional thumb, which he perceives is on ulnar side of the long finger.

Fig. 31.21 Parkes–Weber syndrome. **(A,B)** Teenager with type C AVM, and his parents wanted to save the hand. Index ray had been resected for uncontrollable pulsatile bleeding. The thumb was ulcerated; patient was suicidal because of unrelenting pain. **(C)** Angiography showed massively tortuous and enlarged axial vessels feeding microfistulous shunts within forearm and hand with involvement of all soft tissue and skeletal structures. **(D)** Later sequence demonstrates extent of shunting and lack of distal digital perfusion. **(E)** Chest radiograph and electrocardiogram confirmed congestive heart failure (Schobinger Stage IV). **(F)** Below elbow amputation followed by predictable recovery, normal adolescent growth spurt, and good function with his prosthesis.

Table 31.2 Diagnostic work-up of vascular anomalies.

Table 31.7 Variations of venous malformations.

Table 31.8 Combined and fast flow malformations.

Access the complete references list online at **http://www.expertconsult.com**

1. Mulliken JB, Glowacki J. Hemangiomas and vascular malformations in infants and children: a classification based on endothelial characteristics. *Plast Reconstr Surg.* 1982;69:412–422.

   This classic article helped clarify the delineation between hemangiomas and vascular malformations. The classification is based on histologic differences in the tissue; these endothelial characteristics are correlated with the natural history of hemangiomas vs vascular malformations.

10. Upton J, Coombs CJ, Mulliken JB, et al. Vascular malformations of the upper limb: A review of 270 patients. *J Hand Surg Am.* 1999;24:1019–1035.

    This is an extremely large series of patients with vascular malformations of the upper limb. The diagnosis and treatment of various types is reviewed in retrospective fashion.

17. Sapp JC, Turner JT, van de Kamp JM, et al. Newly delineated syndrome of congenital lipomatous

overgrowth, vascular malformations, and epidermal nevi (CLOVE syndrome) in seven patients. *Am J Med Genet Am.* 2007;143:2944–2958.

    This is a presentation of the newly described CLOVE syndrome.

19. Upton J, Carty MJ. Macrodactyly. *Clin Plast Surg.* 2011; In press.

21. Tan WH, Baris HN, Burrows PE, et al. The spectrum of vascular anomalies in patients with PTEN mutations: Implications for diagnosis and management. *J Med Genet.* 2007;44:594–602.

24. Parkes Weber F. Right-sided hemihypertrophy resulting from right-sided congenital spastic hemiplegia with a morbid condition of the left side of the brain revealed by radiogram. *J Neurol Neurosurg Psych.* 1922;37:301–311.

26. Upton J, Mulliken JB, Murray JE. Classification and rationale for treatment of vascular anomalies in the upper extremity. *J Hand Surg Am.* 1985;10:970.

29. Kilcline C, Frieden IJ. Infantile hemangiomas: how common are they? A systematic review of the medical literature. *Pediatr Dermatol*. 2008;25:168–173.

33. Frieden IL, Drolet BA. Propranolol for infantile hemangiomas: promise, peril, pathogenesis. *Pediatr Dermatol*. 2009;26:642–644.

    Propranolol is a newly proposed treatment for hemangiomas. This paper discussed early results, with discussion of possible risks and mechanisms of action.

39. van der Horst CM, Koster PH, de Borgie CA, et al. Effect of the timing of treatment of port-wine stains with the flash-lamp-pumped pulsed-dye laser. *N Engl J Med*. 1998;338:1028–1033.

    Treatment of flat capillary vascular malformations is optimally treated with the flash-lamp pumped pulsed-dye laser. This is because the wavelength of hemoglobin is targeted. This article discusses optimal dosing and timing of treatment.

60. Halsted W. Congenital arteriovenous and lymphaticovenous fistulae: unique clinical and experimental observations. *Proc Natl Acad Sci USA*. 1919;5:76–79.

32

Peripheral nerve injuries of the upper extremity

Simon Farnebo, Johan Thorfinn, and Lars B. Dahlin

SYNOPSIS

- Nerve regeneration after injury is orchestrated by delicate processes in neurons, nonneural cells, and other cells at various levels from the periphery to the central nervous system.
- The clinical effects of a nerve injury include not only impaired sensory and motor function, but also symptoms such as impaired dexterity, sensitivity to cold, and pain. Therefore, they have a severe impact on activities of daily living.
- Correct diagnosis and classification of the injury are crucial for appropriate treatment.
- The surgical approach and technique, as well as timing of surgery, are factors of detrimental importance for outcome.
- The type of injury, condition of the wound, and the vascularity of the wound bed are key factors influencing surgical decision-making.
- Various techniques for nerve repair are described, including epineurial, fascicular, and end-to-side repair, and techniques for nerve reconstruction.
- Factors of importance for outcome, such as age, delay before repair, and level of injury are discussed, as well as means of evaluation after surgery.

Introduction

A nerve injury may have a profound impact on the patient's activities of daily living, with subsequent effects on professional life and leisure time. Patients may have to change profession, or be left with a permanently impaired ability to work. Nerve injuries may, therefore, generate not only costs for society within the healthcare system for treatment and rehabilitation, but also outside the healthcare system resulting from lost production.[1] Nerve injuries most commonly affect the upper extremity. The incidence of injuries to the hand has been calculated as 7–37/1000 inhabitants/year in Europe.[2] Similar data are available for children (incidence 2.7/1000

children/year). Most hand injuries are minor, but injuries to the nerves (that account for about 3% of hand injuries) usually impair hand function.[2,3] Few reports exist about the specific incidence of nerve injuries, but the incidence has been reported to be 13.9/100000 person/year.[4] Most of the injuries to the hand (10%) and the wrist (63%) required less than a week in hospital. However, few inpatient and outpatient data have been reported. The incidence of a digital nerve injury is estimated to 6.2/100000 inhabitants/year. The general pattern of distribution of both hand and nerve injuries between the sexes is that it is usually young (median age 29 years) men (up to 75%) who are injured. The incidence of a radial nerve injury associated with a fracture of the shaft of the humerus is around 0.12/10000 inhabitants and year.[5] Based on these reports one may estimate that 70000 and 29000 patients in the European Community and in the US, respectively, injure a nerve trunk annually.

The costs of treatment and rehabilitation, including those for loss of production, after a nerve injury, may be substantial. The costs for injuries to a median and an ulnar nerve are roughly $70000 USD and $45000, respectively[1]; 87% of these costs are the result of lost production. Costs are higher for patients with coexisting tendon injuries (≥4 tendons). In addition, costs within the healthcare sector are higher for patients who had to change jobs after the injury and in patients in whom both the median and the ulnar nerves were injured. Up to 69% of patients with an ulnar or median nerve injury are back in fulltime work by 1 year after the nerve injury.[1,6,7] Age is one important factor for outcome after nerve repair,[1,8] which is probably based on better cerebral adaptation to the injury, particularly in young children. The clinical effects of a nerve injury include not only subjective impaired sensory and motor functions, but also subjective complaints such as impaired dexterity, cold sensitivity, and pain[9]; thus, having a severe impact on activities of daily living. Altogether, nerve injuries can cause considerable problems for individual patients and costs for society. In the present chapter the principles for repair and reconstruction of nerve injuries are outlined, with emphasis on the fact that such injuries should be treated promptly.

Basic science and natural history

Anatomy

Gross anatomy: the upper extremity

The brain and the spinal cord (central nervous system) are connected to targets by the peripheral nervous system, which consists of cranial nerves, spinal nerves with roots and rami, and peripheral nerve trunks with the peripheral components of the autonomic nervous system. The anterior and posterior nerve roots (that emerge from rootlets attached to the spinal cord) merge into the spinal nerve, where the anterior primary rami form the brachial plexus in the upper extremity *(Fig. 32.1)*. The posterior primary ramus runs posteriorly, and supplies the muscle and skin of the posterior part of the neck and trunk; it does not enter the extremity. The anterior primary rami of the cervical nerve roots C5–8 and the ramus of T1 form the brachial plexus, from which the upper extremity receives its innervation through various branches.

C5–6 form the upper trunk of the brachial plexus, C7 forms the middle trunk, and C8–T1 form the inferior trunks. These trunks divide into anterior and posterior divisions in which the lateral and medial cords are formed from the anterior division while the posterior divisions form the posterior cord, which mainly innervates the extensor muscles in the upper extremity. In contrast, the lateral and medial cords innervate the flexor muscles in the extremity. The musculocutaneous nerve originates from the lateral cord. The median nerve is formed by the joining of the lateral and medial cords, whereas the ulnar nerve branches from the medial cord together with

the medial cutaneous nerves to the arm (brachial) and forearm (antebrachial). The radial and axillary nerves originate from the posterior cord. There is a segmental pattern of sensory and motor innervation *(Fig. 32.2)*.

The anatomy of the plexus and the nerve trunks may vary considerably from person to person. Variations are seen in the forearm, where a "Martin Gruber" anastomosis may be found in as many as 15%, particularly between the anterior interosseous nerve and the ulnar nerve. A similar anastomosis may also be present more distally – Riche–Cannieu (branch between the motor branch of the ulnar nerve and the thenar branch of the median nerve in the thenar region in the hand: *Fig. 32.3*).

The neuron and supporting cells

The cell bodies of the motor and sensory neurons are located in the spinal cord and in the dorsal root ganglia, respectively, with their axons extending out to their respective targets in the periphery. The sensory neuron is pseudounipolar, with one branch of the axon extending into the posterior part of the spinal cord. The transition from the central to the peripheral nervous system takes place in the rootlets (or less often, in roots of the nerves) of the transitional zone, which are almost cone-shaped.[10] In the central part, the neurons are surrounded by oligodendrocytes and astrocyte processes, whereas in the peripheral nervous system axons are closely associated with Schwann cells. In myelinated nerve fibers, each axon is embraced by a series of continuous Schwann cells that create the myelin sheath. The border between individual and enwrapping Schwann cells is called the node of Ranvier *(Fig. 32.4)*. Each nerve fiber is enclosed in a basal lamina (or basement membrane). In contrast, several thinner axons run in troughs in one Schwann cell – nonmyelinated nerve fibers. Each Schwann cell therefore embraces several axons. The diameter of nerve fibers varies, and extends from 0.4 to 1.25 µm (nonmyelinated) and from 2 to 22 µm (myelinated).[11] The number of nerve fibers also varies with nerve trunks. In addition, the number of nerve fibers decreases with age: as many as 26% of the nerve fibers may disappear between the second and eighth decades.

The nerve trunk

A number of nerve fibers are enclosed in bundles around which there are flattened supporting cells and layers of collagen that form the perineurium. These bundles of fibers surrounded by the perineurium are called fascicles, which are embedded in loose connective tissue (called epineurium); this is composed of collagen fibers and fibroblasts *(Figs 32.4 and 32.5)*. The space inside the fascicles is called the endoneurial space, in which the pressure is slightly positive (endoneurial fluid pressure); it consists of collagen fibrils, and cells such as fibroblasts and occasional macrophages and mast cells. Lymphocytes (CD4+ and CD8+) and macrophages are not generally found in the endoneurium (except after injury), but may be present in the epineurium. The amount of connective tissue varies among nerve trunks, and also within the same nerve trunk. More abundant connective tissue is therefore located in the nerve trunk at sites where extra protection is needed (such as joints and superficial nerve trunks). The term "mesoneurium" refers to the additional loose areolar tissue

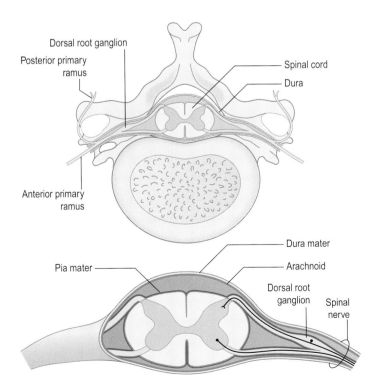

Fig. 32.1 The anterior and posterior nerve roots, which emerge from rootlets attached to the spinal cord.

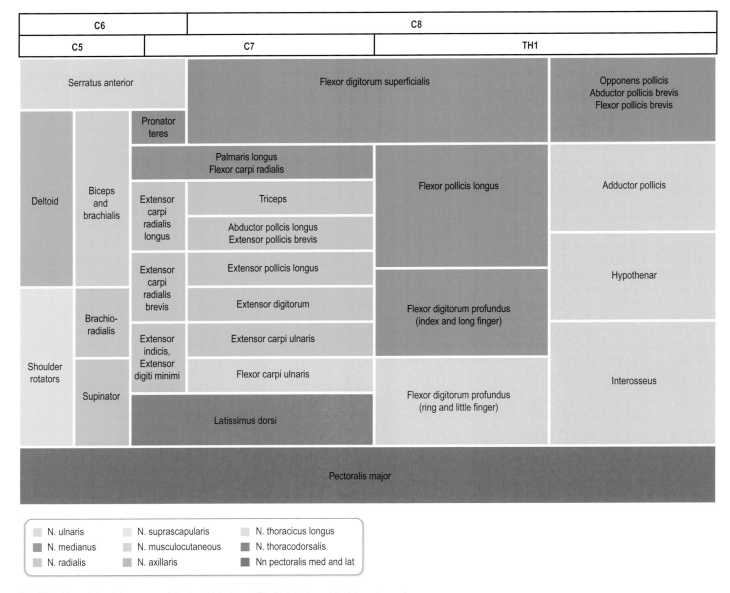

Fig. 32.2 The origin of the nerves of the brachial plexus (C5–Th1, top), and their target muscles.

that is located superficially to the epineurium. This tissue allows for the gliding of the nerve trunk (excursion) during movements of the extremity.

There is topographical segregation of fascicles and nerve fibers in the nerve trunks, particularly in their peripheral parts.[12,13] The latter anatomical feature permits dissection of a bundle of fascicles that can be used in nerve transfers.

Blood supply

Nerve trunks receive their blood supply from segmental blood vessels *(Fig. 32.6)*, which branch into plexuses in the epineurium, perineurium, and in the endoneurial space. The blood vessels inside the fascicles consist mainly of capillaries, which are provided by circulation through blood vessels that pierce the perineurium obliquely. The epineurial blood vessels are more susceptible to trauma than the endoneurial vessels

and so epineurial edema develops more easily than endoneurial edema. Because of the extensive reserve capacity of the intraneural blood supply it is possible to mobilize a nerve over an extended length without disturbing the blood supply. In addition, the blood vessels adjacent to the nerve trunks have a coiled appearance that allows excursion of the nerve trunk. In addition to the vasa nervorum, there are also nervi nervorum, such as free nerve endings in the epineurium, perineurium, and endoneurium.

Physiology

To allow for propagation of the action potential, ions are exchanged between the axon and the extracellular space at the nodes of Ranvier *(Fig. 32.4)*. As this exchange occurs only at the nodes of Ranvier in myelinated nerve fibers, the conduction velocity jumps from node to node. In myelinated nerve

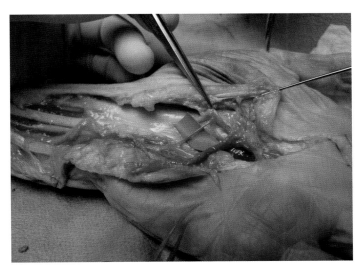

Fig. 32.3 An anatomical preparation of the Riche–Cannieu anastomosis in the palm. This highly variable, although common, anastomosis between the median nerve motor branch and the deep ulnar nerve provides a potential pathway for enormous variation in intrinsic muscle innervation.

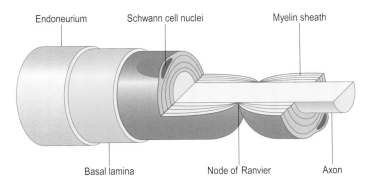

Fig. 32.4 Close-up of myelinated axon and the node of Ranvier.

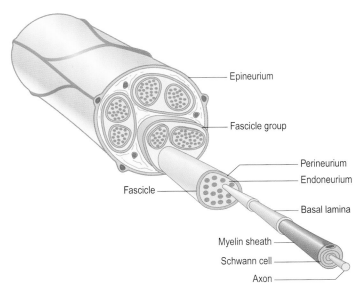

Fig. 32.5 Schematic presentation of a peripheral nerve. Colors for identical structures are the same as in *Figure 32.4*.

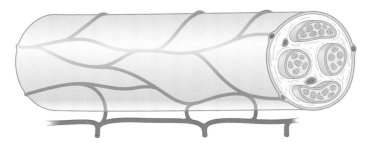

Fig. 32.6 Principal blood supply of nerve segment, highlighted in red.

fibers this saltatory conduction induces high conduction velocity. In contrast, the propagation of impulses is more continuous in nonmyelinated nerve fibers. After a nerve has been injured the process of Wallerian degeneration (see below) takes some time in humans, which explains why it is possible to record propagation of an impulse in an injured nerve by electrical stimulation at neurography for many days after the injury. It is generally agreed, therefore, that neurography should be done no earlier than 3–4 weeks after the injury if signs of degeneration are to be found.

The cytoskeleton of the axon contains neurofilaments and centrally located microtubules. Essential molecules are transported along the microtubules both from the cell body down to the periphery (anterograde) and from the periphery up to the cell body (retrograde) with energy-dependent axonal transport. This transport has several functions, such as recycling of materials that are not used in the periphery, provision of membrane constituents, neurotransmitters, and necessary cytoskeletal components to the axon. Transfer of important molecules is essential for survival and signaling both in the normal state and after nerve injury. After cellular injury these signals are rapidly initiated from the environment by translation into intracellular messengers or commenced in the axon at the site of injury. These changes involve profound alterations in transcription, translation, and posttranslational processes in the cells after the injury.

Degeneration and regeneration

After a nerve injury, deep and intense processes are initiated in the injured neurons and their axons and in the nonneuronal cells, particularly the Schwann cells. In the cells a number of temporary and spatially orchestrated mechanisms guide survival and regeneration. In addition, there are mechanisms that lead to apoptosis of the cells. The signal transduction processes are not clarified, and this is a target of intense research. After the peripheral nerve trunk has been injured by transection or avulsion, the proximal part of the axon is resealed to form a new surface on the tip of the axon – a process that is influenced by the presence of calcium. There is usually a slight retraction of the proximal axon, which is related to the number of injured Schwann cells. At the tip of the axon, signals are formed in the signal transduction processes and transferred to the nucleus of the neuron where the functions are changed from maintenance to survival and growth.

The distal nerve segment

Schwann cells are extremely important for the function of the peripheral nerve, both in the normal state and after injury. After injury there is disintegration of the axons and the myelin sheath in the distal nerve segment, the latter released by Schwann cells. It is important to remove myelin and the disintegrated axon to allow and prepare a conducive environment for the regenerating axons. Both macrophages and Schwann cells can therefore contribute to the cleaning-up mechanisms, where their relevance varies over time.

The timing of nerve repair is of crucial importance for a successful outgrowth of axons after injury,[14,15] which can be related to a large number of factors that are up- and down-regulated by Schwann cells after nerve injury. After the Schwann cells have been activated they proliferate along the inside of their basal lamina, and form the bands of Büngner.

Neurotrophic factors and their receptors are up-regulated in Schwann cells after injury, and these may include neurotrophins (such as nerve growth factor and brain-derived neurotrophic factor), fibroblast growth factors (such as β-fibroblast growth factor), neuropoietic cytokines (such as ciliary neurotrophic factor and leukemia-inhibitory factor), and other groups of factors, such as insulin-like growth factor, transforming growth factor, and interleukins.

Apoptosis (programmed death) of various cells, such as macropahges and Schwann cells, an event that is initiated by release of proapoptotic molecules from the mitochondria (intrinsic pathway), can be activated through the death cell surface receptors (extrinsic pathway; like Fas and tumor necrosis factor receptor 1). The number of apoptotic Schwann cells in the distal nerve segment is increased if the transected nerve is repaired after a delay.[16]

All these changes in the injured neuron and its axon and in the Schwann cells have the common goal of regrowth of the axons into the distal nerve segments down to their targets. Regrowth is a delicate process in which numerous sprouts emerge from the distal part of each axon. On the tip of each sprout there is a growth cone, which is formed as a small hand on which the "finger-like" filopodia palpate the environment with the purpose of finding guidance structures *(Fig. 32.7)*. Intricate mechanisms direct rate and direction of extension of the growth cones, where actin filaments are polymerized and organized.[17,18] Microtubules are polymerized in the growth cones. The growth is a dynamic process, where the filopodia/growth cone is repulsed or attracted depending on the local mechanisms and the structure of the environment.

The extracellular matrix is extremely important for the outgrowth and advancement of the growth cone. Proteins, such as laminin, fibronectin, galactins, tenascin, and collagens, stimulate outgrowth. Laminin exerts its stimulatory effect through cell surface glycoproteins called integrins, which interact with the intracellular actin in the growth cone and in the filopodia, thus, navigating outgrowth of the axon. Precise knowledge about how axons grow and how growth is directed is still limited.

Diagnosis and presentation

Formal classification of injury

Nerve injuries can be divided into two main groups: those that will temporarily block nerve conduction without loss of axonal architecture, and those with severe damage that will result in axonal degeneration distal to the injury *(Fig. 32.8)*.

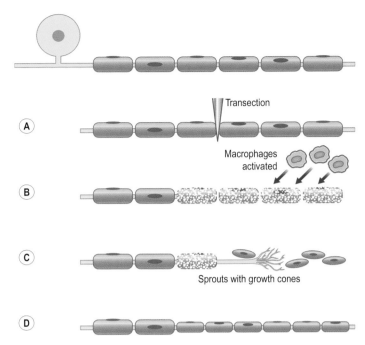

Fig. 32.7 As the nerve is severed **(A)**, activated macrophages and Schwann cells will immediately start the removal of myelin and remnants of the disintegrated axon, to allow for a conducive environment for the regenerating axons **(B)**. Within just a few hours numerous sprouts emerge from the distal part of each axon and form the sprout growth cone that will guide the regeneration process distally **(C)**, until nerve regeneration is complete **(D)**.

This may be one useful clinical way of approaching nerve injuries, but more formal classifications have been presented to describe the complexity of the lesions further, in particular the Seddon classification,[19] in which injuries were divided into three groups of increasing severity (neuropraxia, axonotmesis, and neurotmesis). This classification was modified by Sunderland[20] and by Mackinnon[21] to include six degrees of injury. In *Table 32.1* we summarize the differences between the three classifications, and the specific neural changes are illustrated in *Figure 32.9*.

Neuropraxia

First-degree injury

In neuropraxia there is a physiological block of conduction, but no disruption of the neural architecture at the site of injury, and there are no degenerative changes within the nerve. The pathogenesis is most often external compression, surgical traction, or local ischemia. Complete recovery is the general rule, and the healing time can vary from a few days to 3–4 months. Tinel's sign is not present over the site of injury.

Axonotmesis

Second-degree injury

In second-degree injuries, true degeneration of axons is initiated. Axonal damage leads to distal (Wallerian) degeneration, although the basal lamina of the Schwann cells remains intact.

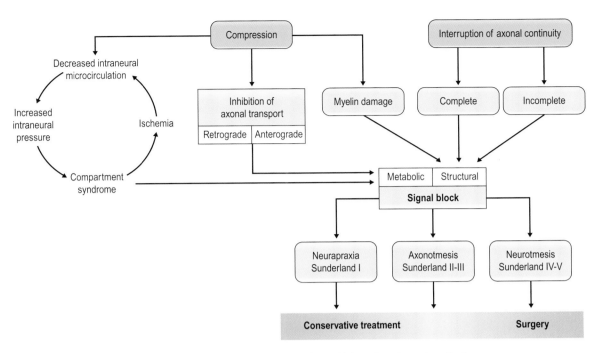

Fig. 32.8 Schematic flowchart of neuronal response to nerve compression and interruption of axonal continuity.

Table 32.1 **Comparison between the Seddon, Sunderland, and MacKinnon classifications of nerve injury**

Seddon	Sunderland	MacKinnon	Description
Neuropraxia	1		Local physiologic block with paralysis but no anatomic disturbance of the nerve. Full recovery is expected
Axonotmesis	2		Nerve injury with degeneration of the distal segment. Intact endoneurium and perineurium. Full recovery occurs at rate of 1.5 mm/day
	3		Endoneurial damage with subsequent scarring and incomplete regeneration. Variable recovery
Neurotmesis	4		Nerve damaged with complete internal structural disorganization. Nerve trunk remains intact. No functional recovery unless operative intervention
	5		Nerve trunk cut completely. Early operative intervention necessary for restoration of some function
		6	Mixed nerve injury

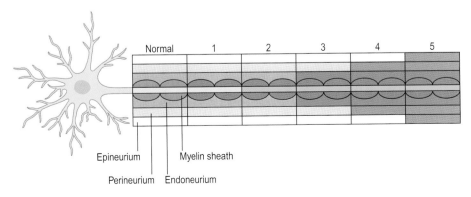

Fig. 32.9 Schematic of damaged structures within an axon according to the classification of Sunderland grades 1–5. Change in color (red) and pattern indicates damage to each structure. Yellow represents an axon and its neuron.

The axons regenerate through their own endoneurial tubes by axonal contact and guidance of the regenerating growth cones at a rate of 1–3 mm/day. No topographical mismatch will occur, and the integrity of sensory and motor nerve fibers remains intact. Tinel's sign is present, and the progress of recovery can by followed by the gradual recovery of motor or sensory function distal to the injury. Full recovery is expected.

Third-degree injury

In a third-degree injury the architecture within the perineurium is disrupted together with axonal damage. The fascicles remain intact, although progression of axonal regrowth will be with less precision as the axonal guidance is impaired and mismatch of fibers will occur. Axonal mismatch follows to a larger extent in proximally based injuries as the fascicular organization is usually of mixed motor and sensory patterns. The clinical outcome is hard to predict, mainly because of subsequent intrafascicular scarring and the failure of some axons to regenerate. Tinel's sign is present and progresses distally with recovery. Microsurgical resection and grafting may not be beneficial in these cases.

Neurotmesis

Fourth-degree injury

In a fourth-degree lesion the epineurium is intact but all other parts of the nerve are damaged. The formation of an intraneural scar impairs both axonal regeneration and reinnervation, and typically forms a neuroma at the site of injury. A more profound retrograde neuronal effect than in a third-degree injury is expected, and this causes a higher incidence of neuronal death. Tinel's sign is usually present over the site of the injury, but there are no signs of recovery, or proximal-to-distal progression of regeneration. The injury requires complete excision of the neuroma and microsurgical nerve repair, usually with nerve grafting.

Fifth-degree injury

In a fifth-degree injury the nerve is completely transected. Recovery of function is dependent on surgical repair, with or without nerve grafting. These injuries are most commonly associated with injuries that include the surrounding structures, such as tendons, muscles, bones, or blood vessels.

Sixth-degree injury

The sixth-degree injury was added by Mackinnon to take account of mixed injuries,[21] for example those that occur after closed traction damage to a nerve, or gunshot or stab wounds that cause partial injuries to a nerve. This type of injury is often referred to as a neuroma in continuity, in which all degrees of nerve injury, from normal to neurotmesis, may coexist within the scarred nerve. A neuroma in continuity typically results from failure of the regenerating nerve growth cone to proceed beyond the injury to reach its peripheral targets. It occurs within an intact nerve with continuity in response to internally damaged axons and fascicles, resulting in a distal portion of the nerve that no longer, more or less, functions properly. Surgical exposure is often necessary and

intraoperative electrodiagnostic studies can help to distinguish fascicles with signs of recovery from those without (grades IV and V).

Clinical examination

A correct diagnosis is crucial. Confirmation of a nerve injury is usually not hard, even though every nerve injury is unique in its character, and highly variable in its symptoms. Lack of active movement, such as against resistance, because of paralysis of the muscles supplied by the nerve, can be seen immediately after the injury if the nerve is completely transected. However, when motor defects are minor or overshadowed by more striking sensory deficits, the diagnosis can sometimes be overseen, particularly in an incoherent patient. The patient's histories, and understanding of the mechanism of the injury, are therefore important for the evaluation of the injury and identification of those that will be improved by operation. It is important that every patient with a dysfunctional nerve and a wound overlying the course of a nerve is regarded as having a transected nerve until proved otherwise (*Fig. 32.10*).

Functional evaluation

Motor and sensory function should be carefully examined and documented in all patients with injured extremities. Motor evaluation should include pinch and grip strength, and assessment of weakness and atrophy of individual muscles. Sensory function should be evaluated with the patient unable to see what the examiner is doing. Acutely, it may be easy to assess the patient's ability to feel pain, such as that applied by forceps, in the innervation area of an individual nerve such as a digital nerve. Assessment of two-point discrimination and the patient's ability to separate sharp and blunt objects for testing of protective sensation can also be used. Loss of sympathetic function, with vasomotor and sudomotor paralysis, gives the loss of ability to produce sweat in the innervated segment of skin, which will look red, dry, and "polished." Tinel's sign is present, and continuous severe pain over the region of injury usually indicates a more severe injury.

Electromyography/neurography

In case of confusing diagnostic signs, electrophysiological studies can help to establish the diagnosis and to identify injured nerve branches, although the results must be interpreted with caution during the first 3–4 weeks. It may take up to 4 or even 6 weeks after the injury before clearly detectable signs of nerve degeneration and muscular denervation can be detected.[22] It is stressed that waiting for an electrophysiological examination should not delay exploration of an injured nerve if indication for surgery is strong.

Intraoperative conduction studies can be of help, particularly in the case of a previously closed injury that has failed to show satisfactory recovery at follow-up. Intraoperative examination enables a higher grade of specificity as the observed nerve or even individual nerve fascicles can be anatomically isolated, and action potentials across the scarred area can be evaluated.[23] If electrical recovery is recorded over the area of interest the patient can be classified as Sunderland

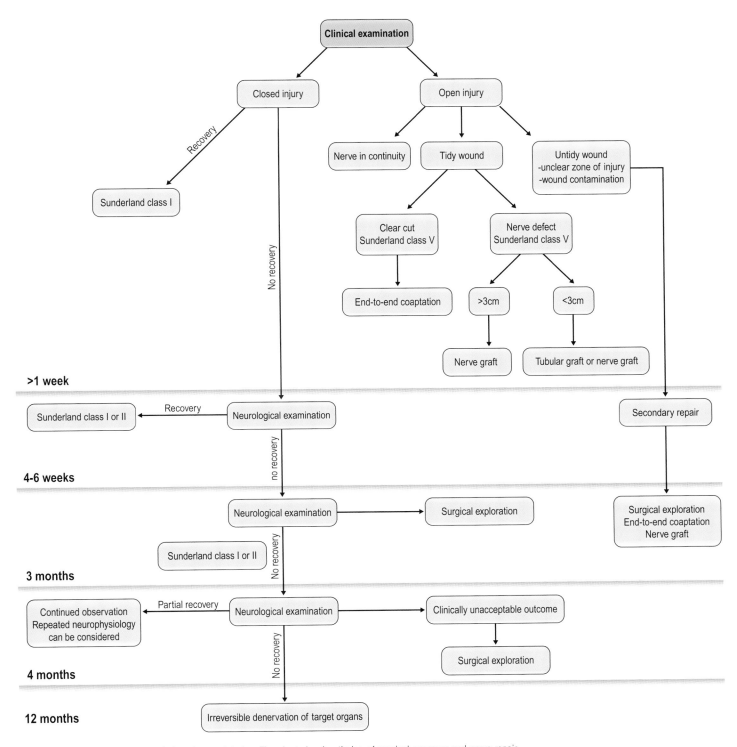

Fig. 32.10 Algorithm for open and closed nerve injuries. Flowchart showing timing of surgical exposure and nerve repair.

grade II or III, in which case spontaneous full recovery is expected. If no electrical recovery can be seen, the patient should be graded Sunderland grade IV and V and will most likely benefit from nerve resection and grafting. However, in the case of a neuroma in continuity (sixth-degree injury), the picture is more complex. Some fascicles will need resection and grafting, whereas others are actually grade II–III and will recover spontaneously. In these cases postoperative outcome may be uncertain and the decision to operate is hard as intervention may result in a tedious and potentially damaging dissection with internal and external neurolysis and resection of damaged sections. However, it may sometimes be possible to distinguish injured fascicles that require nerve grafting from intact healthy fascicles preoperatively. Preoperative electrophysiology is therefore warranted and extremely helpful in decision-making during the procedure.

Wound inspection

Peripheral nerve transections rarely occur in isolation. Depending on the extent of the injury, surrounding structures may be crushed, lacerated, avulsed, or otherwise damaged. Extensive tissue damage and an unclear zone of injury together with a contaminated wound are factors that influence management and may result in delayed neural repair. Extensive debridement and cleaning of the wound are essential for a satisfactory final outcome, and to decrease the risk of a complicating infection and subsequent scarring.

Sharply transected nerves are easier to manage than crushed or avulsed ones. In a sharp transection the zone of injury is limited, and the nerve can usually be prepared and repaired at the primary operation. If, however, the nerve is seriously crushed or longitudinally avulsed, the zone of injury is harder to establish and delayed excision of the damaged nerve followed by repair may improve outcome.

Ideally the repaired nerve should be surrounded by a well-nourished soft-tissue bed, muscle, or fat. In severe cases, this implies that the damaged soft tissues surrounding the injured nerve need to be replaced by a soft-tissue transfer to reconstitute a gliding surface either before secondary reconstruction or in connection with the primary reconstruction.

Patient selection

All patients with a suspected nerve injury should be judged individually as a number of factors must be considered before the decision to explore is made *(Fig. 32.10)*. When one is considering sharp lacerations, traction injuries, blast injuries, or a combination, some key factors must be considered that will be of decisive importance in the timing of operation and the approach, including the type of injury and condition of the wound, and the vascularity of the wound bed.[24,25]

Type of nerve injury

In cases where there are clinical signs of nerve injury but there is no wound, the treatment should be conservative for the first 4–6 weeks, when clinical signs of recovery of function can be investigated. If at this point there has still not been a complete spontaneous recovery, electrophysiological examination can be done. This may be repeated if there is only partial, but insufficient, recovery before any operation is considered. In case of a closed injury where no recovery has been seen at all after 3 months, clinical and electrophysiological examination should be considered.[26] If there are no signs of spontaneous recovery during this period, exploration of the injured nerve is indicated. However, if there is partial recovery during the first 3 months, regular re-evaluation may be indicated for up to another 3 months.[27] The important point is to see if any recovery at all is present.

Nerve injuries with open wounds should always be explored. If the nerve is in continuity it should be treated as a closed injury, and the clinical and electrophysiological function should be evaluated for up to 3 months. In contrast, a clear-cut injury with the nerve ends closely approximated is suitable for immediate repair, whereas a crush injury usually is not. In the latter case, there might be difficulties in distinguishing between viable and nonviable tissue, which would call for careful debridement before any nerve repair is tried. In addition, when the patient presents with signs of an incomplete injury for which there is a chance that spontaneous recovery can yield a better outcome than immediate repair, reconstruction is preferred at a later stage only if the clinical results of conservative treatment are not satisfactory. Therefore, one of the most challenging aspects of a nerve injury will be the decision-making regarding timing of nerve exploration and reconstruction in complex cases, such as open crush injuries or gunshot wounds. In these cases the primary goal should always be to go for careful debridement and viable tissue coverage. Nerve reconstruction can thus only be considered when the surrounding tissue provides a viable environment for the nerve (see Condition of the wound, below). In case of an open injury, where the patient presents with a sensory and/or motor function deficit, but with a macroscopically intact nerve upon surgical exposure, a close follow-up is essential for assessment of the nerve function. Such cases, which include open wound crush injuries and gunshot wounds, should, as the surrounding tissue envelope has healed, be treated the same way as closed traction injuries *(Table 32.2)*. Neurological examination is performed regularly, sometimes together with recurrently performed

Table 32.2 Differing treatments for different types of nerve injury

Type of nerve injury	Neurography/EMG	Exploration	Revision	Repair or reconstruction
Sharp transection	–	Immediate	Immediate	Immediate
Open wound – nerve crush injury	4–6 weeks§	Immediate	Immediate	Immediate* Delayed†
Closed traction injury	4–6 weeks	Delayed	–	3–4 months‡
Open wound –gunshot wound	4–6 weeks§	Immediate	Immediate	Immediate* Delayed†

EMG, electromyogram.

*If there is macroscopic nerve discontinuity on exploration, repair or reconstruction should be performed after repeated revision to ensure that the wound is tidy.

†If there is nerve continuity on exploration, the nerve injury should be treated as a closed injury so that repair or reconstruction is performed only when there is no sign of nerve regeneration (Tinel sign), e.g., for some injuries, exploration after 3–4 months.

‡Repair or reconstruction is performed after 3–4 months if there are no clinical signs of nerve regeneration or reinnervation.

§If the nerve is in continuity on exploration, neurography/EMG can be performed in the same manner as for closed injuries.

neurophysiological testing, and surgery is usually performed if no signs of regeneration or reinnervation occur (e.g., for some injuries, exploration after 3 or 4 months). It is, however, important to stress that all open wounds, where the patient presents with a sensory or motor loss, should be explored in the acute setting, in order to obtain the best outcome.

Condition of the wound

The state of the wound is important. A clean wound calls for an early repair, whereas an untidy wound needs careful debridement to remove nonviable tissue before any nerve reconstruction is undertaken. In severe cases, there may be a need for multiple debridements. In these cases, the nerve repair is better planned as a secondary reconstruction that can be done when other structures have healed with better chances of satisfactory soft-tissue coverage of the reconstructed nerve. Such a reconstruction is preferable within 3 weeks. At the time of re-exploration, the zone of injury is likely to be better defined, and scar tissue can more easily be extracted.

Treatment and surgical techniques

Immediate compared with delayed nerve repair

General principles

Any nerve injury may be repaired immediately, or after a certain delay. If the conditions are favorable, immediate primary suture is the method of choice, resulting in the most favorable outcome,[61] as based on the neurobiological temporally diverse events outlined above. One of the most important prerequisites for primary repair is that it must be completed with little or no tension,[29,30] otherwise a nerve graft should be considered.[31] Several authors have argued that more than 80% of all nerve lesions can be sutured immediately with a primary end-to-end coaptation.[32,33] In these studies, it had to be possible to adapt the nerve endings with a single 9/0 nylon suture, without either separating the endings from each other or tearing the epineurium, to qualify for a primary end-to-end suture.

Primary immediate repair is technically easier than delayed repair, as approximation by rotation of the distal and proximal ends is more obvious when the epineurial vessels are present and clearly visible.[34] The elastic recoil of nerve endings that inevitably occurs as the nerve is injured is also easier to overcome in the acute phase. As time passes, the nerve endings will become embedded in fibrous scar tissue and end-to-end coaptation will be more difficult without tension or more extensive mobilization.

Hints and tips

- Ensure optimal condition of the wound bed
- Careful debridement of injured and lacerated tissue is imperative
- If the zone of injury of the nerve is unclear, go for secondary nerve reconstruction

Timing

Immediate repair is preferable within the first 48 hours, but some authors have suggested that it may also be done successfully during the first 1–3 weeks[35]; however, recent experimental neurobiological data have clearly pointed out the advantage of early nerve repair. This implies that patients who present with uncomplicated open nerve injuries that happened more than 48 hours previously benefit from nerve repair that is delayed in the sense that it is done after the wound has healed completely. Practically, the implication is that the nerve should be repaired as soon as possible, preferably within 2–3 weeks of the injury. The rationale for this approach is to reduce the risk of iatrogenic infection secondary to operation on a contaminated wound. A longer delay will also cause difficulties in doing primary repair due to scar formation and retraction of nerve endings, but most importantly, injured parts of the nerve ends should be resected to obtain viable nerve ends for optimal coaptation.

More than 3 weeks after the injury delayed repair usually involves using a nerve graft, and it can be done several months later, but the regenerative response of neurons and Schwann cells decreases over time (see sections on physiology, above, and autografts, below).

Hints and tips

- Open wounds should always be explored as soon as possible, if a nerve injury is suspected
- Delay in nerve repair or reconstruction causes impaired functional outcome
- If the nerve is in continuity it should be treated as a closed injury

Surgical approach

The incisions follow the general principles of plastic surgery in that the main objective is to prevent contractures and scars in areas of maximum sensory perception (*Fig. 32.11*). Wide exposure is often recommended to obtain a detailed anatomical overview, and it offers a safer dissection as the area of injury can be approached from healthy tissue outside the zone

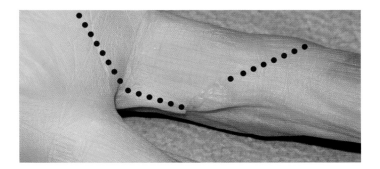

Fig. 32.11 Small stab wound on the radial side of the index finger. Loss of sensation distal to the wound calls for exploration. A modified Bruner incision is used.

of injury. This often means that the traumatic wound needs to be extending proximally and distally, which is particularly important in secondary reconstructions.

Hints and tips

- Wide exposure and careful dissection to obtain well-vascularized tissue flap are vital for nerve coverage
- Approach the nerve injury from viable tissue – thus, "from the known to the unknown"
- Use of a tourniquet is always advised

Principles of nerve repair

General principles

Video 1

Video 2

Proper and thorough microsurgical technical skills are crucial in nerve repair. An atraumatic approach with minimal tissue damage, using microsurgical instruments under either loupe magnification or a microscope, is essential.

Firstly, the injured nerve ends must be identified. Nonviable tissue must be resected, preferably with a surgical blade or using microsurgical scissors, to allow visualization of healthy fascicles that help the adaptation in primary nerve repair (*Figs 32.12–32.14*). When repairing a nerve it is preferable to align the nerve according to its fascicular pattern, which may help topographical arrangement and improve outcome. If later reconstruction is planned (secondary reconstruction), the nerve ends may be tagged with a nonresorbable suture, and sutured to other structures in the wound. This is primarily to prevent the retraction of the nerve that inevitably happens after transection, but also to facilitate identification at a secondary procedure. If the nerve is allowed to retract, it will become tethered in fibrous scar tissue and lose its elasticity and normal excursion. The normal longitudinal excursion of the nerve needs to be taken into consideration, as the immediate demand for suitable length will depend on it. The normal excursion of the median and ulnar nerves is thought to be around 1.5 cm at the wrist when taking the wrist from full extension to full flexion.[36,37] This length should preferably be added to the nerve deficit when estimating the total defect and assessing whether a nerve graft is needed or not. In a primary repair, the longitudinal extension is retained and the nerve can therefore be approximated with minimal tension.

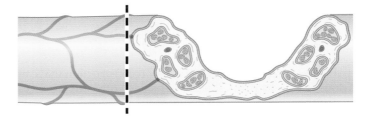

Fig. 32.12 A lacerated nerve and the cut-off line for debridement. The dashed line illustrates suggested resection line to reach healthy nerve tissue.

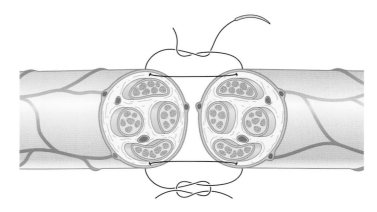

Fig. 32.13 Standard epineurial repair with nylon sutures. To get proper fascicular alignment, nerve endings are aligned based on the pattern of the blood vessels within the epineurium.

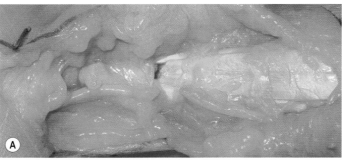

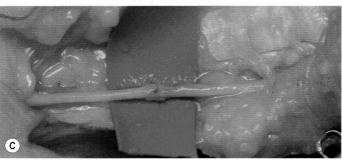

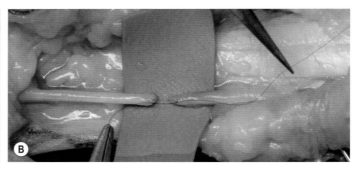

Fig. 32.14 Peripheral nerve repair of a digital nerve using standard epineurial end-to-end coaptation. **(A)** Nerve injury with minimal gap. **(B)** Epineurial suture. **(C)** Complete coaptation with minimal tension.

Secondly, the ultimate aim is a tension-free repair to enable the nerve to heal in optimal conditions. Usually, some dissection of the nerve trunk is necessary to achieve this. Even a small elongation through longitudinal traction will have a potentially devastating effect on the vascular supply to the nerve endings, as stretching of a nerve trunk has been shown to impair intraneural microcirculation.[38] Nerve blood flow decreases approximately 50%, with substantial recovery in 30 minutes after 8% elongation, whereas 15% elongation produced approximately an 80% reduction in blood flow with minimal recovery.[29] Some dissection of the nerve trunks proximal and distal to the injury is therefore often needed to alleviate tension, and this can be done without interfering with the segmentally approaching blood vessels. Other means of alleviating tension, such as transposing the ulnar nerve anteriorly, and therefore increasing excursion over the elbow, can be considered to enable a tension-free direct suture. It is, however, important to bear in mind that mobilization by dissection can theoretically impair the blood supply to the nerve endings. This issue has been an issue of debate,[39–41] although clinical experience from ulnar nerve transposition points to the fact that intraneural microcirculation can resist considerable mobilization, and that gentle handling of the nerve can be acceptable.[40,41]

As complete lesions almost always result in some retraction of the nerve endings there is in most instances a gap between the ends that makes a completely tension-free suture rare. The nerve endings generally need trimming, which means that some nerve tissue has to be resected to reach viable parts. Under the microscope this is seen as "mushrooming" of the fascicles together with slight retraction of the epineurium from the neural stumps (Fig. 32.15B). It is hard to give a general rule for how much tension is acceptable in each individual case, but if flexion of a joint is necessary to shorten the distance between the nerve ends, the resulting tension will usually be too great, and further dissection or nerve grafting should be considered (Figs 32.16A and 32.17A).

Thirdly, the nerve endings should be rotated to their correct positions by matching fascicles, branches, or the longitudinal epineurial vessels of the two nerve endings, which decreases the risk of mismatch between bundles of axons (Figs 32.15A and 32.18). Correct coaptation facilitates a good postoperative outcome.

Nerve endings are commonly coapted with interrupted 9/0 or 10/0 nylon sutures. It is generally thought that a minimal amount of suture material is preferable, and the number of sutures should be no greater than the minimum number required to ensure coaptation of the nerve stumps. It is important that the nerve ends are not closed too tightly so that the fascicles become malaligned and crumple in the process.[42] Outward-pointing fascicles are sometimes found, and should be cut with microscissors. They are then able to retract to within the coaptation and will subsequently probably be able to regenerate sufficiently.

Other means, apart from nylon sutures, of maintaining the primary repair can be considered, particularly if the repair is to be made by a relatively inexperienced surgeon. The use of fibrin glue as an alternative, or as an adjunct, to epineurial sutures has been evaluated in rats after transection of the sciatic nerve.[43,44] The results showed that fibrin glue is as good as suturing in experienced hands, and superior to sutures when the surgeon is inexperienced[43].

Hints and tips

- Proper magnification, appropriate equipment, and microsurgical skills are crucial
- Resect nonviable tissue carefully, possibly stepwise, to visualize healthy nerve endings – look for mushrooming
- Important with tension-free coaptation – if flexion of joints is needed, consider nerve reconstruction
- Aim at fascicular match – look for intraneural vessels to help the alignment in repair and reconstruction

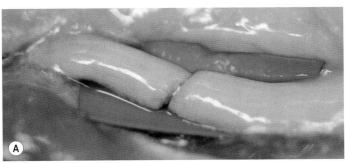
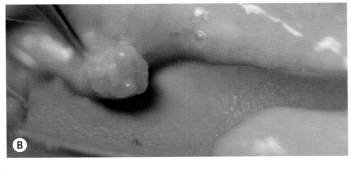
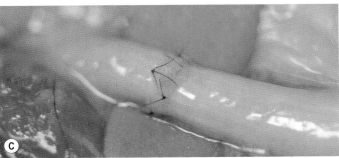

Fig. 32.15 Patient with a median nerve injury that is repaired with standard epineurial end-to-end coaptation at minimal tension. (A) Nerve injury with minimal gap. (B) Mushrooming seen when healthy nerve tissue is reached after resection. (C) Complete coaptation with minimal tension.

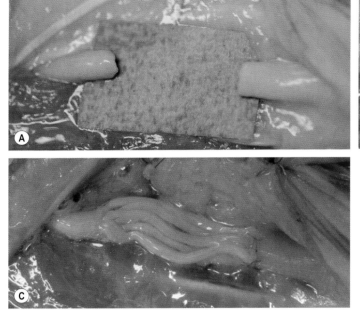

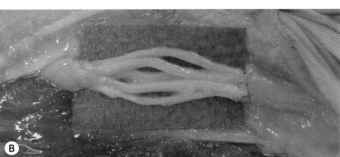

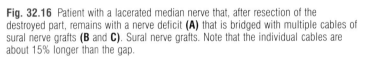

Fig. 32.16 Patient with a lacerated median nerve that, after resection of the destroyed part, remains with a nerve deficit **(A)** that is bridged with multiple cables of sural nerve grafts **(B** and **C)**. Sural nerve grafts. Note that the individual cables are about 15% longer than the gap.

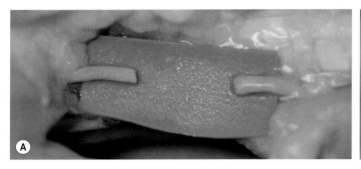

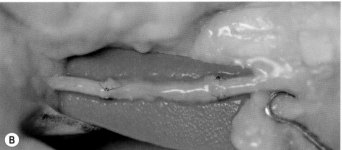

Fig. 32.17 **(A)** Digital nerve laceration. **(B)** The nerve gap was bridged with a single autograft from the lateral cutaneous antebrachial nerve.

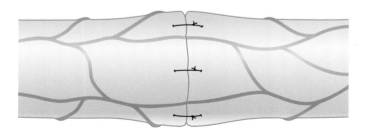

Fig. 32.18 End-to-end coaptation. Note that the epineurial vessels match.

Epineurial compared with fascicular repair

The nerve trunks may be adapted either at the level of the epineurium *(Fig. 32.12)* or the fascicles *(Fig. 32.19)*. Which method is preferable has been a matter of debate, probably because the scientific evidence is not entirely clear as the data are based on experimental studies in rats and primates with their inherent methodological problems.[45,46]

The theoretical advantage of the fascicular repair over the epineurial repair is that it facilitates regeneration with a better chance of keeping the axonal specificity to sensor or motor end organs. However, fascicular repair requires a more

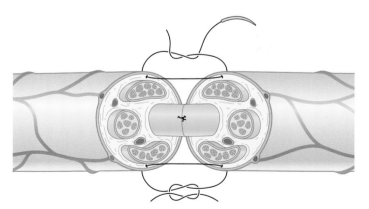

Fig. 32.19 Group fascicular repair with nylon sutures. Corresponding groups of fascicles are sutured through the interfascicular epineurium.

profound dissection to identify the individual fascicles at the two ends, which in turn may increase the risk of compromising the vascular supply. An epineurial repair with careful rotation of the nerve trunks is therefore thought to be as effective, particularly more distally. The dissection is technically more difficult as the individual fascicles are hard to identify

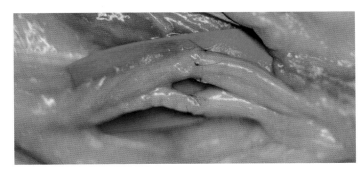

Fig. 32.20 Ulnar nerve injury at the wrist level. Note how the motor and sensory fascicles are anatomically separated. A group fascicular coaptation is performed.

clearly distally. A group fascicular adaptation is preferable, for example with lesions of the ulnar nerve at the wrist. Great care should be taken to make sure that sensory and motor fascicles are located both proximally and distally through dissection, and coapted separately *(Fig. 32.20)*.

End-to-side nerve repair

When conventional surgical methods are unavailable, particularly if the proximal stump is absent, or after injuries to nerve proximally in the extremity (such as in high ulnar nerve injuries), the distal end of an injured nerve can be attached to an "uninjured" donor nerve.[47,48] Collateral or terminal sprouting of donor nerve axons occurs, and donor site morbidity associated with the harvest of a nerve graft is avoided. In addition, the distance traveled by regenerating axons to reach their targets is shortened. Theoretically this implies that a single neuron possesses the ability to innervate two targets, but one of the branches is probably pruned away.[48] Several studies have indicated that the outgrowth of axons from the donor nerve requires an axonal injury to induce sprouting.[49] At present, experimental and clinical experience with end-to-side coaptation has at best achieved mixed results, depending on the type of reinnervated nerve and donor nerve. More extensive clinical and laboratory experiments are presently produced, which is required before end-to-side suturing generally can be included with the more established techniques of nerve repair.[50] However, for reinnervation of muscles from motor donor nerves the end-to-side technique have been reported to be useful.[51]

Wound closure and immobilization

The wound should be closed with interrupted sutures and a local anesthetic may be given before dressing. It is preferably given through a blunt cannula inserted between the stitches. Sharp needles should be avoided to reduce the risk of

neurovascular damage proximal to the injury if the site of repair/reconstruction is located superficially.

A plaster should be applied, primarily to restrict excessive movement, avoiding tension in the repair, and still allow some range of movement for controlled early mobilization. The plaster should position the extremity in such a way that it both releases tension and prevents excessive movement. For digital nerve injuries, the wrist is immobilized at 30° of flexion and the metacarpophalangeal joints at 70°. The splint is usually extended just past the proximal interphalangeal joints to prevent hyperextension. Immobilization with plaster of Paris, with controlled restricted range of movement, is usually maintained for 3 weeks before full range of movement is allowed in digital nerve repairs. In repairs of larger nerve trunks a prolonged protection of the suture line may be recommended up to 6 weeks postoperatively, to avoid extensive extension of the wrist or elbow.

Nerve reconstruction

Autografts

Nerve reconstruction involves the use of a nerve graft to overcome a lack of continuity after an injury *(Figs 32.16 and 32.17)*. The use of autologous grafts is still the method of choice despite the fact that other strategies, such as nerve and muscle allografts, or synthetic materials, have been proposed, but they demand a more complex approach than a primary nerve repair to be successful.

The rationale for using a nerve autograft in reconstruction is to alleviate all tension at the site of suture. If tension is completely avoided, axonal sprouting to cross the two sites of repair will be easier than over a primary repair site under unfavorable conditions.[52] The axonal outgrowth through the nerve graft depends on the diameter of the graft and the vascularity of the tissue bed. The selection of donor nerve will therefore be much influenced by size, as survival is dependent on diffusion from the surrounding tissues. Neovascularization will occur through capillary ingrowth from the periphery and nerve ends.[52,53] Smaller nerves (for example, the sural, and the medial and lateral antebrachial cutaneous nerves) will therefore revascularize easily, and thicker nerves will carry the risk of central necrosis and scarring as a result of poor diffusion. Only one cable is needed when smaller nerves, such as digital nerves, are bridged *(Fig. 32.17)*, whereas multiple cables may be needed to bridge the gap in larger damaged nerve trunks *(Figs 32.16 and 32.21)*.

Approach and preparation

The initial steps in preparing the nerve tissue are no different from those for primary nerve repair. However, when the ends are being resected to create a clean-cut surface, it is important

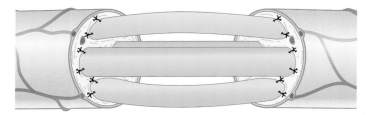

Fig. 32.21 Schematic presentation of autograft repair. Each segment is coapted to the corresponding group of fascicles of the nerve endings. Note how the individual grafts are applied quite loosely.

Table 32.3 Common nerves used as autografts

Donor nerve	Length (cm)	Sensory defect
Sural nerve	30–40 cm	Dorsal aspect of lower leg and lateral foot
Medial antebrachial cutaneous nerve	10–12 cm* 8–10 cm†	Medial forearm
Lateral antebrachial cutaneous nerve	10–12 cm	Lateral forearm
Superficial sensory branch of the radial nerve	25 cm	Radial dorsal hand

*Above elbow.
†Below elbow.

to expose the nerve carefully, including the whole zone of injury. This enables proper evaluation of the viability and vascularization of the nerve and surrounding tissues. In crush or high-velocity injuries, this principle is central. As with all tissue injuries in which the zone of injury is not clear, late effects on viability call for second looks and re-evaluations. When the nerve is explored after the surrounding tissue has healed, it is important to remove any scar tissue carefully, or preferably to approach the nerve lesion through a separate incision. This includes raising a flap that at closure of the wound will enable good tissue coverage.

Nerve ends

A good way to find out whether the nerve endings are viable is to look for "mushrooming" (*Fig. 32.15B*), which is a sign of transected viable axons that will be able to sprout after reconstruction from the resection site, indicating that the nerve is a suitable recipient for a nerve graft.

The gap

To harvest a proper graft it is essential to calculate the maximum gap that is going to be bridged, and this has to be done in relation to any movement of a joint that might occur later on.

Length of graft

Because the graft may shrink slightly, it should be about 15% longer than the maximum gap.[54] Nerve excursion must be considered, and length is best assessed with all adjacent joints fully extended (or in certain cases such as radial nerve injury at upper arm, in a flexed position).

Harvest of the graft

The size of the nerve trunk to be bridged is the main factor to be considered when deciding which donor nerve will be most suitable to use as a graft. Donor site morbidity and functional deficit also have to be considered when choosing the proper donor nerve (*Table 32.3*). Patients should be well informed about these aspects before the harvest. The most common grafts are the sural nerve, the medial antebrachial cutaneous nerve, the lateral antebrachial cutaneous nerve, or the terminal branch of the posterior interosseous nerve.

Gentle handling is of great importance and must follow the same principles as handling of all nerves. As the graft is harvested, great care must be taken that it is kept moist in a gauze soaked in saline. The grafts are sharply cut to proper length

and a few millimeters of extra epineurium is removed from the ends of the graft.

Coaptation and maintenance

The nerve graft is preferably reversed at the time of placement to decrease the risk of diversion of regenerating axons through these cut-off branches. Depending on the size of the nerve trunk, the whole nerve or individual fascicles can be sutured using 9/0 or 10/0 nylon, if possible with fibrin glue as an adjunct. A sufficient number of fascicles are used to bridge the defect, preferably with one cable for each severed group of fascicles (*Figs 32.16C and 32.21*). The coaptation should not be too tight, as this can easily lead to crumpled nerve endings. Fibrin glue may be interposed to reinforce and lessen the risk of separation between the graft and nerve endings. Fibrin glue may also give an instant better match between the graft and the nerve end. The number of sutures should be kept to one or two. If multiple cables are used, the individual grafts are positioned so that they do not adhere too closely to each other. This is to allow diffusion of oxygen and other nutrients, and allow for rapid revascularization from the recipient bed. It must be stressed therefore that the viability of the tissue bed is of crucial importance for optimal survival of Schwann cells and successful axonal regeneration.

Donor nerves

Sural nerve

The sural nerve is often thought to be the main donor nerve for free grafting, because it can easily be harvested in lengths between 30 and 40 cm[55]; it originates from the tibial nerve dorsal to the knee joint (*Fig. 32.22*), and it has communicating branches from the peroneal nerve at levels distal to this. These communicating branches need to be identified and transected before the nerve is pulled out.

The sural nerve is identified through a short longitudinal incision halfway between the lateral malleolus and the Achilles tendon. If the nerve is gently pulled distally, the proximal course of the nerve can be palpated and extracted through 3–5 small transverse incisions that usually pose a minor aesthetic problem for the patient (*Fig. 32.23*).

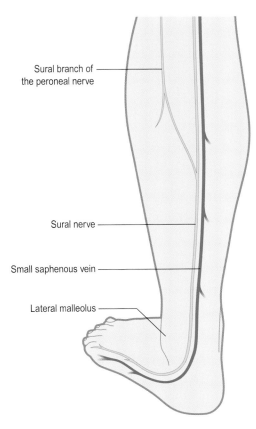

Sural branch of
the peroneal nerve

Sural nerve

Small saphenous vein

Lateral malleolus

Fig. 32.22 Course of the sural nerve in the lower leg, shown in orange.

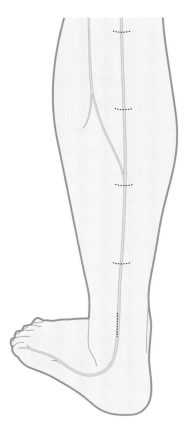

Fig. 32.23 Incisions to enable harvest of the sural nerve, shown by dotted lines.

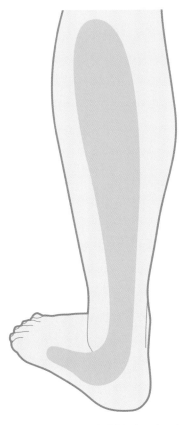

Fig. 32.24 Area of diminished or absent sensation after harvest of the sural nerve.

Alternatively a long dorsal incision can be used, which enables an easier dissection of the nerve and its small branches. It is preferable to cut the nerve beneath the fascia to reduce the risk of a troublesome neuroma. Nerve strippers can be used and endoscopic harvest has been suggested to reduce aesthetic morbidity at the donor site.[56] The area of diminished or absent sensation after the graft has been harvested is shown in *Figure 32.24*, but is usually considered to be of minor importance to the patient.

Medial and lateral antebrachial cutaneous nerves

The medial cutaneous nerve can be harvested from the distal border of the axillary groove to below the elbow (10–12 cm). In the forearm it is located medially (8–10 cm), close to the brachial vein, where it divides into three branches *(Fig. 32.25)*. These branches correspond well in size to digital nerves. The consequences are usually of minor importance to the patient *(Fig. 32.26)*.

The lateral cutaneous nerve (10–12 cm) is the terminal branch of the musculocutaneous nerve. It is identified at the lateral border of the biceps tendon where it parallels the cephalic vein *(Fig. 32.27)*.

A few short incisions are generally sufficient to harvest these nerves adequately. The consequences are usually regarded as more troublesome for the patient after lateral antebrachial cutaneous nerve harvest than after harvest of the medial antebrachial cutaneous nerve *(Figs 32.28 and 32.29)*.

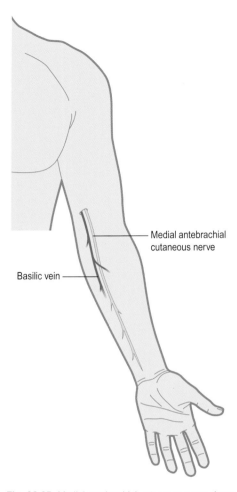

Fig. 32.25 Medial antebrachial cutaneous nerve shown in orange, and basilic vein.

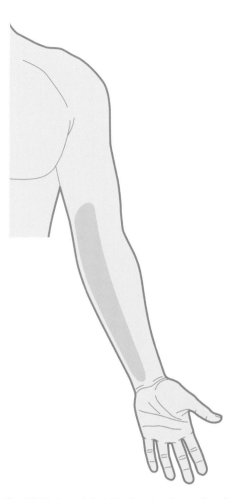

Fig. 32.26 Area of diminished or absent sensation after harvest of the medial antebrachial cutaneous nerve.

The terminal branch of the posterior interosseous nerve

The terminal branch of the posterior interosseous nerve is simple to harvest dorsally just proximal to the wrist, lying on the interosseous membrane. Generally, one can harvest a 4–5-cm long segment (1–3 fascicles), which may fit into a small digital nerve defect. Harvest causes no complications or loss of function.

Superficial sensory branch of the radial nerve

The superficial sensory branch is formed as the radial nerve is divided into a deep (the posterior interosseous nerve) and a superficial branch at the elbow level. The superficial branch runs beneath the brachioradialis muscle to surface distally about 8 cm from the tip of the radial styloid between the tendon of brachioradialis and the tendon of extensor carpi radialis *(Fig. 32.30)*. It provides a 25-cm-long nerve graft, but is rarely used because it tends to cause painful neuromas. It is primarily used when large quantities of nerve grafts are needed in brachial plexus injuries. In the presence of a median or ulnar nerve injury it is considered a relative contraindication to use it as a donor for nerve grafts *(Fig. 32.31)*.

Other

The saphenous nerve (40 cm) has been used primarily in plexus injuries and as a vascularized nerve graft. The lateral femoral cutaneous nerve (20 cm) can be used as a last choice, but has the disadvantages of comparatively large sensory loss, and painful neuromas.

Tubular repair and artificial conduits

Autologous nerve grafts are still considered to be the gold standard for bridging defects in nerves. The superiority in outcome is thought to be mainly the result of their ability to provide a biocompatible scaffold that contains both Schwann cells and their basal lamina. These factors promote regeneration through natural production of growth factors and adhesion molecules, which will help stimulate neurite elongation and direction on site.[57] However, there are disadvantages with autografts, some of which have been mentioned above. Harvesting requires an extra surgical incision to obtain an otherwise healthy sensory nerve. There are limited sources of graft material, and the injured nerve and donor nerve may be mismatched at grafting.[58]

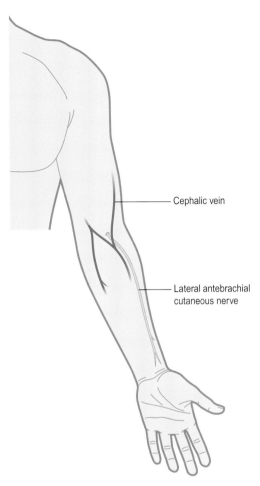

Fig. 32.27 Lateral antebrachial cutaneous nerve shown in orange and cephalic vein.

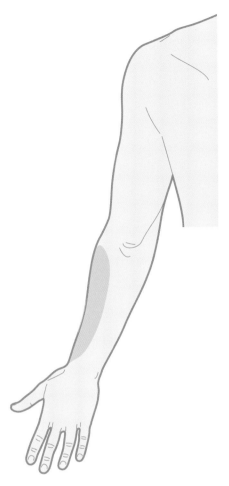

Fig. 32.28 Area of diminished or absent sensation after harvest of the dorsal aspect of the lateral antebrachial cutaneous nerve.

Our present inability to gain full functional recovery with autografts has been the main driving force behind the development of alternative means to bridge nerve defects. Tissue engineering has in recent years offered the opportunity to develop biodegradable guiding materials with tailored properties that imitate normal biological features. Structural stability is enabled, and both growth factors and supportive cells, such as Schwann cells or stem cells, can be added to give physical guidance to the regenerating axons. However, the latter procedure is far from clinical practice, but may be a possibility in the future. Formation of a longitudinally oriented fibrin matrix and accumulation of various tropic and trophic factors will ensue within the conduit, and this will further improve the physical conditions for nerve regeneration. Obviously, donor morbidity after graft harvest will be eliminated.

Biological conduits

The first attempt to bridge a nerve defect with a tube was published by Glück, who used a piece of decalcified bone to bridge a nerve gap.[59] Since then several biological scaffolds have been used, including veins,[60,61] arteries,[62] muscles,[62] tendons,[63] and combinations such as vein–muscle grafts,[64,65] and acellular nerve allografts,[66–68] with variable outcomes. The main theoretical advantage of using biological constructs with a core matrix is the availability of a longitudinally oriented basal lamina and extracellular matrix components that direct and improve the regeneration of axons. In contrast, bridging methods using only tubular material such as vein grafts or nondegradable or degradable nerve conduits (several are commercially available) lack this function and may be less attractive, at least theoretically. The use of composite biological conduits, such as combinations of veins and muscles, has therefore been explored. The main rationale for using this combination, apart from it being of autologous origin, has been that a collapse of the vein is prevented by filling the lumen, and that the vessel wall prevents the risk of axons sprouting outside the muscle. Nerve regeneration is propagated along the longitudinally oriented muscle fibers and no foreign material is used in the bridging process. Another approach reported is to use decellularized chondroitinase-processed nerve allografts, which are also commercially available.[67–69]

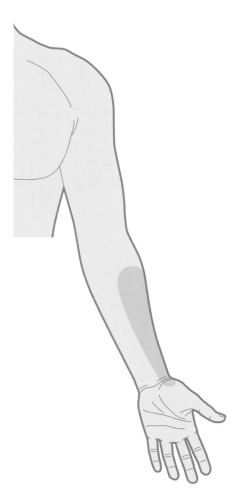

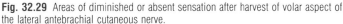

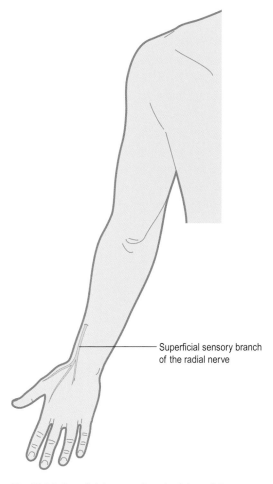

Superficial sensory branch of the radial nerve

Fig. 32.29 Areas of diminished or absent sensation after harvest of volar aspect of the lateral antebrachial cutaneous nerve.

Fig. 32.30 Superficial sensory branch of the radial nerve.

Nondegradable conduits

The first artificial conduits used in preclinical and human trials were composed of nonresorbable polymers based on silicone and polytetrafluoroethylene[70,71] *(Fig. 32.32)*. Silicone was chosen because of its inert material properties and because it is tolerated well by the recipient.[72] It has been used successfully in hand surgery for arthroplasty and two-stage tendon-grafting procedures for the last two decades. As silicone tubes are nondegradable and impermeable to large molecules, they also provide the necessary biological isolation from scar-forming elements of the wound and allow for accumulation of growth factors. A longitudinally oriented fibrin matrix containing macrophages is formed and there is migration of Schwann cells, ingrowth of axons, and neovascularization of the newly formed nerve trunk. Silicone tubes were used in a clinical prospective randomized study that compared tube repair and microsurgical nerve repair in median and ulnar nerve injuries.[73] Results showed no significant differences in outcome between the two methods, except for a decrease in cold intolerance in the conduit group at the 5-year follow-up.[74] The authors concluded that tubular repair may be preferable in the future when appropriate bioresorbable materials are available. However, utilization of a silicone tube is not an alternative when there is a nerve defect.

Biodegradable conduits

Increasing interest has turned towards the use of biodegradable materials as conduits. Ideally, the material from which the tube is made should be highly biocompatible and allow degradation to nontoxic end products. They should be mechanically stable, yet still flexible and porous to ensure supply of nutrients and provide a microenvironment that allows for the production of functional tissue.[57,75,76]

Polymer-based materials, such as collagen, polyglycolic acid polymer, and polylactide-caprolactone polymer and other available materials, offer a high degree of flexibility in chemical and physical properties and are available commercially. Future inclusion of fillers, such as Schwann cells, or incorporation of biologically active substances in the polymers that are released as the tube is degraded are areas of massive research. Yet, presently, clinical experience in terms of randomized trials is lacking,[77] although increasing numbers of studies have reported promising results regarding recovery of both sensory[78–80] and motor function.[81,82]

of cellular components, such as Schwann cells[84] and stem cells,[85] can further be used to improve the regeneration by creating a more optimal microenvironment. In the future, it is possible that "off-the-shelf" conduits may be filled with autologous supporting cells that are harvested and immediately prepared from the patient's injured nerve segments.[86]

Other techniques

Preclinical studies have indicated that shorter digital nerve defects can be bridged by applying longitudinal resorbable sutures that will act as a guide for the fibrin matrix that is formed to fill the defect. Schwann cells and axons will follow this matrix and thereby overcome the defect. The newly formed nerve trunk, which can be made in a branched pattern, is subsequently surrounded by a new perineurium-like structure and provides functional recovery.[87]

Nerve transfers

In recent years there has been an increasing interest in the use of nerve transfers in nerve reconstruction. This technique has primarily been used in brachial plexus injuries, and is based on the assumption that less important nerves can be sacrificed, transected, and rerouted to be attached to a functionally more important nerve segment.[88,89] It can also be used after other proximal nerve injuries, and the procedure transfers a proximal nerve injury to a distal one. The topic is further discussed in Chapter 33.

Postoperative care

General aspects

The role of early active mobilization after microsurgical nerve repair has been debated. It has been hypothesized that it may cause a change in tension at the site of nerve repair, which in turn will result in impaired functional outcome.[90,91] Experimental studies have indicated that intraneural scarring at the repair site can impede revascularization and reduce axonal regeneration across the suture line as a result of tension.[30,92] However, immobilization may result in an increase in scar tissue that surrounds the reconstructed nerve. Tethering of the nerve by scar tissue may lead to additional pain on movement.[93] Maintenance of full range of movement of the neuromuscular unit and preservation of movement of small joints are of importance in the postoperative phase. Intermittent, controlled mobilization in a protected splint is therefore thought to be beneficial for the patient. Most importantly, the nerve grafts should be applied at minimal tension with joints in an extended position and in a manner that allows subsequent full range of motion without causing tension over the repair sites. Surgeons should supervise physiotherapy, check advancement of Tinel's sign and return of muscle function, which is recovered during rehabilitation.

Postoperative movement training

Dorsal splinting may be maintained for 3 weeks in a manner that allows intermittent early gentle mobilization within a protected range without putting the microsurgical repair at

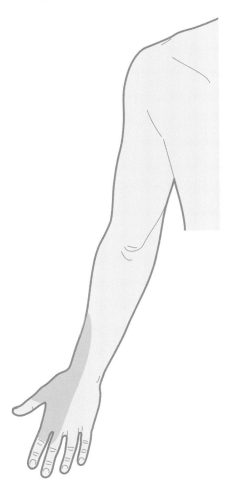

Fig. 32.31 Area of diminished or absent sensation after harvest of the superficial sensory branch of the radial nerve.

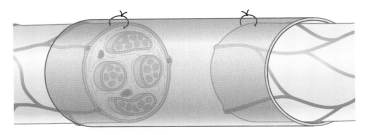

Fig. 32.32 A nerve defect bridged by a nerve conduit.

Fillers

The main purpose of inserting filler structures in the conduits, whether in the form of guidance channels, hydrogels, or others, is to apply haptotatic cues (contact-mediated) to support axonal regeneration or chemotactic cues (diffusible) to guide the regenerating axons.[83] The most commonly used haptotatic cues are extracellular matrix proteins, such as collagen, laminin, and fibronectin. Neurotrophic factors, such as nerve growth factor, glial-derived neurotrophic factor, and neurotrophin NT-3, are additives that act as chemotactic cues that will promote neuronal regrowth and sprouting.[57] Addition

risk or tension. Although some authors have advocated that the nerve should be allowed to rest for 8 days before active and passive mobilization,[31] an earlier start to training may be appropriate within the limits of bandages and restrictive splinting. It is thought that early active movements may reduce the risk of the nerve being tethered in scar tissue,[54,93] which is a possible effect if rigid immobilization is adopted. Elevation of the hand is recommended for the first week postoperatively. Sutures and plaster are usually removed at 3 weeks and active exercises of the fingers can then be initiated. Prolonged protection of the suture line may be recommended up to 6 weeks postoperatively, to avoid extensive extension in the wrist. These general principles apply for digital nerves as well as major nerve trunks and nerve grafts.

Sensory re-education

Cortical reorganization

After an acute nerve transection the brain must compensate for the loss of sensory input. First, a gross decrease in the number of fibers is seen, as well as a topographical mismatch. A "silent area" is created in the nerve's representational area in the brain. However, adjacent cortical areas expand instantly and occupy this former nerve territory.[94–97] These changes are mediated by the unmasking of normally inhibited synaptic connections in the vicinity of this "silent area," and a reorganization of the somatosensory cortex occurs through processes of brain plasticity. This period is referred to as phase 1 during rehabilitation – before any reinnervation has occurred in the hand. During this phase some training may be initiated.

Because of the mismatch and misdirection of the regenerating axons that happens at the repair site, areas of skin in the hand and muscles will not be reinnervated by their original axons to a large extent.[98] The original well-organized hand representation in the sensory and motor cortex alters into a distorted and mosaic-like pattern with disappearance of, and overlapping of, fingers.[94] As a result of misdirection and remapping of the representation of the cortical hand, "the hand speaks a new language to the brain" (phase 2 during rehabilitation). A sensory relearning program that helps the brain to decipher the signals may assist it in interpreting the new language, which works well and improves outcome.[99] Recent data have indicated that it is beneficial for this process to begin when the reorganization in the sensory cortex has already started (phase 1)[96] and that this should not be postponed until touch can be perceived in the hand, as was earlier believed. Effectiveness in the relearning process is probably greatly influenced by the individual motivation of each patient. Coping strategies that are individualized for each patient should be considered, as adaptation to the condition is an evolving process by which the patient's own resources can be used to overcome problems in daily activities.

Sensory re-education in phase 1

During the early postoperative period (phase 1), various "baby-sitting" methods can be used until the hand becomes reinnervated by the outgrowing axons. Functional similarities exist between perception and imagery (the premotor cortex can be activated by just imagining a movement – so-called motor imagery). The corresponding phenomenon for sensory function is "sensor imagery." Imagining touching of the hand activates the same cortical areas as if the hand is really being touched.

Activation of "mirror motor neurons" in the premotor cortex by mere observation of hand motor actions by others plays a fundamental part in action, imitation, and action understanding.[100] Reading or listening to action words related to hand movements activates hand representational areas in the motor cortex and observation of touching a hand activates the corresponding representational areas in the sensory cortex. The patient's observation of the denervated hand being touched is already initiated during the first days postoperatively, which may activate the cortical hand area as a result of visuotactile interaction.

In early sensory training, the multimodality of the brain is activated; the cortical audiotactile interaction is used to activate cortical sensory areas by listening to the sound of touch. A sensor glove, provided with minimicrophones at its fingertips, can be applied to the denervated hand.[101] Active touch of items is associated with a specific "friction sound," depending on the texture touched, which is transmitted to earphones. The patient can "listen to what the hand feels." If the sensor glove is used in the early phase after nerve repair, tactile discrimination may be improved considerably.

Improving effects of sensory re-education – phase 2

A relearning process is required to adapt to the new and distorted afferent sensory input caused by axonal misdirection when familiar objects are touched. For this purpose, sensory re-education is routinely used in phase 2, when the hand has started to reinnervate, to regain tactile gnosis. Ways of touching, and the capacity to localize touch, are trained, followed by touching and exploration of items, presenting shape and textures of varying and increasing difficulty with eyes open and closed. Vision assists training and improves the deficient sense.

Repeated sessions of cutaneous anesthesia of the forearm increase the effects of sensory re-education and result in expansion of representation of the cortical hand[102] *(Fig. 32.33)*. The hand is given more "brain space," which enables the improved processing of sensory impulses. Repeated application of a cutaneous anesthetic cream (lidocaine/prilocaine: EMLA), combined with intensive sensory re-education, increases the effects of sensory re-education with a considerable improvement in tactile gnosis (functional sensibility) in patients with repaired median nerves.[103]

Outcome

Assessment of outcome

Final evaluation of sensory and motor function should not be made until after rehabilitation has finished. Depending on the type of injury, the rehabilitation period may last for 12–24 months postoperatively to allow for reinnervation and sensory re-education,[104] although some authors claim that a follow-up time of at least 3 years is necessary to evaluate the final outcome.[105]

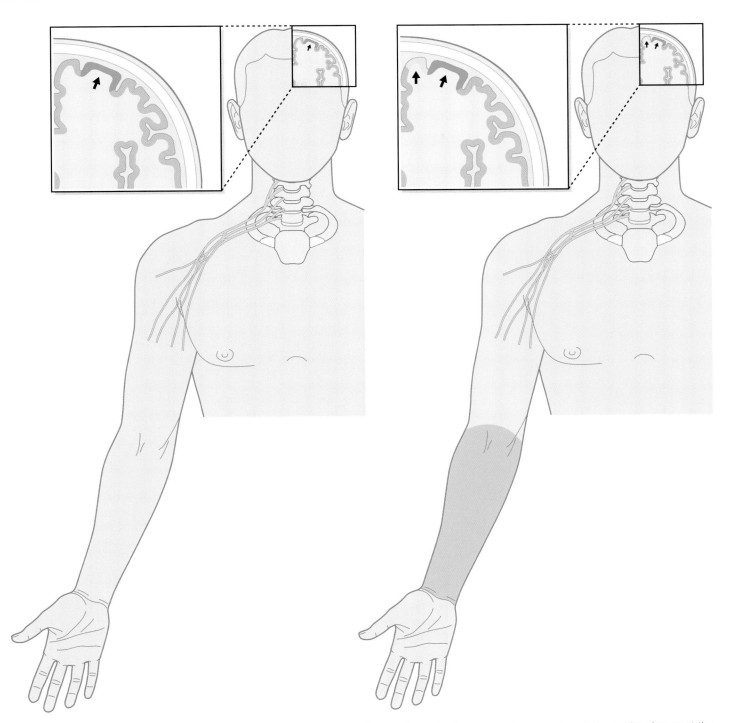

Fig. 32.33 Brain plasticity. Repeated sessions of cutaneous anesthesia of the forearm increase the effects of sensory re-education and result in expansion of representation of the cortical hand. The hand is given more "brain space," which enables the improved processing of sensory impulses.

General aspects

Even though extensive amounts of data have been published on the results of nerve repair, there is no consensus on how to evaluate the outcome in a standardized manner. Different protocols for assessing the outcome have been proposed,[104,106–108] but none has been adapted uniformly. The evaluation instrument most widely accepted is the Highet Scale from 1954, adopted by the British Medical Research Council (*Table 32.4*).

The outcome after nerve repair depends on to what extent the regeneration of the axons is successful, and how many of the axons reach their end target. Several factors that influence the results after nerve repair have been documented.

Table 32.4 The Highet Scale from 1954, adopted by the British Medical Research Council (MRC)

Motor grade	Level of recovery
M0	No recovery
M1	Perceptible contraction in proximal muscles
M2	Perceptible contraction in proximal and distal muscles
M3	Contraction possible against gravity
M4	Contraction possible against resistance
M5	Full recovery in all muscles
Sensory grade	Level of recovery
S0	No recovery
S1	Recovery of deep cutaneous sensibility
S1+	Recovery of superficial pain and sensibility
S2	Recovery of superficial pain and some touch
S2+	S2 recovery with hypersensitivity
S3	Recovery of pain and touch without hypersensitivity
S3+	S3 recovery with localization and some two-point discrimination
S4	Complete recovery with normal two-point discrimination

BMRC

Several modifications of the British Medical Research Council's scale (BMRC) for nerve recovery have been described,[109] and the modification by Dellon et al. is probably the most used.[110] The sensory function is evaluated according to how the patient describes levels of recovery *(Table 32.1)*. Critics claim that the BMRC scale is based on subjective findings without any attempt to standardize defined methods of evaluation, which complicates our ability to compare different sets of patients as well as results from different observers.

The Rosen score

To enable improved interpretation of patients' functional outcome after nerve repair (median and ulnar nerves), Rosen and Lundborg presented a protocol that illustrated patients' functional limitation in activities of daily living.[107] This protocol is based on previous studies that investigated what methods are most effectively used to study the temporal aspects of the outcome after nerve repair.[104] Three domains of function were described: (1) sensory; (2) motor function; and (3) pain and discomfort. A total score is calculated that correlates significantly with the BMRC scale, which was shown in a study of 70 patients who had been treated for nerve transection at the wrist or distal forearm level. The total score also correlated strongly with the patients' overall estimation of the impact of the injury on activities of daily living.[107]

Factors that affect outcome

General aspects

Ruijs et al. presented an excellent meta-analysis of 23 papers based on data from individual patients about motor and sensory recovery after microsurgical repair of the median and ulnar nerves.[105] Prognostic factors that have an impact on outcome varied for motor and sensory recovery. For motor recovery, age, delay before repair, level of injury, and type of injured nerve were important, and for sensory recovery, age and delay before repair were the most important.

Age

In several studies of digital nerve repairs, there was a close positive correlation between the age of the patient and the recovery of sensation.[111–113] For more proximal injuries of the median, ulnar, or radial nerves in the forearm, age also seems to be the factor that played the most important part in the outcome. Children (mean age 6 years) that were evaluated a minimum of 1 year after primary repair of injury to the median nerve were all considered to have regained normal function.[114] In comparison, 95 patients (age 15–55 years) with primary or secondary repair, or grafting, of injuries of the median and ulnar nerves[28] showed that only the younger patients who had primary distal repair had excellent results, with normal sensitivity and motor function. These findings are supported by other authors in similar case series.[106,115–117] Patients under 16 years are four times more likely to have satisfactory outcome in motor recovery, and also a significantly increased chance of satisfactory sensory recovery, with lower age.[105]

The superior results in children can to some extent be explained by better peripheral nerve regeneration and shorter regeneration distances. However, it is likely that a greater adaptability of the brain is of predominant importance for the functional outcome in children.[118,119] This hypothesis is partly confirmed by recent data that showed that early sensory re-education programs improve functional outcome in adults because of improvements in training-induced plasticity.[120]

Digital nerves

In several studies of primary repair of the digital nerves the results of immediate repair of digital nerves were "normal," "excellent," or "good" in 37–68% of the nerves repaired after a follow-up of 8–32 months.[111–113,121,122] In terms of static two-point discrimination (S2PD), "normal" sensory function has been defined in these studies as the equivalent to the uninjured digit or S2PD of 5 mm or less, whereas "excellent" function has been defined as a S2PD of 7–10 mm. To summarize, after microsurgical repair of a digital nerve injury, about half improve to have normal or fair sensation.

Nerve trunks

The motor outcome of lesions to the larger nerve trunks seems to be dependent on their target organ. This is indicated by the results in a series of 1837 nerve lesions that outcome after repair (primary suture, secondary suture, or graft repair) of the median nerve was superior to the outcome of repair of lesions to the radial nerve, which in turn was better than that after ulnar nerve repair.[123] The better outcome of motor function in median nerves than in ulnar nerves is also supported by others.[105,124,125] Recovery of sensation, on the other hand, has not been shown to differ between the median and ulnar nerves,[105] and combined median and ulnar nerve injuries.[105,126,127] The theoretical explanation may be that the ulnar nerve innervates the delicate intrinsic muscles of the hand, and the demand of an accurate innervation is theoretically greater than that of the median or radial nerves that innervate muscles that do not undertake delicate movements to the same extent. However, it is difficult to compare the outcome after injury to various nerve trunks due to their individual characteristics.

Level of injury

Lesions that are more proximal have a worse outcome than more distal lesions.[117] This may probably be explained by the fact that a proximal injury induces a more severe impact on the individual neuron, with higher risk of neuronal cell death, and that the axons have to regenerate over a large distance to reach the targets.[128,129]

Type of repair

In a study of 654 lesions of the ulnar nerve, the functional outcome (grade 3 or better) after suture repair (72%) was superior to that after graft repair (67%).[123,130] In the same series, neurolysis was done for patients with ulnar entrapment, and in comparison these patients achieved a functional outcome of grade 3 or better in 92% of the repairs, indicating the importance of preserving the continuity of nerve trunks if possible. A nerve repair therefore achieves better results than a nerve graft.[131]

Type of injury

Injuries with the nerve in continuity have a good prognosis, and so a nerve crush leads to better functional recovery than a transected nerve trunk. However, a transection injury can often be treated by a primary repair whereas a crush injury, if it does not recover spontaneously, may require a nerve graft, which will lead to an impaired outcome.

Postoperative dysfunction

General aspects

Peripheral nerve injuries often have a dramatic impact on a person's capacity to function adequately, as the functional outcome often fails to reach the level of motor or sensory function present before the injury, at least in adults.[117,132] As most nerve injuries in the upper extremity are seen in young men[32,133] there is a high probability of disability and subsequent social consequences.[7] The accompanying amount of posttraumatic stress after hand and forearm injuries has been evaluated and shown to be comparable with the psychological distress found among survivors of big disasters.[134] Other symptoms, such as pain, dysesthesia, and cold intolerance,[9]

may also affect the outcome, and cause lifelong impairment of hand function. However, patients may have different strategies to cope with their injuries, whether it is a nerve injury or another serious hand injury.[135]

Complex regional pain syndrome

Complex regional pain syndrome (CRPS) is a clinical diagnosis that involves regional pain together with autonomic dysfunction, functional impairment, and atrophy. According to the classification, CRPS type 1 occurs with no evidence of peripheral nerve injury, whereas CRPS type 2 requires known damage to nerve structures. CRPS can be a disabling condition in many cases, and about half of patients with untreated symptoms for more than a year will have extensive residual dysfunction. Cigarette smokers and women are at increased risk of CRPS, and even though it may occur at any age, most patients are around 45 years. During operation, common sites of injury to peripheral nerves that may elicit CRPS are damage to the dorsal branch of the ulnar nerve, the palmar cutaneous branch of the median nerve, and the superficial branch of the radial nerve. However, CRPS may be initiated after any type of nerve injury. The symptoms are pain that is often described as burning or aching, and it is usually induced by a small stimulus that in the normal patient would not result in such a response to pain. It may affect the tissues surrounding the area of injury, or the whole extremity. In addition, there may be some kind of trophic changes, such as edema and stiffness, together with changes of the skin, nails, and hair. The limb may be perceived as different in temperature from the opposite side.

Other

Numbness, weakness, and abnormal pain with or without discoloration after exposure to mild to severe pain can be problematical after peripheral nerve injury.[136–138] In fact, cold intolerance is regarded by many authors as the most disabling symptom after nerve repair or other trauma to the upper extremity.[9,139–141] The mechanism behind hypersensitivity to cold is not known, but its presence has been inversely correlated to sensory recovery.[142–144] In addition, predictors associated with cold intolerance are coexisting injury to major vessels,[143,145,146] crush injury,[146,147] early postoperative pain,[138,148] and the level of the nerve injury.[140]

In a study by Ruijs et al. on 107 patients with median or ulnar nerve injury, or a combination of the two, numbness was reported as the most frequent symptom (80%). Other symptoms were stiffness (77%), weakness (72%), pain (63%), change in skin color (50%), and swelling (33%). Most of the patients (59%) were considered to have abnormal cold intolerance. In this group, a larger proportion (70%) had combined ulnar and median nerve injuries, whereas isolated nerve injuries were less common (median nerve 57% and ulnar nerve 56%). Even though there was no difference in sensory recovery between women and men, cold intolerance was more common in women than in men. Importantly, time since injury did not correlate with the presence of cold intolerance (follow-up time 2–10 years).[144] This is also supported by other investigators,[141] indicating that cold intolerance is a stationary condition when the maximum sensory recovery has been achieved.

There is currently no treatment available that is specifically directed against cold intolerance, although possible effects of treatment by Pavlovian conditioning, a behavioral treatment for digital cold sensitivity where whole-body cold exposure becomes associated with warm hands, has been reported recently in patients with hand injuries.[149] In addition, CRPS may be a severely disabling condition that may be treated with substances like gabapentin and pregabalin[150] and other strategies.[151] This poses a pedagogic challenge to the treating physician when addressing the patient's expectations of the final outcome after nerve repair.

Future perspectives

Nerve injuries, extending from minor digital nerve injuries up to severe injuries to the brachial plexus in the upper extremity as well as less common injuries in the lower extremity, represent one of the most challenging clinical problems for the treating surgeons and physicians. A variety of factors influence outcome and each individual nerve injury is unique in its entity; thus requiring also consideration of factors such as motivation for rehabilitation and coping strategies of the patient. Efforts to improve diagnostic tools and treatment strategies have to be directed against all components. In the future, improved imaging techniques, like three-dimensional high-resolution magnetic resonance imaging with diffusion tensor imaging and tractography and pre- and peroperative high-resolution sonography, may improve the diagnostic accuracy. Appropriate evaluation systems are needed to examine fully new surgical and rehabilitation techniques, such as the nerve transfers, end-to-side repair and the EMLA concept (see above), respectively. In addition, a continuous search for the secrets of intracellular signaling in neurons, Schwann cells, and other cells may give knowledge needed for the introduction of pharmacological treatment, not only of any neuropathic pain, but also to improve regeneration as an adjunct to surgical repair and reconstruction. Whether the nanomic era, in analogy with the genomic and proteomic development, may lead to improved repair and reconstruction strategies, with or without utilization of stem cells, will be clarified in the future.[152]

Acknowledgments

Financial support for this work was received from the Swedish Research Council (MEDICINE). We appreciate all the help from Professor Jørgen Tranum Jensen and his colleagues at the Panum Institute, University of Medicine and Dentistry, Copenhagen, Denmark.

Access the complete references list online at **http://www.expertconsult.com**

2. Rosberg HE, Dahlin LB. Epidemiology of hand injuries in a middle-sized city in southern Sweden: a retrospective comparison of 1989 and 1997. *Scand J Plast Reconstr Surg Hand Surg*. 2004;38:347–355.

14. Sulaiman OA, Gordon T. Role of chronic Schwann cell denervation in poor functional recovery after nerve injuries and experimental strategies to combat it. *Neurosurgery*. 2009;65(suppl):105–114.

34. Dahlin LB. Techniques of peripheral nerve repair. *Scand J Surg*. 2008;97:310–316.

    A comprehensive review of various techniques to repair and reconstruct injured peripheral nerve trunks.

52. Millesi H. Techniques for nerve grafting. *Hand Clin*. 2000;16:73–91, viii.

    The principles of nerve grafting provided by one of the pioneers in peripheral nerve surgery.

73. Lundborg G, Rosen B, Dahlin L, et al. Tubular versus conventional repair of median and ulnar nerves in the human forearm: early results from a prospective, randomized, clinical study. *J Hand Surg Am*. 1997;22:99–106.

    One of the few prospective randomized studies comparing microsurgical and tubular nerve repairs in humans.

77. Weber RA, Breidenbach WC, Brown RE, et al. A randomized prospective study of polyglycolic acid conduits for digital nerve reconstruction in humans. *Plast Reconstr Surg*. 2000;106:1036–1045; discussion 1046–1038.

94. Merzenich MM, Jenkins WM. Reorganization of cortical representations of the hand following alterations of skin inputs induced by nerve injury, skin island transfers, and experience. *J Hand Ther*. 1993;6:89–104.

    A classic paper from the 1990s describing reorganization of the cerebral cortex by various manipulations such as nerve injury.

105. Ruijs AC, Jaquet JB, Kalmijn S, et al. Median and ulnar nerve injuries: a meta-analysis of predictors of motor and sensory recovery after modern microsurgical nerve repair. *Plast Reconstr Surg*. 2005;116:484–494; discussion 495–486.

107. Rosen B, Lundborg G. A model instrument for the documentation of outcome after nerve repair. *J Hand Surg Am*. 2000;25:535–543.

    A specific evaluation instrument to evaluate outcome after median and ulnar nerve repairs, enabling a score and suitable for follow-up of the individual patient and particularly in clinical trials.

110. Dellon AL, Curtis RM, Edgerton MT. Reeducation of sensation in the hand after nerve injury and repair. *Plast Reconstr Surg*. 1974;53:297–305.

135. Cederlund RI, Ramel E, Rosberg HE, et al. Outcome and clinical changes in patients 3, 6, 12 months after a severe or major hand injury – Can sense of coherence be an indicator for rehabilitation focus? *BMC Musculoskelet Disord*. 2010;11:286

33

Nerve transfers

Kirsty U. Boyd, Ida K. Fox, and Susan E. Mackinnon

SYNOPSIS

- Nerve injuries are often devastating, with associated pain and impaired function.
- Motor nerve injuries must be managed expeditiously, because regenerating axons must reach target muscle prior to degeneration and fibrosis – "time is muscle".
- Nerve transfers offer an advantageous method of reconstruction by delivering regenerating nerve fibers to the target end organ more quickly, thus converting a proximal injury to a more distal injury.
- Nerve transfers allow for dissection outside the original zone of injury, providing a safer and more technically straightforward procedure.
- Unlike tendon transfers, the muscle–tendon biomechanical structure is preserved, thus excursion, origin, insertion, and length–tension relationships are undisturbed.
- Nerve transfers require time for the nerve to regenerate and extensive physical therapy for retraining.
- Intraneural dissection is technically demanding, and nerve transfers require intimate knowledge of nerve topography.

 Access the Historical Perspective section online at
http://www.expertconsult.com

Key points

- Nerve transfers are a relatively recent development in peripheral nerve surgery.
- Nerve transfers can be performed to restore sensory or motor deficits.
- Nerve transfers essentially convert a proximal injury to a distal injury, providing a source of regenerating axons in close proximity to the end target.
- Nerve transfers are associated with minimal to no downgrade in donor function.

- Nerve transfers preserve the original biomechanical muscle–tendon relationship.
- Nerve transfers may provide superior results to tendon transfer, with the ability to restore individual and separate muscle function.
- Nerve transfers are replacing other techniques as the gold standard for brachial plexus and other peripheral nerve injury in the authors' practice.

Introduction

Peripheral nerve reconstruction is an evolving field, and nerve transfers are an exciting addition to the surgical options. As our understanding of internal nerve topography improves, we are able to recognize redundant or nonessential potential donor nerves and fascicles. Recent contributions in basic science are broadening options for nerve transfer with new and improved techniques. This chapter will outline the history and principles of nerve transfers as they pertain to upper extremity nerve reconstruction. The recent literature as it relates to current techniques, debates, and advances in nerve transfers will be reviewed. Current commonly performed nerve transfers are detailed with focus on both motor and sensory nerve transfers, their indications, rehabilitation and postoperative protocols, and a basic overview of selected surgical techniques (see key points, above).

Basic science

There have been dramatic increases in our knowledge of nerve injury, healing, and regeneration. The majority will be touched on in Volume 1, Chapter 22 and Chapter 32 of this volume. The most relevant recent basic science advances pertaining to nerve transfers relate to end-to-side transfers (*Fig. 33.1*). End-to-side neurorrhaphy involves the coaptation of the

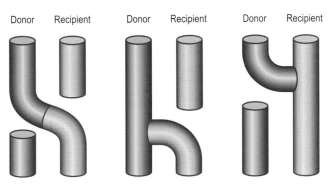

Donor   Recipient   Donor   Recipient   Donor   Recipient

Fig. 33.1 The various options for coaptation in nerve transfer. **(A)** End-to-end coaptation between the donor nerve (red) and the recipient nerve (blue). **(B)** End-to-side coaptation, where the distal end of the divided recipient nerve (blue) is transferred to the side of the intact donor nerve (red). In this transfer, fascicles from the donor will "sprout" into the distal donor nerve. The recipient nerve essentially "pulls" the donor fascicles into the distal nerve. **(C)** Reverse end-to-side coaptation. In this transfer, the donor nerve (red) has been divided and transferred to the side of the intact recipient nerve (blue). The donor essentially "pushes" regenerating fascicles into the distal donor nerve.

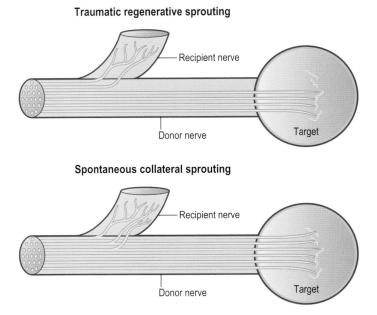

Traumatic regenerative sprouting

Recipient nerve

Donor nerve

Target

Spontaneous collateral sprouting

Recipient nerve

Donor nerve

Target

Fig. 33.2 The difference between regenerative and collateral sprouting. Traumatic regenerative sprouting occurs following injury to the proximal nerve. The damaged axons degenerate and then regenerate at the rate of 1 mm/day into the distal recipient nerve. Collateral sprouting occurs spontaneously, and does not require proximal nerve injury. Axons from the donor nerve simply sprout into the distal end of the recipient nerve. Only sensory nerves will undergo spontaneous collateral sprouting. Motor nerves require an axonotmetic injury to facilitate regenerative sprouting.

distal end of an injured recipient nerve into the lateral aspect of an intact nerve, which serves as a proximal source of axons to regenerate into the injured nerve. Reports of end-to-side transfers occurred as early as the late 1800s and then made a resurgence in the 1990s.[10] There has, however, been controversy regarding the success of these transfers, and sensory recovery has typically been more impressive than motor recovery.[11–15] The sprouting of axons in an end-to-side coaptation, thus eliminating the need for a proximal nerve stump, makes nerve transfers an option for proximal nerve injuries and has been well demonstrated in the literature.[16–19] While sensory nerves are able to sprout spontaneously (collateral sprouting), donor nerve axonotmetic injury is required for motor neuronal regeneration (regenerative sprouting) across the end-to-side repair *(Fig. 33.2)*.[15,17,17,20,21] An epineurotomy in the donor nerve is required, and partial axotomy will result in more significant regenerative sprouting into the recipient nerve, albeit at the potential expense of a measurable downgrade in donor nerve function.[17]

Reverse end-to-side nerve transfers involve the complete transection of the donor nerve, which is then coapted into the side of the intact recipient nerve. This maximizes the potential number of available motor axons from the donor nerve. This procedure does not interrupt any recovery in the injured recipient nerve because the nerve remains in continuity; however the additional axons recruited from the donor nerve improve distal target reinnervation, a concept known as "supercharging."[22–24] In a proximal nerve injury, with a long distance required for reinnervation, this technique can protect target muscles from denervation atrophy and fibrosis.[22]

Hints and tips

The end-to-side transfer can be considered as the recipient nerve "pulling" regenerating axons out of the intact donor, whereas the reverse end-to-side transfer can be considered as the donor nerve "pushing" regenerating axons out into the intact recipient.

Diagnosis and patient presentation

The value of a complete history and physical examination in the patient with a potential brachial plexus or proximal nerve injury of the upper extremity cannot be overstated. Patients should be evaluated promptly after injury, both to provide a baseline for future serial examinations and to facilitate timing of surgical intervention where necessary.

History

On history, details of the mechanism and timing of injury are crucial. The mechanism of injury will determine timing of intervention, with prompt exploration of penetrating sharp trauma, and more expectant management of closed injuries and gunshot wounds. Specific patient symptoms such as loss of function, both sensory and motor, and pain should be precisely elicited, as this will help focus the subsequent physical examination. The pain diagram and questionnaire are particularly useful for eliciting this information *(Fig. 33.3)*. Other factors, such as patient age, handedness, occupation, and comorbidities, will factor into management decisions. When seeing a patient in a delayed fashion, it is also useful to ascertain any interval recovery of function.

Text continued on page 725

Pain Questionnaire

Name: _____   Date: _____

Age: ____   Sex: Male ____ Female ____   Dominant Hand: Right ____ Left ____   Diagnosis: _____

1. Pain is difficult to describe. Circle the words that best describe your symptoms:

Burning	Throbbing	Aching	Stabbing	Tingling	Twisting	Squeezing
Cramping	Cutting	Shooting	Numbing	Vague	Stinging	Indescribable
Pulling	Smarting	Pressure	Coldness	Dull	Other:	

Level of symptoms: place a mark through the line to indicate the level of your pain, if zero is no pain and the end of the line is the most severe pain you can imagine having.

2. Mark your average level of pain in the last month

No pain   Most severe pain

3. Mark your worst level of pain in the last week

Right   No pain   Most severe pain

Left   No pain   Most severe pain

4. Where is your pain? (Draw on diagram)

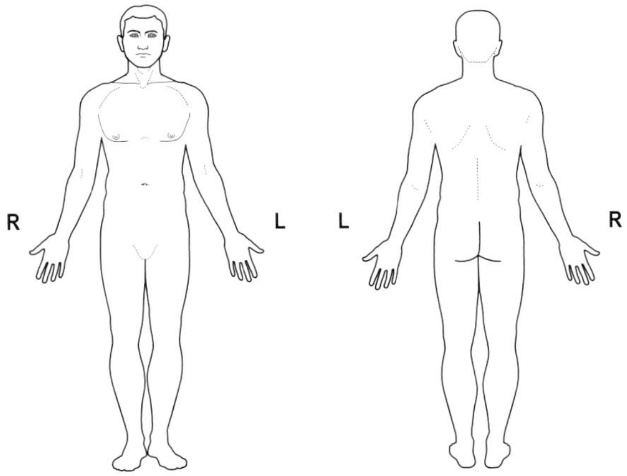

R   L   L   R

Mark on this scale how your pain has affected your quality of life:

0%   100%
Very little   A large amount

%. Mark on this scale how depressed you currently feel:

0%   100%
Not at all   A large amount

(A)

Fig. 33.3 The pain questionnaire is a valuable tool for qualifying and quantifying patient pain and the impact their injury is having on their life. This has uses both in obtaining baseline information, and also in tracking progress as patients recover. This questionnaire is filled out by every nerve patient at each office visit.

5. Mark your average level of stress in the last month?

At home   0 |————————————————————————————————| 10

At work   0 |————————————————————————————————| 10

6. How well are you able to cope with that stress?

At home   Very well |————————————————————————————| Not at all

At work   Very well |————————————————————————————| Not at all

7. **How did the pain that you are now experiencing occur?**
    a. Sudden onset with accident or definable event
    b. Slow progressive onset
    c. Slow progressive onset with acute exacerbation without an accident or definable event
    d. A sudden onset without an accident or definable event

8. **How many surgical procedures have you had <u>in order to try to eliminate the cause of your pain?</u>**
    a. None or one
    b. Two surgical procedures
    c. Three or four surgical procedures
    d. Greater than four surgical procedures

9. **Does movement have any effect on your pain?**
    a. The pain is always worsened by use or movement
    b. The pain is usually worsened by use and movement
    c. The pain is not altered by use and movement

10. **Does weather have any effect on your pain?**
    a. The pain is usually worse with damp or cold weather
    b. The pain is occasionally worse with damp or cold weather
    c. Damp or cold weather have no effect on the pain

(B)

Fig. 33.3, cont'd

11. Do you ever have trouble falling asleep or awakening from sleep?
  a. No – Proceed to Question 12 b. Yes – Proceed to 11A & 11B

11A. How often do you have trouble falling asleep?
  a. Trouble falling asleep every night due to pain
  b. Trouble falling asleep due to pain most nights of the week
  c. Occasionally having difficulty falling asleep due to pain
  d. No trouble falling asleep due to pain
  e. Trouble falling asleep which is not related to pain

11B. How often do you awaken from sleep?
  a. Awakened by pain every night
  b. Awakened from sleep by pain more than 3 times per week
  c. Not usually awakened from sleep by pain
  d. Restless sleep or early morning awakening with or without being able to
    return to sleep, both unrelated to pain

12. Has you pain affected your intimate personal relationships?
  a. No   b. Yes

13. Are you involved in any legal action regarding your physical complaint?
  a. No   b. Yes

14. Is this a Workers' Compensation case?
  a. No   b. Yes

15. Are you receiving receiving or have you ever received psychiatric/psychological treatment?
  a. No   b. Presently receiving psychiatric treatment   c. Previous psychiatric treatment

16. Have you ever thought of suicide?
  a. No   b. Yes   c. Previous suicide attempts

17. Have you a victim of emotional abuse?
  a. No   b. Yes   c. No comment

18. Have you a victim of physical abuse?
  a. No   b. Yes   c. No comment

19. Have you a victim of sexual abuse?
  a. No   b. Yes   c. No comment

20. Are you a presently a victim of abuse?
  a. No   b. Yes   c. No comment

(c)

Fig. 33.3, cont'd

21. If you are retired, a student or homemaker, proceed to Question 21B

21A. Are you still working?
a. Works every day at the same pre-pain job
b. Works every day but the job is not the same as the pre-pain job with reduced responsibility or physical activity
c. Works occasionally
d. Not presently working

21B. Are you able to do your household chores?
a. Does same level of household activities without discomfort
b. Does same level of household chores with discomfort
c. Does a reduced amount of household chores
d. Most household chores are now performed by others

22. What medications have you used in the past month?
a. No medications
b. List medications: _____

_____

_____

23. If you had three wishes for anything in the world, what would you wish for?

a. _____

b. _____

c. _____

(D)

Fig. 33.3, cont'd

Physical examination

A complete physical examination of the upper extremity includes assessment of sensory and motor function, deep tendon reflexes, joint suppleness, and range of motion. Particularly in patients with late presentation, the presence of fixed joint contractures may preclude functional recovery. Perfusion, bony pathology, presence of edema, scar, previous incisions, and other soft-tissue trauma are factors that influence treatment choices.

Function should be graded at each joint. Shoulder function should be assessed by examining deltoid, supraspinatus, infraspinatus, trapezius, latissimus dorsi, serratus anterior, and pectoralis major. The patient's ability to abduct/adduct, flex/extend, and internally/externally rotate must be assessed. The elbow should also be assessed for flexion and extension. Here it is important to differentiate between flexion secondary to biceps brachii and brachialis (musculocutaneous nerve) and brachioradialis (radial nerve). The forearm and wrist should be assessed for flexion/extension and pronation/supination. Palpation of the individual tendons with wrist flexion is essential to determine which nerves are involved, as well as the level and degree of injury. In the hand, a complete examination of extrinsic and intrinsic function again helps to delineate the level of injury.

Sensation should be examined by both dermatome and peripheral nerve distribution, and can be helpful in distinguishing these injuries. The authors advocate the use of both two-point discrimination and the ten-test to evaluate sensory loss in the hand.[25] A Tinel's sign, the tingling sensation elicited with percussion over a regenerating nerve, will help to localize the level of nerve injury, and may also be followed on serial clinical examination to check for signs of advancement, indicating spontaneous recovery. An advancing Tinel's sign distal to the site of injury quite often precedes clinical motor recovery.

For completeness, the presence of Horner's syndrome and dysfunction of nerve branches that come off the proximal brachial plexus (dorsal scapular nerve to rhomboids, long thoracic nerve to serratus anterior) indicate a very proximal level of injury.

The scratch collapse test is useful primarily for patients with nerve compression pathology, but also has a role in evaluating the patient for potential nerve transfer procedures, as it can provide additional confirmation of the level of nerve injury (video 1). The test is performed by having the patient sit facing the examiner with the shoulders adducted, elbows held in 90° of flexion, neutral prosupination, and wrist and fingers extended. The examiner will then lightly scratch the area of the presumed nerve injury and exert force to the patient's arms in the direction of internal shoulder rotation as the patient resists. Nerve injury at the test site is indicated by the inward collapse of the arm on the side ipsilateral to the injury.[26,27]

One of the most important components of the physical examination is the simple determination of what is functioning, and what function has been lost. Not only does this help to determine the level of injury, it can guide future surgical planning. In the presence of an injury requiring surgical intervention, it is important to examine the patient for putative nerve donors, both intraplexal and extraplexal (spinal accessory, medial pectoral, and thoracodorsal).

Imaging

Imaging is primarily useful for confirming level of injury in more complex closed-mechanism nerve injury patients. For example, imaging such as computed tomography myelogram and magnetic resonance imaging provides additional confirmation of a nerve root avulsion pattern. Additional X-rays, such as shoulder films that demonstrate scapular notch-level trauma, may provide information of localized trauma that would make proximal transfer to the suprascapular nerve ineffective due to the extensive zone of injury. Other plain films such as chest X-ray might be used to evaluate pathology such as rib fractures or diaphragm dysfunction that might make the use of intercostal and phrenic nerves as donor nerves less palatable, although the former is debatable.[28]

Electrodiagnostic testing

Electrodiagnostic testing, performed by an experienced person, can be a useful adjunct to physical examination for serial assessment of reinnervation in closed nerve injuries. Electromyography records the electrical activity of muscle fibers, tested both at rest and activity, by the insertion of needles into the muscle. Denervated muscles will demonstrated fibrillations and positive sharp waves on needle insertion; however the findings are not reliable until approximately 4 weeks after injury.[29] Initial electrodiagnostic testing should be deferred until a minimum of 6–8 weeks postinjury to assess for signs of both axonal injury and root-level avulsion. Serial testing will reveal signs of reinnervation with nascent potential and motor unit potentials in the affected muscle groups, often prior to clinical evidence of recovery. Conduction velocity is used to measure the integrity of a peripheral nerve (sensory nerve action potentials (SNAP) or compound motor action potentials (CMAP)).[29] A severed nerve will lose the ability to conduct a signal as wallerian degeneration occurs; however, if measured too early, the distal aspect of the nerve will still conduct, leading to an inaccurate assessment. This is another reason for delaying initial electrodiagnostic studies. Preganglionic injuries will be associated with a loss of sensation but an intact SNAP and an absent CMAP.[29] Thus the level of injury can be confirmed with electrodiagnostic studies.

In patients with no evidence of recovery 3 months after a closed nerve injury, the balance should tilt towards consideration of surgical intervention.

Overall, the complete picture, including history, physical examination, and adjunct testing, should facilitate surgical decision-making. Appropriate treatment for open injuries with nerve dysfunction begs for timely management with surgery on an urgent or semiurgent basis. For these injuries, direct exploration and repair have historically been the treatment of choice, but in very proximal injuries, distal nerve transfer can allow for more timely and successful reinnervation. In closed nerve injuries or in gunshot wounds, appropriate management demands a more measured approach and surgery should be delayed to allow for spontaneous recovery, which is often superior to that seen in patients treated with hasty surgery. These patients in particular may benefit from "supercharging" with reverse end-to-side nerve transfer procedures, which can more quickly deliver regenerating axons to the appropriate end organ, while still allowing slower spontaneous recovery.[22]

Patient selection

Nerve transfers have become increasingly popular for a number of reasons, the most compelling of which is the "time is muscle" issue.[24] The biggest challenge facing peripheral nerve surgeons is that with increasing time since injury, the ability to achieve good motor function becomes increasingly limited. In fact, for any nerve injury where there is complete discontinuity with the motor end organ, no reinnervation procedure will be able to restore muscle once denervation and fibrosis have occurred, a process which occurs as early as 1 year.[24] Nerve transfers, by bringing the regenerating motor fibers closer to the target end organ more rapidly, essentially convert a more proximal-level injury to a more distal-level injury, thus increasing the chance of achieving meaningful muscle function.

Another advantage of nerve transfers is that they enable surgical reconstruction outside the zone of the original injury, avoiding complex dissections and limiting injury to critical neurovascular structures. In patients with brachial plexus trauma, the proximity of vital structures (great vessels, thoracic duct, lung) makes the occurrence of potentially life-threatening complications a real possibility. In other cases, such as concomitant vascular injury, previous blast injury, or soft-tissue deficits requiring flap reconstruction, the ability to avoid doing a complex nerve exploration in the setting of dense fibrotic scar is particularly advantageous.[24]

Nerve transfers allow for a very targeted intervention in cases of partial nerve injury such as in treatment of a sixth-degree or neuroma-in-continuity injury, where transfer can be done distal to the site of injury specifically to the nonfunctioning nerve branch. This allows for preservation of all intact function and restoration of only missing function. In addition, the ability to "supercharge" a recovering nerve is invaluable when it is unclear whether the nerve transfer or intrinsic recovery will be more beneficial.[14,30]

Unlike tendon transfers, nerve transfers require only minimal immobilization (7–10 days), which is especially valuable in patients presenting with significant baseline stiffness. Nerve transfers also preserve the biomechanical properties of the musculotendinous unit, such as end organ origin, insertion, excursion, and length–tension relationships. Finally, nerve transfers can restore unique function such as pronation, which is incredibly difficult to restore by traditional surgical techniques.[31]

Table 33.2 Indications for nerve transfer

- Proximal brachial plexus injuries where grafting is not possible
- Proximal peripheral nerve injuries requiring long distance for reinnervation of distal targets
- Severely scarred areas with risk of damage to critical structures
- Segmental nerve loss
- Major upper extremity trauma
- Partial nerve injuries with functional loss
- Delayed presentation with inadequate time for reinnervation of distal targets with grafting
- Sensory nerve deficits in critical regions

Thus nerve transfers are indicated in a number of situations *(Table 33.2)*, for example, in proximal brachial plexus injury where grafting is not possible or the required distance for reinnervation will not allow motor axons to reach the target motor before denervation and fibrosis have occurred. In situations of extreme scarring, or major upper extremity trauma, a nerve transfer is preferable to risking damage to critical structures within the scarred region. Nerve transfers are also indicated in segmental nerve loss, and in partial nerve transfers with functional loss. Patients presenting in a delayed manner with inadequate time to reinnervate the distal targets are good candidates for distal nerve transfers. Also, patients with sensory nerve deficits in critical regions should be considered for nerve transfer to restore sensation.

The main reason a nerve transfer should not be performed is similar to the contraindication for any other traditional nerve repair/graft intervention, namely end organ unresponsiveness. An old peripheral nerve injury will not respond to the new "magic" of nerve transfers. Muscle that is in complete discontinuity with the nerve for greater than 1 year will not be reinnervated no matter the elaborate reinnervation strategy employed.

More relative contraindications for nerve transfer include issues such as the time required for regeneration, challenges of the surgery, the anatomic knowledge required, and problems of postoperative retraining and therapy as these techniques are less familiar to hand therapists. There are some patients, such as the young manual laborer with a radial nerve injury, who may prefer the more rapid recovery associated with tendon transfer at the expense of the independent fine motor control that could be achieved through the use of nerve transfers. The surgery itself is challenging because of the detailed knowledge of internal nerve topography required. Most surgeons are not formally trained in the intraneural dissection techniques required to perform nerve transfers and the results are not apparent until months down the line. This requires a significant leap of faith for surgeons who are more used to immediate gratification and a clear result in weeks, not months or years!

Direct nerve repair and nerve grafting also remain valuable tools for the peripheral nerve surgeon and should continue to be the treatment of choice in a variety of scenarios. These include cases of multiple nerve injuries where there is a paucity of nerve donor material for nerve transfer. Also, in distal single-function nerve injuries, direct or graft repair is preferable to nerve transfer because one-to-one function is preserved, no retraining is necessary, no donor function is sacrificed, and the distance to the end target is short.

Patient general health, comorbidities, and associated injuries factor into the decision to perform nerve transfers. These procedures can be lengthy, and are not without significant risk from anesthesia in the fragile patient. In addition, patient compliance is an integral part of the recovery process, and patients require education preoperatively about the prolonged recovery and therapy times associated with nerve transfer.

Examples of nerve transfer procedures for specific injury patterns

Hints and tips

- Avoid, or use short-term paralytics with anesthesia induction to allow for nerve stimulation
- Minimize or avoid tourniquet time to avoid interference with nerve stimulation
- Use plain epinephrine in proximal incisions to minimize blood loss without lidocaine paralysis
- Obtain wide surgical exposure to identify nerves and appropriate branches
- Choice of optimal nerve donor is based on quantity of motor axons, proximity to target muscles, synergy of muscle function, and donor expendability
- Conduct neurolysis with your "eyes" except at the site of actual transfer to avoid prolonged dissection and increased trauma to nerve branches
- Confirm no intraoperative stimulation in putative recipient before dividing donor
- Divide donor nerve distally and recipient nerve proximally
- Use 9-0 nylon and the operating microscope to perform tension-free epineurial repair
- Use bupivacaine block at end of case for postoperative pain control

Upper plexus injury

Specific patient exam findings

Upper plexus injuries involve injuries at the C5, C6, and/or C7 root or upper trunk level. Injuries of this type commonly include deficits of the dorsal scapular, the long thoracic, suprascapular, axillary, and musculocutaneous nerves. The dorsal scapular nerve innervates the rhomboid muscles and the levator scapulae muscles, which contribute to scapular adduction, retraction, and elevation. The long thoracic nerve innervates the serratus anterior muscle, which abducts the scapula, permitting the full range of shoulder flexion past 90°. The suprascapular nerve innervates the supraspinatus and infraspinatus muscles. These muscles are rotator cuff muscles. The supraspinatus contributes to shoulder abduction with the deltoid muscle. The infraspinatus contributes to shoulder external rotation with the teres minor. The axillary nerve comes off the posterior cord, receiving innervation from C5 and C6. The axillary nerve supplies the deltoid and teres minor muscles, which provide shoulder abduction and external rotation respectively. It also provides cutaneous innervation over the lateral shoulder. The musculocutaneous nerve arises from the lateral cord and is primarily innervated by C5, C6, and occasionally C7. This nerve innervates coracobrachialis, biceps brachii, and brachialis, which power elbow flexion. The biceps is also the primary forearm supinator. The lateral antebrachial cutaneous (LABC) nerve is a terminal branch of the musculocutaneous nerve, and provides cutaneous innervation to the lateral forearm.

Patients with upper plexus injuries present with glenohumeral joint subluxation, loss of shoulder abduction and external rotation, and absent or weakened elbow flexion depending on the involvement of C7. Numbness over the lateral shoulder and forearm is noted.

Reconstruction techniques

Hints and tips

Priorities for upper plexus injuries include restoration of shoulder external rotation and abduction, as well as elbow flexion. Standard transfers include: (1) spinal accessory to suprascapular nerve; (2) medial triceps to axillary nerve; and (3) double fascicular nerve transfer.

Use of spinal accessory nerve (cranial nerve XI) to suprascapular nerve transfer (motor)

Restoration of shoulder stability and external rotation are facilitated by transferring the spinal accessory nerve (cranial nerve XI) to the suprascapular nerve. This transfer can be conducted by either an anterior or a posterior approach. In the posterior approach, the patient is positioned prone and surface landmarks are used to approximate the position of the nerves (Fig. 33.4). The spinal accessory nerve runs parallel to the border of the trapezius and is localized 44% of the way along a line connecting the acromion to the dorsal midline at the level of the superior border of the scapula (Fig. 33.5). The suprascapular nerve is located midway between the medial border of the scapula and the acromion as it runs through the suprascapular notch.[32,33] These nerves are accessed through an incision located slightly obliquely just above the superior border of the spine of the scapula. Dissection is carried through the trapezius in a muscle-splitting fashion and an end-to-end coaptation, sparing the upper trapezius nerve branches, is performed.

For the anterior approach, an incision is designed 2 cm superior to and parallel to the clavicle extending laterally from the posterior border of the sternocleidomastoid (Fig. 33.6). The upper trunk is identified between the anterior and middle scalene muscles. The suprascapular nerve is a distinct branch of the upper trunk that sits on the superolateral aspect. The spinal accessory nerve is located in the posterior aspect of the incision on the deep surface of the trapezius muscle. Although an end-to-end transfer can be performed, the end-to-side approach with a partial neurectomy of the donor accessory nerve is preferred as this preserves some donor function. In the end-to-side transfer, a short interpositional graft from the recipient suprascapular nerve to the donor spinal accessory nerve is required to avoid tension. A proximal crush injury to the donor nerve encourages axonal sprouting such that regeneration into the recipient suprascapular nerve occurs without loss of significant donor nerve trapezius function.[14]

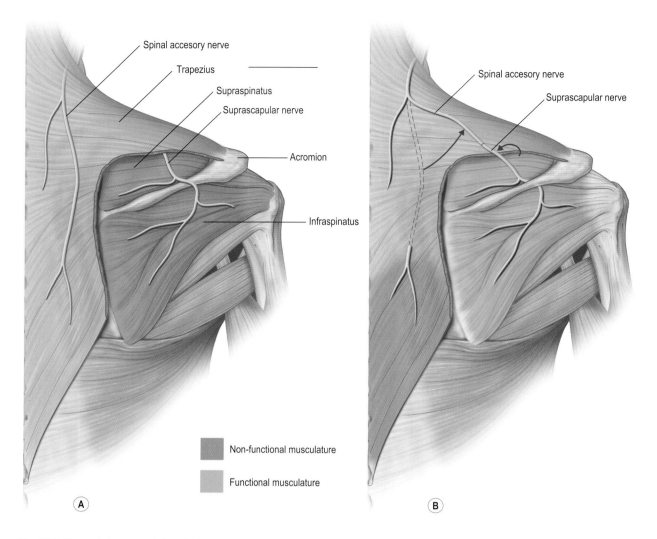

Fig. 33.4 The posterior approach for spinal accessory to suprascapular nerve transfers. **(A)** The nerves can be seen in their original orientation. **(B)** The end-to-end transfer has been completed. The transfer includes the functional spinal accessory nerve (donor) being transposed and coapted to the nonfunctional suprascapular nerve (recipient).

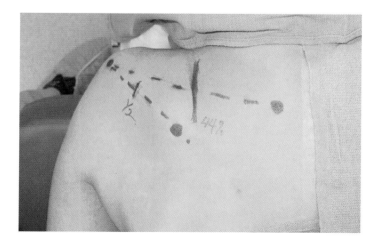

Fig. 33.5 Surface markings for posterior approach to spinal accessory to suprascapular. The spinal accessory nerve is located 44% of the way along a line connecting the dorsal midline to the acromion. The suprascapular nerve is located at the halfway point between the medial border of the scapula and the acromion on an obliquely oriented line at the superior aspect of the scapular spine. It runs in the suprascapular notch.

Use of triceps to axillary nerve transfer (motor component)

Additional reduction of glenohumeral subluxation and abduction of the shoulder are provided by transferring a branch of the triceps, usually from the medial head, to the axillary nerve *(Fig. 33.7)*.[33,34] Better results in upper plexus injury patients are achieved by reinnervating both the suprascapular and axillary nerves.[35] This transfer is performed with the patient positioned prone through a longitudinal incision on the posterior surface of the arm that extends in a curvilinear fashion above the posterior axillary fold *(Fig. 33.8)*. The axillary nerve is identified in the quadrangular space and dissected proximally to include the branch to teres minor, then divided proximally. The natural cleavage plane between the lateral and long heads of the triceps is identified and blunt dissection is conducted to expose the donor radial nerve running along the humerus. The branch to the medial triceps sits superficially and medially on the surface of the radial nerve as a distinct branch. The donor triceps nerve is dissected as far distally as possible and then coapted to the axillary nerve *(Fig. 33.9)*.

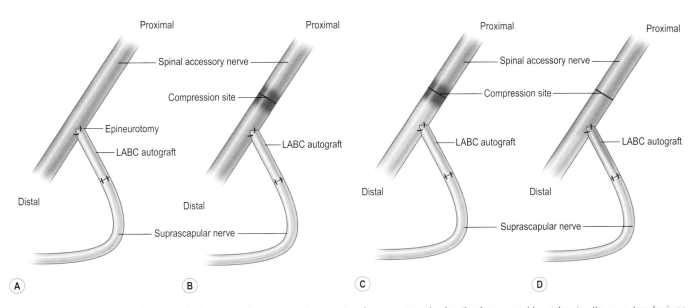

Fig. 33.6 In the anterior approach to the spinal accessory to suprascapular nerve transfer, upper trapezius function is preserved by performing the nerve transfer in an end-to-side manner. **(A)** To inset this transfer with no tension, an interpositional lateral antebrachial cutaneous nerve (LABC) nerve graft is used. **(B)** To facilitate regenerative sprouting, injury to the donor nerve is required proximally. This is accomplished by "crushing" the nerve with a hemostat to cause a second-degree nerve injury. **(C)** Wallerian degeneration occurs distal to the site of compression. **(D)** Axons regenerate from the level of the crush injury, with some axons following the donor nerve and restoring function to the upper trapezius muscle, and some axons diverting into the distal recipient nerve via the LABC graft.

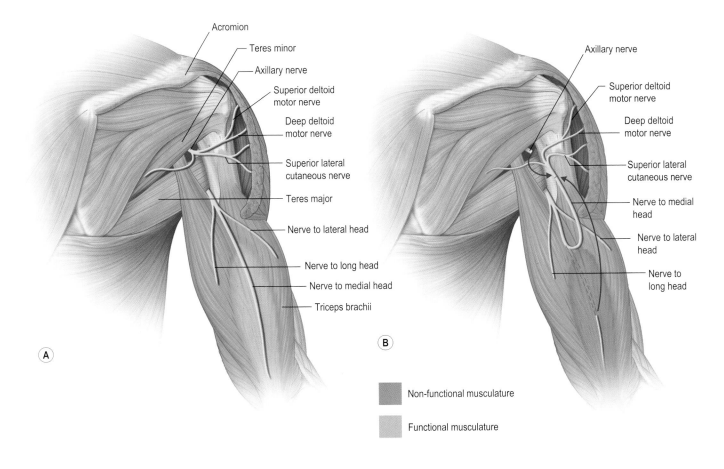

Fig. 33.7 The triceps to axillary nerve transfer via a posterior approach to the upper arm. **(A)** The axillary and radial nerves in their normal anatomical position. **(B)** The branch to the medial head of the triceps (donor) is transposed to meet the divided end of the axillary nerve (recipient). The branch to the medial head is coapted end to end to the axillary nerve.

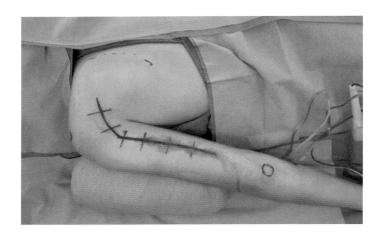

Fig. 33.8 Set-up and incision for triceps to axillary. The patient is positioned in the prone position and draped with the entire extremity free and the medial border of the scapula exposed. A line connecting the olecranon and the acromion is drawn on the posterior aspect of the arm and then extended in a curvilinear fashion just above the posterior axillary fold. Positioning is facilitated by placing a "bump" beneath the anterior shoulder preventing internal rotation and anterior subluxation. The arm is draped free so that distal function can be assessed with intraoperative nerve stimulation.

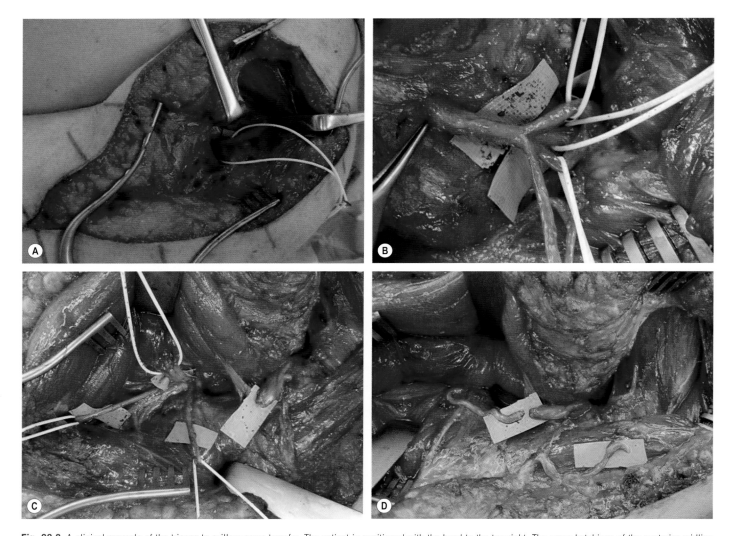

Fig. 33.9 A clinical example of the triceps to axillary nerve transfer. The patient is positioned with the head to the top right. The cross-hatchings of the posterior midline incision in the upper arm are visible and the quadrangular space is exposed. **(A)** The intact nerve *in situ* prior to division. A white vessel loop surrounds the entire nerve at that level. **(B)** The divided nerve transposed caudally with the proximalmost aspect held by the forceps. The branches are clearly visible with vessel loops around motor branches. The superiormost branch is the branch to teres minor. The sensory branch is the most inferior branch (no vessel loop) and can be visualized heading more superficially than the other branches. **(C)** The cut end of the recipient axillary nerve is visible on the most proximal blue background. The radial nerve is visualized at the base of the wound, with vessel loops around branches to the medial, long, and lateral heads of triceps. **(D)** The divided branch to the medial head (donor) is transposed proximally and coapted to the recipient axillary nerve.

Use of the double fascicular (ulnar/median redundant branches to biceps brachii and brachialis branches of the musculocutaneous) nerve transfer (motor)

Restoration of elbow flexion is achieved with the double fascicular nerve transfer *(Fig. 33.10)*. This transfer reinnervates the biceps brachii and brachialis muscles using redundant fascicles from the ulnar and median nerves.[36,37] As visualized, a longitudinal incision in the bicipital groove facilitates exposure of the musculocutaneous, median, and ulnar nerves.[38] An intramuscular dissection at the underside of the biceps brachii muscle allows exposure of the musculocutaneous nerve. The biceps brachii branch is the more proximal branch and is located about halfway between the shoulder and elbow exiting the nerve from the lateral side. The brachialis branch exits the musculocutaneous branch on the medial side of the arm approximately 13 cm proximal to the medial epicondyle, usually under a leash of crossing vessels *(Fig. 33.11)*.[8] These branches are divided and draped over to the median and ulnar nerves to determine best donor–recipient pairings. Confirmation of a tension-free inset with elbow range of motion is mandatory. The ulnar and median nerves are then neurolyzed at the appropriate level, and redundant fascicles to the flexor carpi ulnaris (FCU: ulnar), flexor carpi radialis (FCR), flexor digitorum superficialis (FDS), or palmaris longus (median) are identified. The redundant fascicles are divided distally and coapted end to end.[36] Reinnervation occurs at approximately 5–6 months postoperatively.[37]

Other potential donors (medial pectoral nerve and thoracodorsal nerve)

Other potential donors that can be used to restore elbow flexion include the medial pectoral nerves and the thoracodorsal nerve. The medial pectoral nerves are identified by making an incision in the deltopectoral groove, dividing the pectoralis major tendon distally, and elevating pectoralis minor from lateral to medial *(Fig. 33.12)*. There are several branches to the pectoralis minor and these can be followed as distally as possible into the muscle to increase available donor nerve length.[39] Often a nerve graft will be required. The thoracodorsal nerves runs along the lateral chest wall and can be exposed through an incision running along the free border of latissimus dorsi.

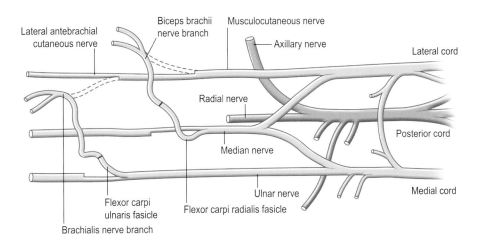

Fig. 33.10 A schematic of the double fascicular nerve transfer. The divided recipient branches of the musculocutaneous nerve (biceps brachii laterally and brachialis medially) are transposed medially to the median and ulnar nerves. In this example, a redundant fascicle to flexor digitorum superficialis (median donor) is transferred to the biceps brachii branch and a redundant fascicle of the flexor carpi ulnaris (ulnar donor) is transferred to the brachialis branch.

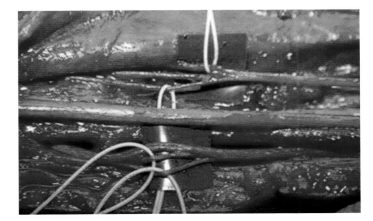

Fig. 33.11 Operative photo of double fascicular nerve transfer. A clinical example of the double fascicular nerve transfer. The superior nerve is the musculocutaneous nerve with vessel loops around the branch to biceps brachii (proximal and lateral) and branch to brachialis (distal and medial). The ulnar nerve is also neurolyzed at the level appropriate for transfer. Redundant fascicles determined by intraoperative nerve stimulation that can serve as potential donors are marked with vessel loops.

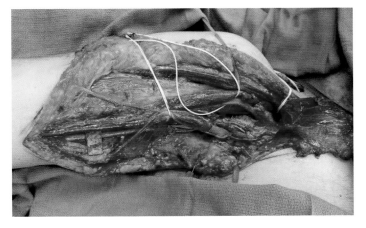

Fig. 33.12 Harvesting the medial pectoral nerve. Clinical photograph of a patient with medial pectoral nerve harvested as a donor. The divided pectoralis major muscle is flipped proximally and lying on the anterior chest wall. The medial pectoral nerves have been dissected from the deep surface of the pectoralis minor and divided distally. They have then been transposed towards the donor nerves in the arm and are lying on the most proximal blue background.

Lower plexus injury

Specific patient exam findings

Lower plexus injuries usually involve damage to C8 and T1 nerve roots or to the lower trunk. Often they are a result of a forceful pull on an abducted arm. The lower trunk contributes primarily to the ulnar nerve, and thus patients have a resultant loss of the intrinsic muscles of the hand, with weakened wrist and finger flexion. Contribution to the median and radial nerves may impact thumb and finger flexion and extension respectively. Involvement of C7 can dramatically influence available options for nerve transfer.

Hints and tips

Priorities for lower plexus injuries include restoration of hand extrinsic function. Restoration of hand intrinsic function is virtually unobtainable except in the very young pediatric patient.

Reconstruction techniques

There are few good options for lower plexus injury reconstruction. Recently the authors have incorporated transferring the nerve to brachialis (a branch of the musculocutaneous nerve) to the anterior interosseous nerve to regain thumb and finger flexion. The details of this technique are described under the median nerve injury section below.

Complete/near-complete plexus injury

Specific patient exam findings

Complete, or near-complete, brachial plexus injury often results from high-velocity, penetrating, or crush-type mechanisms and result in devastating loss of function. These patients will typically have an insensate, flail upper extremity with glenohumeral joint subluxation and a positive sulcus sign. Most will lack shoulder stability, abduction, rotation, flexion and extension, elbow flexion and extension, wrist flexion and extension, finger flexion, extension, and intrinsic function.

Reconstruction techniques

Hints and tips

Priorities for complete plexus injuries are to restore function in the following order of priority: (1) elbow flexion; (2) shoulder stability/external rotation; and (3) hand extrinsic function/grasp. Techniques include extraplexal to intraplexal nerve transfers and free functional muscle flap reconstruction. Contralateral C7 and phrenic nerve transfers are also described with modest results.

Use of spinal accessory and intercostal nerves as donors (motor)

Reconstruction in this scenario has very different goals and outcomes from less traumatic injuries. Priorities include restoring elbow flexion, shoulder stability/external rotation,

and hand extrinsic function/grasp. The extremity will often be a "helper" extremity at best. The severe damage to the brachial plexus means that options for nerve transfers are limited, and that extraplexal donors must be considered. Specifically, available extraplexal nerve donors include the spinal accessory, medial pectoral, thoracodorsal, and intercostal nerves.

Donor nerves are isolated as follows. The spinal accessory nerve is harvested as described previously. Intercostal nerves are harvested through an L-shaped incision extending from the anterior axillary fold and curving anteriorly below the nipple–areolar complex. Rib periosteum is incised and peeled down to expose the neurovascular bundles running along the posterior inferior surface of each rib *(Fig. 33.13)*. The motor nerves are smaller and sit more superiorly than the sensory nerves. Often several are required. These are dissected as far medially as possible and then divided.

These extraplexal donor nerves can be transferred to a variety of potential recipients, depending on surgical goals. They can be used to establish shoulder stability and external rotation (suprascapular and axillary nerves), elbow flexion (musculocutaneous), or even to recreate elbow extension or finger flexion by neurotizing one or two free-functioning gracilis flaps.[40] This is often accomplished as a two-stage procedure.

Discussion of cross C7 transfer, phrenic nerve transfers (motor)

Contralateral C7 transfer has been described as a safe option in the literature[41–46] and has been met with varying levels of success and controversy. The phrenic nerve has also been used,[47] with some studies documenting no significant impact on respiration and others reporting decreased pulmonary capacity that goes on to improve.[48] The senior author no longer uses either the phrenic nerve or the contralateral C7 as a potential nerve donor as results are at best Medical Research

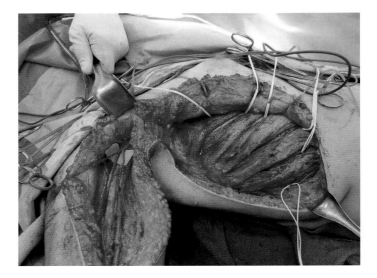

Fig. 33.13 Harvesting intercostal nerves. Clinical photograph of a female patient undergoing intercostal to musculocutaneous nerve transfer. The anterior subcutaneous flap has been turned over medially to expose the anterior chest wall. White vessel loops are around intercostal nerves at the inferior border of each rib. The recipient nerve is visualized in the upper arm on a blue background.

Council (MRC) grade 3 of 5 after several years for limited elbow flexion or poor finger flexion.

Median nerve injury

Specific patient exam findings

The median nerve is a mixed motor and sensory nerve that is derived from C5, C6, C7, C8, and T1. There are no branches in the arm as the nerve courses lateral to the brachial artery and then passes over brachialis in the antecubital fossa. In the forearm, the median nerve proper supplies pronator teres (PT), FCR, palmaris longus, and FDS. The nerve then divides. The anterior interosseous nerve innervates flexor pollicus longus, flexor digitorum profundus (FDP) to the index finger and sometimes long finger, and pronator quadratus (PQ). The remainder of the nerve is largely sensory, with a small motor component contributing to the recurrent motor branch, which innervates the thenar muscles (abductor pollicus brevis, opponens pollicus, and the superficial head of flexor pollicus brevis) and the two radial lumbricals. The sensory contribution is to the volar surface of the thumb, index, long, and radial half of the ring and to the dorsal aspect of those digits distal to the distal interphalangeal joint.

Patients presenting with a median nerve injury will have numbness in the distribution of the median nerve, as described above. Depending on the level of injury, motor deficits will vary.[49] With an injury to the distal forearm, the primary deficits will be thumb abduction and opposition. In more proximal injuries, the patient will also have loss of pronation, thumb flexion and index (and possibly long) finger flexion. Flexion of the wrist will be present with ulnar deviation, due to the intact FCU function provided by the ulnar nerve. Similarly, finger flexion to the ring and small fingers will be retained because of the ulnarly innervated preserved FDP function.

Hints and tips

Priorities with median nerve injury are to re-establish anterior interosseous nerve (AIN) function, thumb opposition, index and long finger flexion, and critical sensation to the first webspace. A combination of nerve and tendon transfers can be done. For reconstruction of proximal median nerve injuries, radial to median nerve transfers are used. For reconstruction of more distal median nerve or isolated AIN injuries, brachialis to AIN branch transfers can be done. This transfer is also useful for patients with lower plexus injuries.

Reconstruction techniques

Use of radial to median branch nerve transfers (motor)

Branches of the radial nerve may be used to restore median nerve function in a proximal median nerve injury.[31] Transfer of the extensor carpi radialis brevis branch (ECRB) of the radial nerve is used to restore PT function. Transfer of the supinator branch is used to restore anterior interosseous nerve (AIN) function (Fig. 33.14). A curvilinear incision is made just distal to the antecubital crease on the volar surface of the forearm. Step lengthening of the PT and release of the deep head will facilitate visualization. The median nerve is

identified and dissected to reveal the AIN and the branch to PT. These recipient nerves are dissected from the main trunk of the median nerve and divided proximally. The nerve to supinator is identified on the posterior aspect of the radial nerve and the ECRB nerve is also identified. There are two fascicles to the ECRB and use of one branch is sufficient to restore pronation. If AIN function is required, the authors recommend using the nerve to brachialis (described below). A disposable nerve stimulator is used for confirmation. The donor nerves are divided distally and a tension-free transfer is then performed.[31] Recovery of pronation occurs approximately 3–4 months postoperatively.[50]

Use of brachialis branch to AIN branch nerve transfer

The brachialis branch of the musculocutaneous nerve may be used to restore AIN function (Fig. 33.15).[51] A curvilinear incision over the anterior aspect of the upper arm is used to expose the median nerve. The LABC nerve is identified traveling with the cephalic vein, and a tug test is used to confirm the identity of this cutaneous nerve. The LABC is followed proximally to its branch point from the musculocutaneous nerve where the nerve to brachialis is identified medially approximately 13 cm proximal to the elbow crease.[8] The donor nerve to brachialis is then followed distally into the muscle as far as possible and divided. It is then transposed over to the median nerve to identify the level for coaptation. Where the nerve to brachialis freely drapes over the median nerve with no tension, an internal neurolysis of the median nerve is performed (Fig. 33.16). Knowledge of the internal topography of the median nerve is crucial to performing this transfer. The lateral aspect of the median nerve is all sensory and the medial aspect is motor. The AIN portion of the nerve is located at the posterior medial aspect of the nerve.[50] First-time users may prefer to dissect the AIN out distally and then visually and, intermittently, physically, neurolyze to confirm that the correct recipient fascicles have been identified. These recipient fascicles are neurotized and divided proximally. Of note, the nerve to the pronator can be included in this transfer to augment AIN function.

Sensory nerve transfer to restore critical sensation to the first webspace is also recommended (see below).

Use of adjunct tendon transfers to augment nerve transfers

Tendon transfers can be utilized to augment nerve transfers in median nerve injury. The most commonly performed tendon transfer would be to restore thumb opposition, as this is innervated by the most distal branches of the median nerve and will be slowest to recover. The authors' preference for restoration of thumb opposition is transfer of extensor indicis proprius tendon to abductor pollicis brevis. Another option is to use extensor digiti minimi.

Ulnar nerve injury

Specific patient exam findings

The ulnar nerve is a mixed motor and sensory nerve that receives contribution from C7, C8, and T1. There are no branches in the arm as the nerve courses medial to the brachial artery, dorsal to the medial intermuscular septum, and

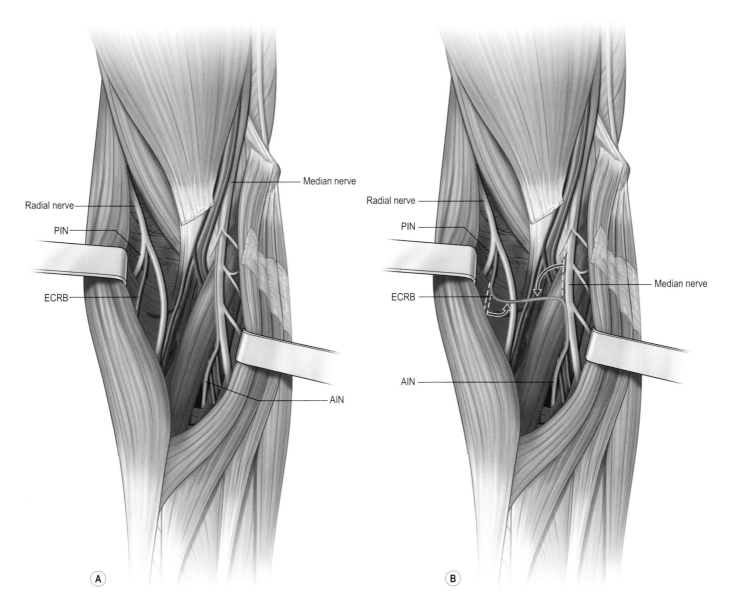

Fig. 33.14 A schematic of radial to median nerve transfers. **(A)** The radial nerve is visualized superiorly as it branches into three branches, from lateral to medial: posterior interosseous nerve (PIN), extensor carpi radialis brevis (ECRB), and radial sensory. The donor ECRB nerve is green. The median nerve is visualized inferiorly, with the nonfunctioning anterior interosseous nerve (AIN) illustrated branching off the lateral aspect of the nerve (red). Note that the AIN is the only branch to exit radially. **(B)** The donor ECRB nerve has been coapted end to end with the distal recipient AIN nerve.

then posteriorly around the medial epicondyle. Branches of the ulnar nerve proper in the forearm include FCU and FDP to the ring and small fingers. The nerve then courses through the forearm deep to FCU and gives off the dorsal cutaneous branch approximately 9 cm proximal to the wrist crease. This branch provides sensation to the dorsal ulnar aspect of the distal forearm and hand. A superficial motor branch provides innervation to palmaris brevis. Then, as the nerve courses into the wrist through Guyon's canal, it divides into a superficial sensory branch, which provides sensation to the small finger and the ulnar aspect of the ring finger, and the deep motor branch, which courses around the hook of the hamate under

the tendinous leading edge of the hypothenar muscles. The deep motor branch innervates the hypothenar muscles (flexor digiti minimi, opponens digiti minimi, and abductor digiti minimi), the palmar and dorsal interossei, the lumbricals to the small and ring fingers, the deep head of flexor pollicis brevis, and the adductor pollicus.[49]

Patients presenting with an ulnar nerve injury will have numbness in the sensory distribution of the ulnar nerve, as described above. Depending on the level of injury, sensation to the dorsum of the hand and wrist may also be affected. The motor deficits associated with ulnar nerve injury are particularly devastating. The deep motor branch of the ulnar nerve

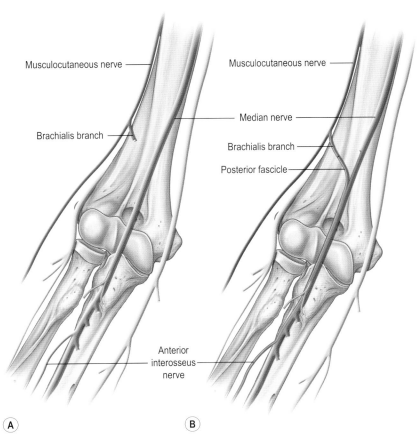

Fig. 33.15 A schematic of the nerve to brachialis to anterior interosseous nerve transfer. **(A)** The median nerve (pink) and musculocutaneous nerve (yellow) are shown in their normal anatomic position. Note that the branch to brachialis exits medially approximately 13 cm to the elbow crease. **(B)** The brachialis branch of the musculocutaneous nerve (donor) is coapted end to end with the divided distal end of the anterior interosseous nerve (recipient), which is located on the posterior medial aspect of the median nerve in the arm.

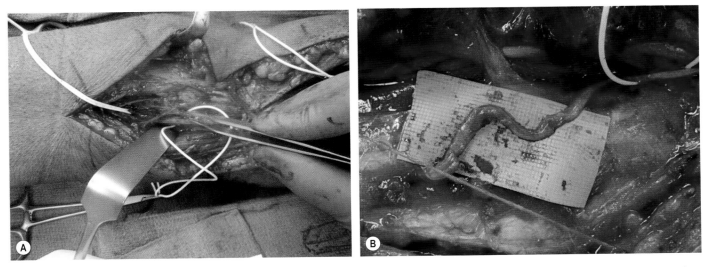

Fig. 33.16 Clinical photos of nerve to brachialis to anterior interosseous nerve. A clinical example of a nerve to brachialis to anterior interosseous nerve (AIN) transfer. **(A)** The median nerve is isolated with a vessel loop. Forceps are used to reveal the AIN nerve branching off the radial aspect of the median nerve. **(B)** A magnified view illustrating the branch to brachialis (marked with a vessel loop) divided and transposed over, to be coapted end to end with the recipient distal AIN.

innervates all of the intrinsic muscles of the hand, and injury results in the inability to pinch, abduct and adduct the fingers, and impairs power grasp. More proximal injuries will also further impair grip, with added losses of FDP to the small and ring fingers and FCU.

Hints and tips

Priorities for ulnar nerve injury are to re-establish intrinsic muscle function, especially pinch, ring, and small finger flexion, and critical sensation to the ulnar border of the hand. A combination of nerve and tendon transfers can be done. For reconstruction of proximal nerve injuries, a direct end-to-end anterior interosseous nerve (AIN) to deep motor branch of ulnar nerve transfer is useful. For incomplete, or partial, nerve injuries where level of recovery is uncertain, reverse end-to-side AIN to deep motor branch "supercharging" should be considered.

Reconstruction techniques

Use of median to ulnar branch nerve transfers (motor)

The median nerve may be used to restore ulnar nerve function, especially following very proximal injuries where time to regenerate to motor end plate becomes an issue. Both sensory and motor nerve transfers are utilized to restore optimal function. The sensory nerve transfers are described later. For restoration of intrinsic muscle function, the distal AIN nerve is transferred to the deep motor branch of the ulnar nerve at the distal forearm level *(Fig. 33.17)*.[24,30] Release of the nerve through Guyon's canal, with particular attention to adequate release of the deep motor branch, is an essential component of this transfer.[16] The donor AIN nerve is identified through a curvilinear incision on the distal volar forearm. The PQ is identified by retracting the flexor tendons radially and the AIN is visualized entering the deep surface of PQ centrally. The nerve is followed distally by dividing PQ until approximately the mid-substance of the muscle, where the nerve begins to branch extensively and is divided just proximal to this branching.[16] The nerve is then transposed over to the ulnar nerve to identify the point where it can be coapted with no tension *(Fig. 33.18)*. The wrist is taken through full range of motion to ensure that wrist motion will not influence the inset tension. At this point, the neurolysis of the ulnar nerve is performed. Within the proximal forearm, prior to the take off the dorsal cutaneous branch, the topography of the ulnar nerve is sensory–motor–sensory. The medialmost sensory portion goes on to become the dorsal cutaneous ulnar branch (DCU) approximately 9 cm proximal to the wrist crease. As the nerve continues, the lateral sensory portion of the ulnar nerve is significantly larger than the more medial motor portion. Microforceps are used to tap along the surface of the nerve until they plunge into the natural cleavage plane between the sensory and motor portions of the nerve.[30] Visual neurolysis from the deep motor branch decompression at the leading edge of the hypothenar muscles confirms this. Once this plane is identified, the recipient motor fascicular group is isolated proximally and divided to allow for the appropriate motor nerve transfer.

Sensory nerve transfer to the ulnar border of the hand is recommended (see below).

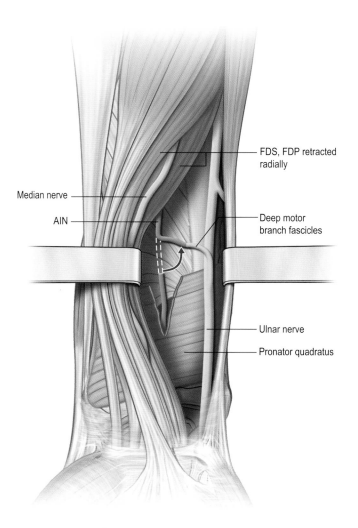

Fig. 33.17 Anterior interosseous nerve (AIN) to deep motor branch of ulnar nerve. A schematic of the distal AIN to deep motor branch transfer. The donor AIN (green) is seen divided under the pronator quadratus muscle and transposed over to the recipient deep motor branch of the ulnar nerve. At this level, distal to the take off the dorsal cutaneous ulnar branch, the motor fascicles are ulnar and the main sensory component of the nerve is radial. The coaptation is performed in an end-to-end manner. FDS, flexor digitorum superficialis; FDP, flexor digitorum profundus.

Use of adjunct tendon transfers to augment nerve transfers

Tendon transfers are frequently performed to augment median to ulnar nerve transfers. The intrinsic muscles are so distal and are so important for function that these tendon transfers are often performed at the same time as the nerve transfers, even though their use might be considered redundant. Tenodesis of the ulnar nerve-powered ring and small FDP tendons to the median nerve-powered index and long FDP tendons is performed. Thumb adduction is also augmented using extensor indicis proprius to adductor pollicus tendon transfer. In patients with a prominent Wartenburg's sign, abductor digiti minimi is transferred to the extensor digitorum communis tendon of the small finger.[30]

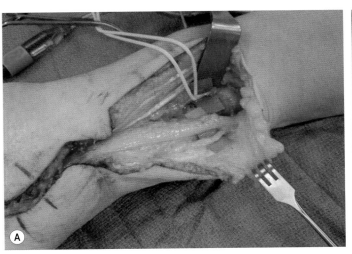 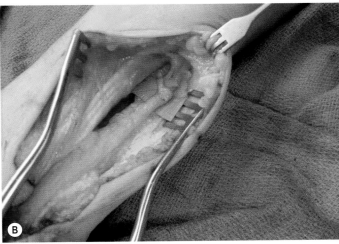

Fig. 33.18 Clinical photos of anterior interosseous nerve (AIN) to deep motor branch of ulnar nerve. Clinical example of an AIN to deep motor branch nerve transfer. **(A)** A vessel loop surrounds the distal AIN. The ulnar nerve is exposed on a blue background. The dorsal cutaneous ulnar branch is illustrated branching off ulnarly. **(B)** The donor AIN is divided distally and transposed over to the ulnar nerve. The dorsal cutaneous branch of the ulnar nerve is now located beneath the blue background, and a motor fascicle from the ulnar aspect of the main nerve is divided as the recipient and coapted end to end to the AIN nerve.

Radial nerve injury

Specific patient exam findings

The radial nerve is a mixed motor and sensory nerve that receives contribution from C5, C6, C7, C8, and T1. In the axilla, the radial nerve gives off the posterior cutaneous nerve of the arm. It then provides innervation to the three heads of the triceps muscle before piercing the lateral intermuscular septum and coursing through the spiral groove. In the distal arm, there are branches to anconeus epitrochlearis and brachioradialis as the nerve crosses the elbow between brachialis and brachioradialis. The extensor carpi radialis longus (ECRL) is the last branch of the radial nerve proper. The nerve then branches into the posterior interosseous nerve (PIN), which continues distally into the arm, passing between the superficial and deep heads of the supinator at the arcade of Froshe, and the radial sensory branch. The radial sensory branch innervates the dorsoradial aspect of the forearm and wrist, and the dorsal aspect of the thumb, index, long, and radial half of the ring finger. The PIN then innervates the remainder of the muscles on the extensor aspect of the forearm, including ECRB, supinator, extensor carpi ulnaris, extensor indicis proprius, extensor digitorum communis, extensor digiti minimi, abductor pollicus longus, extensor pollicus longus, and extensor pollicus brevis. Of note, the ECRB branch can occasionally come off the radial nerve proper or branch off along with the radial sensory nerve, meaning that wrist extension can be variably affected in injuries at this level depending on individual anatomy.

Patients presenting with radial nerve injuries will have sensory defects in the distribution of the radial nerve, as described above. Motor deficits will depend on the level of injury. Injury at the level of the PIN will result in the patient's inability to extend thumb and fingers, with weak, radially deviated wrist extension powered primarily by the ECRL. Injury more proximally will result in complete loss of wrist extension in addition to loss of thumb and finger extension.

Reconstruction techniques

Use of median to radial branch nerve transfers

The deficit created by radial nerve injury can be corrected with median nerve transfers. Primary goals include restoration of wrist, finger, and thumb extension. The most commonly performed transfers include using redundant fascicles to FDS or FCR as donors to provide innervation to PIN and ECRB *(Fig. 33.19)*.[52,53] A curvilinear incision is made over the proximal volar forearm, often beginning just proximal to the antecubital fossa. The lacertus fibrosus is identified and incised to improve exposure. The radial artery and accompanying vena comitantes are identified between PT and brachioradialis. Step lengthening of the PT may be performed to improve visualization. The median nerve is identified on the ulnar aspect of the radial vessels, and exposure of the nerve distally is performed by releasing the tendinous leading edge of the FDS. Again, knowledge of the internal topography of the median nerve is essential for this transfer, as protection of the branches to PT and AIN is mandatory. The most proximal branches, of which there are usually two, are to PT. Then, a branch to FCR and PL departs from the ulnar side of the nerve. The next two branches will be to the FDS and also depart ulnarly. The AIN departs from the median nerve on

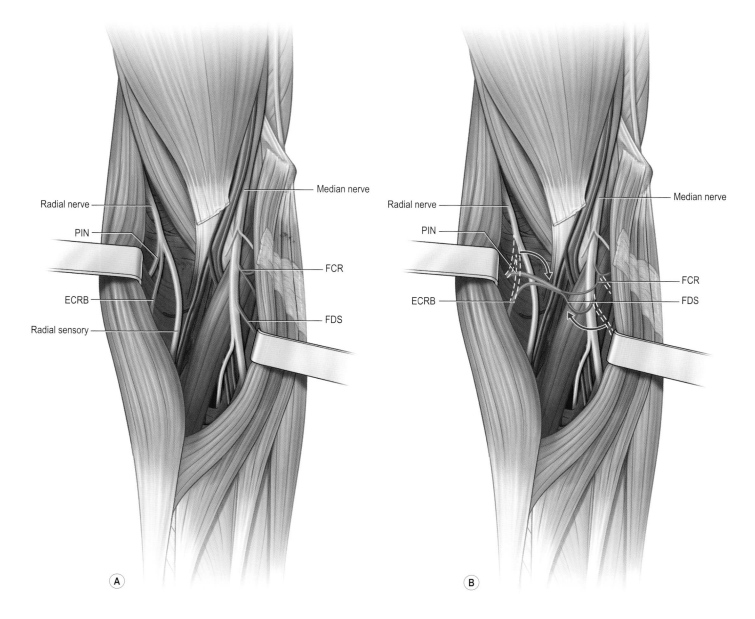

Fig. 33.19 Median to radial nerve transfers. A schematic diagram of median to radial nerve transfers. The redundant fascicles to flexor carpi radialis (FCR) and flexor digitorum superficialis (FDS) (donors) are transferred to the extensor carpi radialis brevis (ECRB) and posterior interosseous nerve (PIN) respectively.

the radial side, and is the only branch to exit radially. This occurs just distal to the leading edge of the FDS, and once AIN has branched off, the majority of the remainder of the median nerve is sensory. Again, a combination of nerve stimulation and identification of natural cleavage planes can facilitate orienting the various components of the median nerve.

The radial nerve branches are identified by retracting the brachioradialis laterally. The first nerve encountered will be the radial sensory branch, followed by the smaller branch to ECRB and the larger PIN located just deep and radial to the sensory branch. These recipient nerves are dissected as proximally as possible and then transected. Mobilization is facilitated by excluding the branch to the supinator, which comes off posteriorly. The recipient nerves are then transposed over

to the median nerve to determine the level for neurolysis. The median nerve is dissected and redundant fascicles to FDS and FCR are divided as donor nerves. Care is taken not to use PT or AIN fascicles, and to ensure through stimulation that median nerve function is not impacted by division of the redundant fascicles.[52] Motor reinnervation occurs at approximately 9–12 months postoperatively.[54,55]

Use of adjunct tendon transfers to augment nerve transfers

The authors suggest augmenting median to radial nerve transfers with tendon transfer of PT to ECRB during the same procedure. This transfer provides earlier restoration of wrist

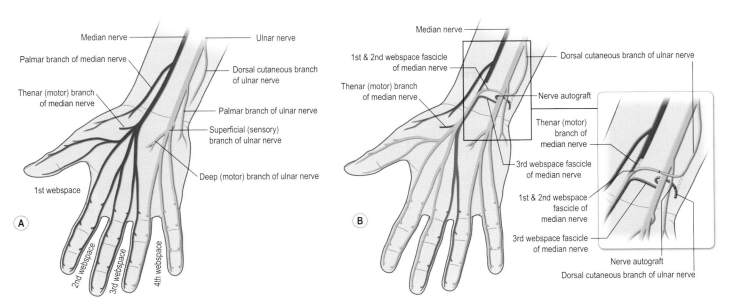

Fig. 33.20 A schematic of the triad of transfers used to restore sensation in a median nerve deficit. **(A)** The nonfunctional median (red) and the functioning ulnar nerve (yellow). **(B)** The triad of nerve transfers from ulnar to median (inset) is a magnification of the transfers showing the dorsal cutaneous branch of the ulnar nerve (donor) coapted end to end to the radial side of the median (recipient) to restore first webspace sensation, the distal third webspace (recipient) end to side to the ulnar sensory (donor), and the distal dorsal cutaneous branch of the ulnar nerve end to side to restore sensation to the donor deficit. The third webspace fascicle is shown in blue.

extension, which is then enhanced once the nerve transfer becomes viable at 9–12 months.[52]

Sensory nerve injury

Restoration of key sensory functions

Restoration of discriminatory sensation in critical areas can be accomplished using noncritical area donors.[24] One of the newer developments in nerve transfer surgery is to maintain some donor territory protective sensation by use of adjunct end-to-side transfers. A number of studies have demonstrated that "collateral sprouting" occurs with an end-to-side sensory repair, and novel axonal regeneration from the donor nerve occurs into the recipient stump.[17,56] Only sensory axons sprout *de novo* without injury, whereas motor nerves require a proximal nerve injury to do so.[17,57] Making use of this principle, efforts are made to restore protective sensation to the donor region with end-to-side coaptation of the distal donor to an intact sensory nerve.

Use of ulnar to median branch nerve transfers (sensory)

Sensory defects associated with median nerve injury include numbness to the radial volar side of the hand, including the first, second, and third webspaces. The first webspace is an area of critical sensation as it is primarily used for pinch. A fourth webspace (ulnar) to first webspace (median) nerve transfer can be performed to restore first webspace sensation only. Alternatively, a triad of nerve transfers from the ulnar nerve can restore more extensive sensation and minimize donor deficits *(Fig. 33.20)*. The DCU is transferred end to end to the radial portion of the median nerve to restore critical thumb and radial index sensation. At this level, the internal topography of the median nerve is such that the nerve to the

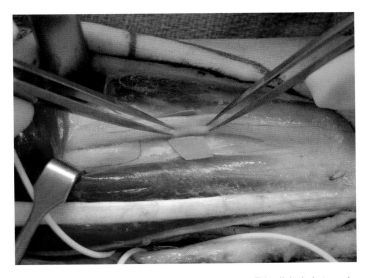

Fig. 33.21 Identifying the fascicle to the third webspace. This clinical photograph demonstrates identifying the third webspace fascicle at the proximal wrist level. Microforceps were walked along the surface of the nerve until they plunged into the natural cleavage plane. The division is also marked with a prominent vessel on the surface of the nerve.

third webspace can be easily identified by tapping across the surface of the nerve and entering this natural cleavage plane. The nerve to the third webspace is the most ulnar portion grouping of fascicles at this level *(Fig. 33.21)*. The third webspace nerve is dissected out from the median nerve and coapted end to side to the main sensory component of the ulnar nerve for restoration of third webspace protective sensation. The distal end of the transected donor DCU is coapted end to side to the ulnar nerve to restore the donor deficit. All

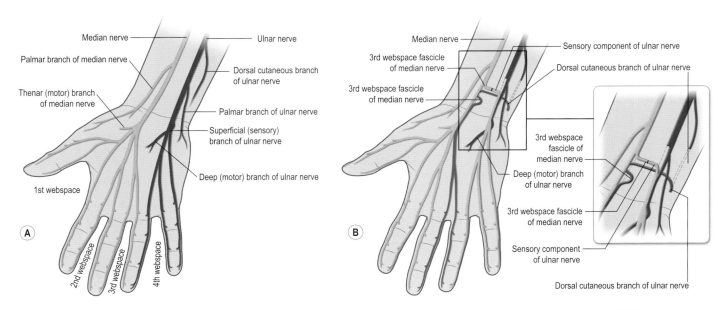

Fig. 33.22 Sensory nerve transfers to restore ulnar nerve deficit. A schematic of the triad of nerve transfers used to restore ulnar nerve sensation. **(A)** The functioning median nerve is shown in yellow and the nonfunctioning ulnar nerve is shown in red. **(B)** The triad of nerve transfers to restore sensation. (Inset) A magnified view of the nerve transfers illustrating the third webspace fascicle (donor) coapted end to end with the ulnar sensory (recipient), the distal dorsal cutaneous branch of the ulnar nerve (recipient) coapted end to side to the sensory side of the intact median nerve (donor), and the distal third webspace nerve coapted end to side to the median sensory to restore donor sensory loss.

of these transfers are conducted through a volar distal forearm curvilinear incision and are accompanied by an open carpal tunnel release.[30]

Use of median to ulnar branch nerve transfers (sensory)

Sensory defects associated with an ulnar nerve injury include numbness to the ulnar aspect of the hand, including the small and ulnar half of the ring finger. In addition, if the take off the DCU is distal to the level of injury, numbness on the ulnar distal forearm and wrist will be present. A third webspace (median) to ulnar small-finger nerve transfer can be used to restore sensation to the ulnar border of the hand. Alternatively, restoration of ulnar nerve sensation can be provided by a triad of nerve transfers from the median nerve *(Fig. 33.22)*. The third webspace fascicle of the median nerve is dissected out and transferred end to end to the main sensory component of the ulnar nerve. The ulnar nerve at this level is oriented in a sensory–motor–sensory alignment. The DCU nerve branches off on the ulnar side of the nerve. The remaining ulnar nerve is approximately two-thirds sensory on the radialmost portion, and one-third motor on the ulnar portion *(Fig. 33.23)*. This motor portion will go on to become the deep motor branch in Guyon's canal. End-to-side coaptation of the dorsal cutaneous ulnar branch to the sensory component of the median nerve is performed more proximally. The distal third webspace (median) donor is then coapted end to side to the remainder of the intact sensory portion of the median nerve to restore protective sensation to the donor defect. Again, these transfers are conducted through a volar distal forearm curvilinear incision and are accompanied by release of both the carpal tunnel and Guyon's canal.

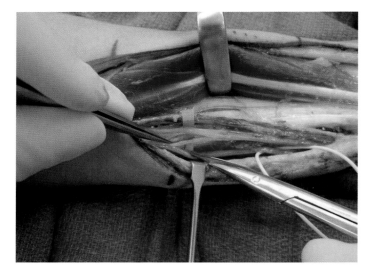

Fig. 33.23 Internal topography of the ulnar nerve in the distal forearm. A clinical photograph illustrating the internal topography of a neurolyzed ulnar nerve at the wrist. The tenotomy scissors are displacing the dorsal cutaneous branch of the ulnar nerve ulnarly, the microforceps are separating the deep motor branch fascicles ulnarly, and the remainder of the radial portion of the nerve is sensory. At this level, the topography of the ulnar nerve is sensory–motor–sensory in a radial to ulnar direction.

Use of median and ulnar nerve transfers to restore first webspace sensation in C5–C6 root level brachial plexus injury (sensory)

In patients with an isolated upper trunk injury, sensation to the first and second webspaces will be absent. A combination of distal transfers at the level of the median and ulnar nerve

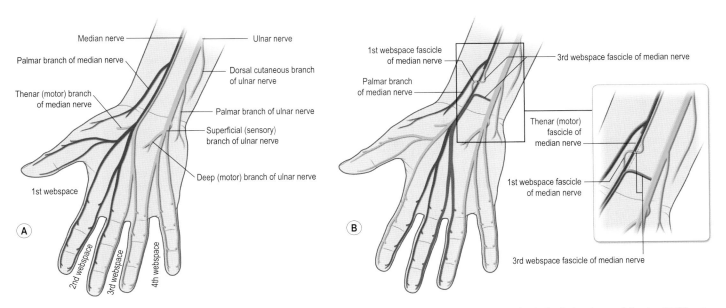

Fig. 33.24 Sensory nerve transfers to restore C5/C6 deficit. A schematic of sensory nerve transfers used to restore sensation to the first webspace following C5/C6 root injuries of the brachial plexus. **(A)** The nonfunctional nerves are visualized in red and the functioning nerves are yellow. **(B)** The ulnar and median nerves are used to restore sensation to the first webspace and the radial border of the thumb. (Inset) A magnified view of the nerve transfers illustrating end-to-end coaptation of the third webspace nerve (donor) to the first webspace nerve (recipient). The distal third webspace nerve is then coapted end to side with the sensory portion of the ulnar nerve to restore sensation to the donor third webspace.

proper can be used to reconstruct this deficit *(Fig. 33.24)*. The third webspace nerve is dissected out from the median nerve, transected, and coapted end to end to the radial aspect of the median nerve to restore thumb and first webspace sensation. The distal end of the transected third webspace is coapted end to side to the ulnar nerve to restore protective sensation of the donor site. This effectively transfers intact sensation that originated from the C7 and C8 roots to the C5 and C6 level at a close-to-target end organ level.

Use of lateral antebrachial cutaneous nerve to radial nerve transfers (sensory)

Patients with radial sensory nerve injury have numbness on the dorsal radial aspect of the hand and wrist. Unfortunately, this injury is also commonly associated with excruciating phantom pain due to this nerve's exquisite sensitivity to denervation. The lateral antebrachial cutaneous nerve runs superficial and medial to the brachioradialis and is in close proximity to the radial sensory nerve. It is also a close size match. Coaptation of the expendable LABC to the denervated radial sensory nerve territory may not restore completely normal sensation, but can significantly interrupt the neuropathic pain cycle.

Use of radial to axillary nerve transfers (sensory)

Patients with axillary nerve injury have numbness on the lateral aspect of the shoulder. The sensory branch of the axillary nerve is always identified when dissecting out the axillary nerve as a recipient for nerve transfer as the most inferior fascicle and can be confirmed with a tug test. To re-establish sensation in this distribution, the axillary nerve can be transferred end to side to a functioning intact nerve such as the radial. At this level, the internal topography of the radial nerve is such that the lateral aspect is sensory.

Postoperative care

Postoperative wound care

Patients are initially placed into a bulky soft dressing and protective splint for distal-extremity transfers, and a shoulder immobilizer for proximal-nerve transfers. An incisional pain pump that delivers continuous bupivacaine 0.5% plain is used, as well as a Blake drain for larger dissections. Bupivacaine is also injected into all surgical sites prior to reversal of anesthesia. Foley catheters are removed and patients are encouraged to ambulate early.

For longer surgeries, proximal-nerve transfer, or patients with any significant comorbidities, a 23-hour observation stay is routine. Patients are instructed to leave their dressings intact for 48 hours, and then return to the clinic for dressing removal, discontinuation of drain and pain pump, and incision check. The majority of incisions are closed with dissolvable sutures; however nondissolvable sutures are removed at 2 weeks. Patients are encouraged to move their extremity early to promote nerve gliding, as all nerve transfers are performed under no tension. Protective splinting for distal nerve transfers is maintained for approximately 7–10 days, although patients come out of their splints for therapy.[24] Concomitant tendon transfers may also dictate splinting and therapy regimens and will supersede the minor restrictions required for post nerve transfer patients. If the insertion of the pectoralis major muscle was disinserted to allow access to the medial pectoral nerve, the tendon is reapproximated and the shoulder is immobilized for a full 4 weeks.[24] Patients are followed at regular intervals depending on the level of their original injury, the type of nerve transfer, and their distance from our surgical center.

Complications

Complications associated with nerve transfers can be divided into general and specific complications. The general surgical complications associated with any surgical procedure include the risk of an adverse event with anesthesia, especially in prolonged surgeries or in patients with concomitant injuries. Other complications include bleeding, hematoma, seroma, pain, scarring, and injury to adjacent structures. Complications specific to nerve surgery include temporary neurapraxia secondary to retraction or manipulation of nerves, neuroma, and inadequate functional recovery. The complication rate associated with nerve transfer should be significantly less than that seen with operating within a scarred and hostile zone of injury. Nerve transfers are performed remote from the time of injury, thus ensuring that patients have been stabilized, appropriately evaluated and educated, serially clinically examined, and perhaps most importantly, that surgery takes place during regular, scheduled hours with a staff familiar with the procedure, as opposed to exploratory repair in a trauma or after-hours situation.

Rehabilitation

All patients are introduced to our hand therapists prior to surgery and referrals for therapy are given at the first postoperative visit. Patients are instructed about wound and scar management, need for protective splinting or sling use, and pain management. Wrist cock-up splints are used in patients with radial nerve injuries until reinnervation occurs. Supportive braces for patients with painful humeral subluxation at the glenohumeral joint due to loss of deltoid function can also be used. Education about their nerve transfer is provided, and retraining is discussed in the early postoperative period, long before clinical recovery will have occurred, to keep the motor cortex prepared for reinnervation.[24,58] The long-term focus of rehabilitation is on re-education, as the cortical command required to initiate target muscle function will differ from before.[59] The patient will "relearn" motor control of the reinnervated target muscle by activating the nerve to the donor muscle, similar to the re-education required following tendon transfer.[4,59] For restoration of sensation, as patients perceive input stimulus from the reinnervated territory, cortical remapping occurs.[4,59] Patients are provided with written instructions about exercises as well as an anticipated time line for recovery.

Many of our patients travel from long distances, therefore our hand therapists are actively involved in directing their local therapists about nerve transfers and retraining. Nerve transfers are such a specialized and unique surgery that many therapists are unfamiliar with them, and we have found that providing written instruction is imperative. In addition, every patient sees our therapist at each return visit in order to check progress and make any necessary adjustments to therapy. Caution is taken to bring patients back to the clinic approximately 1 month before we would anticipate reinnervation to be noted clinically in order to review again the instructions for therapy. Prior to reinnervation, the focus is on maintaining full active and passive range of motion and on prevention of pain syndromes related to musculoskeletal imbalances associated with lost or impaired muscle strength.

Therapists also work to optimize strength of uninvolved and donor muscles following transfer.

Once reinnervation has occurred, therapy is focused on strengthening. Maintaining full passive range of motion throughout is paramount.[24] Patients may start by "strengthening the donor" and then advance to co-contracture activities as reinnervation proceeds. For example, this would include finger and wrist flexion with elbow flexion in double fascicular nerve transfer patients. Specific strategies involve repetitive motor co-contraction of the donor and recipient muscles, with and without passive assistance. The incorporation of resistance into the exercises is progressive as tolerated, starting with gravity completely eliminated and then against gravity, and finally against resistance. Place-and-hold exercises facilitate strengthening. Resisted exercises are introduced much later, after good movement against gravity is obtained, to avoid overfatiguing the transfer and discouraging the patient.

In severe injuries, hand therapists can instruct patients in adaptive strategies for handedness retraining and performing activities of daily living with their impaired extremity. We have found that hand therapy is an integral part of the success of our nerve transfers.

Outcomes and prognosis

Video
2,3

The evaluation of outcomes following brachial plexus and peripheral nerve reconstruction lacks standardization and objectivity, largely given the extent and variation of nerve injuries.[24] In addition, the expected outcomes vary with the initial injury, given that nerve transfer for a partial, distal nerve defect would be anticipated to have near-complete function following surgery compared to a panplexus type of injury presenting with a flail extremity, where expectations are significantly less. Due to these difficulties, it is difficult to compare different surgical approaches with regard to patient outcome and prognosis; however there have been numerous articles reporting favorable outcomes on an increasing number of nerve transfer options (video 2).

Shoulder function is best improved by reinnervation of both suprascapular and axillary nerves, confirmed in a large meta-analysis of 1088 nerve transfers.[35] In a recent study by Garg et al. the use of dual nerve transfers to restore shoulder and elbow function in C5/C6 level injuries was superior to the results of traditional nerve grafting.[60] In a clinical series of 7 patients undergoing nerve transfer from triceps to axillary nerve, all patients recovered MRC grade 4 of 5 deltoid function, 6/7 patients recovered MRC grade 4 of 5 shoulder external rotation, and the last patient regained MRC grade 3 of 5.[34]

The double fascicular nerve transfer has been evaluated with long-term follow-up in more than one study, and all patients were noted to achieve at least MRC grade 4 of 5 function with no appreciable donor deficit.[37,61] Innervation was noted at a mean of 5.5 months postoperatively.[37]

In medial pectoral to musculocutaneous nerve transfers with an interpositional lateral antebrachial cutaneous nerve graft, 3 of 4 patients achieved MRC grade 4 of 5 elbow flexion, and the last MRC grade 3 of 5. Reinnervation was first noted at 6–8 months postoperatively.[8]

Recently, our experience with nerve transfer to triceps for recovery of elbow extension was evaluated. Four patients underwent transfer, 2 with FCU fascicles as a donor, 1 with thoracodorsal as a donor, and 1 using a radial nerve fascicle to ECRL as a donor. The patients received MRC grade 5, 4+, 4, and 4 out of 5 respectively.[62]

Restoration of radial nerve function in the forearm using expendable branches of the median nerve has demonstrated predictable results, with MRC grade 4 of 5 wrist and finger extension by 1 year.[54,55]

In another series, 8 patients undergoing transfer of the distal AIN to the deep motor branch of the ulnar nerve were evaluated. All patients had reinnervation of the ulnar intrinsic muscles facilitating grip and lateral pinch strength. No patient required anticlaw procedures. None of the patients had a deficit in pronation associated with AIN transfer. A single patient required a secondary tendon transfer to improve small-finger adduction.[16]

Inevitably, the literature contains much controversy regarding the outcomes following nerve transfers, and longer follow-up is required to assess the success of these novel procedures. It seems clear, however, that the exponential increase in publications related to nerve transfers demonstrates that nerve transfers can no longer be considered experimental, and are rivaling other procedures in the treatment of severe brachial plexus and many other peripheral nerve injuries.

Secondary procedures

Given the devastating nature of brachial plexus and proximal nerve injuries, it is inevitable that nerve transfers are not successful in every circumstance. Where concern exists regarding the likelihood of functional recovery, adjunct procedures are performed to augment the nerve transfer.

In the event of a failed nerve transfer, and the necessity of further secondary procedures, there are several important considerations. When planning nerve transfers, one must consider the possible salvage procedures required should the transfer fail. Thus, when deciding on donor nerve, it is prudent to ensure that options are left for later (for example, avoiding the harvest of redundant fascicles to both flexor carpi radialis and FCU). A donor for tendon transfer requires MRC grade 5 of 5 strength because following transfer it will be downgraded by a minimum of one grade.[49] This becomes especially challenging in patients with multiple nerve injuries, and illustrates the importance of an accurate and detailed physical examination at preoperative assessment.

Hints and tips

Avoid using a donor nerve that may be required for a secondary procedure such as a tendon transfer down the road. Prior to cutting a donor nerve, make sure the rest of the nerve performs all essential functions with fastidious intraoperative nerve stimulation.

Tendon transfers have the benefit of not being restricted by time, given that distal motor denervation and fibrosis do not affect the outcome. For this reason, there is no harm in attempting a nerve transfer as a primary procedure, and reserving the tendon transfer for a secondary procedure if the functional outcome is less than desired.

Nerve transfers should not be attempted if there are not suitable, redundant, available donors, as in the setting of a multinerve injury. In this setting, nerve grafting combined with tendon transfer, or even arthrodesis, may be warranted.

In our experience, secondary procedures are rarely required following nerve transfer. However we are diligent about considering options when planning our initial procedure.

Access the complete references list online at **http://www.expertconsult.com**

17. Hayashi A, Pannucci C, Moradzadeh A, et al. Axotomy or compression is required for axonal sprouting following end-to-side neurorrhaphy. *Exp Neurol.* 2008;211:539–550.

    This study demonstrated that sensory nerves would collaterally sprout from a normal nerve into a distal end-to-side-positioned nerve spontaneously. By contrast it showed that a motor nerve needed an injury in order to sprout (traumatic sprouting). This is a significant paper in that it shows that if you want to get some sensory recovery, then the end-to-side will work, but if you want motor, you need to injure the motor nerve traumatically in order to get it to sprout in an end-to-side fashion.

22. Kale SS, Glaus SW, Yee A, et al. Evaluation of the reverse end-to-side nerve transfer in an animal model. *J Hand Surg.* 2011 (in press).

24. Tung TH, Mackinnon SE. Nerve transfers: indications, techniques, and outcomes. *J Hand Surg Am.* 2010;35:332–341.

27. Cheng CJ, Mackinnon-Patterson, B, Beck, JL, et al. Scratch collapse test for evaluation of carpal and cubital tunnel syndrome. *J Hand Surg Am.* 2008;33:1518–1524.

29. Kozin SH. Injuries of the Brachial Plexus, In Iannotti JP, Williams GR, eds. *Disorders of the Shoulder: Diagnosis and Management.* Philidelphia, PA: Lippincott Williams & Wilkins; 2007:1087–1130.

30. *Brown JM, Yee A, Mackinnon SE. Distal median to ulnar nerve transfers to restore ulnar motor and sensory function within the hand: technical nuances. *Neurosurgery.* 2009;65:966–977; discussion 977–8.

    This is an up-to-date description of the technical nuances of transfer from the distal anterior interosseous nerve to the motor component of the ulnar nerve. This anterior interosseous nerve to deep motor branch of ulnar nerve was first done by the authors in 1991 and is generally accepted as a procedure of choice for high ulnar nerve problems.

52. Brown JM, Tung TH, Mackinnon SE. Median to radial nerve transfer to restore wrist and finger extension:

technical nuances. *Neurosurgery.* 2010;66(3 Suppl):75–83; discussion 83.

53. Ray WZ, Mackinnon SE. Clinical Outcomes Following Median to Radial Nerve Transfers. *J Hand Surg Am.* 2010;36:201–208.

   This manuscript describes the outcome of a number of patients undergoing median to radial nerve transfer and provides the technical nuances and the pearls and pitfalls of this nerve transfer.

56. Ray WZ, Mackinnon SE. Management of nerve gaps: autografts, allografts, nerve transfers, and end-to-side neurorrhaphy. *Exp Neurol.* 2010;223:77–85.

This summary review article outlines the key challenges in the reconstruction of nerve gaps, with critical points on the use of nerve autografts, allografts, nerve repairs, nerve transfers, and end-to-side repair.

58. *Mackinnon SE, Novak CB. Nerve transfers. *Hand Clin.* 2008;24:319–490.

This Hand Clinics is a multiauthored text covering all aspects of nerve transfers from surgical techniques to physical therapy.

34

Tendon transfers in the upper extremity

Neil F. Jones

SYNOPSIS

- Tendon transfers in the upper limb are indicated to restore function to paralyzed muscle and tendon following nerve injury, traumatic muscle or tendon injury, and to restore balance to hands affected by neurological disease.
- In selecting a donor muscle–tendon, the surgeon has to consider expendability of the muscle-tendon unit, the relative strength of donor and paralyzed muscles, and the amplitude and direction of transfer of the muscle.
- The timing of tendon transfers can be classified as early, conventional or late.
- Upper extremity nerve injuries can be subdivided into radial nerve palsy, low and high median nerve palsy, low and high ulnar nerve palsy, and combined nerve injuries.

Introduction

Tendon transfers are reconstructive techniques that will restore motion or balance to a hand impaired by absent function of the extrinsic or intrinsic muscle-tendon units. In a typical tendon transfer, the tendon of insertion of a functioning muscle is detached, mobilized and reattached to another tendon or bone to substitute for the action of a nonfunctioning muscle-tendon unit. Occasionally, both the tendon of origin and the tendon of insertion are detached and reattached. Unlike a tendon graft, the transferred donor tendon remains attached to its parent muscle. Unlike microsurgical free muscle transfer, the neurovascular pedicle to the muscle of the transferred tendon remains intact.

There are three general indications for tendon transfers in the upper extremity:

1. To restore function to a paralysed muscle due to injuries of the peripheral nerves, the brachial plexus or the spinal cord

2. To restore function following closed tendon ruptures or open injuries to the tendons or muscles

3. To restore balance to a deformed hand due to various neurological diseases.

Tendon transfers are best conceptualized as a means to restore a lost "function", rather than a means of substituting for a specific muscle, i.e., restoring strong pinch as opposed to restoring function of the flexor pollicis longus (FPL). Tendon transfers are performed predominantly following peripheral nerve injuries and therefore will be discussed according to the three specific nerve palsies. However, the general principles described in this chapter apply to all transfers (*Table 34.1*).

Basic science

Bone and soft tissue healing

Steindler[1] recognized that tendon transfers cannot glide through edematous or scarred soft tissues nor can they flex or extend stiff metacarpophalangeal (MCP) and proximal interphalangeal (PIP) joints. He advocated that tendon transfers be delayed until "tissue equilibrium" had been restored. Before a tendon transfer is performed, all fractures should be healed. Chronic scarred skin and subcutaneous tissues or skin grafts in the line of pull of a tendon transfer should be excised and the defect resurfaced with a flap that is itself allowed to heal with mature scars. If secondary tendon transfers are necessary, initial split thickness skin grafting, simply to achieve a healed wound, should be avoided. Instead, a pliable flap of skin and subcutaneous tissues should be considered as a delayed primary coverage using pedicled flaps or free flaps. Occasionally, silicone rods can be placed at the time of flap coverage, either beneath or through the subcutaneous fat of a transferred flap to create a smooth tunnel through which a tendon transfer may be later passed. The span of the thumb-index finger web space should be maintained by splinting especially following median nerve injuries. If a secondary

Table 34.1 Basic principles of tendon transfers

Soft tissue equilibrium
Full passive range of motion of involved joints
Adequate amplitude of donor muscle
Adequate strength of donor muscle
Direct line of pull
Single function for each transferred tendon
Synergy of transfer

adduction contracture has developed, this should be released by a Z-plasty, skin grafting or transposition flap and release of the adductor pollicis, prior to opposition tendon transfer. Full passive range of motion of the MCP and PIP joints should be achieved by physical therapy and dynamic splinting prior to tendon transfer. Preliminary capsulotomies of the MCP and PIP joints or tenolysis of adherent flexor or extensor tendons may occasionally be required if dynamic splinting fails to achieve adequate joint mobility.

Selection of donor muscle-tendon

Expendability

The donor muscle-tendon unit must be expendable. Its sacrifice must not create an important new deficit. For example, the ring finger flexor digitorum superficialis (FDS) tendon may be used to correct MCP hyperextension (claw deformity) in patients with a low ulnar nerve palsy, but it is not expendable in patients with a high ulnar nerve palsy who have no functioning flexor digitorum profundus (FDP) tendon to the ring finger. The selection of a muscle-tendon unit as a tendon transfer may also be influenced by the patient's occupation. For example, the flexor carpi radialis (FCR) may be a more appropriate transfer to provide finger extension in a working man rather than the more conventional flexor carpi ulnaris (FCU) transfer since the FCU provides the important function of flexion and ulnar deviation of the wrist needed in work activities such as hammering. More importantly, if multiple tendon transfers are required, a minimum of one wrist flexor, one wrist extensor, and one extrinsic flexor and extensor tendon to each digit should always be retained.

Strength

In selecting the most appropriate donor muscle-tendon, the surgeon must consider not only the strength of the muscle to be transferred, but also the relative strength of the now paralyzed muscle or muscles and the strength of the antagonist muscle. Brand[2,3] has emphasized that the maximum potential force of a muscle is directly proportional to its physiologic cross-sectional area. It has been calculated that a muscle can produce a force of 3.65 kg/cm^2 of its cross-sectional area. This potential force is maximal when the muscle is at its resting length which is defined as the position mid-way between the length at maximum passive stretch and when it is fully contracted.

Amplitude

The potential excursion of a donor muscle-tendon unit must be sufficient to restore the specific lost function. The finger

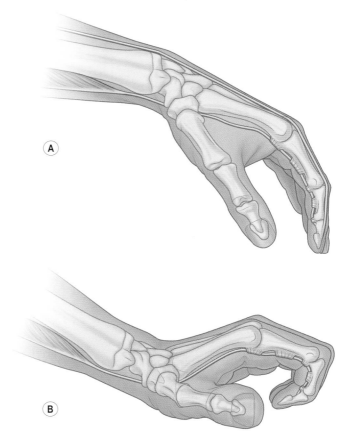

Fig. 34.1 The wrist tenodesis effect: **(A)** Wrist flexion may increase the potential amplitude of a tendon transfer to restore finger extension by 25 mm. **(B)** Similarly wrist extension may increase the potential amplitude of a tendon transfer to restore finger flexion by 25 mm.

flexors have an amplitude of 70 mm, the finger extensors 50 mm and the wrist flexors and extensors 33 mm. The tenodesis effect of wrist flexion or extension may also increase the effective amplitude of a tendon transfer by 25 mm *(Fig. 34.1)*. Excursion of a donor muscle may also be increased by extensive release of its surrounding fascia and is exemplified by transfer of the brachioradialis (Br) muscle. The distal portion and tendon of the Br muscle are surrounded by dense fascia. Division of these fascial attachments will add an additional 2–3 cm of passive excursion.

Direction of transfer and integrity

A tendon transfer should pass in a direct line from the origin of the donor muscle to its new insertion. Unless early tendon transfers are being performed, when there is still a chance of reinnervation following nerve repair, the recipient tendons should be divided proximal to the site of the tendon juncture to create a more direct line of pull (end-to-end) rather than producing a Y-shaped end-to-side juncture. Tendon transfers should only act across one joint and perform one single function. This maintains the "integrity" of the muscle. However, a transfer may be inserted into several recipient tendons as long as they each perform the same function in adjacent digits. Finally, the donor muscle selected should preferably be synergistic with the function of the muscle to be restored or at least be potentially retrainable.

The surgeon has to determine the specific functions to be restored, select the appropriate donor muscle-tendon units and decide on the timing of the tendon transfer. To make this selection, every muscle in the forearm and hand should be tested by manual muscle testing to document which are functioning and their strength graded. From this list of functioning muscles, only those that are expendable are available as donor transfers. The specific functions of the hand that need to be restored are then listed in order of priority. The final step is to match the available donor muscles with the functions that need to be restored, based on the force, amplitude and direction of the various muscles available. Arthrodesis of a more proximal joint such as the wrist may occasionally need to be considered to release a wrist flexor or extensor tendon for transfer. Transfers that require postoperative immobilization with the wrist in flexion are usually performed at a first stage. Those transfers requiring postoperative immobilization with the wrist in extension are performed at a second stage.

Timing of tendon transfers

Timing of tendon transfers may be classified as early, conventional or late. A conventional tendon transfer is usually performed after reinnervation of the paralyzed muscle fails to occur by three months after the expected time of reinnervation based on the rate of nerve regeneration of one millimeter per day. Brand,[2] Omer[4] and Burkhalter[5] have advocated "early" tendon transfers in certain circumstances, in which a tendon transfer is performed simultaneously with the nerve repair or before the expected time of reinnervation of the muscle. This "early" tendon transfer therefore serves as a temporary substitute for the paralyzed muscle until reinnervation occurs, by acting as an internal splint. If reinnervation is sub-optimal the "early" tendon transfer acts as a helper to augment the power of the muscle and if reinnervation fails to occur it then acts as a permanent substitute.

Surgical technique

The success of any tendon transfer depends entirely on preventing scarring or adhesions along the path of the transferred tendon. Incisions should be carefully planned prior to elevation of the tourniquet so that the final tendon junctures lie transversely beneath skin flaps rather than lying immediately beneath and paralleling the incisions. The donor muscle should be carefully mobilized to prevent damage to its neurovascular bundle which usually enters in the proximal third of the muscle. The transferred tendon should glide in a tunnel through the subcutaneous tissues and not cross bone devoid of uninjured periosteum or through small fascial windows. Only the distal end of the tendon should be grasped with surgical instruments and care taken to prevent desiccation of the tendon. Tendon junctures are performed using a Pulvertaft weave technique where possible. The donor and recipient tendons are sutured under normal tension and after one or two nonabsorbable sutures have been inserted, the tension of the transfer is checked by observing the flexion and extension of the digit during tenodesis of the wrist. Postoperatively, the

hand is immobilized in the desired position for 3 to 4 weeks, at which time gentle active range of motion exercises are started, usually under the supervision of a therapist, but the hand is protected for a further three weeks in a light-weight protective splint.

Radial nerve palsy

Patient selection

The functional motor deficit in radial nerve palsy consists of inability to extend the wrist, inability to extend the fingers at the MCP joints and inability to extend and radially abduct the thumb *(Fig. 34.2)*. However, the most significant disability is that patients are unable to stabilize their wrist so that transmission of flexor power to their fingers is impaired resulting in marked weakness of grip strength.

Tendon transfers are therefore required to provide wrist extension, extension of the fingers at the MCP joints and extension and radial abduction of the thumb. Unlike the median and ulnar nerves, sensory loss following radial nerve injury is not functionally disabling unless the patient develops a painful neuroma.

Timing of tendon transfers for radial nerve palsy remains controversial. The two options are either to perform an "early" tendon transfer simultaneously with repair of the radial nerve to act as an internal splint to provide immediate restoration of power grip; or more conventionally, to delay any tendon transfers until reinnervation of the most proximal muscles, brachioradialis and ECRL fails to occur within the calculated time limit. The more proximal the nerve injury, the less likely that functional muscle reinnervation will occur.[4,5] If the nerve remains in-continuity, most surgeons would suggest that three months of observation are indicated to await spontaneous recovery in peripheral nerve palsies. Ring et al.[6] reviewed 24 patients with a complete radial nerve palsy associated with a high energy humeral fracture. Six of 11 open fractures had a transected radial nerve and none of the five patients who underwent primary repair of the radial nerve recovered any function.

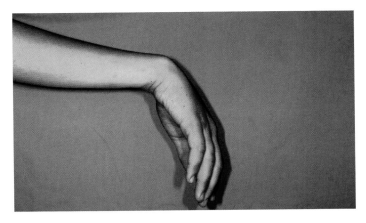

Fig. 34.2 The typical posture of the hand and wrist of a patient with a high radial nerve palsy. The wrist cannot be extended. The fingers are extended through the tenodesis effect.

All eight intact explored nerves and nine of 10 unexplored nerves recovered completely, with initial signs of recovery at an average of 7 weeks and full recovery at an average of 6 months. The authors concluded that primary repair of a transected radial nerve associated with a high energy humerus fracture was very poor, but the prognosis for full recovery of an intact radial nerve, whether the fracture is open or closed was very good. Mayer and Mayfield[7] reported 39 cases of posterior interosseous nerve (PIN) neurorrhaphy with complete recovery in 28 and partial recovery in 11 patients. Young et al.[8] studied 51 patients with PIN palsy of whom only 11 had resolved by 3 months. Of the remaining 40 patients, 20 of the 23 who underwent neurolysis and 10 of the 12 who underwent nerve grafting had excellent or good results. A conflicting study of radial nerve injuries demonstrated useful function in 65%, but only 38% of patients who underwent nerve grafting obtained useful motor function.[9] These studies demonstrate that injury and repair of the radial and PIN nerves can provide significant return of function and should be considered. With extensive nerve gaps or associated soft tissue injuries or in older patients, the chances of successful reinnervation are much less predictable and it may therefore be more appropriate for these patients to undergo the full set of tendon transfers early.[10] In a patient awaiting return of nerve function, it is important to maintain supple MCP joints capable of full extension and adequate radial abduction of the thumb with appropriate splinting and therapy.

Treatment/surgical technique

Franke provided one of the earliest descriptions of tendon transfers for radial nerve palsy using the FCU to extensor digitorum communis (EDC) transfer through the interosseous membrane.[11] Capellen in 1899 described the FCR to extensor pollicis longus (EPL) transfer. The pronator teres (PT) to extensor carpi radialis longus (ECRL) and the extensor carpi radialis brevis (ECRB) transfer for wrist extension was first reported in 1906 by Sir Robert Jones. Zachary[12] emphasized the importance of retaining at least one wrist flexor, preferably the FCR to facilitate wrist control. Other authors have suggested that FCU is not an expendable tendon and therefore prefer to use the FCR as the donor tendon to restore finger extension.[13] The advantage of using FCR is that it preserves the important moment of flexion and ulnar deviation of the wrist which is so important for power grip in a working man. This is particularly true in the patient with a posterior interosseous nerve (PIN) palsy in which ECRL function is preserved, but extensor carpi ulnaris (ECU) activity is lost. This leads to radial deviation of the wrist with attempted wrist extension. Use of the FCU in this setting will increase the radial deviation of the wrist, since only radially deviating wrist motors are preserved.

Several different tendon transfers have been reported for radial nerve palsy but three patterns of transfer have evolved. The use of pronator teres (PT) to provide wrist extension has become universally accepted, the only remaining controversy being whether to insert pronator teres into extensor carpi radialis brevis (ECRB) alone or into both extensor carpi radialis longus (ECRL) and brevis. The three patterns of tendon transfer differ therefore only in the technique of restoring finger extension and thumb extension and radial abduction (*Table 34.2*).[12,14–16]

Standard flexor carpi ulnaris transfer

Treatment/surgical technique

In the patient with a radial nerve palsy, the FCU transfer is the author's preferred technique; in the patient with a PIN palsy, the FCR transfer is preferred. Through an inverted J-shaped incision over the ulnar-volar aspect of the distal forearm, the flexor carpi ulnaris (FCU) tendon is transected at the wrist crease and released extensively from its fascial attachments up into the proximal third of the forearm, taking care not to damage the neurovascular pedicle, using a second incision in the proximal forearm if necessary (*Fig. 34.3*). Through the same distal incision, the palmaris longus (PL) tendon is transected at the wrist crease and the muscle mobilized into the middle third of the forearm (*Fig. 34.3*). An S-shaped incision is then made beginning over the volar-radial aspect of the middle third of the forearm and passing dorsally and ulnarly over the radial border of the forearm (*Fig. 34.4*). The tendon of pronator teres is elevated from the

Table 34.2 Tendon transfers for radial nerve palsy

Standard FCU transfer	FCR transfer	Boyes superficialis transfer
PT to ECRB	PT to ECRB	PT to ECRB
FCU to EDC	FCR to EDC	FDS of ring finger to EDC middle, ring, and small fingers
PL to EPL	PL to EPL	FDS middle finger to EIP and EPL FCR to APL & EPB

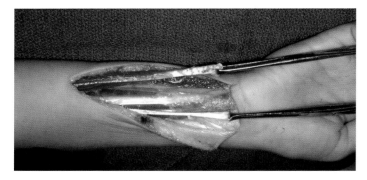

Fig. 34.3 The FCU tendon and distal muscle are dissected. In this case, a palmaris longus was present and its tendon is dissected for later transfer to the EPL.

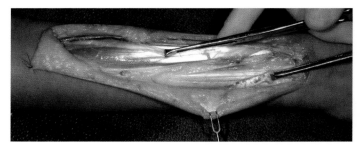

Fig. 34.4 A dorsal incision exposes the wrist and finger extensors. The FCU tendon has been brought from palmar to dorsal, around the ulnar border of the forearm.

radius in-continuity with a 2–3 cm strip of periosteum (*Fig. 34.5*). The ECRB is transected at its musculotendinous junction if there is no chance of future reinnervation of the wrist extensors. The pronator teres is then re-routed around the radial border of the forearm superficial to the brachioradialis and ECRL in a straight direction to its insertion into ECRB (*Fig. 34.5*). The FCU tendon is passed through a subcutaneous tunnel made with a Kelly clamp from the dorsal incision around the ulnar border of the forearm into the proximal incision used to mobilize FCU to lie obliquely across the EDC tendons proximal to the extensor retinaculum. Alternatively, the FCU tendon may be passed from the palmar incision to the dorsal incision through a window in the interosseous membrane.[17] If no return of EDC function is to be expected, the EDC tendons can be transected at their musculotendinous junctions so that a more direct line of pull can be achieved (*Fig. 34.6*). Otherwise an end-to-side juncture is performed. The extensor pollicis longus (EPL) tendon is divided at its musculotendinous junction, removed from the third dorsal extensor tendon compartment, and passed through a subcutaneous tunnel from the base of the thumb metacarpal to the volar wrist incision (*Fig. 34.7*). If the PL is not present, the EPL tendon is included with the tendons of the EDC and the FCU provides for both finger and thumb extension. To prevent a collapse flexion deformity at the carpometacarpal joint of the thumb, tenodesis of the APL will be necessary. After transection of the APL tendon in the distal forearm, it is looped around the brachioradialis proximal to the radial styloid and sutured to itself with the thumb metacarpal held in extension with the wrist in 30° of extension.

The proper tension in radial nerve tendon transfers should be tight enough to provide full extension of the wrist and digits but without restricting full flexion of the digits when the wrist is fully extended. The pronator teres at resting tension is woven through the ECRB tendon with the wrist in 45° of extension. The distal ends of the four EDC tendons to the index, middle, ring and small fingers are sutured to the FCU tendon proximal to the extensor retinaculum. The EDM is usually not included unless there is still an extensor lag when proximal traction is applied to the EDC tendon to the small finger. With the wrist in neutral and FCU under maximal tension, each individual EDC tendon is sutured to provide full extension at the MCP joint, starting with the index finger and finishing with the small finger. Appropriate tension is then evaluated by checking that all four digits extend synchronously when the wrist is palmar flexed and most importantly that all four digits can be passively flexed into a fist when the wrist is extended. Finally, PL and EPL are interwoven over the radio-volar aspect of the wrist with both tendons under resting tension with the wrist in neutral. The wrist is immobilized in 45° of extension in a volar splint with the MCP joints positioned in slight flexion and the thumb in full extension and abduction.

Postoperative care

Active flexion and extension of the fingers and thumb are started at 3.5–4 weeks and active exercises of the wrist begun at 5 weeks. Protective splinting is continued until 6–8 weeks' postoperatively (*Fig. 34.8*).

Flexor carpi radialis transfer

Treatment/surgical technique

The skin incision begins from the radio-volar aspect of the mid-forearm and extends dorsally over the third and fourth extensor tendon compartments. The pronator teres is transferred to the ECRB and the PL is transferred to the EPL exactly as described in the standard FCU transfer. The FCR is divided at the wrist crease and mobilized approximately to the level of the mid-forearm and rerouted around the radial border of the forearm. The four EDC tendons, and if necessary, the EDM may be woven through the donor FCR tendon proximal to the extensor retinaculum, but more usually the extensor tendons need to be re-routed superficial to the extensor retinaculum to obtain a straighter line of pull (*Fig. 34.9*). To prevent a bulky tendon juncture, the small finger EDC and EDM may be

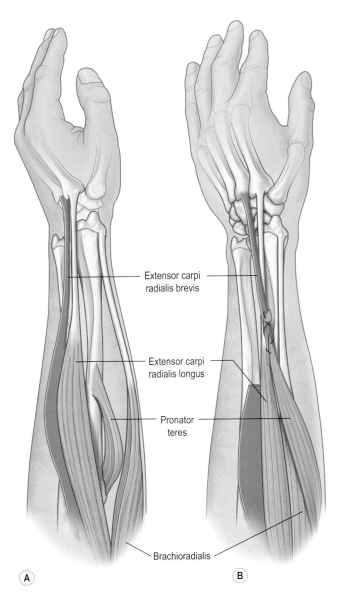

Extensor carpi radialis brevis

Extensor carpi radialis longus

Pronator teres

Brachioradialis

(A)   (B)

Fig. 34.5 (A) The relatively short tendon of insertion of the PT can be extended by elevating a strip of periosteum. **(B)** The PT will be woven into the tendon of the ECRB.

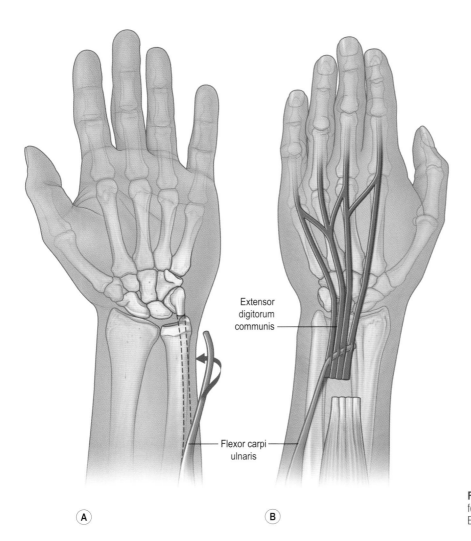

Extensor
digitorum
communis

Flexor carpi
ulnaris

(A)   (B)

Fig. 34.6 The FCU is brought around the ulnar border of the forearm (A,B) and woven into the combined tendons of the EDC.

sutured side-to-side to the ring finger EDC and the index finger EDC sutured side-to-side to the middle finger EDC under appropriate tension. Then only the two EDC tendons to the middle and ring fingers require weaving through the FCR tendon. As with the standard FCU transfer, these tendon junctures are performed with the wrist in neutral and the MCP joints in full extension with the FCR tendon under maximal traction. Post-operative management is similar to that for the FCU transfer. Chandraprakasam et al.[17] described a modification of the modified Jones transfer in which the pronator teres is transferred to ECRB; the FCR is transferred to the finger extensors and the palmaris longus transferred to EPL; all through a single incision along the radial aspect of the distal third of the forearm curving obliquely to end at Lister's tubercle.

Boyes superficialis transfer

Treatment/surgical technique

Boyes[14] was the first to suggest that neither FCU nor FCR have sufficient amplitude (30 mm) to produce full excursion of

the digital extensor tendons (50 mm) without the potential increase in amplitude obtained with the tenodesis effect of wrist flexion. He therefore advocated using the superficialis tendons to the middle and ring fingers which have an amplitude of 70 mm to act as donor tendons to restore finger extension.[14,15] The advantages of the Boyes transfer are that this transfer will potentially allow simultaneous wrist and finger extension. Second, it may allow independent thumb and index finger extension and finally it does not weaken wrist flexion. However, the middle and ring fingers are deprived of superficialis function and this may result in weak grip. Harvesting of the superficialis tendons may also lead to the subsequent development of either a "swan neck" deformity or a flexion contracture at the PIP joint.

The superficialis tendons to the middle and ring fingers are exposed between the A1 and A2 pulleys either through one transverse incision at the base of the fingers or two separate longitudinal incisions. The superficialis tendons are divided just proximal to their decussation and then withdrawn proximally into a longitudinal incision over the volar aspect of the middle third of the forearm. The tendon of pronator teres can be transected and re-routed through this same incision as

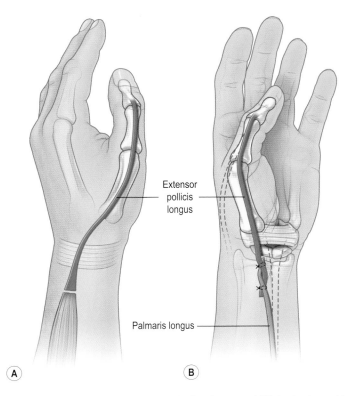

Extensor
pollicis
longus

Palmaris longus

(A) (B)

Fig. 34.7 The PL, if present, can be attached to the rerouted EPL tendon to provide both thumb extension and some radial abduction.

described previously. Blunt dissection on either side of the FDP muscles allows a window to be excised in the interosseous membrane just proximal to the pronator quadratus. *(Fig. 34.10)*. This window should be made as large as possible at least 4 cm long and as wide as the interosseous space, so that the muscle bellies of the two superficialis tendons can be passed through this window to minimize the development of adhesions. It is important to pass the superficialis tendons of the ring and middle fingers to their respective sides of the median nerve to prevent scissoring over the nerve and compression.

Thompson and Rasmussen[18] prefer to transfer the two superficialis tendons through subcutaneous tunnels around the radial and ulnar borders of the forearm. Through a J shaped incision passing transversely across the dorsum of the wrist and then extending proximally along the dorsum of the ulna, the extensor tendons are isolated as well as ECRB. In Boyes' original description, pronator teres was sutured to both ECRL and ECRB,[14] but in order to prevent excessive radial deviation, pronator teres should only be woven end-to-end into ECRB with the wrist in 30° of extension. The middle finger superficialis is then passed to the radial side of the profundus muscles and the ring finger superficialis to the ulnar side through the interosseous window into the dorsal incision. After transection of the EPL and EIP tendons, they are woven end-to-end into the middle finger superficialis tendon. Similarly, the transected EDC tendons to the index, middle, ring and small fingers are woven end-to-end into the ring finger superficialis tendon, although this arrangement can be reversed. The tendon junctures are performed proximal to the extensor retinaculum with resting tension in the donor superficialis tendons and full extension at the MCP joints.

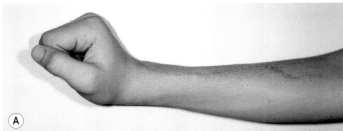

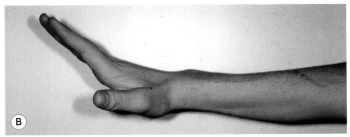

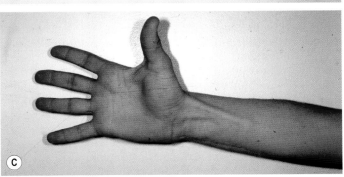

Fig. 34.8 A patient 3 years following PT to ECRB, FCU to EDC and PL to EPL transfers. **(A)** Wrist extension and finger flexion; **(B)** Full finger extension; **(C)** Excellent thumb extension and radial abduction.

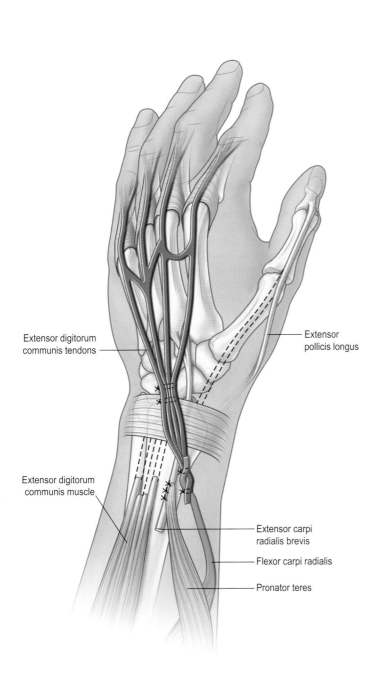

Fig. 34.9 Transfer of the FCR to the combined tendons of the EDC.

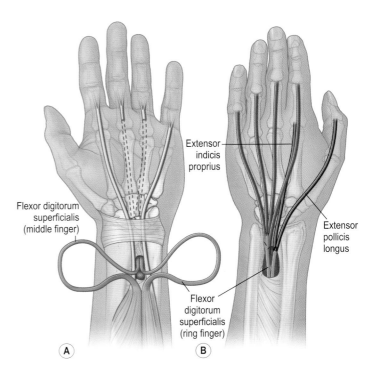

Fig. 34.10 Transfer of the middle and ring finger superficialis tendons (FDS$_L$, FDS$_R$) through a window in the interosseous membrane **(A)** to restore function to the extensor digitorum communis (EDC) tendons and extensor indicis proprius (EIP) and extensor pollicis longus (EPL) **(B)**.

Outcomes, prognosis, and complications

Tendon transfers for radial nerve palsy are generally predictable. Tsuge[19] described the evolution of his technique in 69 patients over a 25-year period. Using the FCU transfer and insertion of pronator teres into both ECRL and ECRB in the initial 41 patients, he reported "fairly satisfactory" results, but felt that there were three problems: development of radial deviation of the wrist, restriction of wrist flexion and marginal thumb abduction. Because of these concerns, pronator teres was transferred only to ECRB and the FCR was transferred through the interosseous membrane for finger extension, leaving the FCU intact leading to good results in 24 of 27 cases. A long-term functional study of the FCU transfer in six patients by Raskin and Wilgis[20] revealed adequate wrist motion and power to perform daily activities and a work simulation protocol showed patients were able to perform tasks without significant difficulty. Problems of inadequate ulnar deviation, grip strength and wrist instability were not seen. A subjective outcome study by Riordan[21] also revealed satisfaction with the standard FCU transfer. Gousheh and Arasteh[22] transferred only the FCU to the finger extensors and EPL in 108 patients. At a mean follow up of 4 years, wrist extension was less than the opposite side, but extension of the fingers was similar to the normal hand and most patients were able to return to their previous job. According to the authors, there was no obvious difference between the results using a single FCU tendon transfer compared to their previous results using the conventional 3 tendon transfers for reconstruction of radial nerve palsy. Altintas et al.[23] compared the long-term results after tendon transfers for radial nerve

If necessary, the APL is transected at its musculotendinous junction and passed through a subcutaneous tunnel from the base of the thumb into the volar forearm incision. Either palmaris longus or FCR are transected at the wrist crease and woven end-to-end with the APL tendon to provide abduction of the thumb and prevent a collapse deformity of the thumb metacarpal. The tourniquet should be deflated prior to the closure of the incisions because of the likelihood of bleeding from the anterior or posterior interosseous vessels.

palsy, using the FCU in 58 patients and the FCR in 19 patients. Wrist extension averaged 73% of the opposite side, finger extension 32% and thumb extension 80%. Grip strength was reduced to 49% and pinch strength to 28% of the opposite hand and the mean total DASH score was 16. 89% of patients remained employed after tendon transfers for radial nerve palsy.

Chuinard et al.[15] studied 21 patients who had undergone the Boyes superficialis transfers with excellent results in 10, good in six, and only a fair result in five patients. Subjectively, 13 patients felt that they had obtained an excellent result and eight a good result. Complications requiring a second procedure were reported in five patients and included adhesions, dehiscence of the transfer, MCP and wrist extension contractures and problems with correct tensioning of the transfers. A report of 13 patients with radial nerve palsy and five patients with PIN palsy by Fujiwara[25] documented generally good results with the Boyes transfers. No patient in either of these studies developed postoperative median nerve compression despite the potential for this complication with this transfer. Krishnan and Schackert[24] evaluated the function of 29 patients who had undergone a Boyes transfer of the sublimis tendons to the middle and ring fingers through the interosseous membrane for radial nerve palsy. Near normal wrist extension was achieved in 22 of 25 patients. Finger extension simultaneously with wrist extension was achieved in 12 patients, but in 17 patients full finger extension was only possible with the wrist in neutral. Selective extension of the index finger and thumb powered by the sublimis tendon from the middle finger was achieved in all patients. Long-term evaluation of the FCU transfer for radial nerve palsy at a mean follow-up of 9.5 years revealed 11 excellent, two good, one fair and one bad result with the main problems being loss of power grip and development of a radial deviation deformity.[26] This has led to an evolution in the authors' technique to use pronator teres to restore wrist extension, FCR to restore finger extension and palmaris longus to restore thumb extension with tenodesis of the APL to brachioradialis to restore thumb abduction.

All three techniques have been reported to yield good results but there are few quantitative studies to substantiate the reported outcomes, and no prospective comparison of the three different techniques. The FCU transfer is perhaps the simplest technique and provides reproducibly good results in patients with radial nerve palsy.

Low median nerve palsy

Basic science/disease process

The functional deficit following injury to the median nerve distal to the innervation of the extrinsic forearm flexor muscles consists primarily of loss of opposition of the thumb and absent sensation over the thumb, index, middle and radial half of the ring finger.

Opposition is a composite motion, which occurs at all three joints to position the thumb pad opposite the distal phalanx of the partially flexed middle finger. Abduction, pronation and flexion occur at the carpometacarpal joint, abduction and flexion at the metacarpophalangeal joint and either flexion or extension at the interphalangeal joint. Approximately 40° of abduction of the thumb metacarpal occurs at the carpometacarpal joint and 20° of abduction of the proximal phalanx occurs at the metacarpophalangeal joint. From a starting position of full extension and adduction, the thumb pronates approximately 90° during opposition to the middle finger. Extension of the thumb interphalangeal joint is required for pulp-to-pulp pinch, whereas slight flexion of the interphalangeal joint allows tip-to-tip pinch. Of the three intrinsic thenar muscles, the flexor pollicis brevis (FPB) muscle typically, although not always, receives a dual innervation from both the median and ulnar nerves. Because the FPB may remain innervated by the ulnar nerve in approximately 70% of median nerve injuries, patients may not notice any significant functional loss, but careful testing will reveal decreased strength of abduction and lack of pronation.

Patient selection

Prior to any opposition transfer, patients with median nerve injuries should be instructed to prevent the development of an adduction or supination contracture of the thumb by a program of passive abduction exercises. A static thumb-index finger web space splint may be used at night but this usually interferes with the already compromised function of the hand if used during the day. Care should be taken to ensure that such splints abduct the thumb metacarpal rather than the proximal phalanx; otherwise the median nerve palsy will be compounded by attenuation of the ulnar collateral ligament of the metacarpophalangeal joint. If patients present with an established adduction or supination contracture of the thumb, release of the thumb-index finger web space skin, fascia over the first dorsal interosseous muscle or even the first dorsal interosseous and adductor muscles themselves may be required prior to any opposition tendon transfer.

Bunnell[27] first emphasized that the pull of an opposition tendon transfer should be in an oblique direction from the thumb metacarpophalangeal joint to the region of the pisiform and secondly that in order to produce pronation, the transfer should be inserted into the dorso-ulnar base of the proximal phalanx. Opposition transfers that are directed along the radial aspect of the palm will produce a greater component of palmar abduction whereas transfers that pass from the pisiform will produce both abduction and pronation. The more distal the transfer passes across the palm, the greater the power of thumb flexion. Several methods of insertion of opposition transfers have been advocated including attachment to the dorso-ulnar base of the proximal phalanx),[27–29] insertion into the APB tendon,[30] dual insertion into the APB and continuation distally into the MCP joint capsule and EPL tendon,[21] insertion into the APB, dorsal joint capsule and adductor pollicis[31] and finally utilization of a distal based EPB tendon.[32] However, a biomechanical study has shown that opposition tendon transfers inserted into the APB tendon alone will produce full abduction and pronation.[33] Therefore the more complex dual insertions should probably be reserved for combined median and ulnar nerve palsies.

Several factors influence the likelihood of useful motor and sensory return following median nerve injury including patient age, level of injury, length of nerve defect and interposition graft and period of preoperative delay. The best results are realized in distal injuries in young patients requiring only primary repair. Associated injuries such as vascular damage, tendon injury, and concomitant ulnar nerve transection portend a worse prognosis. The chances of reinnervation of the thenar muscles following group fascicular repair of a distal median nerve laceration should be reasonably optimistic. Therefore, conventional timing of an opposition tendon transfer may only be required in those patients who fail to demonstrate signs of reinnervation within the usual calculated time interval. For older patients or those with poor prognostic comorbid factors, early tendon transfers should be considered.

Careful observation of thumb function following either a low or high median nerve palsy will reveal whether an "early" tendon transfer for thumb opposition is necessary. FPB remains innervated by the ulnar nerve in approximately 70% of median nerve injuries so that thumb function may not be significantly compromised. Consequently an "early" opposition transfer may not be necessary. Other patients however will adapt to their loss of opposition and abduction by substitution of the APL to provide thumb abduction, but this can only be achieved with the hand positioned in pronation. This places the patient at an even greater disadvantage in that not only do they have absent sensation in the median nerve distribution, but with the forearm in pronation they cannot even see the palmar surface of their hand to compensate for their loss of sensation. Therefore, if the surgeon or therapist observes the patient attempting to grasp objects by radial abduction of the thumb with the forearm in pronation, an "early" opposition tendon transfer should be strongly considered. If however, the patient is able to pick up an object with the forearm in neutral or grasp an object with the forearm in supination, it is likely that FPB remains innervated by the ulnar nerve and consequently the decision for performing an "early" opposition tendon transfer can be delayed.

Burkhalter extensor indicis proprius transfer

Treatment/surgical technique

The extensor indicis proprius (EIP) transfer[34] is the author's preferred technique *(Fig. 34.11A,B)*, except in elderly patients with thenar atrophy secondary to severe carpal tunnel syndrome The EIP tendon is transected through a small transverse incision just proximal to the MCP joint of the index finger. The distal stump of the EIP tendon is then repaired to the EDC tendon of the index finger to prevent extensor lag at the metacarpophalangeal joint. The EIP tendon is mobilized through two small transverse incisions one proximal and one distal to the extensor retinaculum and the muscle belly mobilized through a longitudinal incision over the ulnar aspect of the dorsum of the mid forearm *(Fig. 34.11C)*. A transverse incision is made just proximal to the pisiform bone and a subcutaneous tunnel developed to connect this incision to the dorsal forearm incision. The EIP tendon is then passed subcutaneously around the ulnar border of the distal forearm superficial to the ECU tendon into the pisiform incision The APB tendon is identified through a small incision over the radial aspect of the MCP joint of the thumb and a subcutaneous tunnel made connecting this incision with the pisiform incision *(Fig. 34.12)*. The tendon transfer is passed obliquely

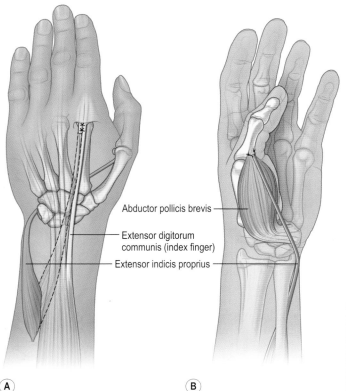

Abductor pollicis brevis

Extensor digitorum communis (index finger)

Extensor indicis proprius

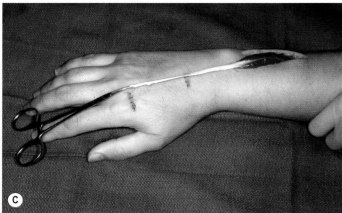

(A)　　　　(B)　　　　(C)

Fig. 34.11 (A,B) The EIP transfer to restore opposition. **(C)** Incisions for harvesting the EIP tendon.

across the palm and woven into the tendon of APB under maximum tension with the wrist in neutral position and the thumb in maximal palmar abduction. The tension of the transfer is then tested by the tenodesis effect of the wrist. Wrist flexion should allow the thumb to be passively adducted. If wrist extension produces excessive flexion or extension of the thumb at the metacarpophalangeal joint, this indicates that the transfer has been inserted either too far volarly or too far dorsally and should be adjusted accordingly. The thumb is immobilized in full abduction with the wrist in slight palmar flexion for 4 weeks, at which time active abduction and opposition movements are begun with protective splinting for a further 3–4 weeks. The only potential disadvantage with this tendon transfer is that the EIP tendon is only just long enough to reach the APB tendon. The postoperative results have been very predictable *(Fig. 34.13)*.

Bunnell ring finger flexor digitorum superficialis transfer

Treatment/surgical technique

In the FDS transfer described originally by Bunnell,[27] the ring finger superficialis tendon is isolated through a small transverse incision just distal to the distal palmar crease *(Fig. 34.14)*.

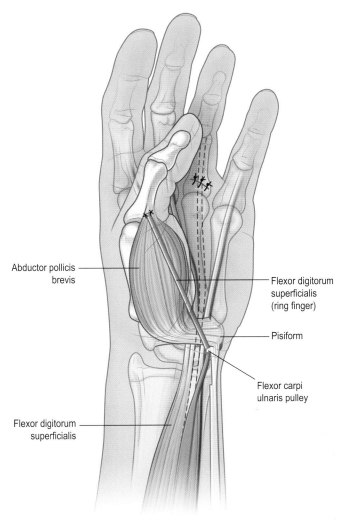

Fig. 34.14 The FDS to APB transfer to restore thumb opposition is depicted schematically.

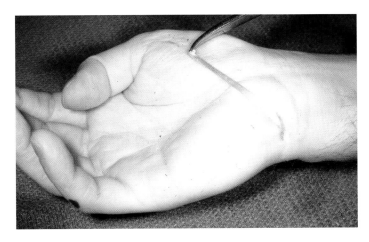

Fig. 34.12 The palmar incision and the direction of the EIP transfer across the palm.

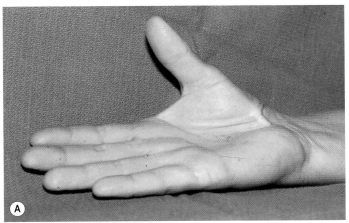

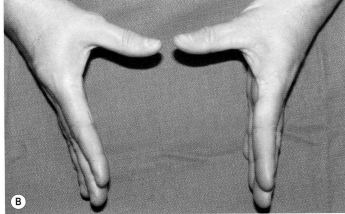

Fig. 34.13 (A,B) Postoperative opposition restored by the EIP transfer.

The tendon is transected between the A1 and A2 pulleys and delivered into a proximal incision made over the volar aspect of the distal forearm *(Fig. 34.15A)*. The FCU tendon is split longitudinally to create a distal-based strip of the radial half of the tendon. This is then passed through a slit in the FCU tendon just proximal to the pisiform and sutured to itself to create a pulley *(Fig. 34.15B,C)*. The distal end of the ring finger superficialis tendon is passed through the pulley and through an oblique subcutaneous tunnel across the palm into an incision over the radial aspect of the MCP joint of the thumb. All the other incisions are then closed and the tension on the tendon transfer adjusted as described previously.

Simple looping of the ring finger superficialis around the FCU tendon rather than using a fixed pulley rapidly becomes ineffective and the transfer becomes converted to a flexor of the MCP joint rather than a true opposition transfer. Other pulleys for the ring finger superficialis transfer include passing the tendon through Guyon's canal or through a window in the transverse carpal ligament.

Compared with the EIP transfer, the ring finger superficialis is relatively stronger and has greater length. However, the ring finger superficialis is not available as a donor tendon in a high median nerve palsy or in low median nerve injuries in which there have been associated injuries to the flexor tendons. The ring finger superficialis transfer should also not be selected in combined low median and high ulnar nerve palsies since the ring finger superficialis is the only remaining flexor tendon in the ring finger. In low median-low ulnar nerve palsies, the ring finger superficialis may be required for correction of clawing. In addition, harvesting of the superficialis tendon may result in either a flexion contracture or a "swan-neck" deformity of the PIP joint of the donor finger. This is perhaps the strongest of the opposition transfers *(Fig. 34.16)*.

Camitz palmaris longus transfer

Treatment/surgical technique

The PL tendon Camitz transfer[35–38] is a simple transfer that will provide abduction of the thumb but little pronation or flexion and is particularly indicated in elderly patients with thenar atrophy due to long-standing carpal tunnel syndrome. A strip of palmar fascia is dissected in-continuity with the distal palmaris longus tendon through a standard carpal tunnel incision in the palm extending proximally into the distal forearm *(Fig. 34.17)*. A subcutaneous tunnel is

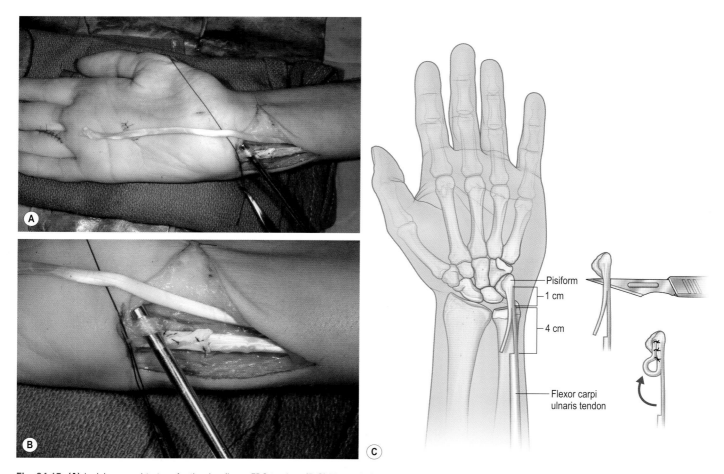

Fig. 34.15 (A) Incisions used to transfer the ring finger FDS tendon. **(B,C)** The technique of using one half of the FCU sutured to itself as a pulley is demonstrated.

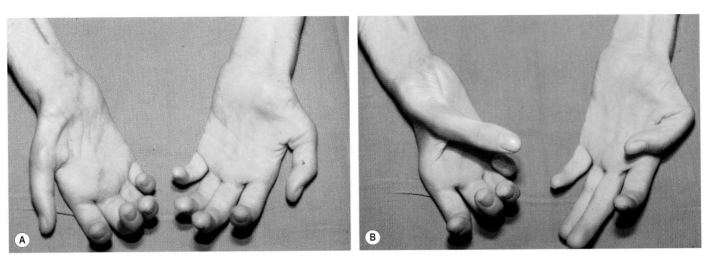

Fig. 34.16 **(A)** Preoperative appearance of a patient who lacks opposition secondary to Charcot–Marie–Tooth disease. **(B)** Postoperatively, opposition has been restored to the operated right hand.

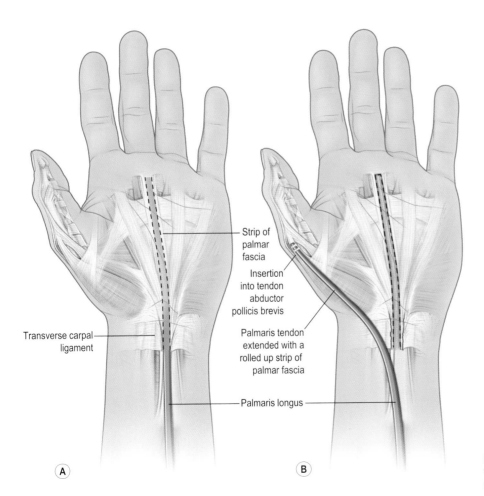

Strip of
palmar
fascia

Insertion
into tendon
abductor
pollicis brevis

Palmaris tendon
extended with a
rolled up strip of
palmar fascia

Transverse carpal
ligament

Palmaris longus

Fig. 34.17 The Camitz transfer using the palmaris longus with its tendon extended by palmar fascia is depicted schematically.

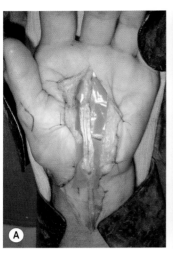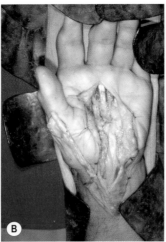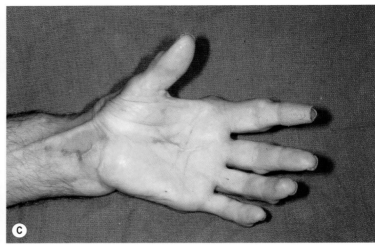

Fig. 34.18 **(A)** A wide strip of palmar fascia is dissected in-continuity with the PL tendon **(B)** This is transferred directly to be inserted into the tendon of APB. **(C)** Postoperative result of the Camitz transfer.

developed from the radial aspect of the distal forearm incision along the thenar eminence into a mid-axial incision on the radial aspect of the MCP joint of the thumb. The fascial extension of the palmaris longus tendon is passed through the subcutaneous tunnel and sutured to the APB tendon under maximal tension with the wrist in neutral position *(Fig. 34.18)*.

Other opposition tendon transfers

Treatment/surgical technique

Huber[39] and Nicolaysen[40] described transfer of the ADM which may occasionally be indicated in patients with a combined median and radial nerve palsy and also in children with congenital anomalies affecting the thumb. Since the muscle originates at the pisiform, this transfer provides excellent flexion and pronation of the thumb but little palmar abduction. The tendinous insertion of ADM is transected from the ulnar lateral band through an ulnar mid-axial incision along the proximal phalanx of the small finger. The incision is then extended proximally along the radial aspect of the hypothenar eminence and the muscle elevated in a distal to proximal direction taking care to protect the neurovascular bundle which enters the muscle just beyond the pisiform. A wide subcutaneous tunnel is dissected between the hypothenar

incision and the insertion of the APB at the MCP joint of the thumb. Hemostasis is achieved after releasing the tourniquet and the entire ADM muscle rotated 180° through the subcutaneous tunnel in the palm and sutured into the APB tendon. This transfer has been compared to turning the page of a book.[39] Cawrse and Sammut[41] described a modification of the Huber transfer in which the ADM is released both distally and proximally so that the muscle is a complete island. This eliminates any compression of the ulnar nerve by the muscle transfer.

Phalen and Miller[32] advocate the use of the EPB tendon activated by ECU. The EPB is divided at its musculotendinous junction in the distal forearm and retrieved through an incision at the metacarpophalangeal joint of the thumb. This distally based tendon may then be passed through a subcutaneous tunnel obliquely across the palm to the area of the pisiform. The ECU tendon is transected at the base of the 5th metacarpal and routed subcutaneously around the ulnar border of the wrist to be interwoven with the EPB tendon *(Fig 34.19)*.

Taylor described the use of the extensor digiti minimi (EDM) as an opposition tendon transfer.[42] This transfer, which was also described by Schneider, re-routes the EDM around the ulnar side of the hand to the thumb MCP joint.[43]

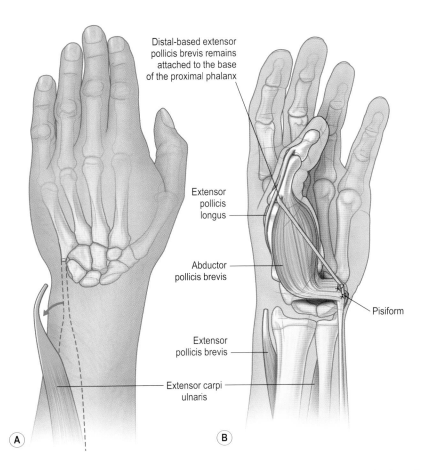

Distal-based extensor pollicis brevis remains attached to the base of the proximal phalanx

Extensor pollicis longus

Abductor pollicis brevis

Extensor pollicis brevis

Extensor carpi ulnaris

Pisiform

(A)

(B)

Fig. 34.19 Phalen and Miller transfer to restore opposition. The ECU tendon is detached and transferred around the ulnar border of the forearm **(A)** and sutured to the distal based EPB tendon **(B)**.

High median nerve palsy

Indications

Patient selection

The functional deficit following injury to the median nerve proximal to its innervation of the extrinsic forearm flexor muscles consists of inability to flex the index finger at the PIP and DIP joints and the thumb at the interphalangeal joint in addition to loss of opposition *(Fig. 34.20)*. This is due to paralysis of all four FDS muscles, the FDP tendons to the index and middle fingers and the FPL muscle. Patients are often still able to flex the middle finger due to interconnections between the profundus tendons to the middle, ring and small fingers in the distal forearm. Therefore the two functions that need to be restored in patients with a high median nerve palsy are flexion at the interphalangeal joint of the thumb and flexion of the PIP and DIP joints of the index and middle fingers, together with a conventional opposition tendon transfer.

Treatment/surgical technique

Flexion of the interphalangeal joint of the thumb may be restored by transfer of brachioradialis to FPL and flexion of the distal joint of the index and middle fingers by side-to-side tenorrhaphy of the FDP II and III to IV and V *(Fig. 34.21)*. The brachioradialis is divided at its insertion on the radial styloid and extensively mobilized from its investing fascia up into the proximal third of the forearm so that the freed muscle can develop approximately 30 mm of excursion. If reinnervation of the FPL muscle is not expected to occur following repair or grafting of the median nerve, the tendon can be divided at its musculotendinous junction and woven end-to-end into the brachioradialis tendon. However, if there is any possibility of reinnervation of FPL, the brachioradialis tendon should be woven end-to-side into the FPL tendon which remains in-continuity.

Through the same volar forearm incision, the profundus tendons to the index and middle fingers can be sutured side-to-side to the ulnar innervated profundus tendons to the ring and small fingers *(Fig. 34.21)*. If power flexion of the index and middle fingers is required, then formal transfer of the ECRL tendon to the index and middle finger profundus tendons may be performed. The ECRL is transected through a small transverse incision at the base of the index finger metacarpal and passed subcutaneously around the radial border of the distal forearm into the volar incision. The profundus tendons to the index and middle fingers are woven into the ECRL tendon so that with the wrist in 30–45° of extension, the tips of the index and middle fingers almost touch the palm. Similarly, with the wrist in full palmar flexion, the fingers will assume an almost fully extended position. Adjusting tension on this transfer using the tenodesis effect of the wrist is absolutely critical because the donor ECRL tendon has only 30 mm of amplitude whereas the profundus tendons normally have 70 mm of excursion. If this transfer is sutured under too much tension, it will result in flexion contractures of these two fingers. The results of these two transfers are also relatively predictable *(Fig. 34.22)*.

The timing of tendon transfers in a high median nerve palsy remains controversial.[5] If a good primary or delayed primary nerve repair can be performed, there is a reasonable

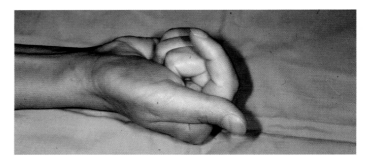

Fig. 34.20 Inability to flex the interphalangeal joint of the thumb and the distal interphalangeal joint of the index finger as a consequence of a high median nerve palsy.

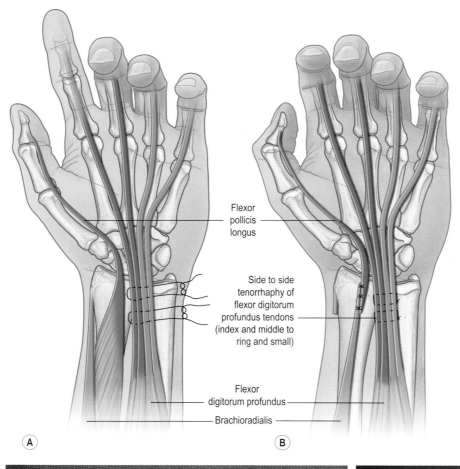

Flexor pollicis longus

Side to side tenorrhaphy of flexor digitorum profundus tendons (index and middle to ring and small)

Flexor digitorum profundus

Brachioradialis

(A)   (B)

Fig. 34.21 Transfer of the brachioradialis to FPL and side-to-side FDP tenorrhaphy.

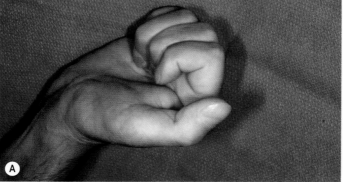

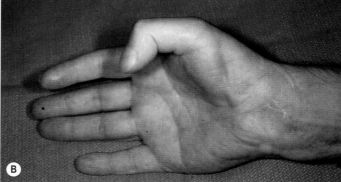

Fig. 34.22 (A) The postoperative finger flexion cascade has been restored by side-to-side tenorrhaphy of the FDP tendons. **(B)** Semi-independent flexion of the IP joint of the thumb following Br to FPL transfer.

chance of reinnervation of the extrinsic flexor muscles in a young patient. Consequently "early" brachioradialis to FPL or side-to-side repair of the index and middle finger profundus tendons to the ring and small finger profundus tendons is not necessary. However, if the patient is seen late and requires secondary nerve grafting of the median nerve, then tendon transfers for restoration of thumb flexion and index and middle finger flexion should be performed simultaneously with the nerve graft.

Outcomes, prognosis, and complications

There is no standard measurement of opposition in the literature. Some authors have developed functional scales to rate outcome, while others have reported subjective patient satisfaction.[44,45] An anatomic and biomechanical study by Cooney et al.[33] showed that the FDS of the ring finger and the ECU were the best transfers at replacing thenar strength, abduction and pronation. They calculated that the ECU and FDS transfers restored 60% and 40%, respectively of required thenar muscle strength. The Camitz transfer provided good abduction, but weak flexion and opposition.

Excellent or good results were obtained in approximately 88% after EIP transfer in patients with nerve deficits secondary to leprosy.[46] Similar results have been reported by other authors, but little data documenting thumb range of motion or rigorous functional outcomes exists. Schwarz and MacDonald[47] performed a retrospective review of 156 opposition tendon transfers primarily using FDS. Objective parameters were rated as good or excellent in 89% and patient satisfaction was rated as good or fair in 93 %. There are few publications containing objective data that discuss the long-term functional outcomes of the Bunnell superficialis transfer. Brandsma et al.[48] reported 32% excellent and 51% good results. Some of the other patients in this study underwent FDS transfers for intrinsic function. Of the 158 donor fingers, swan-neck deformities were seen in 15%, DIP flexion contractures in 29%, and PIP flexion contractures in 18%. Groves and Goldner[49] reported 75% success in 16 patients with high median nerve or brachial plexus lesions reconstructed with superficialis opposition transfers.

While Phalen and Miller[32] reported good results with the ECU transfer, another study described the development of significant radial deviation in one-third of cases.[50] These authors cautioned that the FCU must have normal strength to maintain proper wrist balance after ECU transfer.

Braun[37] reported good results in 28 patients who underwent the Camitz transfer. Foucher et al.[38] reported 91% good long term results in 73 Camitz transfers performed at the same time as carpal tunnel release. Terrono et al.[51] retrospectively reviewed their experience with 33 Camitz transfers for severe median nerve compression in patients with a mean age of 65 years. Some 94% of the patients felt that their thumb dexterity and speed were improved by the operation, only two patients were unhappy with the results. No objective biomechanical data are available for this transfer.

Table 34.3 catalogs some of the clinical studies of opposition tendon transfers. Success is defined differently in each study and thus a cohesive evaluation and enlightened recommendation is difficult to make. Data on high median nerve palsy reconstruction are even more scarce.

Table 34.3 Opposition tendon transfers for median nerve palsy

Technique	Etiology	Author	Success rate (%)
Huber	Trauma Neurologic disease	Wissinger[51a] (1977)	80
Camitz	Nerve compression	Terrono et al. (1993)[51]	94
		Foucher et al. (1991)[38]	91
EIP	Leprosy	Anderson et al. (1991)[46]	88
	Trauma	Burkhalter et al. (1973)[34]	88
Bunnell	Leprosy	Brandsma et al. (1992)[48]	83
	Leprosy	Palande[63] (1975)	94
	Trauma	Kirklin[45] (1948)	85
	Trauma	Groves and Goldner (1975)[49]	75
EDQ	Trauma	Schneider (1969)[43]	80

Low ulnar nerve palsy

Patient selection

Injury to the ulnar nerve distal to the innervation of the ring and small finger FDP and FCU muscles produces a functional deficit consisting of paralysis of all seven interossei, the ulnar two lumbricals, the hypothenar and the adductor pollicis (AP) and part of the flexor pollicis brevis (FPB) muscles. This results in an imbalance of the flexor and extensor forces at the MCP, PIP and DIP joints of the fingers. Since the interossei are the main flexors of the MCP joints, extension of the proximal phalanges at the MCP joints by the extrinsic extensor tendons is unopposed and MCP joint hyperextension occurs to the extent allowed by the volar plates. Because the extrinsic extensor tendons concentrate their extension at the MCP joints and the interossei are unable to actively extend at the PIP and DIP joints, the increased tension in the flexor tendons that occurs as the MCP joints begin to hyperextend will be unopposed at the PIP and DIP joints. This therefore results in the typical claw hand with hyperextension at the MCP joints and reciprocal flexion at the PIP and DIP joints (*Duchenne's sign*) *(Fig. 34.23)*. Imbalance between the extrinsic extensor and flexor tendons leads to asynchronous flexion of the fingers and weak grip strength. The MCP joints do not flex until after the interphalangeal joints have become completely flexed, resulting in curling of the tips of the fingers into the palm with loss of ability to grasp large objects. In a low ulnar nerve palsy, the clawing and loss of integrated MCP and interphalangeal joint flexion are confined to the ring and small fingers and to a lesser extent the middle finger, since the lumbricals to the index and middle fingers remain innervated by the median nerve. However, with a combined median and ulnar nerve palsy, all four fingers are affected. Fowler[52] has shown that the

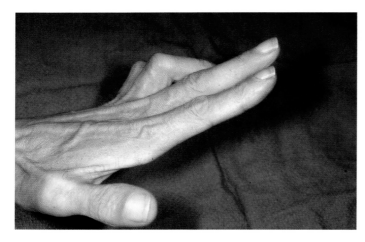

Fig. 34.23 The typical posture of the ulnar "claw" hand characterized by MCP hyperextension and reciprocal PIP and DIP flexion.

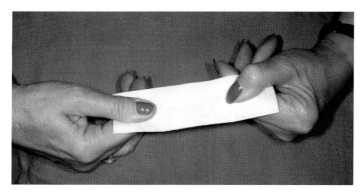

Fig. 34.24 The left thumb in ulnar nerve palsy. In the absence of the AP and FPB, the FPL must provide all the power of thumb flexion. As the prime flexor of the IP joint, it preferentially flexes this joint, leading to IP hyperflexion (*Froment's sign*) and occasionally hyperextension at the MCP joint (*Jeanne's sign*).

Table 34.4 Tendon transfers for ulnar nerve palsy	
Function to be restored	**Preferred tendon transfer**
Clawing of the ring and small fingers	Ring finger or middle finger FDS, 2 slips to the radial lateral bands, proximal phalanges or A2 or A1 and A2 pulleys of the ring and small fingers
Clawing of all 4 fingers	EF4T or PL4T transfers to the radial lateral bands of the middle, ring and small fingers and the ulnar lateral band of the index finger; or to the combined interosseous tendon insertion
Thumb adduction	ECRB + tendon graft to adductor pollicis
Index finger abduction	Accessory APL to first dorsal interosseous
Severe thumb MCP joint hyperextension	MCP joint fusion
Fixed thumb IP joint contracture	IP joint fusion
Weak DIP joint flexion ring and small fingers	Side-to-side tenorrhaphy of the ring and small finger FDP tendons to the middle finger FDP tendon

PIP joints can be extended by the extrinsic extensor tendons provided that the MCP joints are stabilized against hyperextension. Both the claw deformity and the asynchronous flexion may therefore be improved either by static procedures to prevent hyperextension at the MCP joints or by dynamic tendon transfers to produce either MCP joint flexion alone or to provide both MCP joint flexion and interphalangeal joint extension.

The other significant impairment in patients with low ulnar nerve palsy is weak thumb–index finger pinch, which may be only 20–25% of normal due to paralysis of the adductor pollicis, one half of the FPB and the first dorsal interosseous muscles. However, in 58% of ulnar nerve injuries, there is dual innervation of the FPB muscle which can to some extent provide thumb MP joint flexion and key pinch to the index finger. Loss of key pinch is usually manifest by compensatory activation of the FPL producing excessive flexion at the interphalangeal joint (*Froment's sign*) *(Fig. 34.24)* and occasionally hyperextension at the MCP joint (*Jeanne's sign*) as the patient attempts forceful pinch. In such patients with weak pinch, tendon transfers will be required to restore adduction of the thumb and abduction of the index finger.

Patients may also develop an irritating ulnar deviation of the small finger in addition to clawing at the MCP joint of the small finger (*Wartenberg sign*) caused by the unopposed action of the EDM tendon due to paralysis of the third palmar interosseous muscle. Occasionally, a tendon transfer may be required to correct this ulnar deviation of the small finger.

Therefore, tendon transfers may be indicated in an ulnar nerve palsy *(Table 34.4)* to correct:

1. Clawing and asynchronous flexion of the fingers
2. Weak thumb–index finger pinch
3. Ulnar deviation deformity of the small finger
4. Weak FDP flexion at the DIP joints of the ring and small fingers.

Timing of tendon transfers for ulnar nerve palsy is primarily dependent on two factors: the probability of motor recovery and the severity of the functional deficit. Primary microsurgical repair of the ulnar nerve at the wrist can be expected to yield useful results in about 75% of patients. Secondary nerve grafting has been reported to provide some functional motor recovery in approximately 40–75% of cases, with a somewhat worse prognosis for sensory recovery. As in other peripheral nerve injuries, younger patients, those with shorter nerve defects, and those without other significant associated injuries have a better chance of obtaining useful results from ulnar nerve repair.

"Early" tendon transfers should be considered for those with a debilitating claw deformity. While clawing should be treated proactively using a lumbrical block splint, some patients may benefit from early static transfers to prevent MCP hyperextension and clawing. Trevett et al.[53] studied the functional results following both high and low ulnar nerve repairs to better define the indications for tendon transfers. They demonstrated continued improvement in intrinsic muscle power, grip strength and sensation for at least 2 years in high and 3 years in low ulnar nerve repairs. The significant conclusion from this study was that early tendon transfers should only be performed in manual laborers who complain of poor grip or key pinch.

Static procedures to correct clawing of the fingers

Treatment/surgical technique

Static procedures to prevent hyperextension of the proximal phalanges at their MCP joints include A1 pulley release, fasciodermadesis at the MCP joint level, capsulodesis and various tenodeses. Capsulodesis of the MCP joint, described by Zancolli,[54] is a very simple technique in which the A1 pulley is first released, the volar plate is incised longitudinally and detached from the metacarpal to create two distally-based flaps, which are then advanced proximally and attached to the metacarpal neck to maintain the MCP joint in approximately 20° of flexion. Omer[55] described creating a distal-based flap of the volar plate by making two parallel incisions on the medial and lateral aspects of the volar plate and excising Burow's triangles distally to allow proximal advancement of the volar plate. The volar plate is anchored to the metacarpal neck with wire sutures through drill holes or by using a bone anchor *(Fig. 34.25)*. Recurrence of clawing has been demonstrated in long term follow-up studies.[56,57]

Parkes[58] has described an effective tenodesis both to prevent hyperextension at the MCP joints and to provide extension at the interphalangeal joints by using tendon grafts sutured to the transverse carpal ligament and passed volar to the deep transverse intermetacarpal (inter-volar plate) ligaments to insert into the radial lateral band of each finger. Omer[55] modified the Parkes tenodesis by attaching one tendon graft to the ulnar lateral band of the ring finger, passing around the deep transverse intermetacarpal ligament and suturing it to the radial lateral band of the small finger, with a second tendon graft from the ulnar lateral band of the index finger around the deep transverse intermetacarpal ligament to the radial lateral band of the middle finger. Fowler attached tendon grafts to the extensor retinaculum, routed them dorsally through the intermetacarpal spaces and then volar to the deep transverse intermetacarpal ligaments and then attached the grafts to the radial lateral bands of the fingers.[52] The Riordan tenodesis employs a similar dorsal route, utilizing two distally-based strips of the ECRL and ECU tendons passed down the lumbrical canals, volar to the deep transverse intermetacarpal ligaments and attached to the radial lateral bands.[21]

The various dynamic tendon transfers that have been described to correct clawing differ primarily as to whether they provide only MP joint flexion or whether they provide both MP joint flexion and interphalangeal joint extension. The surgeon can determine which general type of transfer is most appropriate by preoperative testing of PIP and DIP joint extension with the MCP joints held passively flexed – the Bouvier manoeuvre. If, with the MCP joints flexed, the extrinsic extensor tendons can produce full extension at the PIP and DIP joints *(Fig. 34.26)* the transfer may only need to produce strong MCP joint flexion by insertion of the transfer either into the A1 pulley[59] *(Fig. 34.24)*, the A2 pulley[60] *(Fig. 34.27C)*, the

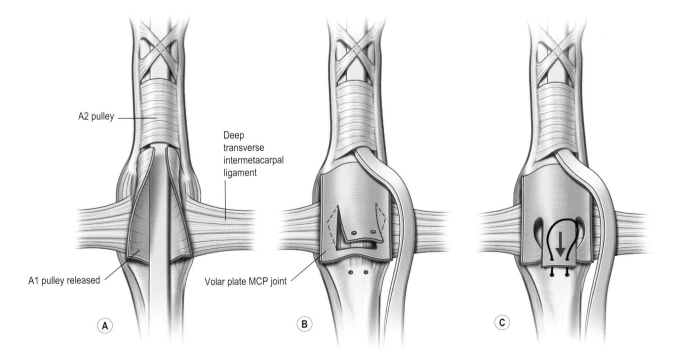

Fig. 34.25 The Omer modification of the Zancolli capsulodesis: **(A)** The A1 pulley is released. **(B)** A distal-based flap is created in the volar plate. **(C)** The distal-based flap of the volar plate is advanced proximally and fixed to the metacarpal neck.

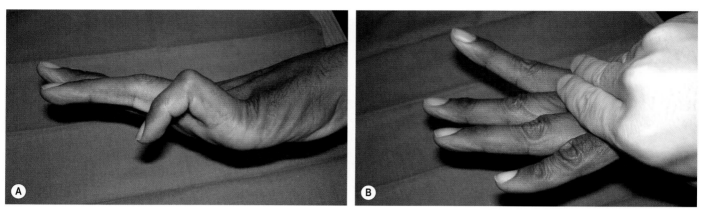

Fig. 34.26 The Bouvier maneuver. **(A)** Typical claw deformity of the small finger and to a lesser extent the ring finger with hyperextension at the MCP joint and flexion at the PIP and DIP joints. **(B)** By preventing hyperextension at the MCP joints, the extrinsic extensor tendons are able to produce full extension at the PIP and DIP joints.

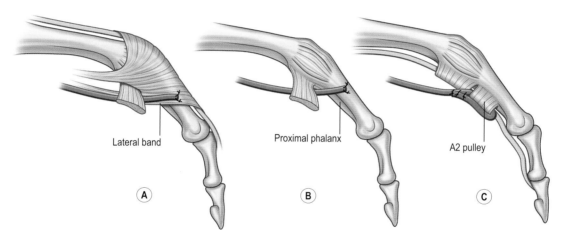

Fig. 34.27 Alternative insertions for tendon transfers to prevent clawing. **(A)** Insertion into the lateral band. **(B)** Burkhalter insertion through a drill hole in the proximal phalanx. **(C)** "Lasso" procedure either into the A1 pulley, (Zancolli) the A2 pulley (Brooks-Jones) or the A1 and proximal half of the A2 pulley (Anderson).

A1 and proximal half of the A2 pulley,[61] or through a drill hole in the proximal phalanx[62] *(Fig. 34.27B)*. However, with long standing flexion deformities of the PIP joints, the central slip of the extensor mechanism may become attenuated. Consequently even with passive flexion of the MCP joints, the patient cannot actively extend the PIP joints using the extrinsic extensor tendons. In these circumstances, the transfer should be inserted into one of the lateral bands *(Fig. 34.27A)*; or into the dorsal base of the middle phalanx; or into the combined interosseous tendons (which Zancolli termed "Direct interosseous activation",[59,63] so that both MCP joint flexion and PIP joint extension can potentially be restored.

If one of the superficialis tendons is used as a donor tendon to produce either MCP joint flexion alone or both MCP joint flexion and interphalangeal joint extension, it does not produce any increase in power grip; whereas adding an extra muscle-tendon unit from outside the hand to activate these transfers, such as a wrist flexor (FCR) or extensor tendon (ECRL, ECRB), will potentially lead to increased grip strength.

Tendon transfers to correct clawing

Treatment/surgical technique

All of the following have been described as the donor muscle-tendon unit in tendon transfers to correct asynchronous finger flexion and clawing in ulnar nerve palsy:

1. Flexor digitorum superficialis
2. Extensor carpi radialis brevis
3. Extensor indicis proprius and extensor digiti minimi
4. Flexor carpi radialis
5. Extensor carpi radialis longus
6. Palmaris longus.

Stiles and Forrester-Brown[64] originally described transfer of one slip of each FDS tendon into the extensor mechanism and this was subsequently modified by both Bunnell[65] and Littler.[30] The Littler modification is referred as the modified Stiles–Bunnell technique and involves transfer of the FDS of the ring finger or middle finger or both fingers, splitting the tendon longitudinally into two slips, passing each slip of the superficialis tendon down the lumbrical canals and attaching them to the radial lateral bands of the fingers *(Fig. 34.28)*.

If the Bouvier manoeuvre confirms that the extrinsic extensor tendons can produce full extension at the PIP and DIP

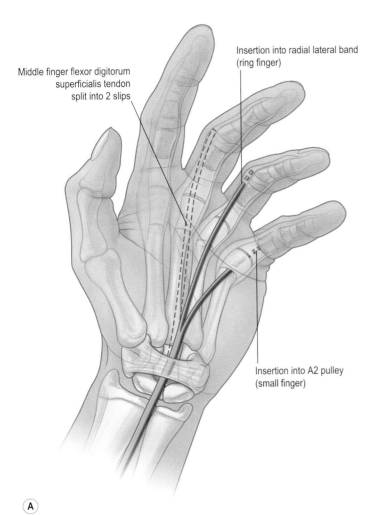

Middle finger flexor digitorum superficialis tendon split into 2 slips

Insertion into radial lateral band (ring finger)

Insertion into A2 pulley (small finger)

(A)

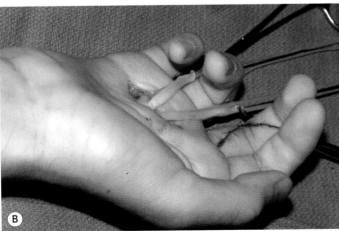

(B)

Fig. 34.28 (A,B) Transfer of the middle finger FDS to the radial lateral band of the ring finger or the A2 pulley of the small finger.

joints with the MCP joints flexed, alternative insertions of the modified Stiles–Bunnell transfer into either the pulleys or the proximal phalanx can be considered in an attempt to prevent the risk of developing a secondary hyperextension deformity at the PIP joint. Zancolli originally described dividing the FDS tendons to the ring and small fingers distal to the A1 pulley between the A1 and A2 pulleys through a distal palmar crease incision. Each tendon is withdrawn from the flexor sheath between the A1 and A2 pulleys, looped around the A1 pulley and sutured back to itself. This has been termed the "Lasso" procedure *(Figs 34.27C, 34.28A)*.[59] In patients with a high ulnar palsy, the ring and small finger superficialis tendons cannot be used and therefore the middle finger superficialis tendon is divided into two slips and each slip is passed under the A1 pulleys of the ring and small fingers and sutured to itself *(Fig. 34.28)*. The superficialis tendon slips are sutured with the wrist in neutral, the MCP joints in 60° of flexion and the wrist is then immobilized in 10° of flexion and the MCP joint in 90° of flexion for 3 weeks, but allowing motion at the PIP and DIP joints. Omer and Brooks-Jones[60] described looping the superficialis tendon around the A2 pulley rather than the A1 pulley and Anderson[61] has described an extended pulley insertion (EPI) by looping the superficialis tendon around both the A1 and the proximal half of the A2 pulleys. Burkhalter[62] recommended insertion of the FDS tendon slips of a modified Stiles-Bunnell transfer into a radial-ulnar drill hole in the proximal phalanx *(Fig. 34.27B)*.

In combined high median-ulnar nerve palsy, all the superficialis tendons are paralyzed and consequently an "indirect lasso" procedure is required. After passing the superficialis tendons around the A1 pulleys, the proximal ends of the superficialis tendons are activated either by ECRL or FCR. Brooks and Jones[60] have described a variant of this transfer in which the ECRL or FCR are elongated with plantaris or toe extensor tendon grafts passed through the carpal tunnel and inserted more distally into the A2 pulley. Burkhalter and Strait[62] have also used the same donor tendons, the ring finger superficialis and ECRL but with insertion through a transverse drill hole in the middle third of the proximal phalanx. The ring finger superficialis is divided at the level of the PIP joint withdrawn into the palm and divided into two slips. Each slip is then passed down the lumbrical canal and drawn into a transverse drill hole on the radial aspect of the middle third of the proximal phalanx of the ring and small fingers.

Modified Stiles–Bunnell transfer

Treatment/surgical technique

In the modified Stiles–Bunnell transfer[30] for patients with an isolated low ulnar nerve palsy, the ring finger FDS tendon is divided just proximal to the PIP joint, withdrawn through a transverse distal palmar crease incision and split longitudinally into two slips. The radial lateral bands of the ring and small fingers are exposed through radial mid-axial incisions and each slip of the superficialis tendon is passed down the lumbrical canals of the ring and small fingers. With the wrist in neutral, each slip is sutured under adequate tension to the radial lateral bands with the MCP joints in 45–55° of flexion and the interphalangeal joints fully extended. Tension is tested using the tenodesis effect of the wrist-with wrist extension, the fingers should assume the "intrinsic-plus" position. The hand is immobilized in a dorsal block splint with the wrist in slight flexion and the MP joints flexed 70° for 3.5–4 weeks. In a high ulnar nerve palsy, the ring finger superficialis tendon is the only extrinsic flexor tendon in the ring finger and therefore the middle finger FDS tendon is used (**Fig. 34.28**). Occasionally, the middle or ring finger superficialis may be split into three slips, should the middle, ring and small fingers need correction. With a total intrinsic palsy, the superficialis tendons to both the middle and ring fingers are each divided into two slips and passed down the lumbrical canals to the radial lateral bands of the index, middle, ring and small fingers. Brand advocates insertion of the slip to the index finger into the ulnar lateral band to provide improved 3-point pinch. However, this may result in scissoring of the index and middle fingers. Zancolli[59] has described insertion of the FDS donor tendon into the combined interosseous tendons rather than the radial lateral bands and termed this alternative technique of restoring MCP joint flexion and IP joint extension as "direct interosseous activation."

One of the disadvantages of the modified Stiles–Bunnell transfer is that the ring finger superficialis is not expendable in a high ulnar nerve palsy or in a combined high median-high ulnar nerve palsy. Second, the transfer may result in progressive over-correction of the claw deformity eventually resulting in a "swan-neck" hyperextension deformity at the PIP joints. A "swan-neck" hyperextension deformity can be prevented by utilizing one of the distal slips of FDS as a tenodesis across the PIP joint. Third, the donor middle or ring finger may develop a flexion contracture at the PIP joint or loss of extension at the DIP joint. North and Littler[66] recommended harvesting the superficialis tendon through a Bruner incision between the A1 and A2 pulleys rather than a midaxial incision at the level of the PIP joint. The modified Stiles–Bunnell transfer should therefore only be used in patients with mild PIP joint flexion contractures or stable fingers without passive hyperextension at the PIP joints.

Brand EE4T transfer

Treatment/surgical technique

Due to his extensive experience of tendon transfers in leprosy patients, Brand[2,67] originally described transfer of the extensor carpi radialis brevis (ECRB), extended with three or four tendon grafts, passed from dorsal to palmar through the intermetacarpal spaces and then down the lumbrical canals to be attached to the radial lateral bands of the middle, ring and small fingers (**Fig. 34.29**) and to the ulnar lateral band of the index finger (EE4T: extensor tendon, extensor route, four-tailed graft). However, during wrist extension, the ECRB and tendon grafts relax which is a relative disadvantage of this dorsal routing of the original Brand transfer. Burkhalter and Strait[62] modified the Brand EE4T transfer, by using ECRL instead of ECRB and by only correcting the ring and small fingers. The ECRL is lengthened with two tendon slips, which are passed through the third and fourth intermetacarpal spaces, down the lumbrical canals, volar to the deep transverse intermetacarpal ligaments and inserted into a drill hole on the radial aspect of the middle third of the proximal phalanges. The wrist is immobilized in forty degrees of extension and the MCP joints in 70° of flexion for four weeks. This

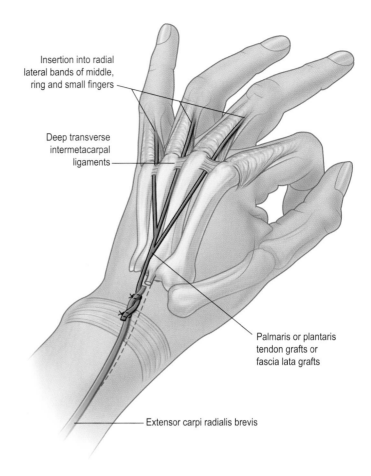

Fig. 34.29 Brand EE4T transfer of ECRB extended by three tendon grafts into the three ulnar fingers.

transfer will only produce MCP joint flexion, but is an alternative transfer for a combined high median-high ulnar nerve palsy when the modified Stiles–Bunnell FDS transfer is not available. Riordan[21] described a similar transfer using flexor carpi radialis (FCR) transferred dorsally around the radial border of the forearm and elongated with tendon grafts passed dorsal-to-palmar through the intermetacarpal spaces volar to the deep transverse intermetacarpal ligaments and inserted into the radial lateral bands. This transfer is mutually beneficial if there is an associated flexion contracture of the wrist.

The dorsal route also forms the basis for the Fowler transfer using both the EIP and EDM tendons. The two tendons are divided just beyond the MCP joints of the index and small fingers and each tendon is split longitudinally into two slips. The four slips are tunnelled subcutaneously to the radial lateral bands of the fingers.[52] The EIP tendon controls the index and middle fingers and the EDM tendon controls the ring and small fingers. In a modification of this Fowler transfer, Riordan has described splitting only the EIP tendon into two slips and passing them from dorsal to palmar through the third and fourth intermetacarpal spaces to insert into the radial lateral bands to correct clawing of the ring and small fingers.[68] A relative disadvantage of the Fowler and Riordan transfers is that the EIP and EDM tendons are only just long enough to reach the radial lateral bands and these transfers are rarely used.

Brand EF4T transfer

Treatment/surgical technique

Brand[67] modified his original dorsal transfer of ECRB by extending ECRL with a four tailed tendon graft or fascia lata graft through the carpal tunnel to the radial lateral bands of the middle, ring and small fingers and the ulnar lateral band of the index finger (EF4T: extensor tendon, flexor route, four-tailed graft) *(Fig. 34.30)*. In an isolated ulnar nerve palsy, this transfer is only attached to the radial lateral bands of the ring and small fingers *(Fig. 34.31A,B)*. Two short transverse incisions are made one over the second dorsal extensor tendon compartment to allow transection of the ECRL tendon which is withdrawn into the second incision over the radial aspect of the mid-forearm *(Fig. 34.31A)*. Either a fascia lata graft or a folded plantaris tendon graft is sutured to the distal end of the ECRL tendon projecting through the radial forearm incision. The elongated ECRL tendon is then passed around the radial border of the forearm into a transverse volar forearm incision just proximal to the wrist crease. Through a 3 cm long incision on the ulnar side of the thenar crease, a tendon tunneling forceps is introduced distal to the superficial palmar arch and passed along the floor of the carpal tunnel to exit on the ulnar side of the volar forearm incision and the tendon grafts or fascia lata graft are then pulled distally through the carpal tunnel into the palmar incision *(Fig. 34.31B)*. The proximal tendon juncture therefore lies distal to the volar forearm incision, but proximal to the transverse carpal ligament. Each of the two plantaris slips are split longitudinally to produce four slips or the fascia lata graft is split into four slips. Through radial mid-axial incisions over the proximal phalanges of the middle, ring and small fingers, the tunneling forceps is passed down each lumbrical canal volar to the deep transverse intermetacarpal ligaments into the palmar incision and the three tendon slips are brought out into each mid-axial incision. The tendon slip to the index finger is tunneled to an ulnar mid-axial incision and attached to the ulnar lateral band. This will produce supination of the index finger and may provide better three point pinch. The hand is positioned on a frame with the wrist flexed 30°, the MCP joints flexed 70° and the interphalangeal joints fully extended. Proximal traction is applied to each lateral band to take up any slack in the extensor mechanism. After taking up the slack in all four plantaris tendon grafts, they are sutured to the lateral bands just proximal to the PIP joints under equal tension. Tension is adjusted in the index finger first, then the small finger and finally the middle and ring fingers. The hand is immobilized with the wrist in neutral, the MCP joints flexed 90° and the IP joints straight for 3 weeks *(Fig. 34.31C)*.

Fritschi PF4T transfer

Treatment/surgical technique

Fritschi[69] has described the palmaris longus as an alternative motor for the Brand EF4T transfer. In the Lennox–Fritschi PL4T (palmaris four-tail) transfer, the palmaris longus tendon is lengthened with a tendon graft or fascia lata graft, which are then passed through the carpal tunnel to the lateral bands in a similar route to the Brand EF4T procedure. However, the palmaris longus is obviously a much weaker donor muscle than the ECRL.

Two alternative insertions have been described for the Brand EF4T and Lennox–Fritschi PL4T transfers, either the common interosseous tendon insertion or the A2 pulley. Zancolli[59] originally described looping the tendon grafts or fascia lata grafts around the common interosseous tendon – a technique described as "direct interosseous activation." In addition to restoring MCP joint flexion, this insertion may potentially provide abduction of the fingers. Palande[63] has also reported using both the ECRL and palmaris longus tendons extended with tendon grafts, inserting them around the common interosseous tendons. ECRL or palmaris longus are elongated with tendon grafts or fascia lata grafts which are then tunneled through the carpal tunnel to emerge distal to the superficial palmar arch through an incision just to the ulnar side of the thenar crease. The first dorsal interosseous tendon, the palmar and dorsal interosseous tendons in the second, third and fourth web spaces and the muscle-tendon junction of the hypothenar muscles are all identified through a transverse incision along the distal palmar crease. The

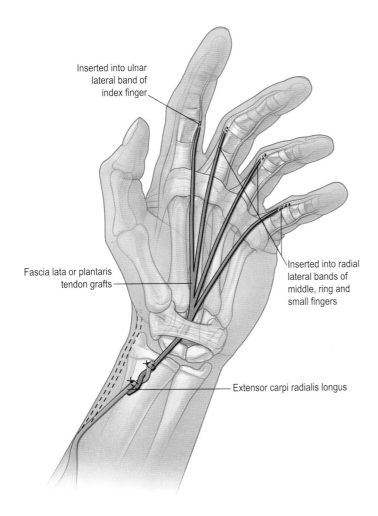

Inserted into ulnar lateral band of index finger

Fascia lata or plantaris tendon grafts

Inserted into radial lateral bands of middle, ring and small fingers

Extensor carpi radialis longus

Fig. 34.30 Brand EF4T transfer of the ECRL extended by four tendon grafts into all four lateral bands in a patient with clawing of all four fingers.

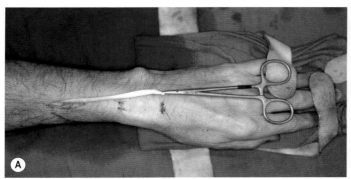

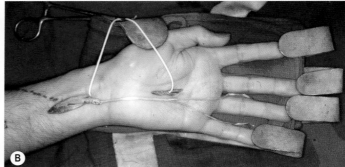

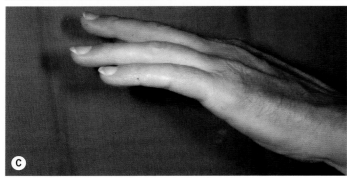

Fig. 34.31 Brand EF4T transfer to correct clawing of the ring and small fingers. **(A)** The ECRL is detached from its insertion into the base of the second metacarpal. **(B)** A palmaris longus graft is attached to the ECRL which has been brought volarly around the radial side of the forearm (or through the interosseous membrane.) **(C)**. Postoperatively, this has corrected the preoperative claw deformity of the 4th and 5th fingers.

plantaris tendon grafts or fascia lata grafts are split into four or five slips. One slip is looped around the muscle-tendon junction of the first dorsal interosseous: one slip around the combined first palmar interosseous and second dorsal interosseous tendons in the index-middle finger webspace: one slip around the combined third dorsal interosseous and second palmar interosseous tendons in the middle-ring finger webspace: one slip around the combined fourth dorsal interosseous and third palmar interosseous tendons in the ring-small finger webspace; and if necessary the final fifth slip can be looped around the muscle-tendon junction of the hypothenar muscles. The hand is positioned with the MCP joints flexed 60° and the interphalangeal joints straight. After slack has been taken up, each of the four of five slips are sutured back onto themselves, starting on the radial side with the index finger, then the slip between the ring and small fingers and finally the slips between the index and middle fingers and between the middle and ring fingers. The correct tension is confirmed by performing a wrist tenodesis maneuver. The hand is immobilized for 3 weeks with the wrist neutral, the MP joints in 90° of flexion and the interphalangeal joints extended.

Brooks and Jones[60] described amalgamating the Brand EF4T transfer with the Zancolli lasso procedure in which the ECRL or FCR tendons are elongated with plantaris or toe extensor tendon grafts and passed through the carpal tunnel and looped around the A2 pulleys of each finger. This variant of the EF4T transfer will only produce MCP joint flexion.

Tendon transfer to correct ulnar deviation of the small finger

Treatment/surgical technique

A variant of the Fowler transfer has been advocated by Blacker et al.[70] to correct the ulnar deviation deformity of the small finger (Wartenberg's sign). The ulnar half of EDM is detached, passed volar to the deep transverse intermetacarpal ligament and sutured into the insertion of the radial collateral ligament of the MCP joint at the base of the proximal phalanx, or if there is associated clawing of the small finger, it is looped under the A2 pulley and sutured back to itself (Brooks insertion). Chung et al.[71] described transferring EIP to the distal radial aspect of the extensor hood of the small finger to correct the persistent abduction deformity of the small finger in an ulnar nerve palsy.

Tendon transfers to provide adduction of the thumb

Treatment/surgical technique

The most successful tendon transfers to restore adduction of the thumb have a transverse direction of pull across the palm deep to the flexor tendons to insert into the tendon of adductor pollicis. Littler[30] has advocated transfer of the ring finger superficialis deep to the flexor tendons of the index and middle fingers parallel and superficial to the transverse fibers of adductor pollicis and inserted into a drill hole just distal to the adductor insertion, and has been able to document an increase in pinch strength to 71% of the opposite hand. Smith[72] described using ECRB extended by a free tendon graft passed through the second intermetacarpal space and tunneled deep to the flexor tendons but superficial to the adductor pollicis to an insertion into the adductor tendon *(Fig. 34.32)*. Other tendon transfers to restore adduction of the thumb have included either the brachioradialis[73] or ECRL[74] elongated with a tendon graft and passed through the third intermetacarpal space to the thumb MCP joint, and the EIP passed through the second intermetacarpal space.[75] Combined transfers to provide both thumb adduction and index finger abduction have been described by splitting the EIP or EDM tendons.[76]

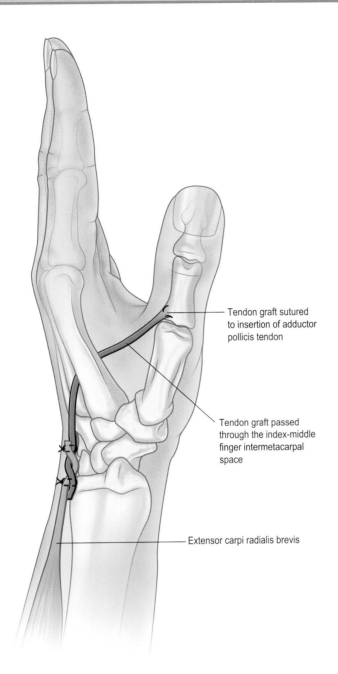

Tendon graft sutured to insertion of adductor pollicis tendon

Tendon graft passed through the index-middle finger intermetacarpal space

Extensor carpi radialis brevis

Fig. 34.32 Schematic representation of the Smith transfer for restoration of thumb adduction. The extensor carpi radialis brevis is extended by a tendon graft through the second intermetacarpal space to the adductor tubercle on the ulnar base of the proximal phalanx of the thumb.

If there is a severe collapse Z-deformity of the thumb with hyperextension at the MCP joint and flexion at the IP joint, or an exaggerated Jeanne's sign when attempting to pinch, arthrodesis of the MCP joint may be necessary.[30,77] The thumb MCP joint is positioned in 15–20° of flexion and 15° pronation and arthrodesis achieved using a dorsal plate, interosseous wiring or tension band wiring. Arthrodesis of the MCP joint may be combined with an adductor transfer or the transfer may be performed secondarily. Occasionally, if there is a severe fixed flexion deformity of the IP joint, arthrodesis of

the IP joint is indicated[78] instead of the MCP joint, combined with an adductor transfer. IP joint arthrodesis is achieved with interosseous wiring or K-wires or a combination of each.

For mild collapse deformities of the thumb without a fixed contracture, a split FPL to EPL transfer may be indicated.[79] Through a volar Bruner incision, the FPL is split longitudinally from its insertion proximally to the distal end of the A1 pulley. The radial half of FPL is transected at its insertion, retracted back proximal to the oblique pulley and passed deep to the radial neurovascular bundle around the radial border of the proximal phalanx into a longitudinal incision on the dorsum of the proximal phalanx. The radial slip of FPL is sutured to the EPL tendon proximal to the IP joint with the MCP joint in 15° of flexion and the IP joint in full extension. The IP joint is fixed with a K wire for four weeks.

Ring finger flexor digitorum superficialis transfer

Treatment/surgical technique

The ring finger FDS tendon is transected between the A1 and A2 pulleys through a short incision at the base of the ring finger.[30] The superficialis tendon is then passed transversely across the palm deep to the index and middle finger flexor tendons to the ulnar aspect of the thumb MCP joint, through a short incision just to the ulnar side of the thenar crease. The transfer is either sutured into the adductor pollicis tendon or passed through a drill hole in the proximal phalanx just distal to the adductor insertion and tied over a button. Tension is set with the wrist in neutral and the thumb adducted against the index finger with the superficialis tendon at its resting length. Appropriate tension is confirmed by tenodesis of the wrist – with wrist flexion, the thumb should be able to be passively abducted. Edgerton and Brand[31] have described a variation of this transfer in which the ring finger superficialis is brought through a window in the palmar fascia and then passed subcutaneously to the abductor insertion. The vertical septum of palmar fascia arising from the middle finger metacarpal acts as a pulley. Obviously, the ring finger superficialis cannot be used as an adductor transfer in patients with a high ulnar nerve palsy since this would deprive the ring finger of its only remaining flexor tendon.

Smith extensor carpi radialis brevis transfer

Treatment/surgical technique

ECRB is transected through a short transverse incision over the second dorsal extensor compartment just distal to the extensor retinaculum and withdrawn through a second transverse incision just proximal to the extensor retinaculum.[72] A small flap is then elevated over the ulnar aspect of the MCP joint of the thumb and a palmaris or plantaris tendon graft sutured to the adductor pollicis tendon. Through a short transverse incision overlying the proximal third of the second intermetacarpal space, a tendon passer is used to tunnel the tendon graft deep to the flexor tendons but superficial to the adductor pollicis, withdrawing it dorsally through the second intermetacarpal space. After passing the tendon graft subcutaneously to the most proximal incision, it is woven into the ECRB tendon with the wrist in neutral and the thumb adducted *(Fig. 34.32)*. Tension is then checked by tenodesis of

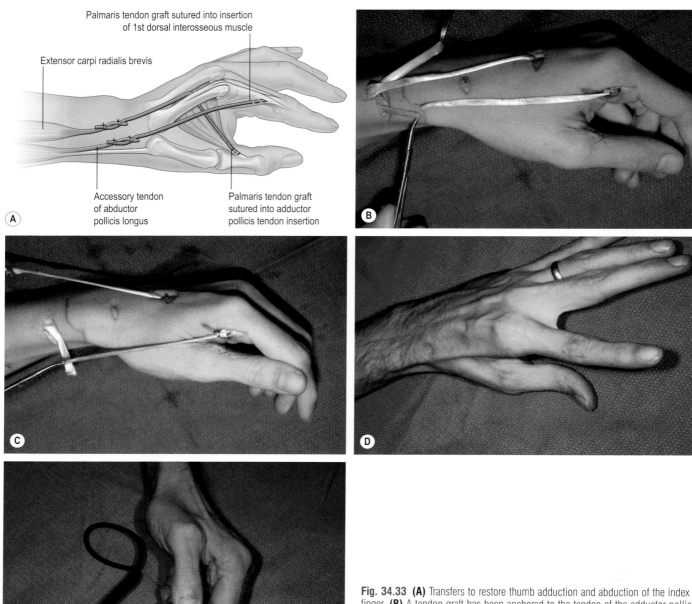

Fig. 34.33 **(A)** Transfers to restore thumb adduction and abduction of the index finger. **(B)** A tendon graft has been anchored to the tendon of the adductor pollicis. It is passed dorsal to the flexor tendons and neurovascular bundles and then from palmar to dorsal through the second intermetacarpal space. A tendon graft has been sutured into the tendon of the first dorsal interosseous **(C)** Traction on these two grafts flexes and adducts the thumb and abducts the index finger at its MCP joint **(D)** Postoperative function following these two transfer **(E)** Pinch strength is significantly improved.

the wrist-with palmar flexion, the thumb should become strongly adducted, whereas wrist extension should allow easy passive abduction of the thumb. Postoperatively the thumb is immobilized for 3 weeks midway between full abduction and full adduction with the wrist in 20–30° of dorsiflexion *(Fig. 34.33)*.

Tendon transfers to provide index finger abduction

Treatment/surgical technique

Restoration of strong abduction of the index finger is the second component required for powerful pinch. Bunnell[65]

described the transfer of extensor indicis proprius (EIP) extended with a short tendon graft and inserted into the first dorsal interosseous tendon. Bruner[80] divided the extensor pollicis brevis (EPB) tendon over the dorsum of the MCP joint of the thumb and tunneled it subcutaneously beneath the EPL tendon into the first dorsal interosseous tendon. Hirayama[81] lengthened the palmaris longus tendon with a strip of palmar fascia (similar to the Camitz transfer) and tunneled it subcutaneously around the radial border of the forearm over the dorsum of the wrist and hand to insert into the first dorsal interosseous tendon. Graham and Riordan[82] transferred the FDS of the ring finger in a similar route around the radial

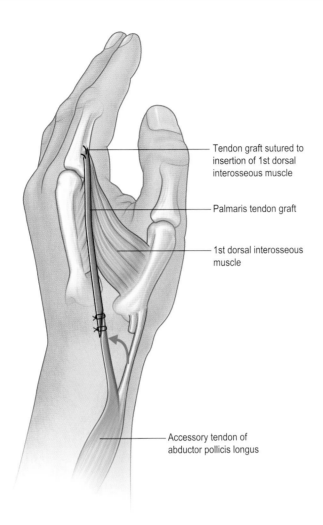

Tendon graft sutured to insertion of 1st dorsal interosseous muscle

Palmaris tendon graft

1st dorsal interosseous muscle

Accessory tendon of abductor pollicis longus

Fig. 34.34 The Neviaser transfer to restore abduction of the index finger. One of the accessory tendons of the abductor pollicis longus is extended by a palmaris tendon graft and sutured to the insertion of the first dorsal interosseous muscle on the base of the proximal phalanx of the index finger.

border of the wrist over the dorsum of the hand to either the first dorsal interosseous tendon or into a drill hole on the radial aspect of the index finger. However, one of the accessory tendons of APL extended with a free tendon graft or attached to the rerouted EDC tendon of the index finger may be the best choice to restore abduction of the index finger *(Fig. 34.34)*.[83]

Neviaser accessory abductor pollicis longus and free tendon graft

Treatment/surgical technique

Neviaser et al.[83] described an accessory APL tendon elongated with a palmaris or plantaris tendon graft transferred to the insertion of the first dorsal interosseous tendon *(Fig. 34.34)*. A small flap is elevated over the radial aspect of the proximal phalanx of the index finger and a tendon graft sutured to the first dorsal interosseous tendon just distal to the MCP joint. The proximal end of the tendon graft is then passed subcutaneously to a transverse incision just distal the first dorsal

extensor compartment. After opening the compartment, one of the accessory APL tendons is transected and interwoven with the tendon graft with the wrist in neutral position and the index finger radially abducted *(Fig. 34.33)*.

High ulnar nerve palsy

Patient selection

Many surgeons fail to realize the significant functional deficit in a high ulnar nerve palsy associated with paralysis of the FCU and FDP tendons to the ring and small fingers. The only remaining tendons on the ulnar side of the hand are the superficialis tendon to the ring finger and the usually diminutive superficialis tendon to the small finger. However, paralysis of the profundus tendons to the ring and small fingers will often be masked by interconnections between these two tendons and the middle finger profundus tendon at the wrist. If there is significant weakness of DIP joint flexion of the ring and small fingers (Pollock's sign), power grip can be restored by side-to-side tenorrhaphy of the ring and small finger FDP tendons to the median-innervated middle finger FDP tendon.[55] This should be performed before tendon transfers to correct clawing are performed, but patients should be warned that this will temporarily exaggerate their clawing and that they should use a lumbrical block splint. To restore independent flexion of the ring and small fingers, the FDS tendon of the middle finger may be used as a donor tendon to activate the FDP tendons of the ring and small fingers. Patients requiring strong ulnar deviation and flexion of the wrist may occasionally need to be considered for transfer of the FCR tendon to FCU.[55]

Outcomes

There are very few reports to substantiate the relative effectiveness of the various transfers to restore synchronous MP flexion and IP extension of the fingers and thumb-index finger pinch. Hastings and Davidson[84] compared four techniques: Zancolli "lasso", Stiles–Bunnell, Brand and Riordan and Fowler transfers to correct the claw deformity in 12 patients with high, 14 patients with low and three patients with mixed high and low ulnar nerve palsy. Successful outcomes were seen in the majority of cases. Most failures occurred in the small finger and transfers utilizing the superficialis tendons were found to further weaken the hand. Only transfers using wrist flexors or extensors have been shown to increase grip strength. A later report examining the effectiveness of the FDS "lasso" procedure showed similar results, with correction of clawing in 19 of 23 digits but no significant improvement in grip strength.[85] The extended pulley insertion for a modified Stiles–Bunnell transfer produced good to excellent correction of clawing in 92% of fingers.[61] Brandsma et al.[48] reported good (57%) or excellent (21%) results using the superficialis transfer to restore intrinsic function. The middle or ring finger superficialis transfer resulted in 95% good or excellent correction of clawing in leprosy patients at an average follow-up of 2 years.[61] The Brand EF4T transfer provided 79–86% good to excellent correction of clawing at a 10-year follow-up.[61] 85% good to excellent results were obtained utilizing the common interosseous tendon insertion technique.[59] PIP hyperextension occurred in 6.25% when the common interosseous tendon insertion was utilized in an EF4T transfer, compared with a 13.75% incidence when the EF4T transfer was inserted into the lateral bands.[61] Therefore, there is less chance of overcorrection producing a PIP joint hyperextension deformity by utilizing the common interosseous tendon insertion. An additional advantage of using ECRL as the motor is that the palmar arch is restored. Ozkan et al.[86] compared the results of three different tendon transfers to restore grip strength and correct the claw deformity in 44 patients with ulnar nerve palsy. A total of 24 patients were reconstructed with a modified Stiles–Bunnell 4-tail procedure, 11 patients with the Brand EF4T transfer, and nine patients with a Zancolli "lasso" procedure. With a recent paralysis, the Zancolli and Brand procedures were the most effective in restoring grip strength, but with long-standing paralysis, the Stiles–Bunnell 4-tail procedure was the most successful in correcting the claw deformity.

Hastings and Davidson[84] showed an approximate doubling of pinch strength in hands treated with the ECRB adductor-plasty transfer, although it is interesting to note that only 18 of the 34 patients in this study felt that pinch strength was compromised enough to warrant a tendon transfer. Robinson et al.[76] evaluated the combination of the ulnar slip of EDM to provide thumb adduction and EIP to restore index finger abduction in six patients and demonstrated an average improvement in pinch strength from 5% to 40–50% of the normal side. Fischer et al.[87] evaluated the results of tendon transfers to restore thumb adduction (ECRL was transferred to adductor pollicis) and index finger abduction (APL was transferred to the first dorsal interosseous) at an average of 6 years postoperatively. Key pinch averaged 73%, pulp-to-pulp pinch averaged 72%, grip strength was 73%, the force of thumb adduction was 63% and the force of index finger abduction was 58% of the normal hand.

Tendon transfers for combined nerve injuries

Patient selection

It is much more difficult to reconstruct the upper extremity affected by multiple nerve injuries. The majority of these patients require multiple reconstructive procedures and tendon transfers. The choice of tendon transfers and the timing of the surgery should be well planned, designed and individualized to address the patient's specific functional needs. It is unwise to adopt a "cookbook" approach for reconstruction of the patient with combined nerve injuries. Basic principles of tendon transfers such as soft tissue equilibrium, full passive range of motion of involved joints, selection of the appropriate donor muscle and direction of transfer as outlined earlier should be carefully considered in preoperative planning.

Before any operation is performed, the patient should be educated about the goals and risks of the procedure and the fact that the injured extremity will never be normal. As a general rule, the results of tendon transfers for combined nerve injuries are inferior to those for a single nerve injury.[88,89]

Adding to the complexity of these problems, the number of donor tendons is limited, more joints need to be mobilized, there is a more profound sensory loss, and the soft tissues may be more scarred in this patient population. Multiple nerve repairs or nerve grafting should be done as soon as clinically appropriate but return of motor function rarely extends beyond two major joints distal to the injury.[90] Reinnervated muscles however, should not be used or only used with great caution as a donor for tendon transfers.

Dynamic tenodesis is an important concept in reconstruction of these combined nerve injuries. Wrist flexion or extension can be used to augment the excursion of any tendon transfer that crosses the wrist. For example, if a wrist flexor such as FCR is used to activate FDP, flexion of the fingers will be enhanced if the patient extends their wrist using the ECRL or ECRB simultaneously with contraction of the FCR transfer. Therefore, if the excursion of a tendon transfer is less than optimal to produce a specific function, increased range of motion can be achieved through wrist tenodesis.[91]

Tendon transfers for low median–low ulnar nerve palsy

Treatment/surgical technique

A low median and low ulnar nerve palsy is the most common combined nerve injury in the upper extremity and is usually the result of a "spaghetti-wrist" laceration.[88] This leads to complete loss of sensation on the palmar surface of the hand and a complete intrinsic motor paralysis that results in a claw hand deformity. A flat transverse metacarpal arch with hyperextension at the MP joints and hyperflexion of the PIP joints accompanied by an abducted small finger are the hallmark of this injury. It is especially important to prevent an adduction contracture of the thumb–index web space.[91] The surgeon should repair or graft the median and ulnar nerves before any tendon transfers are performed in order to restore some protective sensibility to the hand. The goals of reconstruction in a low median-low ulnar nerve palsy are to restore thumb adduction, thumb abduction and opposition, abduction of the index finger and improved extension of the PIP joints of the fingers.

Thumb adduction for key pinch can be restored by transfer of the ECRB extended by a tendon graft through the second intermetacarpal space and inserted into the adductor tubercle of the thumb metacarpal[72] or alternatively by transfer of the superficialis tendon from the ring finger to the adductor insertion.[30] The best option for reconstruction of thumb opposition is the EIP transfer rerouted around the ulnar border of the hand and inserted into the APB tendon.[34,92] This transfer can be combined with arthrodesis of the MCP joint of the thumb to allow for maximum stability.[93] Index finger abduction for strong pinch can be restored by transfer of one of the APL tendon slips extended by a tendon graft to the first dorsal interosseous insertion.[83] Finally, clawing of the fingers can be corrected by using ECRL or palmaris longus[67] extended by four tendon grafts and inserted either into the radial lateral bands or the A2 pulleys as previously discussed. Alternatively, if the patient has developed a flexion contracture of the wrist, by involuntarily trying to prevent clawing by flexing their wrist, the FCR tendon may be used to motor the four tendon grafts.[21]

If the patient still has poor palmar sensibility despite nerve repair or nerve grafting, consideration should be given to transfer of a superficial radial nerve innervated flap to the thumb or nerve transfer of the superficial radial nerve to the distal median nerve.

Tendon transfers for high median-high ulnar nerve palsy

Treatment/surgical technique

This is a very severe injury in which there is no active flexion of the fingers and thumb and loss of thumb opposition and key pinch in addition to the loss of palmar sensibility. Initially, the fingers may be fully extended even at the interphalangeal joints despite the intrinsic paralysis. However, once tendon transfers are completed to provide active finger flexion, the fingers gradually assume a claw-posture. Tendon transfers for reconstruction of a high median-high ulnar nerve palsy have to be performed in two or three stages. The goals are to restore finger and thumb flexion, thumb-index finger pinch, abduction and opposition of the thumb and correct the later development of clawing of the fingers.

Thumb adduction and key pinch can be achieved by transfer of ECRB with a free tendon graft through the second intermetacarpal space to the adductor pollicis insertion.[72,94] Finger flexion can be restored by transfer of ECRL to the four FDP tendons.[55] This can be combined with tenodesis of the DIP joints of the three ulnar fingers.[88] Flexion of the thumb can be restored by transfer of the brachioradialis to FPL through the same palmar incision.[55] The brachioradialis muscle must be mobilized and elevated off the radius into the proximal third of the forearm. A Pulvertaft tendon weave is then performed between the brachioradialis and FPL in the distal third of the forearm.[74,88] As in a low median-low ulnar nerve palsy, the most reliable procedure for thumb opposition is transfer of the EIP to the APB insertion.[34] If the IP joint of the thumb tends to assume a flexed position, the EIP transfer should be inserted both into the APB insertion and then into the EPL tendon just proximal to the IP joint.[21] If thumb pinch remains unstable with MP extension and IP joint flexion, arthrodesis of the MP joint should be considered. A useful procedure that avoids the need to fuse the IP joint of the thumb involves longitudinal splitting of the FPL tendon, detaching the radial half from its insertion into the distal phalanx and transfer of this tendon slip dorsally where it is attached into the EPL tendon proximal to the IP joint of the thumb.[79] This results in a dynamic stabilization of the IP joint when the transfer pulls through the FPL.

If after finger flexion has been restored, the fingers begin to adopt a clawed position, there are no expendable wrist extensors (ECRL and ECRB) remaining to provide integration of MP flexion and IP joint extension, static tenodesis techniques may be necessary. Free tendon grafts can be placed from the deep transverse metacarpal ligaments to the lateral bands[58] or from the dorsal carpal ligament to the lateral bands.[21] Alternatively, hyperextension can be prevented by Zancolli capsulodesis or the PIP joints can be arthrodesed. Finally, abduction of the index finger for pinch can be restored using an accessory APL tendon extended with a free tendon graft to the first dorsal interosseous[83] or alternatively by using EPB.[80]

The importance of restoring sensibility to the radial side of the hand in a high median-high ulnar nerve palsy cannot be overstated, either by secondary nerve repair or nerve grafting. A sensate hand is the prerequisite for performing the tendon transfers mentioned above. If sensation cannot be restored, Omer has advocated a fillet flap of the index finger to resurface the thumb-middle finger web space with dorsal skin innervated by the superficial radial nerve.[88] Alternatively, a first dorsal metacarpal artery flap innervated by the superficial branch of the radial nerve can be transferred to the palmar surface of the thumb or the superficial radial nerve itself transferred to the distal median nerve.

Tendon transfers for reconstruction after trauma

Treatment/surgical technique

Tendon transfers are an excellent method of restoring active motion to the hand and wrist following traumatic injuries of the muscles and tendons of the forearm, wrist and hand. If there has been segmental loss of tendon, a tendon graft is often used instead of a tendon transfer. With more severe trauma (industrial or motor vehicle accidents, blast, missile and explosion injuries), associated damage to the soft tissues will leave a scarred bed which is unsuitable for tendon grafts, since a tendon graft is more likely to become adherent to the scarred surrounding tissue than a tendon transfer. If a forearm muscle itself has been badly damaged, a tendon graft will be unable to restore active motion and a tendon transfer will be necessary.

Time is another important consideration in reconstruction of the post-traumatic upper extremity. Myostatic contracture and atrophy are the unavoidable fate of injured muscle if there has been a long delay between the traumatic event and the reconstructive procedure, again making a tendon transfer a more suitable option for reconstruction.

Tendon transfers to restore thumb extension

Treatment/surgical technique

Rupture of the EPL tendon occurs in approximately 1 in 200 distal radius fractures, classically at Lister's tubercle and may happen at any time from several weeks to several months after the fracture. Ischemia of the tendon due to swelling and edema of the tenosynovium and attrition over the roughened dorsal radial cortex have been postulated as the etiology for this tendon rupture.[95–98] Patients present with weakness or loss of extension at the interphalangeal joint or paradoxically with incomplete extension at the MP joint as well as inability to raise the thumb dorsal to the plane of the hand (*Fig. 34.35A*).

Video 1

The optimal choice for restoration of thumb extension is the EIP to EPL transfer which can be performed under local anesthesia (*Fig. 34.35B*). The EIP tendon is harvested through a short transverse incision just proximal to the index finger MP joint and its distal stump is then sutured end-to-side to the EDC tendon of the index finger to prevent extensor lag of this finger. The EIP is retrieved through a second transverse incision just distal to the extensor retinaculum. A third incision is made over the distal third of the thumb metacarpal and the EIP is channeled subcutaneously to this incision. The distal end of the EIP is sutured to the distal end of the EPL

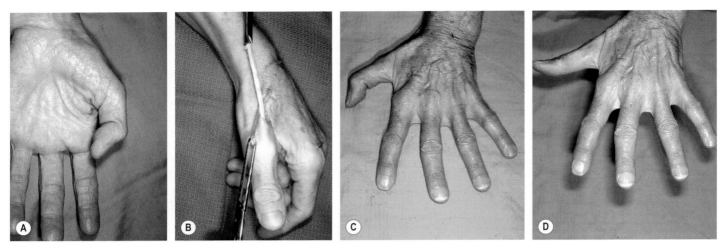

Fig. 34.35 (A) Rupture of the EPL **(B)** Transfer of the EIP to the EPL **(C)** Preoperative thumb extension **(D)** Postoperative thumb extension.

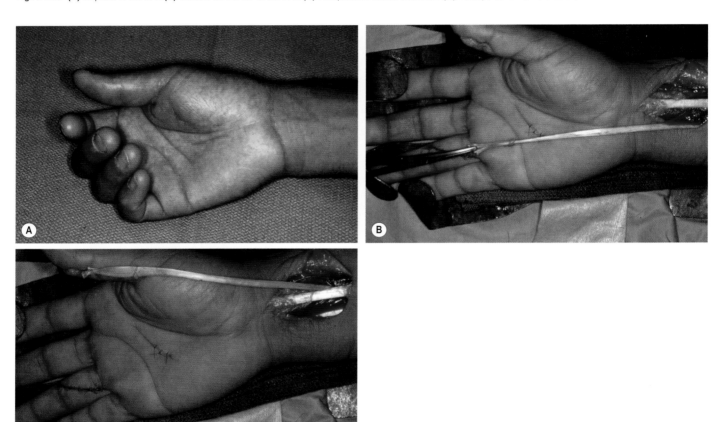

Fig. 34.36 (A) Laceration of the FPL tendon. **(B)** First stage insertion of a silastic rod permits the development of a smooth gliding bed for the transfer of the ring finger FDS tendon. **(C)** The FDS tendon is prepared for passage into its new sheath.

with the wrist held in neutral and the thumb fully extended and parallel or just volar to the plane of the palm.[99] The tension of the transfer can be checked by tenodesis of the wrist. With wrist flexion, the thumb should move dorsal to the plane of the palm and with wrist extension the thumb should be able to be placed in full passive abduction and opposition. The patient is even able to activate the transferred EIP to extend the thumb on the operating table. Postoperatively, the wrist is immobilized in 40° of extension with the thumb

in abduction and extension for 3–4 weeks. A removable splint is used for an additional 3–4 weeks and there is usually no need for retraining *(Fig. 34.35C,D)*.

Tendon transfers to restore finger extension

Treatment/surgical technique

Restoration of finger extension after trauma can be accomplished by tendon transfers similar to those used for radial nerve palsy. Those transfers were discussed in detail earlier in this chapter and include transfer of either of the wrist flexors (FCU or FCR) to the EDC or the Boyes transfer of the FDS of the middle and ring fingers to the EDC.

Tendon transfers to restore thumb flexion

Treatment/surgical technique

Acute lacerations or ruptures of the flexor pollicis longus (FPL) tendon can be treated by primary or delayed primary repair or tendon grafting. However, with missed diagnosis, the muscle fibers undergo significant shortening, atrophy and fibrosis within 6 months to a year from injury. In these situations it is preferable to restore thumb flexion using a tendon transfer, usually the FDS of the ring finger *(Fig. 34.36)*.[100] The ring finger superficialis is harvested through a transverse incision at the base of the proximal phalanx and retrieved through a second incision in the proximal palm. It is then passed through the FPL sheath to the base of the distal phalanx through an open incision or attached to a fine rubber catheter or feeding tube and withdrawn distally through the sheath. The ring finger FDS to FPL tendon transfer can be performed in one or two stages if the bed is scarred with initial placement

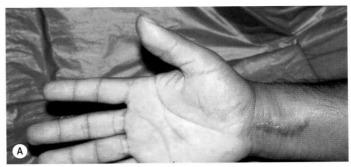

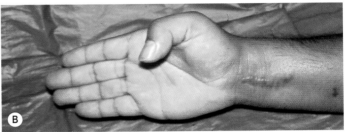

Fig. 34.37 (A) Postoperative extension **(B)** Postoperative flexion.

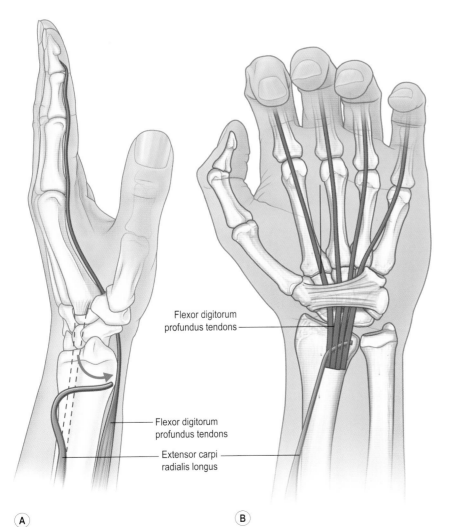

Flexor digitorum profundus tendons

Flexor digitorum profundus tendons

Extensor carpi radialis longus

(A) (B)

Fig. 34.38 Tendon transfer to restore flexion of the fingers. The extensor carpi radialis longus tendon is transected from the base of the index finger metacarpal, transferred subcutaneously around the radial border of the forearm and sutured to the flexor digitorum profundus tendons to the index, middle, ring and small fingers in the distal forearm proximal to the carpal tunnel.

of a silastic tendon rod *(Fig. 34.36).*[100] If necessary, a pulley can be reconstructed using the old FPL tendon remnant or with a palmaris longus graft.[91] The tendon is sutured to the distal phalanx of the thumb using a pullout suture fixed over a button. The tension of the transfer can be checked by wrist tenodesis. With the wrist in full flexion, the thumb should extend completely and with wrist extension the thumb tip should overlie the ring finger MP joint *(Fig. 34.37).*

Tendon transfers to restore finger flexion

Treatment/surgical technique

Occasionally, patients may present with severe crushing or avulsion injuries involving the forearm flexor muscles. The options for secondary reconstruction of finger flexion are either a tendon transfer of the ECRL to all four FDP tendons or a functioning free gracilis muscle transfer. The ECRL is transected at the base of the index finger metacarpal and mobilized through a longitudinal incision on the dorsum of the forearm. It is then tunnelled subcutaneously around the radial border of the forearm to a palmar incision over the distal forearm *(Fig. 34.38).* Great care has to be exercised in adjusting the tension when suturing the ECRL to all four FDP tendons, since the ECRL only has 30 mm amplitude and the

FDP tendons require 70 mm of excursion for full finger flexion. Inserting the transfer too tightly will prevent full finger extension. The wrist tenodesis effect is vitally important in this transfer-wrist extension should cause the fingers to flex down to the palm, whereas wrist flexion should allow the fingers to come out to full extension. If the FPL is also nonfunctioning, thumb flexion can be restored by transferring brachioradialis to FPL through the same palmar incision.

Summary

If carefully selected and performed meticulously, tendon transfers will provide a gratifying functional improvement to the hand affected by radial, median, ulnar or combined nerve palsies as well as severe trauma affecting the extrinsic flexor and extensor muscles and tendons. Quantitative outcome data is lacking for many of the tendon transfers described, but surgeons and patients can attest to the benefits derived from them. Comparative studies must be designed in the future to document the effectiveness of the various transfers and their ultimate impact on hand function and return to work.

Access the complete reference list online at **http://www.expertconsult.com**

2. Brand PW. *Clinical mechanics of the hand.* St Louis: Mosby; 1985.

    This is the definitive reference book detailing the biomechanics of tendon transfers.

14. Boyes JH. Tendon transfers for radial palsy. *Bull Hosp Joint Dis.* 1960;21:97.

    The original description of the Boyes transfer for radial nerve palsy, using the flexor digitorum superficialis tendons from the middle and ring fingers transferred through the interosseous membrane to restore independent index finger and thumb extension.

27. Bunnell S. Opposition of the thumb. *J Bone Joint Surg.* 1938;20:269.

34. Burkhalter W, Christensen RC, Brown P. Extensor indicis proprius opponensplasty. *J Bone Joint Surg Am.* 1973;55:725–732.

    The original description of the Burkhalter transfer to restore thumb opposition in a low median nerve palsy using the extensor indicis proprius tendon.

65. Bunnell S. Surgery of the intrinsic muscles of the hand other than those producing opposition of the thumb. *J Bone Joint Surg.* 1942;24:1.

67. Brand PW. Tendon grafting illustrated by a new operation for intrinsic paralysis of the fingers. *J Bone Joint Surg.* 1961;43B:444–453.

    This paper describes the dorsal route of the extensor carpi radialis brevis tendon extended with free tendon grafts and the palmar route of the extensor carpi radialis longus tendon extended with free tendon grafts to correct the clawing in ulnar nerve palsy due to leprosy.

70. Blacker GJ, Lister GD, Kleinert HE. The abducted little finger in low ulnar nerve palsy. *J Hand Surg Am.* 1976;1:190–196.

72. Smith RJ. Extensor carpi radialis brevis tendon transfer for thumb adduction – a study of power pinch. *J Hand Surg Am.* 1983;8:4–15.

91. Brand PW. Tendon transfers for median and ulnar nerve paralysis. *Orthop Clin North Am.* 1970;1:447–454.

94. Smith RJ. *Tendon transfers of the hand and forearm.* Boston: Little Brown; 1987.

    This classic monograph, unfortunately out of print, is an excellent reference source describing tendon transfers for nerve injuries, trauma, rheumatoid arthritis, congenital anomalies, cerebral palsy and spinal cord injuries.

35

Free-functioning muscle transfer in the upper extremity

Isaac Harvey and Gregory H. Borschel

SYNOPSIS

- Free-functioning muscle transfer involves the transfer of a muscle from a distant location to replace a lost function.
- It is a complex procedure that requires a highly motivated patient.
- The procedure involves microvascular anastomoses and neural coaptation.
- Meticulous attention must be paid to proper positioning and tensioning of the transferred muscle.
- Postoperatively, a highly structured rehabilitation program is required for a prolonged period, often up to 2 years.
- In the appropriate patient, reliably good results can be achieved for patients with otherwise devastating injuries.

 Access the Historical Perspective section online at
http://www.expertconsult.com

Introduction

Key points

- This is a complex procedure for use where no simpler alternative is available.
- Meticulous attention to microsurgical technique is required; thrombosis leads to muscle loss.
- Attention to muscle placement and tensioning is also critical.
- This technique is applicable to restoration of finger, thumb, and wrist flexion and extension, elbow flexion and extension, and shoulder flexion.

Free-functioning muscle transfer involves the microneurovascular transfer of a functioning muscle from its donor site to a recipient site in the upper limb. The aim of the procedure is to restore functionality that has been lost as a result of trauma or disease. It is a complex procedure that was developed for situations where no simpler alternative is available. Most muscles in the body have been assessed for their usefulness for tissue transfer, and many have been identified as expendable and suitable for microvascular transfer. Most of these muscles have a long pedicle of suitably large caliber. The viability of the muscle is maintained by microvascular anastomosis between the muscle's artery and vein and a suitable artery and vein in the recipient area. Neural coaptation of the transferred muscle's motor nerve to a suitable nerve in the recipient area provides the ability of the muscle to contract, giving functionality to the transfer. This functionality is dependent on viability of the muscle and neural regeneration as well as correct technical placement, positioning, and rehabilitative programs. The common indications for free functional muscle transfer include direct trauma with muscle loss, Volkmann's ischemic contracture, nerve injury such as brachial plexus injuries, and oncologic resection.

Free muscle transfers to the upper limb have been used to reconstruct functional deficits in finger flexion, finger extension, thumb abduction, elbow flexion and extension, and shoulder flexion. Key planning issues include: the choice of appropriate muscle for a given function, the choice of an appropriate local nerve to motor the transferred muscle, and/or creation of such a nerve via nerve grafts.

Although function is able to be restored, patients must be counseled to be realistic about their expectations of outcome from this type of surgery.

Basic science/disease process

The basic functional purpose of a muscle is to provide both static tension and functional shortening. To understand its functioning, one must understand the structure of a muscle *(Fig. 35.1)*. A skeletal muscle is composed of parallel muscle cells called myofibers. Each muscle cell is composed of smaller parallel myofibrils. These myofibrils are further subdivided into thin and thick filaments containing actin and myosin.[6]

Within each muscle cell the myofibrils are arranged within functional compartments known as sarcomeres. These sarcomeres are made up of interdigitating fibers of actin and myosin that interact at a subcellular level *(Fig. 35.2)*. When a muscle is stimulated to contract, the actin and myosin fibers move over one another by the flexing action of myosin cross-bridges.[7]

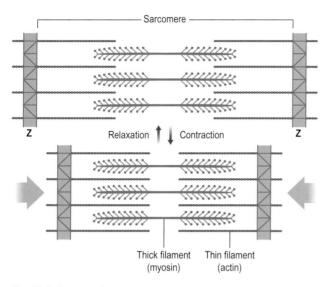

Fig. 35.1 Structure of muscle.

The amount of overlap of the actin and myosin fibers determines the number of side chains that are in contact and therefore able to contribute to force generation. When a muscle is overstretched there are fewer side chains in contact. When a muscle is overcontracted the myosin chains crumple and cannot contract further.[8]

This relationship leads to a length–tension relationship that provides for maximal force generation when the muscle is at its native physiological length *(Fig. 35.3)*. The total force exerted by a muscle is the sum of the passive force provided by the elastic properties of the muscle fibers and surrounding tissues and the active force produced by the contraction of actin and myosin filaments.[6] The relationship of length to contractile force generation is described by a bell curve with decreasing ability of force generation further from the physiological resting state corresponding with less overlap of the actin and myosin fibers. For this reason, determination of the resting length of the donor muscle is critical prior to transfer, such that this length can be reconstituted after transfer at inset of the muscle and maximal contractile force can be generated.[8]

There are many morphological types of muscle in the body. They can be divided into two major types, strap muscles and pennate muscles, or a combination of the two *(Fig. 35.4)*. In a strap muscle the muscle fibers are arranged in parallel to the long axis of the muscle. This is important from a functional standpoint, as the excursion of a strap muscle is directly proportional to its length. It has been demonstrated that at maximal contraction a strap muscle can contract up to 65% of its resting length.[6] In a pennate muscle, the muscle fibers are

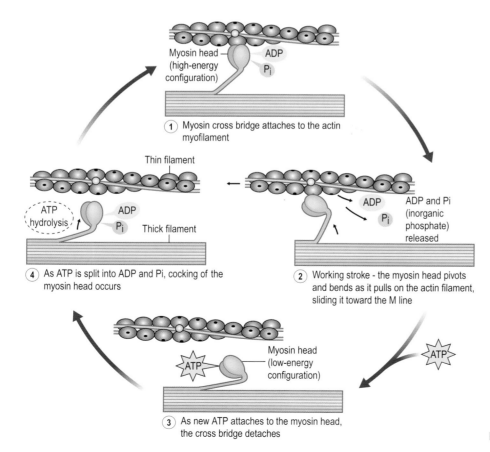

Fig. 35.2 Myosin cross-bridges in action.

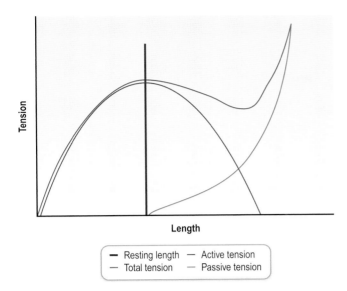

Fig. 35.3 The length–tension relationship.

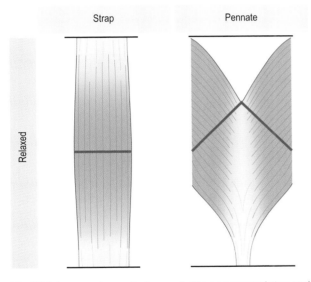

Fig. 35.5 In a pennate muscle the muscle fibers are arranged at an angle to a central tendon.

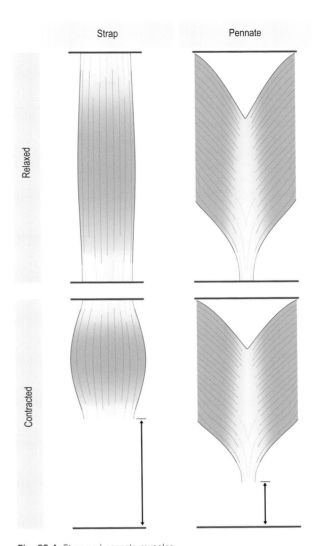

Fig. 35.4 Strap and pennate muscles.

arranged at an angle to a central tendon (*Fig. 35.5*). As a result, the individual fibers in a pennate muscle usually do not run the entire length of the muscle. The excursion achieved by a pennate muscle is proportional to the length of the muscle fibers, not the length of the entire muscle. As such a pennate muscle will usually yield lesser excursion than a strap muscle.[8]

The pennation angle, or angle of pull of the muscle in relation to the tendon, affects both force generation and excursion. Muscles with a lesser pennation angle (a straighter angle between the fibers and the tendon) produce a greater excursion with contraction but less power than those with a greater pennation angle.

The force generated by a muscle is proportional to its total cross-sectional area. Whether this is due to a greater number of muscle fibers or hypertrophy of a smaller number of fibers, the maximal force generation has been calculated in mammals to be approximately $4 \, \text{kg}/\text{cm}^2$.[6] The cross-sectional area is calculated perpendicular to the direction of the muscle fibers. In a strap muscle this is perpendicular to the muscle as a whole and perpendicular to the tendon. In a pennate muscle this is perpendicular to the fibers and oblique to the tendon and muscle as a whole, resulting in a greater cross-sectional area and thus a greater potential for force generation.

The contraction of an individual muscle fiber is an all-or-none phenomenon: when a weak contraction is required, only a few fibers within the muscle are stimulated to contract.[7] When a forceful contraction is required a greater number of muscle fibers are stimulated to contract. Each muscle is innervated by a motor nerve. The motor nerve joins the muscle via its motor endplates at the neuromuscular junction. A given nerve fiber within the nerve will have a defined number of motor endplates, each of these innervating specific fibers within the muscle. A muscle is thus composed of functional motor units, multiple muscle fibers innervated by the same nerve fiber. Depending on the muscle this may be as few as five muscle fibers such as in the extraocular muscles, or as many as several hundred, as is the case with most major skeletal muscles. This relationship is important in relation to

Table 35.1 **Principles of tendon transfer applicable to free-functioning muscle transfer**

- An elective tendon/muscle transfer should never be performed in the presence of unhealed wounds
- Full passive joint motion must be restored before tendon/muscle transfer
- The transfer should not pass through areas of scar tissue or under skin grafts. Furthermore, surgical incisions should not be placed directly over the transfer
- Whenever possible, cutaneous sensibility should be restored before tendon/muscle transfer
- The normal function of the transferred muscle must be expendable
- Synergism between the muscle's original and new actions facilitates rehabilitation (in the case of free muscle transfer this principle could be applied to the function of the donor motor nerve)
- The transferred muscle must have sufficient amplitude and power to perform its new function; thus, reinnervated muscles should be used only in exceptional circumstances

(Adapted from Anastakis D, Manktelow R. Free functioning muscle transfers. In: Green's operative hand surgery, 5th edn. Philadelphia: Elsevier, 2005.)

reinnervation and the number of axons provided by a given donor motor nerve. A muscle with smaller muscle units may provide finer control but less power for a given number of axons, and vice versa – a muscle with larger motor units requires fewer axons for greater force generation.

Individual muscles considered for transfer have been assessed with regard to their internal architecture, vascular anatomy, motor innervation, and characteristics relevant to desired function. Ideally the transferred muscle should have a single dominant vascular pedicle (Mathes and Nahai type 1)[9] of sufficient length to allow easy anastomosis after transfer without the need for vein grafts. The muscle should possess a single motor nerve of sufficient length and in the correct orientation to allow for primary coaptation of the nerve to the donor motor nerve. The muscle and the limb into which it is to be transferred should possess the appropriate characteristics to allow the muscle to perform its desired function *(Table 35.1)*. These characteristics have been well described for tendon transfers in the upper limb, but apply equally to free functional muscle transfer.

Diagnosis/patient presentation

Free functional muscle transfer is applicable to patients who have sustained a major loss of skeletal muscle in the upper limb resulting in a significant functional disability. Free functional muscle transfer is indicated to replace lost function where no easier local option is available. This may be seen following direct trauma, in the setting of Volkmann's ischemic contracture *(Fig. 35.6)*, following tumor ablation such as sarcoma resection, and in long-standing nerve injury such as brachial plexus lesions. Other rarer indications include electrical burns and post gas gangrene and postreplant patients.[10]

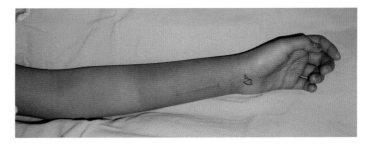

Fig. 35.6 Appearance of arm with Volkmann's ischemic contracture.

Each of these indications presents its own special set of considerations.

Of particular note, in the setting of brachial plexus reconstruction, local donor nerves to power the muscle transfer may be limited or completely unavailable. In this case, careful consideration must be given to the choice of donor motor nerve. In some cases, it is necessary to perform nerve grafts as a preliminary procedure to bring viable motor axons into the denervated limb.[11,12] A similar picture can be found in the setting of Volkmann's ischemic contracture; however here the anterior interosseous nerve of the forearm is often spared and can be available as a motor donor nerve.[13] This will be discussed further later in the chapter in the section on choice of donor motor nerve.

Patient selection

Probably the most important decision to be made is whether to proceed with free muscle transfer at all. This is a highly involved surgical procedure that requires a motivated patient who is aware of the potential of the procedure and who is fully equipped and prepared to undertake the oftentimes intensive pre- and postoperative rehabilitation that is required for a successful outcome. The patient must understand that the maximal outcome of the procedure will not be realized inside 1–2 years.[14] The importance of having a cooperative patient cannot be overemphasized. The ideal patient is stable, intelligent, and motivated to regain function and return to work, with no medical comorbidities. Inappropriate candidates are unfortunately common among patients with injuries who might otherwise benefit from this procedure. Head injuries may often accompany brachial plexus injuries in motor vehicle and motorcycle accidents.

Multiple physical factors must be taken into account prior to muscle transfer. The patient must have stable skeletal structure, including functional joints. He or she must have normal or near normal range of motion in the hand, wrist, and elbow. There must be adequate soft-tissue cover over the planned tendon-gliding site. If there is insufficient unscarred soft tissue to cover the planned site, soft-tissue reconstruction in the form of tissue expansion or local flaps may need to be performed prior to muscle transfer. Sensation in the hand should be normal to achieve optimal results, though this is not an absolute requirement.[10] There must be sufficient evidence that there are suitable recipient artery and veins in the arm to vascularize the transferred muscle. Preoperative Doppler ultrasound or angiography can be very helpful in this regard.[8] Also a suitable donor nerve must be available to power the transferred muscle. There should be adequate antagonist function in the arm to allow the transfer to be of use, for example in performing a transfer to replace long finger flexor function and restore grip, there must be adequate finger extensor function to oppose the new action of the transferred muscle and to release the grip *(Table 35.2)*.

Multiple muscles have been used for free transfer in the upper limb. The gracilis muscle *(Fig. 35.6)* has been the most widely used as it fulfills many of the criteria for the "ideal" muscle transfer.[15,16] Other transfers have included latissimus dorsi,[17,18] rectus femoris,[19,20] serratus anterior,[21–32] gastrocnemius,[24] hemisoleus,[25] flexor hallucis longus,[26] flexor carpi ulnaris,[27] pectoralis major,[28,29] pectoralis minor,[22] and tensor fascia latae.[23]

The principles governing the choice of muscle for free functional transfer are similar to those that have been well described for tendon transfer. Additionally the muscle ideally will have a singular dominant vascular pedicle and a single motor nerve available for transfer.

Table 35.2 **Requirements for free functional muscle transfer**

- Available, undamaged motor nerve, artery, and vein at the site of muscle transplantation
- Adequate skin coverage for the distal half of the muscle
- Supple joints and gliding tendons
- Good hand sensibility and intrinsic function
- Adequate antagonist muscle function
- Good patient motivation
- No simpler solution for the patient's problem

(Adapted from Anastakis D, Manktelow R. Free functioning muscle transfers. In: Green's operative hand surgery, 5th edn. Philadelphia: Elsevier, 2005.)

Treatment/surgical technique

Selecting the appropriate muscle for transplantation is key to the success of the procedure. The ideal muscle to transfer will vary depending on which function it is intended to replace. Important considerations are the length, excursion, and power that are required for the given deficit, e.g., finger flexors normally have an excursion of ~7 cm and finger extensors ~5 cm. A transplanted muscle must be able to generate a sufficient force over the appropriate range of motion to be of functional value. The muscle must be expendable from its donor site with minimal functional deficit from its harvest. The muscle ideally should be easy to harvest, and should have a singular dominant vascular pedicle for ease and reliability of microvascular transfer. Ideally, the muscle should have a single easily identifiable motor nerve. Additionally a strong tendon allows for ease of inset with reduced chance of dehiscence of the muscle insertion. Muscle fibers of uniform length make the procedure technically much easier.

Multiple muscles have been used as functional transfers in the upper limb. For most applications in the upper limb, the gracilis muscle comes closest to satisfying the above criteria.[8,10] It is a fusiform muscle with longitudinally arranged fibers in the proximal portion. It has a single vascular pedicle easily accessible in the upper thigh with a single motor branch from the obturator nerve. Its functional range of motion can be up to 12–16 cm. The donor scar from the gracilis harvest on the inner thigh often widens but is placed in a relatively inconspicuous location for most patients. An additional advantage of the gracilis muscle is that the nerve is often arranged in 2–3 motor fascicles,[8,10] which stimulate discrete portions of the muscle. As such it is possible to use the muscle split into two components for dual functionality with separate motor innervations.[30,31]

The gracilis muscle is a long slender strap-like muscle in the adductor compartment of the thigh *(Fig. 35.7)*. It is the

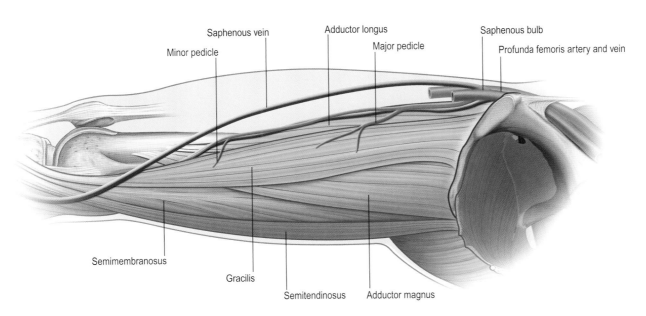

Fig. 35.7 The gracilis muscle.

most superficial of the adductor muscles. It is thickest in its proximal portions and narrows to a tendon in its distal quarter. The gracilis originates from the body and inferior ramus of the pubis. Distally it narrows into a tendon which passes behind the femoral condyle and inserts on the medial aspect of the tibia adjacent to the tibial tuberosity. McKee *et al.*[31] studied the muscle fiber anatomy of the gracilis in fresh and preserved cadavers. They described the muscle as fusiform with fibers of varying length. The shorter posterior fibers were found to insert more proximally into the gracilis tendon, whereas the longer more anterior fibers insert more distally. They also found that the fibers were parallel in the proximal three-fifths, whereas distally the fibers converge on to the tendon. The average fiber length within the gracilis muscle is 24 cm. The action of the gracilis is as a weak adductor of the leg and weak flexor of the knee joint. It also produces slight medial rotation of the tibia on the femur. Several authors have reported on harvest of the gracilis, finding that it does not result in a significant functional deficit.

The gracilis muscle may be harvested by a second team concurrent with preparation of the arm. The two-team approach significantly reduces operative time. For gracilis harvest the markings are made along a line from the posterior aspect of the medial femoral condyle to the pubic tubercle. This line approximates the position of the adductor longus muscle. The gracilis muscle is found 2–4 cm posterior to the palpable margin of the adductor longus. An incision is planned in the upper thigh 2 cm behind the previously marked line. The patient is draped with the entire leg exposed and free-draped in the abducted and externally rotated position *(Fig. 35.8)*. This allows movement of the limb intraoperatively.

An incision 8–10 cm long is made in the junction of the upper and middle third of the thigh. The gracilis muscle is identified beneath the deep fascia. For the inexperienced operator, it can be useful to extend the knee to aid with identification of the gracilis muscle. The gracilis becomes taut on knee extension; the tension of the other adductors is unaffected. The fascia overlying the gracilis muscle is split longitudinally. This layer is preserved for later repair to prevent muscular herniation, a not uncommon problem if this layer is not repaired. The muscle is dissected proximally and distally. The

vascular pedicle is found approximately 10–12 cm inferior to the pubis in adults and proportionately the same distance in children (approximately 25% of the length of the thigh), usually entering the muscle from the posterior medial surface. The pedicle courses deep to the adductor longus muscle, which can be retracted to expose the pedicle. Muscular branches are given off to each of the adductors, which need to be divided. The origin of the pedicle is usually from the profunda femoris artery and it can be traced to here with relative ease in most cases. This usually yields a pedicle length of 6–8 cm. The nerve supply to the gracilis is from a branch of the anterior division of the obturator nerve (L2–3). This can be located taking an oblique course in the plane between adductor longus and magnus and entering the posterior medial surface of the muscle 1–3 cm above the vascular pedicle. This is traced superiorly as far as required to obtain sufficient length for transfer. This may be as much as 10 cm.[14] It is preferable to perform the nerve coaptation as close to the transferred muscle as possible, so a shorter nerve is preferable. A tension-free nerve coaptation is necessary; a single nerve coaptation is always preferable over a nerve graft, so harvest of a longer motor nerve is performed where required. It is necessary to mark the length of the muscle with the leg in full abduction prior to release of either the origin or insertion. 5-0 silk sutures placed at 5-cm intervals will ensure that a correct muscle length–tension relationship is re-established *(Fig. 35.9)*.

If required, it is possible to perform intraneural dissection to identify discrete motor fascicles within the motor nerve that innervate separate portions of the muscle. In 90% of cases it is possible to identify a single fascicle that innervates the anterior 20–50% of the muscle.[8,29,32] Once these functional muscle subunits have been identified, it is possible to separate and inset them individually to the flexor pollicis longus and flexor digitorum profundus (FDP) tendons to recreate independent function of finger and thumb function.[15]

The gracilis is usually harvested as a muscle-only transfer. If it is to be used with a cutaneous paddle, care must be taken in orientation of the skin paddle over the proximal two-thirds of the muscle as the skin paddle becomes unreliable more distally. The operating surgeon must avoid injury to the musculocutaneous perforators, which are almost always located

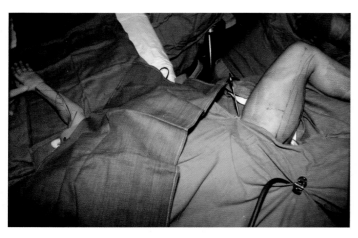

Fig. 35.8 Patient draped for simultaneous gracilis harvest and forearm dissection.

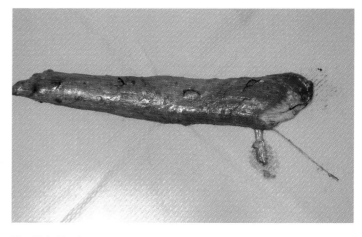

Fig. 35.9 Marking the length of the gracilis muscle with sutures placed 5 cm apart.

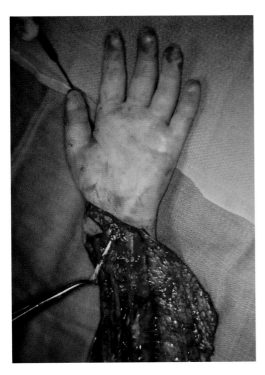

Fig. 35.10 Incisions planned to avoid the gliding path of tendons.

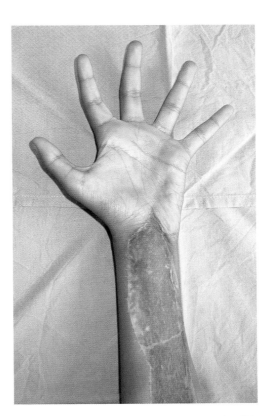

Fig. 35.11 Transferred muscle skin grafted where insufficient coverage is available from local tissue (graft ideally would not be required for distal portions of the muscle).

directly over the dominant muscular pedicle. It is useful once the skin paddle has been incised to suture the skin edge to the gracilis fascia to prevent shearing of the musculocutaneous pedicle.

Preparation of the arm is an integral part of the procedure. Prior to embarking on a muscle transfer the surgeon should be satisfied that there is available a suitable vascular pedicle with which to vascularize the transferred muscle. Assessment of the vascularity of the limb should be performed clinically prior to any operation. In equivocal cases, imaging of the vascular system can be of assistance. A preoperative Doppler ultrasound examination or angiogram can be used.[15] However the final decision to proceed with muscle transfer should be made intraoperatively once a suitable vascular pedicle and donor motor nerve have been identified. The choice of motor nerve is discussed further in the section on choice of donor motor nerve, below.

Incisions should be planned such that they do not cross the path of gliding tendons *(Fig. 35.10)*. Wound closure can often be a problem. In adding the bulk of a transferred muscle and with intraoperative swelling, it is often not possible to close the arm completely. In this case, skin grafts are required to cover the remaining skin defect *(Fig. 35.11)*. This should be planned for with the incisions, so that any areas that require skin grafting are over the more proximal portions of the transferred muscle that undergo less excursion with contraction.

Choice of donor motor nerve

A nerve must be selected that provides motor axons for reinnervation of the transferred muscle. For replacement of long finger flexor musculature the preferred motor nerves are the anterior interosseous nerve, branches of the median nerve that previously supplied the flexor digitorum superficialis or

branches of the ulnar nerve previously supplying the FDP. For reconstruction of the finger and wrist extensors, branches of the radial nerve are used. For biceps reconstruction, branches of the musculocutaneous nerve are used; for the triceps, branches of the proximal radial nerve are used; and finally, for the deltoid, motor branches of the axillary nerve are selected.

Hints and tips

The anterior interosseous nerve may be found arising from the median nerve 3–6 cm distal to the elbow in adults. It courses through the pronator teres and then passes dorsally toward the interosseous membrane, lying next to the flexor digitorum profundus and flexor pollicis longus.

It is important to ensure that an undamaged motor nerve is available for use. This is usually apparent by clinical examination. When uncertainty exists, a preliminary exploration and biopsy of the nerve ends may be used. The biopsy specimen is sent for neurohistology to confirm the presence of motor axons in the resected nerve end. Once the presence of suitable motor nerve is confirmed, the surgeon may proceed with confidence. In the absence of a suitable motor nerve in the upper limb, e.g., in total brachial plexus avulsions, it is possible to perform nerve grafts as a preliminary procedure to introduce a donor source of motor axons into the upper limb. Once a sufficient period of time has elapsed to allow ingrowth of motor axons and there is evidence of regeneration along the nerve, such as a Tinel's sign at the distal end, the surgeon may then proceed with functional muscle transfer.

Muscle transfer to the flexor aspect of the forearm

Muscle transfers to replace long finger flexion are the most common indication for free muscle transfer in the upper limb. It is commonly required following trauma resulting in direct damage to the muscle or from ischemic necrosis following compartment syndrome. Where the extensor compartment remains undamaged it may be more appropriate to perform a tendon transfer such as extensor carpi radialis longus (ECRL), as this is a less involved procedure with a faster recovery. However evidence suggests that a free gracilis transfer is able to provide greater excursion and range of movement compared with an ECRL transfer.[8,10,29]

The forearm must satisfy all the previously mentioned requirements for transfer. If these are satisfied and suitable vessels and nerve are available, transfer may proceed. The gracilis has proven the most useful muscle for this location. The known location of the neurovascular hilum in the donor muscle is matched to the available recipients in the forearm. The length and orientation of the muscle are planned. Incisions are planned to provide good exposure of neurovascular structures and to provide cover of the musculotendinous junction in the distal forearm. As such it is important that primary skin coverage is provided for the distal half of the muscle transfer. It is possible to harvest the gracilis muscle with a cutaneous pedicle to provide extra skin coverage in the forearm. In the majority of patients this cutaneous paddle is too thick, resulting in suboptimal cosmetic appearance. Many patients later request revision of this skin paddle. Alternatively, the muscle can be transferred as a muscle-only flap and the proximal half can be skin-grafted. This solves the problem of the bulky skin paddle. The skin graft in the proximal half does not interfere with gliding and excursion of the transfer. If it will not be possible to provide coverage of the distal muscle and musculotendinous junction, it will be necessary to perform preliminary procedures to provide this. These procedures may include tissue expansion, or local and distant flaps such as groin or abdominal flaps. Once incisions are planned, dissection begins usually from proximal unscarred tissue to distal injured tissue. In dissecting the neurovascular structures, it is important that meticulous technique is used to avoid inadvertent damage to important structures *(Fig. 35.12)*. The medial epicondyle is exposed in anticipation of suturing the proximal end of the transferred muscle. The FDP tendons are explored and checked for their gliding ability.

Hints and tips

Placing a small bean bag or gel roll under the ipsilateral hip permits greater exposure. A headlight is valuable for visualization. The incision must be carried quite proximally in order to visualize the neurovascular bundle adequately. There are usually two veins surrounding a single artery. A small set of perforating vessels may be seen entering the skin at the same level as the vascular pedicle deep to the muscle. A malleable retractor placed deep (posterior) to the pedicle assists in its dissection.

Once the forearm is dissected the muscle may be transferred. The neurovascular structures are aligned and the nerve positioned to allow nerve coaptation as close to the muscle as possible *(Fig. 35.13)*. While the proximal portion is held to the

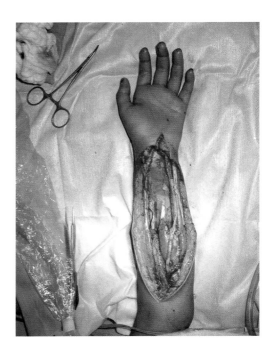

Fig. 35.12 The dissected forearm.

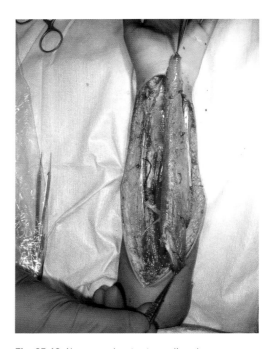

Fig. 35.13 Neurovascular structures aligned.

medial condyle, the distal portion of the muscle is stretched to simulate finger flexion and extension. The neurovascular pedicle is observed during this movement to ensure that no tension will be placed on the repair during finger movement. Tacking sutures are then placed in the muscle to hold it to the forearm and prevent contraction during neurovascular repair. Microvascular repair is then performed under the operating microscope. Once vascular flow is re-established, the muscle is observed for bleeding from cut ends and the re-establishment of a "pink color." The distal portions of the muscle will

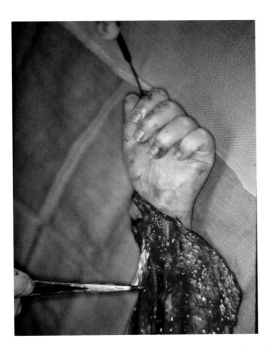

Fig. 35.14 Flexor tendons sutured to provide mass flexion effect.

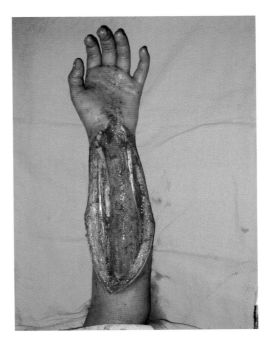

Fig. 35.15 Muscle *in situ* with recreation of original resting tension.

typically take some minutes to regain their color. Any area that fails to appear adequately revascularized can be excised. This does not present a problem as the tendon of the gracilis extends intramuscularly for some way and the cut ends of resected muscle fibers can be rejoined to the intramuscular portion of the tendon without affecting function. The neural repair is performed as a fascicular repair using 10-0 or 11-0 suture, as the nerve to gracilis contains approximately 60% fatty connective tissue. This ensures proper alignment of the fascicles.

When a single muscle is to be used to provide flexion to all of the fingers, they should be positioned such that they flex together, giving simultaneous contact with the object being gripped. A side-to-side tenodesis of the FDP tendons is performed distally in this position with each finger slightly more flexed than the previous. This provides a balanced mass flexion effect of all the fingers together *(Fig. 35.14)*. Where FDP is to be included with a single muscle function, it should be positioned such that the thumb closes slightly later than the fingers. This results in a useful pinch grip for the patient. Alternately the muscle may be separated into its functional components to provide separate finger and thumb flexion.

Hints and tips

Most side-to-side tenodeses between adjacent distal tendons can be readily performed with mattressed 3-0 or 4-0 polyester sutures. A tendon weaver is not generally needed.

The muscle is inserted into the FDP tendons in such a way as to recreate its optimal functional length and excursion. Prior to transfer, the gracilis is placed on maximal physiological stretch by placing the thigh in maximal abduction. Sutures are then placed in the muscle every 5 cm. Once the muscle is

transferred, the origin is fixed to the common flexor origin from the medial epicondyle. The wrist and fingers are then placed in maximal extension. The gracilis is then stretched distally to recreate the 5-cm distance between marking sutures *(Fig. 35.15)*. The intersection of the FDP and gracilis muscle and tendons is then marked. The hand is then relaxed and a tendon weave is performed under no tension at the pre-marked site. This technique ensures that, once the procedure is completed, the transfer will allow a full range of finger and wrist extension and will allow finger flexion within the maximal force-generating range of the muscle. The principles of this technique are applicable to muscle transfers in all locations.

The limb is rested with the wrist and fingers slightly flexed so as to relieve any tension on the musculotendinous junction. Postoperatively at the 3-week mark, a program of passive mobilization and stretching is instituted. This helps prevent any myoclonic contracture and promotes gliding at the musculotendinous junction. Once the muscle regains innervation it is very important to institute an active mobilization program. Once a functional range of motion is regained, a graduated weight-training program can be instituted to improve strength. This should be pursued for at least 1 year following regaining a useful range of motion. This should be incorporated into the patient's work and activities of daily living to maintain patient interest and participation.

In the correct patient good flexion *(Fig. 35.16)* can be expected including, where planned, independent finger and thumb flexion *(Fig. 35.17)*.

Muscle transfer for finger extension

Muscle transfer for finger extension follows the same basic pattern as for finger flexion, though a marginally lesser degree of excursion is required. The gracilis muscle has also been

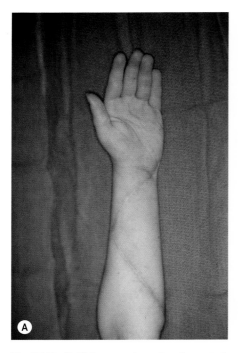 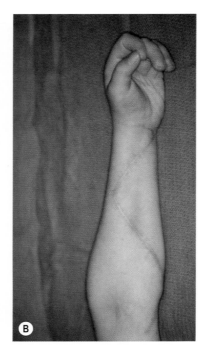 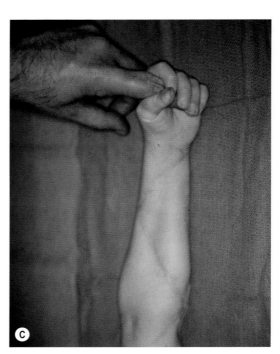

Fig. 35.16 (A–C) Postoperative patient demonstrating good finger flexion.

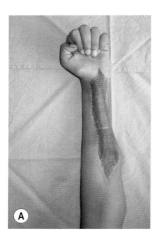 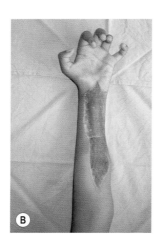 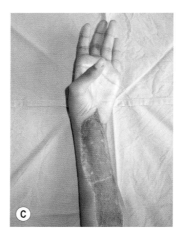 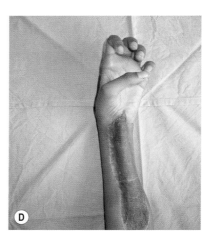

Fig. 35.17 (A–D) Postoperative patient demonstrating independent finger and thumb flexion after separation of gracilis into independent functional units.

used most widely for this application. The choice of motor nerve for reinnervation is crucial. The posterior interosseous nerve has been used most commonly. The most appropriate site for identification and use of the nerve is as it emerges from supinator. At this point it is possible to identify the branches innervating finger, thumb, and wrist extensors. The ideal branches to use are those to the finger extensors; wrist extensor branches are less ideal. Identification of the nerve at this level is particularly useful if there are remnants of extensor motor function. In this case the nerve branches can be individually stimulated to select the appropriate branch or branches. The arterial anastomosis may be to any available artery. The posterior interosseous artery has been used,

though this may be scarred or insufficient. In this case the radial artery has been used in an end-to-side fashion, or the radial recurrent artery may be used. Similar attention as with the flexor reconstruction must be paid to achieving an appropriate physiological length. The distal extensors are joined together with a side-to-side tenodesis with the fingers in a normal cascade. After proximal fixation of the muscle and establishment of vascularity, the wrist and fingers are maximally flexed. The muscle is stretched to recreate the 5-cm distance between marking sutures. The distal insertion is marked after attachment of the muscle has been performed. This allows fixation of the muscle at its maximal physiological length. Postoperatively, the wrist is splinted in neutral with the digits in the safe position. This relieves tension on the muscle during the initial healing period. A mobilization program similar to that used with flexor reconstructions is initiated.

Muscle transfers for elbow flexion (biceps reconstruction)

The loss of elbow flexion can be a devastating injury. Fortunately both the biceps and brachialis can accomplish this function in the absence of the other. Loss of both these muscles is rare. Loss of innervation of these muscles is, however, much more common in the setting of brachial plexus injuries. Many authors have reported on the use of free functional muscle for reconstruction of elbow flexion in this setting.[14,16] The principles are the same as for the previously described transfers. The acromion and bicipital aponeurosis are exposed for attachment of the transferred muscle. End-to-side vascular anastomosis to the brachial artery is performed and, if available, the musculocutaneous nerve is used for neural coaptation. The choice of nerve in brachial plexus cases may be more difficult and is based on preoperative examination and intraoperative findings. In this case, donor nerves can be intercostal nerves (ideally three nerves), motor fascicles of the ulnar or median nerves, or occasionally the spinal accessory or thoracodorsal nerve. Similar attention to length and tension of inset must be paid as previously described.

Transfers have been described for elbow extension, shoulder flexion, and thumb opposition, in which similar principles are applied.

Complications

Complications can be divided into early or late. As the procedure is long and complicated, care must be taken during the intraoperative period to protect the patient with particular attention to care of pressure areas and appropriate use of thromboprophylaxis. The most feared early complication is vascular insufficiency of the transferred muscle. After a period of 4–5 hours sufficient ischemic damage is sustained by the muscle as to make salvage impossible. In this circumstance, a new free muscle transfer is required. Though not a common complication, this is unfortunately more common than

detecting the vascular compromise in time to salvage the muscle. Vascular insufficiency may be due to thrombosis or technical problems with the anastomosis such as kinking or external pressure. Infection is also a risk as the procedure is often performed through a heavily scarred bed and involves open wounds for a prolonged period. The routine use of pre- and intraoperative antibiotics is necessary. Delayed wound healing is a not uncommon complication but should not delay a rehabilitative program.

Late complications include inadequate power and adhesions. Insufficient power can be due to insufficient motor reinnervation either from an insufficient nerve or problems with the neural coaptation. In the setting of adhesions a tenolysis may be required to allow improved function. If this is to be done, it is wise to wait for complete reinnervation of the muscle so that an aggressive postoperative mobilization program can be instituted. Wrist flexion contractures have been noted as a late complication after transfers for finger flexion. As the transferred muscle regains power, it may overpower the extensors, resulting in a flexion deformity. This can be overcome by early splinting programs but, even with appropriate treatment, further serial casting or surgical procedures may be required.

Secondary procedures

Unfortunately, some patients will not regain function following transfer. This can be due to technical problems, loss of the muscle due to ischemia, failure to reinnervate the muscle, tendinous adhesions, or co-contraction of antagonist muscles. In each case, a reason must be sought individually to explain the poor outcome. In the case of tendinous adhesions, a simple tenolysis may be sufficient. Inadequate or excessive tension on the muscle may result in a functioning muscle with incomplete or weak range of motion. In these cases, it may be possible to reposition the musculotendinous junction, or to perform repositioning of the muscular origin from the common flexor origin. These are both difficult procedures and are best addressed by attaining the correct tension at the primary procedure. In the case of muscle loss or failure of reinnervation, where a reason for the failure can be addressed, it is reasonable to perform a second free-functioning transfer with the expectation of a good functional result.

Access the complete references list online at **http://www.expertconsult.com**

2. Tamai S, Komatsu S, Sakamoto A, et al. Free-muscle transplants in dogs with microsurgical neurovascular anastomoses. *Plast Reconstr Surg*. 1970;46:219–225.
   This paper represents the pioneering work on free functional muscle transplantation. Rectus femoris muscles were microvascularly transplanted and analyzed with light and electron microscopy and electromyography. The authors demonstrated viable muscles with normal thresholds for stimulation by 3 months postoperatively.

5. Harii K, Ohmori K, Torii S. Free gracilis muscle transplantation with microneurovascular anastomoses

   for the treatment of facial paralysis. *Plast Reconstr Surg*. 1976;57:133–143.
   This is the original description of gracilis transfer as applied to facial nerve palsy, and includes the authors' technique and two case reports.

15. Zuker RM, Manktelow RT. Functioning free muscle transfers. *Hand Clin*. 2007;23:57e72.
    This is an excellent review of the current status of functioning muscle transfer from a highly respected unit covering both their adult and pediatric experience.

29. Manktelow RT, Zuker RM. Muscle transplantation by fascicular territory. *Plast Reconstr Surg.* 1984;73:751–755.
The authors describe the fascicular functional anatomy of the gracilis muscle and the ability to separate the functioning muscle into its component parts. A single case report is presented.

31. McKee NH, Fish JS, Manktelow RT, et al. Gracilis muscle anatomy as related to function of a free functioning muscle transplant. *Clin Anat.* 1990;30: 87–92.
This is an excellent description of the anatomy of the gracilis muscle in relation to its use as a functional transplant.

36

Brachial plexus injuries: Adult and pediatric

David Chwei-Chin Chuang

SYNOPSIS

■ Complexity of brachial plexus injury (BPI): BPI is characterized by many complex problems and remains a dilemma to many reconstructive microsurgeons. These complexities include: (1) diverse injury patterns; (2) disrupted anatomy; (3) unpredictable nerve degeneration and regeneration; (4) difficult physical examination and diagnosis; (5) challenging nerve surgery; (6) long rehabilitation; (7) different palliative surgeries for sequelae deformity; (8) no consensus of outcome evaluation; and (9) difficult pain management. Many reconstructive microsurgeons show great interest but are greatly frustrated by this field.

■ Differences between adult and pediatric BPI: BPI can occur in adults and children. Although the anatomy is the same, there are many differences, including mechanism of injury, type and degree of injury, preoperative evaluation and diagnosis, surgical options, postoperative management and rehabilitation, palliative surgery for sequelae deformities, outcomes evaluation, and pain management *(Table 36.1)*. Therefore, these two different entities will be discussed separately.

Introduction

- Brachial plexus injury has many complex problems, such as complicated anatomy and pathophysiology
- To avoid confusion, the site of brachial plexus injury is described in term of level, from 1 to 4
- Timing of nerve exploration is dependent upon the degree of nerve injury

Complexity of anatomy

Gross anatomy

The brachial plexus is formed by the anterior primary rami of the lower cervical (C5–8) and the first thoracic (T1) spinal nerves, which give motor innervation to muscles of the shoulder, including all anterior and posterior chest muscles related to glenohumeral joint movement, muscles of the entire upper limb, and sensory innervation of the entire upper limb, except the skin on some part of the medial aspect of the upper arm. In the "prefixed brachial plexus" C4 provides a significant contribution to C5, but T2 does not contribute. In the "postfixed brachial plexus" T2 has significant contributions to T1, but C4 does not. Clinically, the prefixed type is more common than the postfixed. A postfixed plexus in adult BPI has been rarely seen, probably because the injuries are either so extensive that further dissection of C8–T1 is hazadous and unnecessary, or the injuries are diagnosed not to involve C8–T1 so that further identification is also unnecessary.

Each spinal nerve is formed by the joining of the ventral root (motor fibers) and the dorsal root (sensory fibers). Each root is formed by a number of rootlets. The dorsal roots carry sensory information to the central nervous system, while the ventral roots convey motor fibers to the muscles. The cell bodies (neurons) of the motor fibers are located in the anterior horn of the spinal cord, while the cell bodies of the sensory fibers reside in the dorsal root ganglion located within the intervertebral foramen, immediately outside the dura mater of the spinal cord. The dorsal and ventral roots unite a few millimeters distal from the ganglion to form a spinal nerve, a mixed nerve, which goes through the interscalene space between the scalene anterior and middle muscles. Just out of the scalene muscles the five postganglionic spinal nerves make a first union to form the three trunks: upper (formed by C5 and C6), middle (C7 itself), and lower trunk (formed by C8 and T1 spinal nerves). Each trunk divides into anterior and posterior divisions just proximal to or directly under the clavicle. The nerves exchange fibers and form the second union, just distal to the clavicle, and are termed "cords." Lateral and medial cords are anterior compartment nerves, passing anterior to the subclavian artery. The posterior cord is a posterior compartment nerve, passing posterior to the subclavian artery. The cords anterior to the subscapularis muscle run further distally behind the pectoralis minor muscle. Each cord has two or more terminal branches to the periphery *(Fig. 36.1)*.

Table 36.1 Differences between adult and pediatric brachial plexus injury

Terminology	Adult brachial plexus injury	Obstetric brachial plexus palsy
Etiology	Trauma (more closed injuries than open) Traction injury, mostly by motorcycle accident	All are closed injuries Traction injury following delivery
Demography	All ages	All are infants and children
Physical examination	Complex (see text)	Difficult but simple (see text)
Horner's syndrome	Reliable and persistent	Not reliable, not persistent
Spontaneous recovery by aberrant regeneration	Less	Many
Intraoperative findings	Level 1–4 injury Most are level 1 lesion	In operated cases, global > Erb's palsy In nonoperated cases, Erb > global palsy All are supraclavicular injury Rarely associated with vascular damage Rupture injury, the gap is short (2–4 cm) (making the nerve regeneration by itself possible) Platysma, very thin or scarce
Surgical techniques	Nerve transfer ≥ nerve graft	Nerve graft ≥ nerve transfer
Postoperative immobilization	3 weeks	4 weeks
Rehabilitation	Good	Poor cooperation
Prognosis Nerve grafts in level 2 rupture injury, time to achieve elbow flexion >M3 C8 and T1 root injury C5 stump in four-root injury(C6–T1) Phrenic nerve transfer Intercostal nerve transfer Contralateral C7 transfer Oberlin transfer Intrinsic recovery following repair	Depending Usually takes 1 year All or none More healthy Quite strong and very often Fair results Often Often Never	High incidence of aberrant regeneration Usually takes 2 years Usually incomplete (especially T1) More impaired Risk for severe respiratory distress Usually good results Rarely applied Rarely applied Often

Disputed anatomy

Various classifications of the level of BPI have been proposed: two levels of injury described by Leffert[1] and Krakauer and Wood[2]; three levels by Terzis et al.[3]; four levels by Millesi,[4] Alnot,[5] and Chuang[6]; five levels by Narakas[7]; six levels by Mackinnon and Dellon[8]; and eight levels by Boome[9] (Table 36.2). These numerous classifications have made the understanding of the anatomy of the brachial plexus complex and confusing. The most confusing aspect is the so-called postganglionic root (Fig. 36.2). Some anatomists term the part in the interscalene space before formation of the trunks to be "roots."[10] However, some call this part "spinal nerve."[11] In fact, after the dorsal root ganglion, both ventral and dorsal roots continue for only a few millimeters (<5 mm) in distance and unite to become a mixed nerve where it is no longer a root (Fig. 36.2). Sunderland[11] has stated that "the term nerve root should be reserved for the paired anterior and posterior nerve roots in the spinal canal," and that "the part of the plexus extending from the union of nerve roots to the formation of the trunks of the plexus should be referred to as a spinal nerve." The author accepts this statement. Therefore,

the components of the brachial plexus are roots, spinal nerves, trunks, divisions, cords, and terminal branches.

Numerous anatomical variations of the brachial plexus do exist[1,5] and should be always kept in mind. For example, the musculocutaneous nerve may sometimes arise from the median nerve and not from the lateral cord. In some rare cases of C5–6 root avulsion, the musculocutaneous nerve is still found to be functional because part of the musculocutaneous nerve derives from the median with its origins from C7.

Microanatomy

The microanatomy or internal topography of the brachial plexus has been extensively studied and described.[12,13] The monofascicular pattern is usually found in regions of: (1) the spinal nerves; (2) anterior and posterior divisions of the upper trunk; and (3) the origin of the suprascapular and musculocutaneous nerve. Marked changes in fascicular topography occur every 10 mm. It is especially true at the level of the upper trunk where interfascicular crossovers are so extensive that direct repair or repair with short nerve grafts will frequently lead to co-contractions due to aberrant regeneration of a group of muscles. This aberrant regeneration is mainly found in obstetrical brachial plexus palsy (OBPP) patients but rarely in adult BPI. In addition, plexus connective tissue is more abundant than neural tissue. All these factors are reasons why the results of brachial plexus nerve surgery are so unpredictable. Knowledge of the internal topography of the plexus can be helpful in connecting corresponding nerve fibers with bridging nerve grafts. However, localization within the spinal nerve to define specific axonal groups to supply specific muscles or specific branches is difficult and not practical.

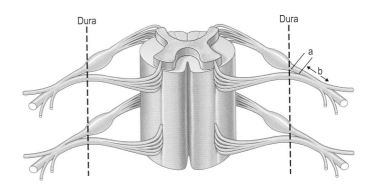

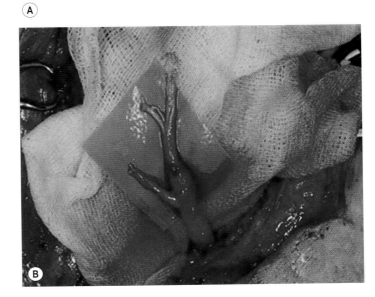

Fig. 36.2 **(A)** The drawing shows that the postganglionic root is part a; postganglionic spinal nerve is part b from the anatomy point of view; **(B)** an avulsion C7 (distal stump) during dissection.

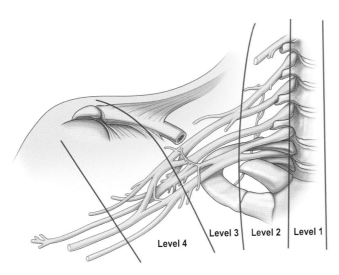

Level 1 Preganglionic root injury
Level 2 Postganglionic spinal nerve injury
Level 3 Pre- and retroclavicular injury (trunks and divisions injury)
Level 4 Infraclavicular injury (cords and terminal branches injury)

Fig. 36.1 Anatomy and numbered level of brachial plexus injury.

Table 36.2 **Classifications for level of brachial plexus injury**

Authors	Levels	Area of injury
Leffert[1]	2 levels	Supraclavicular injury (supraganglionic, infraganglionic, and sub- or retroclavicular) and infraclavicular injury
Krakauer and Wood[2]	2 levels	Supraclavicular (roots, trunks and divisions), infraclavicular (cords and branches)
Terzis et al.[3]	3 levels	Root, supraclavicular postganglionic, infraclavicular
Millesi[4]	4 levels	Supraganglionic root, infraganglionic root, trunk, and cord
Alnot[5]	4 levels	Preganglionic root, postganglionic root, supra- and retroclavicular, and infraclavicular
Chuang[6]	4 levels	Preganglionic root, postganglionic spinal nerve, pre- and retroclavicular, and infraclavicular
Narakas[7]	5 levels	Supraganglionic root, infraganglionic spinal nerve, infraganglionic trunk, retroclavicular and terminal branches
Mackinnon and Dellon[8]	6 levels	Root avulsion (preganglionic and postganglionic), trunk injury, lateral cord, posterior cord, medial cord, terminal cord branch injury
Boome[9]	8 levels	C5–6, C5–7, C5–7 posterior division, C8–T1, C5, C6, lateral and medial cord, posterior cord

Anatomy with level of injury

To avoid anatomical confusion, we have described brachial plexus lesions in terms of the level of injury 1–4 *(Fig. 36.1)*. A total of 819 cases of adult BPI were included (1986–2003) in this new classification[14] and the incidence at different levels was determined:

- Level 1 injury: inside the (vertebral) bone (preganglionic root) injury, including spinal cord, rootlet, and root injury – 70% (574 cases)
- Level 2 injury: inside the (scalene) muscle (postganglionic spinal nerve) injury, located at the interscalene space proximal to the suprascapular nerve – 8% (65 cases)
- Level 3 injury: pre- and retroclavicular injury, including trunks and divisions – 5% (45 cases)
- Level 4 injury: infraclavicular injury, including cords and terminal branch injury proximal to the axillary fossa – 17% (135 cases).

There are some relationships among the levels of injury:

1. An extended-level injury on the same nerve is frequently observed: for instance, C7 injury from the root level down to the interscalene space (level 1 and 2 injury).

2. A combined-level injury on different nerves is common: for instance, C5 and C6 spinal nerve rupture injury (level 2) accompanied with C7–T1 root avulsion (level 1).

3. A skip-level injury is rare: for instance, a longitudinal skip-level injury in which C5 and C7 are injured (avulsion or rupture) but C6 is intact; a horizontal skip-level injury in which level 1 and level 3 are injured, but level 2 is grossly intact.

4. Level 4 injuries are usually isolated, located infraclavicularly, and rarely show upward extension.

5. The term "supraclavicular BPI" will cover a large zone of injury, including level 1, 2, or 3 lesions.

There are two types of characteristic lesions seen in BPI: avulsion and rupture *(Fig. 36.3)*. Both are traction injuries but with different characteristics. Avulsion refers to the nerve being torn from its attachment (proximal avulsion occurs at the spinal cord, distal avulsion at the muscle). Rupture is a nerve injury involving a traction force on an incompletely divided nerve, causing a complete division with irregular proximal and distal ends *(Fig. 36.3C)*. In avulsion injury, only one disrupted end with a coiled spring-like appearance can be seen in the operative field in the acute stage *(Fig. 36.3A or Fig. 36.4A)*, or a fusiform pattern (glioma) in the chronic stage *(Fig. 36.3B or Fig. 36.4B)*. If a surgeon attempts to locate the other disrupted end, a second operative wound is usually required. However, in rupture injury the two nerve ends can be visualized in the same operative wound in the acute stage, or within a big neuroma noted in the chronic stage.

Root avulsion is very common in BPI due to its weak supporting structures consisting of dura and dentate ligaments. A novel approach of performing spinal cord implantation with or without nerve graft[15,16] showed unsatisfactory clinical results. This implies that in avulsion injury only one end (distal end) is available, while the other end (proximal) end is absent or unsuitable for repair. "Root injury" is an obscure term which may mean avulsion from the cord (true avulsion), or rupture or stretch at rootlets or roots. Root avulsion in BPI is usually accompanied by dura tearing and a cerebrospinal fluid leak with cyst formation, called pseudomeningocele. However in some cases the root can be avulsed at its origin with an intact dura cone (called "avulsion *in situ*"). The nerve root may remain inside the spinal canal or at the dural orifice, giving a grossly normal appearance or loosening with curvature of the spinal nerve at the time of surgical intervention despite established paralysis. Most often, however, the entire avulsed root, including ventral, dorsal roots, and ganglia, retracts and migrates downward to the interscalene or preclavicular region.

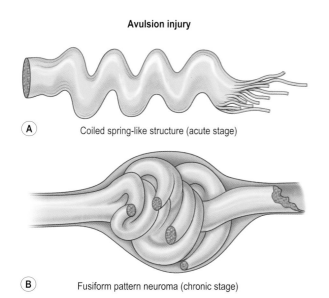

Avulsion injury

(A) Coiled spring-like structure (acute stage)

(B) Fusiform pattern neuroma (chronic stage)

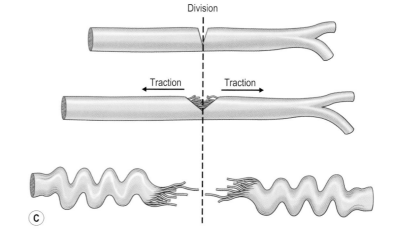

Rupture injury

Division

Traction   Traction

(C)

Fig. 36.3 The mechanism of **(A,B)** avulsion injury versus **(C)** rupture injury.

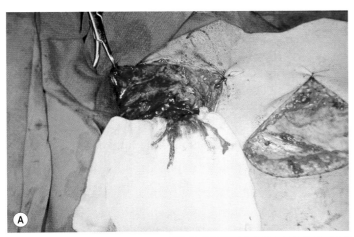

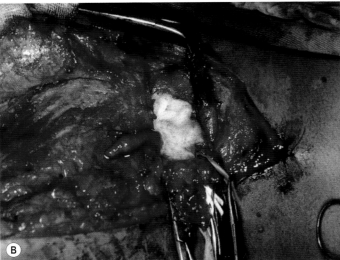

Fig. 36.4 (A) Coiled spring-like structure with irregularity of stumps of C5 and C6 avulsion (acute stage); **(B)** fusiform pattern neuroma (or glioma) of the distal C7 stump (chronic stage) during dissection.

Pathophysiology and degree of nerve injury

Timing of nerve exploration is dependent upon the degree of nerve injury. The degree of peripheral nerve injury can be classified into neuropraxia, axonotmesis, and neurotmesis (Seddon classification[17]) or grade 1–5 injury (Sunderland classification[18]). Seddon's axonotmesis or Sunderland's second-degree injury starts to have wallerian degeneration at proximal and distal stumps. Seddon's neurotmesis or Sunderland's third- to fifth-degree injury has the potential for aberrant reinnervation after nerve regeneration. In Sunderland's fourth- or fifth-degree injuries, only nerve repair can succeed in restoring continuity, but in first-, second- or third-degree injuries, spontaneous recovery, complete and incomplete, may occur.

There is rarely an argument for immediate exploration after penetrating injury by sharp objects for direct nerve repair. Some surgeons also advocate exploration of the BPI as early as possible[19,20] for adult closed BPI for its advantages, including easy diagnosis of root avulsion and avoidance of difficult dissection through scarring. However, such early exploration

is not recommended by most brachial plexus surgeons.[2–6] In cases of closed BPI, the degree and extent of injury are difficult to judge soon after injury and are often underestimated. The benefits of waiting usually outweigh the advantages of early surgery.

Over 1500 adult and 500 pediatric brachial plexus palsy patients have been treated by the author since 1985. The following will deal with the author's experience regarding to adult and pediatric BPI.

Adult brachial plexus injury

Introduction

- Numerous etiologies can cause adult brachial plexus injury
- Clinical evaluation is still the most important step in establishing the site of injury, estimating the degree of injury and determining the surgical treatment and prognosis
- Imaging studies such as magnetic resonance imaging or computed tomography myelography are very helpful for diagnosing level 1 and/or level 2 injury
- Neurolysis, nerve repair, nerve grafts, nerve transfers, and functioning free muscle transplantation are all possible options for brachial plexus reconstruction. Different levels of injury have different reconstructive strategies
- There are many landmarks and key points for supraclavicular and infraclavicular brachial plexus dissection
- Brachial plexus reconstruction involves the use of palliative techniques for long-term sequelae
- Outcome evaluation should be unified to assess the success of the reconstructive technique and to report and share experiences which may help to improve current reconstructive techniques

Etiology of adult BPI

BPI may be caused by trauma (open or closed type), compression, tumor, infection, inflammation, toxins, and other etiologies.

Patient history

Patient history should include mechanism of injury, conscious level at the time of trauma, associated injury (such as head injury, fracture, open wound, chest injury, vascular injury), kinds of previous surgical intervention (such as chest intubation, cervical spine surgery), and characteristics of pain. This information helps to determine the degree and extent of injury and the need for surgical intervention. Mechanism of injury (e.g., upward or downward traction and with or without rotation) is not easily detected due to the patient's loss of consciousness or amnesia for the accident. A history of shoulder dislocation or glenoid fracture may have a high incidence of level 4 injury, whereas a history of cervical spine injury or fracture may cause a level 1 root injury. Artery rupture and repair imply the site of nerve injury. For instance, arm traction by rolling machine or conveyor belt often causes an open wound in the axilla, extensive ecchymosis around the shoulder and chest (due to rupture of axillary vessels), and level 4 BPI. Segmental thrombosis of the subclavian artery is usually associated with C8–T1 root injury. History of rib fracture and chest intubation may preclude intercostal nerve transfer because of a higher failure rate.[21] Extreme causalgia is often seen in cases of root avulsion in lower-root (C8–T1) avulsion as they contain the richest sympathetic fibers.[22] Extreme causalgia is also a major factor for poor outcome due to poor rehabilitation.

Preoperative evaluation and diagnosis

Most adult BPIs are closed injuries. Accurate assessment of the extent and severity of the injury in closed BPI is difficult. Clinical evaluation is still essential and is the most important step in establishing the diagnosis of site and degree of injury, and determining the treatment and prognosis. A brachial plexus chart (left and right formats, *Fig. 36.5*) outlining the

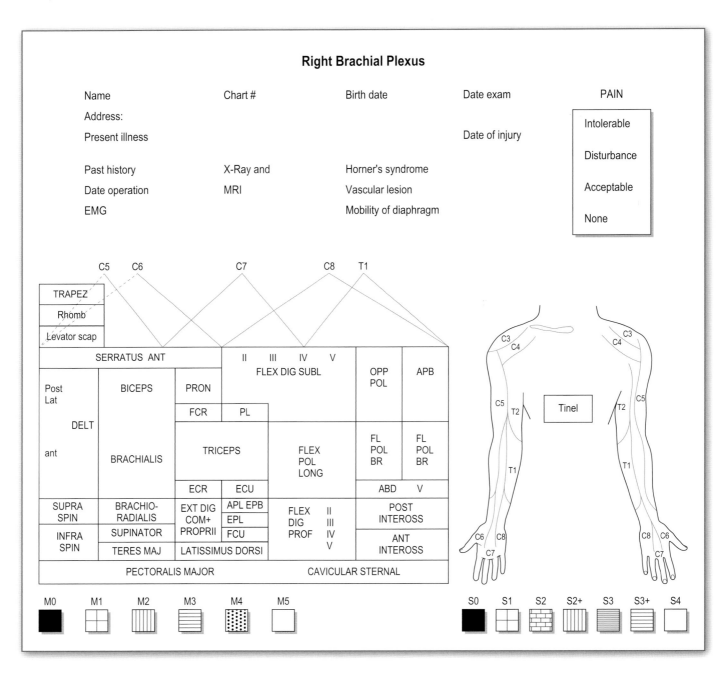

Fig. 36.5 Special charts for the evaluation of the brachial plexus-injured patient **(A)** for the right and **(B)** for the left upper limb.

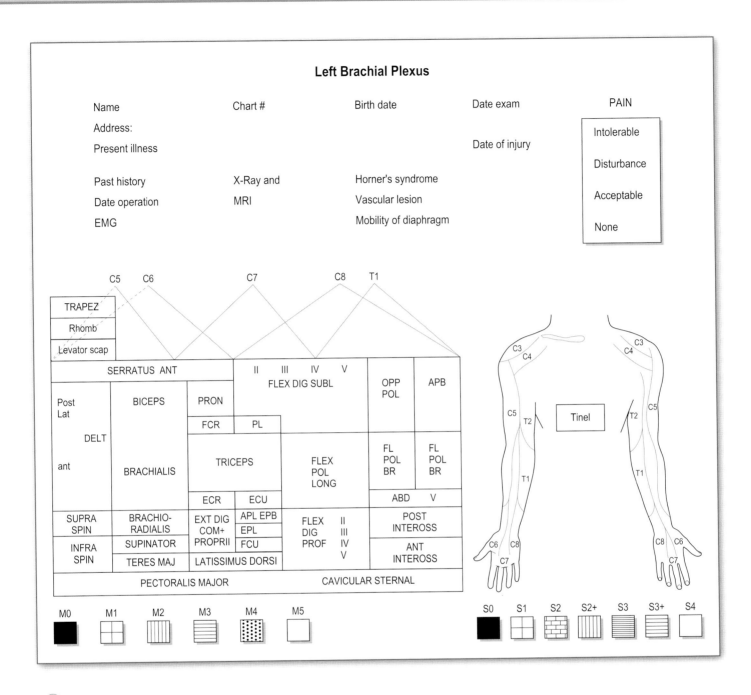

Fig. 36.5, cont'd

Motor examination

possible injury should be completed before definite brachial plexus surgery. This chart is filled at the initial examination, usually performed at 2 months after injury. The chart is also useful for follow-up evaluations allowing comparison of clinical pictures.

Muscle by muscle examination should be completed in a distal-to-proximal fashion and recorded, using the British Medical Research Council (MRC) scale (M0–5).[23] We have modified the motor evaluation system, adding more detailed differentiation: M5, strength against four fingers (examiner) resistance; M4, against one finger, resistance for longer than 30 seconds; and M3, against gravity *(Table 36.3)*. M4 is recognized as useful muscle strength. The action of each muscle should be examined separately in relation to the movement of a single joint. Although there is no single muscle innervated by a single spinal nerve, some muscle palsy can give specific information related to the level of the injury. For instance,

Table 36.3 British Medical Research Council (MRC) scale and Chuang modification

British MRC scale	
Motor scale	**Sensory scale**
M0 No contraction	S0 No sensation
M1 Flicker (trace of contraction)	S1 Pain sensation
M2 Active movement with gravity eliminated	S2 Pain and some touch sensation
M3 Active movement against gravity	S3 Pain and touch with no overreaction
M4 Active movement against gravity and resistance	S3+ Some two-point discrimination
M5 Normal (full) power	S4 Normal sensation

Chuang modification	
Motor scale	**Sensory scale**
M4 Active movement against examiner's one-finger resistance ≥30 seconds	S2+ pain and touch with overreaction

1. Diaphragm palsy implies C4 and very proximal C5 (level 1) injury.

2. The levator scapulae muscle lies anterior to the trapezius muscle in the neck, and can be more easily detected than the rhomboid muscles, which are covered by the trapezius muscle. Both levator scapulae and rhomboid muscles are innervated by the same nerve (dorsal scapular nerve, or C4 and C5). Preservation of its function in upper plexus or total plexus injury may imply C5 rupture injury (level 2) after branching to the muscle.

3. Serratus anterior muscle: The long thoracic nerve has two portions: the upper portion originating from C5 and C6, and the lower portion from C7. The upper portion is responsible for scapular protraction, and the lower portion is important for scapular stabilization.[24] Positive anterior traction of the scapula (shoulder protraction test) shows that at least C5 is ruptured after branching to the long thoracic nerve, so the proximal C5 is available for transfer. Scapular winging is observed only when the lower portion is denervated, but isolated C7 root avulsion is rarely seen in adult BPI. In pure C5–6 level 1 injury, the lower part of the muscle is still functional.

4. Clavicular and sternal portions of the pectoralis major muscle: The major pectoral muscle can be separated into two parts: clavicular and sternal parts. The clavicular part is innervated by upper and middle trunks or its divisions, while the sternal part is innervated by the lower trunk. A functional clavicular portion of the pectoralis major muscle may imply an infraclavicular (level 4) injury.

Sensory examination

Sensory evaluation should include sensory tests and elicitation of a Tinel's sign. Sensibility tests include pain and temperature appreciation, static and moving two-point discrimination, constant touch, and vibration. However, performing complete sensory tests in BPI is both unnecessary and illogical because we are examining the dermatomal distribution from spinal nerves, not the cutaneous distribution. Pinprick test from areas of normal to abnormal sensation to map out the area of sensory disturbance is sufficient for most brachial plexus-injured patients. Sensory grading is based on the British MRC scale (S0–4),[23] modified by adding a grade for sensory overreaction (S2+) *(Table 36.3)*. Such sensory evaluations can give some clues about the level and degree of BPI.

Tinel's sign

The Hoffman–Tinel's sign is an important clinical sign to determine the location of a neuroma or to track the regeneration of the injured nerves. Palpation or percussion at the neck, at the supraclavicular Erb's point (clavicular insertion of the sternocleidomastoid muscle), at the infraclavicular coracoid process of the scapula, or at the route of different nerves along their course may induce an electric current sensation (like pins and needles) running down to the shoulder or the hand (positive Tinel's sign). If the Tinel's sign remains at a fixed point, which means retardation of its progression, surgical exploration is warranted. If the Tinel's sign advances from supraclavicular to infraclavicular and distally to the arm or forearm at successive examinations, observation is recommended, as this may indicate a Sunderland third-degree lesion. A weak or absent Tinel's sign in the neck region usually indicates total root avulsion.

Horner's syndrome

Horner's syndrome (miosis, ptosis, enophthalmos, and anhidrosis) is a sign of sympathetic nervous system disturbance. It indirectly implies avulsion of the T1 and C8 roots because the sympathetic fibers from the T1–2 sympathetic ganglia are quite close to the preganglionic fibers of T1 and C8. This syndrome may regress with time. It is a more reliable sign in adult BPI, but less accurate in obstetric traction injury.

Plain X-ray and imaging studies

Plain X-rays of the chest and cervical spine are required. The chest X-ray should include inspiration and expiration views to exclude diaphragmatic palsy. Cervical spine X-rays are evaluated for any fracture of the transverse process, spinous process, or vertebrae body.

Cervical myelography and computed tomography (CT) myelography can provide valuable information related to the level 1 injury of the brachial plexus.[25] However, in recent years these studies have been gradually replaced by noninvasive magnetic resonance imaging (MRI).[26] The most useful MRI technique for the evaluation of a possible level 1 lesion is the three-dimensional (3D) fast imaging employing steady-state acquisition (FIESTA). These 3D source data are reconstructed along the planes of ventral and dorsal rootlets using a curve planar reformat technique to demonstrate the respective rootlets in a better perspective. Other MR techniques help in the imaging of the whole brachial plexus, notably of level 2 *(Fig. 36.6)*.

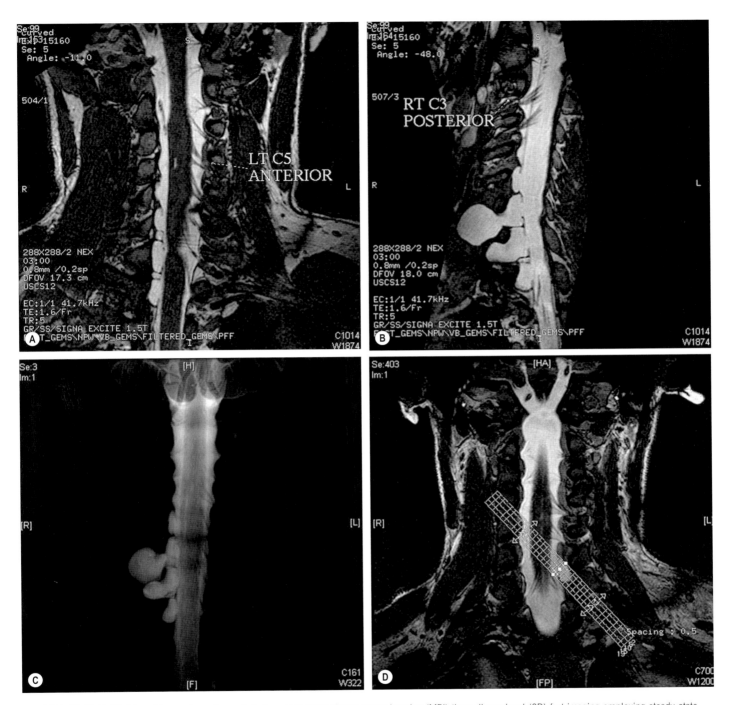

Fig. 36.6 (A) Right C5–T1 avulsion cysts on the ventral view using magnetic resonance imaging (MRI) three-dimensional (3D) fast imaging employing steady-state acquisition (FIESTA) technique; **(B)** dorsal view, using MRI 3D FIESTA and curve planar reformat techniques; and **(C)** MRI cervical spine myelogram on the same patient; **(D)** MRI 3D, coronal view, avulsion cyst of the left C7, and

Electrodiagnostic studies

Electrodiagnostic studies, mainly consisting of nerve conduction studies (NCSs) and needle electromyography (EMG), are used to localize the lesion and to assess its severity. For the NCS, only amplitudes of the sensory nerve action potentials (SNAPs) and compound muscle action potentials (CMAPs) are of value. Both SNAP and CMAP amplitudes provide a good indication of the degree of axon loss, or in contrast, the number of survival axons capable of conducting impulses.[27,28] Sensory NCSs assess the function of the postganglionic portion of the sensory pathway. Therefore, abnormally low SNAP amplitudes indicate a ganglionic or postganglionic lesion. Conversely, SNAP amplitude remains normal in a pure preganglionic lesion such as root avulsion. A combination of unelicitable CMAPs with abnormal low SNAP amplitudes

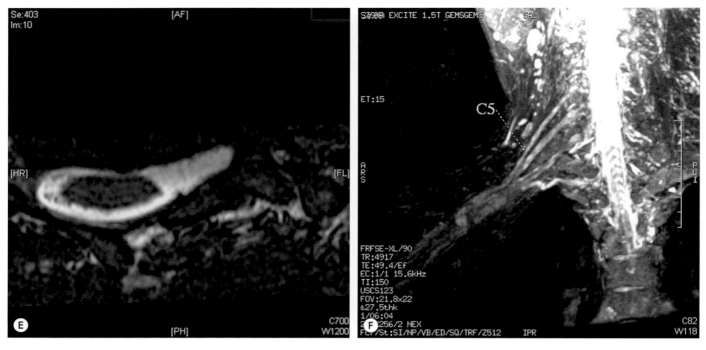

Fig. 36.6, cont'd (E) axial view for comparison; **(F)** MRI 3D diffusion-weighted imaging techniques to see the level 2 spinal nerves.

suggests a combined preganglionic and postganglionic lesion. To assess the major elements of the brachial plexus, NCSs of multiple nerves are usually required. These include sensory NCSs of the lateral antebrachial cutaneous, median, ulnar, radial, and axillary nerves, as well as motor NCSs of the median, ulnar, radial, musculocutaneous, and axillary nerves. The positive pick-up sensory action potentials taken from a paralyzed limb are evidence of preganglionic root lesion. The presence of fibrillation potentials on needle EMG may suggest that the lesion is at least axonotmesis. The reduction of amplitude of compound muscle action potentials during motor NCS is more reliable than the presence of fibrillation potentials to indicate axonal loss rather than a neurapraxia lesion.

Needle EMGs can detect a minimal amount of motor axon loss. For a comprehensive evaluation of the brachial plexus, adequate EMG sampling of muscles is critical. In addition to muscles innervated by major terminal nerves, examination of those supplied from or proximal to the brachial plexus can help to localize the lesion. These include the rhomboid major, serratus anterior, pectoralis major (both the clavicular and sternocostal parts), latissimus dorsi, teres major, and cervical paraspinus muscles. Needle EMG can also reveal evidence of early reinnervation and chronicity of the lesion. Presence of denervation potentials (i.e., fibrillation potentials and positive sharp waves) is the most sensitive indicator of motor axon loss. However, they require about 3 weeks to develop after axon injury.[27]

Percutaneous somatosensory evoked potentials (SEPs) provide far less information than comprehensive NCSs and needle EMG studies in most patients with BPI. Thus SEPs are not routinely performed. Intraoperative SEPs may be useful to determine the continuity of individual segments of the brachial plexus and roots.

Vascular injury

Absence or weakness of pulsation of the radial artery at the wrist indicates a possible vascular injury of the axillary or subclavian artery. It may further indicate the extent and severity of the trauma. Subclavian artery occlusion may indicate a level 1 injury, while axillary artery occlusion may be associated with a level 4 lesion. Vascular injury should be taken into account when considering the use of a vascularized ulnar nerve graft for reconstruction because the ulnar artery is transferred with the ulnar nerve.

Surgical treatment and techniques

Neurolysis (external neurolysis), nerve repair, nerve grafts (free nerve grafts or vascularized ulnar nerve grafts), nerve transfer, and functioning free muscle transplantation (FFMT) are surgical options for brachial plexus reconstruction. The following pages detail our experience with BPI treatment in terms of the level of injury.

Level 1 injury: inside the (vertebral) bone (preganglionic root) injury, including spinal cord, rootlet, and root

The incidence of level 1 lesions is 70%. Nerves may be avulsed from the spinal cord (true avulsion), or ruptured at the preganglionic roots and rootlets. Partial Brown-Séquard syndrome is an example of true avulsion.[22] One to all five roots may be avulsed. Root avulsion injuries lack central connection and are considered irreparable. Nerve transfer, pedicled muscle transfer, and FFMT provide the only possibilities for functional restoration.

Nerve transfer

Nerve transfer is a surgical option which intentionally divides a physiologically active nerve (with low donor morbidity) and transfers it to a distal, more important but irreparable paralyzed nerve. The procedure is best done within a golden time period, within 5 months of the injury,[6] in order to reactivate the paralyzed muscle(s) effectively (aiming for M4). Nerve transfer can be broadly classified into four categories: (1) extraplexus; (2) intraplexus; (3) close-target nerve transfer; and (4) end-to-side neurorrhaphy nerve transfer.

Extraplexus nerve transfer

Extraplexus nerve transfer involves the transfer of a brachial plexus neighboring nerve (from either the ipsilateral or contralateral neck) to the avulsed brachial plexus for neurotization of a paralyzed nerve. The reported donor nerves in common use are mostly aimed at motor reinnervation.[29] These donor nerves include the phrenic (Ph) nerve, spinal accessory (XI) nerve (accessed by an anterior neck approach), deep motor branches of the cervical plexus (cervical motor branches, CMB), hypoglossal nerve (XII), and the contralateral C7 (CC7) spinal nerve. Extraplexus sensory nerve transfer such as supraclavicular sensory nerve to median nerve transfer is sometimes used to provide sensation to the paralyzed hand.

Intraplexus nerve transfer

Intraplexus nerve transfer is applicable in cases of nonglobal root avulsion, in which at least one of the spinal nerves is ruptured and still available for transfer – not to its original pathway, but to other more important nerves. For example, in a case of C5 and C6 rupture injury (level 2) in which the C5 stump is healthier than the C6 stump, the C5 fibers are intentionally transferred to C6 (or the anterior division of the upper trunk) for elbow flexion. The distal C5 (or the posterior division of the upper trunk and suprascapular nerve) is then innervated by the partially injured C6. This strategy acknowledges that elbow flexion has priority over shoulder reconstruction. Intraplexus nerve transfer is individualized depending upon the intraoperative findings, the surgeon's philosophy, and the patient's condition and requirements. Extraplexus and intraplexus nerve transfers are both considered as proximal nerve neurotization.

Closed-target nerve transfer

Closed-target nerve transfer is a procedure that provides a direct coaptation at a more distal site, closer to the neuromuscular junction, thus achieving faster recovery of motor outcomes. Closed-target nerve transfer is defined as a procedure outside the supra- and infraclavicular fossa. Examples include spinal accessory (XI) nerve transfer to the suprascapular nerve via a posterior approach; partial ulnar nerve transfer to the biceps nerve; partial median nerve transfer to the brachialis nerve; long head of triceps branch transfer to the axillary nerve; intercostal nerve transfer to the biceps nerve, the musculocutaneous nerve, or the nerve of the long head of triceps; anterior interosseus nerve transfer to the radial or posterior interosseus nerve; and branch of the anterior interosseus nerve transfer to the deep motor branch of the ulnar nerve in the forearm. Closed-target nerve transfer is considered as distal nerve transfer.[30] Selecting proximal or distal nerve transfer as a reconstructive strategy is now a subject of much debate (*Table 36.4*). Proximal nerve transfer (extraplexus and intraplexus nerve transfer) is traditionally still the main reconstructive procedure.

End-to-side neurorrhaphy nerve transfer

End-to-side neurorrhaphy (terminolateral neurorrhaphy) is a technique to transfer the distal end of a paralyzed and irreparable nerve to the side of an intact nerve with an epineurotomy

Table 36.4 Proximal nerve transfer versus distal nerve transfer in adult brachial plexus injury

	Proximal nerve transfer	Distal nerve transfer
Philosophy	Traditional	New strategy
Donor nerve	Supraclavicular, far from the target muscle	The nearby nerve close to the target muscle
Advantages	Diagnostic and treatment Proximal nerve(s), powerful Nerve cut, fewer functional deficits	A treatment procedure, but not diagnostic No scars, easy dissection Shorter operation time Nerve-cut stumps: healthy, no scar Direct repair; no need to graft nerve Short rehabilitation, faster recovery
Disadvantages	More scars, difficult dissection Health of cut stumps is unpredictable May need long nerve grafts Longer operation time Longer rehabilitation period	Nerve cut, risk of causing deficits Risk of iatrogenic injury May need multiple incisions
Indication	All kinds of avulsion/rupture injury of brachial plexus injury	Not global injury After brachial plexus neurofibroma (C5 and C6) resection Intrinsic palsy of the hand

Table 36.5 Induction exercises recommended with different nerve transfers

Donor nerve	Induction exercise
IC nerve	Aerobic exercise (e.g., run, walk, or climb hill), causing deep breathing
Ph nerve	Aerobic exercise
XI nerve	Shoulder moves up or back with resistance or shoulder lateral abduction with resistance
XII nerve	Tongue to palate push-up exercise
CC7	Shoulder adduction or grasp exercise of the healthy limb
Partial Un or Mn	Hand grasp exercise

IC, intercostal; Ph, phrenic; XI, spinal accessory; XII, hypoglossal; CC7, contralateral C7; Un, ulnar nerve; Mn, median nerve.

or perineurotomy window for both motor and sensory reconstruction.[31] The author has never used this technique for BPI.

Induction or motivation exercise is an important muscle exercise for patients with nerve transfer. The original function of the donor nerve must be practiced to induce movement in the target muscles newly innervated by the transfer. For example, patients who have undergone intercostal nerve transfer must increase their deep-breathing rate to induce movement in their target muscles. An induction exercise is commenced when movement of the innervated muscles is palpable (M1). The action is comparable to an internal electric stimulator. Various nerve transfers have different induction exercises *(Table 36.5)*.

Reconstructive strategies with nerve transfer for different targets

Different injury patterns have different reconstructive strategies *(Table 36.6)*. Proximal nerve neurotization is traditionally the main reconstructive procedure.

Shoulder

Reconstruction for shoulder abduction in a level 1 lesion should take priority over shoulder adduction. If the supraspinatus, infraspinatus, and deltoid muscles are innervated simultaneously, results are predictably better. The Ph and XI are the main donor nerves for shoulder abduction. The XII nerve, CMB, part of C5 or C6, long thoracic nerve, branch to the long head of triceps, medial pectoral nerve, intercostal nerves, and CC7 have also been reported as the donor nerve for shoulder abduction. The recipient nerves for shoulder abduction in order of priority are the distal C5 (not include the anterior division), suprascapular nerve, dorsal division of the upper trunk, then axillary nerve.[29] A study of a series of patients operated on between 2000 and 2003 demonstrated that triple nerve transfers produced the best and most consistently reliable results for shoulder elevation: an average of 160° shoulder abduction was achieved following triple nerve transfers, but 85° following double nerve transfers and 65° following single nerve transfer.[32]

Elbow

In level 1 injury, reconstruction for elbow flexion is always the first priority. Reported donor nerves for elbow flexion include intercostal nerve, XI nerve with a nerve graft, Ph nerve with or without nerve graft, partial ulnar nerve, partial median nerve, pectoral nerve, thoracodorsal nerve, and CC7. The recipient nerve is the musculocutaneous nerve (mixed nerve), biceps nerve, or brachialis nerve. Elbow extension is usually a lower priority for reconstruction. Ph nerve transfer to the distal C5 or to the posterior division of the upper trunk, or to the radial nerve with a nerve graft, can often yield elbow extension, usually in the third year of rehabilitation. Some authors describe transferring two or three intercostal nerves to the branch of the long head of triceps to achieve elbow extension.[28]

Finger

Video 1

In global (C5–T1) level 1 injury, reconstructive priority for finger function depends on the procedure used: nerve transfer or FFMT. Traditionally reconstruction for finger flexion is preferable to finger extension which can sometimes be helped by a dynamic extension splint. In C5 rupture with C6–T1 four-root avulsion, transfer of C5 to the median nerve (video 1) or in a total root (C5–T1) avulsion, transfer of the CC7 to the median nerve *(Fig. 36.7)* can be performed to achieve finger and wrist flexion as well as finger sensation. Each procedure requires a vascularized ulnar nerve graft. In total root avulsion or four-root avulsion with C5 rupture, nerve reconstruction first versus FFMT first is a subject of much debate *(Table 36.7)*. Nerve reconstruction first is a strategy of proximal-to-distal reconstruction, while FFMT first is a strategy of distal-to-proximal reconstruction. Nerve reconstruction first by multiple nerve transfers aims to achieve a one-stage full reconstruction for shoulder, elbow, and hand function.[6,29] In these cases, FFMT is used predominantly as a secondary adjuvant reconstruction to enhance results at a later stage. However, FFMT first is an alternative approach[33]: a long FFMT (usually gracilis muscle) from the clavicle down to the extensor digitorum communis, innervated by the XI nerve, is performed in the first stage, followed by a second long FFMT from the second rib to the flexor digitorum profundus, innervated by intercostal nerves in the second stage. In these cases, nerve reconstruction such as C5 transfer, contralateral C7 transfer, or intercostal transfer is an adjunctive procedure for shoulder function. Comparison between proximal-to-distal reconstructive strategy (nerve reconstruction first, FFMT later) and distal-to-proximal reconstructive strategy (FFMT first, then nerve reconstruction) in total roots avulsion (level 1) is illustrated in *Table 36.7*.

Pedicled muscle transfer

Pedicled muscle transfer is indicated in nonglobal BPI such as C5–6 root avulsion with intact C7–1. Local latissimus dorsi muscle transfer for elbow flexion or finger flexion, or even for shoulder abduction, local pectoralis major muscle transfer, or local pectoralis minor transfer for elbow flexion, part deltoid transfer for elbow extension, or forearm flexor transfer for wrist or finger extension; and forearm muscle transfer for intrinsic palsy are examples of pedicled muscle transfer. Using a reinnervated muscle transfer as a pedicled muscle transfer is also an issue of debate. Preoperative muscle strength

Table 36.6 Reconstructive strategies for different numbers of root avulsion

Condition	Nerve reconstruction	Late reconstruction

Five-root (C5–T1)
Level 1 injury
	Ph → distal C5 for shoulder elevation
	IC → musculocutaneous nerve for elbow flexion
	  contralateral
	CC7 → median nerve for hand
		Wrist and thumb fusion, FFMT for EDC
		  and elbow (XI)

Four-root injury (C5 level 2, C6–T1 level 1)	C5 →median nerve for hand IC →musculocutaneous nerve for elbow flexion Ph → distal C5 for shoulder elevation	Wrist and thumb fusion, FFMT for EDC and elbow (XI)
Three-root injury		
1. C5, C6 level 2, C7–T1 level 1	C5 →SS + PD of UT for shoulder C6 →C8 or median nerve for hand IC →musculocutaneous nerve for elbow flexion	Variable
2. C5–7 level 1, C8–T1 intact	Ph +XI → distal C5 for shoulder elevation part ulnar → biceps br part median → brachialis br for elbow	Variable
Two-root injury		
1. C5–6 level 1, C7–T1 intact	Ph + XI → distal C5 for shoulder elevation part ulnar → biceps br part median → brachialis br for elbow	Variable
2. C6–7 level 1, C5 level 2, C8–T1 intact	Ph + XI → distal C5 for shoulder elevation C5 → AD of UT for elbow	Variable
3. C8–T1 level 1, C5–7 level 2 injury	C5 nerve grafts for shoulder C6→median nerve for hand C7 nerve grafts to C7	Variable
4. C8–T1 level 1 injury, others intact	No nerve reconstruction	ECRL→EDC for finger extension FCR → FDP for finger flexion Br for opponensplasty Thumb IP fusion
Single-root injury		
1. C5 level 1 injury	Ph + XI + CMB →distal C5	
2. C6 level 1, usually C5 level 2 injury	C5→C6 or AD of UT for elbow Ph + XI + CMB →distal C5	
3. C7 level 1, C5–6 level 2 injury	C5, C6 nerve grafts itself	

Ph, phrenic nerve; IC, intercostal; XI, spinal accessory nerve, CMB, cervical motor branches; FFMT, functioning free muscle transplantation; EDC, extensor digitorum communis; SS, suprascapular nerve; PD, AD, UT, posterior division, anterior division of the upper trunk; br, branch; ECRL, extensor carpi radialis longus; FCR, flexor carpi radialis; FDP, flexor digitorum profundus; IP, interphalangeal joint

examination is very important. Before a reinnervated muscle can be used it should be at least M4 muscle strength. Otherwise many of these transfers are useless and wasted. For example, using a local latissimus dorsi muscle transfer for elbow flexion in C5 and C6 (±C7) avulsion injury usually results in M3, but not M4 muscle strength, compared with latissimus dorsi transfer for the traumatic loss of biceps and brachialis, which always results in M4 muscle strength. The reason for this difference in outcome is the state of the thoracodorsal nerve which originates from C6–8. In the former example, the thoracodorsal nerve is actually an injured nerve, but in the latter example of traumatic muscle loss, the thoracodorsal nerve is an uninjured one. Local pedicled muscle transfer, although an alternative restorative option, is often not reliable due to the presence of a partial nerve injury.

Functioning free muscle transplantation

FFMT is the transfer of a muscle utilizing microvascular anastomoses for revascularization and microneural coaptation to the recipient motor nerve for reinnervation. The use of FFMT in brachial plexus reconstruction is one example of the application of nerve transfer (including extraplexus, intraplexus, and closed-target nerve transfer).[34] It has been shown to be effective and has become increasingly popular. The gracilis myocutaneous FFMT is the most common and best choice of

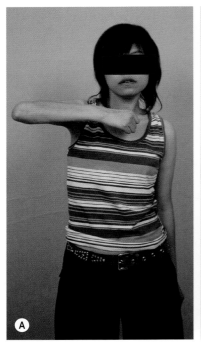
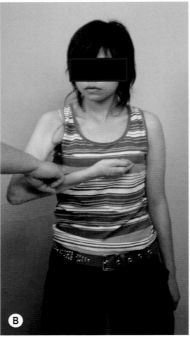
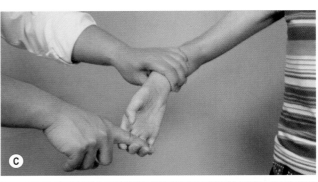
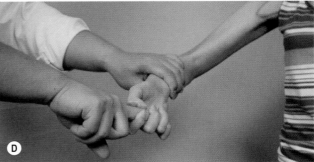

Fig. 36.7 Example of results of one-stage surgery for total root avulsion 5 years after: (1) left contralateral C7 transfer to the median nerve using a vascularized ulnar nerve graft for finger flexion and sensation; (2) three intercostal nerves (T3–5) transfer to the musculocutaneous nerve for elbow flexion; and (3) phrenic nerve transfer to the suprascapular nerve for shoulder elevation: **(A)** 90° shoulder elevation; **(B)** M4 elbow flexion; and **(C, D)** M3 finger flexion.

donor muscle in brachial plexus reconstruction.[35] The commonly used donor nerves include the XI, the intercostal, the Ph nerve, the CC7 nerve, part of the ulnar nerve, part of the median nerve, or more proximally from the infra- or supraclavicular nerve which requires nerve elongation (with a nerve graft in the first stage) and then FFMT in a two-stage procedure. The results from FFMT are more satisfactory than those achieved with a local muscle transfer. It is especially useful for elbow and hand function restoration in global plexopathy. Indications for FFMT in BPI include acute or chronic root avulsion, root injury with failed nerve transfer (muscle strength less than M3), or BPI with associated Volkmann's contracture of the forearm.

Level 2 injury: inside the muscle (postganglionic spinal nerve) injury located at the interscalene space proximal to the suprascapular nerve

Level 2 injury is defined as an injury distal to the dorsal root ganglion (or outside the intervertebral foramen) but between the scalene muscles and proximal to the suprascapular nerve. If the suprascapular nerve is intact, the lesion will be in level 3–4 and not in level 2. The incidence of a pure level 2 injury is approximately 8%. Disruption of the spinal nerve with neuroma formation and dense scar tissue involving the scalene muscles (especially the middle scalene muscle) are the main findings in this type of injury. Nerve rupture may occur at one or multiple spinal nerves. The clinical differential diagnosis between preganglionic root (level 1) and postganglionic spinal nerve (level 2) injury is of great importance with regard to the surgical approach and

prognosis. Segmental resection of the anterior scalene muscle is usually required to approach the healthy proximal stump. Reconstruction for this level of injury includes neurolysis, nerve repair, nerve grafts, and nerve transfer if associated with level 1 lesion in other spinal nerves, and palliative reconstruction.

Level 3 injury: pre- and retroclavicular injury (trunks and divisions)

Level 3 injury involves the trunks and divisions. In our series, only 5% of patients were injured purely in this zone. Nerve rupture with neuroma formation and dense scars were the most common findings. Bypass nerve grafting is required to re-establish the connection between the supra- and infraclavicular brachial plexus. A clavicle osteotomy is often required for wound exposure, especially for injuries involving the lower trunk, to allow grafting or direct neurolysis. Multiple nerve grafts are required and need to be harvested from different locations. A C-loop vascularized ulnar nerve graft is sometimes helpful to reduce the amount of nerve grafts, especially in cases of extensive injury.

Level 4 injury: infraclavicular brachial plexus injury

Level 4 BPI involves the cords and their terminal branches. The incidence is high (17%), second after level 1 injury. Level 4 injury is commonly limited to this zone only and rarely has proximal level involvement. Level 4 injuries are mostly encountered with nerve ruptures and rarely with nerve

Table 36.7 Comparison between proximal to distal and distal to proximal reconstructive priority for total root avulsion

	Proximal to distal	Distal to proximal
Philosophy	Traditional	New strategy
Reconstruction priority	Shoulder, elbow first, then finger	Finger and elbow first, then shoulder
Reconstructive method	Nerve first, then FFMT	FFMT first, then nerve surgery
Brachial plexus exploration	Yes	Maybe not
Nerve reconstruction		
for shoulder	Yes	May or may not be needed
for elbow	Yes	Need FFMT
for finger	Yes	Need FFMT
Stage requirement for full reconstruction	One stage	Multiple stages
Rehabilitation period	At least 4 years	2 years
Patient selection	Highly motivated and intelligent patient	Less intelligent and impatient patient
Predict outcomes		
Shoulder elevation	Better (≥60°)	Shoulder fusion (10–30°)
Elbow flexion	Usually better (M4)	M3–4
Finger flexion	M2–4	M2–4
Finger extension (EDC)	M0	M2–3
FFMT, functioning free muscle transplantation; EDC, extensor digitorum communis.		

avulsion. Any nerve avulsion here is distal avulsion at the bone margin (suprascapular nerve avulsion at the scapular notch, or axillary nerve at the humeral neck, or radial nerve at the spinal canal inlet), or at the muscle attachment (such as the musculocutaneous nerve from the biceps surface). In closed level 4 injury, the nerve damage is variable, ranging from simple isolated nerve injuries (axillary, musculocutaneous, or radial nerve) to lesions of all cords or all terminal branches. Level 4 injury has particular characteristics with specific challenges in surgical dissection and repair due to dense scarring. Nerve grafts are more frequently used with less aberrant reinnervation and better prognosis. There is a high incidence of vascular injury, rupture or segmental occlusion of the subclavian or axillary artery – about 30%. For ease of dissection, detachment of the insertion of the pectoralis major muscle by Z-lengthening incision is often required. For penetrating injuries, vascular and nerve repairs are usually performed simultaneously.

The golden time for primary direct repair of a divided nerve without nerve grafts in penetrating injury is within 2 weeks. Traction injuries in level 4 are usually associated with

fracture of the proximal humerus or the glenoid scapula. The nerve segments have been extensively damaged. Long nerve grafts are usually required to bridge the nerve gap, commonly more than 8 cm in length. Sometimes a C-loop vascularized ulnar nerve graft is harvested from the paralyzed forearm and utilized for median and radial nerve reconstruction. The results are usually good. In nerve avulsion from the muscle, nerve grafting of the proximal nerve stump and direct implantation into the muscle (nerve-to-muscle neurotization) yield fair results (around M3). As described previously, FFMT is another option of reconstruction for such cases.

Surgical technique for exploration of the brachial plexus

A linear incision from the midpoint between the mastoid process of the temporal bone and the jugular notch, going along the posterior border of the sternocleidomastoid muscle, and curving laterally parallel to and above the clavicle (a C-curved incision) is a popular incision for the supraclavicular approach. For the infraclavicular approach, the incision is just along the deltopectoral groove and extends upward to meet the supraclavicular incision, or downward to the medial sulcus of the biceps. Other additional incisions may be required: extended neck incision for accessing the spinal accessory nerve; chest semicircular incision for the intercostal nerve; inframental incision for the hypoglossal nerve; medial arm incision for the biceps nerve and brachialis nerves; and a contralateral neck C-curved incision for contralateral C7 spinal nerve dissection and transfer (*Fig. 36.8*).

Landmarks and key points for supraclavicular dissection

1. A platysma musculocutaneous flap is elevated with the C-curved incision.

2. Dissection beneath the sternocleidomastoid muscle to the internal jugular vein is made but should never go beyond the internal jugular vein. The suprascapular sensory nerves are the uppermost landmark, and one should never go above them.

3. The omohyoid muscle just behind the sternocleidomastoid muscle is identified and spared if possible as it is an important landmark for possible secondary exploration.

4. Below the omohyoid muscle, there is an abundance of adipofascial tissue containing rich lymphatic ducts, lymph nodes, and the transverse cervical vessels. A similar C-shaped incision along the internal jugular vein medially and subclavian vein inferiorly is made and a superiorly based adipofascial flap is elevated. All the lymph tissues, including the ducts coming from the deep plane of the internal jugular vein, should be coagulated or ligated before division to avoid postoperative lymph leakage. The phrenic nerve and anterior scalene muscle are identified following adipofascial flap elevation.

5. The transverse cervical artery and vein in the inferior plane of the adipofascial tissue are preserved if possible as they are potentially required as the recipient vessels for a vascularized ulnar nerve graft. The subclavian artery just beneath the scalene anterior muscle is carefully protected.

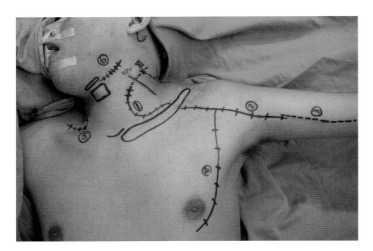

Fig. 36.8 Multiple incision lines for different purposes: (1) for supraclavicular brachial plexus exploration; (2) for infraclavicular brachial plexus exploration; (3) for Oberlin or Mackinnon method of nerve transfer; (4) for intercostal nerve dissection; (5) for contralateral C7 dissection; (6) for hypoglossal nerve dissection.

6. The fibrotic scalene anterior muscle can be segmentally or totally excised depending on the necessity to expose the more proximal spinal nerve in level 2 injury for intraoperative diagnosis and nerve manipulation.

7. Other anatomical landmarks are also helpful for localization:

- The nerve beneath the transverse cervical artery is usually C5 or the upper trunk.
- The nerve beneath the subclavian artery is C8 or the lower trunk.
- The first branch from the upper trunk is the suprascapular nerve, exiting from the plexus and traveling backward. The division beside the suprascapular nerve is the posterior division of the upper trunk, which travels in a posterior plane, while the anterior division of the upper trunk travels in an anterior plane.
- The spinal accessory (XI) nerve can be found through two ways: (1) dissection between the adipofascial tissue and platysma skin flap down to the trapezius muscle where the XI nerve lies in front of the trapezius muscle; or (2) extending the incision upward across the supraclavicular (sensory) nerves to locate the great auricular nerve, when the XI nerve will be seen within about one finger-breadth above the great auricular nerve, and beneath the sternocleidomatoid muscle. This can be confirmed by a nerve stimulator.

Landmarks and key points for infraclavicular dissection

- Chuang's angle (*Fig. 36.9*) is an angle shaped by the main branch of the cephalic vein on one side and the clavicle on the other side. Some of the deltoid and the clavicular part of pectoralis major muscle attachments can be detached to increase the angle zone. Under the clavicle is the subclavius muscle, and under the subclavius muscle is a space where the posterior cord, lateral cord, and suprascapular nerve can be seen. From this, the

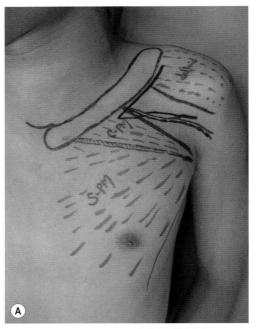

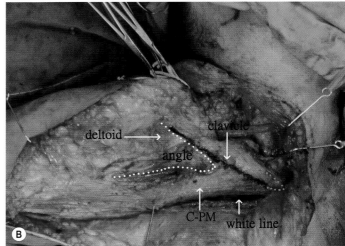

Fig. 36.9 (A, B) Chuang's angle: see text.

supraclavicular and infraclavicular fossa can be connected through this avascular plane which can be created by a finger dissection without fracturing the clavicle. The clavicle and the subclavius muscle are lifted together by a rolled gauze.

- The "white line" is an intermuscular septal line between the clavicular and sternal parts of pectoralis major muscle. Opening the line, the underlying pectoralis minor muscle and infraclavicular brachial plexus can be visualised. Some anatomical landmarks are also helpful for anatomical localization infraclavicularly. The first cord encountered beneath the proximal pectoralis minor muscle is the lateral cord. Y-shaped limbs from lateral and medial cords will become the median nerve. The subclavian artery can be easily found between the Y-shaped limbs. The posterior cord lying posterior to the subclavian artery has two terminal branches: the larger one is the radial nerve, and the smaller one is the axillary nerve.

- In the upper arm, the musculocutaneous nerve can usually be found between the biceps and coracobrachialis muscles. The musculocutaneous nerve will penetrate the proximal coracobrachialis muscle. Sometimes it has anatomical variation and comes from the median nerve.
- The axillary nerve in the axilla can be found at the humeral neck, above the tendinous portion of the teres major, accompanied by the lateral circumflex humeral artery.

Postoperative management and rehabilitation

Immediate postoperative splinting for 3 weeks is required after nerve grafts or nerve transfer. Thereafter, retraining and rehabilitation should start, including physiotherapy (to avoid joint stiffness), muscle stimulation (to delay muscle atrophy), brain cognition, biofeedback, and occupational therapy. Patients should be followed periodically by the surgeon (every 3–4 months) and the physical therapist (twice a month). Patients are encouraged to have electric muscle stimulation at home (twice a day). In cases of intercostal nerve transfer, passive shoulder elevation remains restricted to less than 90° for 6 months. Regular follow-up in the rehabilitation center and outpatient clinic is tremendously important, and should be explained to patients before and emphasized again after surgery. Induction exercises are important muscle exercises for patients with nerve transfer. Realizing the importance of these exercises is crucial. This explains why good results are commonly achieved by psychologically strong and ambitious patients who cooperate well in terms of their rehabilitation program, while poor results are often obtained by uncooperative patients. Permanent external orthosis to extend the interphalangeal joints of the fingers is always required for intrinsic palsy of the hand to improve the final result of surgical reconstruction and long rehabilitation programs.

Palliative reconstruction for sequelae deformities

Palliative reconstruction procedures include local muscle or tendon transfer, FFMT, tenodesis, and arthrodesis, or alternatively the use of orthotics and prosthetics. Palliative reconstruction can be considered when the injury involves C8 and T1 level (Klumpke's palsy in adults), or when deformities persist after maximum recovery either with or without nerve reconstruction.

Outcome evaluation

Although the British MRC scale provides the possibility of homogeneity and consensus in motor evaluation, a considerable degree of heterogeneity exists in the evaluation of functional recovery of the shoulder, elbow, and digits. In the author's opinion, establishing an international consensus on motor evaluation of different movements is vital and imperative for the advancement of our understanding and mutual comparison. The British MRC scheme is used for individual muscle evaluation in plexus injuries, or for evaluation

of the transferred muscle in FFMT. Both are evaluated by target joint movement.

Conclusion

Closed traction injuries of the brachial plexus are devastating injuries. For someone who has nothing, a little is a lot. Patients, especially those with total root avulsion, should be encouraged to recognize their disabilities and make use of the regained but not completely recovered limb. This may be shoulder elevation of 60°, M4 elbow flexion strength, and M2–3 strength of finger flexion. In a failed reconstruction, or if the patient perceives the injured limb as a useless dead weight, amputation may be considered as a last option.

Pediatric brachial plexus injury (obstetric brachial plexus palsy)

SYNOPSIS

- OBPP has two distinct phases: (1) infant OBPP (I-OBPP); and (2) sequelae OBPP (S-OBPP). There are significant differences in management and prognosis for the two phases, which should be discussed separately
- I-OBPP includes risk factors, clinical presentation, preoperative evaluation, timing of nerve surgery, surgical exploration of the brachial plexus, reconstructive strategies for nerve surgery, postoperative management, and outcomes assessment
- S-OBPP includes aberrant reinnervation, shoulder reconstruction, elbow reconstruction, and forearm and elbow reconstruction.

Introduction

Key points

- Obstetric brachial plexus palsy (OBPP) is an obstetric trauma: risk factors include overweight babies (>4000 grams) in cephalic presentation, underweight babies (<2500 grams) in breech presentation, or fetal distress (such as septicemia) with loss of protective muscular tone during cesarean section
- Infant OBPP focuses on nerve surgery, timing of surgery, and results from nerve surgery
- The sequelae of OBPP focus on palliative reconstruction for shoulder, elbow, and hand deformities

Pediatric BPI is termed OBPP. OBPP almost always results from obstetric trauma.

Overweight babies (>4000 grams) in cephalic presentation, underweight babies (<2500 grams) in breech presentation, and fetal distress (such as septicemia) with loss of protective muscular tone during cesarean section are all susceptible to BPI following delivery. It is caused by traction force during delivery which widens the angle between neck and shoulder and induces plexal nerve damage. The term "palsy", not "injury," as in adult BPI, has been used to describe obstetric BPI since the beginning of the 20th century: Thorburn described "obstetrical paralysis" in 1903,[36] and Kennedy described "birth palsy" in 1903.[37]

There are many differences between OBPP and adult BPI. The incidence of stretch (neurapraxia or axonotmesis) and incomplete rupture is more common in OBPP than in adult BPI, in which complete rupture or avulsion is often seen. Often there is paresis (incomplete paralysis) rather than flaccid paralysis (complete paralysis) in OBPP. Even when there is complete rupture, the gaps are short and spontaneous regeneration is still possible, while in adult BPI the gaps are long and the scars are dense, which makes spontaneous regeneration impossible. In OBPP, most are Erb's palsy (upper plexus injury), and the lesion is always supraclavicular. Mixed complex neuroma of the upper and middle trunk is frequently seen and motor recovery with misdirection (or aberrant reinnervation) often occurs in OBPP, particularly in the muscles innervated by the upper and middle trunks. Aberrant reinnervation causes abnormal co-contraction of multiple muscles, especially in the shoulder and elbow. Aberrant reinnervation diminishes function significantly, even in those patients considered to have had complete spontaneous recovery. This is why consequent deformities develop in OBPP and many require reconstruction. In adult BPI, the location of injury varies. Aberrant reinnervation occurs only in cases of penetrating injury of the upper trunk where trunk-to-trunk repair is performed directly or indirectly with short nerve grafts.

Furthermore, for the purpose of treatment, OBPP can be subdivided into two distinct phases: (1) I-OBPP, and (2) S-OBPP (or late OBPP with deformity).[38] These patients may present at any time and have a wide variation in clinical presentation. All stages have different management and prognosis. I-OBPP refers to the infant's brachial plexus that has been paralyzed following delivery. Some require early nerve surgery, and some do not. Reconstruction is focused on primary nerve surgery. S-OBPP refers to the sequelae deformities resulting from I-OBPP with or without previous nerve surgery. Many S-OBPP patients require surgical correction for the shoulder, elbow, forearm, and hand.[39–41] Reconstruction in S-OBPP is focused on palliative surgeries on bone or joint, tendon or muscle, and no longer on nerve surgery of the brachial plexus.

Infant obstetric brachial plexus palsy

Although the evolution of microsurgical nerve repair has significantly allowed surgeons to perform early intervention for I-OBPP, many rehabilitation therapists[42,43] and even some surgeons[44,45] continue to argue against early nerve surgery. Arguments against early surgery include high rates of spontaneous recovery (70–92% in the literature), high risks of surgery and postoperative care at an early age, and lack of significant functional improvement. Nevertheless, following developments in operative magnification (loop and microscope), refinements in nerve grafting and nerve transfer, comprehension of the brachial plexus anatomy, and pathophysiology of nerve degeneration and regeneration, more microsurgeons[46–50] have begun to choose early nerve surgery as the treatment of choice for I-OBPP. This group found that the rate of spontaneous recovery was actually low (7–50%), and early nerve surgery may potentially decrease or eliminate the late sequelae. The results from the author's

series[50] support that early nerve surgery, when indicated, is still the treatment of choice for I-OBPP patients. In addition, the reconstructions performed in the late group were found to be difficult, and required complex procedures to achieve reasonable results.[39–41]

Risk factors for I-OBPP during cephalic delivery include high birth body weight (>4000 grams), shoulder dystocia, cephalopelvic disproportion, forceps or vacuum suction delivery, or poor technique of delivery. I-OBPP may also occur during difficult breech presentation or in fetal distress (such as septicemia) during cesarean section. Associated injuries with birth palsy can be seen, including fracture (ipsilateral or contralateral clavicle, humerus, femur, or ribs), respiratory insufficiency (asphyxia) due to diaphragm palsy, ecchymosis (neck, chest, face, or upper back), and torticollis. Although the cause of I-OBPP is still subject to debate, (some believe it can be of intrauterine origin), the author believes that it is caused by obstetric trauma and not due to intrauterine compression neuropathy. All of the author's intraoperative findings in I-OBPP have been similar to adult brachial plexus traction injury (avulsion, rupture with neuroma, and mixed with muscles), not like pictures of compression neuropathy which present with pseudoneuroma and are rarely mixed with muscle fibers.

Clinical presentation

Determining the relationship between I-OBPP and S-OBPP and predicting the progressive changes in I-OBPP with age is a great challenge. Different surgeons have different opinions about clinical presentation of the I-OBPP: Adler and Patterson (three types),[51] Zancolli[52] (three types for I-OBPP and four types for S-OBPP), Narakas[53] (four groups, related to Sunderland's degree of nerve injury), Grossman et al.[54] (three types), Hentz[55] (three groups), or Kawabata[56] (four types related to mode of delivery and type of paralysis). A more detailed evaluation system for I-OBPP should be made in the future to predict the natural history of I-OBPP. It can also be an important reference for decision-making to treat conservatively or to operate primarily.

In unoperated cases, Erb's palsy (Fig. 36.10) is much more common than global palsy. Many Erb's palsy patients initially show global palsy, but over time this becomes Erb's palsy. However, in operated cases, this is reversed, and global palsy is more common than Erb's palsy. Klumpke's palsy is rarely seen, in only about 1% (Fig. 36.11). In about 1% of I-OBPP cases, the injury is bilateral but predominantly on one side, and it is frequently seen in breech delivery or cesarean section with fetal distress.

Clinical examination

Newborns are difficult to examine thoroughly. A precise muscle or sensory examination of an infant is impossible. The evaluation chart used for adult BPI (Fig. 36.5) is not practical. Evaluation should include parents' observation at home, especially during bathing or dressing, and examiner's observation in clinic. The infant is placed in the lateral decubitus position with the normal side down. The examiner then tickles the baby (tickling test: Fig. 36.12A), or covers the infant's face with a towel (towel test: Fig. 36.12B) and uses this to evaluate dynamic movements of the infant's shoulder, elbow, and

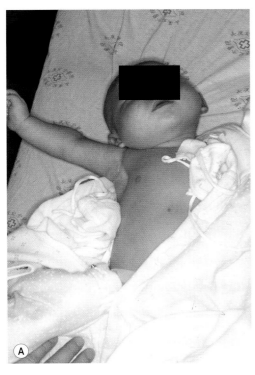
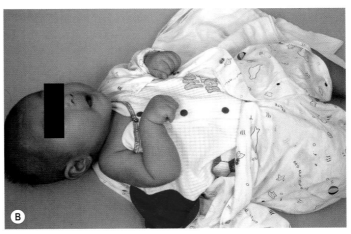

Fig. 36.10 (A) A 2-month-old infant showed improving shoulder abduction of his right upper limb; **(B)** a 3-month-old infant shows improving elbow flexion of her right upper limb. Both were cases of Erb's palsy without primary nerve surgery.

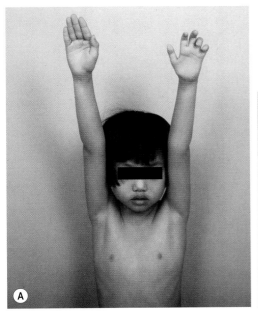
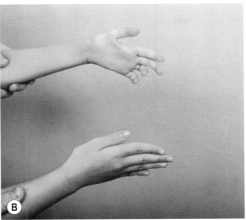

Fig. 36.11 (A, B) A 4-year-old girl shows Klumpke's palsy of her right upper limb.

hand. An M2 muscle strength score (movement with weight eliminated) in a newborn infant is sufficient to predict a good result when the infant grows. In I-OBPP, there is no need to see M4 or M5 muscle strength, as in adult BPI.[46] Horner's sign with ptosis or miosis may disappear with time, indicating that the T1 has a stretch but not an avulsion injury, or that T1 has a good connection with T2 (postfixed brachial plexus). An ipsilateral clavicle fracture is usually a good prognostic sign due to traction force divergence. However, a contralateral clavicle fracture is usually a bad prognostic sign, as this indicates a high-energy traction force. Ideally the infant should be followed up after birth and then at 1-month intervals until the decision to operate or not is made.

Neurodiagnostic studies are not performed routinely. EMG in I-OBPP is usually positive and too optimistic, and may not be accurate enough to predict useful function. Even

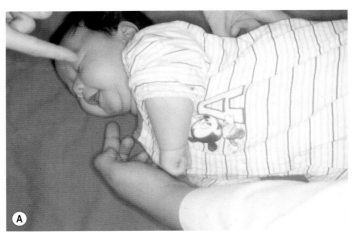
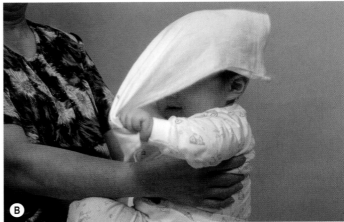

Fig. 36.12 **(A)** Tickling test; and **(B)** towel test to examine infant obstetric brachial plexus palsy.

intraoperative EMGs can be misleading. Improving techniques of MRI are now useful to evaluate level 1 and 2 lesions as in adult BPI, and are becoming our routine investigation for preoperative imaging *(Fig. 36.13)*. CT myelograms can also be useful.

Timing of surgery

Gilbert[57] recommends surgical intervention for infants without evidence of elbow flexion by 3 months. Clarke and Curtis[58] advocate that failure to perform a "cookie test" to place a cookie in the mouth by 9 months of age is an indication for exploration. Terzis and Papakonstantinou[59] emphasize that the presence of total palsy with Horner's syndrome warrants earlier surgical intervention at 2 months of age. Our results[50] indicate that shoulder and elbow recovery were not different when surgery was performed at 2 months or at 11 months of age. Even patients who received primary nerve surgery beyond 1 year of age also showed significant improvement in shoulder and elbow function, but no improvement at all in hand function. In addition, our previous results showed similar improvement of shoulder function in late palliative reconstructions for late OBPP patients compared to those who underwent primary early nerve surgery for I-OBPP.[39] However, recovery of hand function with secondary reconstructive methods was far inferior to those who had early nerve surgery for hand function.[41] The ideal opportunity for improving hand function is by performing nerve surgery early. Our results demonstrate that Gilbert's "rule of 3 months" overestimates the poor results of shoulder and elbow function.[57] However, Clarke and Curtis's "rule of 9 months" underestimates the poor results of forearm and hand function.[58] The presence of poor shoulder and elbow function in I-OBPP is not an urgent indication for surgery. However, hand palsy is an urgent condition, indicating early surgical intervention. Therefore, our recommended timing of surgery falls between that of Gilbert and Clarke. A global palsy with absence of biceps function and little or no hand function is an indication for early exploration within 3 months. However, in the presence of wrist extension and finger flexion, an additional 3 months of observation is recommended. If by 6 months of age

there continues to be no improvement in elbow flexion, then exploration is indicated. If poor shoulder or elbow function persists by 1 year of age, surgery is indicated too. However, poor hand function at this late age is not an indication for exploration as it is too late. The observation of M2 wrist extension or interphalangeal extension on clinical examination may imply that C7 may be injured (more often with avulsion), but C8 and T1 are intact, warranting an additional 3-month period of observation till the child reaches 6 months.

Preoperative preparation

Treating an OBPP patient is treating the whole family. A thorough explanation of the risks and benefits of surgery to the patient's family is very important, including preoperative diagnosis, surgical risks, postoperative care and rehabilitation, long-term follow-up, possible outcomes, and possible subsequent operations. After intubation, central venous pressure and arterial lines with long catheters should be secured in the femoral vessels. Those two vessel lines are crucial during the operation and for the first 3 days of postoperative care.

Surgical technique

Incision lines, dissection, and brachial plexus exploration are all similar to adult BPI, except:

1. The platysma in infants is very thin and scarce, resulting in an incision directly superficial to the surface of the sternocleidomastoid muscle.

2. The phrenic nerve should be isolated and well protected. Care should be taken during the operation to avoid excessive traction as this may prolong the extubation time due to transient palsy of the diaphragm.

3. The scalenus anterior muscle is usually excised, permitting exposure of the level 2 spinal nerves and release of compression of the subclavian artery.

4. All spinal nerves, C5–T1, should be identified and examined.

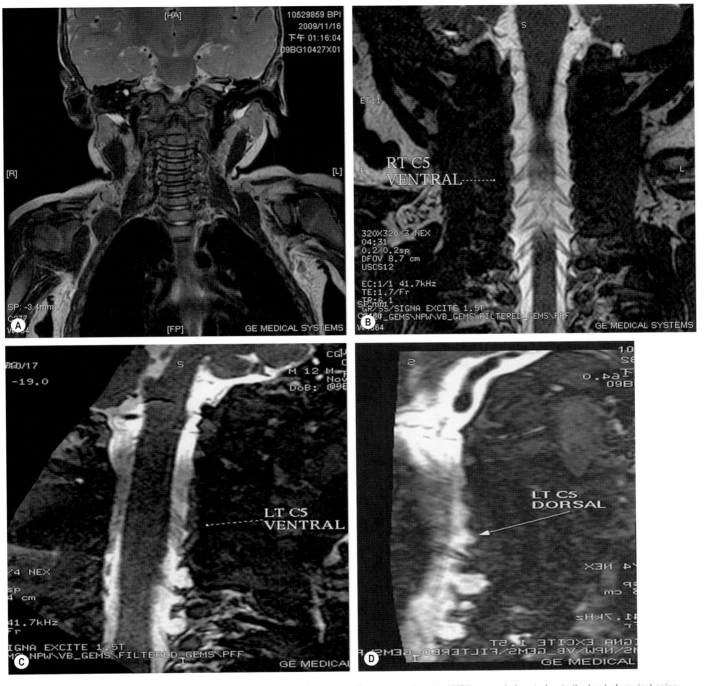

Fig. 36.13 A 3-month-old infant with obstetric brachial plexus palsy. **(A)** T2 magnetic resonance imaging (MRI), coronal view: to locate the level of cervical spine; **(B)** three-dimensional (3D) MRI, coronal view, T2: normal on right side; 3D MRI: fast imaging employing steady-state acquisition and curve planar reformat techniques: **(C)** ventral roots and **(D)** dorsal root showing left C7–C8–T1 root avulsion.

5. Lesion-in-continuity of the upper and middle trunks is commonly seen, requiring microneurolysis to evaluate the severity of scarring and judge the degree of nerve injury. If the scar is dense, resection of the neuroma and nerve grafts are required.

6. When the lesions are more distal involving the divisions (level 3 injury), the incision is then extended to the deltopectoral groove, exposing Chuang's angle *(Fig. 36.9)*.

The supra- and infraclavicular fossa are connected by opening the space under the subclavius muscle. The clavicle can be elevated easily without clavicle osteotomy.

7. Nerve grafts are commonly harvested from the both sural and saphenous nerves. If necessary, the medial cutaneous nerve of the arm, superficial radial nerve, and lateral antebrachi cutaneous nerve from the injured limb are other sources.

Reconstructive strategies

Two groups of spinal nerve injury are classified based on intraoperative findings: (1) pure rupture injury (40%, 47/118); and (2) rupture injury associated with root avulsion (60%, 71/118) *(Table 36.8)*. C5 and C6 tend to be ruptured; but C8–T1 tend to be avulsed *(Table 36.9)*. If C8 is avulsed, T1 tends to be avulsed also, but only partially. Once C8–T1 avulsion occurs, a ruptured C7 tends to have more proximal avulsion injury too. In global palsy, the incidence of three-trunk rupture is about 5% (6/119). Preoperative MRI can be very helpful as a diagnostic tool to visualize level 1 or 2 injury.

Pure rupture injury

Except 6 patients who had rupture of all three trunks, the majority of patients (41 patients, 41/47, 87%) had rupture injury involving the upper and/or middle trunk. The reconstructive procedures consisted of microneurolysis and nerve grafts. Reconstructive strategies in these pure rupture injury groups varied based on intraoperative findings and judgment. The majority of patients received C5 nerve grafting to the suprascapular nerve and posterior division of the upper trunk for shoulder function, and C6 nerve grafting to the anterior division of the upper trunk for elbow function instead of proximal upper trunk nerve grafting to the distal upper trunk. Four to six cable nerve grafts (2–3 cm in length) are usually required for coaptation. A ruptured C7 has a high incidence of accompanying avulsion. The proximal stump of C7 was therefore routinely repaired to the distal stump of C7 via nerve grafts. There were few patients who received longer nerve grafting (4–6 cm in length) from supraclavicular spinal nerves to the infraclavicular selected target nerves (posterior

and lateral cord). *Table 36.10* shows our reconstructive strategies for pure rupture injury.

Rupture injury associated with root avulsion

A total of 72 patients (60%) were included in this series. Once avulsion occurs it tends to involve at least two roots (75%). This type of reconstruction depends on the number of root avulsions, and the remaining proximal neural resources. In global palsy, restoration of hand function becomes the first priority, followed by elbow flexion and then shoulder function. C5 is usually ruptured, not avulsed *(Table 36.9)*. The proximal C5 stump can be a source for selective neurotization to the C8 or lower trunk (intraplexus neurotization). The frequency of nerve transfers increases if associated root avulsion increases, including intercostal nerve transfer for elbow or finger flexion, XI nerve transfer for the shoulder, or intraplexus transfer from C5 or C6 to the C8 or median nerve for hand function in three- or four-root avulsion. Intercostal nerve transfer, either to the musculocutaneous nerve for elbow, or to the median nerve for hand function, is an effective procedure in infant patients (much better than in adults). Few patients require contralateral C7 transfer, branch of ulnar nerve transfer (Oberlin method[60]), or combined branch of median nerve (Mackinnon method[61]) transfer. *Table 36.11* shows our reconstructive strategies for rupture injury associated with root avulsion.

In this series of patients, 10 cases of I-OBPP were operated on later, at 1 year of age or older (range, 1 year to 2 years 6 months). Most of these patients had shown poor spontaneous recovery of shoulder and/or elbow function prior to surgery. Primary nerve surgery for these late operative cases showed encouraging results in shoulder and elbow function recovery, but few gained recovery of hand function.

Postoperative management

A rigid premade neck splint is placed on every patient immediately postoperatively *(Fig. 36.14)*. Total operative time is on average 8 hours, with a range of 6–10 hours. Postoperatively, the patient is transferred to the intensive care unit after extubation. The patient is cared for in the head-up position to avoid dyspnea due to any temporary palsy of the diaphragm. The patient is kept in the intensive care unit for 3–5 days, and

---

Table 36.8 Intraoperative findings of obstetric brachial plexus palsy (1992–2004, Chang Gung Memorial Hospital)

Ruptured injury alone		47 (40%)
Rupture of UT	17	
Rupture of UT and MT	24	
Rupture of UT, MT, and LT	6	
Rupture and avulsion injury		72 (60%)
One-root avulsion	18	
Two-root avulsion	28	
Three-root avulsion	17	
Four-root avulsion	9	
Total		119

UT, upper trunk; MT, middle trunk; LT, lower trunk.

Table 36.9 Incidence of type of injury on different spinal nerves (1992–2004, Chang Gung Memorial Hospital)

	Rupture	Avulsion
C5	117	12
C6	95	42
C7	49	79
C8	9	71
T1	8	39

Table 36.10 Reconstructive strategies for isolated rupture injury

Trunk rupture	Nerve reconstructive strategy
Upper trunk	C5-ng-SS and PD C6-ng-AD
Upper and middle	C5-ng-SS and PD C6-ng-AD C7-ng-C7
Upper and middle and lower	C5-ng-SS and PD C6-ng-AD C7-ng-C7 LT-ng-LT

UT, upper trunk; ng, nerve graft; SS, suprascapular nerve; PD, posterior division; AD, anterior division of the upper trunk; LT, lower trunk.

Table 36.11 Nerve reconstructive strategy for rupture injury associated with root avulsion

Root avulsion		Nerve reconstructive strategy		
		For shoulder	For elbow	For hand
One	C5	XI-SS	C6-ng- (major) AD and (minor) PD	
	C7	C5-ng-SS and PD	C6-ng- AD	C5, C6 (minor)-C7
	C8	C5-ng-SS and PD	T3–5 ICN-MCn	C6-ng-C8 (C7-ng-C7)
	T1	C5-ng-SS and PD	C6-ng-AD	C7-ng-C7; C8-ng-C8
Two	C5 and C6	XI-SS	T3–5ICN-MCN	C8-ng-C8
	C6 and C7	XI-SS	C5-ng-C6	C6-ng-C8
	C7 and C8	XI-SS	T3–5ICN-MCN	C6-ng-C8 (or median)
	C8 and T1(8)	XI-SS	T3–5ICN-MCN	(C7-ng-C7)
Three	C5–7	XI-SS	T3–5ICN-MCN	
	C6–8	XI-SS	T3–5ICN-MCN	C5-ng-median
	C7, C8, and T1	C6-ng-SS and PD	T3–5ICN-MCN	C5-ng-median
Four	C6–T1	C5-ng-SS and PD	T3–4 ICN- MCN	T5–7ICN-median
		C5-ng-SS and PD	T3–5ICN-MCN	CC7T-ng-C8

XI, spinal accessory nerve; ng, nerve graft; SS, suprascapular nerve; MCN, musculocutaneous nerve; PD, posterior division; AD, anterior division of the upper trunk.

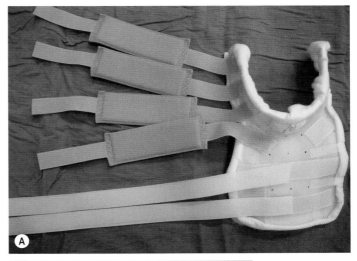

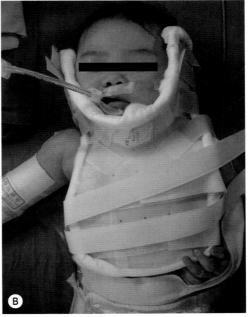

Fig. 36.14 (A, B) Postoperative neck splint.

then transferred to the general ward for an additional 2 days. Total hospitalization is approximately 1 week.

The neck splint is kept in place for 4 weeks. Follow-up at regular intervals (the first month postoperatively and then every 4 months afterwards) is performed for a minimum of 4 years. Home electrical muscle stimulation (twice daily for 15–20 minutes each) is started 4 weeks after surgery and performed for approximately 1 year or until muscle function reaches M2 level.

There are two important exercises for prevention of shoulder adduction contracture and forearm supination contracture: pull-up bar exercise (stretching exercise) and swimming (dynamic exercise), where both upper limbs are exercised simultaneously.

Outcome assessment

There is a lack of consensus with regard to the optimal method of assessing results. This is partly due to the complexity of the lesions (i.e., aberrant reinnervation), complexity of the repair (i.e., different surgical strategies), complexity of limb involvement (shoulder, elbow, forearm, and hand), and finally, the young age of the patients, which makes cooperation difficult. The reported methods of functional assessment include MRC muscle grading system, Gilbert and Tassin muscle grading system, Clarke and Curtis active movement scale, Narakas' grading system, and others.[58] The following are the author's methods of outcomes assessment. All patients should be followed for a minimum of 4 years. The results are categorized as "good", "fair," or "poor" based on the degree of shoulder abduction, external rotation, elbow flexion and extension, and finger flexion (*Table 36.12*).

Results

The overall results in C5 nerve grafting, especially to the suprascapular nerve and posterior division of the upper trunk for shoulder, and C6 nerve grafting to the anterior division of the upper trunk for elbow function, were consistently good

(Fig. 36.15): shoulder abduction averaged 132° (90–180°), shoulder external rotation averaged 67° (50–90°), and elbow flexion was mostly M3. More than half of the patients (71/118: 60%) had rupture injury associated with at least one nerve root avulsion; 75% had at least two-root avulsion. Intraplexus nerve transfer from C5, or C6 to C8 or to the median nerve, resulted in improvement of hand function. Extraplexus nerve transfer by intercostal nerve transfer to the musculocutaneous nerve or median nerve and spinal accessory nerve transfer to the suprascapular nerve have proved useful for restoring shoulder abduction and elbow and finger flexion *(Fig. 36.16)*.

Table 36.12 Postoperative functional assessment of obstetric brachial plexus palsy

	Good	Fair	Poor
Shoulder abduction	>120°	90–120°	<90°
Shoulder external rotation	>90°	60–90°	<60°
(hand to occiput movement)	(occipital line)	(ear line)	(preface or prechest)
Elbow flexion			
Hand to mouth movement	Easy (M = 3)	Difficult (M = 2)	Impossible (M < 2)
Elbow extension	Easy (M = 3)	Difficult (M = 2)	Impossible (M < 2)
Finger flexion	Easy (M = 3)	Difficult (M = 2)	Impossible (M < 2)

Sequelae obstetric brachial plexus palsy

Aberrant regeneration (due to misdirection of regenerated axons), muscular imbalance, and growth are the three main causes of shoulder and elbow deformity following primary OBPP with or without nerve surgery. Flaccid paralysis of the shoulder and elbow is rare, but flaccid paralysis is commonly seen in the forearm and hand due to root avulsion of C7–T1 without aberrant regeneration. Aberrant reinnervation more frequently occurs in the shoulder and elbow and less in the hand. Therefore, contractures (or hypertrophy) of the teres major, pectoralis major, brachialis and biceps muscles are frequently seen and cause the deformity of the shoulder and elbow. In addition, growth is another factor in shoulder and elbow deformities, often found in the form of concomitant skeletal deformity.

There are four main types of co-contractions resulting from aberrant reinnervation causing different types of deformities of the shoulder and elbow:

1. Co-contraction between shoulder abductors (supraspinatus, infraspinatus, and deltoid) and adductors (mainly teres major and pectoralis major). This will result in limitation of shoulder elevation. Shoulder adduction contracture (or internal rotation) will develop when growing.

2. Co-contraction between elbow flexors (biceps and brachialis) and elbow extensors (triceps). In the mild type, patients are unable to perform elbow flexion normally, such as pulling up trousers, hand-to-flank or hand-to-spine movement. In the severe type, patients cannot even perform a hand-to-mouth movement. Flexion contracture of the elbow eventually develops.

3. Co-contraction between elbow flexors (mainly brachialis) and shoulder abductors (mainly deltoid). When asked to

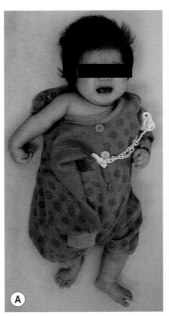
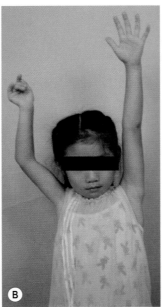
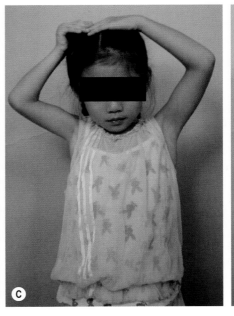
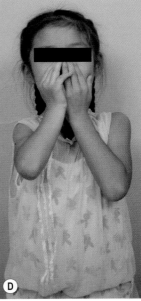

Fig. 36.15 Example of rupture of upper and middle trunks. A 3-month-old infant had right brachial plexus injury **(A)**, receiving nerve grafts from C5 to the suprascapular nerve and posterior division of the upper trunk for the shoulder, C6 to the anterior division of the upper trunk for the elbow, and C7 to C7 due to rupture injury of the upper and middle trunks without C8–T1 avulsion. Six years after, she shows good shoulder abduction **(B)**, good shoulder external rotation **(C)**, and M4 elbow flexion **(D)** following one-stage early nerve surgery. There is no aberrant reinnervation between shoulder and elbow.

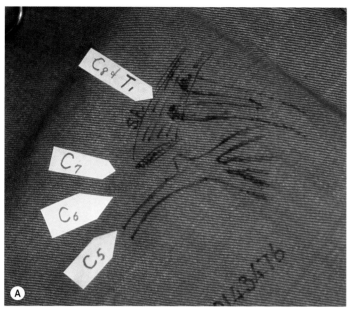

Fig. 36.16 Example of C5 rupture and C6–T1 root avulsion. **(A)** A 3-month-old infant had right brachial plexus injury, receiving primary nerve surgery with nerve grafts from C5 to the suprascapular nerve and posterior division of the upper trunk, nerve transfers from T3–4 two intercostal nerves to the musculocutaneous nerve for elbow, and T5–8 four intercostal nerves to the median nerve. Seven years after he shows **(B)** acceptable shoulder elevation, **(C)** M4 elbow flexion, and **(D, E)** M3 finger flexion.

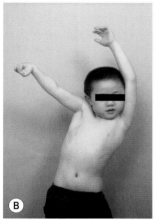
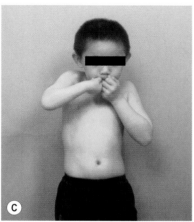
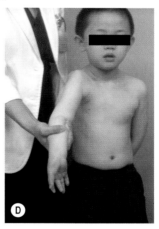
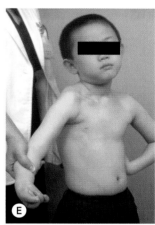

perform a hand-to-mouth movement, the shoulder will be involuntarily elevated, similar to blowing a trumpet (trumpet sign). With this deformity if the arm-to-body angle is less than 40°, mild cross-innervation is present; if the angle is more than 80°, severe cross-innervation is predicted.

4. Co-contraction among shoulder abductors, elbow flexors, and forearm flexors. When asked to perform shoulder elevation, the elbow and fingers flex involuntarily.

A chart for S-OBPP examination *(Table 36.13)* should be completed before planning the reconstructive strategy for the sequelae deformities of shoulder, elbow, and hand. For motor recovery with aberrant reinnervation, release of contracted muscles and augmentation of paretic muscles form the basis of surgical intervention.[39,40]

Shoulder deformity reconstruction

Before 1968, palliative reconstruction for S-OBPP with shoulder deformity was focused on the anatomical deformity (subluxation or posterior dislocation of the shoulder). Osteotomy of the humerus, or release of the contracted internal rotator muscles (concept of muscle fibrosis due to delivery trauma), such as the subscapularis, pectoralis major, or long head of biceps,[62–64] was preferred, but the results were disappointing. These techniques improved only the patient's cosmetic appearance, but not the function. Some authors performed transfer of local muscles such as the trapezius or levator scapulae muscles, to restore some shoulder abduction,[48] using the concept of dynamic reconstruction for muscular imbalance. However, the concept of aberrant reinnervation has now been well accepted by the author as the main cause of shoulder deformity in S-OBPP.[39] All reconstructive methods should be aimed at minimizing the influence of aberrant reinnervation. If preoperative physical examination demonstrates the existence of muscle recovery by aberrant regeneration, the author's studies demonstrate that the following procedures are useful for shoulder abduction: (1) release of antagonistic muscles (pectoralis major and teres major muscles); and (2) augmentation of paretic muscles (transferring teres major to the infraspinatus muscle,

Table 36.13 Special Chart for S-OBPP Examination

Name: Chart No: age:

Address:

Date of exam: History:

Site of injury: R   L

Shoulder Function

Shoulder Abduction (Deltoid, SS): _____degree ; M_____ (muscle strength)

Cross innervation: PM, TM (+ LD); Biceps, Triceps; Forearm (Flexors, extensors)

Shoulder External Rotation (IS, T minor): (without support)_____ degree

(with support)_____ degree

Shoulder Internal Rotation (PM, TM, Subscapul): M_____

Elbow Function

Elbow flexion (Biceps, Brachialis): M_____ , degree_____

   Cross innervation: Deltoid, Triceps, Forearm flexors

Brachioradials : M_____; Triceps function: M_____

Forearm supination: _____degree; Forearm pronation: _____degree

Hand to occipital (forearm pronation, elbow flexion, shoulder abduction and external rotation) Pre-chest; Pre-face; Pre-ear; Ear; Postauricular

Hand to mouth (forearm supination, elbow flexion, shoulder abduction and external rotation) Chest; chin; mouth

Trumpet sign: marked (>80°); partial (40 – 80°); mild (< 40°)

Hand to abdomen (forearm neutral, elbow flexion, shoulder internal rotation)

   not possible   difficult   easy

Hand to spine (forearm pronation, elbow flexion, shoulder post flexion and abduction)

   not possible   difficult   easy

Hand to flank

   not possible   difficult   easy

Hand to object (forearm pronation, elbow extension, shoulder ant flexion)

   not possible   difficult   easy

Hand Function

Wrist Extension: (ECRL, ECRB, ECU)

Flexion : (FCR, PL, FCU, Finger flexors)

Finger Extension (EDC): mass, individual: 2nd, 3rd, 4th, 5th

Finger Extension (Intrinsic mm): 2nd, 3rd, 4th, 5th

Finger Flexion (FDS, FDP): active, passive;

     mass, individual: 2nd, 3rd, 4th, 5th

Thumb: FPL

    EPL

    APL

    Lateral pinch (when pronated forearm) (ulnar)

    Opposition (median): partial, full

Sensation disturbance: ☐ No

      ☐ Yes _____

Others: dislocation of shoulder, proximal radial head, proximal ulnar head, distal radials, distal ulna

Contracture: _____

		Lesioned	Intact
Length:	Acromion-lateral epicondyle	———-	———
	lateral epicondyle-radial styloid	———-	———
	radial styoid-long finger tip	———-	———
Circumference:	deltoid prominence	———-	———
	midarm	———-	———
	upper forearm prominence	———-	———
	midpalm	———-	———

Planning:

rerouting both ends of the clavicular part of the pectoralis major muscle laterally). In addition, latissimus dorsi transfer to the teres minor insertion (or lateral humerus) is beneficial for shoulder external rotation. The ideal age for the reconstruction is between 4 and 10 years. The average shoulder abduction following the muscle transposition was 151° (average gain 77°), and that of external rotation was 72° (average gain 48°). Comparing with the S-OBPP patients who had no surgery and with early nerve surgery for I-OBPP, the outcomes of our reconstructive strategy for the shoulder appear to be significantly improved.[39]

Elbow deformity reconstruction

The common deformities of the elbow in S-OBPP include: (1) aberrant reinnervation between elbow flexors and extensors, which causes weak elbow extension and weak elbow flexion; (2) aberrant reinnervation between shoulder abductors and elbow flexors, resulting in a severe "trumpet sign" with angles greater than 80° between the medial arm and trunk on hand-to-mouth movement; and (3) no motor recovery with muscle paralysis or paresis of biceps and brachialis muscles.[40] Traditionally, elbow flexion is always the top priority and triceps-to-biceps transfer is a commonly used method for achieving elbow flexion. However, this will result in loss of elbow extension, a significant functional problem for a growing child and which is especially frustrating when shoulder elevation has been restored after shoulder correction. In addition, the loss of muscular imbalance at the elbow frequently leads to progressive flexion contracture (40°, range, 30–70°) and/or dislocation at the elbow. Restoration of elbow extension following triceps-to-biceps transfer has been disappointing, whether performed by regional muscle transfer (such as latissimus dorsi transfer) or by free muscle transplantation. Because of these drawbacks, we have discontinued use of the triceps-to-biceps transfer. For motor recovery with aberrant reinnervation between elbow flexors and extensors, reconstruction of elbow extension should precede that of elbow flexion. This is achieved either by biceps-to-triceps transfer (with preservation of an intact brachialis muscle) or by brachialis-to-triceps transfer (with preservation of an intact biceps when elbow shows flexion contracture).[40] Half of our patients can achieve acceptable elbow flexion and extension in a single-stage procedure. The other half require a second-stage procedure either by FFMT or by a Steindler flexorplasty. Existence of brachioradialis muscle power is a determining factor. A powerful brachioradialis can decrease the need for the second procedure.

In patients with a paralyzed biceps due to C5–7 root avulsion, Steindler flexorplasty or FFMT[65] is the option for restoration of elbow function. When shoulder–elbow co-contraction is a major issue, the anterior half of the deltoid is transferred to the distal biceps tendon with a fascia lata graft for biceps augmentation to decrease the "trumpet angle." However, patients with intrinsic deformities of the elbow joint (i.e., dislocation of the radial and/or ulnar head) are not good candidates for the above-mentioned regional elbow muscle transfer. Altered joint anatomy and abnormal joint biomechanics may create instability of the elbow joint, which contributes to untoward results in these patients. In patients with deformities of the shoulder and elbow due to motor recovery by aberrant

regeneration, simultaneous reconstruction of the shoulder and elbow can be safely performed (video 2).

Forearm and hand deformity reconstruction

S-OBPP in the forearm and hand includes weakness or absence of wrist or metacarpophalangeal or interphalangeal joint extension; weakness or absence of finger flexion; forearm supination or, less commonly, pronation contracture; ulnar deviation of the wrist; dislocation of the radius or ulna; thumb instability; or sensory disturbance of the hand.[41] Palliative reconstruction of these forearm and hand problems is more difficult than for the shoulder or elbow because of the lack of powerful regional muscles for transfer. The phenomenon of aberrant reinnervation is less significant. Continuous physical therapy with a rehabilitation program to optimize the residual muscle strength in the forearm and hand is vital for later management. Surgical treatment is highly individualized. The optimal age for forearm and hand reconstruction is therefore usually later (school age, 6–13 years old) than for shoulder and elbow reconstruction (preschool years, 4–6 years old).

Multiple procedures for forearm and hand function are often performed. Sometimes they are done simultaneously with reconstructive procedures to improve shoulder and/or elbow function. Traditional tendon transfer techniques do not provide satisfactory reconstruction for these deformities. Many of the author's patients required more complex techniques such as FFMT[66] to augment traditional techniques of tendon and/or bone management.

For wrist and metacarpophalangeal joint extension, powerful wrist or finger flexors and/or pronator teres can be useful donor muscles for flexor-to-extensor transfers. Sometimes two wrist flexors, flexor carpi radialis and palmaris longus, are woven together, becoming a more powerful unit, and are transferred to the extensor digitorum communis to achieve both wrist and finger extension. For forearm supination contractures, rerouting the biceps muscle, as described by Zancolli and Zancolli,[67] is effective for mild cases. For weakness or absence of finger flexion, wrist extensors are usually too weak to be transferred. FFMT for flexor digitorum profundus replacement using intercostal nerves as the donor nerve is required. Sensory disturbance of the forearm and hand in late OBPP seems a minor problem and further sensory reconstruction is unnecessary.

Conclusion

In I-OBPP, early primary nerve surgery provides therapeutic advantages. Surgery within 3 months is strongly indicated in patients with total palsy, but only relatively indicated for patients without elbow flexion but good hand function. Better results can be achieved when numerous short nerve grafts are used for rupture injuries. Cases associated with multiple root avulsions benefit from intraplexus nerve transfer for hand function and extraplexus nerve transfer for shoulder and/or elbow function. This approach provides patients with a one-stage functional reconstruction of the upper limb.

In S-OBPP, secondary reconstruction for shoulder and elbow deformities can achieve acceptable function. For forearm and hand deformities, surgical treatment and outcomes are highly individualized, and multiple procedures are often required.

Access the complete references list online at **http://www.expertconsult.com**

5. Alnot JY. Traumatic paralysis of the brachial plexus: preoperative problems and therapeutic indications. In: Terzis JK, ed. *Microreconstruction of Nerve Injuries*. Philadelphia: WB Saunders; 1987:331.

   The author describes brachial plexus injury in detail, including anatomy, diagnosis, and treatment. For a novice surgeon who is interested in brachial plexus treatment, this is a good article to read and understand.

6. Chuang DCC. Adult brachial plexus injuries. In: Mathes SJ, Hentz VR, eds. *Plastic Surgery*. Philadelphia: Saunders Elsevier; 2006:515.

   The author describes brachial plexus injury in great detail including anatomy, diagnosis, treatment, and conclusion. There are multiple useful surgical tips. To a beginner who is interested in brachial plexus treatment, this is a good article to read in order to gain confidence.

12. Slingluff CL, Terzis JK, Edgerton MT. The quantitative microanatomy of the brachial plexus in man. Reconstructive relevance. In: Terzis JK, ed. *Microreconstruction of nerve injuries*. Philadelphia: WB Saunders; 1987:285.

   This is an important article because quantitative microanatomy of the brachial plexus is described. After reading it, many questions related to brachial plexus anatomy will be answered.

14. Chuang DCC. Adult brachial plexus reconstruction with the level of injury: review and personal experience. *Plast Reconstr Surg*. 2009;124(suppl):359e.

   This article presents a simple classification system in terms of numbered levels. This easy system may become a universal classification of brachial plexus injury.

58. Clarke HM, Curtis CG. Examination and prognosis. In: Gilbert A, ed. *Brachial Plexus Injuries*. London: Martin Dunitz; 2001:159–172.

   The authors describe birth palsy in detail, including initial evaluation and assessment, classification, prognosis for recovery, indications for surgery, and assessment of surgical results.

37

Restoration of upper extremity function in tetraplegia

Catherine Curtin and Vincent R. Hentz

SYNOPSIS

- For people with tetraplegia, restoration of independence is the primary goal.
- Treatment must be individualized because neurologic deficits vary greatly between patients and within individuals (one arm is different from the other).
- The hands of people with tetraplegia represent a critical residual resource.
- Restoration of function requires a multifaceted approach combining physical therapy, assistive devices, and surgery. including tendon transfer, tenodesis, functional electric stimulation and arthrodesis.
- These procedures have been shown to improve functional independence.[1,2]
- These procedures are underutilized.[3]
- Strengthening connections between spinal cord injury specialists and upper limb surgeons represents an opportunity to improve access to this care.

Introduction

Surgery on the upper limb of people with tetraplegia requires special consideration because the hand represents a critical residual resource.[4] Their upper limbs take on new functions different from any other patient in that they must "walk on their hands." Given the importance of the upper limb, surgery must be carefully planned and be the culmination of a long rehabilitative process involving a team. The patient must understand what can be accomplished and realize that the functional improvements will not result in a "normal arm" but as Dr Sterling Bunnell, the father of upper limb surgery in the United States said, "for those who have nothing a little is a lot."[5]

Basic science/disease process

Today, the most common mechanisms of cervical spine injury (SCI) are motor vehicle accidents, falls, especially in the elderly, and sports injuries. The functional consequences are primarily determined by the anatomic level of and the completeness of the injury. Modern acute care of these injuries has so progressed that almost all survive their injury and thus face a lifetime in a greatly altered state of existence. Every tetraplegic patient suffers some loss of upper limb function and for most, their upper limbs represent, aside from their brain, their most important functional asset.

Though the upper limb surgeon often does not participate in the initial management of the SCI patient, the acute rehabilitation focuses on the upper limbs. Special care is taken to prevent the onset of contractures of fingers, wrist, or elbow. Even a relatively mild elbow contracture can inhibit independent transfers.[6] Fortunately, well-educated therapists are aware of the need for protective splinting right after injury. The shoulder must also be protected as the patient learns to adjust to their injury. Pulling patients, poor posture, or falls can result in shoulder injuries that ultimately limit independence. Indeed the majority of people with tetraplegia have shoulder pain at the end of their acute rehabilitation.[7] Early attention to the upper limb provides the best long-term function.

Classification of the tetraplegic upper extremity

Cervical spinal cord injury has been classified in many ways, including by the skeletal level of injury or according to the most distal remaining functioning cervical root. However, this classification system is too general for hand surgeons because no two patients are exactly alike. Injury pattern can differ between those with the same skeletal level of injury and each patient often has different function between the right and left

Table 37.1 International classification for surgery of the hand in tetraplegia

Sensibility	Motor	Description
O or Cu group	Characteristics	Function
0	No muscles below elbow suitable for transfer	Flexion/supination of elbow
1	Br	
2	ECRL	Extension of wrist (weak or strong)
3	ECRB	Extension of wrist
4	PT	Extension and pronation of wrist
5	FCR	Flexion of wrist
6	Finger extensors	Extrinsic extension of fingers, partial or complete
7	Thumb extension	Extrinsic extension of the thumb
8	Partial digital flexors	Extrinsic flexion of the fingers, weak
9	Lacks only intrinsics	Extrinsic flexion of the fingers
X	Exceptions	

Caution: it is not possible to determine ECRB strength without surgical exposure.
Br, brachioradialis; ECRL, extensor carpi radialis longus; ECRB, extensor carpi radialis brevis; PT, pronator teres; FCR, flexor carpi radialis.

arm. In order to develop useful recommendations for treatment of the upper limb, it was necessary to develop a more precise method for classifying the upper limb in the tetraplegic patient. From these needs arose the International Classification, which is based on the limb's remaining useful motor and sensory resources *(Table 37.1)*. The motor function assesses the number of strong muscles under volitional control below the elbow. To be counted, the muscle must have grade 4 or 5 Medical Research Council strength. The grade 4 level was chosen because a grade 4 muscle can be transferred with the expectation that it will be able to perform useful work. A grade 3 muscle loses so much of its power in transfer that it cannot be reliably expected to do useful work after transfer.

Moberg[8,9] also encouraged a consideration of remaining sensory resources as well. If sufficient proprioception remains in any part of the hand (typically the thumb and index fingers), the patient can control his hand without having to keep it in view. If the hand lacks proprioception, the patient can rely on his eyes to direct his hands. However, lack of proprioception limits the patient in performing bi-manual activities. Today static 2-point discrimination of less than 12–15 mm is acknowledged as indicating the presence of proprioception. The International Classification recognizes the presence or absence of proprioception by including codes to indicate whether afferent control resides in the hands, termed "cutaneous, or Cu" or only in the eyes of the patient, termed "ocular, and abbreviated as "O."

Later, the International Classification scheme was extended to include a determination of the presence or absence of active elbow extension. This system was adopted by the International Federation of Hand Surgery Societies[10] and it is used by essentially all surgeons involved in the care of the upper extremities of these patients.

Patient presentation and patient selection

Forming a team

Moberg stressed the need to develop a "critical mass" of like-minded professionals into a team that should include physiatrists involved in the rehabilitation and long-term care of people with tetraplegia. Critical to the success of an upper limb team are well-trained therapists, either physical therapists or occupational therapists (preferably both). The hand and upper extremity surgeon provides the technical expertise. Others including social workers and psychologists may offer additional support to the team. The patient's support group including family or attendant is the key to success. The central member of the team is the patient.[11–13]

The role of the professionals in this team is relatively clear. The physiatrists assist in determining the appropriateness of the patient for surgery as well as when to time surgery relative to overall rehabilitation goals and schedules. The therapist frequently serves as the patient's advocate. He or she knows the patient better than anyone else and most importantly, the patient's expectations voiced or not.

For the patient, upper extremity surgery can have a large emotional impact. Some patients are concerned about altering their anatomy because they are waiting for the cure for SCI. While the goal of surgical reconstruction for the upper extremity is greater function, the patient must be willing to lose temporarily some of their hard won independence during the postoperative rehabilitation. For family and attendants this greater period of dependence translates into more inconvenience and effort. All the team members must play a role in the decision-making process and must share in the frustrations as well as the rewards.

The hand and upper extremity team should become part of the routine evaluation of even newly injured patients. The cervical cord injured patient arrives at a rehabilitation facility or spinal cord injury unit usually with fairly supple upper limbs though with no or only minimal volitional movement. Once the patient's vertebral injury has become stabilized and the patient can be up in a wheelchair, an assessment by the upper extremity team takes on new meaning. By the 3rd or 4th month following injury, the eventual functional level is usually clearly established for the majority of patients.[14] At this time, the patient's upper limb function is assessed and the therapist help decide what assistive devices are appropriate.[15–17] For some patients early use of a functional orthosis such as a wrist-driven flexor hinge splint will advance the rate of rehabilitation. For patients with early but weak recovery of wrist extension, the wrist-driven flexor hinge splint represents an excellent exercise therapy directed towards strengthening wrist extensors so that they may eventually actuate a surgically reconstructed pinch or grip.

Hand or upper extremity surgery is rarely indicated during the initial months of rehabilitation following injury. The patient needs time to experience neurologic, psychologic, and social stability. From a practical standpoint, there are simply too many more important rehabilitation activities going on. On the other hand, a dogmatic philosophy embracing tired dicta such as "never operate on a patient before 12 months" has no basis in science. Some patients are clearly candidates for surgery prior to this calendar date. For example, early surgical intervention to relieve the pathologic effects of a fixed elbow flexion contracture may allow a patient to participate more vigorously in necessary rehabilitation activities.[6] Early release of a fixed elbow flexion contracture can be done with a simultaneous transfer of the contracted biceps muscle to the triceps. This removes a pathologic or deforming force and reinforces or restores some power to the antagonist. Botox is another important tool in the early rehabilitation armamentarium. It is especially helpful for patients with concomitant brain injury who may not comply with splinting or therapy and have increased tone.

Once the patient has achieved neurological and psychological stability, a formal evaluation to establish the appropriateness of upper extremity surgery can be accomplished by the team. The evaluation should focus on both tangible evidence of recovery by assessing remaining motor and sensory resources and the important intangibles such as motivation and intelligence. There is increasing recognition of the co-occurrence of traumatic brain injury with spinal cord injury and the impact of brain injury on rehabilitation.[18] Cognitive deficits need to be understood before embarking on upper extremity reconstruction given the intensive post-surgical therapy. The initial patient assessment should include an evaluation on how the patient accomplishes tasks of daily living with particular attention to how he or she performs transfers and pushes a wheelchair *(Fig. 37.1)*. Tendon transfers may alter the position of the hand and fingers. After reconstruction wheel chair propulsion and bed transfers must be performed in a safe manner to prevent stretching of the repairs *(Fig. 37.2)*. It is best for patients to learn safe transfer and propulsion techniques before surgery.

The upper limb examination includes assessment of residual motor groups as well as the identification of pathologic conditions such as contracted, painful, or unstable joints. There is also a sensory evaluation, which includes measuring 2-point discrimination in the digits to assess proprioception. The currently used grip patterns are assessed *(Fig. 37.3)*. Occasionally, spinal cord injured patients will have focal areas of severe neuropathic pain that will make the exam painful and potentially limit surgical results.

The patient's current functional status is assessed. Is he dependent or independent in bed mobility? How are transfers performed? Does he use a manual or electric wheelchair? What adaptive devices are used for dressing? … grooming? … feeding? If surgery is to be performed, is there sufficient

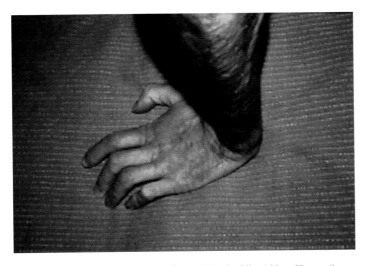

Fig. 37.1 Transfers performed on the flattened hand, while stable, will, over time, destroy the collateral ligaments about the thumb and the MP joints. Furthermore, if continued after functional surgery, this posture will stretch-out tenodeses and break down joint fusions. A similar fate awaits the thumb in this patient who uses his thumb to push the "quad-knobs" of the wheelchair. Patients with these postures must be retrained to perform safer transfers and propulsion maneuvers prior to considering surgical reconstruction.

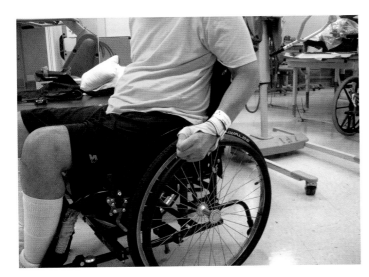

Fig. 37.2 A patient pushing his wheelchair after pinch reconstruction.

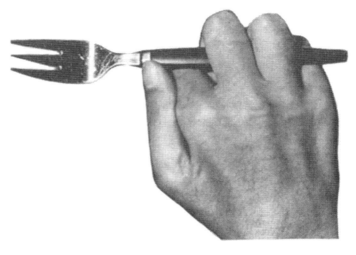

Fig. 37.3 A patient threading a fork through his fingers to grasp.

support to get the patient through a period of greater functional dependence or will be the extra burden of care result in the patient's attendant quitting. For many patients, upper extremity surgery means restriction to an electric-driven chair. Can this be made available? Does the home situation permit the use of an electric wheelchair? Are the controls of the chair mounted on the nonoperated side? The patient's primary therapist plays the most important role in determining these issues. Preparation before surgery will prevent complications such as pressure sores and social consequences such as divorce.

Finally, the patient's goals for surgery are reviewed. It is often helpful for a specific task to be identified, e.g., "I want to eat the triple decker sandwich at Joe's by myself." This was an achievable goal for this patient. This discussion helps the surgeon understand if the patient has reasonable expectations and can help tailor the procedures.

Treatment/surgical technique

General guidelines for reconstruction

Four surgical procedures are applicable for improving upper limb function in tetraplegia:

1. Arthrodesis: permits stabilization of joints lacking muscle stabilization

2. Tenodesis: performed either to stabilize a joint or more commonly so that another, typically more proximal movement, e.g., wrist extension, will result in the tightening of the tenodesis and movement of a more distally located joint

3. Tendon transfer: the transfer of the power of an expendable muscle-tendon unit under good volitional control to compensate for the absence or ineffectiveness of function of another muscle-tendon unit.

4. Functional electrical stimulation or FES: this technique utilizes the residual contractile properties of upper motor neuron paralyzed muscles when stimulated by an extra neural source. FES allows for more the use of more residual muscles in the reconstructive plan. At this time, FES is not commercially available.

Tendon transfers are the workhorse procedures for reconstruction of the upper extremity in tetraplegia. These techniques have been refined over the last 80 years and several basic principles have evolved. (1) First is *correction of any joint contracture*. Tendon transfers are often biomechanically disadvantaged and will not be able to overcome a contracted joint. (2) The *donor muscle must have adequate strength*. Transferred muscles will generally lose a grade of strength after transfer. Therefore it must be strong preoperatively to be able to perform functional tasks postoperatively and should have a MRC >4. (3) The *donor muscle must be expendable*. (4) *Straight line of pull*, for the best biomechanical advantage most effective routing of muscle insertion to origin is a straight line. (5) The *soft tissue bed must be stable*. These surgeries must be performed in a supple bed with adequate skin coverage. Scarred beds will prevent tendon gliding and impair the result. (6) The *donor muscle should have adequate excursion* to perform the desired function.

For people with tetraplegia, spasticity must also be considered. The donor muscle must have volitional control and not have too much tone. Overall level of spasticity can be improved with physical therapy and medications. A small amount of spasticity and tone is acceptable and sometimes beneficial to reconstructive procedures. The surgeon should assess the level of spasticity and make sure it is optimized before intervention.

The remainder of this chapter is devoted to a discussion of the role of surgery for improving function at the elbow, wrist, and fingers. The challenge of this discussion is that a clear linear treatment algorithm cannot be designed. For these procedures it is critical that each patient, and indeed each upper extremity, be evaluated and then each treatment plan individualized.

For high cervical spinal cord injuries, there are no expendable muscles available for transfer in the arm. For patients with lower injuries such as a C7 injury, many potentially expendable, and thus transferable, muscles of grade 4 or 5 power exist. Thus reconstructive possibilities range from procedures to simplify the mechanics of the hand, such as arthrodesing a wrist joint to eliminate the need for an external stabilizing orthosis, to complex multi-staged procedurals involving many muscle-tendon transfers. The choice of procedure depends primarily on the residual resources and, secondly, on the many intangibles such as patient desires, motivation and support. The surgical techniques used in tetraplegia are the same procedures as reconstructions after peripheral nerve injuries, but the difference between these procedures is the preoperative preparation and matching the patient to the correct procedure. A cautious approach while one gains experience pays great dividends in terms of obtaining the acceptance of team members and patients that surgery can promote greater independence for these patients. A poor outcome early in the team's experience creates a tremendous hurdle.

Surgical reconstruction

Elbow extension

Erik Moberg brought to our attention the importance of active elbow extension for the spinal cord injured patient. The individual who uses a wheelchair depends upon good shoulder and elbow power and stabilization to push a manual wheelchair, transfer from bed to chair, and to perform pressure releases to prevent pressure sores. For the person with tetraplegia lack of a functional elbow extension results in a much-reduced functional environment. If surgery can increase the reachable space by an additional twelve inches there is then 800% more space the hand can reach.

Without active elbow extension, the tetraplegic's hands frequently fall into his face when lying supine, which makes eating and daily hygiene challenging *(Fig. 37.4)*. One cannot push a manual wheelchair up any incline without triceps function. Even as simple a task as turning on a room light switch may be impossible without active elbow extension. There are two surgical procedures advocated for restoring active elbow extension, biceps to triceps and deltoid to triceps transfer.

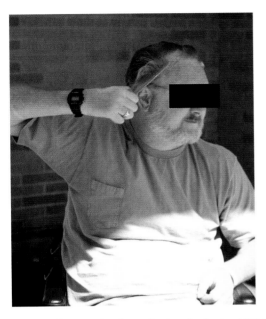

Fig. 37.4 Postoperative elbow extension allowing for stabilization of the arm to assist with combing the hair

Biceps to triceps transfer

This procedure[19–21] has become increasingly popular.[22] It is the procedure of choice when there is a pre-existing flexion contracture of the elbow greater than 45°. In this case, the biceps is usually a deforming force that must be addressed. The advantages of biceps to triceps transfer include no need for an interposition graft and only one tendon repair site. Disadvantages include a more challenging rehabilitation program and the potential for loss of elbow flexion strength.

Surgical technique

The biceps tendon is detached from its insertion on the greater tuberosity of the radius, the muscle-tendon unit routed either medially[23] or laterally,[24,25] and the tendon attached to the triceps aponeurosis or directly into the olecranon.

The incisions that are employed depend in large measure on whether a wide exposure to the anterior aspect of the elbow joint is needed to allow adequate release of contracture. The distal extent of the incision should allow complete dissection of the tendon of the biceps so that it can be detached as close to its point of insertion on the bicipital tuberosity of the radius *(Fig. 37.5A)*.

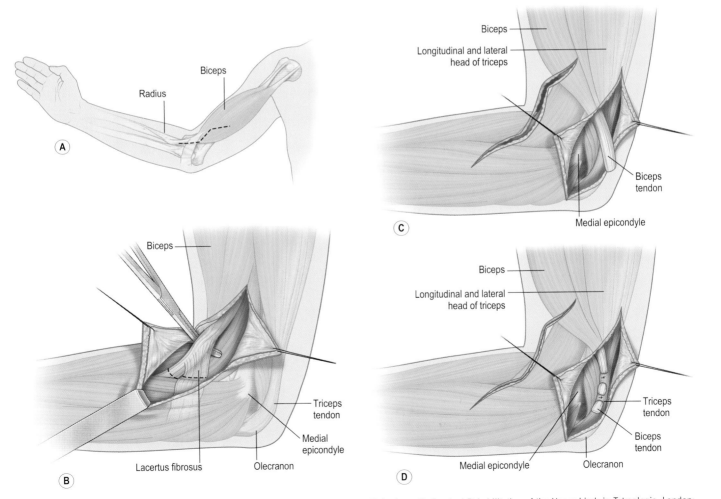

Fig. 37.5 Biceps to triceps transfer by the medial route **(A–D)**. (Redrawn from Hentz V, Leclercq C. Surgical Rehabilitation of the Upper Limb in Tetraplegia. London: Harcourt Health Sciences; 2002, with permission.)

The incision is carried through the subcutaneous tissue, protecting the large tributaries of the basilic and cephalic veins. The soft tissues overlying the lacertus fibrosis are elevated and the lacertus is either divided off the primary tendon or dissected distally as far as possible to provide another point of fixation to the triceps *(Fig. 37.5B)*.

The primary tendon of the biceps is dissected to its point of insertion on the radius. Flexing the elbow and supinating the forearm assists in this exposure. The tendon is sectioned as far distally as possible. The biceps muscle is dissected proximally from within its dense investing fascia, the dissection proceeding proximally until the cutaneous portion of the musculocutaneous nerve is identified as it courses between the overlying biceps and the deeper brachialis muscle. This nerve is protected while dissection of the biceps proceeds proximally until the most distal motor branches coming from the musculocutaneous nerve are visualized.

Both medial and lateral routing of the transfer have been described. Since the ulnar nerve is typically nonfunctional in this population, we have preferred to route the biceps medially. It is necessary to dissect widely the arcade of Struthers and all other fascial communications about the medial intermuscular septum. One must be concerned about compression of the radial nerve when the lateral route is chosen.

A second incision located posteromedially is made in order to expose the medial aspect of the triceps insertion. Through this incision, the medial border of the triceps is elevated and dissected to its insertion on the olecranon. The biceps muscle and tendon are then passed from the anterior to the posterior incision through the widely dissected subcutaneous tunnel *(Fig. 37.5C)*. The anterior incision may be closed at this point.

The biceps tendon typically just reaches the tip of the olecranon but there is infrequently sufficient tendon length to permit a strong attachment into the olecranon. Instead, the tendon of the biceps is woven into the medial border of the triceps tendon and anchored in multiple locations with stout sutures *(Fig. 37.5D)*. We have judged that the proper tension is achieved when the biceps is pulled distally enough to permit the end of the tendon to touch the olecranon with the elbow in about 20° of flexion. Once the tendon-to-tendon junctures are made, the elbow is fully extended to relax the site of approximation.

Postoperative care

Regardless of the technique chosen, the elbow is immobilized in full extension using a light plaster or fiberglass cylinder cast for 3.5 weeks. An overhead, chair-mounted sling is fitted to their wheelchair and is used whenever the patient is in the wheelchair and until the cast is removed.

The initial cast is left undisturbed for 3.5 weeks if the elbow had essentially normal passive extension preoperatively. If the elbow had a preoperative flexion contracture between 15° and 30°, the elbow is extended as much as possible at the time of surgery and casted in that position. This cast is removed between 10 and 14 days postoperatively. Great care must be taken to keep the elbow extended during this maneuver. Typically, the elbow can then be further extended at this time by slow stretch and the arm is recasted, now typically in near full or even full extension. After removal of the cast, the elbow

is exercised for several additional weeks by allowing progressively greater elbow flexion in a specially designed flexion-stop brace *(Fig. 37.6)*. Although the biceps seems to be an antagonist to elbow extension, by teaching the patient to conjointly supinate the forearm and extend the elbow, the patient can be reeducated to use the supinator function of the biceps to extend the elbow. Electrical stimulation and biofeedback therapy has been used on occasion with improved results. Some months of cautious use are necessary to prevent overstretching of the transfer and many months pass before maximal strength is obtained.

Deltoid to triceps transfer[26]

Surgical technique

Hints and tips
1. Detach the deltoid from the humerus with as much fascia and fibrous insertion as possible, including some of the fascial origin of the brachialis muscle.
2. Attach the deltoid to the triceps at maximum tension with the shoulder abducted 30° and the elbow flexed at 30°
3. Cast elbow in full extension and keep the arm abducted at the shoulder during healing.

The surgical landmarks *(Fig. 37.7A)* at the level of the shoulder include the tip of the acromion superiorly, the interval between the posterior margin of the deltoid and the triceps muscle posteriorly, and the estimated point of insertion of the deltoid on the humerus. The landmark at the level of the elbow is the tip of the olecranon. The surgeon should keep in mind the neurovascular anatomy of the region including the course of the axillary nerve and the circumflex humeral artery and the radial nerve and its relationship to the insertion of the deltoid *(Fig. 37.7B)*.

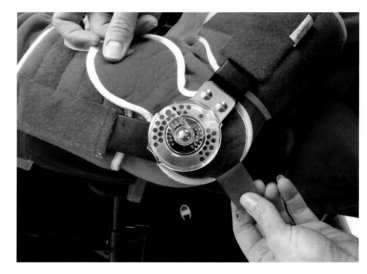

Fig. 37.6 Hinged orthosis to protect the repair across the elbow. The degree of flexion is gradually flexed over time.

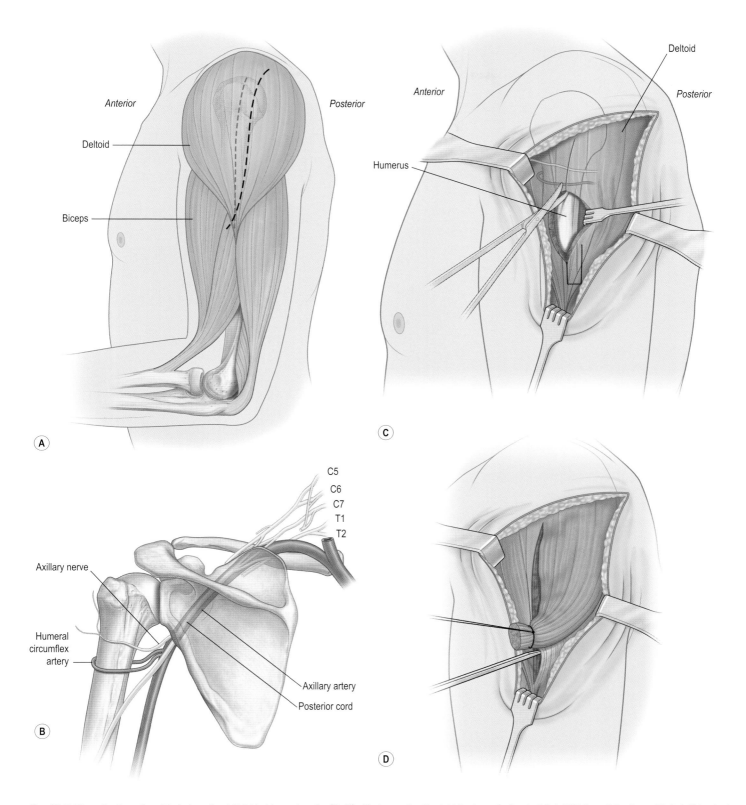

Fig. 37.7 The author's preferred technique for deltoid to triceps transfer **(A–H).** (Redrawn after Hentz V, Leclercq C. Surgical Rehabilitation of the Upper Limb in Tetraplegia. London: Harcourt Health Sciences; 2002, with permission.)

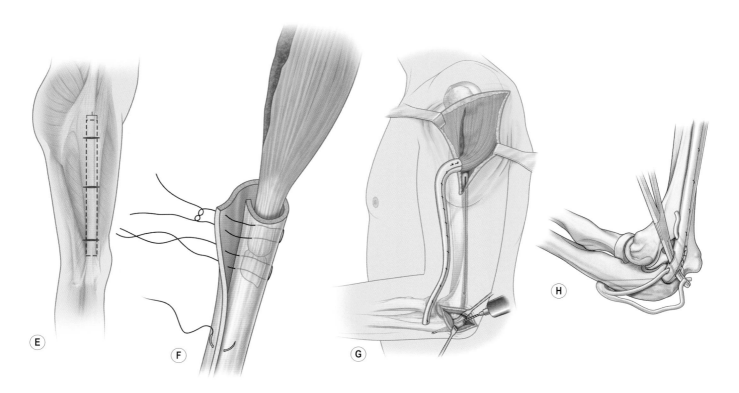

Fig. 37.7, cont'd

The upper incision is centered half way between the mid-axial line of the humerus and the posterior margin of the deltoid *(Fig. 37.7A)*. The skin incision is carried to the level of the muscle fascia and the skin and subcutaneous tissues are elevated anteriorly to just past the mid-axial line of the humerus. Posteriorly, the skin flap is elevated to the confluence of deltoid and the long head of the triceps *(Fig. 37.7C)*. The plane between these two muscles is developed by sharp or finger dissection. As the finger strikes the humerus, the fingertip tip can be insinuated upward through the fibers of the deltoid, separating the muscle into relatively equal anterior and posterior halves.

Detaching the insertion of the posterior half of the muscle from its point of insertion onto the humerus is done by sharply incising a rectangle of periosteum at the point of attachment and elevating the periosteum and the fibers of attachment off the humerus. We include as much fascia and fibrous insertion as possible, including some of the fascial origin of the brachialis muscle. The radial nerve will be emerging from behind the humerus several centimeters distal to this point. Injury to this nerve has been reported as a rare but devastating complication of this procedure.

A suture is placed in the fibrous origin of the posterior half of the deltoid muscle and the dissection is carried superiorly until the branches of the axillary nerve are visualized *(Fig. 37.7D)*. The superior dissection should stop at this point.

Several methods have been proposed to attach the posterior deltoid to the triceps or olecranon including:

- Autogenous tendons such as toe extensors,[27] tibialis anterior tendon,[9] or extensor carpi ulnaris[28]

- A turned up strip of the central part of the triceps tendon with synthetic reinforcement[29]
- Bone to bone attachments[30]
- Various synthetic materials.[31]

We prefer the patient's own fascia lata, especially in the patient whose triceps tendon is relatively short or insubstantial.[32]

The fascia is harvested through several transverse incisions placed over the iliotibial band *(Fig. 37.7E)*. The ideal width is about 2.5 cm. The fascia lata is encircled about the fibrous insertion of the deltoid using mattress sutures of nonabsorbable braided suture *(Fig. 37.7F)*, tubed over its remaining length and tunneled subcutaneously to the olecranon.

The olecranon is exposed just distal to the insertion of the triceps. The triceps tendon is split longitudinally to further expose the tip of the olecranon and a 5 mm drill bit is used to create an oblique tunnel through the olecranon *(Fig. 37.7G)*. A Bunnell tendon-stripper is a useful instrument to "polish" this channel so that the tubed fascia lata can be passed smoothly in a proximal to distal direction *(Fig. 37.7H)*.[33] The fascia lata is passed into the distal exposure, separated into two tails and the tails are passed through the bone channel.

The shoulder is abducted about 30° and the elbow is flexed about 30°. The two fascia lata tails are then pulled to *maximally* tense the transfer and these tails are turned proximally and woven into the fascia lata tube and anchored with nonabsorbable sutures. Once suturing is complete, the fascial tube should be under moderate but definite tension. The wounds are closed and a cylinder cast is placed as is described in the biceps to triceps transfer with the elbow fully extended.

Postoperative care

Postoperative care is quite similar to the biceps to triceps transfer. For deltoid to triceps transfer, shoulder position is more of a concern. The shoulder is kept somewhat abducted and the patient and other care-givers are cautioned to not allow the shoulder to accidentally flop across the chest. The wheelchair frame is critical because it holds the arm somewhat elevated preventing distal edema and helps keep the arm somewhat abducted from the body, a position that relaxes the deltoid.

Complications are rare provided the patient follows the exercise protocol and does not overstretch the transfer by too rapidly regaining full elbow flexion. Reconstruction of elbow extension has been the single most satisfying reconstruction for our patients. Even though the rehabilitation can be relatively lengthy, the functional gain is substantial, predictable, and easily appreciated by the patient.

Surgical reconstruction for the weaker (IC groups 0, 1 and 2) patients

For the IC group 0 patient with no muscles functioning at the grade 4 or greater level distal to the elbow, few reconstructive possibilities exist. For the majority of these patients, some type of functional orthosis must suffice. Rarely for the IC group 0 patient, fusion of the wrist might permit the patient to employ a less cumbersome functional orthosis; e.g., a self-donned universal cuff rather than a long opponens splint, for which the patient needs assistance in donning and doffing. Surgery may also be useful in repositioning a badly positioned part. For example, osteotomy of the radius may be useful in placing the hand in a more favorable pronated position. This might permit easier manipulation of the joy stick control for an electric wheelchair than can be accomplished by a hand that is perpetually supinated.

For these weakest patients Brummer[34] introduced a clever procedure that uses supination of the forearm to create a weak but perhaps useful pinch. The procedure is illustrated in *Figure 37.8*.

Improving wrist extension: the IC group 1 and 2 patient

In the IC group 1 patient, the brachioradialis is typically the only muscle with grade 4 strength distal to the elbow. However, grade 2+ to grade 3+ radial wrist extensor function is typically present as well. The patient may be able to extend the wrist against gravity but cannot generate useful force between digits and thumb through any existing natural tenodesis effect or cannot utilize a wrist-driven flexor hand splint unless it is equipped with a ratchet mechanism lock and release. For this patient, wrist extensor strength can be augmented by transferring the power of the brachioradialis into the more central of the radial wrist extensors, the extensor carpi radialis brevis (ECRB) tendon.[35–37] From several biomechanical studies[38,39] it has been determined that the brachioradialis becomes a more effective wrist extensor following transfer if the patient can stabilize the elbow in space. If no active elbow extension is present, the brachioradialis may

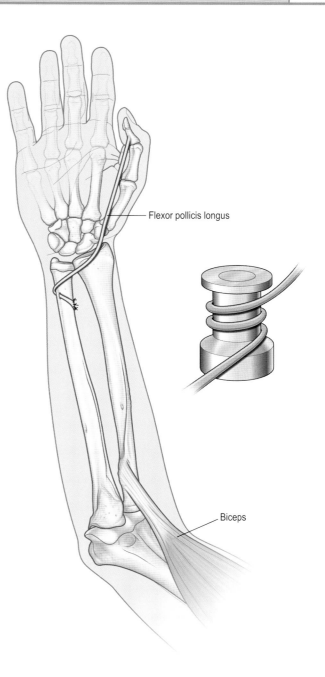

Flexor pollicis longus

Biceps

Fig. 37.8 The Brummer "winch" operation. The tendon of the FPL is divided at the muscle-tendon junction and is passed deep to the flexor tendons and neurovascular bundles toward the ulna. The IP joint of the thumb must be stabilized, either by fusion, pinning, or the split FPL to EPL procedure described in ***Figure 37.9***. With the forearm in full supination, the tendon of the FPL is anchored to the ulna under sufficient tension to create key-pinch between the pulp of the thumb and the radial side of the index finger with the wrist stabilized in a neutral position. Forearm pronation should allow the grip to relax. (Redrawn after Hentz V, Leclercq C. Surgical Rehabilitation of the Upper Limb in Tetraplegia. London: Harcourt Health Sciences; 2002, with permission.)

waste some of its excursion and power by flexing the elbow rather than in extending the wrist. For this reason, we prefer first to reconstruct active elbow extension and occasionally will combine deltoid to triceps and brachioradialis to ECRB transfer.

A wide dissection of the distal muscle and tendon from its insertion at the radial styloid up to the very proximal forearm level is necessary to obtain the most effective excursion of the muscle. The tension on the brachioradialis should be adjusted to re-establish the normal resting length of the muscle with care taken not to overstretch this muscle. In adjusting the tension, it is important to place the elbow in some flexion while tension is set at the junction. Moberg[9] recommended that the elbow be set at about 40° of flexion and we have followed this guideline. This is done so that the transfer does not lose significant power as the elbow if flexed. The wrist is splinted in near full extension to relax the tendon to tendon juncture for approximately 4 weeks.

Postoperative care

The cast is removed at the 4th week and a removable orthosis is fitted. The orthosis is designed to maintain the wrist in some extension to further protect the tendon to tendon juncture. The orthosis is removed initially under the supervision of the therapist. The patient and attendant are instructed in the exercise protocols. The orthosis is replaced between exercise sessions. It is best worn at night for many additional weeks.

Until about postoperative week 6, the patient utilizes the orthosis except when exercising. Beginning about postoperative week 6, the orthosis is removed during much of the day and the patient begins to strengthen the transferred muscle by actively contracting the brachioradialis against no resistance.

The transfer is protected against resistance for an additional 3–4 weeks, depending on whether or not this procedure has been combined with additional procedures such as a key grip procedure or reconstruction of elbow extension by deltoid or biceps to triceps transfer. At this time, the patient can resume weight-shifts and transfers in and out of the wheelchair.

Restoring key pinch: the IC group 1 and 2 patient

Hints and tips
1. Do not release the A1 pulley of the thumb if the MP joint flexes beyond 45°.
2. Routinely perform the split FRL to EPL transfer.
3. If the thumb collapses into supination as the wrist is extended, perform the Brand modification of Moberg's procedure, described later.

Patients at the IC group 2 level, or IC group 1 patients following BR to ECRB transfer can actively extend the wrist against some resistance and are potential candidates for creation of a lateral or key pinch as described by Moberg.[26] Conceptually, this is a very simple operative procedure and, importantly, is essentially totally reversible should the patient decide he was more functional before surgery. The key pinch procedure may be combined with brachioradialis to ECRB transfer if greater wrist extensor power is deemed

advantageous. It represents an automatic pinch in that the tendon of the thumb flexor, the flexor pollicis longus (FPL), is anchored to the palmar surface of the radius under such tension that with wrist extension the thumb tip is pulled against the side of the index finger. The other fingers are usually left supple and the patient frequently must learn to roll these digits into some flexion in order to provide a platform against which the thumb can act. Gravity is needed to flex the wrist, releasing tension on the tenodesed FPL and allowing opening of the grip. Preoperative prerequisites include:

- Adequate passive wrist mobility
- Voluntary wrist extension of grade 4 or greater
- Supple thumb joints
- Adequate flexibility in the remaining digits
- Appropriate transfer and weight shift techniques to prevent over-stretching the tenodesis following surgery.

Provided that wrist extension power is adequate, the key steps of the procedure have evolved to currently include:

- Stabilization of the interphalangeal joint of the thumb by splitting the flexor pollicis longus insertion and transferring half the tendon dorsally where it is attached to the tendon of insertion of the extensor pollicis longus
- Fixation of the tendon of the flexor pollicis longus to the radius at the correct tension
- Stabilization of the thumb's metacarpophalangeal joint against excessive flexion (necessary if this joint can be passively flexed more than 45°), or against excessive extension (necessary if the joint passively hyperextends beyond 10°.)

The procedure is carried out preferably under regional arm block. Depending on the status of the thumb's metacarpophalangeal joint, either four or five small incisions are planned in addition to the incision on the radial aspect of the forearm for transfer of the brachioradialis to the radial wrist extensor, if this is to be done. If this transfer is indicated, it is performed as the initial operative step.

The first step is stabilization of the interphalangeal joint of the thumb. Initially this was performed with pin stabilization as described by Moberg[27] but there were multiple hardware complications. Thus the split flexor pollicis longus transfer as described by Mohammed et al.[40] has been adopted. This technique eliminates the need for long-term hardware and preserves some active and even greater passive interphalangeal joint movement.

Split FPL to EPL interphalangeal stabilization

For an optimum result, the critical pulleys, including the oblique pulley of the flexor sheath of the thumb must be preserved. The procedure may be carried out using the incisions outlined in figure *(Fig. 37.9A)*, or using just one incision along the radial mid-axis of the thumb.

The zig-zag incision is made and the neurovascular bundle on the radial side of the digit is dissected. The neurovascular bundle is included within the skin flap to protect it. Frequently, there is a small annular ligament or pulley located

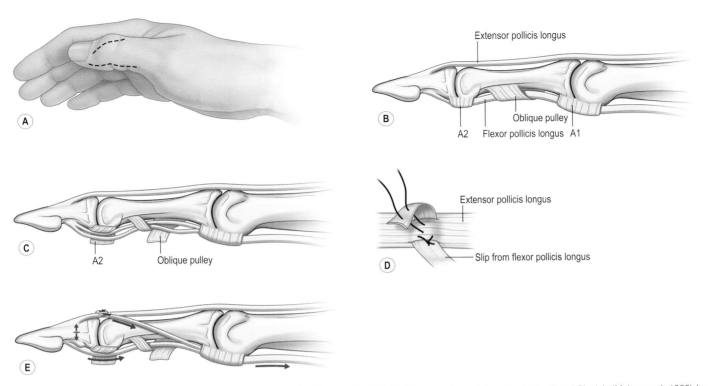

Fig. 37.9 A very effective method to stabilize the IP joint of the thumb without making it rigid. This procedure, attributed to Rothwell and Sinclair (Mohammed, 1992) has become universally accepted. (Redrawn after Hentz V, Leclercq C. Surgical Rehabilitation of the Upper Limb in Tetraplegia. London: Harcourt Health Sciences; 2002, with permission.)

at the level of the interphalangeal joint. This can be incised to visualize the flexor pollicis longus tendon *(Figs 37.9B, C)*.

A blunt probe is used to find the naturally occurring midline split in the tendon's structure. This split is lengthened both distally and proximally. When the distal dissection reaches the insertion of the tendon, the radial half of the split flexor pollicis longus tendon is divided at its bony insertion. The tendon end is delivered into the wound and by pulling distally on the tendon, some additional as yet unsplit flexor pollicis longus is visualized. The proximal split is extended. Finally, a small window into the flexor sheath is created just proximal to the oblique pulley and the detached radial half of the tendon is brought through this window.

If a second incision is used, it is located on the mid-dorsum of the thumb, over the course of the extensor pollicis longus. The radial half of the flexor pollicis longus is tunneled under the intervening skin, deep to the radial digital nerve and brought out the dorsal incision.

The tendon slip is passed under the tendon of the extensor pollicis longus and then brought back over onto itself *(Fig. 37.9D)*. The thumb interphalangeal joint is temporarily stabilized in about 20° of flexion with a 0.045 Kirschner wire placed across the joint. The transferred slip of tendon is pulled distally until a noticeable slackening of the remaining tendon half is noted and then relaxed slightly so that there is equal tension on the slip of transferred tendon and on the original remaining half of the tendon *(Fig. 37.9E)*. Pinning the interphalangeal joint before final adjustment of tension makes this step much more practical and more easily

accomplished. The transferred half of the tendon is sutured to itself and to the extensor pollicis longus with absorbable 4–0 sutures.

Flexor pollicis longus (FPL) tenodesis

The tendon of the FPL is to be anchored to the distal radius. Moberg's original procedure left the FPL within its natural bursa. He and Brand later modified the technique to include routing the FPL across the palm deep to the finger flexors before passing it into the forearm via Guyon's canal. Moberg's original method is technically easier but Brand's modification provides, according to his biomechanical analysis, a more favorable FPL flexor moment. We continue to utilize both routs of FPL transfer and frequently will test each method to determine which rout seems to provide a more stable thumb posture in the key pinch position when the FPL is placed under tension.

The Moberg–Brand FPL tenodesis procedure requires three incisions. The first is designed along the radial aspect of the thumb and exposes the flexor sheath of the thumb from the interphalangeal joint to the level of the A1 pulley at the metacarpophalangeal joint. The second incision is made in the palm at the level of the hook of the hamate. Through this incision, access is gained to Guyon's canal. The third incision will be located on the on the radio-volar side of the distal forearm. The three volar incisions are illustrated in *(Fig. 37.10A)*. The fourth small incision will be made last and is to be located on the dorsum of the distal aspect of the forearm.

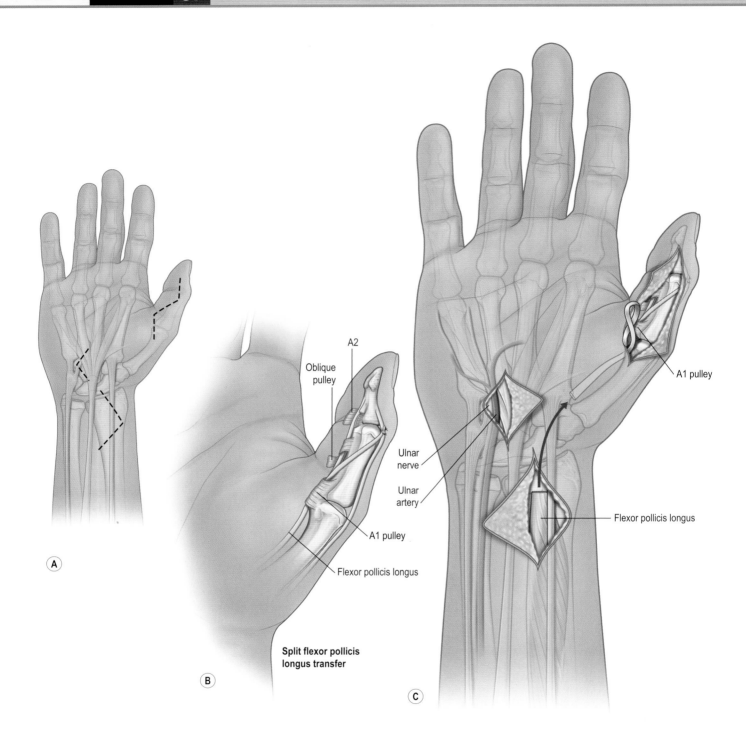

Fig. 37.10 The Moberg–Brand modification of Moberg's original key pinch procedure. (Redrawn after Hentz V, Leclercq C. Surgical Rehabilitation of the Upper Limb in Tetraplegia. London: Harcourt Health Sciences; 2002, with permission.)

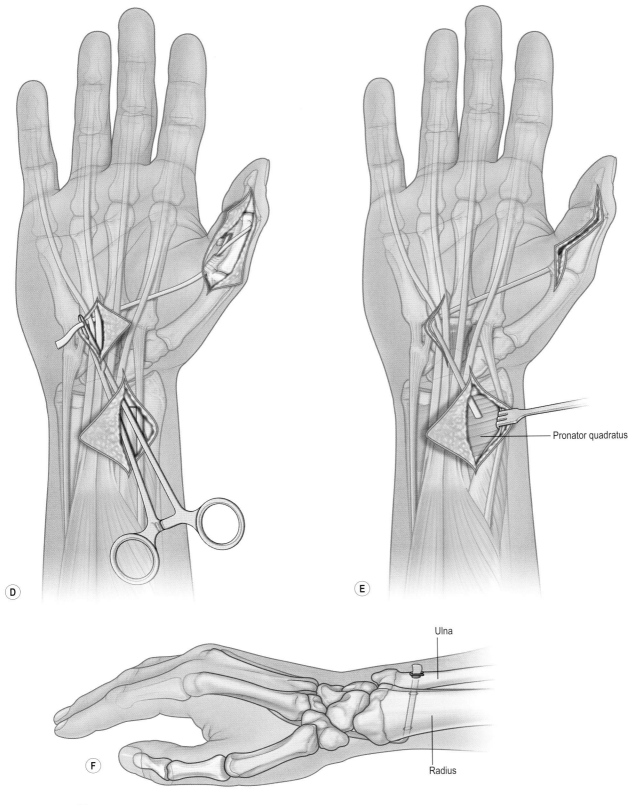

Pronator quadratus

Ulna

Radius

Fig. 37.10, cont'd

After the FPL-EPL transfer is performed, the FPL tendon is identified just proximal to the A1 pulley of the thumb *(Fig. 37.10B)*. This pulley should be preserved, especially if the thumb metacarpophalangeal joint can be passively flexed more than 30° on preoperative testing. A small probe is placed under the FPL tendon just proximal to the A1 pulley.

The volar forearm incision is made and the interval between the FCR and the PL tendons dissected. Just deep to this interval will be the muscle-tendon junction of the FPL. The tendon is identified and the muscle-tendon junction divided as far proximal as possible. The FPL tendon is brought into the thumb incision *(Fig. 37.10C)*.

The third (palmar) incision is made and the dissection is carried down through the hypothenar fat and the palmaris brevis muscle, the ulnar neurovascular bundle located, and retracted ulnarward to expose the flexor tendons to the little and ring fingers. A curved tendon passing forceps is tunneled dorsal to the adjacent flexor tendons and neurovascular structures to the ring, middle and index fingers and is then directed toward the thumb incision. The tendon of the FPL is delivered into the hypothenar incision *(Fig. 37.10D)*.

The same tendon passing forceps is then introduced into the volar forearm incision to exit at the hypothenar incision *(Fig. 37.10E)*. The tendon of the FPL is grasped and withdrawn into the forearm incision.

The final part of this procedure involves the firm fixation of the FPL tendon to the radius at the proper tension. A 3 or 4 mm drill point is then used to drill a hole from volar to dorsal through the radius, avoiding interfering with the radial wrist extensor tendons. The site where the drill point exits the dorsal aspect of the radius is the location for the final incision *(Fig. 37.10F)*. A loop of 30 gauge (3–0) monofilament wire is passed through the drill hole in a dorsal to palmar direction and the tendon of the FPL placed in the loop and then drawn through the radius and into the small dorsal incision. All the skin incisions are closed with absorbable skin sutures or subcuticularly placed sutures. The tendon of the FPL that exits the skin on the dorsum of the forearm is grasped firmly in a large clamp. By pulling on the tendon, the tension can be adjusted so that the pulp of the thumb just contacts the radial side of the flexed index finger when the wrist is in the neutral position. When the wrist is flexed, the tension of the FPL is relaxed and the thumb ray will extend in response to the dorsal tenodesis/viscoelastic forces. As the wrist is brought from the flexed to the neutral position, the thumb will contact the index finger. As the wrist is further extended, the thumb exerts greater and greater force against the side of the index finger.

After satisfactory tensioning of the FPL tendon, a large vascular clip is fixed across the tendon at the level of the skin and one or two final skin sutures are placed to close the small dorsal wound *(Fig. 37.10F)*. By properly positioning the thumb or wrist in the cast, the correct tension of the re-routed FPL is maintained

The position of postoperative immobilization depends on whether or not the brachioradialis was transferred as part of this procedure. If this transfer has been performed, the wrist is immobilized in the neutral position and the thumb is flexed at the carpometacarpal joint to relax tension of the FPL. If this transfer has been unnecessary, the wrist may be immobilized

in 15–20° of flexion, again to relax tension on the FPL tenodesis site.

Postoperative care

Typically, the hand and wrist are immobilized for 4–5 weeks and cautious use is required for an additional 1–2 months to allow firm adherence of the tenodesis. Unless there is a very effective preoperative finger tenodesis effect, the patient must learn to roll the fingers into flexion in order to provide a platform for the pulp of the thumb. We have performed this procedure on more than 50 hands and the results have been very satisfying. We can measure the gain in pinch strength and it is typically proportional to the strength of the wrist extensor power but somewhat depends on the stability of the thumb and finger joints. Pinch strengths between 1–5 kg have been uniformly achieved. We have not had any patient ask to have his operative procedure reversed.

Restoring active key pinch by brachioradialis to FPL transfer: IC group 2 and some IC group 3 patients

Hints and tips
<ul><li>Arthrodese the thumb CMC joint in minimal palmar abduction.</li><li>Avoid arthrodesing the CMC joint if there is little MP joint passive flexion.</li></ul>

After gaining experience with Moberg's key pinch procedure, we have chosen to modify the key pinch operation for the patient with very strong wrist extension, meaning a strong IC group 2 or group 3 patient. These patients do not require augmentation of wrist extension. Instead of tenodesing the FPL to the radius as described above, in a single stage procedure the following steps are accomplished *(Fig. 37.11)*:

1. The carpometacarpal (CMC) is evaluated and if there is excess laxity a CMC arthrodesis is performed to preposition the thumb tip to contact the index finger middle phalanx.

2. The extensor pollicis longus (EPL) tendon is anchored to the extensor retinaculum on the dorsum of the wrist.

3. The brachioradialis is transferred to the tendon of the FPL.

4. The split FPL to EPL transfer is performed.

Operative procedure

The operative steps are carried out via one longer and three or four smaller incisions as illustrated in *Figure 37.11A*. An FPL to EPL interphalangeal joint stabilization procedure is completed as illustrated in *Figure 37.11B*. If needed the CMC joint is then exposed through an incision made along the juncture of the glabrous and hair-bearing skin over the

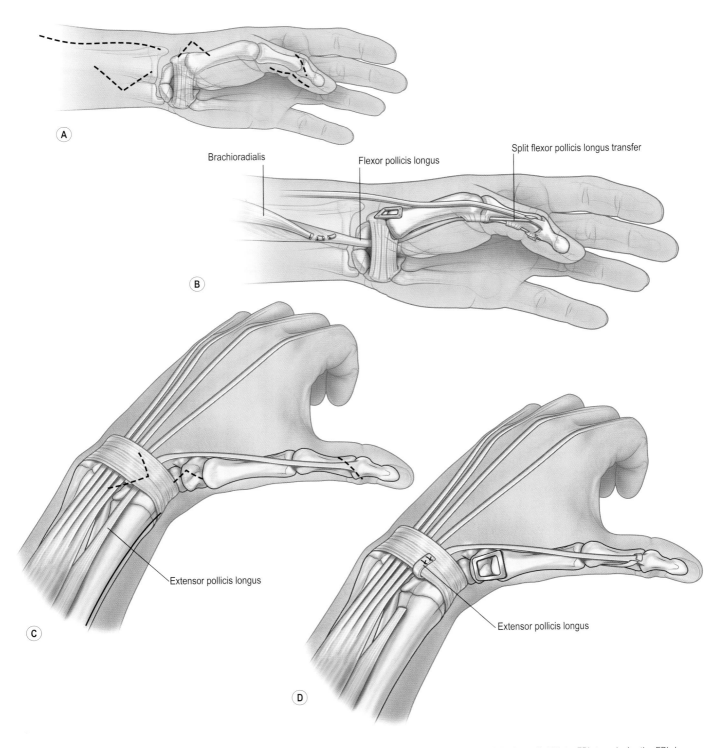

A

B

Brachioradialis

Flexor pollicis longus

Split flexor pollicis longus transfer

C

Extensor pollicis longus

D

Extensor pollicis longus

Fig. 37.11 A procedure to restore active key pinch. The CMC joint of the thumb is stabilized by fusion, the thumb IP joint by split FPL to EPL tenodesis, the EPL is tenodeses to the radius so that the thumb extends with wrist flexion and the BR is transferred to the FPL to provide potential voluntary pinch irrespective of wrist position. (Redrawn after Hentz V, Leclercq C. Surgical Rehabilitation of the Upper Limb in Tetraplegia. London: Harcourt Health Sciences; 2002, with permission.)

palmar-radial aspect of the thumb's thenar eminence. The thenar muscles are reflected off the capsule of the CMC joint and the capsule opened. The adjacent joint surfaces are prepared for arthrodesis by sharp excision of all cartilage and by perforating the dense subchondral bone in several areas on the metacarpal base and the face of the trapezium. Bone is removed with a small osteotome, curette or powered burr equally from both sides of the joint. This maintains the relative contours of metacarpal base and trapezium and good bone-to-bone contact between the two surfaces.

The angles of palmar and radial abduction for the CMC fusion are determined somewhat by the preoperative digital flexor tenodesis pattern and the passive range of motion at the thumb's MP joint. The goal is to have the pulp of the thumb contact the radial side of the index finger over the middle phalanx as the wrist is extended. Opening of the grip is affected by wrist flexion and occurs almost exclusively at the MP joint. The ideal candidate has a well-preserved digital flexor tenodesis pattern and passive MP flexion that exceeds the range of CMC extension. For such a patient, the thumb ray should be positioned in only about 20° of palmar abduction, and almost maximum radial abduction. A thumb ray fused in great palmar abduction will interfere with transfers and pressure relief efforts and will be subject to great stress when the patient performs these maneuvers. If the patient demonstrates very poor finger flexion as the wrist is extended, the CMC joint should be arthrodesed in a slightly less palmarly abducted posture. If the range of passive MP flexion is small, the CMC joint should be fused in less than maximal radial abduction. If too radially abducted, the patient with a poorly flexible MP joint will not be able to effect firm contact between pulp of thumb and index finger.

The CMC joint is temporarily pinned with a 2 mm Kirschner wire to test the preoperative hypothesis. If the position seems ideal, the joint is further stabilized. A small 4-corner plate as illustrated) has provided sufficiently rigid bone-to-bone contact. Bone staples also provide excellent immobilization at the fusion site.

The third step involves creating a firm tenodesis of the extensor pollicis longus (EPL) to the dorsal surface of the radius. Since the CMC joint is now fused, no particular EPL re-routing is needed. Through a transverse incision made just proximal to Lister's tubercle, the tendon of the EPL is located and divided at its muscle-tendon junction. The end of the tendon brought over the extensor retinaculum, and then passed under the EPL tendon just distal to the retinaculum. The wrist is flexed to 45° and the EPL is tensioned so that the thumb extends maximally. Several nonabsorbable sutures are used to anchor the EPL to itself and to the dense extensor retinaculum. The wrist is then passively flexed and extended and the thumb's motion observed. The thumb should reach maximum extension as the wrist reaches 45° of flexion but the pulp of the thumb should contact the radial side of the index finger as the wrist is extended to reach the neutral position.

The last procedure involves brachioradialis to FPL transfer. The FPL is identified in the volar forearm, either through the same incision used to dissect the brachioradialis or through a separate volar incision. The FPL is divided at its muscle-tendon junction and the two tendons are directed in as straight a line as possible toward one another. The ends of both tendons are passed through one another several times,

interweaving them. The ideal tension for the transfer is established as described for brachioradialis to ECRB transfer. The juncture is created with the elbow in 40° of flexion, the wrist in a neutral position and the index finger held flexed at MP and PIP joints. The brachioradialis is pulled distally to a point midway between maximum passive stretch and fully relaxed (zero-tension) tension and the FPL tendon is pulled proximally so that the pulp of the thumb just touches the radial side of the index finger. The assistant maintains this posture of both tendons while the surgeon joins together the two tendons with three or four nonabsorbable sutures. Once this tendon-to-tendon juncture is secure, the tension of the FPL transfer and the EPL tenodesis is tested by gently moving the wrist between 45° of flexion and 45° of extension. It is important that the thumb still fully extend at the MP joint with wrist flexion after brachioradialis transfer. The wounds are closed and the limb solidly immobilized in a below elbow cast that maintains the wrist in a neutral position, and the thumb MP joint in some flexion. We typically place the thumb in contact with the flexed index finger.

Postoperative care

The immobilization is continued for four weeks and then a plastic splint is constructed that keeps the initial position of postoperative immobilization. The splint is removed for exercises and the initial exercises are directed at regaining the preoperative range of wrist movement. At the beginning of the fifth postoperative week, the patient is encouraged to begin practicing grasping small, light objects, and for these exercises, the therapist constructs a small hand based splint to protect the CMC fusion. These exercises progress until the beginning of the eighth week when greater resistance is permitted. The splint is then only worn at night for four additional weeks. Weight-bearing precautions including no transfers out of the splint are continued for eight weeks. The fused thumb CMC joint requires that the patient's transfer mechanics be closely monitored by the therapist.

The BR provides stronger pinch if elbow extension is present and we try to perform elbow reconstruction before transferring the BR.[41]

Restoring both grasp and release in two operative stages: the IC groups 3, 4 and 5 patients

For our tetraplegic patients who possess additional motor resources distal to the elbow, more complicated reconstructions are possible but not always indicated. These patients are, of course, also candidates for either procedure described above if reversibility seems an important consideration. In the early years of our experience, only key pinch reconstruction for IC groups 3, 4 and even 5 patients was offered. As we have gained confidence in being able to achieve a reliable outcome, we have extended the risk-benefit equation to include more complex procedures in these IC group.

The strong IC group 3 patient

The very strong IC group 3 patient will have at least one of the two radial wrist extensors at MRC grade 5. The other will

Video 1

probably be MRC grade 4. They commonly have some function (MRC grade 2–3) of the pronator teres and this assists them in pronating their wrists

For these patients, a two-stage procedure that takes advantage of the presence of two expendable muscles for transfer, the extensor carpi radialis longus and the brachioradialis may be performed. The initial procedure is directed at obtaining a reliable opening posture of the hand and is referred to as the extensor phase. Prerequisites for surgery include near normal passive wrist movement and reasonably flexible fingers. These patients may possess useful triceps function. If not, this function should be restored and this can be done as part of the initial extensor phase.

The extensor phase

The operative steps for the initial extensor phase include:

- Assessing the strength of the ECRB
- Identifying any accessory radial wrist extensors[42]
- Passive tenodesis of the extensor tendons of the fingers (EDC) and of the thumb (EPL)
- Thumb CMC joint arthrodesis (described above)
- Split FPL to EPL transfer (described above).
- It is critical to be certain of the true strength of the ECRB before transferring the ECRL.

Robbing the patient of strong wrist extension is a grave error and this is a risk since it is impossible to isolate the ECRB in preoperative testing. Therefore, in the strong IC group 3 patients, the ERCB tendon is exposed just distal to the extensor retinaculum under local anesthesia as the initial operative step. A probe is slipped under the tendon and the patient is asked to forcefully extend the wrist. The surgeon then tries to displace the now tightened tendon with the probe. This is essentially impossible if the muscle is MRC grade 4 or 4+. If the ECRB is judged to be sufficiently strong, we proceed to perform the split FPL to EPL tenodesis, and then arthrodes the carpometacarpal joint of the thumb to preposition the thumb ray for pinch, as described above. The tendons of the extensor digitorum communis and extensor pollicis longus are fixed into a window excavated from the dorsum of the radius. Tension of this transfer is adjusted so that the fingers and thumb begin to extend as the wrist reaches the neutral position.

The arm is casted for 4 weeks and then exercised, avoiding any resistance to finger and thumb extension. Now, with gravity-assisted wrist flexion, the fingers and thumb extend. This is a very natural and synergistic motion and is easily learned.

The flexor phase

The second phase, centered on activation of the flexor tendons to the thumb (FPL) and fingers (FDP), is termed the "flexor phase." It includes:

- Transfer of ECRL to the deep finger flexors
- Transfer of BR to FPL
- Intrinsic stabilization.

Through the long dorsal incision described for BR transfer, the ECRL and BR tendons are mobilized and then passed volarward where the tendons of the BR and FPL are passed through each other and sutured. The tendons of the FDP are grouped together and the normal finger cascade is *reversed* somewhat by suturing the radial two FDP tendons under slightly tighter tension than the ulnar two. The tendon of the ERCL is woven back and forth through the now combined tendons of the FDP in the manner of Pulvertaft.[45] Tension of this transfer is adjusted so that a relatively natural posture of the fingers is achieved with wrist flexion and extension. It may be preferable to tension this transfer after intrinsic stabilization is performed (see below.) The BR to FPL transfer is tensioned so that with the wrist in neutral, the thumb pulp just touches the side of the flexed index finger. If an accessory radial wrist extensor has been identified during the extensor phase, it can be transferred to the FPL and the BR can be transferred to the FCR to provide better wrist flexion.

Intrinsic stabilization

For the nontetraplegic person, the multiple functions of the intrinsic muscles are made more apparent when they no longer function. The strength of grip is considerably weakened. The fingers can no longer be widely spread apart at the metacarpophalangeal joint during finger extension. Even though the long flexors of the fingers have excursion sufficient to flex all the intervening joints, in the absence of the synchronizing effect of the intrinsic muscles, the finger tips in full flexion usually touch only to the bases of the fingers rather than fully into the center of the palm. Digital flexion begins at the distal joint under the influence of the long flexors and the finger tips roll into flexion rather than sweeping broadly and expansively along the spiral that the normally innervated finger tip follows. This rolling up of the fingertip will tend to push large objects out of the grasp.

The second major biomechanical function of the intrinsic muscles is also manifest in their absence. In the normal hand, the extrinsic extensors lift the proximal phalanges into extension, and are assisted in extending the interphalangeal joints by the action of the intrinsic muscles. In the absence of intrinsic muscle activity, the action of the extrinsic muscles at the metacarpophalangeal joint is unopposed. In hyperextending the metacarpophalangeal joint, the extrinsic extensor forfeits the excursion that might allow it to extend the interphalangeal joint. Furthermore this metacarpophalangeal hyperextension increases the visco-elastic tone of the long flexors, and induces some flexion at the interphalangeal joints. This imbalance gives rise to a particular posture termed the "claw hand" characterized by metacarpophalangeal hyperextension and interphalangeal joint flexion.

In the majority of tetraplegic patient, the absence of intrinsic muscle function may also result in an imbalance between the paralysed extrinsic flexors and extensors. The preoperative tetraplegic hand of IC groups 1–5 possesses only residual passive tenodesis grasp and release. For these patients, the tendency for the finger to claw as the wrist is flexed may represent only a cosmetic annoyance. However, operative procedures designed to improve digital flexion and extension in IC groups 3 and higher may accentuate the clawed posture by adding tone to both extrinsic extensors and flexors. In this circumstance, the claw deformity frequently becomes a significant functional liability in addition to further detracting from the appearance of the reconstructed hand. The deformity restricts the ability of the hand to open as widely as possible and reduces the range of objects easily grasped.

House and Walsh[46] presented convincing evidence that some type of intrinsic substitution results in a better and stronger grasp in the tetraplegic patient who is a candidate for the two-stage grasp-release procedure. Since most tetraplegic patients do not possess sufficient numbers of transferable muscles to allow intrinsic substitution by standard tendon transfer procedures, static procedures must typically suffice. One of two procedures, the first attributed to Zancolli[43] and termed the "lasso" procedure and the other described by House et al.[44] may be utilized for the tetraplegic patient.

Zancolli "lasso" procedure

In IC groups 3, 4 and 5, the flexor digitorum superficialis muscles are paralysed, typically at the upper motor neuron level. As such, they retain some stretch reflexes through the intact spinal reflex arc and relatively normal visco-elastic properties. Zancolli[43] proposed using these paralysed muscles as an elastic tenodesis to reduce metacarpophalangeal joint hyperextension and lessen the clawed posture of the tetraplegic's hand. For each finger that exhibits significantly troublesome clawing, the superficialis tendon is inserted under some tension, into the flexor sheath at the distal margin of the A1 pulley or even slightly more distally into the proximal part of the A2 pulley *(Fig. 37.12)*. The superficialis tendon is redeployed from its role as the primary flexor of the proximal interphalangeal joint to become the prime flexor of the metacarpophalangeal joint. This achieves the principal goal of surgery, providing a proper balance between the flexor and extensor muscles.

The mechanical basis for this dynamic tenodesis procedure is debated. Zancolli believes that the transfer must be fixed under significant tension in order to still provide MP flexor tone even with the wrist near maximally flexed. He believes that the transfer may assist in initiating some MP flexion as a consequence of wrist extension triggering some reflexive FDS contraction.

This procedure may be performed as part of either the extensor (release) or flexor (grasp) phase of reconstruction. It is more difficult to judge the proper tension of the transfer if performed at the time of the extensor phase. If performed as part of the flexor phase, it is preferable to perform the "lasso procedure" before adjusting the tension of the finger flexor transfer.

House intrinsic tenodesis

This procedure, described by House et al.,[44] is a modification of Riordan's tenodesis procedure.[47] In the tetraplegic patient, it is frequently performed for only the index and middle finger, since these fingers are the most critical in grasp and release functions. However, the procedure *(Fig. 37.13A)* can be performed on all four fingers as well. In this procedure,

a free tendon loop is anchored at the level of the head of the metacarpal. The free ends of the tendon graft may be anchored to one of several sites on the extensor mechanism at or proximal to the proximal interphalangeal joint, depending upon the finding of the preoperative examination. If the preoperative examination demonstrates that the interphalangeal joints are extended by the EDC tenodesis (with the examiner preventing MP joint hyperextension, then the graft may be anchored into the lateral band. If this test indicates that the extensor mechanism has become overstretched at the central slip area, the graft should be anchored into the base of the middle phalanx as demonstrated in *Figure 37.13B–H*.

The Zancolli procedure may be chosen when preoperative testing demonstrates that the interphalangeal joints are extended by the EDC tenodesis performed at the initial stage. If the extensor mechanism over the PIP joint has become overstretched, this joint will not be extended by the EDC tenodesis. In this case, the procedure described by House should be chosen.

Postoperative care

The hand is casted with the wrist in slight flexion, the metacarpophalangeal joints in moderate flexion and the interphalangeal joints in very slight flexion. After 4 weeks of immobilization, the cast is removed and an orthosis fitted to protect the MP joints against full extension for several more weeks. No resistance is allowed for 8 weeks.

The IC group 4 and 5 patient

In IC group 4 the pronator teres (PT) is strong and available for transfer. In IC group 5 the flexor carpi radialis (FCR) is strong, but experience has shown that it should not be used as a transfer. Therefore, the surgical options are similar for both IC groups 4 and 5.

The pronator teres is the only functioning pronator muscle in these IC group 4 and 5 patients. However it can be transferred and yet retain most of its pronator function if the direction of the transfer does not differ much from its original direction. In this respect, it can be safely use to activate the FPL. The BR is then available for another function. As stated above it can be transferred to the finger extensors provided there is enough volar stabilization of the wrist. This is achieved if FCR is graded MRC 3 or above. Otherwise the results of the transfers may be unpredictable.

Alternative procedures for IC groups 4 and 5 include various combinations of procedures already described. Since patients differ, it is important to be able to plan for variations in patient presentation and individual functional objectives. For example, it has been our experience that patients who have had different procedures performed for each arm have been pleased with their differences. They preferentially use one hand for certain activities, such as grasping large objects and the other for different tasks, e.g., manipulating smaller objects. The greatest variation in hand use has been a consequence of the management of the thumb's CMC joint. A fused CMC joint, while predictably pre-positioning the thumb, does

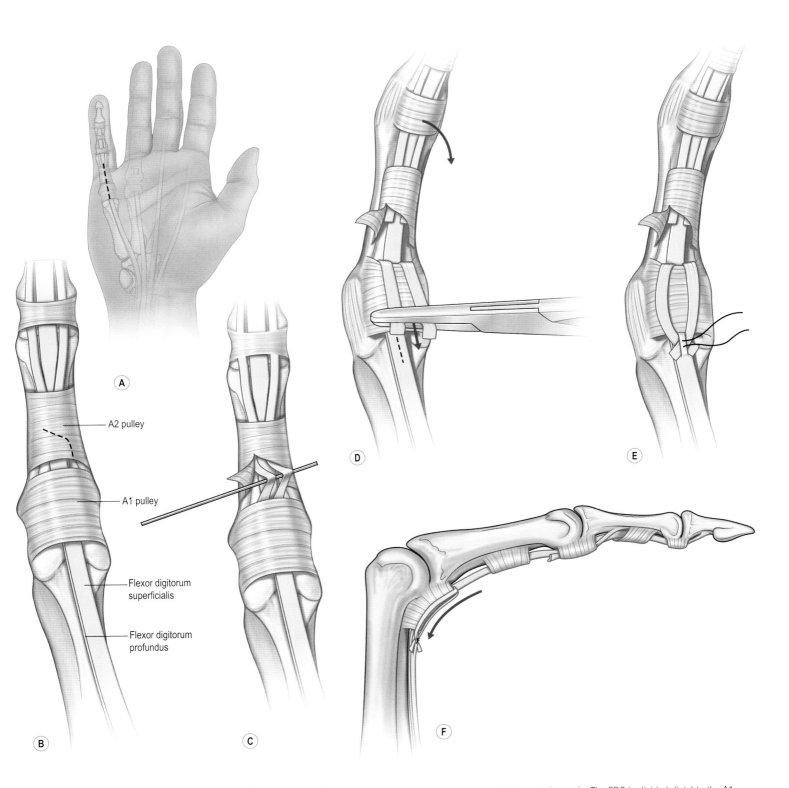

Fig. 37.12 The Zancolli "lasso" procedure **(A–F).** Either several longitudinal incisions or one longer transverse incision can be made. The FDS is divided distal to the A1 pulley, looped about the pulley and sutured to itself proximal to the pulley under strong tension. If the MP joints remain nearly fully flexed with the wrist in neutral, proper tension has been achieved. (Redrawn after Hentz V, Leclercq C. Surgical Rehabilitation of the Upper Limb in Tetraplegia. London: Harcourt Health Sciences; 2002, with permission.)

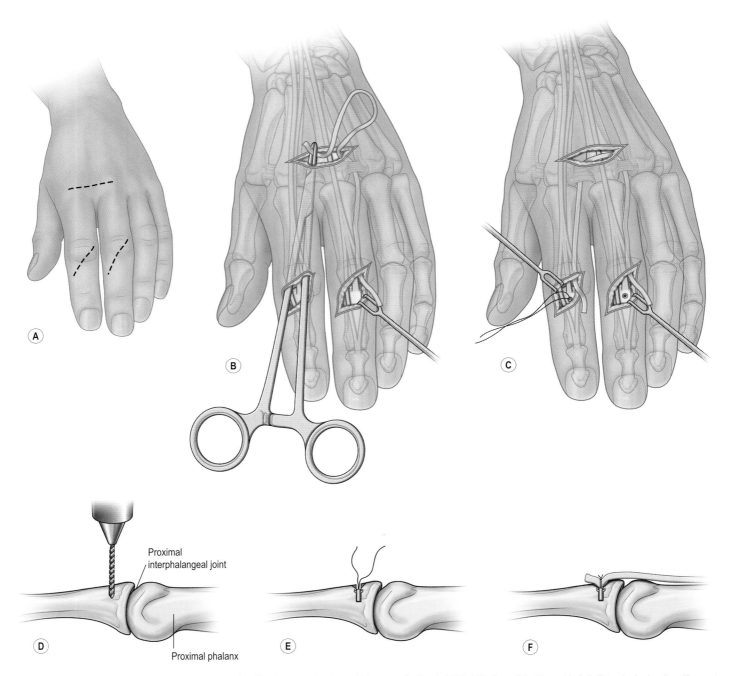

Fig. 37.13 The House intrinsic substitution procedure **(A–H).** (Redrawn after Hentz V, Leclercq C. Surgical Rehabilitation of the Upper Limb in Tetraplegia. London: Harcourt Health Sciences; 2002, with permission.)

limit the size of objects easily grasped within the first web space. If the CMC joint is left mobile, the postoperative position of the thumb ray is less predictable, sometimes significantly so, but larger objects can be pushed into the first web space and held.

We have based decisions regarding these alternatives in large part on the preoperative presentation of the thumb's CMC joint. If the joint is completely unstable, meaning time

and poor transfer mechanics have resulted in slackening of all CMC ligaments, we prefer to fuse the CMC joint. Other options include fusing or leaving flexible the thumb's CMC joint and options regarding the number of transfers directed at strengthening thumb function, typically carried out during the flexor phase. Surgery is performed in two stages, as in IC group 3 with the extensor phase performed before the flexor phase.

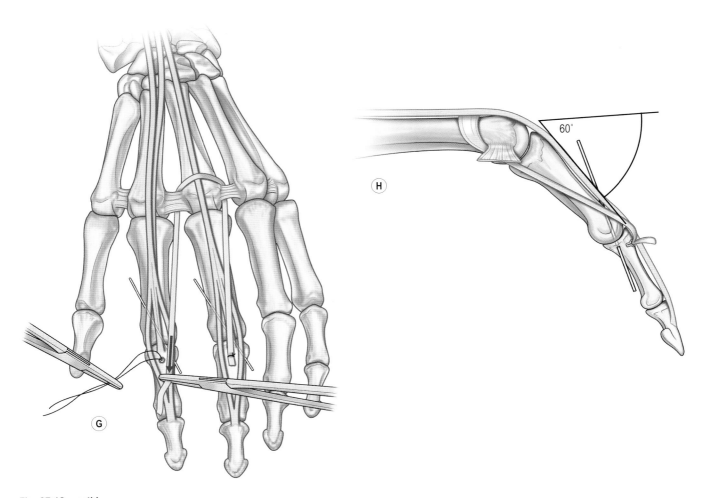

Fig. 37.13, cont'd

The unstable CMC joint

Extensor phase

If the flexor carpi radialis is weak (less than MRC grade 3, IC group 4, the extensor phase is identical to IC group 3:

- Tenodesis of EDC and EPL to the radius
- Thumb CMC joint fusion
- Split FPL to EPL tenodesis.

If the FCR is graded MRC 3 and above (typically an IC 5 arm), the fingers and thumb extensors can be activated by the brachioradialis. The procedure then includes:

- Transfer of BR to EDC and EPL
- Thumb CMC joint fusion
- Split FPL to EPL tenodesis.

If BR to EDC/EPL is chosen, tension is set with the elbow in 40° flexion, the wrist in a neutral position, and the MP joint in about 20° of flexion. Tension should be such that, during passive flexion of the wrist, the MP joints start extending when the wrist reaches neutral from an extended position. The tension on the EPL tendon should be adjusted last and its tension is typically set slightly looser than that of the EDC. The fingers should exhibit full passive flexion when the wrist is fully extended.

After 4 weeks in the cast, rehabilitation of active finger extensors is directed toward developing active extension of the MP joints.

Flexor phase

The second stage is performed once the patient has been able to demonstrate active thumb and finger extension. The operative steps include:

- Transfer of ECRL to finger flexors (FDP)
- Transfer of either BR or PT to FPL
- Intrinsic stabilization, if not performed at the extensor phase.

Transfers of ECRL to FDP and BR to FPL have been described. An interpositional tendon graft may be needed if the PT is chosen to power the FPL. The tension is adjusted so that with the wrist in neutral the thumb rests against the lateral aspect of the index finger.

Postoperative care

Postoperatively, the wrist and fingers are immobilized with the wrist in slight flexion, and the fingers in 60° of MP and 45° of PIP flexion. At 4 weeks, the cast is removed, and physiotherapy is conducted in the same manner as in IC group 3. The use of a manual wheelchair and shifting of the body weight on to the hands are restricted for one more month.

Stable thumb CMC joint

Extensor phase

For this patient, the extensor phase typically includes the following operative steps:

- Tenodesis of EDC to the radius
- Tenodesis of the re-routed EPL
- Split FPL to EPL thumb IP stabilization.

In this case, the tendon of the EPL is divided at its muscle-tendon junction, withdrawn at the level of the MP joint, passed proximally and under the tendons of the first dorsal compartment, and then toward the third compartment where it is anchored. This provides an extensor-abductor vector when the wrist is flexed. Postoperative immobilization, rehabilitation and precautions have been addressed above.

Flexor phase

The flexor phase can be carried out once passive mobility and muscle strength has recovered to its maximum potential. The goals of this phase include transfers to provide both positional control and a powerful thumb pinch, a transfer to restore active finger flexion, and intrinsic balance. The operative steps include:

- Transfer of the ECRL to FDP (fingers in reverse cascade position)
- Transfer of pronator teres to FPL
- Brachioradialis, extended with ring FDS tendon, transferred across the palm to restore thumb flexion/abduction *(Fig. 37.14)*.
- Intrinsic substitution procedure, either lasso or House method, if not performed in extensor phase.

Tension is assessed by gently passively flexing the wrist and determining that the fingers and thumb can be opened almost fully and by gently extending the wrist and judging the cascade of the fingers and the posture of the thumb. The wrist and fingers are splinted with the wrist in very slight flexion; the fingers are nearly fully flexed at the metacarpophalangeal joints and the thumb relatively widely abducted, with the tip of the thumb touching the tip of the index finger. Immobilization is maintained for approximately four weeks followed by rehabilitation. The tendon junctures must be protected against great force for some additional weeks particularly in the wheelchair-bound patient. Transfers and pressure relief activities are restricted for a full 8 weeks.

Strong grasp and refined pinch: IC groups 6, 7 and 8

Video 2

Patients classified at the OCu-6 level possess active digital extension but lack thumb extension. They require only adding an extensor force for the thumb and, at the same operation, multiple tendon transfer to achieve balanced thumb pinch and strong finger grasp. Therefore, only one procedure is necessary and their period of dependence is minimal.

Patients with even greater number of remaining resources, such as patients in IC groups 7 and 8, can be reconstructed similar to patients with a lower peripheral nerve injury. The surgical procedures performed for these patients are directed at reconstructing some aspects of hand intrinsic muscle function and balance. There are relatively few tetraplegic patients in this category compared to the OCu-2 or OCu-5 categories and we have operated on insufficient numbers to draw useful conclusions.

Other presentations

Some injury patterns do not fit easily into the international classification. Patients with so-called central cord injuries have hands that defy classification. These patients require prolonged studies and frequent re-examination before formulating a surgical plan. Temporary nerve blocks have been particularly helpful in determining the procedure of choice.

Functional neuromuscular stimulation

Functional electrical stimulation (FES) is an exciting adjuvant for improving arm function in these patients. The initial commercially available system was eight epimysial electro-channels device called the Freehand System. This system allowed patients with very high spinal injury to activate and control a pre-program sequence of muscle contractions and thus achieve a useful grasp for one hand.[48–51] Research continues on this system and current models have the ability to stimulate 12 muscles.[52] These systems of electrodes placed on predetermined upper motor neuron paralyzed muscles is often the only option to restore useful function in limbs heretofore deemed useless and unreconstructable by standard surgical techniques. We hope that as further research proceeds, these may again become commercially available *(Fig. 37.15)*.

Outcomes and complications

These procedures have evolved overtime and can provide predictable improvement in function. A recent systematic review gives data on the average outcomes for the most common of these procedures posterior deltoid to triceps transfer and procedures to restore pinch. For the deltoid to triceps the average postoperative strength was 3.3 MRC. This would certainly allow stabilization of the arm in space. Complications were not infrequent at 25% with the most frequent being rupture or stretching of the repair. Pinch reconstruction procedures were divided into those with active motors, such as a BR, or those that were simply a FPL tenodesis or Moberg procedure. The mean postoperative strength after both types of pinch surgery was 1.9 kg. The mean postoperative after FPL tenodesis was 1.17 kg and for those using an active motor postoperative strength was 2.32 kg. There was a 40% rate of complications in this review. The most common complications were flexion contracture of the elbow or of the thumb, stretching or rupture of repair, and loosening of pins across the thumb IP joint. Two of these complications, flexion contracture of the thumb and loosening of pins, are no longer applicable as the procedures have evolved to address these

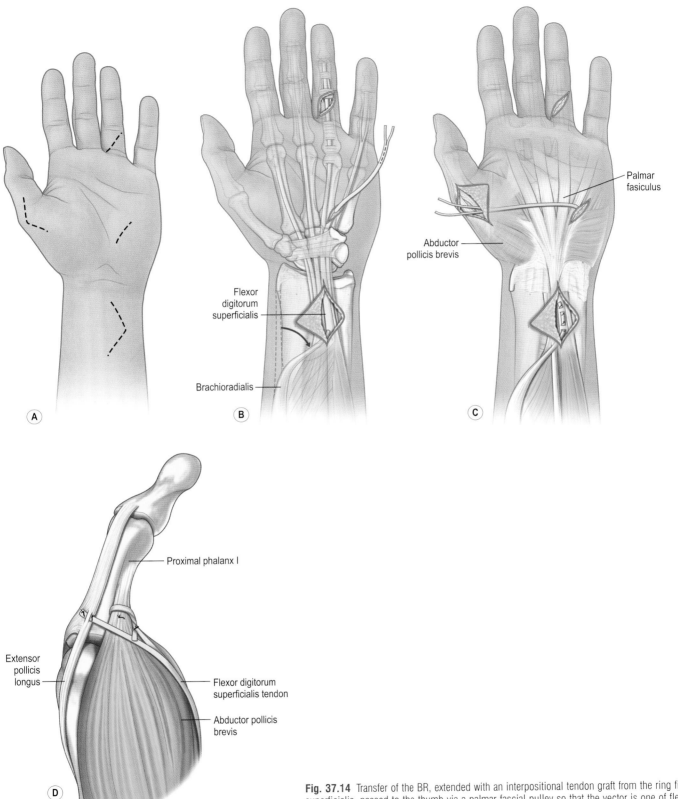

Fig. 37.14 Transfer of the BR, extended with an interpositional tendon graft from the ring finger superficialis, passed to the thumb via a palmar fascial pulley so that the vector is one of flexion-abduction **(A–D).** (Redrawn after Hentz V, Leclercq C. Surgical Rehabilitation of the Upper Limb in Tetraplegia. London: Harcourt Health Sciences; 2002, with permission.)

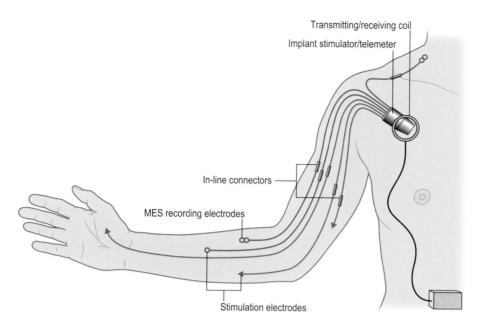

Fig. 37.15 A multichannel functional electrical stimulation (FES) system. (Redrawn after Kilgore KL, Hoyen HA, Bryden AM, et al. An implanted upper extremity neuroprosthesis utilizing myoelectric control. J Hand Surg Am 2008; 33:539–550.)

complications (we no longer fuse the IPJ and do not release the A1 pulley) *(Fig. 37.16A–C).*[53]

These procedures are also very durable. We examined 45 patients who had been operated at least 10 years prior to evaluation. We analyzed these patients according to the proposed major preoperative goals. A total of 21 of these patients had undergone elbow extensor reconstruction; 15 patients had posterior deltoid to triceps transfer and 10 had bilateral transfers. All 15 had required a motorized wheelchair as their primary means of movement before surgery. Ten years following surgery, nine now used a pushchair as their standard chair and four others used a push-chair at least some of the time. There were three patients who had undergone bilateral posterior deltoid to triceps transfer who, were able to self-transfer in the early postoperative period. All three continued to be able to perform this monumental, for a tetraplegic, task. In the six patients having biceps to triceps transfer (all needing contracture release), two could use a push-chair, but not exclusively so. None had developed a recurrence of elbow contracture.

The second goal was the restoration of pinch for the weaker patients and pinch and grasp, as well as the ability to open the hand for the stronger patients. IC group 2 patients typically had key grip fashioned by tenodesis of the flexor pollicis longus to the radius. Seven were evaluated for greater than 10 years. Five had maintained pinch strength essentially equivalent to that demonstrated 6–12 months following surgery.

IC group 3 patients typically had transfer of brachioradialis to flexor pollicis longus to restore dynamic voluntary key pinch. Six were evaluated and all had maintained useful power, which averaged 20 Newtons. Thumb interphalangeal joint instability seemed to play a strong role in the diminished

power seen in several of the BR-FPL patients. We now routinely employ the split FPL attachment described by Mohammed et al.[40] to provide thumb interphalangeal stabilization, thus avoiding IP joint fusion.

Of the IC group 4 and 5 patients, the strong patients, 18 were re-examined. Almost all had undergone two stage procedures, and half had elected bilateral reconstruction. Flexor power was by active transfer of extensor carpi radialis longus, brachioradialis or pronator teres or accessory wrist extensor, always in some combination to the thumb and digital flexors. Six had undergone some type of additional surgery in the period between their initial surgery and the date of long term evaluation, typically, adjustment of the flexor to one or another finger (usually the index) or release of a contracted proximal interphalangeal joint (usually the ring or little.) Grip power had not deteriorated in these patients compared to value measured at the 6–12 months evaluation post their initial surgery. Pinch force averaged 34 Newtons. We found, as did House and Walsh,[46] that those patients who had had some type of intrinsic stabilization, either by Zancolli[43] lasso or by House et al.'s[44] intrinsic reconstruction procedure, had, on average, more powerful grasp. This may be a product of preselection however, the stronger patients selectively chosen for intrinsic substitution.

Conclusions

Carefully planned upper limb reconstructive procedures in tetraplegia are both effective and durable *(Fig. 37.17).* Systematic post-injury evaluation of their upper limbs should

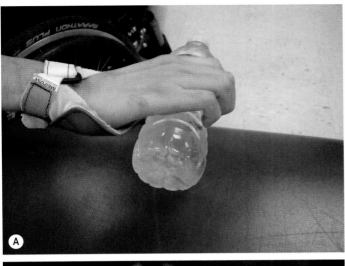

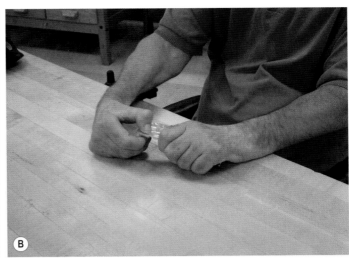

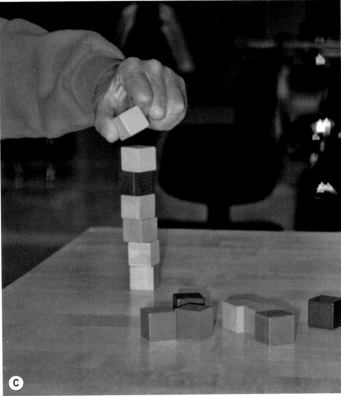

Fig. 37.16 (A–C) Postoperative results after pinch reconstruction.

becomes a standard part of the more generally studied systems such as renal and bladder function, blood pressure and pulmonary status. Aside from their brain, the upper limbs remain the most important residual resource for people with tetraplegia.

The rewards for surgeons, rehabilitation medicine specialists, and therapists are best expressed by one of our patients who replied to a question requesting his feelings on his outcome, "it's not as much as I hoped for, but it's much more than I ever had."

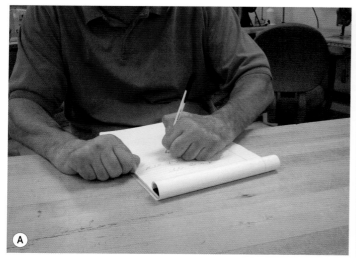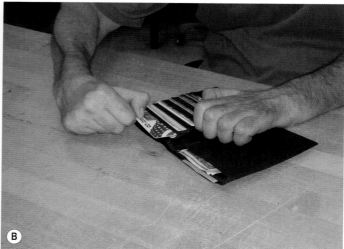

Fig. 37.17 (A,B) Postoperative results after pinch reconstruction.

Access the complete reference list online at **http://www.expertconsult.com**

4. Hentz VR, Leclercq C. *Surgical Rehabilitation of the Upper Limb in Tetraplegia*. London: Harcourt Health Sciences; 2002.

    This is the most up-to-date monograph devoted to the field of upper extremity reconstruction for tetraplegia. It delves into all of the nuances of these procedures.

10. McDowell CL, Moberg EA, Smith AG. International conference on surgical rehabilitation of the upper limb in tetraplegia. *J Hand Surg Am*. 1979;4:387–390.

22. Kozin SH, D'Addesi L, Chafetz RS, et al. Biceps-to-triceps transfer for elbow extension in persons with tetraplegia. *J Hand Surg Am*. 2010;35(6):968–975.

    This article presents the key technical details for biceps to triceps transfer. The illustrations simplify the procedure. The postoperative regimen is clearly described.

26. Moberg E. Surgical treatment for absent single-hand grip and elbow extension in quadriplegia. *J Bone Joint Surg Am*. 1975;57(2):196–206.

    This is the classic article that must be read by anyone contemplating operating on a tetraplegic patient. It describes two key procedures, the Moberg key pinch and deltoid to triceps transfer.

36. Freehafer AA. Gaining independence in tetraplegia. Cleveland technique. *Clin Orthop*. 1998;355:282–289.

    This article represents a summary of techniques and pearls gathered over a 30 year career.

39. Waters RL, Stark LZ, Gubernick I, et al. Electromyographic analysis of brachioradialis to flexor pollicis longus tendon transfer in quadriplegia. *J Hand Surg Am*. 1990;15:335–339.

44. House JH, Gwathmey FW, Lundsgaard DK. Restoration of strong grasp and lateral pinch in tetraplegia due to cervical spinal cord injury. *J Hand Surg Am*. 1976;1(2):152–159.

46. House J, Walsh T. Two stage reconstruction of the tetraplegic hand. Master techniques in orthopaedic surgery. In: Strickland JW, ed. *The Hand*. Philadelphia: Lippincott; 1998.

48. Mulcahey MJ, Smith BT, Betz RR, et al. Functional neuromuscular stimulation: Outcome in young people with tetraplegia. *J Am Paraplegia Soc*. 1994;17:20–35.

51. Wuolle KS, Van Doren CL, Thrope GB, et al. Development of a quantitative hand grasp and release test for patients with tetraplegia using a hand neuroprosthesis. *J Hand Surg Am*. 1994;19(2):209–218.

53. Hamou C, Shah NR, DiPonio L, et al. Pinch and elbow extension restoration in people with tetraplegia: a systematic review of the literature. *J Hand Surg Am*. 2009;34(4):692–699.

    Review. This systematic review provides information on what the average results and most common complications are for pinch and elbow reconstruction.

38

Upper extremity composite allotransplantation

Vijay S. Gorantla, Stefan S. Schneeberger, and W. P. Andrew Lee

SYNOPSIS

- Composite tissue allografts are composed of multiple tissue components of variable immunogenicity such as skin, lymph nodes, bone marrow and nerves, vessels, muscles, and bone.

- In nonsalvageable upper extremity loss, transplantation can restore the appearance, anatomy, and functionality by replacing and restoring missing tissue without donor site morbidity or multiple reconstructions.

- Composite tissue allotransplantation is not life saving but significantly enhances quality of life. Unlike in solid organs, recipients are otherwise healthy without co-morbidity. Risk-benefit consideration for patients must include the potential side effects from drug treatment necessary for graft survival.

- The conventional immunosuppression protocols used in upper extremity allotransplantation are similar to solid organ transplantation and have prevented early graft loss but not acute rejection at the expense of complications.

- Acute rejection in composite tissue allotransplants can be monitored visually which allows for timely intervention. Topical therapies of skin potentially allow reduction or supplementation of systemic therapy. Repetitive acute rejection of the skin, when properly treated, does not appear to impact long term allograft function or survival.

- During the past decade, more than 100 reconstructive transplant procedures have been performed around the world, including over 70 upper extremity allotransplantations with encouraging intermediate to long-term functional and graft survival outcomes.

- The overall goal is to further reduce immunologic risk and maximize functional outcomes by implementation of novel immunomodulatory approaches that integrate bone marrow cellular therapies with minimization of maintenance immunosuppression.

Access the Historical Perspective sections and Figure 38.1 online at **http://www.expertconsult.com**

Introduction

Millions of individuals each year sustain major trauma, have tumors surgically excised or are born with congenital defects that require complex reconstructive surgeries to repair the resulting large tissue defects. Conventional management of such tissue deficiencies with prosthetic rehabilitation or surgical reconstruction (with autologous tissues) may not achieve optimal outcomes. Current surgical procedures are limited by available tissues for reconstruction, morbidity from extensive surgery, prolonged rehabilitation and costs of multiple surgeries. For such complex injuries not amenable to conventional reconstruction, composite tissue allotransplantation can achieve near perfect primary restoration of tissue defects with improved functional and aesthetic outcomes. Composite tissue allotransplantation is among the newest of transplant areas and combines the time-tested techniques of reconstructive microsurgery with the immunologic principles of transplantation. The overall goal of composite tissue allotransplantation is to improve the quality of life of patients who have significant tissue defects.

Upper extremity transplants are vascularized composite tissue allografts because they are modules of distinct tissues, including skin, muscle, ligament, tendon, nerve, blood vessel, bone, joint and cartilage, bone marrow, and lymph nodes.[1] In the United States alone, the numbers of extremity amputations are estimated to be around 1285000 per year.[2] In 2005, there were approximately 1.6 million people living with limb loss, in the US.[3] Of these, nearly 540000 individuals had upper extremity amputations – 34000 individuals had major limb loss. Even if 1% of those with major upper limb loss were deemed candidates for hand transplantation, this would entail over 300 procedures. However, only 50 patients have undergone upper extremity allotransplantation in the world over the past 12 years. The reason for this disparity in numbers has largely been due to skepticism of the immunological feasibility[4] and concern for immunosuppression-related complications in upper extremity allotransplantation.[5] Despite their obvious advantages, the adverse effects of prolonged immunosuppression necessary for graft survival have limited the routine clinical use of these procedures. These risks include infection, cancer, and metabolic derangement and greatly affect recipient quality of life, alter the risk profile and jeopardize the potential benefits of upper extremity transplantation. Notably, unlike in solid organs, clinical success is dictated not only by graft acceptance and survival but also by nerve regeneration, which determines ultimate functional outcomes. Novel strategies such as cellular and biologic therapies that integrate the concepts of immune regulation with those of nerve regeneration have shown promising results in small and large animal models. Clinical translation of these insights to upper extremity reconstructive transplantation could further minimize the need of immunosuppression and optimize functional outcomes; enabling greater feasibility and wider application of these procedures as an option for upper extremity amputees.

Evolution of upper extremity allotransplantation

Immunology of composite tissue allografts

Much knowledge concerning the immunologic aspects of composite tissue allografts has been gained from studies in small and large animal models. Animal research has confirmed that each tissue in a composite tissue allograft has its own distinct degree of antigenicity and is rejected by different mechanisms. This is because each of the component tissues is characterized by different antigen expression and presentation mechanisms.[69] The components of a composite tissue allograft express different amounts of major histocompatibility complex (MHC) antigens and tissue-specific antigens, which are primarily responsible for the elicitation of the recipient's cellular mediated response.[70] Antigen recognition and targeting by the recipient immune system also differ among the allograft tissue elements owing to their different vascular and lymphatic supply. Altogether, these facts explain a pattern of differential rejection observed in whole limb transplanted allografts. For example, transplanted muscle elicits mainly a cell-mediated immune response, whereas skin elicits both cellular and humoral responses.[71] In general, skin and bone marrow appear to reject earlier and more aggressively than muscle, bone, cartilage or tendon. The knowledge of relative antigenicity can lead to the development of strategies intended to decrease the antigenicity of a specific component. In addition, a better understanding of this relative antigenicity of allograft components enables the concept of tailored immunosuppression, targeting only specific cellular and humoral components of rejection. This would limit the amount of immunosuppression used and the consequent related complications of opportunistic infections and malignancies. Thus, it is logical to presume that to prevent rejection; the most effective immunosuppressive strategy would be a combination of agents that affect different pathways of the immune response through different mechanisms.[72] Ideally, this combination of drugs must be selective, specific, and synergistic, free of toxic reactions, easy to administer, and inexpensive. Most of the information regarding potential immunosuppressive

regimens has been derived from small animal (rat) and large animal (porcine, canine, and primate) composite tissue allograft models.

Experimental background and scientific basis

In early rodent limb transplant studies (pre-cyclosporine A era), recipients treated with various combinations of immunosuppressive doses of 6-mercaptopurine or its derivative azathioprine and prednisone all died from drug-induced side-effects before the onset of macroscopic signs of rejection.[73] Even high doses of cyclosporine A did not improve limb or animal survival.[74–78] The incidence of side-effects and morbidity/mortality was significant. Indeed, cyclosporine A monotherapy has been uniformly unsuccessful in prolonging composite tissue allograft survival not only in small animal but also in nonhuman primate models, which have been considered to be representative of the human immune system and the best predictors of success in clinical trials.[79] Remarkably, composite tissue allograft rejection in nonhuman primates cannot be prevented unless trough levels of cyclosporine A are 3–4 times the level achieved in human solid organ transplantation resulting in peri-transplant infections and malignancies.[80–83]

None of the above-mentioned studies attempted to combine a calcineurin inhibitor and an antimetabolite drug (such as mycophenolate mofetil) with or without steroids. None of the above studies could consistently demonstrate long-term limb allograft survival. In 1996, Benhaim and colleagues demonstrated that a combination of cyclosporine with mycophenolate mofetil could successfully prolong rat hind limb allograft survival.[84] For the first time, predictable long-term, functional limb allograft survival was achieved. Using a similar regimen, the only large animal model that demonstrated long-term survival of fully mismatched composite tissue allografts was the swine model.[85,86] It should be noted that like the nonhuman primate, swine and humans share immunological similarities. These include the structure of MHC and the expression of MHC class II antigens (on endothelial cells, epithelial cells, and dendritic cells).[87] Therefore, there was sufficient sound evidence in both a small (rodent)[88,89] and large animal composite tissue allograft model,[85,86] implying that the experimental basis of human extremity composite tissue allotransplantation was feasible.[90]

The success in rodent and swine models did not translate to primate studies. This was because modern combination immunosuppression (tacrolimus or cyclosporine A with mycophenolate mofetil ± steroids) has never been tested in a nonhuman primate composite tissue allograft model.[79] However, given the marked success of the early hand transplant experience (95% graft survival with 100% 1- and 2-year patient survival) using standard combination therapy, the lack of a pre-clinical primate model may now only be semi-relevant.

Extensive experience with organ transplantation has provided us with valuable information about the immunologic consequences of organ allografting and the efficacy and toxicity of immunosuppressive drugs. The field of transplantation evolved from transplanted kidneys[91] and hearts[92,93] to livers,[94] lungs,[95] pancreas,[96] small bowel,[97] multiple abdominal viscera,[98] bone marrow,[99] and, most recently, composite tissue allografts.[100,101] The initial results of graft and patient survival after organ transplantation in the 1960s were poor. Editorials in major clinical journals,[102] including the *New England Journal of Medicine*,[103–105] questioned the feasibility and ethical basis of these procedures. There was great concern for the adverse effects of chronic immunosuppression, especially the risk of opportunistic infections and malignancies. During the next four decades, because of the improvements in immunosuppression and in the management of post-transplant complications, this pessimism abated. Remarkably, however, attempts at hand transplantation,[106,107] after three decades of quiescence since the first attempt in Ecuador,[46,47] met with vigorous opposition. Paradoxically, most of the criticism came from hand surgeons.[108–114] They argued that the risks of immunosuppressive therapy were justifiable in potentially life-saving organ transplants, but not in quality-of-life-enhancing transplants such as hand transplants. Furthermore, many hand surgeons thought that the immunological, ethical,[115,116] and psychological[117] issues associated with hand transplantation needed to be addressed.[118]

The rationale for proceeding with clinical trials of hand transplantation using modern immunosuppression, has been based on scientific progress on several fronts: (1) the availability of novel immunosuppressive drugs that have improved efficacy and lower risk profiles; (2) improved prophylaxis and treatment of opportunistic fungal or viral infections (such as *Pneumocystis carinii* and *Cytomegalovirus*); 3) improved therapies for post-transplant malignancies (such as rituximab for post-transplant lymphoproliferative disorder, PTLD); (4) better expertise with drug dosing and fine-tuning of immunosuppressive drug combinations based on years of experience with solid organ transplantation, and, most importantly (5) all individual component tissues of the hand, including skin, muscle, tendons, vessels, nerve, bone and joint, were successfully transplanted in humans before the modern era of hand transplantation.[119]

Chronology of clinical upper extremity allotransplantation

In September 1991, the first conference on composite tissue allotransplantation was held in Washington, DC to "determine the clinical feasibility of transplanting limbs in patients with limb loss" and the "direction in which clinically oriented limb transplantation research should head."[120] In November 1997, the 1st International Symposium on Composite Tissue Allotransplantation was convened in Louisville, Kentucky to discuss the "scientific, clinical and ethical barriers standing in the way of performing the first human hand transplant." International experts at the meeting predicted that limb allotransplantation was not far from "becoming a clinical reality."[121] Within the next 22 months; 34 years after the first hand transplant,[46,47] surgeons in Lyon, France, performed the world's second unilateral hand transplant in September, 1998.[106,107,122,123] In January 1999, the first unilateral hand transplant in the United States was performed in Louisville, Kentucky.[124,125]

Following these attempts, over the past 12 years, seven centers in Europe, five centers in China and five centers in the US have performed over 70 upper extremity allotransplantations. These were predominantly wrist to mid-forearm amputations, except for two partial hand grafts in China, one partial hand graft in the US, and two cases of above elbow transplantation. The first American patient has the longest surviving transplant, at 12 years, in January 2011.[126,127]

Experience with upper extremity allotransplantation

Program, patient, procedural and protocol-related considerations

Program establishment and implementation

Starting a hand transplant program poses tremendous challenges.[128,129] Solid organ transplantation and hand replantation are time-tested procedures and are now the standard of care. Hand transplantation is the amalgamation of the scientific principles of reconstructive surgery and the concepts of organ transplantation. Thus, for any hand transplant program to be successful, it must be collaboration between a multidisciplinary team comprised among others of a core group of hand (plastic or orthopedic) and transplant surgeons. The transplant process is well established but is bound by tight regulation. This is not well known to most outside the field and often comes as a surprise to reconstructive plastic/hand surgeons who wish to start a hand program. The logistics of upper extremity allotransplantation can often be overwhelming and challenging for a new program. This is where the experience of the solid organ transplant members of the group helps in negotiating through the process. Such a joint effort can overcome the challenges that are inherent in a complex therapeutic option that integrates multiple specialties during the planning, procedural, and post-transplant phases.

Donor and recipient selection

The overall success of composite tissue transplantation relies on many factors. One could argue that it is the technical expertise of the team and effective postoperative care of the recipient that plays a significant role in transplant outcomes. However, it is the proper evaluation, selection and management of donors and potential recipients that is probably more important. Decades of experience with solid organs have allowed us to establish criteria for donor and recipient selection. In a novel field like hand transplantation, parameters for inclusion and exclusion of donors and recipients have not yet been conclusively defined nor standardized.[130,131] *Tables 38.1 and 38.2* highlight the general selection criteria in upper extremity transplantation and compares them to those of solid organ transplantation. Patients below the age of 18 are not considered to be adults, and, therefore, there are issues of informed consent in an experimental procedure. Furthermore, pediatric patients are more likely to develop immunosuppressive related complications like PTLD, than adults.[132] Patients over the age of 65 are excluded because of increased immunosuppression-related complications; limited years of potential gain from the transplant; and decreased nerve regeneration. Medical screening of recipients includes a complete medical history and physical examination; routine laboratory studies; blood typing and cross-matching; human

Table 38.1 Donor considerations in upper extremity transplantation versus solid organ transplantation

Upper extremity transplantation	Solid organ transplantation

Demographic and phenotypic characteristics
   Skin color, tone, and texture match
   Limb size and dimension (bone length and diameter match)
   Age, sex, race and ethnicity match if possible
	Organs from older/marginal donors may be considered. No other demographic or phenotypic exclusions

Donors must be deceased (brain death declared)	Donors may be deceased or living-related in particular organ transplants
Donor limb dissection and procurement must not interfere with organ recovery. Limb usually prepped first, perfused under isolated tourniquet, dissected after cross clamp and retrieved in sequence with heart and lung recovery. This minimizes overall ischemia time	Organs are dissected and procured in order of importance or in tandem by multiple teams. Sensitivity of organ to ischemia may be a consideration in timing or recovery
Donor family consent includes a discussion of cosmetic prosthesis for open casket funerals	No such consideration
History of malignancy (recent or remote) may be an exclusion	Donors with some malignancies (CNS tumors) may be considered
Paralysis of ischemia or traumatic origin, inherited peripheral neuropathy, infectious, post infectious or inflammatory neuropathy, toxic neuropathy (i.e., heavy metal poisoning, drug toxicity, industrial agent exposure) or mixed connective tissue disease, severe deforming rheumatoid or osteoarthritis in the limb may be exclusions	No such consideration

Table 38.2 Recipient considerations in upper extremity transplantation versus solid organ transplantation

Upper extremity transplantation	Solid organ transplantation
Subjects can be of any race, color, ethnicity in good health	Subjects usually have extensive co-morbidity
Age range for eligibility is variable but usually over 18 years and under 65 years	Age range is broader and related to organ failure or need for organ replacement
Subjects with congenital defects (e.g., transverse arrest) are currently not candidates due to the unknowns related to lack of pre-existing cortical recognition	Congenital (structural/genetic/metabolic) organ defects are candidates
Blindness is an exclusion in some programs due to complicated rehabilitation and lack of visual feedback that is critical for functional recovery	Blindness is not an exclusion
Rigorous psychosocial assessment mandatory to determine motivation for transplantation, emotional and cognitive preparedness for the procedure, body image adaptation, level of realistic expectations regarding post-transplant outcomes, anticipated comfort with the transplant, personality organization/risk of regression, history of medication compliance/substance abuse, potential for compliance, and social support system/family structure	Psychosocial screening performed but not rigorous or as exhaustive in nature
Use or attempted use of prostheses prior to transplant is a suggested requirement	No such consideration

leucocyte antigen (HLA) typing; testing for panel-reactive antibodies; and serology for Epstein–Barr virus, cytomegalovirus, HIV, and viral hepatitis. Other tests include radiography (to plan for osteosynthesis), angiography (to exclude abnormal vascular patterns), electromyography, nerve conduction velocity, and functional magnetic resonance imaging (fMRI).

Procedural aspects

Donor limb procurement

The organ procurement organization (OPO) will ensure that selection of potential hand donors is completely in accordance to study criteria. If the donor is unstable, the hand dissection is performed following organ dissection. However, before cross clamping of aorta, the hand team commences dissection and retrieves the limb prior to organ retrieval. The limb is perfused under isolated tourniquet by cold Histidine–Tryptophan–Ketoglutarate (HTK, Custodiol) solution through a brachial artery cannula prior to disarticulation. Upon completion of hand retrieval *(Fig. 38.2)*, the donor stump is closed *(Fig. 38.3)* and the body can be fitted with a cosmetic prosthesis *(Fig. 38.4)*, allowing the family the option of an open-casket funeral. Following retrieval, the limb (wrapped in moist sterile gauze and placed in a polyurethane bag) is transported in a sterile container (provided by the OPO) with

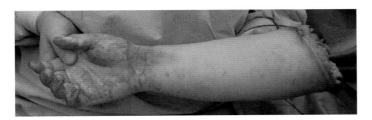

Fig. 38.2 Donor graft after isolated perfusion and disarticulation.

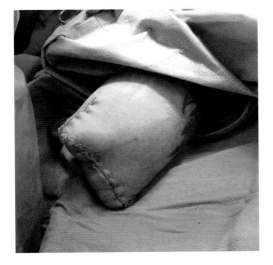

Fig. 38.3 Donor stump following closure.

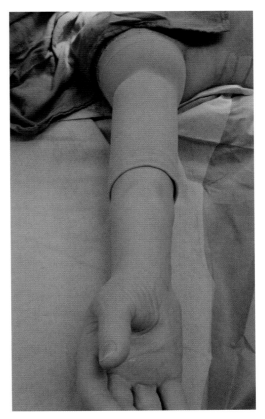

Fig. 38.4 Donor stump fitted with a cosmetic prosthesis to facilitate open casket viewing.

iced water at 4°C–6°C. Donor spleen and lymph nodes are collected and cell suspensions cryopreserved for future immune assays.

Recipient surgery

After confirming donor match, the recipient undergoes placement of regional blocks, preparation for general anesthesia and induction therapy (most commonly with basiliximab, Simulect; anti-thymocyte globulin, ATG, or alemtuzumab, Campath 1H). Hand transplantation does not differ greatly from replantation. Instrumentation and technique are similar. A two-team approach is used. The donor team prepares the donor limb once received on the back table, tailoring the graft to the needs of the recipient and tagging the structures *(Fig. 38.5)*. The two main hand transplant surgeons and assistant hand transplant surgeons (dissecting the donor limb), are assisted by one scrub nurse per extremity, two circulators per room, and at least one anesthesiologist. Based on the preoperative assessment of the recipient, tissue requirements from the donor will be known. The team dissecting the recipient must know exactly what measurements are necessary for the donor team to proceed. The recipient team will need to clearly identify the amount of nerve, artery and veins required for transplantation *(Fig. 38.6)*. The sequence of tissue repair is to minimize ischemia time and could depend on surgical preference. Commonly, it includes bony fixation → artery repair → vein repair (revascularization) → tendon repair → nerve

repair → skin closure *(Fig. 38.7)*. Intraoperative biopsies should be taken of all tissues to serve as baseline controls.

Protocol-related considerations

Maintenance immunosuppression

The current immunosuppressive protocols applied to upper extremity transplantation are extrapolated from regimens used in solid organ transplantation. The overall amount of immunosuppression required to ensure graft survival is comparable with that used in renal transplantation. Such conventional immunosuppression has resulted in 100% patient and graft survival at 1 year after upper extremity transplantation; an outcome that has not been achieved in any other field of transplantation.[126] The majority of hand transplant patients received either polyclonal (antithymocyte globulins, ATGs) or monoclonal (alemtuzumab, basiliximab) antibody preparations as induction therapy followed by high-dose triple-drug combination for maintenance therapy including tacrolimus, mycophenolate mofetil (MMF), and steroids, although the doses and trough levels of each drug differed between some centers. Such regimens have proved sufficient to prevent early immunologic graft loss but were not able to prevent acute rejection. Some programs follow steroid avoidance regimens, while others rely on monotherapy immunosuppression. Successful reversal of acute rejection episodes *(Fig. 38.8)* has been achieved using topical clobetasol or tacrolimus ointment with or without short-term bolus steroid doses.[133,134]

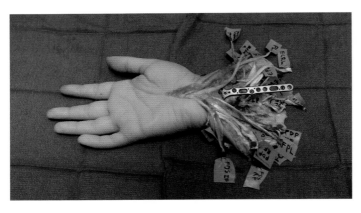

Fig. 38.5 Tagging of structures in the donor graft following back-table dissection. Proper identification of donor tendons, nerves and vessels expedites the surgery, improves technical success and reduces ischemia time.

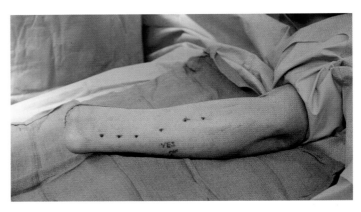

Fig. 38.6 Recipient stump marking for planning skin incisions, orientation of donor and recipient flaps, and identification of superficial veins.

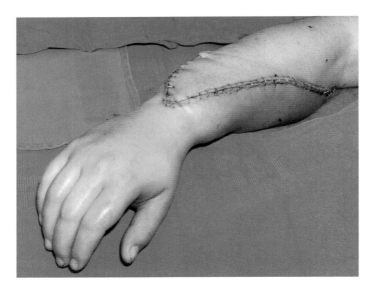

Fig. 38.7 Recipient post-transplant showing flap orientation.

Rehabilitation and functional assessment after hand transplantation

Rehabilitation and functional assessment are integral components of successful upper extremity allotransplantation.[135] The hand therapist is involved in the entire process from initial screening of prospective patients through final discharge. The goal is functional integration of the transplanted hand into the patient's daily activities. Successful rehabilitation for the hand transplant patient follows guidelines similar to replant protocols. There are several significant differences, however, such as screening for an ideal candidate and monitoring for signs of rejection.

Preoperative evaluation includes patient acceptance of the amputation, attempted prosthetic use and set realistic goals for surgery and outcomes. This includes a full history and physical exam to document the range of motion (ROM) of the available joints; manual muscle testing (MMT) of available muscles; response of the residual forearm musculature to electrical muscle stimulation; documentation of pain and sensitivity

complaints; scar quality; level of amputation; sensation; edema; skin and soft tissue integrity; and circumference of the forearms at varying levels, as well as length of the forearms. Different tests, questionnaires or instruments can be used to evaluate preoperative functional level and the status of residual muscles that will power the transplanted hand. As appropriate, electrical muscle stimulation, as well as isometric exercise can help in preoperative strengthening of these muscles.

The goals of postoperative therapy, bracing and splinting are similar to replantation. Knowledge of the exact level of nerve repair; type of osteosyntheses; and details of tendon repairs are essential in planning of splinting and therapy. Uniquely, the hand therapist can help monitor for signs of rejection as the patient spends considerable time in rehabilitation after surgery. It is also common for the patient to feel significant fatigue initially while adjusting to the immunosuppressive medications.

A rigorous rehabilitation regimen has to be implemented in all patients with 3–6 h of supervised therapy 5 days a week during the first 3–6 months or even longer, depending on the nature and level of the transplant. Therapy must consist of passive and active ROM exercises with appropriate static and dynamic splinting to allow gentle active flexion/extension and limit adhesions and promote healing. Hand-based splints such as dynamic extension outrigger splints *(Fig. 38.9)* and anti-claw splints should be used in all patients. The outrigger allows for an intrinsic-plus position, protects flexors and extensors, and enables constant tension throughout the range of controlled motion. Compression gloves are useful in patients with lymphedema. Qualitative and quantitative tests for hand and upper extremity function such as the Carroll score,[136] DASH[137] score and the Hand Transplantation Score System[138] may be utilized along with standard tests for evaluation of motor and sensory recovery (Tinel's, Semmes–Weinstein monofilaments, 2PD, dynamometry, peg board tests, etc.) to enable assessment of graft functional and quality of life outcomes as well as the ability to take part in activities of daily living. After discharge 3–6 months postoperatively, communication and coordination with a certified local therapist is critical to ensure follow-up continuity of an intensive regimen and a home therapy exercise routine that is paramount to achieving functionality.

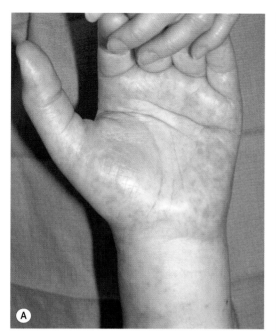
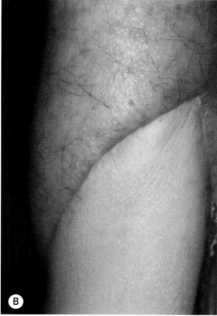
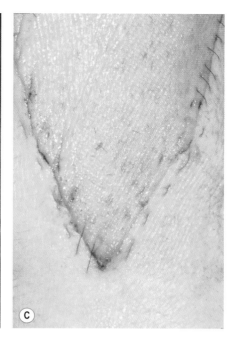

Fig. 38.8 (A–C) Clinical manifestations of acute skin rejection. These can range from discrete or diffuse maculopapular rash with or without edema and palmar involvement.

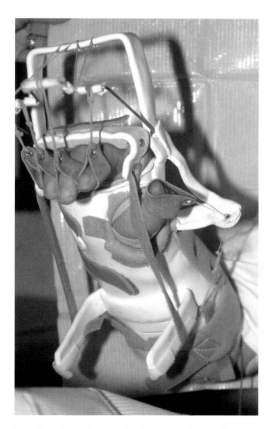

Fig. 38.9 Dynamic extension (crane) outrigger splint.

Table 38.3 Banff grading scale

Grade	Histopathology of skin
Grade 0	None. Rare inflammatory infiltrates
Grade I	Mild. Mild perivascular lymphocytic and eosinophilic infiltration. No involvement of the overlying epidermis
Grade II	Moderate. Moderate-to-severe perivascular inflammation with or without mild epidermal and/or adnexal involvement (limited to spongiosis and exocytosis)
Grade III	Dense inflammation and epidermal involvement with epithelial apoptosis, dyskeratosis and/or keratinolysis
Grade IV	Necrotizing acute rejection. Necrosis of single keratinocytes and focal dermal-epidermal separation

Reproduced with permission from Cendales LC, Kanitakis J, Schneeberger S, et al. The Banff 2007 working classification of skin-containing composite tissue allograft pathology. Am J Transplant. 2008;8(7):1396–1400.

Assessment for rejection (host versus graft reaction)

Acute rejection (AR) is a T-cell and/or antibody mediated attack of the transplant by the recipient's immune system resulting in damage and ultimately loss or the graft. The skin has been demonstrated to be the prime target of rejection and monitoring of the skin by inspection is therefore considered most important for monitoring. Protocol graft-skin biopsies must be routinely performed until the first year plus whenever clinically indicated (visible signs of rejection such as a maculopapular rash). Biopsy samples may be analyzed by means of histology and immunohistochemistry (staining for CD3, CD4, CD8, CD20, and CD68) for quantification and characterization of cellular infiltrates. Scoring for severity of acute rejection is accomplished using established standard grading criteria such as the Banff classification *(Fig. 38.10, Table 38.3)*.[139,140] Important clinical characteristics of AR include edema, erythema, escharification, and necrosis. Atypical rejection in the form of scaling, leuconychia or nail dystrophy can also occur *(Fig. 38.11)*.[134] Biopsies must also

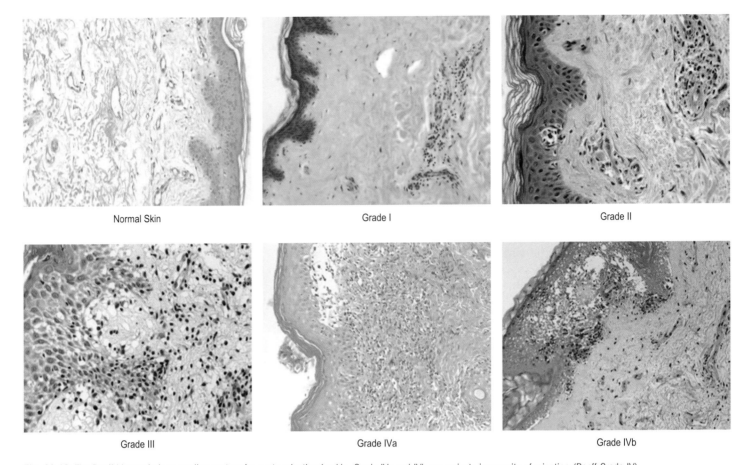

Normal Skin   Grade I   Grade II

Grade III   Grade IVa   Grade IVb

Fig. 38.10 The Banff histopathology grading system for acute rejection in skin. Grade IVa and IVb are variants in severity of rejection (Banff Grade IV).

be examined for evidence of chronic rejection (CR), including intimal hyperplasia and sub-intimal foamy histiocytes in the vessels of the skin or muscle and tissue fibrosis *(Fig. 38.12)*.

Immunomonitoring

Recipient and donor cells must be typed pre-transplant for human leucocyte antigens (HLA).[141,142] Additional DNA samples from recipient/donor must be stored for future typing for MICA (MHC Class I Chain A related) genes in those patients in whom anti-MICA antibody is detected. All sera should be screened by antihuman globulin-enhanced complement-dependent cytotoxicity assays (AHG-CDC), by ELISA (to identify IgG anti-HLA Class I- and Class II specific antibodies independently) and by Luminex® (allows for the identification of anti-MICA antibodies, as well as ascertainment of their donor specificity). The MICA and MICB antigens are expressed on surface of endothelial cells and epithelial cells and elicit a strong antibody response in recipients of solid organ transplants. Cell mediated immunity may be measured by the ImmuKnow® (Cylex) assay that detects adenosine triphosphate (ATP) synthesis in CD4 cells. Immune responses are reported in ng/mL of ATP and categorized as strong (>525) moderate (226–524) or low (<225). The desirable target zone for all transplant recipients is 280 ng/mL ATP, with a 96% negative predictive value for rejection or infection.

World experience and outcomes (graft and patient survival, function, and complications)

The International Registry of Hand and Composite Tissue Transplantation (IRHCTT) (www.handregistry.com) tracks upper extremity allotransplants around the world. The 2008 and 2010 reports[126,143] indicate that the average age of recipients is 32 years (range 19–54 years), usually male, with time from injury to transplant ranging between 2 months and 34 years. Follow-up ranged from 1 month to 11 years. Patient survival following hand transplantation stands at 100% in the United States. Long-term graft survival among patients in Europe and the United States is >94%, with two graft losses. The first French patient underwent amputation following irreversible graft rejection secondary to medication non-compliance. One American patient lost the graft due to ischemia secondary to vascular intimal hyperplasia. Fibro-intimal hyperplasia can be a manifestation of chronic rejection as described in solid organs.[144]

In hand transplant recipients compliant with immunosuppressive medication and rehabilitation, early and intermediate functional outcomes are highly encouraging, superior to those secondary to prosthesis and in quite a few cases comparable with what can be achieved after replantation. Such excellent functional results are dependent on intensive and continuous rehabilitation. Protective sensation was achieved in all patients within 12 months. Hand transplants have

Video
1

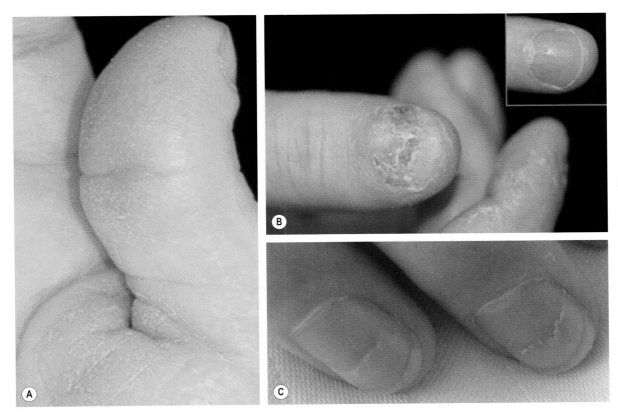

Fig. 38.11 Atypical manifestations of acute rejection: **(A)** palmar scaling, **(B)** nail dystrophy, and **(C)** pitting and leuconychia.

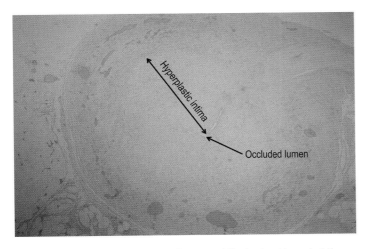

Fig. 38.12 Intimal hyperplasia of the ulnar artery following hand transplantation. (courtesy of Dr Warren Breidenbach, Christine M. Kleinert Institute)

the hand and fingers. The return of motor power and grip strength has also been observed. Electrophysiologic testing has confirmed clinical evidence of motor return in the transplanted intrinsic muscles of the hand, and, in a few cases, true recovery of partial intrinsic function has been observed. Results of early objective testing using the Carroll test after hand transplantation also show that functional return with hand transplants mirrors that after replantation and is consequently superior to that of prostheses.[145,146]

Immunosuppressive protocols currently used in solid organ transplantation have proved to be sufficient to prevent rejection after hand transplantation. However, adverse effects reported include opportunistic infections (including cytomegalovirus, *Clostridium*, herpes, cutaneous mycosis) and *Staphylococcus aureus*-mediated ulnar osteitis; metabolic complications such as hyperglycemia, hyperlipidemia, impaired renal function, arterial hypertension, and aseptic hip necrosis requiring bilateral hip replacement. Of note, no life-threatening complications or malignancies have been observed in the world experience thus far.[126]

Upper extremity transplantation versus replantation

Upper extremity transplantation allows for the planned procurement of the donor hand that is modified to match the site-specific needs of the recipient. Since the recovery/

restored abilities not otherwise afforded by prostheses.[145,146] These include abilities like grasping small objects, pouring water from pitchers, tying shoe laces, playing chess, throwing a ball and using hands in activities of daily living and professional tasks. Recipients have demonstrated rapid progression of their Tinel's sign and early return (at 1 year) of temperature, pressure sensation, touch localization, and pain sensation in acquisition of the donor hand is a planned procedure, warm ischemia times can be reduced to minutes. The cold ischemia time is variable both in transplantation and replantation. Upper extremity replantation has the advantage of dealing with unscarred, acutely injured tissue. Upper extremity transplantation has the disadvantage of a recipient with marked muscle contracture, motor atrophy, and longstanding absence of distal motor and sensory axonal re-innervation. Replants may lack potential structures such as tendons or nerves, thereby necessitating immediate or later grafting. Transplants have the advantage that structures missing in the recipient may be bridged by similar donor tissues obtained from the allograft. Replantation normally allows end-to-end tendon repair. Transplantation has the advantage of stronger tendon repair with Pulvertaft weave using extra donor tendon length. Upper extremity replantation sometimes requires immediate soft tissue coverage such as emergency free-tissue transfer. Upper extremity transplantation is able to avoid the problems of soft tissue coverage by the extra donor tissue derived from the allograft. In summary, except for scarring of the graft bed, technically there are many advantages to transplantation.

In both replantation and transplantation, reintegration of the hand into the neural circuitry of the pre-motor cortex occurs with time. Common factors that may affect functional outcome after replantation or transplantation include a higher level of amputation, ischemia times, the age of the patient, co-existing medical conditions and psychosocial issues.

Unique aspects of composite tissue allotransplantation

Unlike solid organs, upper extremity transplants allow continuous visual monitoring of the graft for skin rejection. This allows for early diagnosis by directed biopsy, unbiased pathologic confirmation of the earliest stages of acute rejection and timely intervention with topical therapies in conjunction with precise and individualized tailoring of systemic medications. When treated adequately and effectively, acute rejection does not seem to impair graft function or long-term survival. Studies from our own group demonstrated that a whole-limb allograft elicited a less intense alloimmune response than did its individual components.[69] In addition, composite tissue allografts contain immunocompetent elements such as bone marrow and lymph nodes that may hasten the rejection processes or result in graft-versus-host disease (GvHD). These factors not only govern the immune reactivity of these allogeneic tissues but also define potential immunomodulating strategies that are different from those currently used in solid organ transplantation.[147,148]

Unlike solid organ transplants that are immediately functional after revascularization, a composite tissue allograft is viable after revascularization of the graft but not functional. The recipient nerves/axons have to regrow and replace donor nerves, which serve as temporary scaffolds, and finally reinnervate the muscles and sensory end organs within the graft. Neuroregeneration represents a unique challenge as, in addition to functional loss caused by lack of innervation, changes occur along the entire route of the nerve from the target end organ to the central nervous system, which might have important implications in recovery and outcome. The use of immunosuppressive drugs like tacrolimus, that is the cornerstone

of regimens in composite tissue allotransplantation has been shown in animal models not only to prolong the survival of limb allografts but also to augment nerve regeneration.[149–151] The early return of function after clinical hand transplantation may reflect the positive neuro-regenerative effects of this drug, but this remains to be scientifically confirmed.

Emerging insights in composite tissue allotransplantation

Cortical plasticity and neuro-integration

A unique phenomenon observed after upper extremity transplantation is the reassignment of portions of the recipient's brain to control the limb. This is called "re-organization" or "plasticity" of the brain. Previous studies have demonstrated that changes in cortical organization occur after amputation. However, the impact of limb transplantation on spatial reorganization of the motor cortex is just now being revealed.[152]

After a hand is amputated, the area of the brain that was receiving signals from the hand is gradually lost and is taken over by other functions. However, after an upper extremity transplant, that area of the brain can re-establish its original function, and the signals from the new hand go back to the area of brain that was used to control the original hand.[153] Such neural integration of the transplant into the pre-motor cortex has been demonstrated using functional magnetic resonance imaging studies and high definition fiber tracking with diffusion tractography. This phenomenon has not been reported after organ transplantation.

Chronic rejection

In solid organ transplantation, chronic rejection is a low-grade injury to the vascular endothelium of the allograft leading to irreversible allograft damage.[144] The hallmark of CR shared by all solid organs is concentric generalized sclerosis and low-grade perivasculitis of graft arteries leading to obliterative arteriopathy. It is known that both immunologic and non-immunologic factors play a role in its pathogenesis.

The possibility of chronic rejection was anticipated after upper extremity transplantation. The first French patient whose hand was amputated due to medication non-compliance induced irreversible rejection, did not demonstrate intimal hyperplasia by skin biopsy or vascular study. Biopsies were also negative for C4D. "Diffuse concentric fibrous intimal thickening and occlusion of graft vessels" was reported in a series of vascularized knee transplantation as well as one case of upper extremity allotransplantation where the graft was lost to ischemia secondary to rapidly progressive vascular intimal hyperplasia (*Fig. 38.12*).

To date, transplant recipients have been monitored for chronic rejection by clinical and functional exams, skin biopsies, donor specific antibodies and standard vascular imaging. These are inadequate to diagnose and monitor for intimal hyperplasia as the primary predictor of chronic rejection. A novel method using high-resolution ultrasound biomicroscopy of graft vasculature is proving to be promising as a

Table 38.4 Recommendations to reduce risk of acute and chronic rejection in hand transplantation

Immunologic factors

1.	Prevention of AR	Use selective, specific and safer immunosuppressive drugs. Potent and targeted induction agents like Campath 1H (alemtuzumab) could maximize AR prevention, allowing monotherapy maintenance and steroid avoidance
2.	Treat steroid resistant or CD20 positive AR	Campath-1H (anti-CD52) or rituximab (anti-CD20)
3.	Monitor and curb medication noncompliance	Suggested methods include electronic measurements of pill container opening, regular monitoring of blood drug levels, frequent clinical examinations, repeated biopsies or immune monitoring
4.	Reduce risk factors	Exclude patients with high PRA, avoid sex/racial mismatch between donor-recipient and exclude hand allografts from CMV^{positive} donors.

Nonimmunologic factors

1.	Choose younger donors and exclude donors with systemic atherosclerosis.
2.	Avoid prolonged cold ischemia.
3.	Treat recipient risk factors aggressively (antidiabetic, antihypertensive, or lipid lowering drugs with dietary or lifestyle changes if necessary).

monitoring tool. At this point, we do not conclusively know if factors that play a role in genesis of chronic rejection in solid organs mediate the phenomenon in upper extremity transplants. With prolonged survival of upper extremity transplants 10 years, we will inevitably see more grafts develop signs of chronic rejection or succumb to chronic rejection. We will then be able to better define, diagnose and grade this condition. Meanwhile, we are limited to minimizing the known risk factors (from solid organ experience) that may contribute to a postulated increase of chronic rejection in upper extremity transplants *(Table 38.4)*.

Tolerance approaches and immunomodulatory strategies

Despite the excellent results thus far, the risks of immunosuppression in composite tissue allotransplantation need to be reduced or eliminated. One potential strategy to achieve this goal is through tolerance induction. A strict mechanistic definition of tolerance is lacking. An "operational" definition would be "the long-term functional survival of an allograft in a patient without the need for maintenance immunosuppression."[154] Such a tolerant state is characterized by hyporesponsiveness to donor tissue with the preservation of the recipient's immune responses to microorganisms (bacteria, viruses) and tumor antigens. The strategies for allograft tolerance can be broadly divided into approaches utilizing donor bone marrow or inducing peri-transplant depletion of recipient T cells.[154a]

When considering development of novel therapeutic strategies for minimization or avoidance of maintenance immunosuppression after upper extremity transplantation, cell-based protocols, including donor bone marrow or stem cells are promising candidates due to the unique nature of these grafts. Fundamentally, when donor bone marrow containing stem cells is transplanted in a treated recipient, the newly developing recipient T cells begin to see donor cells as "self." Therefore, the recipient perceives an organ from the same marrow donor as "self" and accepts it without immunosuppression. The ATG

model consists of depleting the T cells in the host with ATG, followed by infusion of donor bone marrow cells.[155] The mixed chimerism model involves induction of allograft tolerance by establishing long-term mixed chimerism, a state in which both donor and recipient hematopoietic cells co-exist.[156] In contrast to the ATG model, it requires engraftment of donor stem cells. Some composite tissue allografts, in particular limb transplants, bring with them vascularized bone marrow in its microenvironment enabling a sustainable, renewable source of donor bone marrow cells that could promote immunoregulation without the need for engraftment.[157,158] In solid organs, infusion of donor bone marrow cells has also been shown to reduce/avoid maintenance immunosuppression required for graft survival.[159] Bone marrow is critical to establish macrochimerism, microchimerism, or mixed chimerism after organ transplantation, which is known as a prerequisite for potential donor-antigen specific tolerance induction[160,161]

Allograft rejection is caused by activated T cells and cannot occur in their absence. Campath-1H (alemtuzumab) is an antibody that binds to the CD52 receptor, critical for T-cell function in humans.[162] Campath-1H leads to peri-transplant depletion of T cells, B cells, and monocytes, but spares bone marrow stem cells. Renal transplant trials with Campath-1H demonstrated that allograft survival could be prolonged but with low doses of maintenance immunosuppression.[163,164] Such a state of tolerance is called "prope-tolerance" or "tolerance-lite." Campath 1H is used as an induction agent in several upper extremity transplant programs toward the goal of minimizing maintenance immunosuppression.

Over the past five decades, more than 50 different methods of tolerance induction have succeeded in small or large animal models. Yet tolerance protocols have not widely replaced immunosuppression in clinical transplantation. The reason for this is straightforward. Many of the tolerance protocols are too risky for clinical application. In other protocols, the risks remain unknown.

Therefore, the transition of experimental tolerance protocols to the clinical transplant arena is fraught with several questions. Can experimental tolerance protocols meet the stringent fail-safe clinical standards of reliability and efficacy? How durable or persistent is the tolerant state? How immunocompetent will the recipient be? What is the universally accepted test or "assay" for tolerance? What are the long-term adverse effects of tolerance induction? The few tolerance strategies that hold future promise are at very early stages of research and application. Until these questions can be answered and true tolerance becomes a reality, routine immunosuppression as used in organ transplantation will remain the "gold standard" in composite tissue allotransplantation.

The future of upper extremity reconstructive transplantation

Preliminary results of upper extremity transplants around the world have demonstrated functional return similar to that of replants. Graft survival after upper extremity transplantation has far exceeded all initial attempts at solid organ transplantation. This procedure holds tremendous promise in the reconstruction of limb defects. However, results with this experimental procedure are still emerging. It is possible, based on solid organ transplant experience, that eventually the majority of upper extremity transplants may be lost to chronic rejection. Therefore, it is important to note that upper extremity transplantation should be limited to specialized centers that have the multidisciplinary expertise in the techniques of reconstructive microsurgery and the practice of organ transplantation, infrastructure, fiscal resources, and institutional regulatory approval. It should be recommended in a select group of patients and must be performed according to universally standardized ethical guidelines. All procedures should be open to professional scrutiny through periodic reporting at scientific forums and to the public through news media. If all these guiding principles are strictly adhered to, upper extremity transplantation may herald a new era in reconstructive and transplant surgery.

Access the bonus content for this chapter online at http://www.expertconsult.com

Fig. 38.1 St. Cosmas and Damian perform the first human extremity allotransplantation. Per mythology, Christian Roman deacon, Justinian, had a malignant growth on his leg and fell asleep while praying for a cure in the Church of Cosmas and Damian in Rome. In his dreams, the saints amputated the diseased limb and transplanted the leg of a Moor, brought to the church for burial. The patient awoke and gratefully observed a now healthy leg, though black in color. (Reproduction with permission from Württembergisches Landesmuseum, Stuttgart.)

Access the complete references list online at http://www.expertconsult.com

20. Carrel A. Results of the transplantation of blood vessels, organs and limbs. *JAMA*. 1908;51:1662.

26. Merrill JP, Murray JE, Harrison JH, et al. Successful homotransplantation of the human kidney between identical twins. *JAMA*. 1956;160:277.

31. Gibson T, Medawar PB. The fate of skin homografts in man. *J Anat*. 1943;77:299.

    This is a classic landmark paper by Thomas Gibson and Sir Peter Medawar that provides the first insights into the immune behavior of skin transplants and laid the foundations for tissue transplantation.

46. Anonymous. Historic cadaver-to-man hand transplant. *Med World News*. 5(6); March 1964;13:60.

69. Lee WP, Yaremchuk MJ, Pan YC, et al. Relative antigenicity of components of a vascularized limb allograft. *Plast Reconstr Surg*. 1991;87(3):401.

    This is a highly cited study that addresses the differential antigenicity of limb transplants, establishing that whole-limb allografts elicit lesser immune response than their individual components (skin, subcutaneous tissue, muscle, bone, and blood vessels) in terms of cell-mediated and humoral immune responses as well as the timing and intensity of rejection.

90. Breidenbach WC, Tobin GR, Gorantla VS, et al. A position statement in support of hand transplantation. *J Hand Surg Am*. 2002;27(5):760.

    This is a comprehensive review of emerging outcomes in upper extremity transplantation with emphasis on the early developments in the field, experimental, scientific, and clinical considerations and the ethical debate surrounding initial human trials.

126. Petruzzo P, Lanzetta M, Dubernard JM, et al. The International Registry on Hand and Composite Tissue Transplantation. *Transplantation*. 2010;90(12):1590–1594.

128. Amirlak B, Gonzalez R, Gorantla V, et al. Creating a hand transplant program. *Clin Plast Surg*. 2007;34(2):279–289.

    This is essential reading to understand the basic requirements to establish an upper extremity composite tissue transplant program. The planning, preapproval, personnel, protocol and public relations related aspects and the program, procedural and patient considerations are discussed.

139. Cendales LC, Kanitakis J, Schneeberger S, et al. The Banff 2007 working classification of skin-containing composite tissue allograft pathology. *Am J Transplant*. 2008;8(7):1396–1400.

154. Starzl TE. Immunosuppressive therapy and tolerance of organ allografts. *N Engl J Med*. 2008;358:407–411.

    Authored by one of the pioneers in organ transplantation, this paper discusses the concepts and clinical applications of immunosuppression, immunomodulation and tolerance, highlighting the paradigm shifts in the field.

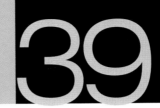

Hand therapy

Christine B. Novak and Rebecca L. von der Heyde

SYNOPSIS

- In optimal situations, hand therapists work closely with hand surgeons to maximize nonoperative and postoperative outcomes for patients with upper extremity conditions.
- Assessment in the area of impairment and body structures includes edema, wound, vascularity, pain, range of motion, strength, and sensibility.
- Following nerve injury and with chronic nerve compression, rehabilitation strategies should be directed not only to the distal recovery but also to re-establishing normal movement patterns and cortical remapping.
- The study of flexor tendon healing over time has demonstrated that early controlled motion is both beneficial to tendon healing and preferable to immobilization.
- Hand fractures are challenging and as such require careful attention to bony integrity and maintenance of the flexor and extensor tendon-gliding systems.

Introduction

Tenets of hand therapy

According to the Hand Therapy Certification Committee (www.htcc.org/about/index.cfm), the specialty of hand therapy is defined in the following manner:

Hand therapy is the art and science of rehabilitation of the upper limb, which includes the hand, wrist, elbow, and shoulder girdle. It is a merging of occupational therapy and physical therapy theory and practice that combines comprehensive knowledge of the structure of the upper limb with function and activity. Using specialized skills in assessment, planning and treatment, hand therapists provide therapeutic interventions to prevent dysfunction, restore function and/or reverse the progression of pathology of the upper limb in order to enhance an individual's ability to execute tasks and to participate fully in life situations.

In optimal situations, hand therapists work closely with hand surgeons to maximize nonoperative and postoperative outcomes for patients with upper extremity conditions. The purpose of this chapter is to provide the plastic surgeon with an overview of the evaluative and rehabilitative approaches for patients with nerve, tendon, skeletal, and soft-tissue conditions as afforded by collaboration with a hand therapist.

Evaluative guidelines

A comprehensive evaluation provides valuable diagnostic and prognostic information to the plastic surgeon and hand therapist prior to intervention, and serves to inform clinical decision-making for management (nonoperative and postoperative) of patients with upper extremity conditions. In concert with the *International Classification of Functioning, Disability and Health*,[1] hand therapists are well versed in the clinical assessment of patients in areas of impairment, activity, and participation.

Assessment in the area of impairment and body structures includes edema, wound, vascularity, pain, range of motion, strength, and sensibility. Edema is most commonly assessed with circumferential measurement. However, it is more accurately assessed using volumetric displacement with a reported test–retest reliability within ±3 mL.[2] Wound assessment is characterized by both descriptive and objective components, including a detailed patient history and observation of wound size, color, drainage, odor, and temperature. Vascularity can be assessed both proximally and distally in the upper extremity using provocation maneuvers. In addition to the Allen's test for circulation via the radial and ulnar arteries at the wrist, vascularity may be assessed more proximally using Adson's maneuver at the subclavian artery; the costoclavicular maneuver and hyperabduction test assessed via the radial pulse; and the elevated arm stress test, as described by Roos.[3–5] Pain, certainly a subjective and multifaceted construct, should be assessed before, during, and after therapeutic interventions. Numeric, verbal, and visual analog scales are commonly used to rate pain intensity and have been identified as having good construct validity.[6] Simple measures which assess only pain intensity may be inadequate to capture and measure the multidimensional aspects of the pain. The McGill Pain Questionnaire and the Short-Form McGill Pain Questionnaire

(SF-MPQ) are the most widely used pain questionnaires to assess the multidimensional qualities of the pain experience and overall have been shown to possess good to excellent psychometric properties.[7–11] The SF-MPQ consists of a visual analog scale pain intensity, the present pain intensity index, and 15 pain adjectives (11 sensory, four affective) to calculate the pain-rating index.

Video 1,2

Goniometric measurement is used to assess passive and active range of motion. While electrogoniometers and costly systems are available for clinical use, standard manual goniometers are easily portable and inexpensive (video 1). In a recent study, high intrarater reliability was found in multiple techniques to assess wrist range of motion, with a dorsal volar approach demonstrating the highest interrater reliability.[12] Ellis and Bruton found composite finger flexion measurements to be as reliable as manual goniometry between raters, with manual goniometry demonstrating increased intrarater reliability for measurement of the proximal interphalangeal joint.[13] Manual muscle testing is employed to isolate strength of individual muscles and often graded using the Medical Research Council (MRC) grade 0–5 classification.[14] In a review, Cuthbert and Goodheart reported good evidence to support the use of manual muscle testing for patients with neuromusculoskeletal dysfunction.[15] Sensory impairment is most often assessed using monofilaments for threshold testing (video 2) and/or two-point discrimination for innervation density.[16–22] Using standardized techniques, good validity and reliability have been shown using these types of assessment tools.[16,17,19,23–25] The Ten Test was introduced as a quick assessment of light touch sensation and has been shown to be a valid measure as compared to monofilament testing.[26,27]

Clinical assessment may also include grip and pinch strength testing.[28–31] A calibrated, hand-held dynamometer is used to measure grip strength in a standard position of glenohumeral adduction, elbow flexion, and neutral forearm rotation.[29] One trial has been identified as equally reliable to the best or average of three trials and elicits less patient discomfort.[28] The influences of hand size and span have also been identified as factors to consider when selecting the grip handle position.[32–34] Calibrated gauges are also used to measure both lateral and tip pinch.

A paradigm shift towards increased incorporation of qualitative and patient-reported data into outcomes assessment is strongly encouraged as a means of assessing participation.[35] Clinical evaluation tools, such as range of motion, which assess physical impairments, have demonstrated poor validity and limited responsiveness as compared to patient self-report measures.[36–39] Research has also shown a weak relationship between patient perception of health-related quality of life and ratings from healthcare providers.[40] Patient perception of ability has been suggested as more valuable than functional evaluations.[41] In addition, patient assessment of the importance of change in health status is preferable to that interpreted by the healthcare professional.[42] Despite numerous tools and support in the literature, the incorporation of self-report outcome measures is inconsistent in clinical practice.[43]

The Disabilities of the Arm, Shoulder, and Hand (DASH), one of the most recognized self-report outcome measures for the upper extremity, was published as a joint effort of the American Academy of Orthopedic Surgery and the Institute for Work and Health.[44] The DASH was created as a tool that would allow comparison of conditions throughout the upper extremity while considering it a single, functional unit.[44,45] Careful development of this tool, including an extensive literature review and consideration of questions and attribution, has made it a popular tool in upper extremity research and clinical practice.

Rehabilitation following nerve injury/surgery

Following nerve injury and with chronic nerve compression, neural changes occur in the peripheral and central nervous system. The primary focus has been on the alterations that occur to the nerve and the distal sensory receptors and muscle fibers. The proximal changes that occur in the central nervous system have been less emphasized. Cortical remapping and cell body changes have been documented with nerve injury and nerve compression. Therefore to optimize outcome, rehabilitation strategies should be directed not only to the distal recovery but also to re-establishing normal movement patterns and cortical remapping. This section will review postoperative management following surgery for carpal and cubital tunnel syndrome, nerve repair, and nerve transfers.

Compression neuropathies

Postoperative care following surgery for compression neuropathies is a balance between protecting the surgical repair site and maintaining neural mobility. To minimize adhesions and scarring, early motion is advocated. However the definition of "early motion" following release of an entrapment site is variable and is determined by the surgical procedure performed and surgeon preference.[46,47] Compared to the historical reports in the literature, the tendency has been to decrease the length of time of immobilization and to use less restrictive postoperative dressings.[25,48] Range-of-motion exercises are instituted and restoration of muscle balance is also a goal of postoperative care.

In the acute postoperative stage, consideration is given to edema control and pain management, and the patient is instructed in strategies to minimize edema and pain. Even in the early stages following surgery, nerve-gliding exercises are instituted with range-of-motion exercises to the distal and proximal joints which are not included in the bulky dressing. These types of exercise will provide some longitudinal movement of the nerve to minimize adhesions.

Carpal tunnel syndrome

Postoperative care

Historically, following release of the carpal tunnel, immobilization was used to protect the wound and to prevent bowstringing of the flexor tendons by restricting motion at the wrist. With recognition of the importance of early motion, the duration and type of immobilization following carpal tunnel release have substantially decreased. In our practice, a bulky dressing is used for restriction of wrist movement and for patient comfort in the immediate postoperative period. Following surgery, the patient is instructed in range-of-motion exercises for the fingers, elbow, and shoulder. Two days following surgery, the bulky dressing is removed and the patient is instructed in range-of-motion exercises for the fingers, wrist, elbow, and shoulder. For patient comfort, a splint in a wrist neutral position may be used at night. The sutures are removed 12–14 days following surgery. Return to work is dependent upon the type of job and specific patient factors. However at 4 weeks after surgery, patients should have full range of motion and may lift up to 2 lb (0.9 kg) and, by 2 months following surgery, full activity without restrictions is expected.[48] Depending on the severity of nerve compression, the time to full sensory and motor recovery may vary.

Cubital tunnel syndrome

With failure of nonoperative treatment, there are numerous surgical procedures performed for the operative treatment of cubital tunnel syndrome, ranging from simple decompression, medial epicondylectomy to various types of anterior transposition.[48] With each procedure, there are numerous protocols for the postoperative management and many vary depending upon surgeon preference. In general, early motion is recommended to minimize adhesions and scarring of the ulnar nerve and surrounding soft tissue.

Postoperative care

There is wide variability in the duration of immobilization following surgery for cubital tunnel syndrome and this depends upon the operative procedure performed and surgeon preference. The period of immobilization is increased for those procedures that involve more complex release of the soft tissue surrounding the ulnar nerve (i.e., least immobilization for simple decompression). In most cases, the postoperative dressing may be removed 2–3 days after surgery and then a postoperative method of immobilization may be used if required. For patient comfort, a sling may be used at night to restrict upper extremity motion while the patient is sleeping. The postoperative care following a transmuscular transposition will be described.[48] In our experience, patients may begin range-of-motion exercises (fingers, wrist, forearm, elbow, and shoulder) when the dressing is removed at postoperative day 2 or 3. Patients are cautioned to perform these exercises slowly and initially to avoid full forearm supination combined with full elbow extension because this motion will place the most stress on the soft-tissue repair. Initially elbow extension is performed with the forearm in pronation and then, as a separate exercise, forearm supination is performed with the elbow flexed at 90°. When the patient is able to move comfortably into full supination, forearm supination is combined with elbow extension. A sling is used at night for patient comfort to avoid rapid elbow extension and may be discontinued when the patient has achieved full elbow extension with full forearm supination. The emphasis in the early postoperative period is to regain full range of motion and it is anticipated that this is achieved within the first 2–3 weeks following surgery. If the patient appears to be progressing slowly, more structured hand therapy is recommended. Strengthening exercises are instituted 1 month following surgery and full activity is permitted at 8 weeks.

Concomitant soft-tissue muscle imbalances and other sites of nerve compression in the upper extremity may require rehabilitation therapy to achieve full recovery. Some patients may also have restricted neural excursion, cervicoscapular discomfort, and/or rotator cuff tendinitis associated with muscle imbalances in this region. Specific exercises to address these more proximal soft-tissue and neural structures will help to ameliorate these types of symptoms in patients with more diffuse upper extremity discomfort, paresthesia, and/or numbness.[49–56]

Nerve repair

Changes in the peripheral and central nervous system begin shortly after injury and continue through recovery. The ultimate functional outcome depends upon reinnervation of the sensory receptors and motor end plates and the appropriate remapping of the motor and sensory cortex. Based upon these proximal changes, rehabilitation is maximized by including strategies directed towards these cortical alterations.

Early postoperative care

In the immediate postoperative period, the primary goal is to protect the nerve repair site. Initially, a bulky dressing is used and, if required by the operative procedure, more rigid support can be utilized. The patient is instructed in edema control and range-of-motion exercises for the joints that are not immobilized by the bulky operative dressing. The initial dressing is removed within a few days following surgery. Immobilization is continued with the use of a custom-made or prefabricated splint or, in some cases, a sling or shoulder immobilizer may provide sufficient support to restrict forces on the repair site. Nerve repairs compared to nerve grafts or transfers are typically immobilized for longer periods of time and in some cases up to 3 weeks. The timing of immobilization will depend upon the location of the nerve repaired and the amount of nerve mobility. In some cases, such as with digital nerve injuries, some have advocated no immobilization after the initial operative dressing has been removed.[57] With a nerve graft or transfer, there is extra nerve length at the repair site and lack of tension associated with these reconstructions and, as such, these types of reconstruction require less rigid immobilization and may be mobilized earlier (7–14 days) compared to nerve repairs. However, other soft tissues (tendons, muscles, or ligaments) which may have been released or repaired in the operative procedure may prolong the period of immobilization. For example, repair of the pectoralis minor with exploration of the brachial plexus may require 4 weeks of immobilization in internal shoulder rotation using a shoulder immobilizer to avoid tension on the soft-tissue repair or, with acute injuries that may involve a tendon repair, a tendon rehabilitation protocol would be followed.

Early postoperative pain resulting from the operative procedure may be controlled with analgesics, edema control, early motion, and hand therapy. However ongoing neuropathic pain may negatively impact outcome and therefore early intervention is recommended.[58,59] Neuropathic pain following trauma may require a comprehensive multidisciplinary approach and as such referral to a pain management team may be warranted.

The use of electrical muscle stimulation is often advocated following nerve injury to prevent muscle degeneration and to protect the muscle fiber until regeneration occurs. However, the literature does not present strong support for the use of this modality following nerve injury.[60,61] Historically, the rationale for electrical stimulation of denervated muscles has been to retain integrity of the muscle fibers while waiting for muscle reinnervation. Studies using animal models of denervated muscles and electrodes implanted directly into the muscle have shown preservation of some normal muscle properties.[62,63] However, no efficacy trials have provided evidence of these benefits in humans. More recent evidence presented in the literature suggests that longer durations of axotomy and Schwann cell denervation are predictive of poor functional outcome.[64-66] Low-frequency stimulation of the nerve following nerve transection and repair in animal models has shown an increase in axonal regeneration into the appropriate neural pathway.[64,67] In patients after carpal tunnel release, 1 hour of low-frequency nerve stimulation resulted in significantly faster motor reinnervation.[67] This evidence provides the impetus for future investigation into the benefits of direct nerve stimulation to improve recovery following a motor nerve injury. However, the use of direct current stimulation for denervated muscles has not been shown to be efficacious in humans and as such is not advocated by the authors.

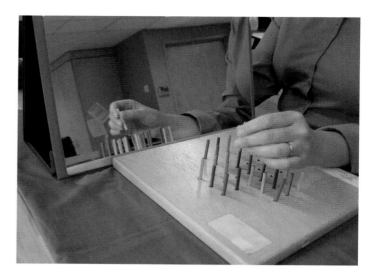

Fig. 39.1 Re-education can be optimized with the use of mirror imagery. This allows the patient to visualize the uninjured hand as the contralateral hand and perform the task. (Courtesy of Christine B. Novak PT PhD.)

Late rehabilitation

In the later phases of rehabilitation, sensory re-education has been recognized as an integral component of therapy following nerve injury; however the importance of motor re-education following nerve injury has been less emphasized. The integration of function between the sensory and motor cortex is essential for restoration of sensorimotor control and to optimize outcome. The concept of cortical plasticity and its importance to recovery following nerve injury have gained increased attention in the past decade.

Sensory re-education

Following sensory nerve reconstruction, sensory re-education is commonly included in the rehabilitation program to improve hand sensibility and function. These strategies have been used to maximize sensory recovery and also to decrease pain and for desensitization related to allodynia and/or hyperalgesia.[68-73] Desensitization exercises using different textures and vibration techniques may be used to decrease allodynia and/or hyperalgesia. The concept of vibration for desensitization relates to the gate control theory of pain and stimulation of large A-beta fibers with vibration.[74] The use of small-amplitude vibration for desensitization is most tolerated by patients and may be obtained by using an electric shaver with the cap on it. This will provide an easy technique for the patient to continue this exercise in a home program. With decreasing sensitivity, the area of allodynia may be challenged with different types of texture to promote sensory re-education and appropriate cortical mapping.

With evidence of reinnervation of the sensory receptors, sensory re-education is advocated.[69] This typically includes a structured program with an emphasis on textures, localization, and discriminatory tasks.[69] The exercises are progressed to challenge the sensory system as the patient's sensation improves, beginning with varying textures, localization exercises, and then discriminatory tasks. However, strategies to enhance and promote cortical remapping have been also advocated in the earlier phases following surgery. Rosen and Lundborg have described re-education programs using mirror imagery, visuotactile training, and audiotactile interaction to enhance the functional reorganization of the sensory cortex in the early phases of recovery before there is evidence of sensory receptor reinnervation.[75]

Mirror visual feedback has been extensively used for treatment in patients following stroke and with amputation injuries and has been more recently reported for use in patients with pain syndromes or nerve injury.[76,77] The concept of mirror visual feedback is that patients observe their reflected image in the mirror, which would appear as the contralateral limb (*Fig. 39.1*) and thus activate the brain. Patients may perform specific exercises or movements with the unaffected hand or extremity and in the mirror it would appear as normal movement to the affected hand or extremity. With improvement in sensory function or decreased pain, more complex activities may be introduced.

Motor re-education

The goals of treatment for motor function are directed towards re-establishment of normal movement patterns and muscle balance. Following nerve injury, motor re-education is not as frequently advocated compared to sensory re-education. Alterations in cortical mapping and motor patterns occur following injury to a motor nerve.[78-80] With reinnervation of the denervated muscles, muscle imbalances will remain due to weakness of the reinnervated muscles compared to the uninjured muscles and also compensatory movement patterns that have performed since the injury. Particularly in patients with brachial plexus injuries, the period of time until muscle reinnervation occurs may be prolonged (12–18 months) and abnormal movement patterns are established. Therefore motor re-education will provide the opportunity to focus on appropriate muscle recruitment and muscle balance. Even in patients with only sensory loss following median nerve injury, there will be alteration of the motor pattern due to compensation in movements as a result of numbness to the sensory distribution of the median nerve. Therefore, the emphasis should be on restoration of the integration of motor and sensory re-education following nerve injury. Sensorimotor control to perform upper extremity tasks requires the coordination of both the sensory and motor systems.[81] Alteration in either motor or sensory function as a result of nerve injury will impact sensorimotor control in the upper extremity. Improvement in hand function may occur with increased use of the hand, but progress may be enhanced with the use of activity-based sensorimotor retraining, emphasis on control, and appropriate feedback learning. As with any new task learning, repetition and feedback are essential and therefore patient education and an effective home program should be emphasized.

Nerve transfers

Historically, motor nerve transfers were used as a salvage procedure when nerve repair or graft was not possible due to avulsion of the proximal nerve source, and there was limited potential for excellent outcome. However, the utilization of nerve transfers has increased, particularly with proximal nerve injuries, where recovery is limited due to the distance from the injury to target muscle fibers and prolonged time for reinnervation.[82–84] Because a nerve transfer can provide a closer innervation source, the distance and time for reinnervation are shorter and the results following these types of transfer have been very encouraging.[85–93] However, optimal results depend not only on the number of regenerating motor axons and reinnervation of muscle fibers but also on cortical plasticity and remapping. Previously established motor patterns and cortical maps are no longer relevant because a new proximal nerve source is used with a nerve transfer. Studies have evaluated cortical mapping following nerve transfers, muscle transfers, and toe-to-thumb transfers.[78–80,94–97] Collectively, these studies have illustrated shifts in the motor cortex following transfers and the importance of effective relearning to optimize outcome. Therefore rehabilitation programs should include not only range-of-motion and strengthening exercises to regain muscle balance, but also motor re-education to promote normal movement patterns and cortical mapping.[98,99]

With nerve transfers, there is alteration of the proximal nerve source, therefore muscle contraction is initially recruited with "contraction" of the muscle from the donor nerve because of the established motor pattern. The new recruitment pattern from the new proximal nerve source from the donor nerve has yet to be recognized. Even with evidence of muscle reinnervation, the newly innervated muscle may not contract with initiation of the intended action, but rather requires "contraction" of the muscle from the donor nerve. To facilitate relearning, contraction of the muscles on the uninjured contralateral side will provide cortical input of a normal movement. The relearning associated with nerve transfers is similar to relearning following tendon transfers. In general, relearning is more straightforward following a transfer (nerve, muscle, or tendon) when the donor is from a muscle with a synergistic action. While it is possible to relearn an action that is from a muscle with an antagonistic action (such as triceps-to-biceps muscle transfer), the relearning is more difficult compared to a synergistic muscle action.

In patients with brachial plexus avulsion injuries, an intercostal to musculocutaneous nerve transfer is often performed

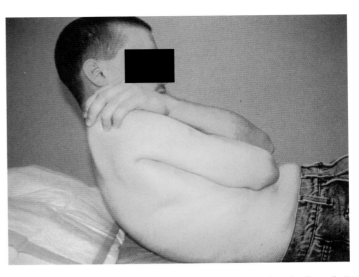

Fig. 39.2 Following an intercostal-to-musculocutaneous nerve transfer, the patient is performing an abdominal crunch to initiate contraction of the intercostal muscles and thus initiate contraction of the biceps and brachialis muscles. (Courtesy of Susan E. Mackinnon.)

to restore elbow flexion. Postoperative education often includes deep-breathing exercises to provide a stimulus to the intercostal nerves for contraction of the biceps and brachialis muscles, which are innervated via the musculocutaneous nerve. While deep breathing does initiate contraction of the newly innervated elbow flexors, it is difficult to provide a prolonged contraction for re-education and strengthening. The abdominal muscles and intercostal muscles are activated with core abdominal exercises. Therefore core-strengthening exercises will also provide contraction of the biceps and brachialis muscles in patients who have had an intercostal-to-musculocutaneous nerve transfer. The muscle activity in the elbow flexors associated with trunk flexion has been shown by Chalidapong and colleagues.[100] Core exercises which use the abdominal and intercostal muscles may begin early in the rehabilitation stages (*Fig. 39.2*) and with early reinnervation will recruit the muscle fibers in the brachialis and biceps.

More recent descriptions of nerve transfers to restore elbow flexion have included donor pectoral nerves and fascicles from the median and ulnar nerves.[87,93] To assist with the retraining following these types of nerve transfer, re-education may begin preoperatively with education on the unaffected extremity and contraction of the muscles from the donor nerve and recipient muscle. In this way, the patient may practice co-contraction of these muscle groups to understand better the re-education that will be required with reinnervation of the denervated muscles. For a medial pectoral-to-musculocutaneous nerve transfer, the patient will simultaneously contract the pectoral and the biceps (and brachialis if included) muscles (*Fig. 39.3*). This is initially done bilaterally and then only to the injured side. Using place-and-hold positioning in 90° of elbow flexion, an isometric contraction is performed. Once the patient is able to hold this contraction against gravity, the degree of flexion may be altered and progressed through a full range of motion. A double fascicular transfer from the median and ulnar nerves to restore elbow flexion will require contraction of the wrist flexors to initiate contraction of the biceps and brachialis muscles (*Fig. 39.4*).

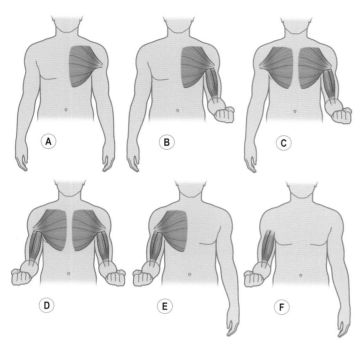

Fig. 39.3 To facilitate understanding and relearning following a motor nerve transfer, re-education begins with a muscle contraction on the unaffected side. **(A)** With a medial pectoral-to-musculocutaneous nerve transfer, the patient begins on the unaffected side with contraction of the pectoralis major muscle and **(B)** then contraction of both the pectoralis major and the biceps muscle. **(C)** This is followed by simultaneous contraction of the pectoralis major muscle on the affected side, **(D)** followed by bilateral contraction of these muscles. **(E)** The contraction is then isolated to the affected side and **(F)** finally dissociation of the donor muscle from the target muscle.

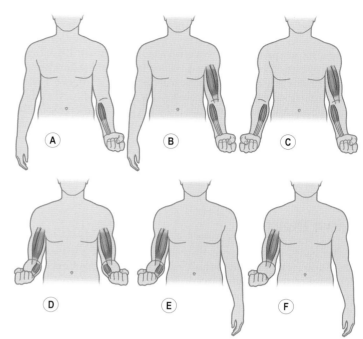

Fig. 39.4 The relearning associated with a partial ulnar and median nerve transfer from the forearm to the elbow flexors is illustrated. Initially, simple grip-strengthening exercises and/or gentle wrist flexion will initiate contraction of the biceps and brachialis muscles. **(A)** The patient begins on the unaffected side with a contraction of the forearm flexors and **(B)** then simultaneously contracts biceps/brachialis muscles and the forearm flexors. **(C, D)** The next step is bilateral contraction of these muscles and **(E)** then the exercise is isolated to the affected side. **(F)** The final exercise is to dissociate contraction of the donor muscle from the target muscle.

To restore innervation to the ulnar nerve intrinsic muscles, an anterior interosseous nerve (AIN) to deep motor branch of the ulnar nerve transfer may be performed.[88] With an AIN to deep motor branch of the ulnar nerve transfer, attempts by the patient to pinch must be combined with forearm pronation to recruit the newly innervated intrinsic muscles from the AIN proximal source *(Fig. 39.5)*. With motor retraining, cortical remapping, and relearned motor patterns, the patient will be able to complete the ulnar motor nerve actions independent of the action of forearm pronation.

As outlined previously in this chapter, the evidence in the literature does not support the efficacy of direct current electrical stimulation with denervated muscles. With evidence of muscle reinnervation, some have advocated the use of electrical muscle stimulation using an alternating current to increase the force of the muscle contraction and thereby increase muscle strength. Theoretically with an innervated muscle, it is possible to use an alternating current to elicit a muscle contraction. However, with a reinnervated muscle, there may be scarcity of reinnervated fibers to produce the intended muscle contraction via electrical stimulation. Passive muscle contraction will not assist in the relearning of motor patterns. Therefore it is our recommendation that these types of modality should not be considered as the primary treatment but may be used as an adjunct to therapy as a "sensory stimulus" for relearning if necessary.

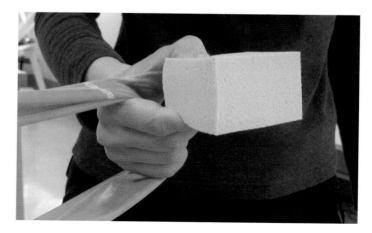

Fig. 39.5 With an anterior interosseus nerve to deep motor branch of the ulnar nerve transfer, forearm pronation is combined with pinching to recruit the innervated intrinsic muscles and facilitate relearning. (Courtesy of Christine B. Novak PT PhD.)

Functional relearning may be facilitated with visual or auditory feedback which can provide immediate response to the patient regarding the muscle contraction. Simple biofeedback units with external surface electrodes may be used to facilitate muscle contraction or to minimize aberrant co-contraction of an antagonistic muscle action. Using a two-channel or four-channel biofeedback unit, the electrodes may be placed on the appropriate muscles to increase or decrease muscle contraction. To facilitate relearning, the action should be performed on the unaffected side first to allow the patient to understand better the strategies necessary to enhance or minimize the intended action. It is also useful to perform these actions simultaneously with the affected and unaffected extremity. This will provide immediate feedback on the "normal" contraction and motor pattern and provide the opportunity for the patient to reproduce the action in the newly reinnervated muscles. With adequate muscle reinnervation, the patient will receive feedback by observing and "feeling" the muscle contraction. Specific exercises to promote muscle contraction without a specific biofeedback unit will allow the patient to perform the exercises more frequently as a home program.

Muscle physiology and biomechanics should be considered when structuring rehabilitation programs following nerve repair or transfer. Because of the weakness and associated fatigue in newly reinnervated muscle, exercise sessions should be of short duration. A slow-onset contraction with a longer duration hold of 10–15 seconds is recommended to increase muscle endurance and strength. To minimize the muscle forces required initially, muscle contraction in midrange is suggested. Place-and-hold exercises or gravity-eliminated positions may be used and then progressed to different degrees of motion as the patient is able to sustain a muscle contraction. With MRC grade 3 strength, progressive resistance exercises can be implemented. The focus of strengthening is to regain muscle balance. Because of the relative weakness between the uninjured and reinnervated muscles, it is important to regain good motor control of the reinnervated muscles before resistance exercises are instituted, otherwise learned compensatory motor patterns will be maintained.

Upper extremity movement requires composite motor patterns involving the glenohumeral and scapular muscles.[52,56] While distal nerve injuries may not include the shoulder complex, strength of uninjured upper extremity muscles may be weakened from disuse or from compensatory movement patterns. Similarly, brachial plexus nerve injuries may not include direct injury to the scapular muscles; however these muscles (such as the middle and lower trapezius and serratus anterior muscles) may be weak from disuse and thus compromise upper extremity function. Assessment of muscle strength and length in the cervicoscapular region should be performed, and then a rehabilitation program to address these muscle imbalances implemented to optimize outcome.

Rehabilitation programs following nerve injury and nerve compression surgery must include sensorimotor re-education and the inclusion of normal movement patterns for appropriate cortical remapping. Bimanual tasks will encourage use of the injured extremity and input normal movement patterns and purposeful movements involving self-care, recreation, and work will facilitate the resumption of normal activities. In some cases, vocational rehabilitation will be necessary to assist in future planning and employment opportunities. Patient education and an effective home program are necessary to optimize learning of new motor/sensory tasks and to optimize outcome.

Rehabilitation following tendon injury/surgery

Flexor tendon injuries

Surgical and rehabilitative approaches following flexor tendon injury can be described as one of the most researched, controversial, and clinically complex aspects of hand therapy. Whereas bench research in this area is advancing towards tissue engineering and the introduction of substances to modulate tendon glide and healing, the need for outcome studies as they pertain to progression of rehabilitation remains. A substantial amount of literature has been published which contributes to clinical decision-making for the management of flexor tendon injuries.

The timing of rehabilitation following flexor tendon repair can readily be identified as a topic of historical and continued controversy. The study of tendon healing over time has demonstrated that early controlled motion is both beneficial to tendon healing and preferable to immobilization.[101–103] Timing of early motion continues to be researched; however, some consistency is evident. Postoperative day 4–5 is suggested as a time during which work of flexion is decreased and preferable for the initiation of rehabilitation.[104–106]

The progression of therapeutic exercise requires careful consideration as it pertains to the force exerted and consequential excursion of the tendon relative to adjacent structures. Studies have suggested that rehabilitative protocols should use the least possible force to achieve tendon excursion that will deter peritendinous adhesions.[104–109] From a rehabilitative perspective, it is important to recognize that tendon excursion occurs in both proximal and distal directions, and can be influenced by both type of exercise and antagonistic musculature.[110–115] A working knowledge of the force and excursion produced by specific exercises facilitates clinical progression following tendon repair (Table 39.1).

A specific challenge in the study of flexor tendon rehabilitation is the multitude of terms describing the range-of-motion exercises used during the early postoperative phase. Descriptors such as "early active motion" and "light active motion" have served to complicate the literature and deter progression of rehabilitative strategies for this diagnosis. Most notably, the work of Urbaniak et al.[114] and Strickland and Cannon[116] has led most surgeons and therapists to avoid the initiation of "active" motion with patients following two- and four-strand flexor tendon repairs.

Place-and-hold synergistic motion is a highly specific exercise which includes passive flexion of the digits followed by active holding of this position, completed with the wrist in extension (Fig. 39.6) (video 3). This exercise has been comprehensively studied using numerous models and is suggested as an optimal exercise to facilitate force and excursion.[117–120] The position of metacarpophalangeal flexion coupled with wrist extension has been suggested to produce the least passive tension in the extensor tendons, thereby decreasing

Video 3

Table 39.1 Analysis of tendon excursion and force

Exercise	Excursion	Force
Passive protected extension	3–8 mm Distal Duran and Houser[110]	200–300 grams Urbaniak et al.[114]
Place-and-hold digital flexion during wrist extension	FDS 26 mm FDP 33 mm Proximal Wehbe and Hunter[115]	900 grams Lieber et al.[112]
Active straight fist	Wrist neutral FDS 28 mm FDP 27 mm Maximum FDS Proximal Wehbe and Hunter[115]	1100 grams Greenwald et al.[111]
Active hook fist	Wrist neutral FDS 13 mm FDP 24 mm Maximum differential Proximal Wehbe and Hunter[115]	1300 grams Greenwald et al.[111]
Active composite fist	Wrist neutral–extension FDS 24–26 mm FDP 32–33 mm Maximum FDP Proximal Wehbe and Hunter[115]	400–4000 grams Schuind et al.[113]
Active, isolated PIP flexion	~13 mm (calculated) FDP Proximal	900 grams Schuind et al.[113]
Active, isolated DIP flexion	~6.5 mm (calculated) FDP Proximal	1900 grams Schuind et al.[113]

FDS, flexor digitorum superficialis; FDP, flexor digitorum profundus; PIP, proximal interphalangeal; DIP, distal interphalangeal.

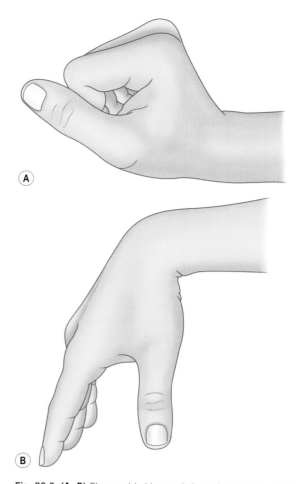

Fig. 39.6 (A, B) Place-and-hold synergistic motion includes passive flexion of the digits, active wrist extension, and a 5-second hold of the digits in the flexed position. This exercise is safe immediately postoperatively for patients with two-strand repairs.

the minimal active tension of the flexor tendons.[119] Synergistic motion has also been observed to create the greatest amount of flexor digitorum superficialis, flexor digitorum profundus, and differential excursion,[117] serve as an effective pulling force to create proximal glide,[120] and result in low force with high excursion.[112,121] Conversely, the literature indicates that asking patients either to perform place-and-hold or active digital motion when the wrist is flexed actually demands more force than the same motions performed with the wrist extended. The most recent addition to the study of synergistic motion was from Amadio, who introduced a passive, modified synergistic exercise.[104] Passive wrist and metacarpophalangeal extension coupled with passive proximal and distal interphalangeal flexion was suggested to produce 100–150 grams of force on the healing tendon and serve as a preparatory exercise for place-and-hold synergistic motion (*Fig. 39.7*).

Early place-and-hold synergistic motion has been suggested as safe following both two- and four-strand repairs and should be considered as a means of optimizing outcomes for this difficult diagnosis. The use of consistent measurement to

assess tendon glide is suggested as a means of progressing exercise, using force and excursion parameters for clinical decision-making (*Table 39.1*). The use of straight fist, hook fist, composite fist, and isolated joint exercises is suggested as a sequential regimen for controlled force once place-and-hold synergistic exercises have been initiated (*Fig. 39.8*). Consistent communication between the therapist and plastic surgeon is essential to both initiation and progression of exercise for the patient following flexor tendon repair, beginning with a detailed operative report outlining the number of strands crossing the repair site and perceived integrity of the repair.

Extensor tendon injuries

Care of the patient following an extensor tendon injury is a far less complicated pursuit compared to flexor tendon injury. Use of standard protocols based on the anatomy and biomechanics of the extensor apparatus has led to consistent and favorable results throughout all zones of the extensor musculature.

A zone I injury is commonly referred to as "mallet finger." Upon clinical examination, patients demonstrate an inability

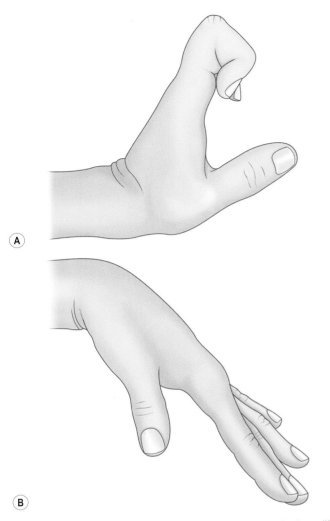

Fig. 39.7 (A, B) The most recent addition to postoperative exercise is modified synergistic motion, described by Amadio.[104]

is resumed and flexion exercises are decreased or discontinued.

Loss of integrity of the central slip in zone III is termed a boutonnière deformity. As the lateral bands sublux volarly, flexion of the proximal interphalangeal joint is unopposed. Flexion contractures are common sequelae of this condition; avoidance of this difficult complication must be pursued early in the treatment process. In addition, extensor forces are transmitted to the distal interphalangeal joint, resulting in hyperextension. Differential diagnosis of a pseudoboutonnière from a true boutonnière is an important component of the evaluative process. In the former, the distal interphalangeal joint remains passively flexible, whereas in the latter, the distal interphalangeal joint cannot be passively flexed. Nonoperative management of the boutonnière deformity includes continual splinting or casting of the proximal interphalangeal joint at 0° extension for 6–8 weeks. The distal interphalangeal and metacarpophalangeal joints do not need to be included in the splint or cast if the therapist is successfully able to maintain the proximal interphalangeal joint at 0° extension, an often difficult undertaking. The splint is continued between exercises until the 10th week.

Evans suggested a short arc motion protocol may be initiated within 48 hours of surgical correction of a boutonnière deformity.[122] A template is fabricated that allows 30° of proximal interphalangeal and 20° of distal interphalangeal joint flexion. The patient is instructed to produce finger flexion to the template and active extension to 0°. This exercise is completed 10–20 times every 1–2 hours with the wrist held in 30° flexion and the metacarpophalangeal joints between 0° extension and slight flexion. The template is adjusted to 40° of flexion after the second week if there is no active extensor lag. It is then progressed to 50° by the third postoperative week and up to 70–80° by the end of the fourth week. The finger is splinted in full extension between exercises and an exercise splint to facilitate isolated distal interphalangeal flexion is also fabricated.

Injuries in zones V–VII can be open or closed, with lacerations and blunt trauma as typical mechanisms of injury. Disturbance of the sagittal bands often leads to long extensor tendon subluxation with resultant metacarpophalangeal extensor lag. Following surgical repair, multiple protocols are considered effective for treating extensor tendon injuries in these zones.

The most conservative protocol includes splinting the wrist in 40–45° extension and the metacarpophalageal joints in 0–20° flexion. A volar interphalageal extension splint is fabricated to support the joints in full extension between exercises and at night as a means of preventing both flexion contractures and an extensor lag. Treatment of edema and scar is critical in this zone as adhesions are likely and will limit both proximal and distal glide of the extensor tendons. Exercises begin at 3–4 weeks postoperatively and include a wrist tenodesis exercise with active metacarpophalangeal flexion and extension as well as continued interphalangeal active motion.

Evans and Burkhalter suggested a dorsal dynamic extension assist splint following injuries in zone VI–VII; this allows 30° active metacarpophalangeal flexion and returns the digits to 0° extension via dynamic traction.[123] The early distal glide afforded by this splint makes it an excellent choice for patients who can manage a more intricate splint design. Individual

actively to extend the distal interphalangeal joint due to detachment of the terminal extensor tendon from the distal phalanx. A mallet finger is characterized by varying degrees of flexion at the distal interphalangeal joint. Nonoperative treatment for a mallet finger includes continuous immobilization of the distal interphalangeal joint in full extension for 6 weeks *(Fig. 39.9)*. The proximal interphalangeal joint is mobilized during this timeframe as a means of maintaining proper alignment of the lateral bands and balance of the flexor and extensor tendons. Fabrication or issuance of two splints is suggested as a means of minimizing maceration of tissues and facilitating skin integrity during daily hygiene activities. After 6 weeks, the therapist initiates a gradual splint-weaning process and the patient begins gentle, composite flexion exercises. The patient is also educated on the avoidance of isolated joint motion that can unnecessarily stress the terminal tendon. Lateral tracing of the digit for daily comparison serves as an effective visual aid to monitor for development of an extensor lag during the splint-weaning process. If an extensor lag develops at any time during this process, extension splinting

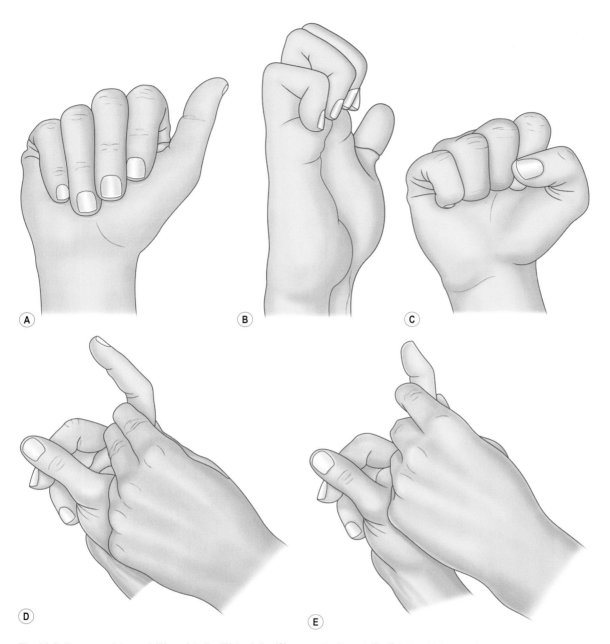

Fig. 39.8 The sequential use of **(A)** straight fist **(B)** hook fist **(C)** composite fist and **(D, E)** isolated joint exercises are suggested as a means of consciously progressing forces on the healing flexor tendon.

proximal interphalangeal extension gutters are added for those patients who demonstrate extensor lags. Howell *et al.* suggest immediate controlled active motion (ICAM) for patients with repairs in these zones.[124] This protocol includes three phases, the first of which can be initiated between 0 and 21 days after surgery. The wrist is splinted in 20–25° extension, while the metacarpophalangeal joint of the affected digit is positioned with a "yoke" splint in 15–20° of hyperextension relative to the other digits *(Fig. 39.10)*. Both splints are to be worn at all times and the patient must achieve full active motion within the ICAM splints before progressing to the next phase. Phase 2 begins 22–35 days after repair, during which

the yoke splint is worn at all times and both splints are only worn for medium to heavy activities. The patient is instructed to relax the digits during wrist exercise. Phase 3 is initiated 36–49 days after repair and includes discontinuation of the wrist splint with the yoke splint or buddy tapes continued during activities. The yoke splint is removed for active motion during the final phase.

Despite the seeming simplicity of extensor tendon as compared to flexor tendon rehabilitation, attention to anatomic specificity is very important as it pertains to final outcomes. Edema collects easily in the dorsal hand and must be managed immediately to avoid tendon adhesions. Attention to both

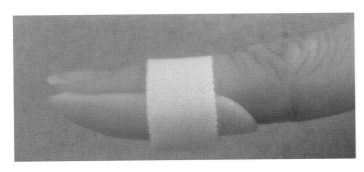

Fig. 39.9 An injury to the extensor tendon in zone I, commonly termed mallet finger, is most often treated conservatively with distal interphalangeal extension splinting at all times for 6 weeks. (Courtesy of Rebecca von der Heyde PhD OTR/L CHT.)

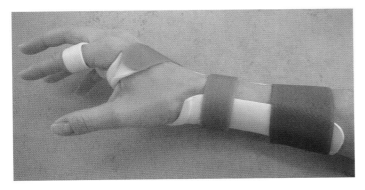

Fig. 39.10 The immediate controlled active motion protocol, as described by Howell et al.,[124] includes a wrist cock-up splint and a yoke splint which effectively creates hyperextension of the affected digit relative to the other digits. (Courtesy of Rebecca von der Heyde PhD OTR/L CHT.)

active and passive motion at all joints provides valuable information for the choice and progression of interventions. A passively mobile joint with an active extensor lag is best managed via active tendon gliding in both proximal and distal directions. Resistive exercises are an excellent method of restoring tendon glide after the eighth week. Perhaps the most important approach is the isolation of specific musculature to produce joint extension – the extensor digitorum communis for metacarpophalangeal extension and the intrinsic musculature for interphalangeal extension.

Tenolysis

Following flexor and extensor tendon repairs, the likelihood of scar adhesions that limit active excursion is unfortunately high. While early motion coupled with continual evaluation and progression can modulate scar formation, confounding factors, including overall health, pain, and compliance, may negatively impact postoperative results. If progress has plateaued at the 3-month interval, patients are often evaluated as candidates for tenolysis.

Proper assessment of tendon gliding includes comprehensive measurement and comparison of active and passive range of motion at all joints of the affected digit(s). The optimal candidate for tenolysis is the patient who

demonstrates full passive motion of the digit and is deemed compliant by the therapist and surgeon. As the postoperative treatment of tenolysis is both painful and time-intensive, thorough education of patient and family is vital to success. A therapy schedule for daily treatment during the first 7 days posttenolysis, including weekend days, should be established preoperatively.

Direct communication between the surgeon and the hand therapist regarding the integrity of the tendon and active motion as accomplished during surgery should be a priority and postoperative treatment should begin on the same day as surgery. It is advisable to allow the patient multiple hours of recovery time, including a full meal and initiation of pain medication if possible to decrease the likelihood of adverse reactions (i.e., fainting) if treatment is promptly initiated. Use of a sterile field and gloves is important to minimize the likelihood of infection as the therapist initiates hourly active exercises to facilitate tendon glide. Edema management and wound care are also carefully addressed as the therapist attempts to find a balance between adequate dressings for drainage absorption that provide minimal physical blockage to active motion. Consistent measurement of active and passive motion is pursued during the first 7 consecutive days of treatment.

Therapy intensity can decrease after the first week for patients who demonstrate compliance with hourly exercise and the ability to complete wound care independently. The outcomes of tenolysis are quickly recognized and difficult to remediate after the first 3–4 weeks of treatment. For this reason, communication between the surgeon and hand therapist and careful selection of patients for this procedure are perhaps the most influential factors influencing final outcome.

Tendon transfers

Rehabilitation following tendon transfers requires careful communication between the plastic surgeon and hand therapist and attention to detail. This detail not only includes surgical specificity, but the unique needs and expectations of the patient coupled with a neuromuscular intervention plan. For the purposes of brevity, the example of a pronator teres (PT) to extensor carpi radialis brevis (ECRB) tendon transfer, as performed in cases of radial nerve injury, will be used throughout this section as a case example.

Patient education should include the purpose of the surgical procedure, expected timeline for rehabilitation, possible complications, and expected outcomes.[125] The patient needs to be informed that functional use will be altered following surgery and that a tendon transfer procedure will not correct for losses in sensation.[126] Prior to surgery, efforts are instituted to strengthen the donor muscle selected for the procedure.[125] If the patient has difficulty isolating the donor muscle, biofeedback and exercise splints may be useful.[125]

Immediately following surgery, the transfer and all involved joints are immobilized in a position that places minimal tension on the newly transferred tendon. An immobilization period of 3–4 weeks is commonly implemented to allow adequate healing and minimize the risk of tendon

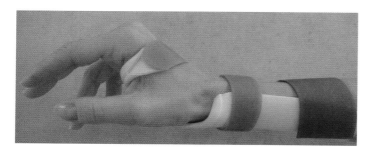

Fig. 39.11 The patient with a pronator teres to extensor carpi radialis brevis tendon transfer is splinted in 45° of wrist extension for 3–4 weeks following surgery. (Courtesy of Rebecca von der Heyde PhD OTR/L CHT.)

rupture upon mobilization of the transfer.[126] During this period, the postoperative dressing is removed and the patient is immobilized in a thermoplastic splint. In the case of a PT-to-ECRB transfer, the patient is immobilized in a wrist cock-up splint at 45° extension *(Fig. 39.11)*. For those cases in which coaptation of the muscles are considered tenuous, a splint that limits forearm rotation while positioning the wrist in extension can be fabricated. During this period, the therapist's focus is centered on the evaluation and treatment of edema, pain, and infection.

In the absence of complications during the immobilization phase, initiation of active motion typically occurs 3–4 weeks postoperatively.[125,126] The therapist initiates neuromuscular re-education exercises, including isolation and activation of the transfer to produce a desired motion. Central to this process is the concept of cortical plasticity, or the capacity of a cortical circuit to reorganize its structure or response subsequent to an experience.[127] As suggested by Sanes and Donoghue, the primary motor cortex exhibits such plasticity as a result of repetition of simple movements.[127] Combination exercises are frequently incorporated to facilitate re-education of a donor muscle, and include training the patient to produce the primary movement of a denervated muscle utilizing a new musculotendinous unit. For instance, if a PT-to-ECRB transfer is performed to restore wrist extension, the patient is instructed to pronate the forearm while simultaneously extending the wrist. Proprioceptive feedback is preferable to visual as it facilitates cortical reorganization and auditory feedback can also be helpful.

The length of time it takes to isolate a transfer effectively is highly variable, depending on the type of transfer and the age and skill set of the patient. Isometric activation can be carefully initiated with those patients who find combination exercises difficult. In the case of a PT-to-ECRB transfer, gentle resistance is provided to the wrist while the patient is producing pronation with wrist extension. As the patient progresses, the goal is isolated activation of the donor muscle in production of the newly desired motion, in this case, wrist extension against gravity without the need to pronate.

At 6–7 weeks postsurgery, the tendon has healed and is able to tolerate functional activities and light resistance. Passive range-of-motion exercises may also be initiated to mitigate any residual tightness incurred during surgery or the immobilization period.[125] At 8 weeks postsurgery, progressive resistance exercises may be incorporated into the exercise regimen.[125]

Rehabilitation following skeletal injury/surgery

Proximal phalanx fractures

Proximal phalanx fractures are challenging and as such require careful attention to bony integrity and maintenance of the flexor and extensor tendon-gliding systems. Therapeutic interventions as outlined in this section are based on the assumption that a patient presents with one of the following: a potentially unstable, yet nondisplaced extra-articular fracture; an inherently stable fracture; or hardware fixation facilitating stability such as an open-reduction internal fixation or closed-reduction external fixation.

According to Feehan, structural strength following a proximal phalanx fracture is influenced by location, pattern and displacement, type of reduction, hardware, concomitant soft-tissue injuries, stage of healing, and the functional demands of the patient.[128] Initiation of early controlled mobilization is based on the surgeon's perception of structural strength and can be altered by choosing the number of joints to be mobilized, active and/or passive motion, a safe arc of motion, and the duration or repetitions of motion.[128] Isolating short arc motion at one or more joints when possible provides tendon glide and lengthening of connective tissue structures that will facilitate final outcomes for patients following proximal phalanx fracture. As the flexor digitorum profundus lies in close proximity to the proximal phalanx, isolated distal interphalangeal motion should be initiated as soon as possible. Moving the joint actively through flexion and extension will also afford some proximal and distal excursion of the extensor mechanism.

Following a proximal phalanx fracture, metacarpophalangeal joint positioning and proximal interphalangeal joint mobilization have been studied as a means of avoiding complications. Metacarpophalangeal joint flexion is the close-packed position of the joint, or the position at which the joint space is minimized, and the joint surfaces of the head of the metacarpal and the base of the proximal phalanx are maximally congruent. In addition, metacarpophalangeal joint flexion moves the extensor hood distally, translates the force of the extensor digitorum to the proximal interphalangeal joint, and creates circumferential compression on the fracture.[129] From a volar perspective, flexion also decreases the proximity of the flexor tendons to the fracture site. Proximal interphalangeal joint range of motion has been suggested to maintain the length of the joint capsule and increase soft-tissue gliding as well as creating a dynamic tension band effect in conjunction with the extensor digitorum to facilitate fracture reduction.[130,131] According to Feehan, the functional and physiologic stresses associated with early controlled mobilization increase the quality and rate of bone healing.[128]

Complications following proximal phalanx fractures are often sequelae of scar tissue that limits all structures in the zone of injury. Typical issues include extensor mechanism adherence and fracture deformity with resultant proximal interphalangeal joint extensor lags.[129,132] In a study by Kurzen *et al.*, 52% of patients demonstrated less than 180° of total active motion following plate fixation of a proximal phalanx fracture.[133] To avoid such outcomes, LaStayo *et al.* recommend

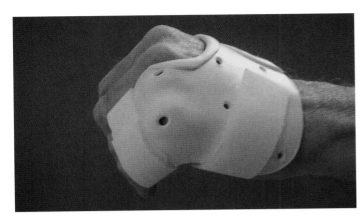

Fig. 39.12 Following a proximal phalanx fracture, splinting the metacarpophalangeal joint in flexion facilitates close-packed positioning, creates circumferential pressure via the extensor mechanism, and decreases the proximity of the flexor tendons to the fracture site. Allowance of proximal interphalangeal joint motion increases the opportunity for differential tendon gliding along the fracture site. (Courtesy of Rebecca von der Heyde PhD OTR/L CHT.)

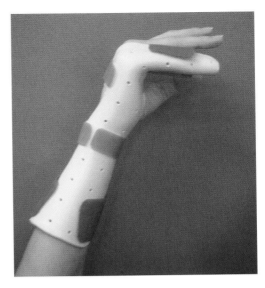

Fig. 39.13 Fractures to the metacarpal head are splinted or casted with wrist extension, metacarpophalangeal joint flexion, and interphalangeal joint extension. (Courtesy of Rebecca von der Heyde PhD OTR/L CHT.)

a progressive program be initiated in the following order: protection or external support, edema management, protected and controlled mobilization of proximal and distal joints, tendon gliding, passive range of motion, and strengthening.[131] The external support, typically a custom-fabricated splint, can either be hand- or forearm-based and dorsally blocks the metacarpophalangeal joints in flexion[129,134] *(Fig. 39.12)*.

Metacarpal fractures

Metacarpal fractures are commonly seen primarily in the fourth and fifth metacarpal and often in adolescent males. From an anatomic perspective, consideration of both the metacarpals and their adjacent tendinous and connective tissue structures directs clinical decision-making. The second through fifth metacarpals are aligned as parallel long bones and serve both mobility and stability functions for the digits. The proximal bases of the second and third metacarpal are firmly affixed to the distal carpal row, more specifically, the trapezoid and capitate. More mobile CMC joints at the thumb and small finger surround this stable center, while the fourth metacarpal demonstrates limited mobility on the hamate. Distally, the deep transverse metacarpal ligament connects the heads of the second through fifth metacarpals. The alignment of the distal carpal row, reinforced by this ligament, creates the transverse arches of the hand that contribute to grasp and function.

According to McNemar *et al.*, metacarpal head fractures are immobilized in the position of safety, with the wrist extended, metacarpophalangeal joints fully flexed, and proximal and distal interphalangeal joints extended, in either a cast or a custom-fabricated splint[135] *(Fig. 39.13)*. This close-packed positioning maintains the length of the collateral ligaments, counteracts the tendency towards a claw deformity, and draws the extensor mechanism distally to support the fracture.[135] For those cases requiring open reduction and internal fixation through an incision of the extensor mechanism, early motion becomes a necessity to avoid tendon adherence.[135]

The more typical metacarpal neck fracture often occurs in the fourth or fifth metacarpal and is typically seen in young males who have been involved in an altercation. A more conservative approach to this injury includes immobilization of the wrist in extension and the metacarpophalangeal joints in flexion, with early mobilization of the proximal and distal interphalangeal joints.[135] For those fractures that are minimally displaced with reasonable stability, a less restrictive regimen of splinting and exercise can be initiated. A cuff splint that creates circumferential pressure around the hand and approximates the metacarpals towards anatomical alignment is fabricated to allow unrestricted motion of the wrist and metacarpophalangeal joints *(Fig. 39.14)*. For additional distal alignment, the proximal phalanx of the affected metacarpal can be taped or strapped to the adjacent digit with which it is optimally aligned lengthwise. Using this approach, the patient is encouraged to perform active exercise while avoiding sustained or forceful grasp during the healing phase.

Complications after metacarpal fractures include rotational deformities, loss of length, and dense adhesions restricting tendon glide of the extrinsic extensor tendons. Rotational deformities lead to scissoring of the digits during active flexion, while metacarpal shortening can lead to active insufficiency of the extrinsic digit extensors and the possibility of decreased grip strength.[135] Extensor adherence can be avoided with early motion protocols emphasizing isolated glide of the long extensors. Composite extension of the digit will not achieve this goal; rather, the patient is instructed in transition from a full fist to a hook fist, which creates maximal, isolated glide of the extensor digitorum communis. These exercises are of increased importance following open reduction and internal fixation of metacarpal head, neck, and shaft fractures.

Thumb carpometacarpal osteoarthritis

Osteoarthritis of the first CMC joint is an extremely common diagnosis addressed by the plastic surgeon and hand therapist; most often observed in women of middle age. This

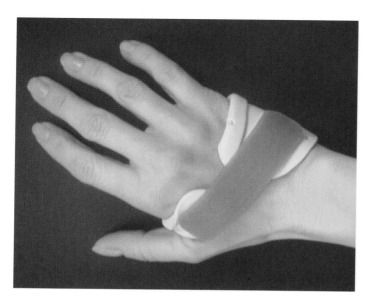

Fig. 39.14 Metacarpal neck and shaft fractures that are minimally displaced can be splinted using a simple cuff which approximates the metacarpals and creates circumferential pressure. (Courtesy of Rebecca von der Heyde PhD OTR/L CHT.)

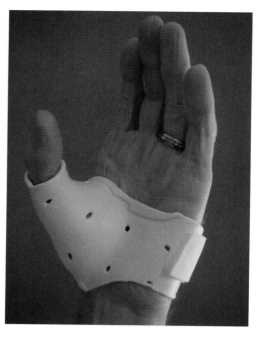

Fig. 39.15 Patients with carpometacarpal osteoarthritis are often immobilized in a hand-based thumb spica splint to relieve pain and provide support and positioning to facilitate functional use. (Courtesy of Rebecca von der Heyde PhD OTR/L CHT.)

diagnosis is the subject of much debate, ranging from anatomy to interventions.

The typical presentation of a patient with CMC osteoarthritis includes marked adduction of the first CMC joint with hyperextension of the metacarpophalangeal joint. This positioning is influenced by numerous musculoskeletal imbalances that are presumed to have both causative and resultant roles. Prolonged adduction of the joint leads to shortening of the adductor pollicis, active insufficiency of the abductor pollicis brevis and extensor pollicis brevis, and decreased stabilization by the first dorsal interossei. The extensor pollicis longus, having the greatest moment arm for metacarpophalangeal extension, subsequently creates compensatory metacarpophalangeal hyperextension to increase the first webspace for grasp and function. Offsetting this compensatory pattern via positioning of the metacarpophalangeal joint in flexion has been noted to unload the palmar surfaces of the CMC joint, suggesting that the more distal metacarpophalangeal joint may play a role in the progression of arthritis at the proximal CMC joint.[136]

A recent systematic review of conservative interventions for osteoarthritis of the hand provides evidence for numerous interventions based on specific patient goals.[137] Moderate evidence was found to support heat, exercise, education on joint protection, and issuance of adaptive equipment as adjunctive methods for pain reduction and increased function. The use of splints to decrease pain and increase function was supported with high to moderate evidence. Numerous splints are available for conservative management of CMC osteoarthritis, both custom and prefabricated. Evidence to suggest the superiority of one splint design from a diagnostic perspective is lacking; however, studies have shown patient preferences towards prefabricated, hand-based splints[137] *(Fig. 39.15)*. The work by Moulton *et al.* supports the inclusion of the metacarpophalangeal joint in the splint, positioned

in flexion as a means of unloading the volar surface of the CMC joint and decreasing forces on the anterior oblique ligament.[136]

For patients with advanced stages of CMC osteoarthritis, or those who have failed nonoperative management, surgical intervention is often recommended. Despite the numerous surgical methods for thumb CMC arthroplasty, generically referred to as ligament reconstruction tendon interposition, postoperative care is relatively straightforward. Emphasis during the rehabilitative phase is placed on the maintenance of stability of the newly reconstructed joint as a means of facilitating painfree thumb function. For this reason, the patient is typically immobilized in a forearm-based thumb spica cast or splint for 4 weeks following surgery. The interphalangeal joint is left free to facilitate tendon gliding of the extensor pollicis longus and flexor pollicis longus across the surgical site. This early motion can also contribute to decreasing edema and hypersensitivity; two common sequelae of this procedure.

After 4 weeks, a program of active circumduction range of motion, scar management, and desensitization is initiated. Active range of motion of the CMC joint is pursued gently, mindful of the influence of proximal stability on distal mobility and overall function of the thumb. Close attention to the balance of musculature about the thumb is also important, especially as it pertains to the length of the adductor pollicis and activation of the extensor pollicis brevis and abductor pollicis longus. Metacarpophalangeal hyperextension should be carefully monitored; blocking the interphalangeal joint of the thumb in slight flexion during active exercise is often effective in controlling the mechanical advantage of the extensor pollicis longus. Scar adhesions and hypersensitivity are common complaints following this procedure and should be addressed with early and progressive massage and desensitization.

While gentle passive motion can be initiated at 6 weeks, splinting between exercise sessions and at night is often continued until the eighth postoperative week. Strengthening should be avoided until pain is no longer a primary complaint, and pursued only within the realm of the function required on an individual basis.

Conclusion

Comprehensive evaluation and multidisciplinary treatment approaches are advocated for patients following hand surgery and optimal outcomes necessitate a collaborative relationship and open communication between the patient, surgeon, and hand therapist.

Access the complete references list online at **http://www.expertconsult.com**

35. Amadio PC. Outcome assessment in hand surgery and hand therapy: An update. *J Hand Ther*. 2001;14:63–68.

76. Ramachandran VS, Altschuler EL. The use of visual feedback, in particular mirror visual feedback, in restoring brain function. *Brain*. 2009;132:1693–1710.

98. Novak CB. Rehabilitation following motor nerve transfers. *Hand Clin*. 2008;24:417–423.

104. Amadio PC. Friction of the gliding surface: Implications for tendon surgery and rehabilitation. *J Hand Ther*. 2005;18:112–119.

112. Lieber RL, Silva MJ, Amiel D, et al. Wrist and digital joint motion produce unique flexor tendon force and excursion in the canine forelimb. *J Biomech*. 1999;32:175–181.

    This study using a canine model suggested that forces exerted on the healing flexor tendon are highly dependent on wrist position. Synergistic motion was noted to result in low passive forces on the flexor tendon with high excursion.

117. Cooney WP, Lin GT, An KN. Improved tendon excursion following flexor tendon repair. *J Hand Ther*. 1989;2:102–106.

    In this cadaveric study, postoperative rehabilitation protocols were compared, including Kleinert, the Brooke Army Hospital modification, and synergistic motion. Synergistic motion yielded the greatest flexor digitorum profundus, flexor digitorum superficialis, and differential excursion.

124. Howell JW, Merritt WH, Robinson SJ. Immediate controlled active motion following zone 4–7 extensor tendon repair. *J Hand Ther*. 2005;18:182–190.

    The protocol described for extensor tendon injuries includes a wrist splint paired with a yoke splint which positions the metacarpophalangeal joint of the affected digit in hyperextension relative to the other digits. Full active motion within the immediate controlled active motion splints is expected prior to progression to the next phase of the protocol.

128. Feehan LM. Early controlled mobilization of potentially unstable extra-articular hand fractures. *J Hand Ther*. 2003;16:161–169.

    This article suggests that functional and physiologic stresses associated with active range of motion increase the quality and rate of healing in potentially unstable extra-articular hand fractures. Control of clinical factors is recommended as a means of incorporating early motion into fracture management.

136. Moulton MJ, Parentis MA, Kelly MJ, et al. Influence of metacarpal joint position on the basal joint loading in the thumb. *J Bone Joint Surg*. 2001;83A:709–716.

    In this cadaveric study, immobilization of the metacarpophalangeal joint was studied as it pertained to forces on the trapezial surface during lateral pinch. Metacarpophalangeal flexion was noted to unload the most palmar aspect of the carpometacarpal joint effectively, decreasing strain on the palmar oblique ligament.

137. Valdes K, Marik T. A systematic review of conservative interventions for osteoarthritis of the hand. *J Hand Ther*. 2010;23:334–351.

40

Treatment of the upper extremity amputee

Gregory A. Dumanian and Todd A. Kuiken

SYNOPSIS

- Upper extremity amputees face many unique challenges in everyday life.
- The surgeon can be an active participant in patient care, both at the time of the amputation and years later to maximize function and use of the residual limb.
- Prostheses may be custom-fit to recreate digits and to make amputations less discernible.
- New techniques in active prostheses may allow better function of traumatized upper extremities.

 Access the Historical Perspective section online at **http://www.expertconsult.com**

Introduction

Upper extremity amputees are different from lower extremity amputees in many aspects. The patients are younger and their amputations are primarily due to trauma and tumors rather than dysvascular conditions. The patients live longer with their residual limbs. Prosthetic concerns for the two groups of patients dramatically differ. Upper extremity prostheses require more control, more movement, and more precision than that for a leg. Fortunately, upper extremity prostheses have less load-bearing and do not support the weight of the body.

The purpose of this chapter is to familiarize the reader with necessary concepts to care for the upper extremity amputee. Handling of soft tissues, bones, and nerves is reviewed for each of the levels of amputation. Prosthetics and prosthetic control will be a necessary accompaniment of this chapter. Recent advancements in the field, including targeted reinnervation, will be introduced.

Aesthetic prostheses

Aesthetic prostheses refer to a device used to camouflage a limb deformity, while functional prostheses refer to devices that are operational.[5] Aesthetic prostheses assist patients in issues of body image and self-esteem, with possible functional gains as well. These secondary functional gains are a due to a newfound social openness and ability to expose the limb, rather than to a subconscious desire to avoid detection of the limb deformity. Patients can appear fairly normal in public with aesthetic prostheses (*Figs 40.1 and 40.2*). Most of these prostheses are custom-made and require a high level of expertise on the part of the prosthetist. Because intact skin is used to secure the prosthetics in place, some amount of sensory feedback of the residual limb will be lost, and this is one drawback to these devices. Osseointegration of aesthetic prostheses into bone has been studied at length because it will improve the tolerance of the soft tissues to the prosthesis, limit the amount of soft tissues covered, and permit the use of stiffer materials in the devices for possible secondary functional gains. The bone–soft-tissue–implant interface for osseointegration of upper limb prosthetics remains problematic.[6]

Control of upper extremity prosthetic devices

A prosthesis is only as good as the control signals that it receives from the user. The goal of any prosthesis is to be moved and positioned in space smoothly, quickly, intuitively, and with minimal exertion and mental fatigue to accomplish this task.[7] Multifunctional prostheses create new unique problems for control, because signaling will need to be directed specifically between one function and another. For example, prostheses with both a terminal device and a prosthetic elbow will need to switch from "hand" to "elbow" and then back to

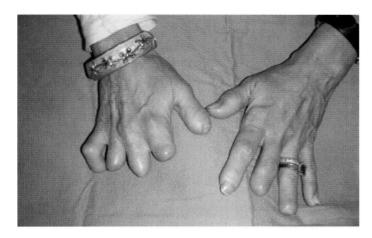

Fig. 40.1 Patient with multiple finger amputations due to sepsis and hypotension.

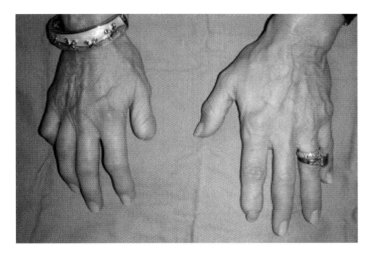

Fig. 40.2 Multiple-digit prostheses for improvement of cosmetic appearance.

considerable complexity. As with body-powered devices, only one joint can be operated at a time with current myoelectric control systems. Multifunctional devices require an additional switch or signal to cause the device to change from one prosthetic "joint" to another. It was a lack of smooth and intuitive control of myoelectric prostheses that impeded any progress on these devices since the 1970s.

Kuiken *et al.* in 1995 demonstrated a new strategy, now called "targeted muscle reinnervation" (TMR), for control of myoelectric prostheses. Rather than using the "wrong" signals from nearby and functionless muscles, nerve transfers were performed to amplify the nerve signal that had previously controlled the limb. After successful neurotization, the muscle would serve to amplify the signal of the amputated nerve, and this EMG signal would be detected transcutaneously.[8] The downside of this approach is that the amputee would need a surgical procedure to perform the nerve transfer, and that the intact EMG signal from that muscle would be lost. Kuiken *et al.* reported this procedure in humans in shoulder disarticulation patients in 2004,[9] and O'Shaughnessy *et al.* reported the same procedure in transhumeral amputees in 2008.[10] Continuing the example of a transhumeral amputee with a myoelectric prosthesis, the median nerve could be transferred to the motor nerve of one segment of the biceps muscle and the distal radial nerve could be transferred to the motor nerve of one segment of the triceps muscle. Segments of the biceps and triceps would be left intact during the surgical dissection to maintain the native innervation from the musculocutaneous nerve and the proximal radial nerve, respectively. Therefore, TMR preserves two control areas for prosthetic elbow function, and creates two new control signals for prosthetic hand function. Targeted reinnervation allows for simultaneous movement of both prosthetic joints. The control paradigm is intuitive, because nerves that previously had controlled native joints have regained their function to control the prosthetic joint. The musculocutaneous nerve activates one head of the biceps to cause prosthetic elbow flexion. One intact branch of the proximal radial nerve serves to extend the prosthetic elbow. After neurotization, the median nerve once again causes the terminal device to close with its signal to a segment of the biceps, and the distal radial nerve causes the terminal device to open after causing a segment of the triceps to contract. TMR has been successfully performed clinically in over 40 patients with proximal arm amputations with very high success rates.

Other strategies for prosthetic control are still in the investigative phase, but show promise. Implantable myoelectric sensor systems that transmit EMG signals out to a detecting device could improve the EMG signal quality and consistency, as well as provide control signals from small muscle bodies such as the individual finger extensors of the forearm.[11] Advanced computer programs are being developed to decode EMG signals and enable intuitive control of multiple functions. Direct signal acquisition from the amputated nerves using a variety of implanted electrodes has been investigated.[12] Prosthetic control using fine wire electrodes was recently demonstrated in an acute experiment in humans.[13] Direct recording and stimulation of the cerebral cortex have been performed in monkeys in order to effect peripheral movement. This brain–machine interface, if successful, could have wide applicability not only for amputees, but also for patients with spinal cord injuries.[14]

"hand" again to accomplish almost every task. This will cause the device to appear jerky and slow in its use.

The problem with body-powered prostheses is that the "wrong" muscles are driving the device. Body-powered prostheses, as previously described, utilize shoulder motions to operate the prosthesis. This is problematic, because muscles that are designed for strong movements, such as the latissimus dorsi and the serratus anterior, are required to move accurately and sensitively to control cables and switches. Body-powered devices use nonintuitive shoulder muscles to control a prosthetic elbow or hand. Those muscles are clumsy and not designed for fine movements. Finally, only one function of the prosthesis can be actuated at one time; a hand, wrist, and elbow must be used sequentially, which is slow and cumbersome.

Myoelectric prostheses, for one-dimensional devices, have a much more intuitive control system. The best example is a myoelectric device for a transradial amputee. Two EMG signals from the amputee are recorded, one from the volar flexors for closing of the terminal device, and one signal from the extensors for terminal device opening. At this point, the control paradigm is still rather straightforward. Adding additional joints (such as in higher-level devices) adds

Prosthetic implications of upper limb amputation surgery

The surgical treatment of patients with unreconstructable upper extremity conditions must consider issues unique to the amputee. The amputation must have durable soft tissues to allow for prosthetic fitting. In all instances, an evaluation is performed in how to preserve intact nerves, and how to manage unavoidable end neuromas. The means by which the prosthesis will be controlled must be considered. With these concepts in mind, a level-by-level analysis of the common levels of upper extremity amputation will be presented.

Finger amputation

Patients undergoing reconstructive upper extremity surgery do best when the surgeon "think[s] nerve."[15] Patients can easily exclude a painless stiff digit, whereas they are greatly troubled by a mobile painful digit with a symptomatic neuroma. Patients with wounds of the fingers should be evaluated as to which nerves are irreparably cut, and which digital nerves are intact. If a major portion of one of the two digital nerves is intact, then a flap should be performed for wound closure, rather than a shortening amputation with division of both digital nerves. The digital nerves to the finger pulp trifurcate approximately 2 mm distal to the volar distal interphalangeal skin crease. A branch travels to the nail fold, one branch travels to the volar tip, and the third branch innervates the volar pad. Amputations at or proximal to the trifurcation have two cut digital nerves, and therefore a revision amputation will not cut a new nerve to achieve wound closure. In *Figures 40.3 and 40.4*, the ulnar digital nerve to the ring finger is intact, while the radial digital nerve is cut. The cross-finger flap is performed to achieve wound closure, but more

importantly, to avoid the necessity of dividing an intact digital nerve in a revision amputation.

Much has been written about more proximal finger amputations. For these patients, a traction neurectomy is performed to keep the nerve from trying to reinnervate the skin laceration area. The surgeon should attempt to achieve a smooth and tapered end to the digit, rather than having a bulbous tip. This requires removal of the condyles for joint disarticulations, and longer skin incisions down the mid-axial lines of the digits.

Partial hand

Again, "think[ing] nerve," loss of the ulnar, radial, or dorsal aspect of the hand with some intact volar nerves should undergo flap reconstruction to obviate the need to divide nerves that are in continuity. Typically, this will be either a free flap, or a pedicled groin flap as a second choice. If the majority of the digital nerves are divided, then the next decision is if there is a functional and stable wrist joint. Maintenance of the wrist will allow the residual limb to be an excellent helper hand without a prosthesis *(Figs 40.5–40.7)*. In some avulsive injuries, the dorsal wrist extensors have been removed by the injury, and it is worthwhile reinserting extensor tendons to the residual carpal bones with bone anchors and a flap for coverage. Muscle flaps are preferable to skin flaps, as the associated eventual atrophy will facilitate the placement of passive finger prostheses that can assist in grasp.[16]

Body-powered and externally powered prostheses exist for partial hand amputations, but have significant size constraints to provide movable components that will not cause the device to be longer than the opposite hand. Suspension of these devices is also difficult in the desire not to impede wrist motion. Rather than prosthetics, improvements in hand function for patients with thumb, multiple digit, or partial hand amputations can be achieved with toe-to-hand transfers.

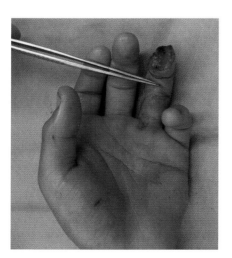

Fig. 40.3 Young adult with injury to half of the pulp of his ring finger. Completion amputation was recommended at an outside institution.

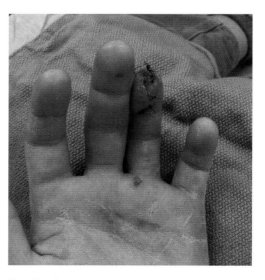

Fig. 40.4 Two weeks after, the cross-finger flap was sewn in place.

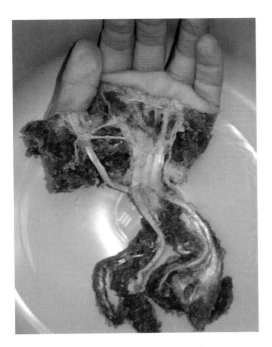

Fig. 40.5 Amputated specimen in young male.

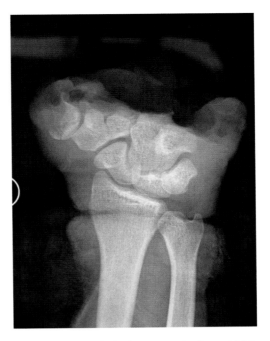

Fig. 40.6 Radiograph showing preserved radiocarpal joint.

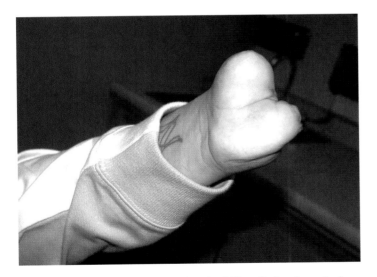

Fig. 40.7 Mobile wrist joint acts as a helper hand. The patient's extensor tendons were reinserted into the carpal bones with bone anchors.

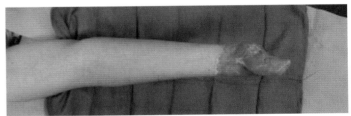

Fig. 40.8 A young worker had skin grafts applied to a proximal hand stripped of almost all soft tissues in an attempt to "save length." He underwent a transradial amputation for treatment of his painful immobile scarred hand.

Wrist disarticulation and transradial amputation

Injuries that strip the soft tissues off the carpal bones and with divided digital nerves should undergo a wrist disarticulation or a transradial amputation, rather than preserving a scarred and immobile hand to "preserve length" *(Fig. 40.8)*. These patients have already suffered a complete division of the median, radial, and ulnar nerves from their injury, and so a more formal amputation with manipulation and redivision of the nerves where the soft tissues are more supple is appropriate.

In the operating room, plans are made for soft-tissue coverage of the residual limb with development of palmar and dorsal skin flaps. A dorsal approach to the wrist identifies the proximal carpal row, and these bones are excised much like a proximal-row carpectomy. The ulnar and radial arteries are doubly ligated. The radial and ulnar styloids are trimmed to allow for easier prosthetic fitting without pressure points, but the triangular fibrocartilage complex is maintained to preserve pronation and supination. When possible, more durable volar skin is used for coverage as opposed to thinner dorsal skin.

Handling of the nerves to prevent a symptomatic mixed major nerve neuroma from developing is important, as a painful neuroma will prevent the patient from wearing any type of prosthesis. The standard treatment is the traction neurectomy, where the nerves are placed on stretch, divided, and allowed to retract away from the incision line. A general concept is that the better "padded" is a neuroma, the less symptomatic. Other treatments supported by both experimental animal surgery and clinical experience include placing the cut nerve ending within immobile muscle, as opposed to simply allowing them to retract.[17,18]

Clinical work with TMR has revealed that major mixed nerves do not form symptomatic neuromas when nerve transfers are performed. Nerve transfers are now often performed at the time of a wrist disarticulation. This is not to obtain new control signals (though this may occur), but rather to prevent symptomatic end neuromas. The median nerve can be transferred to the anterior interosseous nerve through a proximal incision, the ulnar nerve can be transferred to a motor nerve innervating the flexor carpi ulnaris, and the radial nerve can be transferred to the motor nerve innervating the pronator quadratus. This strategy has been successful because the motor nerves that are cut to receive the transfer serve no function due to the distal amputation. Also, as demonstrated clinically with every muscle flap harvest, cut motor nerves in humans do not form symptomatic neuroma.

If the patient is unlikely to wear a prosthesis, a wrist disarticulation with good soft coverage will give the patient a longer and more functional residual limb. Wrist disarticulation prostheses do well in capturing the distal bony structures for wrist rotation; however room is limited for prosthetic components and the devices tend to look bulky. A long transradial amputation generally enables a better prosthetic fitting, allowing more room for prosthetic components and providing better cosmetic appearance.

A lack of soft tissue may require a transradial amputation as opposed to a wrist disarticulation. In these instances, the shorter lever arm will place more stresses on the residual soft tissues for movement of the prostheses. Pronation and supination will not be as easily translated into prosthetic movement and positioning. Patients undergoing transradial amputations will have similar treatments of the arteries and nerves of the forearm. The radial nerve will be divided and allowed to retract underneath the brachioradialis. A myoplasty of the extensor and flexor muscles over the cut ends of the radius and ulna will stabilize the muscle masses, and facilitate later prosthetic fitting. Drill holes through the bones for passage of suture are useful to prevent muscle movement over the end of the residual limb. At least 5 cm of ulna is necessary to retain elbow movement, but in these instances of very short residual limbs the insertion of the biceps tendon may need to be transferred to the ulna. Preservation of length of bone may require a soft-tissue flap taken from the flank.[19] This pedicled flap is divided after 3 weeks, but provides thick soft tissue and a smoother soft-tissue envelope for prosthetic fitting *(Figs 40.9 and 40.10)*. The function of a transradial amputation is much greater than a transhumeral amputation, thus aggressive treatment to save the elbow and reasonable forearm length is warranted.

Elbow disarticulation and long transhumeral amputation

Nonreconstructable and nonreplantable injuries at the elbow level require removal of the ulna and radius. The elbow disarticulation residual limb is a more functional level than a higher amputation. For example, the limb is long enough to reach a table in sitting and thus is easier to use for moving and stabilizing objects. The condyles in an elbow disarticulation can also be useful in suspension of the prosthesis and for humeral rotation. However, they preclude the use of myoelectric prostheses and require a bulkier body

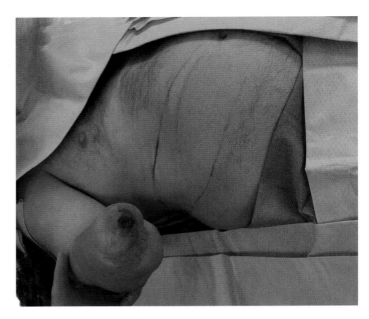

Fig. 40.9 Patient with previous transradial amputation plagued by poor soft-tissue coverage of residual limb.

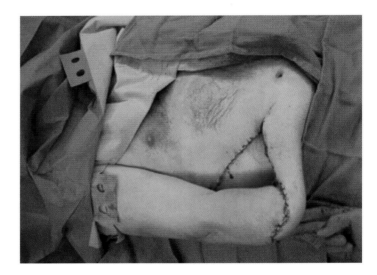

Fig. 40.10 Pedicled periumbilical perforator flap is transferred to the end of the limb after excision of skin-grafted area, and divided 3½ weeks later.

power prosthesis to fit around the distal residual limb. A transhumeral amputation 5–6 cm above the olecranon allows room for a more cosmetic prosthetic elbow, including a myoelectric elbow. With long transhumeral amputations an angulation osteotomy of the distal humerus is also an option. It can similarly provide a lever arm for suspension and for rotational control of the prosthesis when the epicondyles have been removed.[20]

In the operating room, anterior and posterior skin flaps are elevated. The level of the bone division is decided, and either the elbow capsule and ligaments are divided sharply, or else the humerus is cut just proximal to the epicondyles. A myodesis of the triceps and biceps to the distal bone is performed utilizing drill holes for several reasons. Good-quality soft-tissue coverage of the distal bone is a necessity. The end of the residual limb should not have too much redundancy and mobility to facilitate application of a socket and donning the prosthesis. Finally, prevention of proximal migration of the muscle mass during contraction is important for later signal detection for a myoelectric prosthesis.

Handling of the neurovascular structures is another important decision branch point. Treatment of the median, ulnar, and radial nerves is quite important at this stage. The standard traction neurectomy is no longer the optimal treatment for these large mixed nerves. The question is if targeted reinnervation should be performed at the time of the amputation, or at a later date. Immediate targeted reinnervation would avoid a second surgery, and the nerve transfers would be performed when the nerves are at their longest length, without neuromas to resect and with a full axon complement. Benefits of immediate targeted reinnervation include a shorter time between amputation and the possibility to have additional control signals for improved prosthetic function. As has been mentioned, nerve transfers are a method of preventing the development of symptomatic neuroma. While it has been hoped that targeted reinnervation would prevent or improve "phantom limb" sensations, this has not been seen clinically. Amputation followed by a later TMR has the advantage of improved patient education and consent, the avoidance of new proximal incisions in a swollen traumatized limb and the ability to thin the subcutaneous fat to improve EMG control. If a decision is made to perform TMR at a later date, then the major mixed nerves should be left long and without additional dissection at the time of amputation.

Transhumeral amputations through the middle third of the humerus still allow for a mobile shoulder joint, and successful fitting of a prosthesis. Often TMR can be still be performed. Pedicled latissimus flaps can be extremely useful to achieve wound closure and maintain length when needed. Short transhumeral amputations can undergo Ilizarov lengthening or even free fibula transfer to achieve a longer lever arm for the prosthesis.

With severe brachial plexopathies resulting in flail limbs, amputation is often considered. Amputation will not relieve neuropathic plexopathy pain, but can relieve traction pain at the shoulder and it clearly removes the inconvenience of having a paralyzed arm. We recommend a transhumeral amputation at 25–30% of humeral length. This removes the weight of the limb, relieving traction pain, and preserves a nice shoulder and upper arm contour for clothing. Fusion of the shoulder to enhance prosthetic fitting is not recommended. Prosthetic fittings with flail residual limbs have extremely poor outcomes and a humerus fused in abduction and flexion interferes with some activities, especially positioning in bed.

Proximal transhumeral and shoulder disarticulation

Loss of the biceps and triceps due to electrical injury or avulsive injuries is best treated with a proximal transhumeral amputation or a shoulder disarticulation. Maintenance of the humeral head in its glenohumeral fossa has cosmetic implications in shirt fitting, and depends on the local soft tissues. Again, traction neurectomies should be avoided to preserve nerve length. As will be discussed, TMR for shoulder disarticulations is a lengthy procedure, and should not be performed at the time of the amputation. Preservation of a small humeral remnant under deltoid motor control can be extremely useful to activate switches via miniature touch pads. The deltoid muscle is typically spared in electrical injuries due to the increased cross-sectional area of the body. In avulsive injuries, the deltoid is spared due to its broad origin on the scapula. The deltoid is pulled inferiorly with sutures, and the chest skin can be mobilized superiorly for closure of the glenohumeral fossa.

Surgery of the residual limb

Soft-tissue improvement

Patients with traumatic amputations often have suboptimal soft tissues for wearing prostheses for the majority of the day. Scars, skin grafts, and skin redundancies compromise the suction fit of prosthetic sockets and liners. Skin breakdown is common, leading to discomfort, more frequent infections, and inability to wear the prosthesis while healing. The prosthetist and physiatrist assess patient comfort with the prosthesis. A risk assessment is performed by the plastic surgeon as to the various possibilities for improvement of the soft tissues. Close collaboration between the specialties allows the amputee to have a residual limb without skin breakdown, painful neuromas, and poorly covered bone. This can include simple advancement flaps, excision of skin grafts, Z-plasties for scar contractures, and circumferential liposuction for thick subcutaneous tissue *(Figs 40.11 and 40.12)*. The patient must be aware that, even after primary skin healing, swelling will take many weeks to resolve, and therefore it will be longer than expected before the prosthesis with revised sockets can be used again.

Skin breakdown can occur from poor prosthetic fit, but it also can occur when skin grafts are used to preserve length and result over pressure points. Both pedicled flaps and free flaps are useful to improve the soft-tissue envelope. The goal is a smooth contour to distribute pressure better. Revision amputations are also possible for poor soft tissues when the

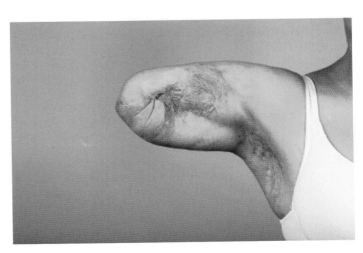

Fig. 40.11 Transhumeral amputee with scarred soft tissues of her residual limb.

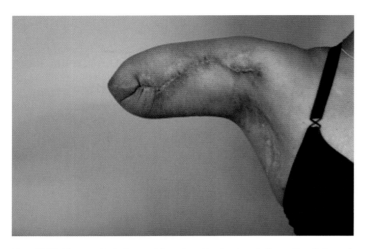

Fig. 40.12 Same patient after excision of previously placed skin graft and closure with advanced skin flap, analogous to a brachioplasty.

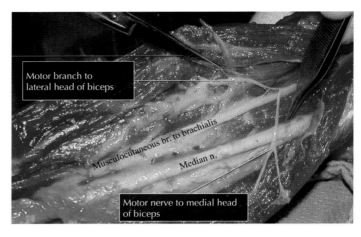

Motor branch to lateral head of biceps

Musculocutaneous br. to brachialis

Median n.

Motor nerve to medial head of biceps

Fig. 40.13 Cadaveric dissection splitting the medial and lateral heads of the biceps to expose the motor points of the musculocutaneous nerve.

prosthetist and physiatrist agree that a shorter residual limb with improved soft tissues will be preferable to a longer amputation covered with skin grafts.

The function of myoelectric prosthetic control can also be improved with soft-tissue revision. The removal of subcutaneous fat will enable surface electrodes to be placed much closer to the residual muscles. This can markedly increase the size of the EMG signals and decrease interference (cross-talk) from neighboring muscles.[21]

Neuroma management

Neuromas are significant problems after upper extremity amputations. Large series from areas of conflict document neuromas and stump pain in over one-quarter of upper extremity amputees.[22–24] Clinically, large mixed neuromas can be very symptomatic, as can superficial sensory nerve neuromas. Divided "pure" motor nerves are less than 50% motor fibers by staining, yet they clinically do not create symptomatic end neuromas when cut. Neuroma pain is described as a localized area of chronic tenderness when pressure is applied, typically with a radiation of discomfort in the area that the nerve had previously innervated. This is in contradistinction to phantom sensations, which are defined as the feeling that a deafferented body part is still present following amputation.[25]

Numerous strategies have been reported to be successful in the management of painful stump neuromas. The simplest method of neuroma excision and traction neurectomy has a documented 70% improvement rate.[26] Neuroma excision with burying the nerve end in muscle,[27] neuroma translocation away from areas of pressure,[28] and the centro-centralization technique of Gorkisch[29] have all been documented to have high levels of patient satisfaction and low recurrence rates. These studies are all limited by being clinical studies. Experimental neuroma work in animal models is hampered by a lack of rigorous criteria of what would constitute a quiet neuroma from a symptomatic one.

Clinically, despite the mismatch in sizes between the donor mixed nerve and recipient motor nerve of TMR, no patient to our knowledge has been re-explored for a symptomatic

neuroma at the nerve coaptation site after 40 cases worldwide and with 2–5 nerve coaptations per case. TMR has been used clinically for symptomatic neuromas in both the forearm (see above, transradial amputation) and the leg.

Targeted muscle reinnervation

As noted above, TMR is a technique that transfers the median, radial, ulnar, and/or musculocutaneous nerve in an amputated arm to nonfunctional residual limb muscles. These reinnervated target muscles then serve as biological amplifiers of the nerve signals providing more EMG control signals for improved operation of motorized prostheses. The TMR surgical procedure was recently reviewed,[30] and demonstrates improved outcomes in comparison to standard prostheses documented.[8] The following is a brief review of surgical techniques.

Transhumeral level

The indications to perform TMR at the transhumeral level include poor prosthetic function using standard body-powered, myoelectric, or hybrid systems despite adequate training. Good candidates are young patients with cortical control of biceps and triceps contraction without plexopathy, supple soft tissues, and without other cardiopulmonary risk factors. Bilateral amputations and long residual limbs also favor the procedure. Patients who have suffered avulsions of the limb at the time of injury or patients with brachial plexopathies are poor candidates for surgery.

On examination, Tinel's signs signifying the ends of the median, ulnar, and radial nerve are marked. Tinel's signs located at the mid-humeral level or distal have long enough nerves to perform nerve transfers. The outlines of the biceps and triceps muscles are carefully marked. The goal of the anterior incision is to transfer the median nerve to the motor nerve of the medial head of the biceps, while preserving the innervation of the musculocutaneous nerve to the lateral head of the biceps *(Fig. 40.13)*. This will add a "hand-closing" signal for the prosthesis, while preserving the "elbow flexion" signal. In the operating room, after raising thin skin flaps, an

Video 1

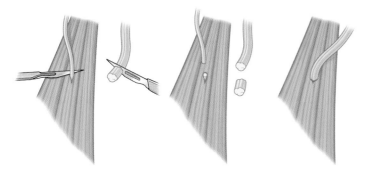

Fig. 40.14 Schematic of targeted muscle reinnervation nerve transfer.

adipofascial flap is elevated and based proximally. This serves to improve later signal detection by thinning the subcutaneous tissue, and the adipofascial flap placed between the medial and lateral heads of the biceps at the close will separate the two muscle bellies axially. The median nerve neuromatous end is identified, cut back to healthy fascicles, and mobilized into the space adjacent to where the musculocutaneous nerve enters the medial head of the biceps. A nerve transfer is performed by dividing the motor nerve to this muscle segment, and coapting the median nerve directly to this 1–1.5-mm motor nerve *(Fig. 40.14)*. The coaptation site should be as near to the muscle belly as possible to decrease innervation times, and also to facilitate a suture placed from the epineurium of the median nerve, through the tiny motor nerve, and catching an aspect of the epimysium for a solid bite. An identical thought process and procedure are performed on the posterior aspect of the arm. The distal radial nerve is transferred to the motor nerve innervating the lateral head of the triceps, while still maintaining the native innervation of the long head of the triceps. This creates a "hand-opening" signal, while still leaving intact the "elbow extension" signal of the proximal radial nerve. After the elevation of a proximally based adipofascial flap, the triceps is split between the long and lateral heads to reveal the motor nerve to the lateral head of the triceps and the distal radial nerve. The distal radial nerve is coapted to the newly divided motor nerve of the lateral head of the triceps. Drains and a mildly compressing dressing are applied. Therapy can begin several weeks after the nerve transfer procedure.[31] A video demonstrating patient selection, marking, and performance of TMR for transhumeral amputees is available at http://www.ric.org and http://drdumanian.com/pages/bionic-arm.html.

Shoulder disarticulation level

TMR at the shoulder level is a long procedure, and should not be performed unless the surgical team has significant knowledge of upper chest and axillary anatomy.[32,33] Patient evaluation begins with a thorough history and physical examination. Patients with brachial plexus injuries are not candidates for the procedure, as the median, radial, and ulnar nerves must elicit action potentials under direct cortical control. Though it may seem obvious, patients cannot undergo TMR unless they have had an amputation, as there is no region of the body to accept the prosthetic arm. The indication for performing surgery is to improve prosthetic function. Painful neuromas and uncomfortable areas of heterotopic ossification have been other relative indications for the procedure. A Tinel's sign over the major three nerves is elicited, as is confirmation that the pectoralis, serratus, and latissimus muscle are under active cortical control. These will be potential recipient targets for the nerve transfers.

An infraclavicular approach to the plexus and proximal nerve branches is performed incising the skin two fingerbreadths below the clavicle and carefully opening the interspace between the sternal and clavicular heads of the pectoralis major *(Figs 40.15–40.19)*. During the approach, thin skin flaps are raised and the thick chest adiposity is thinned for improved signal detection in a region 10 cm in superior-to-inferior dimension, and from the medial chest to the anterior axillary line. The motor nerves to the clavicular head of the pectoralis off the lateral cord are located at the midpoint of the clavicle and tagged. Motor nerves to the sternal head pectoralis are identified next and come in three clusters: (1) a motor nerve that is near the thoracoacromial vessels and travels to the central aspect of the muscle; (2) a motor nerve that travels through the pectoralis minor or is just medial to the pectoralis minor; and (3) a motor nerve that is on the lateral aspect of the pectoralis. The origin of these motor nerves does not matter, as only the size and location of these motor point nerves as they reach the muscle (where the transfers will be performed) are important. What major mixed nerve can reach which motor nerve? Next, either medial or lateral to the pectoralis minor tendon, the brachial plexus and the musculocutaneous, median, ulnar, and radial nerves emanating from it are identified. The radial nerve is stimulated to make sure there is no triceps remnant to leave in continuity. The identity of the nerves is made by their branching pattern off the brachial plexus. The axillary nerve is not seen with this dissection. Deep to the plexus, the proximal thoracodorsal nerve is identified as a potential target.

Typically, there are four nerves to transfer and there must be four recipients *(Table 40.1)*. The most common transfers are the musculocutaneous nerve to the clavicular head of the pectoralis, the median nerve to the largest motor nerve innervating the sternal head of the pectoralis, and the radial nerve to the thoracodorsal nerve. The recipient for the ulnar nerve is generally the motor nerve found on the lateral aspect of the pectoralis minor. Alternatives for the ulnar nerve include the long thoracic nerve, or the nerve innervating the pectoralis minor. If the pectoralis minor is used, it will need to be mobilized laterally, and the insertion of the pectoralis major divided (if present) so that it moves medially for better signal detection of the deeper muscle. When the pectoralis major receives more than one innervation, it can be divided along its fibers based on its vascular and motor nerve anatomy. Segments should be at least 4–5 cm in diameter for adequate signal detection. The target muscle should be completely denervated during these transfers so that the previous pectoral EMG signal is eliminated. Nerve coaptations are performed as close to the entry point of the motor nerve into the muscle as possible to decrease the time of reinnervation. The adipofascial flap is placed between the pectoral heads to reduce aberrant reinnervation and to separate the muscle bellies from each other, thereby improving EMG signal detection. The skin is closed over drains after placement of quilting sutures to decrease seromas. The patient may resume wearing his/her original prosthesis when there is adequate wound healing.

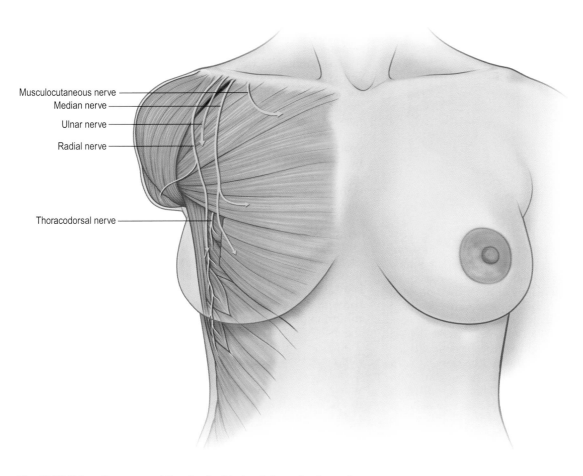

Musculocutaneous nerve

Median nerve

Ulnar nerve

Radial nerve

Thoracodorsal nerve

Fig. 40.15 Schematic nerve coaptations for shoulder targeted muscle reinnervation.

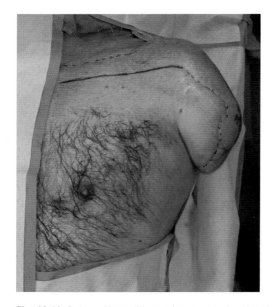

Fig. 40.16 Patient with small humeral remnant undergoing shoulder-level targeted muscle reinnervation. The clavicle is dotted, and the incision is drawn.

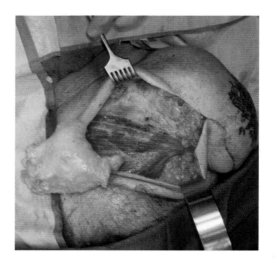

Fig. 40.17 Adipofascial flap is raised, exposing the interspace between the clavicular and sternal heads of the pectoralis major.

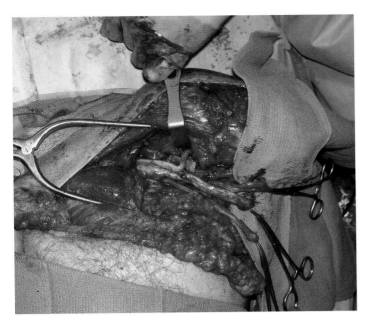

Fig. 40.18 The radial, median, and ulnar nerves are dissected free with hemostats holding them laterally. The musculocutaneous nerve is visible just inferior to the army-navy retractor.

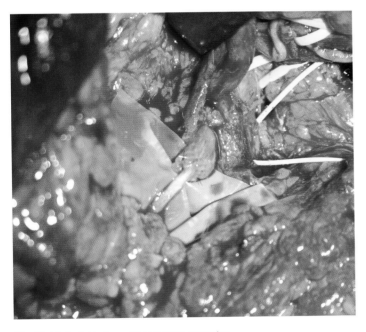

Fig. 40.19 Radial to thoracodorsal nerve coaptation.

Table 40.1 TMR for shoulder disarticulations

Nerve	Possible recipient
Musculocutaneous	Clavicular head of pectoralis major
Median	Largest motor nerve innervating sternal head of pectoralis major
Radial	Thoracodorsal or long thoracic
Ulnar	Lateral motor nerve innervating sternal head of pectoralis major or minor

Prosthetic fitting for new control sites will occur in 3–6 months. The latissimus muscle, being farthest away from the coaptation site, will take the longest to come under cortical control.

Special evaluation of the radial nerve should occur at the time of surgery. Though not consistently seen, a posterior group of fascicles can be discerned that had been the proximal aspect of the radial nerve innervating the triceps, and a more anterior aspect of the nerve innervating the forearm and finger extensors. If these two groups of fascicles can be separated, this perhaps allows another nerve transfer to be performed. In this situation, the pectoralis major sternal head can be divided into three segments, or else both the pectoralis minor and the serratus muscles will need to be used for an additional target.

Targeted sensory reinnervation is also possible; the afferent fibers of the transferred nerves will reinnervate any denervated skin overlying the target muscle. When this reinnervated skin is touched, the patient feels that his or her missing hand is being touched, providing cortical feedback to the "hand" aspect of the brain. All modalities of cutaneous sensation are restored, including pressure, vibration, and thermal. In the future special devices termed "tactors" may provide feedback from the prosthesis to the brain in the correct part of the brain for position or pressure applied by the terminal device. In doing so, targeted motor and sensory reinnervation will "close the loop" for prosthetic function. Sensory nerves, including the supraclavicular nerve and the lateral intercostal nerve, can be coapted end to end of the medial and ulnar nerves to provide targeted sensory reinnervation.

Transradial level

TMR has been performed for patients with transradial amputations, but for neuroma control, rather than improved prosthetic function. These transfers are described above in the "wrist disarticulation and transradial amputation" section. The EMG signals for these transradial nerve transfers are not currently contributing to the control of myoelectric prostheses. However, some day the additional EMG information on intrinsic hand muscle activation may help control multifunction prosthetic hands using computer-decoding algorithms.[34]

Comparison of prosthetics with composite tissue allotransplantation

There have not been any direct comparisons between improved function with prosthetics and composite tissue allotransplantation (CTA). Both have significant benefits and drawbacks. Having performed TMR and currently developing a CTA program, we have had the opportunity to consider the ideal patients for both procedures.

The best patient for TMR is an above-elbow amputee, because standard prosthetic function is so poor. Without TMR, the amputee will not be able to move the prosthetic elbow and hand intuitively or at the same time. There is ample room within the prosthesis for both motors and battery packs considering the length of prosthesis available between the mid-humerus and the terminal device. Transplantation above the elbow, in comparison, would be problematic due to the large amount of transplanted tissue, long reinnervation distances and times, and the inability to use a functional prosthesis during the recovery time. A poor candidate for TMR is an amputee at the distal forearm level or an amputation across the hand. Devices for long transradial amputations have little room for the batteries and motors; the prostheses are generally bulky and often the arm is longer than it should be. CTA, on the other hand, is ideal in the distal forearm, where there is little muscle mass in the transplanted piece, and nerve topographic anatomy is defined. Reinnervation distances, and therefore the time before meaningful sensory recovery is returned, would be short. The total transplant load is relatively low, and salvage of the patient from a failed transplant would be facilitated by its distal location. The patient would still be left with a useful transradial amputation. With current technology both for prosthetics and for CTA, we expect that proximal amputees would do better functionally with targeted reinnervation, and distal amputees potentially better with CTA.

Access the complete references list online at **http://www.expertconsult.com**

9. Kuiken TA, Dumanian GA, Lipschutz RD, et al. The use of targeted muscle reinnervation for improved myoelectric prosthesis control in a bilateral shoulder disarticulation amputee. *Prosthet Orthot Int.* 2004;28:245–253.

   This is the initial report of TMR in a shoulder disarticulation patient. Objective testing before and after the nerve transfer procedure is presented.

25. Watson J, Gonzalez M, Romero A, et al. Neuromas of the hand and upper extremity. *J Hand Surg.* 2010;35A:499–510.

   Review article regarding the current knowledge on the physiology and treatment of symptomatic neuromas of the upper extremity.

30. Dumanian GA, Ko JH, O'Shaughnessy, KD, et al. Targeted reinnervation for transhumeral amputees: Current surgical technique and update on results. *Plast Reconstr Surg.* 2009;124:863–869.

   Current technique with additional images and outcomes for TMR in transhumeral amputees. The entire surgical technique is well illustrated in this article.

33. Kuiken TA, Miller LA, Lipschutz RD, et al. Targeted reinnervation for enhanced prosthetic arm function in a woman with a proximal amputation: a case study. *Lancet* 2007;369:371–380.

   Illustrated case of TMR in a shoulder disarticulation patient, with additional diagrams of targeted sensory reinnervation.

Index

Note: **Boldface** *roman numerals indicate volume. Page numbers followed by f refer to figures; page numbers followed by t refer to tables; page numbers followed by b refer to boxes.*

*Note: **Boldface** roman numerals indicate volume. Page numbers followed by f refer to figures; page numbers followed by t refer to tables; page numbers followed by b refer to boxes.*

Note: **Boldface** *roman numerals indicate volume. Page numbers followed by f refer to figures; page numbers followed by t refer to tables; page numbers followed by b refer to boxes.*

Note: **Boldface** roman numerals indicate volume. Page numbers followed by f refer to figures; page numbers followed by t refer to tables; page numbers followed by b refer to boxes.

Note: **Boldface** *roman numerals indicate volume. Page numbers followed by f refer to figures; page numbers followed by t refer to tables; page numbers followed by b refer to boxes.*

*Note: **Boldface** roman numerals indicate volume. Page numbers followed by f refer to figures; page numbers followed by t refer to tables; page numbers followed by b refer to boxes.*

Note: **Boldface** roman numerals indicate volume. Page numbers followed by f refer to figures; page numbers followed by t refer to tables; page numbers followed by b refer to boxes.

Note: **Boldface** roman numerals indicate volume. Page numbers followed by f refer to figures; page numbers followed by t refer to tables; page numbers followed by b refer to boxes.

Note: **Boldface** *roman numerals indicate volume. Page numbers followed by f refer to figures; page numbers followed by t refer to tables; page numbers followed by b refer to boxes.*

*Note: **Boldface** roman numerals indicate volume. Page numbers followed by f refer to figures; page numbers followed by t refer to tables; page numbers followed by b refer to boxes.*

Note: **Boldface** roman numerals indicate volume. Page numbers followed by f refer to figures; page numbers followed by t refer to tables; page numbers followed by b refer to boxes.

Note: **Boldface** roman numerals indicate volume. Page numbers followed by f refer to figures; page numbers followed by t refer to tables; page numbers followed by b refer to boxes.

Note: **Boldface** roman numerals indicate volume. Page numbers followed by f refer to figures; page numbers followed by t refer to tables; page numbers followed by b refer to boxes.

craniofacial surgery (Continued)
 etiology
  embryologic craniofacial development, III:702f, 704–705
  failure of fusion theory, III:705–706
  neuromeric theory, III:706
  FOXE1 (Forkhead box protein E1) mutation, III:510–511
  general discussion, III:509–511
  inadequate growth, III:509–510
  IRF6 (interferon regulatory factor) gene, III:511
 median craniofacial dysraphia
  anterior encephaloceles, III:703–704
  characteristics, III:703–704
  number 0 cleft, III:709
  skeletal involvement, III:709
  soft-tissue involvement, III:709
  true median cleft, III:703
 median craniofacial hypoplasia (tissue deficiency or agenesis)
  holoprosencephalic spectrum (alobar brain), III:702
  median cerebrofacial hypoplasia (lobar brain), III:702
  median facial hypoplasia, III:702
  microform variants, III:702–703
  number 0 cleft, III:703t, 708–709, 708f
  skeletal deficiencies, III:708–709, 708f
  skeletal excess, III:709
  soft-tissue deficiencies, III:708, 708f
  soft-tissue midline excess, III:709
 number 0 cleft
  characteristics, III:706–709
  median craniofacial dysraphia, III:709
  median craniofacial hyperplasia (tissue excess or duplication), III:709
  median craniofacial hypoplasia, III:703t, 708, 708f
  treatment strategies, III:722f–723f
 number 1 cleft
  characteristics, III:709
  skeletal involvement, III:709, 710f
  soft-tissue involvement, III:709, 710f
 number 2 cleft
  skeletal involvement, III:711
  soft-tissue involvement, III:709–711, 710f
  treatment strategies, III:723f
 number 3 cleft
  characteristics, III:711
  skeletal involvement, III:711, 711f
  soft-tissue involvement, III:711, 711f
  treatment strategies, III:724f
 number 4 cleft
  characteristics, III:712–713
  skeletal involvement, III:712f, 713
  soft-tissue involvement, III:712, 712f
 number 5 cleft
  characteristics, III:713–714
  skeletal involvement, III:713f, 714
  soft-tissue involvement, III:713, 713f
 number 6 cleft
  characteristics, III:714
  skeletal involvement, III:714, 714f
  soft-tissue involvement, III:714, 714f

craniofacial surgery (Continued)
 number 7 cleft
  characteristics, III:714–715
  skeletal involvement, III:715, 715f
  soft-tissue involvement, III:714–715, 715f
 number 8 cleft
  characteristics, III:715–716, 715f–716f
  skeletal involvement, III:715–716, 716f
  soft-tissue involvement, III:715
 number 9 cleft
  characteristics, III:716–717
  skeletal involvement, III:716–717
  soft-tissue involvement, III:716, 717f
 number 10 cleft
  characteristics, III:717
  skeletal involvement, III:717
  soft-tissue involvement, III:717, 717f
 number 11 cleft
  characteristics, III:717–718
  skeletal involvement, III:717–718
  soft-tissue involvement, III:717, 718f
 number 12 cleft
  characteristics, III:718
  skeletal involvement, III:718, 718f
  soft-tissue involvement, III:718, 718f
 number 13 cleft
  characteristics, III:718–719, 719f
  skeletal involvement, III:718–719
  soft-tissue involvement, III:718
 number 14 cleft
  characteristics, III:719
  skeletal involvement, III:719, 720f
  soft-tissue involvement, III:719, 720f
 number 30 cleft
  characteristics, III:719–720, 721f
  skeletal involvement, III:720
  soft-tissue involvement, III:720
 orbital hypertelorism, III:686–700
  Apert syndrome, III:689
  craniofrontonasal dysplasia, III:689
  Crouzon syndrome, III:688, 688f
  embryology, III:686
  faciocraniosynostosis, III:688–689
  median facial clefts, III:687
  oculomotor disorders, III:699
  outcomes and complicatons, III:698
  pathogenesis, III:686–689
  patient presentation and diagnosis, III:687–688
  patient selection, III:689
  Pfeiffer syndrome, III:688–689
  postoperative care and follow-up, III:695–696
  recurrences, III:699–700
  secondary procedures, III:698–700, 698f
  surgical technique and treatment, III:689–695
  Tessier cleft classification system, III:687–688, 687f
 outcomes and complicatons, III:725
 patient selection
  number 0 cleft, III:706–709
  number 1 cleft, III:709
  number 2 cleft, III:709–711
  number 3 cleft, III:711
  number 4 cleft, III:712–713
  number 5 cleft, III:713–714

craniofacial surgery (Continued)
  number 6 cleft, III:714
  number 7 cleft, III:714–715
  number 8 cleft, III:715–716
  number 9 cleft, III:716–717
  number 10 cleft, III:717
  number 11 cleft, III:717–718
  number 12 cleft, III:718
  number 13 cleft, III:718–719
  number 14 cleft, III:719
  number 30 cleft, III:719–720
  Tessier cleft classification system, III:687–688, 687f, 706, 707f
 research summary, III:725
 transforming growth factor-β (TGF-β) superfamily, III:509, 509f–510f
 treatment strategies
  basic procedure, III:721–725
  number 0 cleft, III:722f–723f
  number 2 cleft, III:723f
  number 3 cleft, III:724f
 Wingless (Wnt) signaling defects, III:509–510
facial injuries, III:49–88
 causal factors, III:49
 condylar and subcondylar fractures, III:83, 83f
 edentulous mandible fractures, III:83–84, 84f
 facial transplantation, III:131
 frontal bone and sinus fractures
  clinical examination, III:51
  complications, III:53
  computed tomography (CT), III:51
  injury patterns, III:51
  nasofrontal duct, III:51, 52f
  surgical technique and treatment, III:52–53, 52f
 gunshot wounds
  delayed versus immediate reconstruction, III:85
  immediate and high velocity gunshot wounds, III:86–87
  low velocity gunshot wounds, III:85–87
  treatment strategies, III:86–87, 86f
 initial assessment
  blunt trauma craniofacial injuries, III:50–51
  clinical examination, III:50–51
  computed tomography (CT), III:51
  general discussion, III:49–51
  timing considerations, III:49–50
 lower facial fractures, III:75
 mandibular fractures
  antibiotics, III:82
  characteristics, III:75
  Class I fractures, III:77–78
  Class II fractures, III:78
  Class III fractures, III:78–80
  classification systems, III:76–77
  clinical examination, III:76
  comminuted fractures, III:78, 79f
  complications, III:82–83
  dental wiring and fixation techniques, III:75–76
  diagnosis, III:76
  displacement direction and extent, III:77

Note: **Boldface** *roman numerals indicate volume. Page numbers followed by f refer to figures; page numbers followed by t refer to tables; page numbers followed by b refer to boxes.*

Note: **Boldface** roman numerals indicate volume. Page numbers followed by f refer to figures; page numbers followed by t refer to tables; page numbers followed by b refer to boxes.

Note: **Boldface** roman numerals indicate volume. Page numbers followed by f refer to figures; page numbers followed by t refer to tables; page numbers followed by b refer to boxes.

Note: **Boldface** roman numerals indicate volume. Page numbers followed by f refer to figures; page numbers followed by t refer to tables; page numbers followed by b refer to boxes.

Note: **Boldface** roman numerals indicate volume. Page numbers followed by f refer to figures; page numbers followed by t refer to tables; page numbers followed by b refer to boxes.

Note: **Boldface** roman numerals indicate volume. Page numbers followed by f refer to figures; page numbers followed by t refer to tables; page numbers followed by b refer to boxes.

*Note: **Boldface** roman numerals indicate volume. Page numbers followed by f refer to figures; page numbers followed by t refer to tables; page numbers followed by b refer to boxes.*

*Note: **Boldface** roman numerals indicate volume. Page numbers followed by f refer to figures; page numbers followed by t refer to tables; page numbers followed by b refer to boxes.*

*Note: **Boldface** roman numerals indicate volume. Page numbers followed by f refer to figures; page numbers followed by t refer to tables; page numbers followed by b refer to boxes.*

Note: **Boldface** *roman numerals indicate volume. Page numbers followed by f refer to figures; page numbers followed by t refer to tables; page numbers followed by b refer to boxes.*

Note: **Boldface** *roman numerals indicate volume. Page numbers followed by f refer to figures; page numbers followed by t refer to tables; page numbers followed by b refer to boxes.*

Note: **Boldface** *roman numerals indicate volume. Page numbers followed by f refer to figures; page numbers followed by t refer to tables; page numbers followed by b refer to boxes.*

Note: **Boldface** *roman numerals indicate volume. Page numbers followed by f refer to figures; page numbers followed by t refer to tables; page numbers followed by b refer to boxes.*

Note: **Boldface** roman numerals indicate volume. Page numbers followed by *f* refer to figures; page numbers followed by *t* refer to tables; page numbers followed by *b* refer to boxes.

Note: **Boldface** *roman numerals indicate volume. Page numbers followed by f refer to figures; page numbers followed by t refer to tables; page numbers followed by b refer to boxes.*

*Note: **Boldface** roman numerals indicate volume. Page numbers followed by f refer to figures; page numbers followed by t refer to tables; page numbers followed by b refer to boxes.*

Note: **Boldface** *roman numerals indicate volume. Page numbers followed by f refer to figures; page numbers followed by t refer to tables; page numbers followed by b refer to boxes.*

Note: **Boldface** roman numerals indicate volume. Page numbers followed by *f* refer to figures; page numbers followed by *t* refer to tables; page numbers followed by *b* refer to boxes.

Note: **Boldface** *roman numerals indicate volume. Page numbers followed by f refer to figures; page numbers followed by t refer to tables; page numbers followed by b refer to boxes.*

Note: **Boldface** roman numerals indicate volume. Page numbers followed by f refer to figures; page numbers followed by t refer to tables; page numbers followed by b refer to boxes.

Note: **Boldface** roman numerals indicate volume. Page numbers followed by f refer to figures; page numbers followed by t refer to tables; page numbers followed by b refer to boxes.

Note: **Boldface** roman numerals indicate volume. Page numbers followed by f refer to figures; page numbers followed by t refer to tables; page numbers followed by b refer to boxes.

Note: **Boldface** roman numerals indicate volume. Page numbers followed by f refer to figures; page numbers followed by t refer to tables; page numbers followed by b refer to boxes.

Note: **Boldface** *roman numerals indicate volume. Page numbers followed by f refer to figures; page numbers followed by t refer to tables; page numbers followed by b refer to boxes.*

*Note: **Boldface** roman numerals indicate volume. Page numbers followed by f refer to figures; page numbers followed by t refer to tables; page numbers followed by b refer to boxes.*

Note: **Boldface** *roman numerals indicate volume. Page numbers followed by f refer to figures; page numbers followed by t refer to tables; page numbers followed by b refer to boxes.*

Note: **Boldface** roman numerals indicate volume. Page numbers followed by f refer to figures; page numbers followed by t refer to tables; page numbers followed by b refer to boxes.

*Note: **Boldface** roman numerals indicate volume. Page numbers followed by f refer to figures; page numbers followed by t refer to tables; page numbers followed by b refer to boxes.*

*Note: **Boldface** roman numerals indicate volume. Page numbers followed by f refer to figures; page numbers followed by t refer to tables; page numbers followed by b refer to boxes.*

Note: ***Boldface*** *roman numerals indicate volume. Page numbers followed by f refer to figures; page numbers followed by t refer to tables; page numbers followed by b refer to boxes.*

Note: **Boldface** roman numerals indicate volume. Page numbers followed by f refer to figures; page numbers followed by t refer to tables; page numbers followed by b refer to boxes.

Note: **Boldface** roman numerals indicate volume. Page numbers followed by f refer to figures; page numbers followed by t refer to tables; page numbers followed by b refer to boxes.

Note: **Boldface** roman numerals indicate volume. Page numbers followed by f refer to figures; page numbers followed by t refer to tables; page numbers followed by b refer to boxes.

Note: **Boldface** roman numerals indicate volume. Page numbers followed by f refer to figures; page numbers followed by t refer to tables; page numbers followed by b refer to boxes.

*Note: **Boldface** roman numerals indicate volume. Page numbers followed by f refer to figures; page numbers followed by t refer to tables; page numbers followed by b refer to boxes.*

Note: **Boldface** *roman numerals indicate volume. Page numbers followed by f refer to figures; page numbers followed by t refer to tables; page numbers followed by b refer to boxes.*

Note: **Boldface** *roman numerals indicate volume. Page numbers followed by f refer to figures; page numbers followed by t refer to tables; page numbers followed by b refer to boxes.*

Note: **Boldface** roman numerals indicate volume. Page numbers followed by f refer to figures; page numbers followed by t refer to tables; page numbers followed by b refer to boxes.

Note: **Boldface** *roman numerals indicate volume. Page numbers followed by f refer to figures; page numbers followed by t refer to tables; page numbers followed by b refer to boxes.*

*Note: **Boldface** roman numerals indicate volume. Page numbers followed by f refer to figures; page numbers followed by t refer to tables; page numbers followed by b refer to boxes.*

---

*Note: **Boldface** roman numerals indicate volume. Page numbers followed by f refer to figures; page numbers followed by t refer to tables; page numbers followed by b refer to boxes.*

Note: **Boldface** roman numerals indicate volume. Page numbers followed by f refer to figures; page numbers followed by t refer to tables; page numbers followed by b refer to boxes.

Note: **Boldface** roman numerals indicate volume. Page numbers followed by f refer to figures; page numbers followed by t refer to tables; page numbers followed by b refer to boxes.

Note: **Boldface** *roman numerals indicate volume. Page numbers followed by f refer to figures; page numbers followed by t refer to tables; page numbers followed by b refer to boxes.*